Every Decker book is accompanied by a CD-ROM.

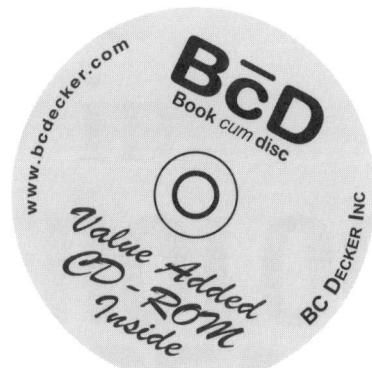

BC Decker Inc is committed to providing high-quality electronic publications that complement traditional information and learning methods.

Advanced Therapy in Gastroenterology and Liver Disease is accompanied by a dual-platform CD-ROM, which features the complete text and full-color images. The fully searchable PDF files facilitate the exploration of need-to-know information. The disc is also ideal for printing pertinent information necessary for patient education.
The book and disc are sold only as a package; neither are available independently, and no prices are available for the items individually. We trust you will find the book/CD package invaluable and invite your comments and suggestions.

Access information. Acquire knowledge. Please visit www.bcdecker.com for a complete list of titles in your discipline. Our innovative approach to meeting the informational needs of healthcare professionals ensures that Decker products belong in your library and on your computer.

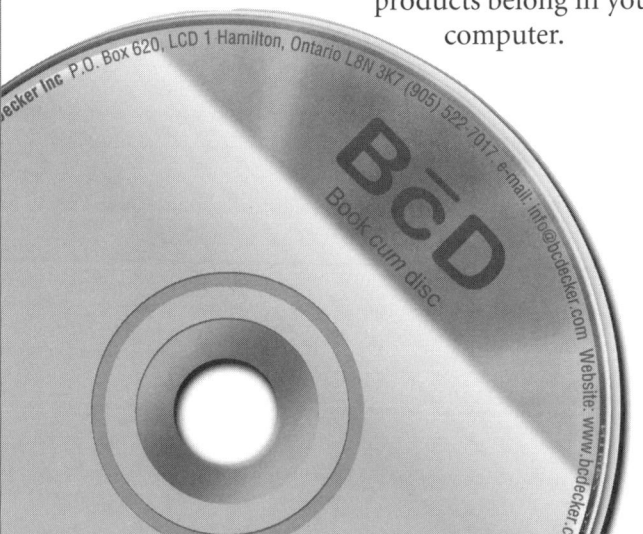

Brian C. Decker
CEO and Publisher

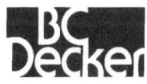

Advanced Therapy in GASTROENTEROLOGY AND LIVER DISEASE

Fifth Edition

Theodore M. Bayless, MD
Professor of Medicine
Johns Hopkins University School of Medicine
Clinical Director
Meyerhoff Digestive-Disease-Inflammatory Bowel Disease Center
The Johns Hopkins Hospital
Baltimore, Maryland

Anna Mae Diehl, MD
Professor of Medicine
Chief, Division of Gastroenterology
Director, Duke Liver Center
Duke University Medical Center
Durham, North Carolina

2005
B.C. Decker Inc.
Hamilton • London

BC Decker Inc
P.O. Box 620, L.C.D. 1
Hamilton, Ontario L8N 3K7
Tel: 905-522-7017; 800-568-7281
Fax: 905-522-7839; 888-311-4987
E-mail: info@bcdecker.com
www.bcdecker.com

© 2005 BC Decker Inc

All rights reserved. No part of this publication may be reproduced, stored in a retrieval system, or transmitted, in any form or by any means, electronic, mechanical, photocopying, recording, or otherwise, without prior written permission from the publisher.

06 07 08 09 10/WPC/9 8 7 6 5 4 3 2

ISBN 1-55009-248-0
Printed in the United States of America

Sales and Distribution

United States
BC Decker Inc
P.O. Box 785
Lewiston, NY 14092-0785
Tel: 905-522-7017; 800-568-7281
Fax: 905-522-7839; 888-311-4987
E-mail: info@bcdecker.com
www.bcdecker.com

Canada
BC Decker Inc
50 King Street East
P.O. Box 620, LCD 1
Hamilton, Ontario L8N 1A6
Tel: 905-522-7017; 800-568-7281
Fax: 905-522-7839; 888-311-4987
E-mail: info@bcdecker.com
www.bcdecker.com

Foreign Rights
John Scott & Company
International Publishers' Agency
P.O. Box 878
Kimberton, PA 19442
Tel: 610-827-1640
Fax: 610-827-1671
E-mail: jsco@voicenet.com

Japan
Igaku-Shoin Ltd.
Foreign Publications Department
3-24-17 Hongo
Bunkyo-ku, Tokyo, Japan 113-8719
Tel: 3 3817 5680
Fax: 3 3815 6776
E-mail: fd@igaku-shoin.co.jp

UK, Europe, Scandinavia, Middle East
Elsevier Science
Customer Service Department
Foots Cray High Street
Sidcup, Kent
DA14 5HP, UK
Tel: 44 (0) 208 308 5760
Fax: 44 (0) 181 308 5702
E-mail: cservice@harcourt.com

Singapore, Malaysia, Thailand, Philippines, Indonesia, Vietnam, Pacific Rim, Korea
Elsevier Science Asia
583 Orchard Road
#09/01, Forum
Singapore 238884
Tel: 65-737-3593
Fax: 65-753-2145

Australia, New Zealand
Elsevier Science Australia
Customer Service Department
STM Division
Locked Bag 16
St. Peters, New South Wales, 2044
Australia
Tel: 61 02 9517-8999
Fax: 61 02 9517-2249
E-mail: stmp@harcourt.com.au
www.harcourt.com.au

Mexico and Central America
ETM SA de CV
Calle de Tula 59
Colonia Condesa
06140 Mexico DF, Mexico
Tel: 52-5-5553-6657
Fax: 52-5-5211-8468
E-mail: editoresdetextosmex@prodigy.net.mx

Brazil
Tecmedd Importadora E Distribuidora De Livros Ltda.
Avenida Maurílio Biagi, 2850
City Ribeirão, Ribeirão Preto – SP – Brasil
CEP: 14021-000
Tel: 0800 992236
Fax: (16) 3993-9000
E-mail: tecmedd@tecmedd.com.br

India, Bangladesh, Pakistan, Sri Lanka
Elsevier Health Sciences Division
Customer Service Department
17A/1, Main Ring Road
Lajpat Nagar IV
New Delhi – 110024, India
Tel: 91 11 2644 7160-64
Fax: 91 11 2644 7156
E-mail: esindia@vsnl.net

Notice: The authors and publisher have made every effort to ensure that the patient care recommended herein, including choice of drugs and drug dosages, is in accord with the accepted standard and practice at the time of publication. However, since research and regulation constantly change clinical standards, the reader is urged to check the product information sheet included in the package of each drug, which includes recommended doses, warnings, and contraindications. This is particularly important with new or infrequently used drugs. Any treatment regimen, particularly one involving medication, involves inherent risk that must be weighed on a case-by-case basis against the benefits anticipated. The reader is cautioned that the purpose of this book is to inform and enlighten; the information contained herein is not intended as, and should not be employed as, a substitute for individual diagnosis and treatment.

Table of Contents

	Contributors	xi
	Preface	xix
1	Using Evidence-Based Medicine in Patient Care	1
	Brooks D. Cash, MD	
2	Decision Analysis in the Management of Digestive Diseases	8
	Amnon Sonnenberg, MD, MSc	
3	Endoscopic Sedation	17
	Anthony N. Kalloo, MD, FACP, Donna Beitler, RN, CGRN	
4	Endoscopic Disinfection	23
	Lawrence F. Muscarella, PhD, Anthony J. DiMarino Jr, MD	
5	Endoscopic Ultrasonography and Fine Needle Aspiration	29
	Kenneth J. Chang, MD	
6	Endoscopic Mucosal Resection	36
	Massimo Conio, MD, Rosangela Filiberti, PhD, Darius Sorbi, MD	
7	Oral Considerations in Patients with Gastrointestinal Disorders	43
	Michael A. Siegel, DDS, MS, Wendy S. Hupp, DMD	
8	Oropharyngeal Dysphagia	49
	Peter J. Kahrilas, MD, John E. Pandolfino, MD	
9	Gastroesophageal Reflux: Medical Therapy	54
	Radu Tutuian, MD, Donald O. Castell, MD	
10	Lifestyle Measures for the Treatment of Gastroesophageal Reflux Disease	59
	William C. Orr, PhD	
11	Management of Extraesophageal Presentations of GERD	63
	Joel E. Richter, MD	
12	Surgery for Gastroesophageal Reflux Disease	69
	J. Andrew Isch, MD, Brant K. Oelschlager, MD, Carlos A. Pellegrini, MD	
13	Endoscopic Therapies for Gastroesophageal Reflux Disease	73
	Reza Shaker, MD, Walter J. Hogan, MD	
14	Barrett's Esophagus	86
	Richard E. Sampliner, MD	
15	Ablative Therapy in Esophageal Disease	90
	Sanjay Jagannath, MD, Marcia I. Canto, MD, MHS	
16	Esophageal Infections	96
	C. Mel Wilcox, MD	
17	Management of Esophageal Strictures	100
	Asyia Ahmad, MD, Faullin Paletsky, MD, James C. Reynolds,	
18	Esophageal Motor Disorders and Chest Pain	107
	Ray E. Clouse, MD	
19	Management of Achalasia	112
	William J. Ravich, MD	
20	Management of Acute Variceal Bleeding	119
	Paul J. Thuluvath, MBBS, MD, FRCP	

21	**Cancer of the Esophagus** 125	
	Michael K. Gibson, MD, Arlene A. Forastiere, MD	
22	**Palliation of Esophageal Cancer** 131	
	Shou-Jiang Tang, MD, Norman E. Marcon, MD	
23	***Helicobacter Pylori*** **and Gastroduodenal Disease** 138	
	Mae F. Go, MD	
24	**Nonsteroidal Anti-Inflammatory Drugs and Gastrointestinal Complications** 142	
	Francis K. L. Chan, MD, David Y. Graham, MD	
25	**Peptic Ulcer Disease** 147	
	Joseph R. Pisegna, MD	
26	**Gastrinoma** 156	
	Chandra Are, MD, FRCS, Charles J. Yeo, MD, FACS	
27	**Management of Stress-Related Erosive Syndrome** 161	
	Jaime A. Oviedo, MD, M. Michael Wolfe, MD	
28	**Upper Gastrointestinal Bleeding** 167	
	Gregory J. Monkewich, MD, FRCPC, Gregory B. Haber, MD, FRCPC	
29	**Chronic Gastritis** 178	
	Wilfred M. Weinstein, MD	
30	**The Management of Nonulcer Dyspepsia** 183	
	Michael P. Jones, MD, FACP, FACG	
31	**Gastroparesis** 190	
	Daniel C. Buckles, MD, Richard W. McCallum, MD	
32	**Percutaneous Endoscopic Gastrostomy** 196	
	Abdul Jabbar, MD, Craig J. McClain, MD, Stephen McClave, MD	
33	**Primary Gastric Lymphoma** 202	
	Luis A. Herrera, PhD, Yinka Davis, MD, Julie Parsonnet, MD	
34	**Gastric Cancer** 207	
	Daniel M. Labow, MD, Murray F. Brennan, MD	
35	**Obesity** 212	
	Lawrence J. Cheskin, MD	
36	**Bariatric Operations** 219	
	Michael G. Sarr, MD, Michel M. Murr, MD, Michael L. Kendrick, MD	
37	**Alcoholism and Associated Disorders** 226	
	Mack C. Mitchell Jr, MD	
38	**Anorexia Nervosa and Bulimia** 232	
	Graham Redgrave, MD, Angela S. Guarda, MD	
39	**The Irritable Bowel Syndrome** 239	
	Robert S. Fisher, MD	
40	**Chronic Recurrent Abdominal Pain in Childhood and Adolescence** 243	
	Marvin E. Ament, MD	
41	**Chronic Abdominal Pain** 249	
	W. A. Hoogerwerf, MD, P. Jay Pasricha, MD	
42	**Exaggerated and Factitious Disease** 255	
	David Edwin, PhD	
43	**Psychotropic Drugs and Management of Patients with Functional Gastrointestinal Disorders** ..260	
	Lin Chang, MD, Douglas A. Drossman, MD	
44	**Role of a Nurse Advocate** 266	
	Lisa Turnbough, RN	
45	**Smoking and Gastrointestinal Disease** 270	
	Michael F. Picco, MD, PhD	

46	Gastrointestinal and Nutritional Complications of Human Immunodeficiency Virus Infection .274
	Donald P. Kotler, MD, Irina Kaplounov, MD
47	Chronic Immunodeficiency Syndromes Affecting the Gastrointestinal Tract 280
	Jimmy Ko, MD, Lloyd Mayer, MD
48	Gastrointestinal and Hepatic Complications of Stem Cell Transplantation 285
	Linda A. Lee, MD, Georgia B. Vogelsang, MD
49	Acute Infectious Diarrhea 292
	Beth D. Kirkpatrick, MD, W. Kemper Alston, MD
50	Traveler's Diarrhea 297
	R. Bradley Sack, MS, MD, ScD
51	*Clostridium Difficile* and Antibiotic-Associated Diarrhea 302
	John H. Kwon, MD, PhD, Ciarán P. Kelly, MD
52	Intestinal Parasites 307
	Amita Gupta, MD, Robert C. Bollinger, MD, MPH
53	Current Management of Whipple's Disease 316
	Axel von Herbay, MD
54	Enteral and Parenteral Nutrition 320
	Mark H. DeLegge, MD, FACG
55	Metabolic Bone Disease in Gastrointestinal and Liver Patients 327
	Maria T. Abreu, MD
56	Dietary-Induced Symptoms 339
	Lawrence R. Schiller, MD, FACP, FACG
57	Gastrointestinal Food Allergy 344
	Sheila E. Crowe, MD, FRCPC
58	Complementary and Alternative Medicine in Gastrointestinal Disease 352
	Robert J. Hilsden, MD, PhD, FRCPC, Maria J. Verhoef, PhD
59	Obscure Gastrointestinal Bleedings 357
	Andrew I. Sable, MD, Jamie S. Barkin MD, FACP, MACG
60	Nonsteroidal Antiinflammatory Drug-Induced Small and Large Intestinal Injury 364
	Ken Takeuchi, MD, Samuel N. Adler, MD, Ingvar Bjarnason, MD, MSc, FRCPath, FRCP, DSc
61	Celiac Sprue and Related Problems 367
	Karoly Horvath, MD, PhD, Alessio Fasano, MD
62	Lactose Intolerance 372
	Johanna C. Escher, MD, PhD, Hans A. Büller, MD, PhD
63	Chronic Intestinal Pseudo-Obstruction 375
	Justin Rosemore, DO, Brian E. Lacy, MD, PhD
64	Short Bowel Syndrome 381
	Alan L. Buchman, MD, MSPH
65	Intestinal and Multivisceral Transplantation 386
	Ernesto P. Molmenti, MD, PhD, Nicholas Pyrsopoulos, MD, Andreas G. Tzakis, MD, PhD
66	Crohn's Disease of the Small Bowel 390
	Chinyu Su, MD, Gary R. Lichtenstein, MD
67	Therapeutic Strategies in Pediatric Crohn's Disease 397
	Anthony P. Olivé, MD, George D. Ferry, MD
68	Surgical Management of Chrohn's Disease 402
	Mark A. Talamini, MD
69	Monitoring of Azathioprine Metabolite Levels in Inflammatory Bowel Disease 406
	C. Cuffari, MD
70	Mesenteric Vascular Ischemia 411
	Awori J. Hayanga, MD, AFRCSI, Eugene P. Ceppa, MD, Gregory B. Bulkley, MD, FACS

71	Management of Diabetic Diarrhea	420

Michael Camilleri, MD, Filippo Cremonini, MD

72	Secretory Diarrhea	425

Fathia Gibril, MD, Robert T. Jensen, MD

73	Reducing Cardiovascular Risk with Major Surgery	430

Michael Y. Chan, MD, Stephen C. Achuff, MD

74	Acute Appendicitis	435

Dorry Segev, MD, Paul Colombani MD, FACS

75	Constipation	439

Onki Cheung, MD, Arnold Wald, MD

76	Management of Abdominal Wall Defects	444

Kurtis A. Campbell, MD, Anthony P. Tufaro, MD, DDS

77	Left-Sided Ulcerative Colitis And Ulcerative Proctitis	447

Philip B. Miner Jr, MD

78	Ulcerative Colitis	453

Kenneth W. Schroeder, MD, PhD, William J. Tremaine, MD

79	Ileoanal Pouch Anastomosis	457

Feza H. Remzi, MD, Victor W. Fazio, MB, MS

80	Crohn's Colitis	465

Miles Sparrow, MD, Stephen B. Hanauer, MD

81	Perianal Complications in Crohn's Disease Patient Management	471

Daniel H. Present, MD

82	Perianal Disease in Inflammatory Bowel Disease	476

David W. Larson, MD, John H. Pemberton, MD

83	Dysplasia Surveillance Programs	485

Teresa A. Brentnall, MD

84	Pregnancy and Inflammatory Bowel Disease	490

Mary Lawrence Harris, MD

85	Intestinal and Colonic Strictures	494

Richard Kozarek, MD

86	Acute Colonic Pseudo-Obstruction	503

Parviz Nikoomanesh, MD, Salim A. Jaffer, MD

87	Microscopic Colitis: Collagenous, Lymphocytic, and Eosinophilic Colitis	506

Marcia Cruz-Correa, MD, PhD, Francis M. Giardiello, MD

88	Fecal Incontinence: Evaluation and Treatment	511

Arden M. Morris, MD, MPH, Robert D. Madoff, MD

89	Rectal Prolapse, Rectal Intussusception, and Solitary Rectal Ulcer Syndrome	518

Anders Mellgren, MD, PhD, Johan Pollack, MD, Inkeri Schultz, MD, PhD

90	Ileoanal Pouch: Frequent Evacuation	525

L. J. Egan, MD, S. F. Phillips, MD

91	Anorectal Diseases	530

Steven D. Wexner, MD, Giovanna DeSilva, MD

92	Hemorrhoids	536

Nir Wasserberg, MD, Howard S. Kaufman, MD

93	Colorectal Polyp and Cancer Screening	541

John H. Bond, MD

94	Colonic Neoplasia: Genetic Counseling	545

Jennifer E. Axilbund, MS, CGC, Francis M. Giardiello, MD

95	Colorectal Polyps and Polyposis Syndromes	550

Robert F. Wong, MD, Randall W. Burt, MD

96	**Colon Cancer** 557	
	Eugene Kennedy, MD, Michael A. Choti, MD	
97	**Colorectal Carcinoma: Adjuvant and Chemotherapy** 563	
	Sharlene Gill, MD, Richard M. Goldberg, MD	
98	**Curative Intent Management of Rectal Cancer** 569	
	Nancy N. Baxter, MD, PhD, David A. Rothenberger, MD	
99	**Palliative Therapy for Rectal Cancer** 575	
	Jeffrey R. Avansino, MD, Matthias Stelzner, MD	
100	**Abdominal Radiation** 579	
	Michael A. Hughes, MD, MS, Ross A. Abrams, MD	
101	**Lower Gastrointestinal Bleeding** 584	
	Carlos G. Micames, MD, Michael F. Byrne, MD, John Baillie, MD, ChB, FRCP	
102	**Transcatheter Management of Upper and Lower Gastrointestinal Tract Bleeding** ... 590	
	Anthony C. Venbrux, MD, Elizabeth A. Ignacio, MD, Amy P. Soltes, RN, MSN, ACNP-BC, Albert K. Chun, MD	
103	**Diverticular Disease of the Colon** 597	
	James W. Thiele, MD, Ira J. Kodner, MD	
104	**Laboratory Evaluation and Liver Biopsy Assessment in Liver Disease** 604	
	F. Fred Poordad, MD	
105	**Acute Hepatitis: Management and Prevention** 611	
	Maria H. Sjogren, MD, MPH	
106	**Chronic Hepatitis B** 616	
	Averell H. Sherker, MD, FRCP(C)	
107	**Chronic Hepatitis C** 621	
	Rudra Rai, MD	
108	**Viral Hepatitis in Children** 625	
	Kathleen B. Schwarz, MD	
109	**Fulminant Hepatic Failure** 629	
	Timothy J. Davern, MD	
110	**Adult Liver Transplantation: Selection and Pretransplant Evaluation** 638	
	Paul J. Thuluvath, MBBS, MD, FRCP, Cary H. Patt, MD	
111	**Liver Transplantation: Surgical Techniques, Including Living Donor** 644	
	Luis Arrazola, MD, Ernesto Molmenti, MD, PhD, Andrew Klein, MD	
112	**Pediatric Liver Transplantation** 650	
	Ruba Azzam, MD, Estella M. Alonso, MD, Karan M. Emerick, MD, Peter F. Whitington, MD	
113	**Ascites and Its Complications** 656	
	Ke-Qin Hu, MD, Bruce A. Runyon, MD	
114	**Hepatic Encephalopathy** 661	
	Challa Ajit, MD, Santiago Munoz, MD	
115	**Alcoholic Liver Disease** 665	
	Christian Mendez, MD, Luis Marsano, MD, Daniell B. Hill, MD, Craig J. McClain, MD	
116	**Nonalcoholic Fatty Liver Disease** 671	
	Brent A. Neuschwander-Tetri, MD	
117	**Portal Hypertension** 675	
	Anne T. Wolf, MD, Norman D. Grace, MD	
118	**Noncirrhotic Portal Hypertension** 682	
	Christos S. Georgiades, MD, PhD, Jean-Francois Geschwind, MD	
119	**Drug-Induced Liver Disease** 689	
	Basuki Gunawan, MD, Neil Kaplowitz, MD	
120	**Liver Disease and Pregnancy** 694	
	Anne M. Larson, MD	

#	Chapter	Page
121	Primary Biliary Cirrhosis	701
	Jordan J. Feld, MD, E. Jenny Heathcote, MD	
122	Chronic Cholestasis and Its Sequelae	707
	Nora V. Bergasa, MD	
123	Primary Sclerosing Cholangitis and Cholangiocarcinoma	715
	Paul Angulo, MD, Gregory J. Gores, MD	
124	Management of Wilson's Disease	720
	Michael L. Schilsky, MD	
125	Hereditary Hemochromatosis	724
	Stephen A. Harrison, MD, Bruce R. Bacon, MD	
126	The Porphyrias	728
	Joseph R. Bloomer, MD	
127	Primary Hepatic Neoplasms	732
	Jorge A. Marrero, MD, MS, Anna S. Lok, MD	
128	Management of Hepatocellular Carcinoma	739
	Timothy M. Pawlik, MD, MPH, Melanie B. Thomas, MD, Jean-Nicolas Vauthey, MD	
129	Metastatic Cancer of the Liver	744
	Michael A. Choti, MD	
130	Laparoscopic Cholecystectomy	748
	Don J. Selzer, MD, Keith D. Lillemoe, MD	
131	Acute and Chronic Cholecystitis	753
	Alexandra L.B. Webb, MD, Aaron S. Fink, MD, FACS	
132	Cholelithiasis	759
	Cynthia W. Ko, MD, MS, Sum P. Lee, MD, PhD	
133	Biliary Strictures and Neoplasms	763
	Sergey V. Kantsevoy, MD, PhD	
134	Endoscopic Management of Bile Duct Obstruction and Sphincter of Oddi Dysfunction	766
	David J. Novak, MD, Firas Al-Kawas, MD	
135	Postcholecystectomy Syndrome	774
	Ayman Koteish, MD, Anthony N. Kalloo MD	
136	Acute Pancreatitis	777
	Anil B. Nagar, MD, Fred S. Gorelick, MD	
137	Chronic Pancreatitis: Surgical Considerations	784
	Oscar Joe Hines, MD, Howard A. Reber, MD	
138	Pancreatitis: Endoscopic Therapy	789
	Lee McHenry Jr, MD, Glen A. Lehman, MD	
139	Chronic Pancreatitis	796
	Peter Draganov, MD, Phillip P. Toskes, MD	
140	Cystic Fibrosis and Other Hereditary Diseases of the Pancreas	803
	Margaret P. Boland, MD, David R. Mack, MD	
141	Pancreatic and Periampullary Neoplasms	813
	Richard D. Schulick, MD	
142	Pancreatic Cancer Therapy	818
	Dan Laheru, MD	
143	Neoplastic Cysts and Other Precancerous Lesions of the Pancreas	823
	Ralph H. Hruban, MD, Michael Goggins, MD, Charles J. Yeo, MD, FACS	
144	Pancreatic and Islet Cell Transplantation	828
	Antonello Pileggi, MD, Camillo Ricordi, MD	
	Index	834

Contributors

Ross A. Abrams, MD
Department of Radiation Oncology
 and Molecular Radiation Sciences
Johns Hopkins University
Baltimore, Maryland

Maria T. Abreu, MD
Department of Medicine
Mount Sinai School of Medicine
New York, New York

Stephen C. Achuff, MD, FACC, FAHA
Department of Internal Medicine
Johns Hopkins University School of
 Medicine
Baltimore, Maryland

Samuel Nathan Adler, MD
Department of Gastroenterology
Bikur Holim Hospital
Jerusalem, Israel

Asyia Ahmad, MD
Department of Medicine
Drexel University College of Medicine
Philadelphia, Pennsylvania

Challa Ajit, MD, MACP
Department of Gastroenterology
Albert Einstein Medical Center
Philadelphia, Pennsylvania

Firas Al-Kawas, MD
Department of Medicine
Georgetown University
Washington, District of Columbia

Estella M. Alonso, MD
Department of Pediatrics
Northwestern University Feinberg
 School of Medicine
Chicago, Illinois

W. Kemper Alston, MD
Department of Medicine
University of Vermont College of
 Medicine
Burlington, Vermont

Marvin E. Ament, MD
Department of Medicine
UCLA Medical Center
Los Angeles, California

Paul Angulo, MD
Department of Medicine
Mayo Clinic College of Medicine
Rochester, Minnesota

Chandra Are, MD, FRCS
Department of Surgery
Johns Hopkins University School of
 Medicine
Baltimore, Maryland

Luis Arrazola, MD
Department of Surgery
Johns Hopkins Hospital
Baltimore, Maryland

Jeffrey R. Avansino, MD
Department of Surgery
University of Washington
Seattle, Washington

Jennifer E. Axilbund, MS, CGC
Department of Oncology
Johns Hopkins University
Baltimore, Maryland

Ruba K. Azzam, MD
Department of Pediatrics
Northwestern University Feinberg
 School of Medicine
Chicago, Illinois

Bruce R. Bacon, MD
Department of Internal Medicine
Saint Louis University School of
 Medicine
St. Louis, Missouri

John Baillie, MB, ChB, FRCP
Departmetn of Medicine
Duke University Medical Center
Durham, North Carolina

Jamie S. Barkin, MD, FACP, MACG
Department of Medicine
University of Miami
Miami, Florida

Nancy N. Baxter, MD, PhD, FRCSC
Department of Surgery
University of Minnesota
Minneapolis, Minnesota

Theodore M. Bayless, MD
Johns Hopkins University School of
 Medicine
Baltimore, Maryland

Donna M. Beitler, RN, CGRN
Department of Gastroenterology
Johns Hopkins Hospital
Baltimore, Maryland

Nora V. Bergasa, MD
Department of Medicine
Columbia University, College of
 Physicians and Surgeons
New York, New York

Ingvar Bjarnason MD, MSc, FRCPath, FRCP, DSc
Department of Medicine
King's College London
London, England

Joseph R. Bloomer, MD
Department of Medicine
University of Alabama at Birmingham
Birmingham, Alabama

Margaret P. Boland, MD
Department of Pediatrics
University of Ottawa
Ottawa, Ontario, Canada

Robert C. Bollinger, MD, MPH
Department of Medicine
Johns Hopkins University School of
 Medicine
Baltimore, Maryland

John H. Bond, MD
Department of Medicine
University of Minnesota
Minneapolis, Minnesota

Murray F. Brennan, MD
Department of Surgery
Cornell University, Wall Medical
 College
New York, New York

Teresa A. Brentnall
Department of Medicine
University of Washington School of
 Medicine
Seattle, Washington

Alan L. Buchman MD, MSPH
Department of Medicine
Northwestern University Feinberg
 School of Medicine
Chicago, Illinois

Daniel C. Buckles, MD
Department of Internal Medicine
Kansas University Medical Center
Kansas City, Kansas

Gregory B. Bulkley, MD, FACS
Department of Surgery
Johns Hopkins University School of
 Medicine
Baltimore, Maryland

Hans A. Büller, MD, PhD
Department of Pediatrics
Sophia Children's Hospital
Rotterdam, The Netherlands

Randall W. Burt, MD
Department of Internal Medicine
University of Utah School of Medicine
Salt Lake City, Utah

Michael F. Byrne, MD
Department of Medicine
University of British Columbia
Vancouver, British Columbia, Canada

Michael Camilleri, MD
Mayo Medical School
Rochester, Minnesota

Kurtis A. Campbell, MD
Department of Surgery
Johns Hopkins University School of
 Medicine
Baltimore, Maryland

Marcia I. Canto, MD, MHS
Department of Medicine
Johns Hopkins University School of
 Medicine
Baltimore, Maryland

Brooks D. Cash, MD
Department of Gastroenterology
Uniformed Services University of the
 Health Sciences
Bethesda, Maryland

Donald O. Castell, MD
Department of Medicine
Medical University of South Carolina
Charleston, South Carolina

Eugene P. Ceppa, MD
Department of Surgery
Duke University School of Medicine
Durham, North Carolina

Francis K. L. Chan, MD, FRCP, FACG
Department of Medicine &
 Therapeutics
The Chinese University of Hong Kong
Hong Kong, China

Michael Y. Chan, MD
Department of Internal Medicine
Johns Hopkins Medical Institutions
Baltimore, Maryland

Kenneth J. Chang, MD, FACG
Department of Medicine
University of California
Orange, California

Lin Chang, MD
Center for Neurovisceral Sciences and
 Women's Health
UCLA Division of Digestive Diseases
Los Angeles, California

Lawrence J. Cheskin, MD, FACP
Department of International Health
Johns Hopkins Bloomberg School of
 Public Health
Baltimore, Maryland

Onki Cheung, MD
Department of Medicine
University of Pittsburgh Medical
 Center
Pittsburgh, Pennsylvania

Michael A. Choti, MD
Department of Surgery
Johns Hopkins University School of
 Medicine
Baltimore, Maryland

Albert K. Chun, MD
Department of Radiology
George Washington University
 Hospital
Washington, District of Columbia

Ray E. Clouse, MD
Department of Medicine
Washington University
St. Louis, Missouri

Paul M. Colombani MD, MBA
Department of Surgery
Johns Hopkins University School of
 Medicine
Baltimore, Maryland

Massimo Conio, MD
Department of Gastroenterology
National Institute for Cancer Research
Genova, Italy

Filippo Cremonini, MD
Department of Neuroscience
Translational and Epidemiological
Mayo Clinic
Rochester, Minnesota

Sheila E. Crowe, MD, FRCPC
Department of Internal Medicine
University of Virginia
Charlottesville, Virginia

Marcia Cruz-Correa, MD, PhD
Department of Medicine
Cleveland Clinic Florida
Weston, Florida

Carmen Cuffari, MD
Department of Pediatrics
Johns Hopkins University School of
 Medicine
Baltimore, Maryland

Timothy J. Davern, MD
Department of Medicine
University of California
San Francisco, California

Yinka K. Davis, MD
Department of Pediatrics
Stanford University
Palo Alto, California

Mark H. DeLegge, MD, FACG
Department of Medicine
Medical University of South Carolina
Charleston, South Carolina

Giovanna DeSilva, MD
Department of Colorectal Surgery
Cleveland Clinic Florida
Weston, Florida

Anna Mae Diehl, MD
Duke University Medical Center
Durham, North Carolina

Anthony J. DiMarino Jr, MD
Department of Medicine
Thomas Jefferson University
Philadelphia, Pennsylvania

Peter Draganov, MD
Department of Medicine
University of Florida College of
 Medicine
Gainesville, Florida

Douglas A. Drossman, MD
Department of Medicine
University of North Carolina
Chapel Hill, North Carolina

David Edwin, PhD
Department of Psychiatry and
 Behavioral Sciences
Johns Hopkins University School of
 Medicine
Baltimore, Maryland

Lawrence J. Egan, MD
Department of Medicine
Mayo Clinic
Rochester, Minnesota

Karan M. Emerick, MD
Department of Pediatrics
Northwestern University Feinberg
 School of Medicine
Chicago, Illinois

Johanna C. Escher, MD, PhD
Department of Gastroenterology
Sophia Children's Hospital Erasmus
 Medical Center
Rotterdam, The Netherlands

Alessio Fasano, MD
Department of Pediatrics
University of Maryland School of
 Medicine
Baltimore, Maryland

Victor W. Fazio, MB, MS
Department of Colorectal Surgery
The Cleveland Clinic
Cleveland, Ohio

Jordan Feld, MD, FRCP(C)
Department of Medicine
University of Toronto
Toronto, Ontario, Canada

George D. Ferry, MD
Department of Pediatrics
Baylor College of Medicine
Houston, Texas

Rosangela Filiberti, PhD
Department of Environmental
 Epidemiology
National Cancer Research Institute
Genova, Italy

Aaron S. Fink, MD, FACS
Department of Surgery
Emory University School of Medicine
Atlanta, Georgia

Robert S. Fisher, MD
Department of Medicine
Temple University School of Medicine
Philadelphia, Pennsylvania

Arlene A. Forastiere, MD
Division of Medical Oncology
The Sidney Kimmel Comprehensive
 Cancer Center at Johns Hopkins
Baltimore, Maryland

Christos S. Georgiades, MD, PhD
Department of Radiology
Johns Hopkins Hospital
Baltimore, Maryland

Jean-Francois H. Geschwind, MD
Department of Radiology
Johns Hopkins Hospital
Baltimore, Maryland

Francis M. Giardiello, MD
Department of Medicine
Johns Hopkins University School of
 Medicine
Baltimore, Maryland

Fathia Gibril, MD
Department of Digestive Diseases
 Branch
National Institutes of Health
Bethesda, Maryland

Michael K. Gibson, MD
Division of Medical Oncology
The Sidney Kimmel Comprehensive
 Cancer Center at Johns Hopkins
Baltimore, Maryland

Sharlene Gill, MD, MPH, FRCPC
Department of Medicine
University of British Columbia
Vancouver, British Columbia, Canada

Mae F. Go, MD
Department of Medicine
University of Utah School of Medicine
Salt Lake City, Utah

Michael Goggins, MD
Department of Pathology and
 Medicine
Johns Hopkins University School of
 Medicine
Baltimore, Maryland

Richard M. Goldberg, MD
Department of Medicine
University of North Carolina at Chapel
 Hill
Chapel Hill, North Carolina

Fred S. Gorelick, MD
Department of Medicine and Cell
 Biology
Yale University
New Haven, Connecticut

Gregory J. Gores, MD
Department of Internal Medicine
Mayo Foundation
Rochester, Minnesota

Norman D. Grace, MD, FACP, FACG
Department of Medicine
Brigham and Women's Hospital
Boston, Massachusetts

David Y. Graham, MD, FACP, MACG
Department of Medicine
Baylor College of Medicine
Houston, Texas

Angela S. Guarda, MD
Department of Psychiatry
Johns Hopkins University School of
 Medicine
Baltimore, Maryland

Basuki Gunawan, MD
Department of Medicine
University of Sothern Califonia Keck
 School of Medicine
Los Angeles, California

Amita Gupta, MD
Department of Medicine
Johns Hopkins University School of
 Medicine
Baltimore, Maryland

Gregory B. Haber, MD, FRCPC
Department of Medicine
University of Toronto
Toronto, Ontario, Canada

Stephen B. Hanauer, MD
Department of Gastroenterology
University of Chicago
Chicago, Illinois

Mary Lawrence Harris, MD
Department of Medicine
Johns Hopkins Medical Institutions
Baltimore, Maryland

Stephen A. Harrison, MD
Department of Internal Medicine
Brooke Army Medical Center
Houston, Texas

Awori J. Hayanga, MD, AFRCSI
Department of Surgery
Johns Hopkins University School of
 Medicine
Baltimore, Maryland

E. Jenny Heathcote, MD
Department of Medicine
University of Toronto
Toronto, Ontario, Canada

Paul Angulo Hernandez, MD
Department of Internal Medicine
Mayo Foundation
Rochester, Minnesota

Luis A. Herrera, PhD
Medician Genómica y Toxicologia
 Ambiental
Universidad Nacional Autónama de
 Mexico
Mexico, DF, Mexico

Daniell B. Hill, MD
Department of Medicine
University of Louisville
Louisville, Kentucky

Robert J. Hilsden, MD, PhD, FRCPC
Department of Medicine
University of Calgary
Calgary, Alberta, Canada

Oscar Joe Hines, MD
Department of Surgery
UCLA School of Medicine
Los Angeles, California

Walter J. Hogan, MD
Department of Medicine
Medical College of Wisconsin
Milwaukee, Wisconsin

W. A. Hoogerwerf, MD
Department of Internal Medicine
University of Texas Medical Branch
Galveston, Texas

Karoly Horvath, MD, PhD
Department of Pediatrics
University of Maryland
Baltimore, Maryland

Brenda J. Horwitz, MD
Department of Medicine
Temple University School of Medicine
Philadelphia, Pennsylvania

Ralph H. Hruban MD
Department of Pathology
Johns Hopkins University School of
 Medicine
Balitmore, Maryland

Ke-Qin Hu, MD
Department of Medicine
University of California, Irvine
Orange, California

Michael A. Hughes, MD, MS
Department of Radiation Oncology
Johns Hopkins University School of
 Medicine
Baltimore, Maryland

Wendy S. Hupp, DMD
Department of Diagnostic Sciences
Nova Southeastern University
Fort Lauderdale, Florida

Elizabeth A. Ignacio, MD
Department of Radiology
George Washington University
 Hospital
Washington, District of Columbia

J. Andrew Isch, MD
Department of Surgery
University of Washington
Seattle, Washington

Abdul Jabbar, MD
Department of Medicine
University of Louisville
Louisville, Kentucky

Salim A. Jaffer, MD
Department of Medicine
Johns Hopkins University School of
 Medicine
Baltimore, Maryland

Sanjay Jagannath, MD
Department of Medicine
Johns Hopkins University School of
 Medicine
Baltimore, Maryland

Robert T. Jensen, MD
Digestive Diseases Branch
National Institute of Health
Bethesda, Maryland

Michael P. Jones, MD, FACP, FACG
Division of Gastroenterology
Northwestern University Feinberg
 School of Medicine
Chicago, Illinois

Peter J. Kahrilas, MD
Department of Medicine
Northwestern University Feinberg
 School of Medicne
Chicago, Illinois

Anthony N. Kalloo, MD, FACP
Department of Medicine
Johns Hopkins University School of
 Medicine
Balitmore, Maryland

Sergey V. Kantsevoy, MD, PhD
Department of Internal Medicine
Johns Hopkins University School of
 Medicine
Baltimore, Maryland

Irina Kaplounov, MD
Department of Medicine
St. Luke's-Roosevelt Hospital Center
New York, New York

Neil Kaplowitz, MD
Department of Medicine
University of Southern California Keck
 School of Medicine
Los Angeles, California

Howard S. Kaufman, MD
University of Southern California Keck
 School of Medicine
Los Angeles, California

Ciarán P. Kelly, MD
Department of Medicine
Beth Israel Deaconess Medical Center
Boston, Massachusetts

Michael L. Kendrick, MD
Division of General and
 Gastroenterologic Surgery
Mayo Clinic
Rochester, Minnesota

Eugene Kennedy, MD
Department of Medicine
Johns Hopkins University School of
 Medicine
Baltimore, Maryland

Beth D. Kirkpatrick, MD
Department of Medicine
University of Vermont College of
 Medicine
Burlington, Vermont

Andrew S. Klein, MD, MBA
Department of Surgery
Cedars-Sinai Medical Center
Los Angeles, California

Ira J. Kodner, MD
Department of Colon and Rectal
 Surgery
Springfield Clinic
Springfield, Illinois

Cynthia W. Ko, MD, MS
Department of Medicine
University of Washington School of
 Medicine
Seattle, Washington

Jimmy Ko, MD
Department of Medicine
Mount Sinai Medical Center
New York, New York

Ayman Koteish, MD
Department of Medicine
Johns Hopkins University School of
 Medicine
Baltimore, Maryland

Donald P. Kotler, MD
Department of Medicine
St. Luke's-Roosevelt Hospital Center
New York, New York

Richard Kozarek, MD
Department of Medicine
University of Washington
Seattle, Washington

John H. Kwon, MD, PhD
Department of Medicine
Beth Israel Deaconess Medical Center
Boston, Massachusetts

Daniel M. Labow, MD
Department of Surgery
Memorial Sloan-Kettering Cancer
 Center
New York, New York

Brian E. Lacy, MD, PhD
Division of Gastroenterology
Johns Hopkins University School of
 Medicine
Baltimore, Maryland

Dan Laheru, MD
Department of Medical Oncology
Johns Hopkins University School of
 Medicine
Baltimore, Maryland

Anne M. Larson, MD
Deparment of Medicine
University of Washington
Seattle, Washington

David W. Larson, MD
Department of Surgery
Mayo Graduate School of Medicine
Rochester, Minnesota

Linda A. Lee, MD
Department of Medicine
Johns Hopkins University School of
 Medicine
Baltimore, Maryland

Sum P. Lee, MD, PhD
Department of Medicine
University of Washington School of
 Medicine
Seattle, Washington

Glen A. Lehman, MD
Department of Medicine
Indiana University
Indianapolis, IN

Gary R. Lichtenstein, MD
Department of Medicine
University of Pennsylvania School of
 Medicine
Philadelphia, Pennsylvania

Keith D. Lillemoe, MD
Department of Surgery
Indiana University School of Medicine
Indianapolis, Indiana

Anna S. Lok, MD
Department of Internal Medicine
University of Michigan
Ann Arbor, Michigan

David R. Mack, MD
Department of Pediatrics
University of Ottawa
Ottawa, Ontario, Canada

Robert D. Madoff, MD
Department of Surgery
University of Minnesota
Minneapolis, Minnesota

Norman E. Marcon, MD
Department of Medicine
University of Medicine
Toronto, Ontario, Canada

Jorge A. Marrero, MD, MSc
Department of Internal Medicine
University of Michigan
Ann Arbor, Michigan

Luis Marsano, MD
Department of Medicine
University of Louisville
Louisville, Kentucky

Lloyd Mayer, MD
Department of Immunology
Mount Sinai School of Medicine
New York, New York

Richard W. McCallum, MD
Department of Internal Medicine
Kansas University Medical Center
Kansas City, Kansas

Craig J. McClain, MD
Department of Medicine
University of Louisville
Louisville, Kentucky

Stephen McClave, MD
Department of Medicine
University of Louisville
Louisville, Kentucky

Lee McHenry Jr, MD
Department of Medicine
Indiana University
Indianapolis, Indiana

Anders Mellgren, MD, PhD
Department of Medicine
University of Minnesota
Minneapolis, Minnesota

Christian M. Mendez, MD
Department of Medicine
University of Louisville School of
 Medicine
Louisville, Kentucky

Carlos G. Micames, MD
Department of Medicine
Duke University Medical Center
Durham, North Carolina

Philip B. Miner Jr, MD
Oklahoma Foundation For Digestive
 Research
Oklahoma City, Oklahoma

Mack C. Mitchell Jr, MD
Department of Internal Medicine
Johns Hopkins University School of
 Medicine
Baltimore, Maryland

Ernesto P. Molmenti MD, PhD
Department of Surgery
Johns Hopkins University School of
 Medicine
Baltimore, Maryland

Gregory J. Monkewich, MD, FRCPC
Department of Medicine
University of Toronto
Toronto, Ontario, Canada

Arden M. Morris, MD, MPH
Department of Surgery
University of Michigan
Ann Arbor, Michigan

Santiago J. Munoz, MD
Department of Medicine
Albert Einstein Medical Center
Philadelphia, Pennsylvania

Michel M. Murr, MD, FACS
Department of Surgery
University of South Florida
Tampa, Florida

Lawrence F. Muscarella, PhD
Custom Ultrasonics, Inc.
Ivyland, Pennsylvania

Anil B. Nagar, MD
Department of Medicine
Yale University
New Haven, Connecticut

Brent A. Neuschwander-Tetri, MD
Department of Internal Medicine
Saint Louis University
St. Louis, Missouri

Parviz Nikoomanesh, MD
Department of Medicine
Johns Hopkins University School of
 Medicine
Baltimore, Maryland

David J. Novak, MD
Department of Medicine
Georgetown University
Washington, District of Columbia

Brant K. Oelschlager, MD
Department of Surgery
University of Washington
Seattle, Washington

Anthony P. Olivé, MD
Department of Pediatrics
Baylor College of Medicine
Houston, Texas

William C. Orr, PhD
Department of Medicine
University of Oklahoma Health
 Sciences Center
Oklahoma City, Oklahoma

Jaime A. Oviedo, MD
Division of Gastroenterology
Boston University School of Medicine
Boston, Massachusetts

Faullin Paletsky, MD
Department of Medicine
Drexel University College of Medicine
Philadelphia, Pennsylvania

John E. Pandolfino, MD
Department of Medicine
Northwestern University Feinberg
 School of Medicine
Chicago, Illinois

Julie Parsonnet, MD
Department of Medicine and Health
 Research and Policy
Stanford University School of
 Medicine
Stanford, California

Pankaj J. Pasricha, MD
Department of Internal Medicine
University of Texas Medical Branch
Galveston, Texas

Cary H. Patt, MD
Department of Medicine
Johns Hopkins University School of
 Medicine
Baltimore, Maryland

Timothy M. Pawlick, MD, MPH
Department of Surgical Oncology
University of Texas M. D. Anderson
 Cancer Center
Houston, Texas

Carlos A. Pellegrini, MD
Department of Surgery
University of Washington Medical
 Center
Seattle, Washington

John H. Pemberton, MD
Department of Surgery
Mayo Graduate School of Medicine
Rochester, Minnesota

Sidney F. Phillips, MD
Department of Medicine
Mayo Clinic
Rochester, Minnesota

Michael F. Picco, MD, PhD
Department of Medicine
Mayo Medical School
Jacksonville, Florida

Antonello Pileggi, MD
Department of Surgery
University of Miami School of
 Medicine
Miami, Florida

Joseph R. Pisegna, MD
Department of Medicine
David Geffen School of Medicine at
 UCLA
Los Angeles, California

Johan Pollack, MD
Department of Surgery
Karolinska Institutet at Danderyd
 Hospital
Stockholm, Sweden

F. Fred Poordad, MD
Department of Medicine
David Geffon School of Medicine at UCLA
Los Angeles, California

Daniel H. Present, MD
Department of Medicine
Mount Sinai School of Medicine
New York, New York

Nicholas Pyrsopoulos, MD
Department of Surgery
Johns Hopkins University School of Medicine
Baltimore, Maryland

Rudra Rai, MD
Department of Medicine
Johns Hopkins University School of Medicine
Baltimore, Maryland

William J. Ravich, MD
Department of Medicine
Johns Hopkins University School of Medicine
Baltimore, Maryland

Howard A. Reber, MD
Department of Surgery
University of California, Los Angeles, School of Medicine
Los Angeles, California

Graham Redgrave, MD
Department of Psychiatry and Behavioral Sciences
Johns Hopkins University School of Medicine
Baltimore, Maryland

Feza H. Remzi, MD
Department of Colorectal Surgery
Cleveland Clinic Foundation
Cleveland, Ohio

James C. Reynolds, MD
Department of Medicine
Drexel University College of Medicine
Philadelphia, Pennsylvania

Joel E. Richter, MD
Temple University School of Medicine
Philadelphia, Pennsylvania

Camillo Ricordi, MD
Department of Surgery
University of Miami School of Medicine
Miami, Florida

Justin Rosemore, DO
Department of Gastroenterology
Johns Hopkins School of Medicine
Baltimore, Maryland

David A. Rothenberger, MD
Department of Surgery
University of Minnesota
Minneapolis, Minnesota

Bruce A. Runyon, MD
Department of Internal Medicine
Loma Linda University
Loma Linda, California

Andrew I. Sable, MD
Division of Gastroenterology
University of Miami Affiliated Hospitals
Miami, Florida

R. Bradley Sack, MS, MD, ScD
Department of International Health
Johns Hopkins Bloomberg School of Public Health
Baltimore, Maryland

Richard E. Sampliner, MD
Department of Medicine
University of Arizona College of Medicine
Tucson, Arizona

Michael G. Sarr, MD
Division of General and Gastroenterologic Surgery
Mayo Clinic
Rochester, Minnesota

Lawrence R. Schiller, MD, FACP, FACG
Department of Internal Medicine
University of Texas Southwestern Medical Center
Dallas, Texas

Michael L. Schilsky, MD
Department of Medicine
New York Weill Cornell Medical Center
New York, New York

Kenneth W. Schroeder, MD, PhD, FACP
Department of Internal Medicine
Mayo Clinic College of Medicine
Rochester, Minnesota

Richard D. Schulick, MD, FACS
Department of Surgery, Oncology, Obstetrics and Gynecology
Johns Hopkins Medical Institutions
Baltimore, Maryland

Inkeri Schultz, MD, PhD
Department of Surgery
Karolinska Institutet at Danderyd Hospital
Stockholm, Sweden

Kathleen B. Schwarz, MD
Department of Pediatrics
Johns Hopkins University School of Medicine
Baltimore, Maryland

Dorry Segev, MD
Department of Surgery
Johns Hopkins University School of Medicine
Baltimore, Maryland

Don J. Selzer, MD
Department of Surgery
Indiana University School of Medicine
Indianapolis, Indiana

Reza Shaker, MD
Department of Medicine
Medical College of Wisconsin
Milwaukee, Wisconsin

Averell H. Sherker, MD, FRCP(C)
Department of Medicine
Washington Hospital Center
Washington, District of Columbia

Michael A. Siegel, DDS, MS
Department of Diagnostic Sciences
Nova Southeastern University of Dental Medicine
Fort Lauderdale, Florida

Maria H. Sjogren, MD, MPH
Department of Medicine
Georgetown University
Washington, District of Columbia

Amy P. Soltes, RN, MSN, ACNP-BC
Department of Radiology
George Washington University Hospital
Washington, District of Columbia

Amnon Sonnenberg, MD, MSc
Department of Medicine
Oregon Health and Science University
Portland, Oregon

Darius Sorbi, MD
Department of Gastroenterology
Mayo Clinic
Scottsdale, Arizona

Miles P. Sparrow, MD
Department of Gastroenterology
University of Chicago
Chicago, Illinois

Matthias Stelzner, MD, FACS
Department of Surgery
University of California at Los Angeles
Los Angeles, California

Chinyu Su, MD
Department of Medicine
University of Pennsylvania School of
 Medicine
Philadelphia, Pennsylvania

Ken Takeuchi, MD
Department of Medicine
GKT Medical School
London, England

Mark A. Talamini, MD
Department of Surgery
Johns Hopkins University School of
 Medicine
Baltimore, Maryland

Shou-Jiang Tang, MD
University of Toronto
Toronto, Ontario, Canada

James W. Thiele, MD
Department of Colon and Rectal
 Surgery
Springfield Clinic
Springfield, Illinois

Melanie B. Thomas, MD, MS
Department of Gastrointestinal
 Medical Oncology
University of Texas MD Anderson
 Cancer Center
Houston, Texas

Paul J. Thuluvath, MBBS, MD, FRCP
Department of Medicine
Johns Hopkins University School of
 Medicine
Baltimore, Maryland

Phillip P. Toskes, MD
Department of Medicine
University of Florida College of
 Medicine
Gainesville, Florida

William J. Tremaine, MD
Division of Gastroenterology and
 Hepatology
Mayo Clinic College of Medicine
Rochester, Minnesota

Anthony P. Tufaro, DDS, MD
Department of Surgery
Johns Hopkins University School of
 Medicine
Baltimore, Maryland

Lisa Turnbough, RN
Department of Medicine
Johns Hopkins University
Baltimore, Maryland

Radu Tutuian, MD
Department of Medicine
Medical University of South Carolina
Charleston, South Carolina

Andreas G. Tzakis, MD, PhD
Department of Surgery
Johns Hopkins University School of
 Medicine
Baltimore, Maryland

Jean-Nicholas Vauthey, MD, FACS
Department of Surgical Oncology
University of Texas MD Anderson
 Cancer Center
Houston, Texas

Maria J. Verhoef, PhD
Department of Community Health
 Sciences
University of Calgary
Calgary, Alberta, Canada

Anthony C. Venbrux, MD
Department of Radiology
George Washington University
 Hospital
Washington, District of Columbia

Georgia B. Vogelsang, MD
Department of Oncology
Johns Hopkins University School of
 Medicine
Baltimore, Maryland

Axel von Herbay, MD
Institute of Pathology
University of Heidelberg
Heidelberg, Germany

Arnold Wald, MD
Department of Medicine
University of Pittsburgh Medical
 Center
Pittsburgh, Pennsylvania

Nir Wasserberg, MD
Department of Surgery
University of Southern California
Los Angeles, California

Alexandra L.B. Webb, MD
Department of Surgery
Emory University School of Medicine
Atlanta, Georgia

Steven D. Wexner, MD
Ohio State University Health Sciences
 Center
Cleveland, Ohio

Wilfred M. Weinstein, MD
Department of Medicine
David Geffen School of Medicine at
 UCLA
Los Angeles, California

Peter F. Whitington, MD
Department of Pediatrics
Northwestern University Feinberg
 School of Medicine
Chicago, Illinois

C. Mel Wilcox, MD
Department of Medicine
University of Alabama at Birmingham
Birmingham, Alabama

Anne T. Wolf, MD
Harvard University School of Medicine
Boston, Massachusetts

M. Michael Wolfe, MD, FACP, FACG
Department of Medicine
Boston University School of Medicine
Boston, Massachusetts

Robert F. Wong, MD
Division of Gastroenterology
University of Utah School of Medicine
Salt Lake City, Utah

Charles J. Yeo, MD, FACS
Department of Surgery
Johns Hopkins University School of
 Medicine
Baltimore, Maryland

PREFACE

This is the fifth edition of a book devoted to the details of medical, endoscopic, surgical, nutritional and supportive management of patients with digestive tract and liver disease. The concept, originally provided by our publisher Brian C. Decker, has been to gather a series of "consultations" on common or troubling disorders, which provide specific and detailed guidelines or recommendations for the physician caring for an individual patient. We have assumed that many of the readers of this text will be experienced and competent digestive and liver disease experts who have already made the correct diagnosis and are now looking for another opinion regarding a new or controversial treatment modality. Dr. Anna Mae Diehl, a leader in liver disease therapy and research, has joined me as Co-Editor.

Just as each of us would be tempted to call the expert on new therapies for Crohn's Disease, on management of Hepatitis C, endoscopic mucosal resection, endoscopic therapy for GERD, psychotropic drugs for functional disorders or abdominal pain, or for the latest on colon cancer chemotherapy, we have persuaded the experts to write a brief chapter on her or his approach to a specific treatment problem. The authors of the 144 chapters have been generous with their insights and recommendations. All have been able to present their views on management and prognosis both clearly and concisely. We want to know what they do and why. This usually goes beyond the results of clinical trials and evidence-based medicine. As in many phases of medicine, there still are a lot of unanswered questions that we as clinicians face almost daily. Most chapters end with a list of supplemental readings. This has been more useful than asking the author to document every opinion. The editors added brief comments to some of the chapters to call attention to other views or other areas of potential interest.

As one looks through the table of contents, they will appreciate the combined medical and surgical approach to common digestive tract problems. Thirty of the authors are surgeons. Common and troublesome patient problems are discussed, at times, by more than one author to present divergent views. New endoscopic techniques and new medications are described by experienced clinicians. There is a strong focus on functional disorders, including recurrent abdominal pain, and the use of psychotropic medications. We are keenly aware of the need for additional laboratory and clinical research in digestive and liver diseases and the authors often point out the unanswered questions. Ensuing editions will chronicle improvements in the management of these important maladies.

We are grateful to our patients who have taught us the importance of many of the issues in this book; to the authors, who shared their views with us; to our colleagues in the Gastroenterology-Liver Division and in the Meyerhoff Digestive Disease-Inflammatory Bowel Disease Center who have participated in the patient care and research that form many of our views of patient management; to our publisher and his staff at BC Decker, including Paula Mucci, Monika Holden and Petrice Custance; and to our editorial assistants Donna Rode and Estelle Boyko. Our profound thanks to our spouses, children and grandchildren, who gave up their time to permit this type of endeavor.

Theodore M. Bayless, MD
Anna Mae Diehl, MD
January 2005

CHAPTER 1

USING EVIDENCE-BASED MEDICINE IN PATIENT CARE

Brooks D. Cash, MD

The practice of evidence-based medicine is the ideal to which all clinicians should aspire. As defined by Sackett and colleagues (1996) evidence-based medicine is "the conscientious and judicious use of current best evidence from clinical care research in the management of individual patients." The "conscientious use" of clinical evidence implies a persistent pattern of review of current and emerging research by clinicians seeking to improve patient-centered outcomes and the efficiency of their practice. The evidence should be the "current best evidence," implying that the studies reviewed are the most methodologically sound studies available, and that clinicians understand and apply criteria for determining the validity and accuracy of the study results. Lastly, the clinician understands that ultimately he or she must use their informed judgment to determine if the results of a particular study apply to their "individual patients," and whether or not their practice habits will be altered by the study findings.

Outcomes Research

Inherent in the practice of evidence-based medicine is the concept of outcomes research, which is the study of "the outcomes of health care services and procedures used to prevent, diagnose, treat, and manage illness and disability" (Agency for Healthcare Policy and Research, 1990). In other words, outcomes research attempts to demonstrate real and tangible effects of the integration of clinical care research into the everyday practice of medicine. Outcomes are often difficult to quantify and may differ depending on one's perspective. Few would argue that the most important outcome for patients is improvement of their health related quality of life, but in an era of increasing financial pressures and access demands, outcomes that are considered from a societal perspective, such as delineating the most cost effective approaches to disease states and minimization of practice variation, have taken on additional importance. In its simplest form, evidence-based medicine is a method of appraising the medical literature to determine the most relevant and accurate studies that will provide an answer to a focused clinical question. Studies about different aspects of a disease state (risk, diagnosis, prognosis, and therapy) necessarily have different designs (Figure 1-1). Similarly, different validity criteria apply to different types of studies (Tables 1-1 through to 1-7).

Evidence-Based Medicine Approach to Therapy

Therapy to Prevent Recurrent Gastrointestinal Bleeding

Many clinical decisions will deal with therapeutic options. For example, a 64-year-old black male is admitted to the intensive care unit after presenting with hematemesis and near syncope. His previous medical history is notable for osteoarthritis, for which he takes a nonsteroidal anti-inflammatory agent bid. He has been adequately resuscitated and an upper endoscopy reveals a 1 cm bleeding gastric ulcer. The lesion is treated endoscopically. The senior medicine resident inquires about the need for acid suppression medications to reduce the risk of recurrent bleeding.

Using an evidence-based medicine approach, the initial focused clinical questions are twofold: Does the use of acid suppression reduce the risk of recurrent bleeding in patients with endoscopically treated bleeding peptic ulcer lesions and, if so, what is the best regimen? Secondly, the fastest routes to finding answers to focused clinical questions are the prefiltered online databases, such as *Best Evidence* or the *Cochrane Collaboration*. Prefiltered databases contain rigorous, systematic reviews of the literature, about particular clinical questions, that are frequently updated. Unfortunately, not all clinical scenarios are included in these databases and one must often use a nonprefiltered database, such as *PubMed*, to search for articles pertaining to a particular clinical scenario. The potential for retrieving many irrelevant citations is sizable using such databases, but various strategies, as reviewed by Greenhalgh (1997) may be used to maximize the results of an individual search.

Methodologic Validity

The clinician needs to consider three questions: Are the results of the trial valid (ie, is the methodology of the study appropriate for the type of trial), what are the results (ie, the degree and accuracy of the differences between approaches), and how will the results affect their practice (ie, are the clinician's patients similar to the patients in the study, and have all important outcomes been measured)? For a valid article about therapy, certain methodologic features should be present (see Table 1-1).

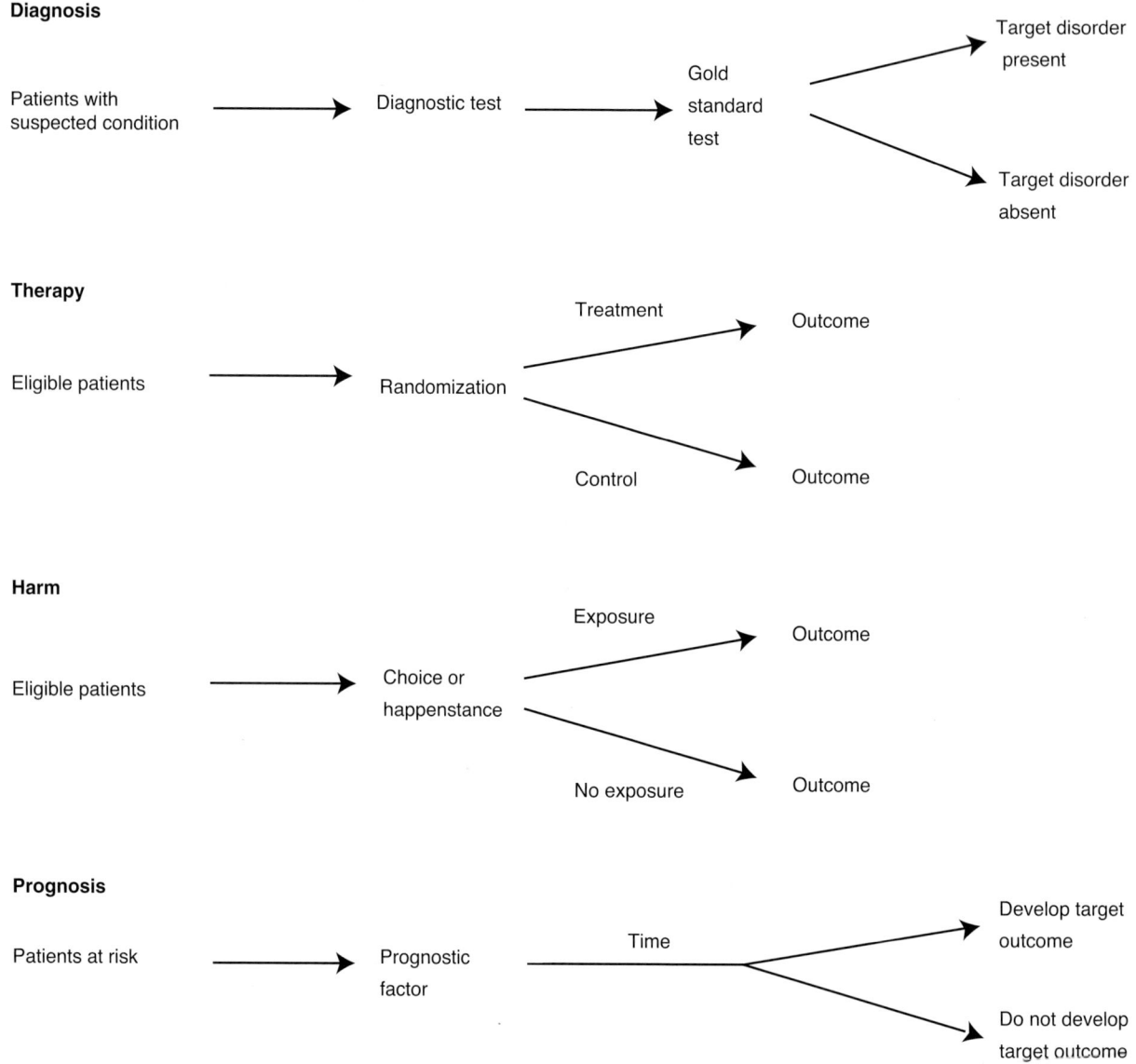

FIGURE 1-1. Clinical design of studies for core clinical questions.

For our case scenario, trials using histamine-2-receptor antagonists indicate that the clinical benefit for reducing recurrent bleeding may not be significantly greater than placebo. However, several trials examining proton pump inhibitors (PPI) do indicate a potential to reduce rebleeding. The most promising of these is by Lau and colleagues (2000) who examined the use of an intravenous (IV) PPI after endoscopic treatment of high risk peptic ulcer lesions, just as in our case scenario. The methods of this study indicate that it was a randomized controlled, double blind trial with concealed allocation, well-defined primary and secondary endpoints, and complete follow-up. It is appropriately powered for the primary endpoint (recurrent bleeding), and the results are reported in an intention to treat fashion, minimizing potential bias due to patient withdrawals or exclusions. The study results indicate a significant decrease in the incidence of recurrent peptic ulcer bleeding after endoscopic treatment, as well as shorter hospital stays and fewer transfusions, as a result of IV PPI administration.

Statistical Analysis

Appropriate statistical analysis is an integral part of any clinical trial in terms of the magnitude of the observed effect and the accuracy of the results. Differences in treatment effect are typically described as relative benefit increase and absolute benefit increase or relative risk reduction (RRR) and absolute risk reduction (ARR). The formulas for RRR and ARR are shown in Table 1-2. The RRR is the risk of the target outcome in one treatment group relative to the risk

TABLE 1-1. Characteristics of a Well-Designed Trial about Therapy

Are the results valid?
  Was the prognosis of patients in each group similar at the start of the trial?
    Was the trial randomized?
    Was the randomization blinded (concealed allocation)?
    Were patients analyzed according to the group to which they were randomized?
    Were patients similar with respect to demographics and known prognostic factors?
  Was the prognosis of patients in each group similar after randomization?
    Was there double blinding (patients and investigators)?
    Was follow-up complete?
What are the results?
  How large is the treatment effect?
  What is the precision of the estimate of the treatment effect?
Can the results be applied to patient care?
  Were the problem, study patients, and interventions similar to your practice?
  Were all outcomes of interest considered?
  Are the treatment benefits worth the potential harm and costs?

of the outcome in the other group. It tells us to what degree patients in the experimental group are more (or less) likely to experience the outcome of interest compared with patients in the control group. What it does not tell us is how often patients in either group will experience the outcome. Although it is true that a larger RRR is associated with a larger treatment effect, even a high RRR may be misleading if the control (expected) rate is very small. Because of this, the ARR may be a more useful basis for clinical decisions. The ARR describes the therapeutic yield of the experimental therapy above and beyond the control (expected) rate. It

TABLE 1-2. Computation of Relative Risk Reduction (RRR), Absolute Risk Reduction (ARR), and Number Needed to Treat (NNT)

	Presence of Rebleeding by Day 30	
	Yes	No
IV PPI	8/120 (a)	112/120 (b)
Placebo	27/120 (c)	93/120 (d)

RRR = (expected rate − experimental rate)/expected rate
   = (c − a)/c = (27/120 − 8/120)/(27/120)
   = (22.5% − 6.6%)/22.5%
   = 15.9%/22.5%
   = 70.6%
ARR = (expected rate − experimental rate)
   = (c − a) = (27/120) − (8/120)
   = 22.5% × 6.6%
   = 15.9%
NNT = 1/(ARR)
   = 1/(c − a) = 1/(22.5% − 6.6%)
   = 1/15.9%
   = 6.3

Adapted from Lau et al, 2000.
PPI = proton pump inhibitor.

describes the additional portion of the experimental group who would benefit as a result of using the experimental therapy rather than the control therapy. The reciprocal of the ARR is the number needed to treat (NNT), which is the number of patients who must be treated with the experimental therapy to achieve one additional outcome of interest. To illustrate this, consider a trial where the outcome is death. Assume that the baseline risk of death is 1 out of 1,000 (0.1%) with the control therapy. If the risk of death with the experimental therapy is 0.05%, then the RRR is 50%, the ARR is 0.05%, and the NNT is 2,000. It is up to the clinician to decide, based upon the cost, potential harms, feasibility and patient acceptance, whether or not pursuing the experimental therapy is reasonable. Additionally, it is important to realize that the NNT only applies to the period of time over which the study was conducted. For the trial by Lau and colleagues (2000), the RRR of 70.6% with IV PPI indicates that these patients are 70.6% less likely to rebleed than patients treated with placebo. The ARR of 15.9% indicates that rebleeding episodes will be decreased to 6.6% with use of an intravenous PPI, down from the baseline risk of 22.5%. The NNT of 6.3 indicates that between 6 and 7 patients need to be treated with IV PPI to prevent one rebleeding episode within 30 days.

The decision whether or not to reject the null hypothesis (that two different interventions do not affect the outcome) is commonly reported as the p value. By convention, we reject the null hypothesis and conclude that different outcomes exist as a result of true differences in interventions if the p value is "statistically significant" or < .05. That is, there is a 99.5% chance that the observed outcome differences are due to differences in intervention rather than due to chance alone. Alternatively, there is a less than 0.5% chance that the outcome differences are due to chance alone. Although statistical significance is an important result, the accuracy of the results and the clinical significance of treatment options are also important considerations. One of the most common ways to report the accuracy of the results is 95% CIs. For the trial in question, the relative risk (RR) of rebleeding with IV PPI relative to placebo was 30%. The 95% CI associated with this RR is 14.5% to 64.7%. This simply means that if the same trial were conducted 100 times, the true RR of rebleeding with IV PPI relative to placebo would be between 14.5% to 64.7%, 95 times out of 100. The 95% CI tells us, within the range of plausibility, how much greater or smaller the "true" effect is relative to the measured effect. The narrower the 95% CI, the closer to the truth the measured effect is.

Although this study offers a concise answer to our question, several other issues must be considered. This study was not adequately powered to demonstrate differences in mortality between treatment groups, was performed in Asian patients, and used a different IV PPI than is available in the United States. It is therefore up to the clinician to determine whether or not these issues are important enough to prevent him or her from using a different, albeit similar, medication in his non-Asian patient. This highlights one of the limitations of evidence-based medicine. Individual patients and scenarios rarely match those of a randomized controlled trial. There is a separate chapter on upper gastrointestinal bleeding (see Chapter 28, "Upper Gastrointestinal Bleeding"). A cost effectiveness analysis is presented in Chapter 2, "Decision Analysis in the Management of Digestive Diseases."

Evidenced-Based Medicine Approach to Diagnosis

Use of Computed Tomography Colonography As Screening

Consider the following scenario: "Executive physicals" with widespread application of computed tomography (CT) scanning to detect a variety of disease states has been gaining popularity. You have been asked by your hospital administration whether or not they should initiate a CT colonography program to screen patients for colorectal cancer.

A search of the literature databases reveals several articles about the use of CT colonography, or "virtual colonoscopy," for the identification of adenomatous neoplasia in the colon. Using the keywords "colorectal cancer screening" and "virtual colonoscopy," and limiting the search to English language articles with abstracts published within the last 5 years, 23 citations are identified. Further refinement of the search identifies 11 clinical trials, the most germane of which was a recent large trial by Fenlon and colleagues (1999) that addressed the diagnostic accuracy of virtual colonoscopy for colorectal polyps. After submission of this manuscript another publication on this topic appeared (Pickhardt et al, 2003).

The steps involved in an evidence-based medicine approach to a study about diagnosis may be found in Table 1-3. The study population consisted of patients with a history of polyps, a family history of colorectal cancer, or clinical symptoms suggestive of cancer. It used an appropriate gold standard comparison test, conventional colonoscopy, and blinded investigators performed the tests independently of one another. Virtual colonoscopy was completed in 87 of 100 patients and conventional colonoscopy was completed in 89 of 100 patients. The reasons for failure to complete colonoscopy or CT colonography were not defined.

As long as study design is appropriate, the results should be credible. Different statistical representations, including sensitivity and specificity, positive and negative predictive values, and likelihood ratios, may be used to report the accuracy of a diagnostic test. Although sensitivity and specificity are commonly reported, these representations fail to define the posttest probability (ie, the probability of disease after the performance of a diagnostic test), which is what the clinician really wants to know. Although positive predictive values (PPV) and negative predictive values (NPV) can provide the posttest probability of disease, these values will vary depending upon the prevalence of a disorder in a specific population. For studies about diagnosis, likelihood ratios are the most clinically helpful representations of accuracy because they facilitate transition from pretest to posttest probability.

Likelihood Ratios

Likelihood ratios are not commonly used in clinical practice, but they offer advantages over sensitivity, specificity, PPV, and NPV. Likelihood ratios do not vary with changes in the prevalence of a disorder and may be used for diagnostic test results that are continuous as well as dichotomous. The likelihood ratio is the probability that a specific test result will be found in patients with the disease divided by the probability that the same test result will be found in patients without the disease. In other words, they quantify the degree to which a given diagnostic test result will affect (positively or negatively) the pretest probability of disease. One can arrive at the posttest probability by applying the likelihood ratio to a nomogram (Figure 1-2), which incorporates a starting point (pretest probability), a modifier (likelihood ratio), and an ending point (posttest probability). A likelihood ratio of 1.0, when applied to the nomogram, will deliver a posttest probability that is equal to the pretest probability. Likelihood ratios > 10 or < 0.1 will typically generate large and often clinically meaningful shifts in pretest to posttest probability, whereas ratios between 1 to 2 and 0.5 to 1 have minimal effects on probability.

The results from the CT colonography article are depicted in Tables 1-4, 1-5. This data can easily be converted to a 232 table, and the sensitivity, specificity, PPV, NPV, and likelihood ratios may be calculated. When analyzed on a per patient basis, virtual colonoscopy has a sensitivity of 84%

TABLE 1-3. Characteristics of a Well-Designed Trial About Diagnosis

When are diagnostic tests necessary?
   Is the pretest probability of a disorder very high or very low?
Are the results valid?
   Was a blinded comparison between the new diagnostic test and a gold standard test performed?
   Was an acceptable alternative used if no gold standard test was available?
   Did all study patients get the gold standard test, regardless of the results of the new diagnostic test?
   Did investigators enroll patients in whom the diagnosis was in doubt?
   Was the frequency of indeterminate test results reported?
Interpreting the results
   Appropriately interpret and apply data about sensitivity, specificity, positive and negative predictive values
   Use likelihood ratios to maximize the utility of data from a diagnostic test study
Can the results be applied to patient care?
   Are your patients similar to the patients examined in this trial?
   Is the test likely to be reproducible with minimal variation in your clinical setting?

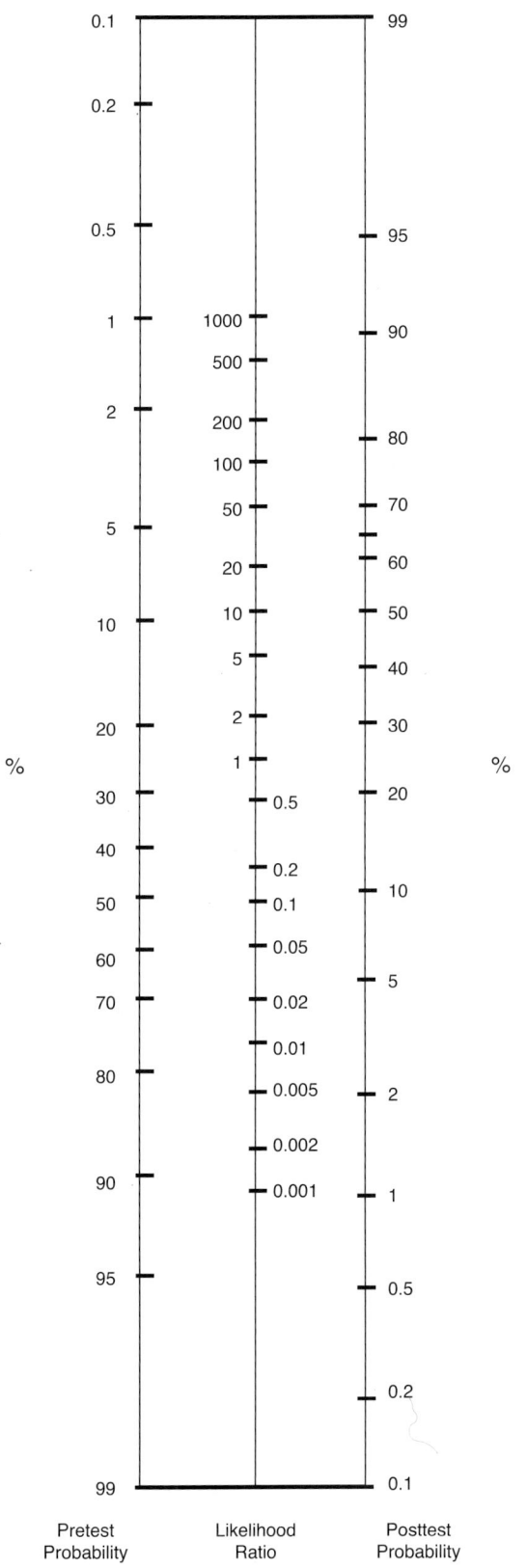

FIGURE 1-2. Nomogram for converting likelihood ratios into posttest probability. Place a straight edge at the pretest probability and draw a line through the likelihood ratio to determine what the posttest probability becomes after a positive or negative test result.

TABLE 1-4. Computation of Sensitivity/Specificity/ Positive Predicted Value (PPV)/Negative Predictive Value (NPV) and Likelihood Ratios

	Colon Polyps (per Patient Analysis)	
	Present	Absent
Positive test (polyp on CT colonography)	42 (TP)	8 (FP)
Negative test (no polyp on CT scan)	9 (FN)	41 (TN)

Sensitivity = TP/(TP + FN) = 42/(42 + 9) = 42/51 = 84%
Specificity = TN/(FP + TN) = 41/(41 + 8) = 41/49 = 82%
PPV = TP/(TP + FP) = 42/(42 + 8) = 42/50 = 84%
NPV = TN/(FN + TN) = 41/(9 + 41) = 41/50 = 82%

Likelihood ratio (positive test)
= Sensitivity/(1 − Specificity) = TP/(TP + FN)/(1 − TN)/(FP + TN)
= 0.84/(1−0.82) = 84%/18% = 5

Likelihood ratio (negative test)
= (1 − Sensitivity)/Specificity = ([1 − TP]/[TP + FN])/ TN/(FP + TN)
= (1 − 0.84)/0.82 = 16%/82% = 0.2

Adapted from Fenlon et al, 1999.
CT = computed tomography; FN = false negative; FP = false positive; TN = true negative; TP = true positive.

TABLE 1-5. Characteristics of a Well-Designed Systematic Review

Are the results valid?
  Did the review address a focused clinical question?
  Were the criteria for study selection appropriate?
  Was the validity of individual studies assessed?
  Was study selection and review performed independently and was it reproducible?
What are the results?
  What are the overall results of the study?
  How precise were the results?
Can the results be applied to patient care?
  Can the results be applied to my patient population?
  Were all clinically relevant outcomes addressed?
  Are the benefits worth the potential harms and costs?

and a specificity of 82% for identifying a polyp. The PPV is 84% and the NPV is 82%. The likelihood ratio for a positive test is 5, and the likelihood ratio of a negative test is 0.2. The prevalence of polyps in this high risk group of patients was 51%. Using this prevalence and these likelihood ratios, a positive CT colonography implies that a patient with a 51% pretest probability has a posttest probability of having polyps in the colon of 81%. A negative CT colonography implies a 17% posttest probability of having polyps in the colon (Stronger data using three-dimensional [3-D] CT is presented in Pickhardt et al, 2003).

The final step in this exercise is applying the results of the study to your scenario. Although this study fulfills the validity criteria for a study about diagnosis and the results are likely accurate, there are some potential limitations. The investigators chose a narrowly defined patient population that had a higher pretest probability of advanced polyps than the "spectrum" of asymptomatic patients over 50 years of age who will be screened for colorectal polyps and cancer. Additionally, this study did not report the interobserver variation associated with CT colonography and other studies that have reported less promising results for the detection of smaller polyps. Thus, because evidence did not support using CT colonography in an average risk screening population, and the data may not be as strong for the detection of small or flat lesions, you advised against initiation of the program until such time as there was evidence to support CT colonography for average risk colorectal cancer screening. There is a separate chapter on colorectal cancer screening (see Chapter 93, "Colorectal Polyp and Cancer Screening") which refers to the more accurate 3-D CT data (Pickhardt et al, 2003).

Evidence-Based Medicine Approach to Prognosis

Prognosis of Hepatitis C

You are the attending in a busy liver clinic. The gastroenterology fellow has just seen a 25-year-old male with chronic hepatitis C (HCV). The patient has liver enzymes that are two to three times the normal level, an elevated HCV RNA, and an HCV genotype of 1b. The fellow expresses a desire to treat the patient aggressively with interferon-based therapy because "he has a worse prognosis than patients with other HCV genotypes." When you ask him to justify his comment, he produces a recent article by Roffi and colleagues in which the influence of HCV genotype on the clinical outcome of liver disease was assessed in 2,307 patients with chronic HCV (Roffi et al, 2001).

Prognosis studies should seek to explain possible outcomes of a disease and define the probability with which they occur. Knowing this information is important for clinicians because it will affect their treatment thresholds and also aid them in discussing options with patients. Studies about prognosis are almost always cohort studies in which patients with similar risk factors for the outcome of interest are identified and followed over time to identify which patients develop the outcome, or case-control studies in which differences are investigated between similar groups with one of the groups consisting of subjects with the outcome of interest. Randomized controlled trials also may provide important prognostic information for each treatment arm.

The first consideration in considering an article about prognosis is determining whether or not the sample of patients included is representative of all patients to whom the results may apply. Referral bias is an example of where this concept may be important. Consider a study about the prognosis of irritable bowel syndrome (IBS). Patients with IBS seen at tertiary care facilities may represent the most refractory and symptomatic patients among the entire spectrum of IBS patients. As such, these patients may have a worse "prognosis" for continued IBS symptoms compared with the majority of patients with IBS who never seek medical attention for their symptoms. Individual patients in a study about prognosis should be reasonably homogeneous in terms of the "stage" of their disease and risk of the outcome of interest. Additionally, other potentially confounding factors (eg, age, gender, or habits) should be analyzed and, if found, adjusted for by the investigators. Follow-up should be sufficiently long and complete to minimize the chances of missing the development of any cases of the outcome of interest. If the outcome of more than 10 to 20% of a study population is unknown, the validity of the results may be compromised. Lastly, the outcome of interest should be as objective as possible, and all subjects should be examined for this outcome equally. If more subjective outcome criteria are used, individuals measuring outcomes should be blinded to the outcome and hypotheses of the study.

Upon reviewing the abstract and methods sections of the study by Roffi and colleagues (2001), you determine that it meets the validity criteria for a study about prognosis (see Tables 1-6 and 1-7). The sample of patients in this trial was representative of patients with chronic HCV who were sufficiently homogeneous with respect to their risk of objective outcomes, such as cirrhosis, hepatocellular cancer (HCC), and death. Investigators took explicit steps to account for potential confounds, such as age, alcohol and IV drug use, methods of HCV transmission, prevalent cirrhosis, and duration of infection in their analysis. Follow-up was sufficiently long and complete at 1,482 cumulative years, so that important outcomes were unlikely to be missed. The outcomes that were measured were done so in an objective and unbiased manner equally in all patients.

TABLE 1-6. Characteristics of a Well-Designed Trial About Harm

Are the results valid?
  Was the prognosis of patients in each group similar at the start of the trial?
    Did the investigators demonstrate similarity in all known determinants of outcome and did they adjust for any differences in the analysis?
    Were exposed patients equally likely to be identified in all groups being compared?
  Was the prognosis of patients in each group similar after randomization?
    Were outcomes measured equally in the groups being compared?
    Was follow-up long enough and sufficiently complete?
What are the results?
  How strong is the association between exposure and outcome?
  What is the precision of the estimate of risk?
Can the results be applied to patient care?
  Were the problem and study patients similar to those in your practice?
  Was the duration of follow-up adequate?
  What is the magnitude of the risk?
  Should the exposure be intervened against?

TABLE 1-7. Characteristics of a Well-Designed Trial About Prognosis

Are the results valid?
   Was a representative sample of patients included in the analysis?
   Were the patients similar with respect to prognostic risk?
   Was follow-up sufficiently long and complete?
   Were objective and unbiased outcome criteria used?
What are the results?
   How likely are the outcomes over time (the cumulative incidence of the outcome)?
   What is the precision of the estimates of the outcome of interest?
Can the results be applied to patient care?
   Were the study patients and management styles similar to the patients that you encounter?
   Did the study account for all important confounders?
   Can the results be used in the management of patients in your practice?

Statistics

Results of studies about prognosis are usually reported as cumulative incidence rates or survival curves. That is, prognostic studies report the number of events occurring over time. A cumulative incidence rate provides an absolute risk of an outcome over a period of time, whereas survival curves can quantify trends in the risk of an outcome over time. The results of this study indicate that the most common HCV genotypes encountered were type 1b and type 2, and that patients with genotype 1 had a significantly worse prognosis regarding survival and the development of HCC compared with patients with other genotypes. The incidence rates of HCC were 5.9 per person per year for patients with genotype 1a, 4.5 for patients with genotype 1b, and 2.8 in patients with nongenotype 1 HCV. Development of cirrhosis and HCC was significantly greater in the genotype 1b group compared with other genotypes. Treatment with interferon, regardless of total dose or response to therapy, was associated with significantly improved survival and a lower incidence of hepatocellular carcinoma in all groups. You conclude that the study results are compelling, and that they offer important prognostic information that may prove useful for the future care of patients in whom the decision whether or not to treat with an interferon-based regimen may be equivocal.

Conclusions

The continued application of evidence-based medicine concepts has been shown by Fritsche and colleagues, (2002) to increase knowledge. By being able to assess the validity of a clinical trial, a clinician using an evidence-based medicine approach can rapidly differentiate between a study that is worth reading versus a study that may, because of methodologic limitations, present flawed or misleading results. Evidence alone, however, is rarely sufficient to affect clinical decision making and must be considered along with other factors, such as potential costs (direct and indirect), risks, inconvenience, and feasibility of the interventions being considered. By incorporating these "best evidence" practices and values, clinicians are more likely to impact upon outcomes that are important to health care consumers and other interested parties, such as payers and society. With the rapid increase of medical information available in both traditional and untraditional formats, being able to discern well-designed trials will give the practicing clinician a distinct advantage with regards to conforming to the evolving standards of care for different conditions and health states. Additionally, the ability to explain the basis of current practice and limitations of knowledge to increasingly informed health care consumers is becoming more important. Using evidence-based medicine to identify and incorporate important new information into daily practice will keep the informed clinician in line with reasonable expectations for continued high levels of health care delivery.

Supplemental Reading

Agency for Health Care Policy and Research. Medical treatment effectiveness research [Agency for Health Care Policy and Research Program note]. Rockville (MD): Department of Health and Human Services, Public Health Service; 1990.

Fenlon HM, Nunes DP, Schroy PC, et al. A comparison of virtual and conventional colonoscopy for the detection of colorectal polyps. N Engl J Med 1999;341:1496–503.

Fritsche L, Greenhalgh T, Falck-Ytter Y, et al. Do short courses in evidence based medicine improve knowledge and skills? Validation of Berlin questionnaire and before and after study of courses in evidence based medicine. BMJ 2002;325:1338–41.

Greenhalgh T. How to read a paper. The Medline database. BMJ 1997;315:180–3.

Lau JYW, Sung JJY, Lee KKC, et al. Effect of intravenous omeprazole on recurrent bleeding after endoscopic treatment of bleeding peptic ulcers. N Engl J Med 2000;343:310–6.

McKibbon A, Hunt D, Richardson WS, et al. Finding the evidence. In: Guyatt G, Rennie D, editors. Users' guides to the medical literature. A manual for evidence-based clinical practice. 1st ed. Chicago: AMA Press; 2002. p. 13–47.

Pickhardt PJ, Choi JR, Hwang I, et al. Computed tomographic virtual colonoscopy to screen for colorectal neoplasia in asymptomatic adults. N Engl J Med 2003; 349:2191–200.

Roffi L, Redaelli A, Colloredo G, et al. Outcome of liver disease in a large cohort of histologically proven chronic hepatitis C: influence of HCV genotype. Eur J Gastroenterol Hepatol 2001;13:501–6.

Sackett DL, Rosenberg WM, Gray JA, et al. Evidence based medicine: what it is and what it isn't. BMJ 1996;312:71–2.

Walt RP, Cottrell J, Mann SG, et al. Continuous intravenous famotidine for haemorrhage from peptic ulcer. Lancet 1992;340:1058–62.

CHAPTER 2

DECISION ANALYSIS IN THE MANAGEMENT OF DIGESTIVE DISEASES

AMNON SONNENBERG, MD, MSc

Although, at a first glance, medical decision analysis appears to be focused primarily on techniques of how to optimize choices among alternative medical tests and therapies, a closer look will soon reveal that it deals with a much broader aspect of medicine. In essence, medical decision analysis constitutes a large assortment of mathematical methods to study the entire theoretical underpinning of medical practice. It tries to solve such questions as: How does a medical test actually function? What is the best test to choose among multiple competing test options? What is the most efficacious sequence of medical tests? How do physicians recognize a disease pattern? How do physicians solve medical riddles, and how do they extract a diagnostic hypothesis from a bewildering array of clinical signs and symptoms? When is it time to stop a diagnostic pursuit and start therapy? In a population of human subjects, who benefits most from what type of medical management? What is the best therapy to choose among alternative therapies? How does one arrange the most efficacious and least expensive medical management strategy? In dealing with such questions, medical decision analysis has adopted techniques from operation research, business management, economics, psychology, probability theory, and statistics.

The armamentarium of decision analysis contains a large variety of tools, including *decision trees, threshold analyses, Markov chains, Bayes analysis, receiver operation characteristics, waiting line theory, compartment models, linear programming, discrete event simulations, Monte Carlo simulations, Monte Carlo Markov Chain modeling, prospect theory,* and many more. In addition to some general textbooks about decision analysis, there are multiple treatises that deal exclusively with individual techniques, such as decision trees, receiver operation characteristics, waiting lines, or linear programming. Most investigators in medical decision analysis use dedicated software to design and execute their mathematical models. It should be obvious from these introductory remarks that a single chapter on medical decision analysis can only present a small piece from a much larger pie.

Decision Models

Most problems addressed by currently published decision analyses are of general relevance to all gastroenterologists. For instance, they concern different management options in *reflux disease, peptic ulcer, dyspepsia, hepatitis C infection, colorectal cancer,* and *Crohn's disease,* to name just a few. The underlying intentions of such decision analyses are to advocate particular health policies that would be then taken up by the majority of gastroenterologists, be endorsed by professional societies, or even become mandated by governmental agencies. Because of their intended general audience and far-reaching purpose, the analyses try to paint a rather detailed and all-inclusive picture of the disease in question, which considers all potential disease scenarios, even if they are only associated with a low probability of occurrence. For these reasons, many such decision models have become rather complex and somewhat difficult to understand. Besides its general application as an instrument to promote a particular health policy, medical decision analysis also plays an important role as a clinical bedside tool to resolve problems of daily patient encounters. Applied in this fashion, it helps physicians derive better decisions by using a more rigorous and quantifiable means of decision making. This chapter tries to teach the reader how to design simple decision models that provide a practicing gastroenterologist with insights into mundane clinical problems. They involve little calculation and they can be done on the backside of the proverbial envelope. In the following sections, various aspects of *peptic ulcer disease (PUD)* are used as clinical background to illustrate the applicability of *decision trees, threshold analyses,* and *Markov chains* to resolve decision problems that arise during routine gastroenterological practice.

Decision Tree

Nonsteroidal Anti-Inflammatory Drug (NSAID)-Induced Ulcer

Consider the example of a 60-year-old man who is treated for his osteoarthritis with 375 mg of naproxen (Naprosen) bid. Because of his epigastric pain and nausea, the patient undergoes an esophagogastroduodenoscopy, which reveals a nonbleeding gastric ulcer with a clear ulcer base. His physician now wonders whether the naproxen should be replaced by a cyclooxygenase-2-selective inhibitor (COX-2), such as 100 mg celecoxib (Celebrex) bid or tid.

As an alternative to COX-2, the physician also considers treatment with a proton pump inhibitor (PPI), such as 20 mg of rabeprazole (Aciphex) once daily or bid. Which treatment option should be given preference?

Figure 2-1 depicts a decision tree to illustrate the current scenario. The initial decision between a COX-2 and a PPI is depicted by the first fork on the left side of the tree and symbolized by the open square at the first branching point. For the time being, the cost numbers in the lower right corner of each box should be ignored; we will deal with them later. The decision in favor of a COX-2 is followed by two chance events, symbolized by the open circle at the next branching point following the COX-2 decision. The patient may fare well on COX-2 and no other events or costs will ensue, or the patient will fail COX-2 treatment, redevelop his ulcer, and require a switch from COX-2 to PPI treatment added to a regular NSAID, such as naproxen. The branches leading off the chance node are assigned the two probability values (p) of .9 and .1. In general, all probabilities emanating from a chance node need to add up to 1.0. The NSAID plus PPI outcome is followed by yet another set of two probabilities. The patient may stay free of recurrent ulcerations on the NSAID plus PPI combination, and drug cost alone will be encountered with a .9 probability, or the patient may develop ulcer complications. The occurrence of future complications under NSAID plus PPI treatment in this patient, given his present ulcer, is given an overall p value of .1. Lastly, three possible complications are considered: pain, hospital admission, and death, with the three respective p values of .9, .09, and .01. The time frame of the analysis is restricted to one year.

A decision tree provides the means to describe the natural disease history and the possible occurrence of future events in terms of a flow diagram. The flow runs from the left to the right side of the tree and ends in a set of final events without further progression. In the tree of Figure 2-1, all boxes indicating final events have been shaded with a light gray. To calculate the tree outcome, the final events need to be described in terms of some commensurable values, the most commonly used descriptor being money. Frequently, however, the events can also be described in terms of other health parameters, such as healthy or pain free days, hospital days, or number of deaths, as long as the same unit of measurement is used to describe all the different outcomes. The physician estimated that episodes of pain would cost overall $500 per year. Similarly, the physician estimated that one hospital admission per year for ulcer complication would cost on the average $3,000. Death was equated with the average annual income in the United States. Lastly the drug costs associated with NSAID plus PPI treatment or COX-2 treatment was estimated based on pharmacy listings.

The tree outcome is calculated from right to left. The cost values of the final outcomes are multiplied by their probability of occurrence and added. The final fork on the right, for example, yields:

$$90\% \times \$500 + 9\% \times \$3,000 + 1\% \times \$30,000 = \$1,020.$$

This process is called averaging out, because it calculates the average expected outcome of a chance fork. It is repeated again at the next fork to the left. For illustrative purposes, however, the drug costs that are still incurred in patients who experience ulcer complications have been left out. Rather than $1,020, the correct value of the box should be listed as $1,020 + $1,800 = $2,820, and the expected value of the next chance fork is actually:

$$90\% \times \$1,800 + 10\% \times \$2,820 = \$1,902.$$

This value also corresponds to the general expected value of PPI, as opposed to COX-2 treatment at the initial decision fork. Rather than redraw this part of the decision tree twice following the box labeled PPI, the detailed tree was executed only once and the expected value was then transferred to the initial PPI box. The identity of the two event boxes is symbolized by their double outline. The process

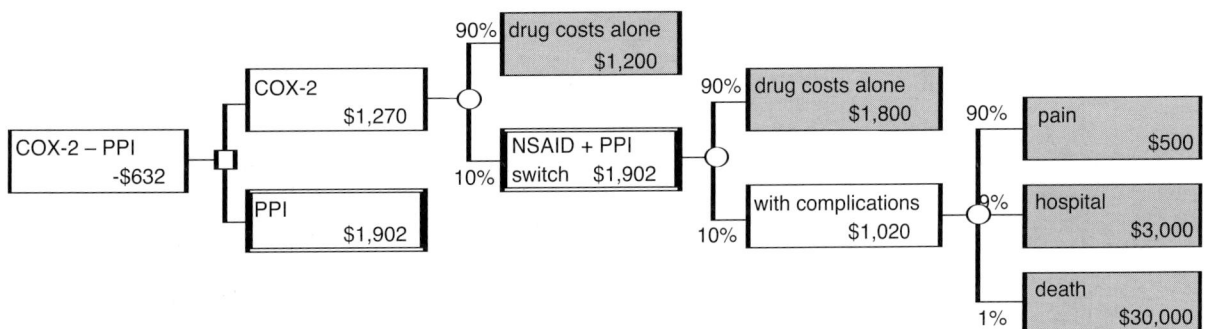

FIGURE 2-1 Decision tree for management of NSAID-induced peptic ulcer. COX-2 = cyclooxygenase-2-receptor antagonist; NSAID = nonsteroidal anti-inflammatory drug; PPI = proton pump inhibitor.

of averaging out is thus carried out from right to left until all boxes have been assigned a value. The first box on the left contains the cost difference of the COX-2 minus PPI treatment strategy. A cheaper COX-2 treatment translates into a negative value for the overall tree. Accordingly, in this patient with active peptic ulcer, preference should be given to the COX-2 treatment strategy.

Sensitivity Analysis

The probabilities and costs entered into the decision tree are based solely on the physician's estimates. The model is not intended to be published, convey absolute truths, or convince anyone but the physician involved in the management of this particular patient. As the example tries to demonstrate, such analysis relies primarily on the clinician's own assessment of the medical issues involved. In most cases the decision could be derived without digressing into an extensive study of the scientific literature or an elaborate cost analysis. The parameters built into a model are supposed to represent only crude estimates of the true values, reflecting the physician's medical understanding and using his or her current knowledge in the best and most efficient fashion. Potential uncertainties about relevant decision parameters can then be addressed by a subsequent sensitivity analysis.

In a sensitivity analysis, all questionable parameters are varied over a wide range to test their influence on the initial decision. The physician may not know, for example, how much the annual treatment with a COX-2 drug actually costs. The current value of $1,200 is only a crude estimate. In the subsequent sensitivity analysis, the drug cost entered into the first gray box on the right is, therefore, varied between $0 and $3,000. The outcome of the analysis is shown in the right panel of Figure 2-2. Negative values of the y-axis represent a cheaper COX-2 than PPI treatment strategy. An increase in COX-2 drug costs shifts the balance towards the PPI branch and changes the decision in its favor. When the COX-2 drug cost exceeds $1,902, the PPI strategy becomes the preferential treatment option.

Two-Way Sensitivity Analysis

Similarly, the physician may have only vague ideas concerning the actual costs of treating the patient with the PPI plus NSAID drug combination. In the middle panel of Figure 2-2, the drug costs of PPI plus NSAID were varied between $0 and $3,000. Again, a negative value on the y-axis indicates a cheaper COX-2 than the PPI plus NSAID strategy. As expected, any increase in PPI plus NSAID cost renders the COX-2 alternative increasingly more advantageous. Only with a PPI plus NSAID cost of less than $1,098 does the PPI plus NSAID treatment strategy represent the preferential treatment option.

As opposed to the *one-way* sensitivity analyses from above, in a subsequent *two-way* sensitivity analysis, one could also vary both types of drug costs simultaneously and check their joint influence on the cost difference between the two treatment options. Let us return to the decision tree of Figure 2-1. In the first step of a two-way sensitivity calculation, one would leave the COX-2 costs fixed at $1,200 and vary the NSAID plus PPI costs until the cost difference between the two treatment strategies (depicted in the first box on the left) becomes zero. This is achieved at NSAID plus PPI costs of $1,098. The pair of COX-2 and NSAID plus PPI costs ($1,200 and $1,098), which yield a zero net difference, are kept in a separate list. In a second step, one would choose a new value for the COX-2 costs, for example $1,600, and then restart the process of varying the NSAID plus PPI costs until the overall cost difference between the two treatment strategies again turns zero. The new pair of COX-2 and NSAID plus PPI costs ($1,600 and $1,498) is added to the list of pairs. These steps are repeated multiple times until a sufficient number of COX-2 and NSAID plus PPI cost pairs have been generated to plot the line shown in the right panel of Figure 2-2. In this particular example, a linear relationship for the COX-2 versus NSAID plus PPI costs is found, although nonlinear associations will frequently characterize other instances of a two-way sensitivity analysis.

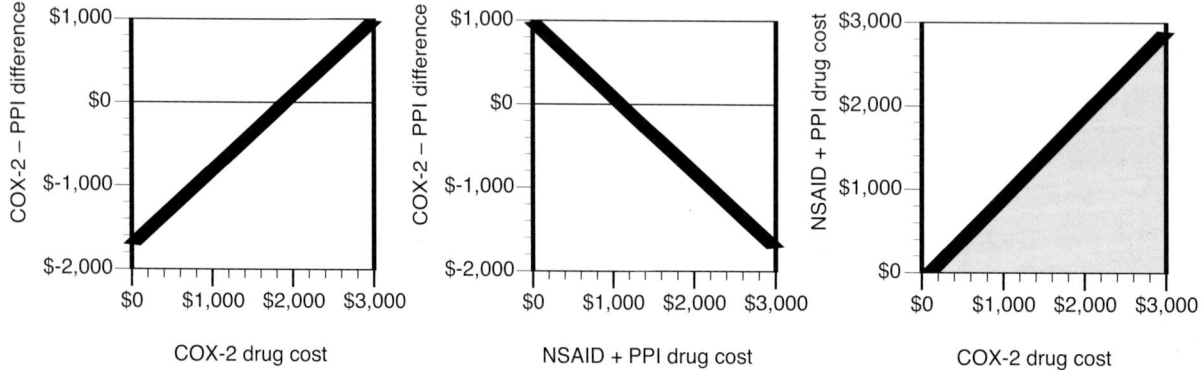

FIGURE 2-2. Sensitivity analysis of ulcer management. One-way sensitivity is shown in the left and middle panel; Two-way sensitivity analysis is shown in the right panel. COX-2 = cyclooxygenase-2-receptor antagonist; NSAID = nonsteroidal anti-inflammatory drug; PPI = proton pump inhibitor.

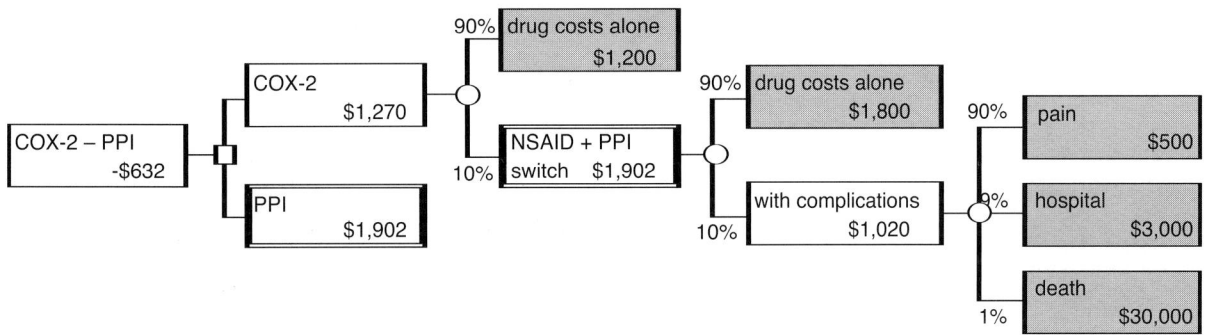

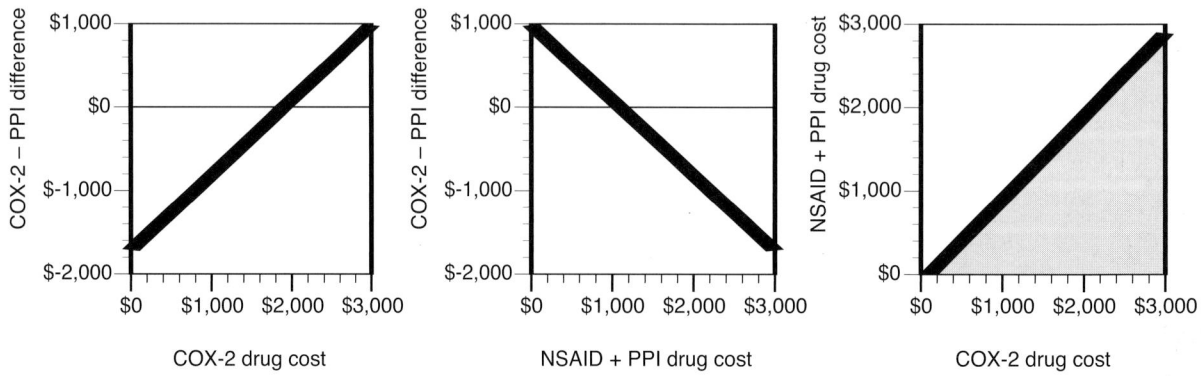

Each point on the line represents a combination of COX-2 and NSAID plus PPI costs, for which the decision tree yields an identical outcome for the two treatment strategies. The area beneath the black line includes all cost combinations of COX-2 and NSAID plus PPI, for which the PPI strategy is cheaper than the COX-2 strategy. This applies, for example, to a large variety of COX-2 and NSAID plus PPI cost pairs, such as $1,500 and $500, $2,000 and $500, or $2,500 and $1500. The white area above the black line represents all possible cost pairs for which the COX-2 strategy provides the cheaper treatment strategy. The line itself in this particular example depicts the equation NSAID + PPI = COX-2 − $102. In other words, the two treatment strategies yield identical outcomes, as long as the combined drug costs for NSAID plus PPI cost $102 less than the COX-2 costs alone.

Where does the $102 come from? Inspection of the original decision tree reveals that the $102 value stems from the 10% probability for the overall occurrence of complications multiplied by their respective expected value of $1,020. To reach equivalence between COX-2 and NSAID plus PPI, the NSAID plus PPI strategy needs to be cheaper by at least $102 to compensate for the additional costs of potential ulcer complications. The original decision tree was designed in such a way that any ulcer recurrence would automatically result in a switch from failed COX-2 to NSAID plus PPI. Obviously, if the COX-2 were to be continued even after instances of ulcer recurrences, and if it were to carry the same risk of future complications, the expected values of future complications in both treatment arms would cancel each other out. The two strategies would become equivalent if NSAID + PPI = COX-2. On the other hand, if COX-2 were associated with different probabilities for the occurrence of complications or different costs for the management of complications, the relationship between the two treatment options would change again. This last example serves as a reminder that the outcome of the decision tree depends on its overall structure and the type of question modeled by the tree.

Besides varying the costs or probabilities of the decision tree, as alluded to in the previous paragraph, one could also redraw parts of the tree or change its overall appearance. How far and how detailed should the medical history and the disease progression be followed into the future? The final outcomes of the present tree may seem somewhat arbitrary in that one could have easily proceeded further and spelled out many more details about the subsequent development of the patient's peptic ulcer. One could, for instance, subdivide pain into different types and severities or associate the hospital admission with far more detailed descriptions of the disease progression, such as ulcer bleeding, perforation, surgery, and their respective clinical outcomes. Because parameters on the far right of the decision tree become multiplied with an ever *increasing* number of probability values, they also tend to exert an ever *decreasing* influence on the initial decision. For instance, in the overall process of averaging out the decision tree from right to left, the cost of death becomes multiplied once by 0.01 and twice by 0.1. In the final analysis, therefore, even doubling the annual cost of death from $30,000 to $60,000 only changes the COX-2 minus PPI cost difference from −$632 to −$659. Many of the parameters of a decision analysis exert little influence on its overall outcome, especially if they are located at the far end of the tree. As a general rule, therefore, it is not advisable to expand the tree too far into the future or include too many events that are associated with an a priori low probability value.

Threshold Analysis

First Threshold Analysis (*Helicobacter pylori* and NSAIDs)

The foregoing analysis addressed only one very specific question: Should a given patient with a newly identified acute NSAID-induced ulcer be switched from treatment with a conventional NSAID to treatment with a COX-2 inhibitor? The analysis did not address the issue of whether all patients on NSAIDs should be generally switched over to COX-2 therapy, or whether presently asymptomatic patients with any remote ulcer history should be given COX-2. It also left the question of *Helicobacter pylori* and its potential role in NSAID-induced ulcers unanswered. Let us assume that the patient from the first example tested positive for *H. pylori*. Should this patient then undergo antibiotic (ABX) therapy to eradicate H. pylori *rather than COX-2 therapy?* A new decision tree, as depicted in Figure 2-3, is needed to analyze this question.

Treatment with ABX is followed by two equally likely outcomes. First, the patient may respond to eradication of *H. pylori*, his ulcer will not relapse, and no other costs will

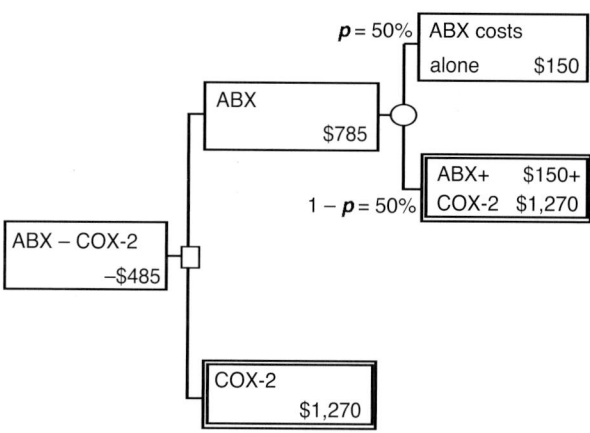

FIGURE 2-3. Threshold analysis of ulcer management with antibiotics (ABX) versus cyclooxygenase-2 receptor antagonist (COX-2).

be incurred. Second, the patient may not respond to eradication of *H. pylori*, and, besides the expenditures for the futile ABX therapy, additional costs will be spent on the continuous treatment with COX-2. The expected costs of a COX-2 strategy (known from the previous example) are entered into the decision at the two instances marked by the double lined box. The costs of ABX therapy are estimated at $150. The negative cost difference indicates that the ABX represent the cheaper and therefore preferential treatment strategy.

As in the previous examples, one could subject the decision tree to a sensitivity analysis and test the robustness of its overall outcome to various cost assumptions. The cost of the COX-2 strategy is about eight times higher than the ABX's cost. It is highly unlikely that any cost combination could ever shift the balance in favor of COX-2 therapy. The p value indicates the likelihood that an NSAID-associated ulcer would respond to ABX therapy. This p value represents a far more interesting parameter to be subjected to a sensitivity analysis. Varying p between 0 and 1.0 (and accordingly $1 - p$ between 1.0 and 0) reveals that the two ABX and COX-2 branches reach equivalence when $p = .125$. Whenever the likelihood for an ulcer cure equals or exceeds the threshold of $p = .125$, ABX therapy becomes the preferred treatment strategy.

Instead of varying the p value over a broad range, one can also derive the threshold value by a simple algebraic manipulation. For the upper and lower branch of Figure 2-3 to be identical the following equation must hold:

$$p - ABX + (1 - p) \times (ABX + COX\text{-}2) = COX\text{-}2$$

Solving the equation for p yields the threshold value $p = ABX/COX\text{-}2$. Because the cost of a one-time ABX therapy is much lower than the cost of COX-2 prescribed over 1 or more years, the p value will be very small. In the present example $p = \$150/\$1270 = 0.125$. The exact costs of ABX or COX-2 become secondary, and the outcome of the threshold analysis can be derived based on comparative estimates and considerations of magnitude alone. In essence, the analysis states that ABXs should be given a trial, because even with low chances of success this one-time strategy will still be much cheaper than long term COX-2 therapy. In general, the result of a threshold analysis is expressed as a p, which forms the threshold between the two choices against or in favor of a particular medical action. A low threshold supports the decision in favor of the action, because the low threshold becomes easily surpassed by the expected outcome, even if the expectations are relatively low to begin with. Compared to cost values and cost benefit or cost effectiveness ratios, a p value is more appealing to the *physician decision maker*, because it pertains to a parameter that the physician is intimately familiar with and that constitutes the currency of his or her daily activities.

Second Threshold Analysis (Nonulcer Dyspepsia [NUD])

The next example serves to further illustrate the powers of threshold analysis and deepen the understanding of its versatility. The clinical scenario represents only a slight deviation from the previous examples of above. Consider the case of a 60-year-old man who presents with symptoms of dyspepsia, nausea, and epigastric pain. An upper gastrointestinal endoscopy has not been performed, but a serologic test for *H. pylori* has returned positive. The patient has had similar symptoms for the past five years and has been diagnosed with NUD. The patient's new physician has to decide whether to continue treating the patient's symptoms with a PPI or start the patient on an empirical trial of ABXs. The decision tree is outlined in Figure 2-4.

The decisions in favor of ABX or PPI are both followed by the same set of possibilities: The patient may suffer from PUD or NUD. The response rates to ABX or PPI therapy (shown in parentheses inside the white boxes) would, of course, vary depending on the type of unknown disease from which the patient actually suffers. The economic outcome was calculated and entered into the analysis, as represented by the set of gray boxes on the far right. For example, a 90% response rate of PUD to ABX leaves a 10% risk for recurrent ulcer associated with complications. The previous analyses yielded an expected value of $1,020 for ulcer-associated complications. Hence,

$$\$150 + .1\ p \times ABX + (1 - p) \times (ABX + COX\text{-}2) = \\ COX\text{-}2 \times \$1,020 = \$252.$$

Similarly, a 40% response rate of NUD to ABX leaves a 60% risk for recurrent pain associated with persistent NUD but no other ulcer-related complications. Based on the previous estimate of $500 spent per year to alleviate ulcer-like symptoms, $150 + .6\ p \times \$500 = \$450$. The contents of the two lower boxes were calculated accordingly.

The outcome of the decision tree can be solved by inspection only, without the need to resort to any type of calculation. The costs inside the two upper boxes are both lower than the costs inside the two lower boxes. No matter what type of value the p assumes, the ABX branch always yields a lower expected cost than the PPI branch. Therefore, the decision in favor of ABX provides the better outcome and the preferred choice.

Third Threshold Analysis

Some physicians may not want to spend the time extracting and estimating cost data, or they may harbor great suspicions against such iffy estimates. The physicians may feel that the clinical success rates of PUD and NUD associated with various treatment modalities have been well established by

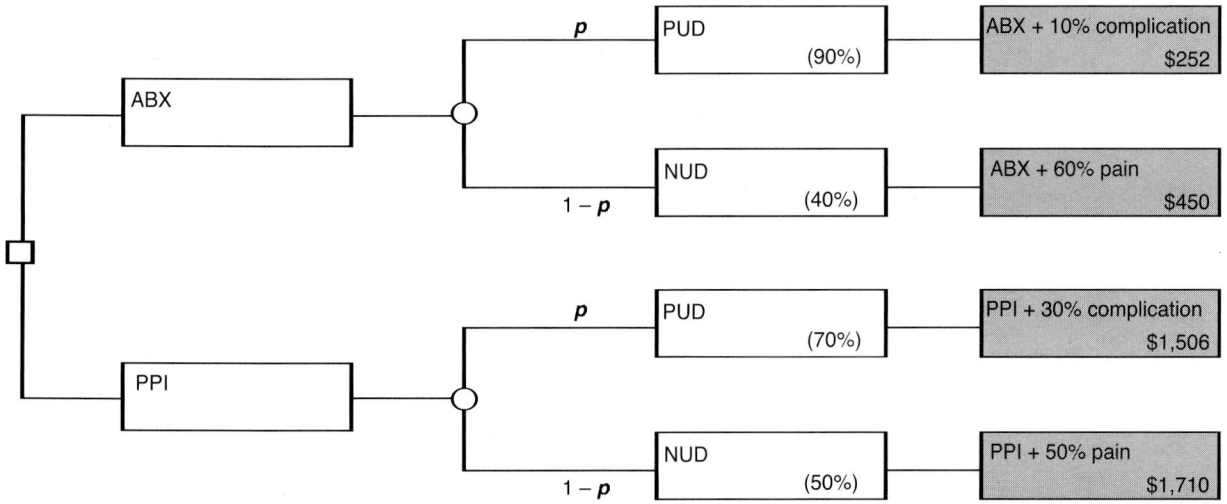

FIGURE 2-4. Threshold analysis of ulcer management with antibiotics (ABX) versus proton pump inhibitors (PPI). NUD = nonulcer dyspepsia; p = probability of PUD; PUD = peptic ulcer disease.

many controlled clinical trials, but that the cost data are far less well substantiated. In essence, they would want to restrict their analysis to medical issues, such as the *success rates* of various therapies shown by the decision tree of Figure 2-5. The success rates from the previous decision tree now change to become the new outcomes of the revised tree. The same type of reasoning and calculation that was used in the first threshold analysis can be used here to extract the threshold value for p. For the upper ABX and the lower PPI branch to be equivalent, the following equation must apply:

$$p \times A + (1 - p) \times B = p \times C + (1 - p) \times D.$$

The letters A through D are used to label the outcomes of the right column of boxes. Again, this equation can be solved algebraically for p to yield the following formula:

$$p = \frac{D - B}{A - B - C + D}$$

The formula applies similarly to all types of threshold analysis. Substituting the actual success rates from Figure 2-5 into the formula yields the following outcome:

$$.33 = \frac{.5 - .4}{.9 - .4 - .7 + .5}$$

If the probability of peptic ulcer exceeds .33, it would be worthwhile to subject the patient to an empirical trial of antibiotics before committing him to any long-term therapy with PPI. This last example serves to illustrate that threshold analysis is not necessarily dependent on cost data and that, in principle, any outcome parameter can be used to calculate a threshold probability. To be phrased as a simple 2 × 2 threshold analysis, a medical problem needs to be shaped into a relatively rigid form. The initial decision against or in favor of a medical action is followed by a set of probabilities (p versus $1 - p$), which govern the occurrence of medical events. The probabilities should be independent of the action taken and, therefore, identical for both decisions, in the present scenario of ABX versus PPI. Each of the final outcomes is determined by the interaction between the action taken (decision made) and the probable medical event. In spite of its striking simplicity, this framework is able to capture and faithfully analyze a large variety of heterogeneous and often perplexing medical problems.

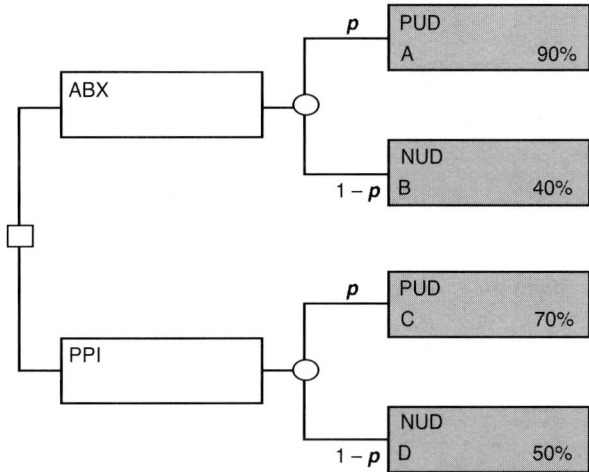

FIGURE 2-5. Threshold analysis of ulcer management with antibiotics (ABX) versus proton pump inhibitors (PPIs). NUD = nonulcer dyspepsia; p = probability of PUD; PUD = peptic ulcer disease. The letters A through D are used to label the outcomes of the right column of boxes.

Markov Chains

In the previous analyses of the NSAID-induced ulcer, the response to therapy with COX-2 was treated as a dichotomous yes–no variable. Patients were considered responders to COX-2 therapy only if they stayed completely free of recurrent ulcerations. In all other instances, COX-2 therapy was regarded a failure and the patients were automatically switched to a combination of a conventional NSAID plus PPI. In clinical practice, however, patients may be maintained on a COX-2 and the therapy would still be considered a success if the number of ulcer recurrences were halved or if the patient stayed ulcer-free for a longer time period than without a COX-2. The Markov chain provides a means to estimate the ulcer-free time and compare the success rates of competing treatment strategies.

Any acute ulcer can go in two directions: It can heal or it can stay acute. Similarly, any healed ulcer can become acute again or stay healed. The natural history of PUD can, therefore, be conceptualized as ongoing transitions between two health states (ie, acute and healed peptic ulcer). All that one needs to know to be able to set up the Markov model are the healing rate (HR) of acute ulcers and the relapse rate (RR) of healed ulcers. For the model of Figure 2-6, it was assumed that during a 1-month time period 40% of all acute ulcers would heal spontaneously and 8% would relapse. Because the entirety of possibilities to exit any given health state needs to add up to 100%, the monthly rate of patients remaining unhealed equals 100% − HR = 60%, and the monthly rate of healed ulcers without recurrence equals 100% − RR = 92%. The same set of transition rates acts on the patient population with acute and healed ulcers every month. In essence, patients are shifted back and forth between the two Markov states of acute and healed ulcers until a steady state is reached. In the example of Figure 2-6, the analysis was started with 100 patients in the state of acute ulcerations. By looking at the numbers of patients in each two boxes of consecutive months, one can appreciate that after 4 months the numbers of patients in the acute and healed ulcer states start to approach some steady state. If the chain is continued for a few more months, a steady state is achieved with 17 patients staying continuously in the acute state and 83 patients in the healed ulcer state. In other words, at any given point in time after the chain has been allowed to settle, about 83% of ulcer patients will be ulcer-free even without medical intervention. One could also say that 83% of the time during the natural history of untreated ulcer disease is spent ulcer-free.

How does ulcer prevention with COX-2 affect its natural history? COX-2 maintenance therapy may half the RR = 4%, but it will probably leave the HR = 40% unaffected. Under these conditions the Markov chain of Figure 2-6 yields steady state conditions of 91% healed and 9% acute ulcers. This outcome represents an overall improvement by 8% compared with the 83% fraction of ulcer-free patients without any therapy at all. How would maintenance therapy with PPI affect the natural history of peptic ulcer? In addition to halving the RR by inhibiting acid secretion, PPI may also double the HR. With a RR of 4% and an HR of 80%, a steady state is reached with 95% of all subjects having a healed ulcer and 5% having an acute ulcer. Compared with no therapy or COX-2 therapy, this represents overall improvements of 12% and 4%, respectively.

It is important to realize that Markov chains address different questions and yield different answers compared to decision trees. Decision trees are centered on the concept of the *expected value* and how to select the best expected value from a multitude of alternative options. In Markov chains, by contradistinction, the analysis is focused on the *average* or *cumulative amount of time* spent in different medical states and how to select a management strategy that provides the most time spent in a healthy state.

Figure 2-6 depicts the *extensive form* of a Markov chain. Although the chain is stopped after 4 months, it could have been continued for an endless time. This type of drawing provides an intuitive explanation for why the analysis is referred to as a "chain," and it also allows the model to be transformed directly into a spreadsheet calculation. From a mathematical perspective, however, all the relevant information necessary to calculate the chain outcome is already contained in the transitions drawn for the first month only. Frequently, this relevant information can be condensed into a *short form* of a Markov chain, as shown in the upper drawing of Figure 2-7. The arrows pointing towards the

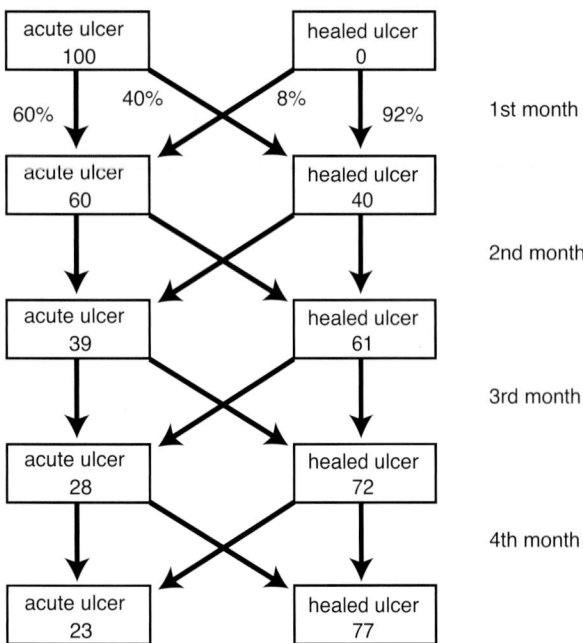

FIGURE 2-6. Markov chain (drawn in extensive form) for the natural history of an ulcer.

same health state, from which they originate, indicate the fractions of patients who remain in the same health states during the monthly cycle. If a Markov chain is made up of more than a few health states, the extensive form becomes cumbersome to draw and difficult to appreciate with its many crisscrossing arrows. The short form lends itself to be used for the depiction of more elaborate Markov chains comprising multiple health states. As an example, in the bottom part of Figure 2-7, the basic model was expanded by two additional health states.

Cost Effectiveness Analyses

To obtain clinical insights and compare different strategies based on their medical performance alone, the Markov chains outlined above may be sufficient. In recent years, Markov chains have been used increasingly to predict the outcomes of medical screening and surveillance, and to assess the amount of lifetime saved through different strategies. Because such questions also touch upon issues of public health and health policy, the comparison of various strategies needs to include costs and assess whether these strategies are economically feasible. The analysis shown in Figure 2-6 could have been expanded further by accumulating the costs that are incurred during each month spent in various states of the Markov chain. For example, if treatment of acute ulcers required additional medical expenses, those would have been multiplied by the fraction of patients with acute ulcers during each month and then added for the entire running period of the Markov analysis. In other more elaborate Markov models, the transitions among various states could also result in cost expenditures that need to be accumulated over the entire running period to estimate the overall costs of competing treatment strategies. Ultimately, such analyses deal with the average costs and lengths of time associated with various health states. The ratio of cumulative cost over time is referred to as the average cost effectiveness ratio ([ACER]; ACER = cost/time). The ACER combines the medical perspective of *health time* with the economic perspective of *costs* spent to make this health time happen.

The first Markov chain from above considered only two health states and a dichotomous grading of time (ie, healthy versus sick time). In more complex Markov models, however, patients are shifted among many more health states and spend various amounts of time in health states associated with varying health quality. Rather than focus solely on the healthiest state alone, the times spent in other less favorable health states also need to be accumulated and accounted for in the final analysis. Time spent in fear of medical disease, time spent in pain, time spent in a medical institution, or time spent after a debilitating medical procedure are all associated with different qualities. To compare and sum such different time periods, the quality of time associated with different health states needs to be

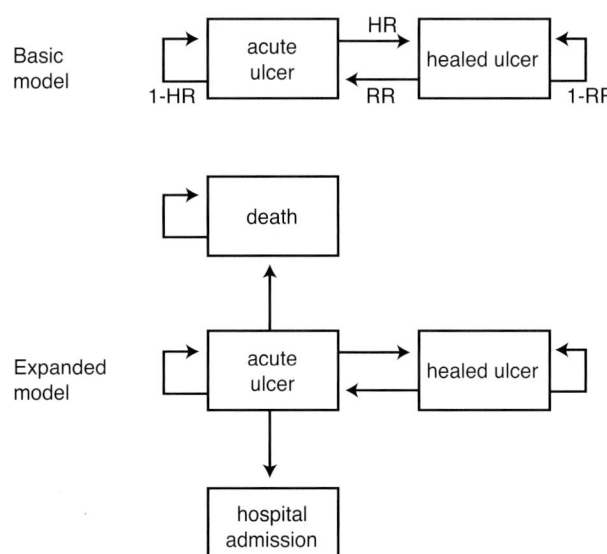

FIGURE 2-7. Basic and expanded Markov chain models for the natural history of an ulcer (drawn in short form). HR = healing rate; RR = recurrence rate.

made commensurable by grading it on a continuous scale from 0 and 1. By definition, death becomes associated with 0 quality and perfect health with a quality value of 1. The quality of time multiplied by the length of time corresponds to the quality-adjusted time, usually expressed as quality-adjusted life years (QALYs). The ACER changes accordingly to a ratio of ACER = cost/QALYs.

Rather than being restricted to the ACER of one particular strategy, most cost effectiveness analyses are now concerned with the comparison of different treatment strategies, for example, no therapy versus COX-2 therapy versus PPI therapy of the present example. Each two strategies can be compared by their incremental cost effectiveness ratio (ICER):

$$\text{ICER} = \frac{\text{cost}_1 - \text{cost}_2}{\text{QALY}_1 - \text{QALY}_2}$$

The indices 1 and 2 refer to the first and second strategy to be compared, respectively. The ICER tells the decision maker how many additional costs would be incurred in trying to achieve more time spent at a healthier state. For instance, how much would it cost to spend 4% more time ulcer-free with PPI as compared with COX-2? This chapter was focused on medical decision analyses that could be used by gastroenterologists as a bedside tool to resolve issues that arise in their daily care of patients. Most cost effectiveness analyses, however, reach beyond this clinical confinement. They require far more elaborate cost analyses and address issues relevant to general health policy rather than routine medical practice.

Conclusions

The emphasis of this chapter was directed towards the clinical application of decision analysis in the management of gastroenterology patients and its use as a bedside tool for optimizing clinical management of common medical problems. The examples were purposefully based on crude cost estimates and restricted to simple models that could be calculated without resorting to dedicated decision software. All models used in this chapter were actually drawn and executed on an *Excel* spreadsheet from *Microsoft Office*. The examples serve to demonstrate that there is still ample room for use of decision analysis as a bedside tool. Frequently the models can be solved without mathematical calculations. Numerical precision is not an issue, because the analysis is not meant to be published but to serve to make the best use of the clinician's current knowledge in deriving the most sensible medical decision.

In general, the decision models to address patient management do not need to be elaborate and can be developed within a short time period. The difficulty resides less with the mathematical analysis and more with the conception of the decision models. The clinician must be able to see within a seemingly large, complex, and multifaceted clinical picture the underlying simple decision problem. The challenge is then to ignore many of the less relevant factors and concentrate on the two or three parameters with the largest impact on the medical outcome. One of the biggest mistakes made by those unfamiliar with decision analysis is to assume that the technique is useless unless good estimates are known for every variable encountered in the model. It is important to understand that, in contradistinction, a sensitivity analysis can account for a wide variation of each variable, and that the decisions often turn out to be rather insensitive to the actual values of many of the variables anyway.

There are no a priori right or wrong models, except for logical inconsistencies built into erroneous models or instances when the *p* values do not add up to 1.0. However, models can be insightful and helpful or they can be overly sophisticated and useless. The number and types of parameters built into a model are left solely to the clinician's discretion, because there are few, if any, absolute rules. The appearance of the model depends largely on the questions the analysis is intended to answer. Seemingly minor variations in the question asked can lead to major variations in the resulting models. Modeling a medical question, therefore, helps to phrase the underlying clinical problem in a more precise fashion and reveal its hidden structure. Decision analysis provides a wonderful tool to spell out different assumptions built into clinical management and clarifies many of the roots of disagreement among controversial management decisions.

Supplementary Reading

Chapman GB, Sonnenberg FA. Decision making in health care: theory, psychology & applications. Cambridge (UK): Cambridge University Press; 2000.

Clemen RT. Making hard decisions: an introduction to decision analysis, 2nd ed. Pacific Grove (CA): Duxbury Press; 1997.

Drummond MF, O'Brien B, Stoddart GL, Torrance GW. Methods for the economic evaluation of health care programmes, 2nd ed. New York: Oxford University Press; 1997. p. 96–138.

Gold MR, Siegel JE, Russel LB, Weinstein MC. Cost-effectiveness in health and medicine. New York: Oxford University Press; 1996.

Lusted LB. Decision-making studies in patient management. N Engl J Med 1971;284:416–24.

Lusted LB. Introduction to medical decision making. Springfield (IL): Charles C. Thomas; 1968.

Pauker SG, Kassirer JP. Decision analysis. N Engl J Med 1987;316:250–8.

Pauker SG, Kassirer JP. The threshold approach to clinical decision making. N Engl J Med 1980;302:1109-17.

Petitti DB. Meta-analysis, decision analysis, and cost-effectiveness analysis, 2nd ed. New York: Oxford University Press; 2000.

Raiffa H. Decision analysis: introductory lectures on choices under uncertainty. Reading (MA): Addison-Wesley Publishing Company; 1968.

Sackett DL, Haynes RB, Guyatt GH. Clinical epidemiology: a basic science for clinical medicine, 2nd ed. Philadelphia (PA): Lippincott Williams & Wilkins Publishers; 1991.

Sonnenberg A. Decision analysis in clinical gastroenterology. Am J Gastroenterol 2003. [In press]

Sonnenberg A. What to do about *Helicobacter pylori*? A decision analysis of its implication on public health. Helicobacter Journal 2002;7:60–7.

Sonnenberg A. Cost-effectiveness of competing strategies to prevent or treat GORD-related dysphagia. PharmEconomics 2000;17:391–401.

Sonnenberg A. Game theory to analyse management options in gastroesophageal reflux disease. Aliment Pharm Ther 2000;14:1411–7.

Sonnenberg A. Timing and scheduling of endoscopic procedures. Gastrointest Endosc 2000;52:204–11.

Sonnenberg A. Waiting lines in the endoscopy unit. Gastrointest Endosc 2000;52:517–24.

Sonnenberg A. Threshold analysis of *Helicobacter pylori* therapy. PharmacoEconomics 1998;14:423–32.

Sonnenberg A. Cost-benefit analysis of testing for *Helicobacter pylori* in dyspeptic subjects. Am J Gastroenterol 1996;91:1773–17.

Sonnenberg A, Gavin MW. Timing of surgery for enterovesical fistula in Crohn's disease: decision analysis using a time-dependent compartment model. Inflammatory Bowel Disease 2000;6:280–5.

Sonnenberg A, Inadomi JM, Bauerfeind P. Reliability block diagrams to model disease management. Med Dec Making 1999;19:180–5.

Sonnenberg A, Inadomi JM, Becker LA. Economic analysis of step-wise treatment of gastroesophageal reflux disease. Aliment Pharm Ther 1999;13:1003–13.

Weinstein MC, Fineberg HV, Elstein AS, et al. Clinical decision analysis. Philadelphia (PA): WB Saunders Company; 1980.

CHAPTER 3

ENDOSCOPIC SEDATION

ANTHONY N. KALLOO, MD, FACP, AND DONNA BEITLER, RN, CGRN

> "We are having the baby (Prince Leopold)
> and we shall have the chloroform"
> Queen Victoria 1853

Adequate sedation for endoscopy is a critical process for successful procedural outcome. The last decade has seen a move to sedation-less endoscopy by the use of ultrathin endoscopes, but this has not gained widespread popularity in the United States mainly because of patient acceptance (Faulx et al, 2002). This chapter will describe the approach to intravenous (IV) sedation in patients having both routine and complex therapeutic procedures in the endoscopy setting. A review of the levels of sedation, the importance of identification of the high risk patient, and the pharmacology of sedating and reversal agents will be presented.

Background

The goal of sedation/analgesia for endoscopic procedures is to relieve anxiety, discomfort, and pain, while minimizing its associated risks (Gross et al, 2002). The appropriate choice of agents and techniques for sedation is dependent on the experience and preference of the practitioner, requirements or constraints imposed by the patient or procedure, and the likelihood of producing a deeper level of sedation than anticipated. In the United States, patients expect to receive sedation for endoscopic procedures other than sigmoidoscopy, and few physicians feel comfortable performing endoscopy without sedation. Thus, most endoscopic procedures require accompanying sedation. At times, these sedation practices may result in cardiac or respiratory depression, which must be rapidly recognized and appropriately managed to avoid risk of hypoxic brain damage, cardiac arrest, or death. Conversely, inadequate sedation may result in undue patient discomfort or injury because of lack of cooperation or adverse physiologic or psychological response to stress.

Moderate sedation, previously known as *conscious sedation*, is the medically controlled state of depressed consciousness that allows maintenance of protective reflexes. The patient retains the ability to maintain their airway while responding purposefully to verbal commands and/or tactile stimuli (Gross et al, 2002). There are four levels of sedation/analgesia that are clinically and medico-legally important because they have different monitoring requirements with an increasing potential for adverse effects (Table 3-1). Although these sedation levels are distinct, they occur on a continuum with the potential for the level of sedation to become deeper than desired. Therefore, practitioners intending to produce a level of sedation should be able to rescue patients whose level of sedation becomes deeper than initially intended. Table 3-2 lists the monitoring and resuscitative equipment that should be available during the sedation process.

Preprocedure Evaluation

It is important to be familiar with sedation-oriented aspects of the patient's medical history, because this may affect the type of sedation administered. These include abnormalities of the major organ systems, *previous personal or family adverse experience with sedation*, drug allergies, current medications, and history of tobacco, alcohol, or substance use or

TABLE 3-1. Continuum of Depth of Sedation

	Minimal Sedation (Anxiolysis)	Moderation Sedation/Analgesia ("Conscious Sedation")	Deep Sedation/ Analgesia	General Anesthesia
Responsiveness	Normal response to verbal stimulation	Purposeful* response to verbal or tactile stimulation	Purposeful* response following repeated or painful stimulation	Unarousable even with painful stimulus
Airway	Unaffected	No intervention required	Intervention may be required	Intervention often required
Spontaneous Ventilation	Unaffected	Adequate	May be adequate	Frequently adequate
Cardiovascular Function	Unaffected	Usually maintained	Usually maintained	May be impaired

*Reflex withdrawal from pain is not considered a purposeful response.

TABLE 3-2. Monitoring and Rescusitation Equipment Required for Moderate Sedation

Procedure Room	Immediately Accessible
Cardiac monitor	Defibrillator
Pulse oximeter	Emergency cart
Oxygen source	Emergency drug box
Ambu bag with facemask	
Suction	
Oral pharyngeal airway	

abuse. The time and nature of last oral intake is important and avoidance of fluids or solid foods for a sufficient period to allow for complete gastric emptying before the procedure (as recommended by the American Society of Anesthesiologists [ASA] "Guidelines for Preoperative Fasting") is essential and has potential medico-legal implications. In urgent, emergent situations, or situations in which gastric emptying is impaired, there is a potential for pulmonary aspiration. Consideration should be given to endotracheal intubation for airway protection in these patients.

Before initiating sedation for endoscopy, patients should have a focused physical examination, including vital signs, auscultation of the heart and lungs, and evaluation of the airway. The need for preprocedure laboratory testing will depend on the patient's underlying medical condition and the likelihood that the results will affect the management of sedation. Informed consent for the sedation and for the procedure should be obtained and witnessed.

Patients who are at increased risk for developing complications related to sedation should be identified. Special precautions are needed in patients with significant underlying medical conditions (eg, extremes of age; severe cardiac, pulmonary, hepatic, or renal disease; pregnancy; drug or alcohol abuse). In patients with significant sedation-related risks factors (eg, uncooperative patients, morbid obesity, potentially difficult airway, sleep apnea), a consultation with an anesthesiologist should be obtained. A useful medical risk classification system used universally by endoscopists is the ASA Physical Status Classification (Table 3-3).

Vascular access is required for all endoscopic procedures requiring sedation. It should be maintained throughout the procedure and until the patient is no longer at risk for cardiorespiratory depression.

TABLE 3-3. American Society of Anesthesiologists Classification System for Physical Status

Healthy patient
Mild systemic disease (slight functional limitation)
Severe systemic disease (moderate functional limitation)
Severe systemic disease (threat to life)
Moribund (not expected to survive without the operation or procedure)

Pharmacology

Benzodiazepines

Benzodiazepines act within the central nervous system (CNS) at specific benzodiazepine receptor sites. Occupation of these receptors results in augmentation of γ-aminobutyric acid, which is an inhibitory neurotransmitter resulting in depression of cortical function. Thus, benzodiazepines result in a dose dependent continuum of effect from mild sedation through drowsiness and sleep to deep sedation. They produce sedation, anxiolysis, and amnesia.

MIDAZOLAM

Midazolam is the preferred benzodiazepine of choice for sedation because of its rapid onset of action (3 to 5 minutes), short half-life (1.8 to 6.4 hours), and better antegrade amnesia properties. Dosing based on an otherwise healthy patient is 0.03 mg/kg as an initial dose over 2 minutes. Initial dosing should not exceed 2.5 mg for patients under 60 years of age, and 1.5 mg for patients over 60 years of age. Additional midazolam may be given in 0.25 to 1 mg to maintain the desired level of sedation. Subsequent doses should be separated by at least 2 to 3 minutes (Johns Hopkins, 2001). A total dose of < 5 mg is usually adequate for sedation in most patients; however, a higher dose may be necessary in longer procedures and in the individual patient. Midazolam is metabolized to 1-hydroxymethyl-midazolam, which is rapidly conjugated in the liver and then excreted renally. Renal insufficiency does not require dose modification. *Smaller doses* should be used in *older, debilitated,* or *chronically ill* patients, and in patients with hepatic insufficiency.

IV midazolam has been associated with *respiratory depression*, especially when combined with a narcotic. Other adverse effects include *hiccoughs, nausea* and *vomiting,* and *tenderness* at the IV site. Paradoxical reactions, such as *agitation, hyperactivity,* and *combativeness,* have been reported in patients with alcohol and substance abuse.

Narcotics

Narcotics affect the CNS via their binding to the μ-opiod receptor, which results in an analgesic effect as well as euphoria. Opiates also cause *respiratory depression* in a dose-dependent manner that may be reversed by narcotic antagonists. Respiratory depression can occur with doses smaller than the dose needed to achieve altered consciousness. Narcotics depress both the hypoxic and hypercarbic respiratory drive.

FENTANYL

Fentanyl is the narcotic of choice for sedation because of its rapid onset of action (almost immediate when the drug is given by IV), as well as shorter duration of action (30 to 60 minutes), and less emetic effect as either meperidine or morphine. The initial dose is 50 to 100 µg administered over a 2-minute period. Titration to desired level of sedation should be performed with adequate time interval (3 to 4 minutes) between doses. Maximum total dose should not exceed 3 µg/kg; however, larger doses may be necessary in long procedures and in the narcotic intolerant patient (Johns Hopkins, 2001). The elderly, debilitated or chronically ill patients, and patients with chronic obstructive pulmonary disease require smaller doses. Fentanyl is primarily transformed in the liver and demonstrates a high first pass clearance with approximately 75% of an IV dose excreted in urine, mostly as metabolites with < 10% as unchanged drug. The risk of *respiratory depression* and *hypotension* is potentiated when fentanyl is *combined* with sedatives such as *midazolam* and *droperidol*.

Meperidine

Meperidine (Demerol) is still widely used as the narcotic analgesic for sedation. Meperidine is a synthetic analgesic structurally very dissimilar to morphine, but with many of the same pharmacologic properties. Its onset of action is 3 to 5 minutes, with duration of action of 2 to 4 hours. The initial dose is 1 to 2 mg/kg, with maximum initial dose of 100 mg, titrating to desired effect with 2 to 3 minute intervals between doses.

Meperidine is metabolized in the liver, resulting in a toxic metabolite of normeperidine, which may cause *seizures*. Other adverse effects include *nausea, vomiting,* and *sphincter of Oddi spasm*. The *elderly, debilitated,* or *chronically ill* patients require *smaller doses*. Meperidine has catastrophic interactions with monoamine oxidase inhibitors. *Respiratory depression* is potentiated when meperidine is combined with sedatives.

Adjunct Medications

Adjunct medications enhance the effects of narcotics and sedatives, especially in the narcotic tolerant patient, and patients with a history of alcohol and substance abuse. Most adjunct medications also have antiemetic qualities. Examples of adjunct medications include *promethazine* (Phenergan), *droperidol*, and diphenhydramine (*Benadryl*). Use of adjunct medications for long procedures will decrease the need for larger amounts of narcotic analgesics, thereby reducing risks associated with these doses. These medications should be given early in the procedure because their onset of action is typically longer than narcotic analgesics and benzodiazepines. Therefore, identification of high risk patients and potential for longer therapeutic procedures is useful for optimal sedation practices. It should be noted that in December 2001 the US Food and Drug Administration issued a "black box" warning for droperidol. This warning is intended to increase the physician's awareness for the *potential of cardiac arrhythmias* during drug administration, and to consider use of alternative medications for patients at high risk for cardiac arrhythmias. The warning states that cases of QT prolongation and/or torsades de pointes have been reported in patients receiving droperidol at doses at or below recommended doses. Some of these cases have occurred in patients with no known risk factors for QT prolongation and have been fatal (USFDA, 2003).

Reversal Agents

Because of the potential for cardiorespiratory complications associated with sedation, the practitioner should have knowledge of the pharmacology and indications for reversal agents.

Naloxone

Narcotic antagonists compete with opiates for the receptor site without causing an opioid effect. At lower doses, *naloxone* (*Narcan*) is used to reverse narcotic induced respiratory depression or hypotension without reversing the analgesic effects. Naloxone should be diluted for sedation reversal because the doses are much smaller than for narcotic overdose. A vial of 0.4 mg should be diluted in 10 mL of normal saline. Administer 1 to 2 mL (0.04 to 0.08 mg) as initial dose (ENDO Pharmaceuticals, 2001). This can be repeated at 2 to 3 minute intervals. As dosage of naloxone is increased, analgesic effects of narcotics are reversed which may result in hypertension, cardiac arrhythmia, and cardiac arrest. The elimination of naloxone is more rapid than that of narcotics and therefore may result in the reappearance of narcosis. Patients should be monitored for a minimum of 2 hours following administration of naloxone. It should be used with caution in patients with narcotic dependency because it can cause acute narcotic withdrawal.

Flumazenil

Flumazenil (Romazicon) is a *benzodiazepine antagonist* that has a high affinity and great specificity for the benzodiazepine receptor and therefore has antagonist activity. Flumazenil should be administered slowly with an initial dose of 0.2 mg over 15 seconds. A second dose of 0.2 mg may be given after 45 seconds. If necessary, the dose of 0.2 mg may be repeated up to a total dose of 1 mg (Johns Hopkins, 2001). Flumazenil has *not* been established in patients as an effective treatment for hypoventilation caused by benzodiazepine administration. It may cause seizures, arrhythmias, and hypertension. Flumazenil has a half-life of 40 to 80 minutes and therefore "resedation" may occur. As with naloxone, patients should be monitored for a minimum of 2 hours following administration of flumazenil. It is very important to recognize that flumazenil may precipitate *acute benzodiazepine withdrawal* when given to patients on chronic benzodiazepine therapy.

Dosing

Combinations of sedative, analgesic, and adjunct agents may be administered as appropriate for the procedure being performed and the condition of the patient. Combination therapy is used to achieve desired level of sedation for longer therapeutic procedures, and in the difficult-to-sedate patient. An initial dose may be a combination of an agent from each drug class in varying doses. When using narcotic adjuncts, they should be given early during the sedation process in order to achieve the desired effects. Once the desired level of sedation is achieved, the practice of alternating administration of a sedative with a narcotic at regular intervals is useful for maintaining satisfactory sedation level for longer procedures. Further administration of drugs should be titrated in incremental doses with sufficient time between doses to allow the effect of each dose to be assessed before subsequent drug administration. Continual assessment of patient response is essential, with the practitioner responding to subtle patient clues such as increases in heart rate and blood pressure. Medications should be administered based on these trends throughout the procedure to avoid "getting behind the eight ball" in level of sedation and patient comfort.

When performing therapeutic procedures, the practitioner should anticipate patient response and dose accordingly. Boluses of medications should be given prior to painful manipulation therapies such as dilation of strictures and before critical portions such as needle knife sphincterotomy or fine-needle aspiration. The use of multiple sedating agents may increase the likelihood of adverse outcomes including ventilatory depression and hypoxemia. Therefore, dosing in combination therapy may need to be decreased for each agent.

Nonchemical sedation or verbal feedback might also help to calm the patient. Continually talking to the patient can potentiate the effects of sedating medications while reducing the patient's anxiety. Tactile methods, such as back rubbing, handholding, and head rubbing, can prove useful. One study by Schiemann and colleagues (2002) reported reduced requirements of analgesia, increased completion of procedures, and shortened examination time in patients receiving music therapy for colonoscopy.

Anesthesiologists

The assistance of anesthesiologists is required for general anesthesia and in most states for use of propofol. It should be considered in patients needing deep sedation such as those having prolonged therapeutic procedures, anticipated intolerance of standard sedatives, and those at increased risk for sedation-related complications as mentioned previously (ASGE, 2002). The presence of one or more of sedation-related risk factors, coupled with the potential for deep sedation, will increase the likelihood of adverse, sedation-related events. In this situation, if the practitioner is not trained in the rescue of patients from deep sedation, then an anesthesiologist should be consulted (Table 3-4).

Propofol

Because of its rapid induction and recovery from anesthesia, propofol has created a niche for itself in the ambulatory setting. In Maryland, this must be administered by an anesthesiologist, nurse anesthetist, or specifically trained and dedicated physician. Propofol is an IV sedative-hypnotic approved by the US Food and Drug Administration in 1989. It has a distribution half-life of 2 to 10 minutes, with a mean induction time of 30 to 40 seconds after a 2.0 to 2.5 mg/kg bolus (Massachusetts Poison Control System, 1997). Discontinuation of propofol anesthesia usually results in a rapid decrease in plasma concentrations and prompt awakening. Longer anesthesia cases may produce higher plasma concentrations and thus prolong awakening time.

There are several "pros and cons" for the use of propofol in the endoscopy setting. The short onset of action and rapid elimination time makes this an ideal drug for *short outpatient procedures*. Faster recovery time has been shown to *improve operational efficiency* of endoscopy units. Propofol provides amnesia and sedation as well as decreasing the hypertensive effects of airway manipulation. The airway management requirements need careful monitoring because the patient can go from breathing independently to apneic in a matter of seconds. Hypotension has been reported and a constant infusion is required to maintain sedation. Propofol may not be ideal for the longer therapeutic procedures as the plasma level increases, awakening time delays. In addition, propofol has no analgesic qualities, therefore narcotics need to be administered concomitantly.

Monitoring

There are no fixed guidelines for the frequency and type of monitoring of patients having sedation for endoscopy. Propofol requires very close monitoring by a single duty

TABLE 3-4. Guideline for Anesthesiology Assistance during Gastrointestinal Endoscopy

Anesthesiologist assistance may be considered in the following situations:
1. Prolonged or therapeutic endoscopic procedure requiring deep sedation
2. Anticipated intolerance to standard sedatives
3. Increased risk for complication due to severe comorbidity (ASA class III or greater)
4. Increased risk for airway obstruction due to anatomic variant

ASA = American Society of Anesthesiologists.

individual. For both moderate and deep sedation, the patient's level of consciousness, ventilatory and oxygenation status, and hemodynamic variables should be assessed and recorded according to institutional guidelines, but should also depend on the type and amount of medication administered, the length of the procedure, and the general condition of the patient. There is controversy in the frequency and type of monitoring needed.

Level of Consciousness

Monitoring of level of consciousness is somewhat difficult because it potentially can disrupt the procedure. It should be done during the noncritical periods of the procedure. Monitoring of patient response to verbal commands should be routine during moderate sedation, unless the patient is unable to respond appropriately (young children, uncooperative patients). During deep sedation, patient responsiveness to a deeper stimulus should be attempted, unless contraindicated, to ensure that the patient has not drifted into a state of general anesthesia. Note that a response limited to reflex withdrawal from a painful stimulus is not considered a purposeful response and signals deep sedation.

Pulse Oximetry

All patients undergoing sedation should be monitored by *pulse oximetry*. Supplemental oxygen should be considered for moderate sedation, patients with significant cardiopulmonary disease, and administered during deep sedation. If hypoxemia develops during sedation, supplemental oxygen should be administered.

Ventilatory Function

Monitoring of *ventilatory function* by observation or auscultation is recommended and required now by many institutions. Ventilation and oxygenation are separate though related physiologic processes; monitoring oxygenation by pulse oximetry is not a substitute for monitoring ventilatory function. *Capnography* or the measurement of exhaled carbon dioxide has been gaining increased popularity in institutions because it reflects ventilation and is more sensitive than pulse oximetry for detecting respiratory depression.

Hemodynamic Monitoring

Hemodynamic monitoring is required during sedation. Its frequency should be dictated by the level of sedation, condition of the patient, and protocols and guidelines set forth by the individual institutions.

Electrocardiogram

Continuous electrocardiography is also recommended, especially in patients with significant cardiovascular disease and dysrhythmias. Sedative and analgesic agents may blunt the appropriate autonomic compensation for hypovolemia and procedure-related stress. On the other hand, inadequate sedation may cause potentially harmful autonomic responses such as hypertension and tachycardia. Blood pressure should be monitored at frequent intervals of 5 to 15 minutes, again dictated by level of sedation, patient condition, and institutional protocols.

Designated Individual

A designated individual, other than the practitioner performing the procedure, should be present to monitor the patient throughout procedures performed with sedation. All physicians administering endoscopic sedation should be trained in basic life support skills. At least one individual capable of establishing a patent airway and positive pressure ventilation should be present whenever sedation is administered. It is recommended that an individual with advanced life support skill be immediately available. As mentioned, in some states, an anesthetist or a nurse anesthetist is required in each room for propofol use.

Postprocedure

Patients may continue to be at significant risk for developing complications even following completion of the procedure. The critical period following procedures is usually the initial 15 minutes after removal of the endoscope. Patients should be observed in an appropriately staffed and equipped area until they are near their baseline level of consciousness and no longer at risk for hypoxemia and cardiorespiratory depression. Discharge criteria should follow the institutional guidelines.

Future Trends

Nurse-Administered Propofol

There have been several recent studies involving the use of nurse-administered propofol in the endoscopy setting. A large study by Rex and colleagues (2002) of 2,000 patients concluded that propofol can be given safely by appropriately trained nurses under the supervision of endoscopists. They reported a reduced mean recovery time by approximately 31 minutes. Results included 5 episodes of oxygen desaturation to < 85% that were treated by brief (< 1 minute) periods of mask ventilation (Ulmer et al, 2003). Currently, in most states, nurses are prohibited from administering propofol, but this may change as more data substantiates its safety and efficacy in the endoscopy setting.

Patient-Controlled Sedation

Another area of increasing interest in the endoscopy suite has been the use of patient-controlled sedation. This method allows the patient to control their own sedation during the procedure, and recent studies have shown an increase in patient satisfaction and safety. One study done by Lee and colleagues (2002) evaluated patient-controlled sedation using propofol with alfentanil versus IV sedation with diazepam and meperidine. This study showed less hypotension and no oxygen desaturation in the patient-controlled sedation group in elderly patients undergoing elective outpatient colonoscopy.

Supplemental Reading

ASGE Standards of Practice Committee. Guidelines for the use of deep sedation and anesthesia for GI endoscopy. Gastrointest Endosc 2002;56:613–7.

ASGE Standards of Practice Committee. Sedation and monitoring of patients undergoing gastrointestinal endoscopic procedures. Gastrointest Endosc 1995;42:626–9.

ENDO Pharamceuticals Inc. Narcan (Naloxone hydrochloride injection, USP) insert; 2001.

Faulx AL, Catanzaro A, Zyzanski S, et al. Patient tolerance and acceptance of unsedated ultrathin esophagoscopy. Gastrointest Endosc 2002,55;620–3.

Gross JB, Bailey PL, Connis RT, et al. Practice guidelines for sedation and analgesia by non-anesthesiologists. Anesthesiology 2002;96;1004–17.

Johns Hopkins Hospital Sedation Task Force. Moderate sedation/analgesia and deep sedation/analgesia for diagnostic, operative, and invasive procedures. Protocol #PAT001. Appendix D: guide to drug dosages, Oct 2001.

Lee DW, Chan AC, Sze TS, et al. Patient-controlled sedation versus intravenous sedation for colonoscopy in elderly patients: a prospective randomized controlled trial. Gastrointest Endosc 2002;56:629–32.

Massachusetts Poison Control System. Clinical toxicology review: propofol. 1997;Vol 19.

Rex DK, Overley C, Kinser K, et al. Safety of propofol administered by registered nurses with gastroenterologist supervision in 2000 endoscopic cases. Am J Gastroenterol 2002;97:1159–63.

Schiemann U, Gross M, Reuter R, Kellner H. Improved procedure of colonscopy under accompanying music therapy. Eur J Med Res 2002;7:131–4.

U.S. Food and Drug Administration. FDA strengthens warnings for droperidol. 2001;T01–62:1–2. Available at http://www.fda.gove/bbs/topics/answers/2001/ans01123.html (accessed Sept 29, 2003).

Ulmer BJ, Hanson JJ, Overley CA, et al. Propofol versus midazolam/fentanyl for outpatient colonoscopy: administration by nurses supervised by endoscopists. Clin Gastroenterol Hepatol 2003;1:425–32.

CHAPTER 4

ENDOSCOPIC DISINFECTION

LAWRENCE F. MUSCARELLA, PHD, AND ANTHONY J. DIMARINO JR, MD

Endoscopic Reprocessing

Endoscope reprocessing, a three stage process that involves *cleaning, high-level disinfection,* and *drying* of endoscopes, breaks a crucial link in the chain of infection and is essential for the prevention of disease transmission during flexible gastrointestinal (GI) endoscopy. Failure to realize the importance of endoscopic reprocessing and to understand its principles, nuances, and the specific steps at each stage can result in nosocomial infection or other adverse patient complications. Several professional organizations, including the American Society for Gastrointestinal Endoscopy (ASGE) and the Society of Gastroenterology Nurses and Associates (SGNA), have published detailed step-by-step guidelines for reprocessing GI endoscopes (SGNA, 2000; Nelson et al, 2003; Walter and DiMarino, 2000).

Cautionary Reports

Although these published endoscope reprocessing guidelines are the result of an evolutionary process and are comprehensive, up-to-date, and effective against the transmission of infectious agents during GI endoscopy, some recent medical and lay reports have called into question the adequacy and safety of these guidelines (CDC, 1999). These reports maintain that the physical designs of GI endoscopes marketed by at least one manufacturer are flawed and feature internal channels that cannot be accessed, cleaned, or receive high-level disinfection as required to prevent disease transmission and ensure patient safety. As a consequence of their publicity, these reports that claim GI endoscopes pose a grave and overlooked public health risk have attracted the attention of state legislators. In New York State, for example, politicians, who had at first proposed introducing a bill mandating new endoscope reprocessing guidelines, decided instead to study current endoscope reprocessing practices to determine whether they are adequate and prevent disease transmission. These politicians, in both the Senate and the Assembly of New York State, deemed their legislative involvement necessary because GI endoscopy is used so frequently to diagnose and treat diseases of the GI tract. In truth, any risk associated with GI endoscopy would have significant and far-reaching public health implications and consequences. Although any study, inspection, or evaluation designed to determine whether current health care standards are safe and effective is certainly welcome—particularly at a time when reports of patient deaths linked to medical errors are all too common—the medical literature is replete with independent studies that indicate current endoscope reprocessing guidelines and practices are adequate and prevent the transmission of infectious agents during GI endoscopy. Although improving current endoscope designs to facilitate reprocessing is certainly encouraged, there are no endoscope models currently on the market that feature internal channels or surfaces that can become contaminated with patient debris during GI endoscopy but that cannot be adequately reprocessed and therefore pose an infection risk.*

The Risk of Exogenous Infection During GI Endoscopy

The potential for infection exists whenever individuals reprocessing GI endoscopes do not follow established guidelines. No cases of nosocomial infection linked to a GI endoscope contaminated with infectious agents from an *exogenous* source (ie, another patient or the environment) have been documented when the endoscope (and biopsy forceps or other reusable endoscopic accessories) was *reprocessed* in *strict accordance* with current reprocessing guidelines and instructions. This finding is *reassuring considering that more than 10 million GI endoscopic procedures* are performed each year in the United States alone. *Colonoscopy,* for example, which is reportedly performed 4.4 million times each year in the United States, is a crucial GI endoscopic procedure used to screen patients for colon cancer, the second leading cause of cancer-related deaths in the United States. Education about the safety and effectiveness of colonoscopy and its reported low risk of infection is crucial to ensure patient compliance with scheduled screenings and exams. As a result of overall adherence to published endoscope reprocessing guidelines over the past 10 years, *only 35 cases of likely* or *possible infection* caused by a contaminated GI endoscope have been reported (Weber et al, 1999; Nelson et al, 2003). Of these 35 cases, disease transmission was suspected or confirmed during colonoscopy in *only five cases.* Based on these num-

---

*Editor's Note: The first author is employed by industry.

bers, the reported risk of exogenous infection from a contaminated GI endoscope in general, and a colonoscope in particular, can be calculated to approximate 1 in 3 million and 1 in 9 million, respectively.

Although a plethora of clinical data indicate that current endoscope reprocessing guidelines are adequate and prevent disease transmission, efforts to educate GI physicians about the required step-by-step instructions provided in several published endoscope reprocessing guidelines remain a centerpiece of GI endoscopy training (DiMarino, 1999; Cheung et al, 1999). Complacency and failure by GI physicians to acknowledge and appreciate the potential for infection during GI endoscopy, although rarely reported, can compromise patient safety and generate appropriate concern by patient advocacy groups and governmental agencies. Development and implementation of a quality assurance (QA) program that, among other considerations, monitors all of the steps of endoscope reprocessing are necessary to maintain the reported low risk of disease transmission during GI endoscopy. It is important that the QA program ensures the endoscope and all of its internal channels (even if not used during the procedure), valves, and removable components are reprocessed in strict compliance with the published endoscope reprocessing guidelines, as well as the reprocessing instructions provided by the endoscope's manufacturer and the manufacturer of the automated endoscope reprocessor (AER), if used.

Breaches in Reprocessing Protocol

Years of experience and data from laboratory testing and both retrospective and prospective clinical studies have resulted in the evolution of endoscope reprocessing guidelines into their current set of refined and comprehensive instructions that are endorsed by several professional organizations. The conclusion that these current guidelines are safe and effective and do not require significant modifications is primarily based on the finding that, without exception, *every documented case* of exogenous infection resulting from a contaminated GI endoscope (or endoscopic accessory) identified as its cause a *breach* of at least one of the instructions published in these guidelines. Common failures or breaches in reprocessing protocols linked to disease transmission during GI endoscopy include *improper cleaning, ineffective high-level disinfection* or *inappropriate use* of a *liquid chemical sterilant (LCS)*, and *insufficient drying* before storage.

Only a few reports of disease transmission via a GI endoscope or endoscopic accessory have been published. There are, nevertheless, some examples that are educational and warrant discussion to highlight the adverse outcomes that can result when reprocessing practices deviate from current endoscope reprocessing guidelines. For example, one report identified *improper cleaning* and *ineffective high-level disinfection* using a LCS as responsible for disease transmission during GI endoscopy (Bronowicki et al, 1997). This report documented patient-to-patient transmission of the *hepatitis C virus* during colonoscopy due to failure to clean the endoscope's suction and biopsy channels using a brush as reprocessing guidelines emphasize. In addition, this report indicated that high-level disinfection of the colonoscope was ineffective because the colonoscope was immersed in 2% glutaraldehyde for only 5 minutes, guidelines recommending an immersion time of no less than 20 minutes not withstanding. This report also indicated that, although mechanically cleaned using a detergent, the biopsy forceps, like the colonoscope, were immersed in 2% glutaraldehyde and not steam sterilized as reprocessing guidelines recommend. (Also contributing to the possibility for disease transmission, the intravenous (IV) lines and needles used on patients discussed in this report were changed, but the syringes used to administer the IV medications were reused and not disposable and single use as guidelines for administration of IV medications recommend.)

Another report identified disease transmission as a result of *ineffective high-level disinfection*. This report documented patient-to-patient transmission of *Campylobacter pylori* during esophagogastroduodenoscopy (EGD) and biopsy due to exposure of the endoscope and its internal channels after cleaning with 70% alcohol for 3 minutes between patient procedures (Langenberg et al, 1990). Seventy percent alcohol is classified as an intermediate-level disinfectant—not a high-level disinfectant as recommended—and, therefore, its use is in violation of endoscope reprocessing guidelines. Disinfection, rather than sterilization, of the biopsy forceps used during EGD also reportedly contributed to the transmission of *C. pylori*.

Improper cleaning and ineffective high-level disinfection are not the only reported causes of exogenous infection during GI endoscopy. *Insufficient drying* of the endoscope has also been blamed for disease transmission. In one case, an outbreak of *Pseudomonas aeruginosa* and Enterobacteriaceae in patients undergoing endoscopic retrograde cholangiopancreatography (ERCP) was reported (Streulens et al, 1993). Failure to dry the endoscope's channels, including the narrow elevator forceps raiser channel, with 70% alcohol followed by compressed or forced air after high-level disinfection (and water rinsing) was identified as the cause of the outbreak. *Terminal drying* of the endoscope's internal channels is recommended by reprocessing guidelines to prevent infection due to gram-negative waterborne bacteria and atypical mycobacteria that may be present in the water used to rinse the endoscope after high-level disinfection. Virtually every report that links patient infection to an inadequately dried GI endoscope contaminated with bacteria occurred during ERCP, suggesting that infection is based on the type of GI procedure performed, among other factors. All of these aforementioned reports underscore the importance of strict adherence to all of the recommended practices and steps provided in current endoscope reprocessing guidelines.

The Three Stages of Endoscope Reprocessing

As discussed, several organizations have published their own set of endoscope reprocessing guidelines. Although each organization's guidelines may be uniquely formatted or organized in a slightly differ manner, each is in general agreement with the other, with a few exceptions that may be clinically significant. For instance, whereas *The Association of periOperative Registered Nurses* (AORN) recommends reprocessing the endoscope in the morning immediately before the first patient, ASGE and SGNA instead recommend drying the endoscope after reprocessing and before storage, a practice that is significantly less expensive and time consuming and prevents patient infection caused by bacterial colonization in the endoscope's channels during storage. AORN's guidelines also do not recommend drying the endoscope after reprocessing it using a specific AER labeled to achieve "sterilization" and to rinse the endoscope with "sterile" filtered water. According to AORN's guidelines (and the manufacturer of the AER), drying the endoscope after reprocessing in this uniquely labeled AER is superfluous and unnecessary. Other organizations, however, suggest a more evidence-based and standardized approach and instead recommend drying the endoscope after completion of each reprocessing cycle irrespective of whether using tap water, bacteria-free water, or sterile water for rinsing. In general, however, differences between published endoscope reprocessing guidelines represent the exception, not the rule. Most published guidelines are in agreement with one another and with the operating instructions provided by the endoscope's manufacturer (and AER's manufacturer).

In general, endoscope reprocessing can be divided into three stages: *cleaning, high-level disinfection,* and *drying (and proper handling and storage)*. If each of these three stages is performed in strict accordance with manufacturers' instructions and organizations' guidelines, the likelihood of disease transmission via a GI endoscope is remote. As discussed, deviations in these guidelines, however slight, can result in exogenous infection during GI endoscopy.

Stage 1 – Cleaning

Cleaning is the first and arguably the most important stage of endoscope reprocessing. Failure to perform this stage properly has been reported to result in cross-infection (Bronowicki et al, 1997). This first stage, which is a prerequisite to high-level disinfection (stage 2), is made up of several manual cleaning steps that significantly reduce the amount of patient debris, including serum, blood, feces, bacteria, and other microorganisms, on the endoscope. Although not intended to completely remove all of the microorganisms on an endoscope, the goal of cleaning is to render the endoscope visibly clean and reduce the number of microorganisms by approximately 3 logs (or 99.9%). As a result, cleaning may shorten the exposure time required to achieve high-level disinfection. Whereas 2% glutaraldehyde is labeled to achieve high-level disinfection of endoscopes that have not been cleaned in 45 minutes (at 25°C), this LCS after manual cleaning is reported to achieve high-level disinfection in 20 minutes (at 20°C). Refer to the endoscope manufacturer's instructions and published guidelines for the specific steps that are required to clean the endoscope, its channels, valves, and its removable components.

Stage 2 – High-Level Disinfection

During this second reprocessing stage, the endoscope is exposed to a LCS to achieve high-level disinfection. This stage, which can be performed either manually or using an AER, destroys potentially pathogenic microorganisms that may remain on the endoscope after cleaning. Immersing the entire endoscope in the LCS and flushing each of its channels with the LCS is necessary to achieve high-level disinfection. If reused, it is important that the LCS be periodically monitored (ie, once a day or more often) using test strips to ensure its concentration has not dropped below the level required to achieve high-level disinfection. Because some LCSs are not effective at room temperature, their temperature may also have to be elevated and monitored. In addition, the amount of time the endoscope is immersed in the LCS requires monitoring to achieve high-level disinfection. Whereas too short an immersion time can result in cross-infection due to ineffective high-level disinfection, too long an immersion time can also result in serious patient complications and adverse reactions. Some instruments, such as the probes used during transesophageal echocardiography, may be constructed of materials that, if immersed in the LCS for a period of time longer than indicated to achieve high-level disinfection, can absorb and retain residues of the LCS that are not easily rinsed off with water and can be toxic to the patient.

After high-level disinfection, the endoscope is rinsed with a large volume of clean water. Most LCSs recommend that the endoscope be rinsed using three separate water rinses to thoroughly remove any remaining chemical residue following high-level disinfection. Whereas during manual reprocessing, tap water or bottled sterile water may be used for rinsing, during automated reprocessing, the AER typically rinses the endoscope with water that has been filtered through a 5.0 μ sediment prefilter and a 0.2 μ bacterial postfilter. Although often overlooked, the quality of the rinse water is crucial to the outcome of the reprocessing procedure. Contaminated rinse water can result in contaminated endoscopes, despite effective high-level disinfection. Because of the significance of the quality of the rinse water, it has been recommended that the rinse water be microbiologically monitored to prevent recontamination of the endoscope, after high-level disinfection, with waterborne bacteria and atypical mycobacteria that could be transmitted to the patient during GI endoscopy. Refer to the endoscope manufacturer's instructions and published guidelines for the specific steps that are required for high-level disinfection, and proper rinsing of the endoscope, its channels, and its removable components.

Stage 3 – Drying

The third and final stage of an effective endoscope reprocessing procedure is as essential to the prevention of patient infection as cleaning and high-level disinfection. Drying can be easily and inexpensively achieved by flushing the endoscope's channels with 70% alcohol (to facilitate drying), followed by forced air. Like a plugged drinking straw, endoscope channels can retain rinse water after reprocessing, providing the ideal environment for waterborne microorganisms to colonize during storage. The transmission of waterborne bacteria via inadequately dried GI endoscopes has been reported. After drying, the endoscope is hung vertically with its valves and biopsy cap removed, to prevent moisture buildup and to permit ventilation of its internal channels. Proper storage of the endoscope in a dry and dust-free environment is recommended. Refer to the endoscope manufacturer's instructions and published guidelines for the specific steps that are required to dry and properly store the endoscope, its channels, and its removable components.

LCSs

There are several LCSs currently on the market that are indicated for reprocessing flexible GI endoscopes. In general, LCSs are sterilants during long exposure times (8 to 10 hours), but achieve high-level disinfection during shorter immersion times of 5 to 20 minutes. As a sterilant, an LCS is capable of destroying high numbers of bacterial spores, an important factor that distinguishes sterilization from high-level disinfection. It is important to note that

TABLE 4-1. A List of Some of the Liquid Chemical Sterilants/Disinfectants Used to Reprocess Flexible Gastrointestinal Endoscopes in the United States

Product (Active Ingredient)	Manufacturer	Trade Name	Sterilant Contact Conditions	High-Level Disinfectant Contact Conditions	Maximum Days of Reuse
0.55% *ortho*phthalaldehyde	Advanced Sterilization Products	Cidex OPA Solution High Level Disinfectant	No indication for sterilization (Passes the AOAC Sporicidal Activity Test in 32 hours at 20°C and 25°C.)	Manual processing: 12 minutes at 20°C AER: 5 minutes at 25°C	14 14
Hypochlorite 650 – 675 parts per million of active free chlorine	Sterilox Technologies, Inc.	Sterilox Liquid High Level Disinfectant System	No indication for sterilization (Passes the modified AOAC Sporicidal Activity Test in 24 hours at 25°C	10 minutes at 25°C.	Single use
1.12% glutaraldehyde, 1.93% phenol/phena	Sporicidin International	Sporicidin Sterilizing and Disinfecting Solution	12 hours at 25°C	20 minutes at 25°C	14
2.5% glutaraldehyde	MediVators, Inc.	Rapicide High Level Disinfectant and Sterilant	7 hours 40 minutes at 35°C	AER: 5 min at 35°C	28
7.35% hydrogen peroxide, 0.23% peracetic acid	Cottrell Limited	EndoSpor Plus Sterilizing and Disinfecting Solution	3 hours at 20°C	15 minutes at 20°C	14
7.5% hydrogen peroxide	Reckitt & Colman Inc.	Sporox Sterilizing and Disinfecting Solution	6 hours at 20°C	30 minutes at 20°C	21
1.0% hydrogen peroxide, 0.08% peracetic acid	Minntech Corporation	Peract 20 Liquid Sterilant/ Disinfectant	8 hours at 20°C	25 minutes at 20°C	14
2.4% glutaraldehyde	Advanced Sterilization Products	Cidex Activated Dialdehyde Solution	10 hours at 25°C	45 minutes at 25°C	14
2.6% glutaraldehyde	Metrex Research, Inc.	Metricide Activated Dialdehyde Solution	10 hours at 25°C	45 minutes at 25°C	14
2.5% glutaraldehyde	Wave Energy Systems	Wavicide –01	10 hours at 22°C	45 minutes at 22°C	30
0.2% peracetic acide	STERIS Corporation	Steris 20 Sterilant	No indication for high-level disinfection	12 minutes at 50–56°C	Single use

Refer to the Food and Drug Administration's (FDA) website for a complete list of liquid chemical sterilants/disinfectants cleared by the FDA as of March 2003: http://www.fda.gov/cdrh/ode/germlab.html.
AER = automated endoscope reprocessors; AOAC = Association of Official Analytical Chemists.

no clinical differences between processes that achieve high-level disinfection of GI endoscopes (and bronchoscopes) and those labeled to achieve sterilization, such as ethylene oxide gas, have been demonstrated. In the endoscopic setting, the clinical outcomes of high-level disinfection and sterilization, although academically distinguished from one another, are virtually identical. As a result, health care facilities that use high-level disinfection on GI endoscopes while sterilizing surgical instruments are not practicing two standards of care. Each LCS on the market is associated with its own unique set of advantages and disadvantages. Factors to consider when selecting a LCS include its exposure time and temperature required to achieve high-level disinfection, its environmental friendliness or associated hazards (eg, bad odor, irritating vapors, or the need for neutralization before disposal), its ease of use, its documented compatibility with the endoscope (and, if used, the AER), its use/reuse life, its tendency to stain the endoscope, its required number of water rinses, and its initial cost and cost per cycle.*

AERs

In the early days, the painstaking and time-consuming task of endoscope reprocessing was exclusively performed manually. In many of today's busy GI endoscopy centers, endoscope reprocessing is often accomplished using an AER. Each of these AERs automates "Stage 2," during which the endoscope is completely immersed in an LCS and its channels are automatically flushed with the LCS. All AERs rinse the endoscope with fresh filtered water after high-level disinfection. Manual cleaning ("Stage 1") of the endoscope, its channels, and removable components is required before automated reprocessing. Manual drying ("Stage 3") of the endoscope's channels is also required after both automated and manual reprocessing. Each AER on the market is associated with its own unique set of advantages and disadvantages. Factors to consider when selecting an AER include its overall reprocessing time, its ability to reduce, if not eliminate exposure of reprocessing staff to the LCS and its odor and vapors, the ease with which it can be operated and connected to complex endoscopes, its size and footprint, whether it has been reported to support bacterial colonization in its internal plumbing and components, its ability to document and record important reprocessing and clinical parameters, its compatibility with different LCSs on the market, its initial cost and cost per cycle, and the cost of required accessories, such as bacterial water filters, which can be expensive.

Conclusions: The Challenges of Encoscope Reprocessing

As in many aspects of medical practice, endoscope reprocessing is an art that requires education, attention, practice, and supervision. When its three stages are performed properly in accordance with published guidelines, there is minimal risk of a GI endoscope transmitting disease from either another patient or from the environment. Strict adherence to all of the recommended practices and steps in these guidelines is essential. Although crucial to the prevention of disease transmission, several factors can contribute to the formidability of endoscope reprocessing. One such factor involves the label instructions of LCSs used to achieve high-level disinfection of GI endoscopes. These label instructions can be confusing if controversial. In general, the labels of all LCSs list the exposure time and temperature required to achieve high-level disinfection (Table 4-1). In accordance with premarketing guidelines established for LCSs by the Food and Drug Administration (FDA), simulated in-use tests using soiled instruments (eg, flexible endoscopes) are performed in a laboratory setting to determine the exposure time and temperature required to achieve a 6 log reduction of resistant mycobacteria, which the FDA uses as the benchmark to define "high-level disinfection." To build in a margin of safety and to make

*Editor's Note: Storage after disinfection is not dilineated in this otherwise comprehensive chapter.

TABLE 4-2. A List of Automated Endoscope Reprocessors Used to Reprocess Flexible Gastrointestinal Endoscopes in the United States

Manufacturer	Trade Name	FDA Label Claim	Compatibility
Advanced Sterilization Products	ASP Automatic Endoscope Reprocessor	Disinfector	Can be used with most liquid chemical sterilants
Custom Ultrasonics, Inc.	System 83 Plus Washer-Disinfector (features a number of different models)	Washer-disinfector	Can be used with most liquid chemical sterilants
MediVators, Inc.	DSD Endoscope Disinfector (features a number of different models	Disinfector	Can be used with most liquid chemical sterilants
	MV-1/MV-2 Endoscope Reprocessor	Disinfector	Can be used with most chemical sterilants
Steris Corporation	Steris System 1	Advertised for sterile processing	Can be used with only one liquid chemical sterilant (0.2% peracetic acid)

FDA = Food and Drug Administration.

these tests more challenging, the FDA does not permit the soiled complex instruments to be manually cleaned before exposure to the LCS. Based on these challenging conditions, most 2% (alkaline) glutaraldehyde formulations, which are LCSs commonly used to reprocess GI endoscopes, list on their labels an exposure time of 45 minutes (at 25°C) to achieve high-level disinfection. This 45-minute exposure time for 2% glutaraldehyde is controversial, because it is arguably not applicable to the clinical setting, where, unlike during simulated in-use premarket testing, cleaning before high-level disinfection is the standard of care. Several studies have shown that manual cleaning, which is required by all endoscope reprocessing guidelines, reduces the amount of bioburden on the endoscope by 3 to 5 logs. Some of these studies have demonstrated that as a result of this log reduction achieved during manual cleaning, although ignored by the FDA, 2% glutaraldehyde should be labeled to achieve high-level disinfection in 20 minutes (at 20°C). This shorter, more desirable, and clinically relevant exposure time is advantageous because without jeopardizing patient safety it lowers reprocessing costs by reducing overall reprocessing times, *exposure of any personnel to LCSs, and* the number of expensive GI endoscopes required in inventory to meet patient demand. Labels of LCS that indicate an immersion time and temperature for sterilization are also controversial. Indeed, the ability of an LCS or other low-temperature agent to sterilize flexible endoscopes, as opposed to high-level disinfect them, will be debated for some time.

Confusion and controversy surrounding the use and application of LCSs in the clinical versus the laboratory setting, although academically of interest, do little to facilitate or simplify the challenging task of endoscope reprocessing. Other factors that can further complicate endoscope reprocessing include a lack of standardization. In general, manufacturers of endoscopes and AERs provide different reprocessing instructions and equipment, such as the adapters, "irrigators," fittings, and connectors. Failure to resolve discrepancies between the endoscope's and the AER's disparate and sometimes contradictory reprocessing instructions has been reported to have caused an outbreak. The complex internal design of GI endoscopes can also pose a formidable challenge to endoscope reprocessing. Because of their different therapeutic applications, different models of GI endoscopes may feature a different number of internal channels. Moreover, some models may feature a specialized channel that is used to, for instance, manipulate an elevator forceps raiser at the endoscope's distal tip during ERCP. Keeping track of all of the different models in inventory, and the unique and specialized internal channels and reprocessing instructions that some GI endoscope models require, can be demanding. As a result, it is essential to routinely review the reprocessing instructions and schematics of every endoscope model in inventory to ensure that after each procedure all of the endoscope's internal channels, including the endoscope's valves and other removable components, are accounted for and reprocessed, even if all of the channels were not used during the procedure. Efforts by the manufacturers of endoscopes and AERs to redesign their respective devices to simplify and further improve endoscope reprocessing are encouraged.

Supplemental Reading

Bronowicki P, Venard V, Botte C, et al. Patient-to-patient transmission of hepatitis C virus during colonoscopy. N Engl J Med 1997;337:237–40.

Centers for Disease Control and Prevention. Bronchoscopy-related infections and pseudoinfections—New York, 1996 and 1998. MMWR 1999;48:557–60.

Cheung RJ, Ortiz D, DiMarino AJ. GI endoscopic reprocessing practices in the United States. Gastrointest Endosc 1999;60:362–8.

DiMarino AJ. GI endoscopic reprocessing: maintaining public confidence in the face of decreasing reimbursements. Gastrointest Endosc 1999;50:585–8.

Langenberg W, Rauws EA, Oudbier JH, Tytgat GN. Patient-to-patient transmission of *Campylobacter pylori* infection by fiberoptic gastroduodenoscopy and biopsy. J Infect Dis 1990;161:507–11.

Muscarella LF. Automatic flexible endoscope reprocessors. Gastrointest Endosc Clin N Am 2000;10:245–57.

Muscarella LF. High-level disinfection or "sterilization" of endoscopes? Infect Control Hosp Epidemiol 1996;17:183–7.

Nelson DB, Jarvis WR, Rutala WA. Multi-society guideline for reprocessing flexible gastrointestinal endoscopes. Infect Control Hosp Epidemiol 2003;24:532–7.

Struelens MJ, Rost F, Deplano A, et al. *Pseudomonas aeruginosa* and Enterobacteriaceae bacteremia after biliary endoscopy: an outbreak investigation using DNA macrorestriction analysis. Am J Med 1993;95:489–98.

The Society of Gastroenterology Nurses and Associates. Standards of infection control in reprocessing of flexible gastrointestinal endoscopes. Gastroenterol Nurs [Serial online] 2000;23:172–9.

Walter VA, DiMarino AJ. American Society for Gastrointestinal Endoscopy-Society of Gastroenterology Nurses and Associates Endoscope Reprocessing Guidelines. Gastrointest Endosc Clin N Am 2000;10:265–73.

Weber DJ, Rutala WA, DiMarino AJ. The prevention of infection following gastrointestinal endoscopy: the importance of prophylaxis and reprocessing. In: DiMarino AJ, Benjamin S, editors. Gastrointestinal Disease—An Endoscopic Approach. Thorofare (NJ): Slack, Inc.; 1999. p. 87–106.

CHAPTER 5

ENDOSCOPIC ULTRASONOGRAPHY AND FINE-NEEDLE ASPIRATION

KENNETH J. CHANG, MD

Endoscopic ultrasonography (EUS) was first developed in the early 1980s by investigators in Japan, Germany, and the United States, predominantly because of the limitations of transabdominal ultrasonography (US) in imaging the pancreas. However, prior to the development of EUS-guided fine needle aspiration (FNA), EUS as an imaging modality (without biopsy or intervention capabilities) had major limitations. For example, EUS alone cannot distinguish high specificity metastatic lymph nodes from benign inflammatory nodes. Likewise, focal chronic pancreatitis can mimic pancreatic cancer on EUS. EUS was also not considered a "therapeutic" procedure. Now, two decades later, many of these limitations have been overcome with the adjunctive capabilities of EUS-guided FNA (Chang et al, 1994; Wiersema et al, 1994) and more recently, EUS-guided fine-needle injection (FNI) (Chang et al, 2000; Hecht et al, 2003; Chang et al, 2004) and other interventional EUS procedures. Thus, EUS has become a powerful tool for gastroenterologists in the diagnosis, staging, and treatment of gastrointestinal (GI), pancreaticobiliary, and pulmonary lesions. I will review the current indications for EUS and FNA.

Indications for EUS and FNA

At our institution, approximately 60 to 70% of all EUS cases result in FNA. EUS-guided FNA is used for the following indications in decreasing frequency:
1. Pancreatic tumors
2. Lymph nodes
3. Cystic lesions
4. Submucosal lesions
5. Ascites or pleural effusion
6. Liver lesions
7. Biliary lesions
8. Mediastinal tumors

We routinely obtain consent from every EUS patient for the possibility of FNA. We find this maximizes efficiency and avoids a second procedure and sedation. This approach, however, makes room time less predictable and scheduling more challenging. During an EUS examination, the decision to perform an FNA is based on whether obtaining a tissue diagnosis of the lesion in question will make a difference in the clinical decision making, management, or prognosis of the patient. For this reason, it is important to discuss with the patient and his/her physician team the algorithm of possible management scenarios in the context of a positive or negative FNA. If the algorithm is unaffected by the result of the FNA, then it should not be performed, unless there is a need for further diagnostic or prognostic confirmation.

Esophageal Cancer

STAGING

Accurate measurement of the depth of tumor and the extent of metastasis are critical factors that determine the therapeutic options and prognosis of patients with carcinoma of the esophagus, and may reduce the cost of care. EUS is currently the most accurate modality available to determine the depth of tumor and the status of regional lymph node involvement. Based on a review of 739 reported cases, EUS is accurate for evaluation of tumor depth in 85% of cases, and of nodal stage in 79% (Rosch and Classen, 1992). EUS staging is more accurate for T3/T4 tumors (> 90%) than for T1/T2 tumors (65%). However, the use of high-frequency (15 to 30 MHz) US catheter probes for staging small T1 and T2 tumors improves this accuracy to 83 to 92%. EUS-guided FNA has further improved the specificity of EUS in diagnosing lymph node metastasis and also provides pathological evidence of metastasis to peritoneal or pleural fluid, or liver.

In patients with malignant esophageal strictures (about 30% of cases), EUS assessment may require dilatation for complete assessment of the abdominal organs and lymph nodes, or remain incomplete. I usually employ dilatation only if absolutely necessary and then only up to three incremental dilator sizes. This helps to minimize perforations (forcing an operation in patients who most likely would benefit from neoadjuvant therapy), which in the literature may be as high as 24%. Adhering to this guideline may at times require a pre-EUS dilatation session. However, this strategy has resulted in successful complete staging in the vast majority of cases with a minimal risk of perforation. An alternative to dilatation may be the use of a 7.5 MHz nonoptical wire-guided tapered esophagoprobe that may traverse the stricture. FNA, however, is not possible with this instrument.

We studied the role of EUS in combination with FNA in guiding the choice of therapy made by patients who had esophageal cancer (EC) who otherwise were surgical candidates (Chang et al, 2003). Among 60 consecutive patients, the accuracy of EUS/FNA in tumor and lymph node staging was 83% and 89%, respectively. Twenty-five patients (42%) had EUS stages I and II and were candidates for curative surgery. Twenty-eight patients (47%) had stage III and 7 (12%) had stage IV. All patients with stage I had surgery, whereas all patients with stage IV had medical therapy. The majority (62%) of patients with stage II had surgery, whereas only the minority (25%) of patients with stage III had surgery. Altogether, 36 patients (60%) decided to have medical therapy. Patients' medical decisions toward surgical or medical therapy correlated strongly to results of their EUS staging ($p = .005$), but not to age, sex, or referring physicians (surgeons versus nonsurgeons). This suggests that EUS plays a significant role in patients' decision making. In addition, EUS-guided therapy had potentially *decreased the cost* of care by $870,564 ($14,509/patient) by reducing the number of thoracotomies.

The general clinical algorithm for staging EC once diagnosed by endoscopy with biopsy is shown in Figure 5-1. A helical computed tomography (CT) scan should be performed to rule out distant metastasis, such as to the liver, lung, and bone. In addition to distant metastatic disease (M1b), careful attention should be placed at looking for T4 disease (direct extension into trachea or aorta) or distant lymph node involvement (M1a), such as celiac/hepatic (in patients with proximal or mid-esophageal tumors) or cervical nodal metastasis in patients with distal esophageal tumors. *Surgical resection* is indicated for all operable candidates who are considered curable (T1N0 or T2N0). Patients with locally advanced disease (T3 or N1) should be offered *neoadjuvant chemoradiotherapy (CRT)* followed by *surgical resection*. Although *adenocarcinoma (AC)* of the esophagus is generally less sensitive to CRT than *squamous cell cancer*, patients with AC experience a greater survival benefit with multimodal therapy before surgical intervention. The chapter on esophageal carcinoma provides details on therapeutic options.

Restaging

TNM restaging by EUS has been found to be inaccurate due to inflammation, fibrosis, and "ghost cells" after CRT. However, a ≥ 50% reduction in the tumor's maximal transverse cross-sectional area has been shown to correlate with both a pathologic tumor regression and with improved clinical outcomes. In addition, finding new metastatic lesions with EUS/FNA would preclude further deliberations about surgery. Likewise, in patients who have apparent complete response on endoscopy with biopsy, an EUS/FNA showing definite residual cancer in the wall of the esophagus or in an adjacent lymph node would confirm the need for resection. Thus, in patients with locally

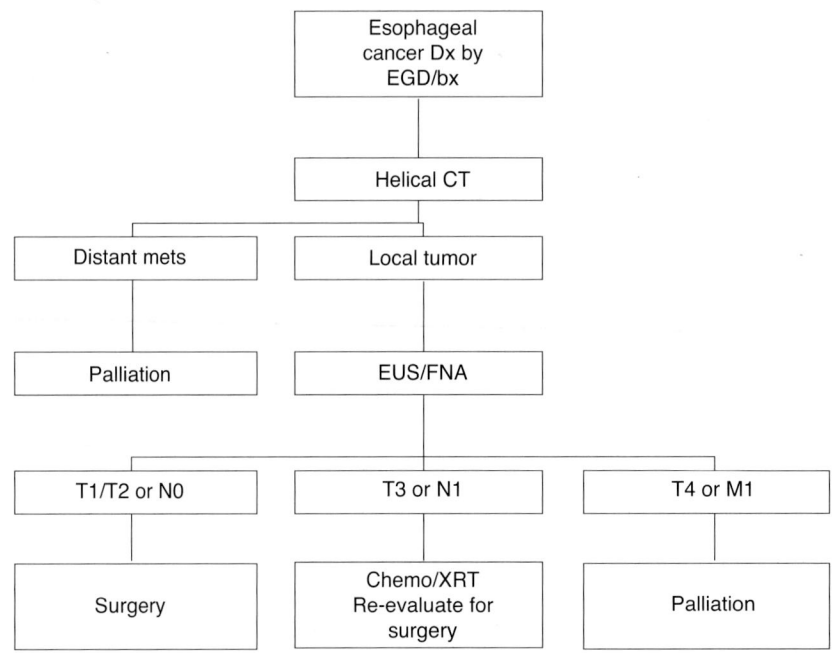

FIGURE 5-1. Algorithm for management of esophageal cancer. bx = <AU/ED: please provide definition>; CT = computed tomography; EUS = endoscopic ultrasonography; FNA = fine needle aspiration.

advanced disease who have completed neoadjuvant chemoradiation, I will usually perform preoperative EUS, especially if the patient is uncertain about surgery.

Pancreatic Cancer

AC of the pancreas is the fifth leading cause for cancer-related death in the United States. Despite improvements in medical and surgical therapy, the overall 5-year survival still remains at 4%. The most favorable outcome is among surgical patients with small tumors without nodal, vascular, or systemic metastasis. These patients have 5-year survivals that range up to 25%. Optimally, earlier detection and precise preoperative staging would best stratify patients who would most likely benefit from surgery while sparing the remaining patients from exploratory or palliative-only surgery.

Detection

EUS is considered as one of the most useful diagnostic procedures among the body imaging tools for detecting pancreatic cancer. EUS was shown to be superior (sensitivity 98%) to other imaging modalities, including CT, in 146 patients with pancreatic cancer (Table 5-1) (Hunt and Faigel, 2002). With the more recent introduction of spiral CT with dual phase contrast, the detection rate for CT is improving. However, recent comparisons between dual-phase spiral CT and EUS still favor EUS.

Diagnosis with EUS-Guided FNA

The ability to obtain cytological specimens by EUS-guided FNA has overcome the difficulty in differentiating between benign versus malignant lesion seen on EUS alone. The application of EUS-guided FNA to the pancreas in particular has great clinical utility. CT- or US-guided percutaneous FNA are the more common methods for diagnosing pancreatic cancer. The sensitivity of percutaneous FNA ranges from 45 to 100%, with a specificity of up to 100%. However, obtaining a tissue diagnosis with CT or US guidance is limited by the ability to visualize the lesion. In our previous multicenter trial, 56% of patients with pancreatic carcinoma had CT scans that did not demonstrate a mass or revealed nonspecific enlargement of the pancreas. Endoscopic retrograde cholangiopancreatography (ERCP) with cytologic brushing also has a relatively low yield, with sensitivities between 30 and 56%. The overall sensitivity, specificity, diagnostic accuracy, negative predictive values, and postive predictive values of EUS-guided FNA for pancreatic cancer were 83%, 90%, 85%, 80%, and 100%. This was superior to CT alone (without FNA) (56%, 37%, 50%, 28%, and 65%, respectively [$p < .05$]). There were 4 complications in 164 patients (2%), including 2 major (perforation, bleeding) and 2 minor (fever). Comparison among the four centers showed that institutions in which a cytologist was present during the procedure had a significantly higher number of passes, cytologic yield, sensitivity, and diagnostic accuracy. Advantages of EUS-guided FNA include procuring a tissue diagnosis while also obtaining additional TN staging information, the avoidance of additional diagnostic testing and/or surgery, and the prognostic information relating to accurate TN staging. A large single institution study of EUS-guided FNA, including 144 pancreatic lesions, had a sensitivity, specificity, and diagnostic accuracy of 82%, 100%, and 85%, respectively. More recently, helical or spiral CT has improved imaging of the pancreas. However, preliminary studies still show superiority of EUS versus spiral CT. The most difficult diagnosis to make for any imaging test, including EUS-guided FNA, is the differentiation between pancreatic carcinoma and chronic pancreatitis. Although a positive FNA is almost 100% accurate, a negative FNA is about 80% accurate.

We believe that all patients thought to have operable disease based on initial CT imaging should undergo EUS ± FNA prior to surgical intervention. At the same time, considering the possibility of a false negative result (up to 20%, especially in the setting of chronic pancreatitis), we believe that surgical intervention should not be precluded in a patient with a high suspicion of resectable pancreatic carcinoma and a negative FNA cytology.

EUS-guided FNA of pancreatic lesions is also worthwhile in patients with a prior negative tissue diagnosis by ERCP or CT of the abdomen. Gress and colleagues (2001) reported his experience with EUS-guided FNA of pancreatic mass lesion in 102 patients who had negative cytological tissue diagnosis by ERCP sampling or CT-guided FNA. Among those patients, 57 of the 61 patients (93.4%) with a final diagnosis of pancreatic cancer had positive cytology results for AC EUS-guided FNA. The false positive results were zero.

We have reviewed a series of 44 consecutive patients who

TABLE 5-1. Detection of Pancreatic Carcinoma by Body Imaging Tools

Size	EUS	US	CT	ERCP	AG
< 20 mm (N = 10)	8/10	3/10	1/10	7/10	3/10
> 20 mm (N = 136)	135/136	104/132	102/136	121/136	77/80
Total sensitivity (%)	143/146 (98)	107/142 (75)	103/129 (80)	128/146 (86)	80/90 (89)

AG = angiogram; CT = computed tomography; ERCP = endoscopic retrograde cholangiopancreatography; EUS = endoscopic ultrasonography; US = ultrasonography.

underwent EUS with or without FNA as part of their pancreatic cancer evaluation. Surgery and further diagnostic testing were avoided in 41% and 57% of patients respectively. A substantial cost saving of $3,300 per patient was calculated. In a series of 216 consecutive patients, the use of EUS with EUS-guided FNA as the initial approach to patients with obstructive jaundice was studied by Erickson and colleagues. EUS/FNA proved useful not only as a diagnostic and staging modality, but also served in directing the need for subsequent therapeutic ERCP, saving approximately $1,007 to $1,313 per patient. In addition, if EUS/EUS-guided FNA were not used at all, an extra $2,200 would be spent per patient. The economic impact of EUS–FNA in the preoperative staging of patients with pancreatic head AC was clearly demonstrated in a decision analysis model by Harewood and colleagues (2002). The use of EUS–FNA prevented 16 surgeries per 100 patients compared with 8 per 100 patients if CT-guided FNA was performed for nonperitumoral lymph nodes (NPT LN). If the frequency of NPT LN was > 4%, then EUS–FNA is the least costly procedure ($15,938) versus ($16,378) for CT–FNA, and ($18,723) for surgery. EUS-guided FNA of the pancreas, unlike CT-guided FNA, can be preformed during the initial endosonographic procedure. The overall complication rate of EUS–FNA was reported to be 0.5 to 2.9%. Several case reports had described malignant seeding of the needle tract after transcutaneous FNA. The true incident has yet to be established. Theoretically, EUS-guided FNA of pancreatic cancers should have lower chance of malignant seeding because of the short needle tract. In pancreatic head lesions, EUS-guided FNA is usually performed from the second portion of the duodenum, a segment resected surgically along with the tumor during Whipple procedure. This is another theoretical advantage in eliminating the needle tract and decreasing the risk of malignant seeding when compared with the percutaneous approach. However, this may not apply to pancreatic body and tail lesions, where the possibility of malignant seeding of the gastric wall could still exist. The ability to detect vascular structures around the targeted lesion by Doppler flow analysis is another advantage as to minimize the bleeding complication rate. Most of the bleeding is self-limited and resolves spontaneously.

EUS Staging

The initial studies on the staging accuracy of EUS for pancreatic cancer were very encouraging. These results showed that EUS had a T-stage accuracy of 85 to 94% and a N-stage accuracy of 72 to 80%. During this time period, EUS T-stage and N-stage accuracy was superior to conventional imaging with either transabdominal US or CT. Thus, in the early 1990s, it was stated that "EUS is the single best modality for the preoperative local staging of pancreatic cancer." However, over the last 5 years, this notion has been challenged. The controversies that have arisen include the following: (1) more recent studies do not confirm the earlier staging accuracies of EUS compared to findings at surgery and (2) EUS is not thought to be useful for metastatic (M) staging, and therefore is restricted to local staging. Therefore, a helical CT is still necessary. As helical CT and magnetic resonance imaging (MRI) studies are improving for local staging, is there still a role for EUS in the staging of pancreatic cancer? In other words, in the year 2004, is CT alone sufficient in staging pancreatic cancer? The T-stage accuracy for EUS in the recent literature (1999 to present) ranges from 69 to 85%. Taking the combined accuracy of these studies, the mean accuracy for EUS T-stage accuracy is 77% (95% CI 70 to 83%) (Table 5-2). The N-stage accuracy ranges from 54 to 72%. The calculated combined nodal accuracy is 69% (95% CI 56 to 71%, Table 5-3).

EUS versus Helical CT

Although the gap is closing between EUS and CT in staging pancreatic cancer, EUS/FNA still remains in many ways

TABLE 5-2. Endoscopic Ultrasonography T-Stage Accuracy for Pancreatic Cancer

Author	Number of Patients Staged by EUS	Number of Surgical Patients	Staging Accuracy	Accuracy (%)
Buscail	73	26	19/26	73
Gress	151	75	64/75	85
Ahmad	?	89	55/79	69
Total	–	190	138/180	77 (95% CI, 70 to 83)

TABLE 5-3. Endoscopic Ultrasonography N-Stage Accuracy for Pancreatic Cancer

Author	Number of Patients Staged by EUS	Number of Surgical Patients	Staging Accuracy	Accuracy (%)
Buscail	73	26	18/26	69
Gress	151	71	51/71	72
Ahmad	?	89	35/67	54
Total	–	186	104/164	63 (95% CI, 51 to 71)

superior to CT in its overall utility in pancreatic cancer. A recent review of studies comparing EUS to helical CT by Hunt and Faigel (2002) is summarized in Table 5-4. This review shows that the pooled data among the four recent studies show superiority of EUS to helical CT in detection of pancreatic tumor (97% versus 73%), accuracy for resectability (91% versus 83%), and sensitivity for vascular invasion (91% versus 64%). Therefore, EUS is still the most accurate modality for tumor detection, with a relatively high accuracy for local staging. In addition, as a single modality, EUS, especially when combined with EUS-guided FNA has been shown to be cost efficient by Harewood and colleagues (2002).

M-Staging by EUS

It has long been thought that EUS cannot be used for metastatic staging of pancreatic cancer. Recent studies are showing that EUS combined with FNA may be quite effective at assessing the majority of the liver, detecting and taking tissue samples of suspected metastatic lesions within both the left and right lobe. In addition, EUS/FNA can also sample scant amounts of ascitic fluid to assess peritoneal metastasis. Newer generation echoendoscopes will be able to penetrate further into the liver and potentially assess the entire liver for possible metastasis. If this occurs, EUS may become even more effective in the diagnosis and staging of these patients. Furthermore, therapeutic interventions with EUS-guided celiac nerve block and/or simultaneous ERCP with stent placement for palliation of jaundice could be performed during the same session. Thus, based on the studies presented, I recommend the algorithm in Figure 5-2 for patients with suspected AC of the pancreas. Patients with suspected pancreatic cancer should first undergo a helical CT with pancreas protocol. If there is an obvious mass with liver metastasis or unequivocal vascular invasion, a CT-guided biopsy should be performed and palliative therapy offered. If the CT shows a mass that appears resectable, or the CT is equivocal or negative, then the patient should undergo

TABLE 5-4. Summary of Studies Comparing Endoscopic Ultrasonography With Helical Computed Tomography for Pancreatic Cancer

Series	Detection		Accuracy for Resectability		Sensitivity for Vascular Invasion	
	EUS	CT	EUS	CT	EUS	CT
Legmann	27/27	25/27	20/22	19/22	6/7	7/7
Midwinter	33/34	26/34	25/30	23/30	13/16	9/16
Tierney	–	–	30/31	25/31	16/16	10/16
Mertz	29/31	16/31	16/16	13/16	6/6	3/6
Total	97%	73%	91%	83%	91%	64%
p value*	< .001	–	.02	–	< .001	–

CT = computed tomography; EUS = endoscopic ultrasonography
*Fisher exact test.

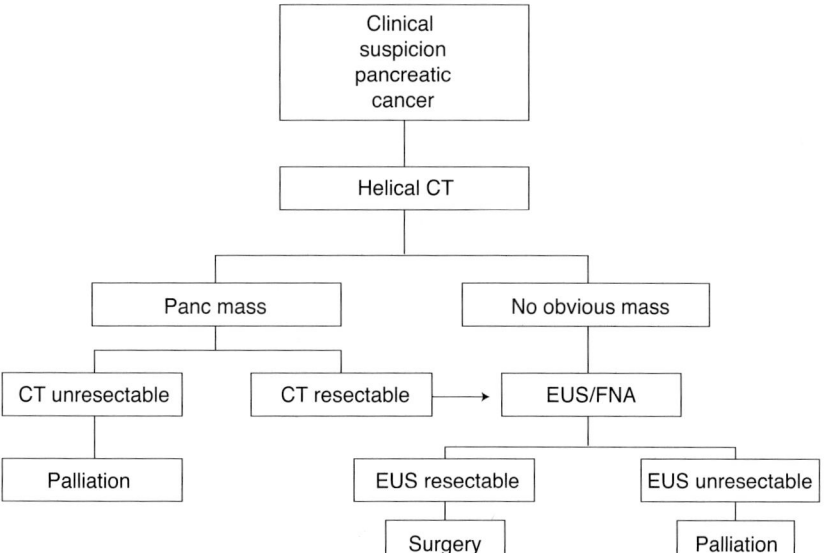

FIGURE 5-2. Algorithm for diagnosis and staging of pancreatic cancer. CT = computed tomography; EUS = endoscopic ultrasonography; FNA = fine needle aspiration.

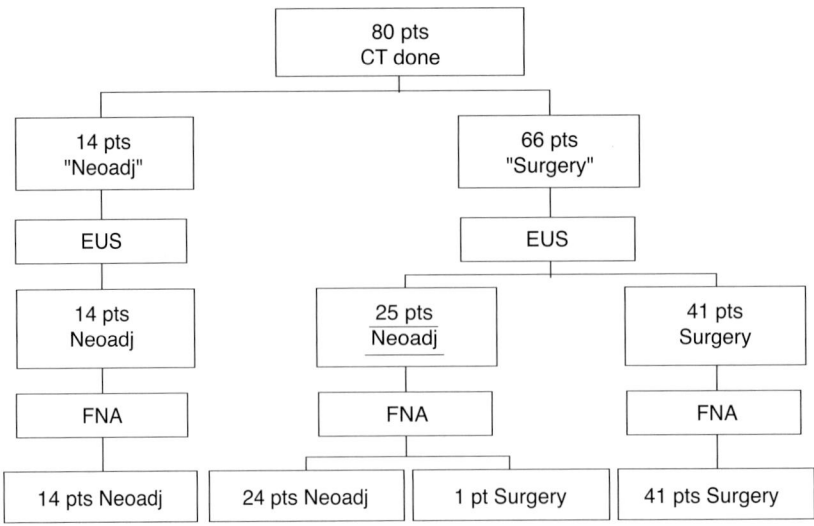

FIGURE 5-3. Outcomes of rectal cancer based on endoscopic ultrasonography (EUS) staging. CT = computed tomography; FNA = fine needle aspiration.

EUS/FNA. The EUS/FNA can further stratify those patients found to be unresectable from those who are resectable. Those who are resectable by EUS/FNA should undergo surgical exploration/resection. Using this algorithm approximately 50% of patients who were assessed as "resectable" by CT were found to be unresectable by EUS. Fourteen of the 23 patients assessed as "resectable" by EUS were able to undergo curative resections at surgery with a significantly longer survival compared to all other groups ($p < .01$). The chapter on pancreatic cancer contains more information on this topic (see Chapter 142, "Pancreatic Cancer Therapy").

Rectal Cancer

The clinical utility of EUS in staging rectal cancer is even greater than in EC. I say this because the treatment of rectal cancer has a number of surgical/presurgical approaches, and stratifying patients to the most optimal therapy can really only be done with very accurate local staging (ie, with EUS). Large tubulovillous adenomas in the rectum can often be treated with *endoscopic mucosal resection (EMR)*. In these cases, EUS can play an important role in ruling out malignancy deep in the rectal wall, or more importantly, in surrounding lymph nodes. Small, early rectal cancers may be optimally managed by transanal full thickness resection followed by possible external beam radiation, thus avoiding a colostomy. Here, EUS is useful to rule out T3 or N1 disease, in which case the transanal approach would not be appropriate. For locally advanced rectal cancers (ie, T3N0 or T3N1), preoperative chemoradiation followed by resection offers the best long term survival. EUS and FNA are very helpful in providing accurate T and N staging to determine if neoadjuvant therapy is indicated. The overall T-stage accuracy of EUS is 80 to 95% and N-stage accuracy is 70 to 75% (Table 5-5). EUS is more sensitive and specific than CT for T and N staging, although CT is still needed to detect liver metastasis. MRI with pelvic surface coils is more accurate than CT for T staging and similar to EUS. However, MRI has a lower specificity for N stage and is more expensive (although less operator dependent) than EUS. A recent outcomes paper examining the role of EUS in rectal cancer staging showed that of 80 consecutive patients with rectal cancer, 66 patients would have gone directly to surgery based on CT alone (Figure 5-3) (Harewood et al, 2002). However, EUS/FNA was able to determine that 24 of the 66 patients (36%) had locally advanced diseased and more appropriately received neoadjuvant chemoradiation. There is a chapter on rectal carcinoma (see Chapter 98, "Rectal Cancer") and on rectal cancer palliation (see Chapter 99, "Rectal Cancer Palliation").

Submucosal Lesions

EUS plays a very important role in the evaluation of submucosal lesions throughout the GI tract because of its abil-

TABLE 5-5. Endoscopic Ultrasonography Accuracy for Rectal Cancer

EUS Stage	Accuracy (%)	Range
T1	85	(33–100)
T2	73	(50–100)
T3	87	(65–100)
T4	100	–
Overall T	–	(80–95%)
N0	76	(70–92)
N1	82	(50–95)
Overall N	–	(70–75%)

EUS = endoscopic ultrasonography.

ity to visualize all five echolayers and determine the layer of origin (Figure 5-4). The first priority is to determine whether the lesion is extramural (ie, a lesion, structure, or tumor that is bulging against the GI wall from the outside) or intramural. Intramural lesions are then stratified by their layer of origin. Mucosal lesions include *gastritis, mucosa-associated lymphoid tissue lymphoma,* or *granular cell tumors.* Lesions arising from the muscularis propria are most likely *gastrointestinal stromal tumors (GIST)*, previously known as *leiomyomas.* True submucosal lesions are further stratified into those that are echo-poor, anechoic, or iso-echoic. Iso-echoic (and sometimes hyper-echoic) lesions are most characteristic of *lipomas.* Lesions that are anechoic are most likely *cysts or vessels.* Echo-poor or hypo-echoic lesions in the submucosal space could represent *carcinoid, lymphoma,* or *pancreatic rest.* Although I will often forgo an FNA in lesions that are anechoic or hyper-echoic, I will usually try to obtain a tissue diagnosis with the echo-poor or hypo-echoic lesions arising from the submucosa. The yield of EUS-guided FNA for submucosal lesion is actually considerably lower than that for extramural lesions. On average, the yield for FNA is approximately 50 to 60%. This, however, depends on the layer of origin and the size of the tumor. We recently performed a retrospective review of 102 consecutive patients over a 2.5-year period with submucosal lesions. The overall sensitivity, specificity and diagnostic accuracy for EUS/FNA were 64%, 50%, and 69%, respectively. Subanalysis comparing the accuracy of FNA between lesions from the fourth echolayer versus the second and third echolayers was 76% versus 47% ($p = .020$, Fisher's exact). There was direct correlation between the size of GIST and diagnostic accuracy on FNA. Larger tumors (≥ 2.66 cm^2 or approximately 1.6 × 1.6 cm) had a diagnostic accuracy of 90% and were 10 times more likely to be diagnosed by FNA than smaller lesions (odds ratio = 9.5, CI = 95%, $p = .014$). We also found that EMR of second/third echolayer lesions appeared to have a higher yield than FNA and may be useful as an adjunct modality for these submucosal infiltrative lesions. The next chapter is on EMR (see Chapter 6, "Endoscopic Mucosal Resection").

Supplemental Reading

Chang KJ, Katz KD, Durbin TE, et al. Endoscopic ultrasound-guided fine-needle aspiration. Gastrointest Endosc 1994;40:694–9.

Chang KJ, Nguyen PT, Thompson JA, et al. Phase I clinical trial of allogeneic mixed lymphocyte culture (cytoimplant) delivered by endoscopic ultrasound-guided fine-needle injection in patients with advanced pancreatic carcinoma. Cancer 2000;88:1325–35.

Chang KC, Senzer N, Chung T, et al. A novel gene transfer therapy against pancreatic cancer (TNFerade) delivered by endoscopic ultrasound (EUS) and percutaneous guided fine needle injection (FNI). Gastrointest Endosc 2004.

Chang KJ, Soetikno RM, Bastas D, et al. Impact of endoscopic ultrasound combined with fine-needle aspiration biopsy in the management of esophageal cancer. Endoscopy 2003;35:962–6.

Gress F, Gottlieb K, Sherman S, Lehman G. Endoscopic ultrasonography-guided fine-needle aspiration biopsy of suspected pancreatic cancer. Ann Intern Med 2001;134:459–64.

Harewood GC, Wiersema MJ, Nelson H, et al. A prospective, blinded assessment of the impact of preoperative staging on the management of rectal cancer. Gastroenterology 2002;123:24–32.

Hecht JR, Bedford R, Abbruzzese JL, et al. A phase I/II trial of intratumoral endoscopic ultrasound injection of ONYX-015 with intravenous gemcitabine in unresectable pancreatic carcinoma. Clin Cancer Res 2003;9:555–61.

Hunt GC, Faigel DO. Assessment of EUS for diagnosing, staging, and determining resectability of pancreatic cancer: a review. Gastrointest Endosc 2002;55:232–7.

Rosch T, Classen M. Gastroenterologic endosonography. Thieme: Stuggart; 1992.

Wiersema MJ, Kochman ML, Cramer HM, et al. Endosonography-guided real-time fine-needle aspiration biopsy. Gastrointest Endosc 1994;40:700–7.

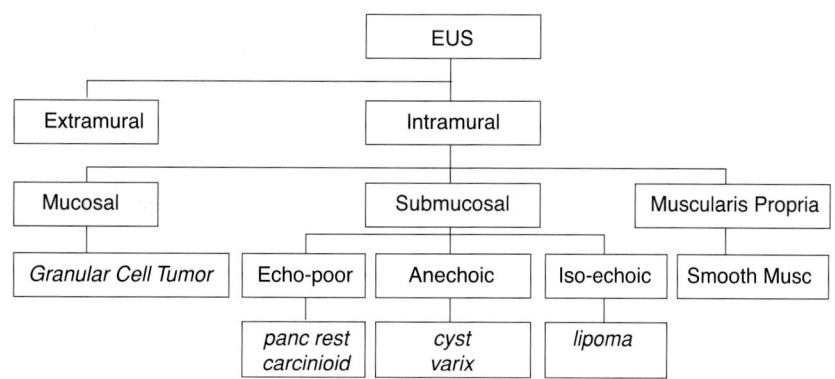

FIGURE 5-4. Endoscopic ultrasonography (EUS) diagnosis of submucosal lesions. GIST = gastrointestinal stromal tumor.

CHAPTER 6

ENDOSCOPIC MUCOSAL RESECTION

MASSIMO CONIO, MD, ROSANGELA FILIBERTI, PHD, AND DARIUS SORBI, MD

Endoscopic mucosal resection (EMR) maximizes histologic assessment of the resected lesion. The aim of EMR is to completely remove the mucosa and submucosa, thus exposing the muscularis propria. The majority of the available data in the literature is from eastern countries, which probably reflects differences in the cancer incidence between eastern and western countries. EMR is becoming popular in western countries, as indicated by the increasing number of publications devoted to this topic (Figures 6-1 and 6-2).

A strategy based on improved instrumentation, greater experience in detecting early cancers, and identification and surveillance of high risk groups would expand the application of EMR.

Indications

EMR is indicated when the malignancy is at an early stage and the risk of lymph node metastasis is absent. The depth of the lesions usually predicts the risk of cancer. However, the pathologic Japanese classification, encompassing three layers of both *mucosa* (m1, m2, m3) and *submucosa* (sm1a, b c, sm2, and sm3), is not applied in western countries. Western pathologists define high grade dysplasia (HGD) by cytologic and architectural changes confined to the mucosa. Malignant lesions are those infiltrating the submucosa, but not reaching the muscularis propria. There are differences in the pathologic interpretation between Japanese and western pathologists. Japanese pathologists base diagnosis of cancer on nuclear, cytologic, and glandular architectural abnormalities, whereas western pathologists require the presence of invasion. In the esophagus, infiltration encompassing m1 and m2 stages can be safely resected.

The rate of lymph node metastasis in patients with early gastric cancer (EGC), ranges between 0 and 3%, but when submucosa infiltration is present the rate ranges between 9 to 19%. ECG are classified as follows:
1. Type I (protruded)
2. Type IIa (superficial elevated)
3. Type IIb (superficial flat)
4. Type IIc (superficial depressed)
5. Type III (excavated)

The exclusion criteria for EMR include the following:
1. Poorly differentiated cancer
2. Presence of an ulceration
3. Diameter greater than 20 mm
4. Type IIc greater than 10 mm
5. Poorly demarcated border
6. Appearance of submucosal tumor infiltration

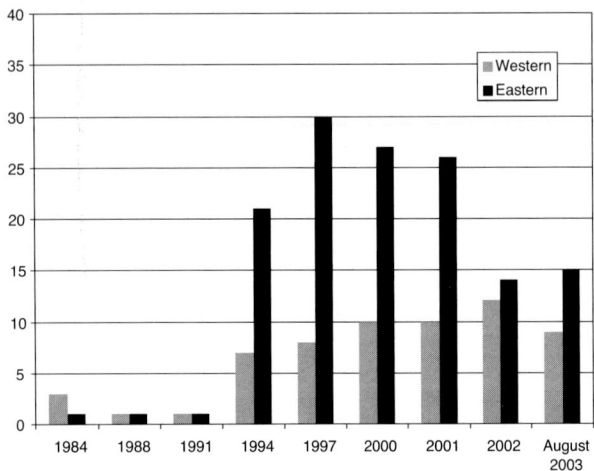

FIGURE 6-1. Articles on endoscopic mucosal resection in eastern and western countries.

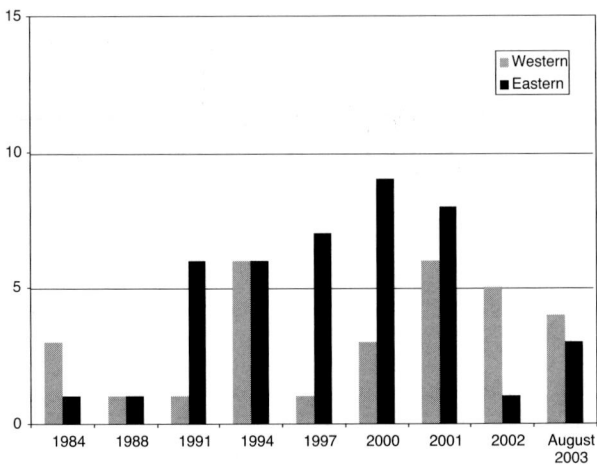

FIGURE 6-2. Articles on colorectal endoscopic mucosal resection in eastern and western countries.

Sessile colorectal lesions, including "laterally spreading tumors" characterized by low height and superficial growth, flat adenomas without central depression, can be removed by EMR. EMR should not be carried out in the presence of ulceration, depressed lesions, or absence of lifting after submucosal injection. When sm1a and sm1b (upper third of the first sm layer) infiltration is detected, the risk of lymphatic invasion ranges between 10.7 and 19.1%, but if vessel invasion is observed, surgery is mandatory.

Techniques

Techniques can be divided into the following two groups: "without suction" (freehand) and "with suction" ("cap" technique) (Table 6-1). Before performing EMR it is recommended to visualize the lesion margins. Chromoendoscopy with indigo carmine, methylene blue, or lugol for squamocellular cancer (SCC), and marking the periphery of the lesion with burn spot performed with the tip of the snare, facilitate EMR. The lesion can be removed in one single piece ("en bloc" resection), or in multiple fragments ("piecemeal"). Piecemeal resection increases the risk of recurrence.

"Strip Biopsy"

After the submucosal injection, the open polypectomy snare is placed around a portion of the lesion and pressed against the mucosa. Excess air is aspirated from the hollow organ to decrease distension and to allow the grasp of the targeted lesion. After snare excision, air is again insufflated to visualize the resected area and the residual tissue to be removed. The size of the specimen obtained with this procedure ranges between 10 to 15 mm and larger lesions must be resected by piecemeal.

This technique was modified by using a double channel endoscope. A polypectomy snare is open around the lesion and the lesion itself is then lifted with a grasping forceps. The use of a monofilament polypectomy snare has been used without submucosal injection. Seven early SCC (5 to 30 mm) were resected, and no local recurrence was observed. Strip biopsy can be difficult to perform in certain parts of the stomach (upper lesser curvature, posterior wall, and cardia) or in removing interhaustral flat polyps of the colon.

TABLE 6-1. Techniques of Endoscopic Mucosal Resection

Without suction
 "Strip-off biopsy" (injection and snaring)
 "Lift-and-cut" with double channel endoscope
 Insulated-tip diathermic knife (IT-knife) (injection + incision + snaring)
 Barbed snare
With suction
 EMR "cap-assisted" (plastic cap, injection, and snaring)
 "Suck-and-ligate" with a variceal ligating device

EMR = endoscopic mucosal resection.

Endoscopic Mucosal Resection "Cap-Assisted" (EMRC)

A transparent, hard plastic cap is preloaded on the tip of a standard front viewing endoscope. The appropriate size and diameter of the cap is selected according to the location where the EMR will be performed. Inside the distal end of the cap is a gutter, which positions the opened polypectomy snare. Removal of a 3 mm segment of the gutter with a blade scalpel before placement on the endoscope tip is recommended. This modification is then aligned with the operative channel of the endoscope to avoid interference with the injection needle or other devices with the gutter. After creation of the submucosal fluid cushion, the cap is applied against the lesion, which is aspirated into it. The opened snare is then firmly secured around the tissue and resection is performed. A monofilament polypectomy snare is used. It should be applied with caution in the gastric fundus, duodenum, and ascending colon. The limited thickness of the muscularis propria can result in its entrapment, leading to a perforation. Injection of a large amount of a submucosal solution is recommended.

A soft cap has been tested to remove large diameter gastric lesions. This cap is deformable and can be introduced into the esophagus. The diameter of the soft cap is 18 mm, whereas the diameter of the hard one is 16.5 mm. The diameter, the depth of the resected specimen, and the rate of "en bloc" resection were compared between the two. With the soft cap the diameter was larger (22.1 mm vs 15.8 mm), deeper (1.54 mm vs 1.08 mm), and the rate of "en bloc" resection was higher (66.7% vs 43.2%) (Matsuzaki et al, 2003).

"Suck-and-Ligate" Technique

EMR can be performed using a variceal band ligator. After submucosal injection, an artificial polyp is created and the resection is performed with a standard polypectomy snare. It has been used for minute gastric cancer with the diameter of the resected mucosa ranging from 10 to 15 mm. The submucosal injection is not always necessary. This technique is cumbersome, because the endoscope has to be introduced twice for each resection. The use of two different endoscopes is mandatory to speed up the procedure and perform multiple resections.

Insulated-Tip Diathermic Knife

The insulated-tip diathermic knife (IT-knife) has a ceramic ball at the top of a conventional diathermic needle to prevent damage to the muscularis propria. After a submucosal injection, a 2 mm incision is made with a diathermic knife to make a hole for the insertion of the ceramic ball. The incision is performed around the lesion. When the circumferential incision has been completed, the resection is performed with a snare polypectomy. The IT-knife technique is difficult and can be associated with bleeding and perforation (Ohkuwa et al, 2001).

Submucosal Injection

The gastrointestinal wall has two components, the mucosal layer and the muscle layer. The two components are attached by a loose connective tissue of submucosa. Injecting a solution into the submucosa, creates a *fluid cushion* between the lesion and the deeper layers of the gut wall before removal. The piecemeal removal of large sessile polyps (SP) without injection can result in deep thermal ulceration. A more durable submucosal fluid cushion may result in safer procedures, avoiding the need for repeated injections. Several solutions have been proposed, including the following: normal saline with or without epinephrine, 50% dextrose, Glyceol (which contains 10% glycerol and 5% fructose), and hyaluronic acid. Hyaluronic acid appears to be the ideal solution for submucosal injection. However, 50% glucose is more readily available and may be a more practical alternative to hyaluronic acid. Yamamoto and colleagues (2002) evaluated the use of sodium hyaluronate in 70 patients with early gastric cancers. "En bloc" resection of 20 mm lesions was successful in 89% of cases and in 48% of cases with greater lesions (Yamamoto et al, 2002).

The effects of hydroxypropyl methylcellulose were studied in the esophagus of pigs (Feitoza et al, 2003). The mean submucosal fluid cushion duration was 36 minutes, without causing tissue reaction. In our endoscopic practice, we elevate the lesion by injecting a large amount (15 to 100 cc) of normal saline plus epinephrine solution (1:60/100,000) into and around the lesion. Normal saline only is used when supplemental injections are required during EMR. Methylene blue is added for visual enhancement of the fluid cushion in contrast to the lesion.

Postprocedure

After *esophageal, gastric and duodenal EMR*, the patient should fast for 24 hours. Liquids are then allowed for 5 days before a normal diet is resumed. In patients who undergo extended esophageal EMR, fasting should be prolonged for 48 hours and the liquid diet for at least 1 week. All patients receive a double dose of a proton pump inhibitor per day orally. Intravenous antibiotics are only administered to patients with pain and fever. After *colonic EMR* (> 30 mm), liquids are given by mouth 24 hours after the procedure. Patients are discharged from the hospital 24 hours after the EMR. Antibiotics, abdominal plain radiography, and 48 hours fasting are advised for patients with abdominal pain due to postcoagulation syndrome.

Histopathologic Assessment

It would be ideal to remove a malignant lesion in one piece, so allowing an adequate histologic evaluation. However, in many instances piecemeal resection is unavoidable. The specimens should be immediately stretched and fixed on a rubber plate, then placed in 10% formalin solution. The surface of the lesion should be reconstructed for the pathologist. If the resected fragments are placed in a tube with formalin, without being fixed, they will retract, and the histologic analysis will be inaccurate.

Esophagus

Superficial Esophageal Cancer

When EMR is applied in patients with *superficial cancer*, the 5-year survival rate is up to 95%. A *preoperative evaluation* of the patients by means of endoscopic ultrasonography (EUS) is desirable to assess the lymph nodes. Neoplastic infiltration may be suspected in lymph nodes larger than 10 mm with hypoechoic pattern. It is possible to detect preoperatively 50 to 80% of infiltrated lymph nodes. High frequency ultrasonography probes of 20 and 30 MHz can improve the evaluation of superficial tumors.

The EMR of 25 superficial esophageal cancers (m1), performed either "en-bloc" (72%) or piecemeal (28%), did not show recurrences after a mean follow-up of 2 years. Shimizu and colleagues (2002) evaluated 26 patients with SCC invading the muscularis mucosa or the submucosa, compared with 44 patients with the same characteristics who underwent surgery. Survival was similar in the two groups (77.4% vs 84.5%) (Bergmann and Beger, 2003).

Barrett's Esophagus

Patients with Barrett's esophagus (BE) are advised to undergo endoscopic surveillance with multiple biopsies to detect HGD and/or early adenocarcinoma (AC). Several endoscopic methods have been used to remove HGD, including photodynamic therapy (PDT) and Argon Plasma Coagulator (APC), but the disadvantage is the lack of final histological assessment. Moreover, PDT with photofrin caused severe esophageal stenoses in 34% of patients. EMR could become a therapeutic alternative to esophagectomy in these patients (Table 6-2).

Most of the published studies report EMR of endoscopically visible areas of HGD or early AC (Table 6-3). EMR changes the pathologic stage in a significant number of patients.

The risk of overlooking simultaneous associated foci of malignancy is greater for patients with long extension of BE. The reported frequency of *undetected cancer* is about 50%. For this reason, the *gold standard* therapy is still represented by *esophagogastrectomy*. However, surgery is associated with a significant mortality rate, ranging between 3 and 5%. When HGD is detected in *tongues* of BE patients (≤ 30 mm), without endoscopic abnormalities, and not involving the entire circumference of the esophagus, EMR can remove all the metaplastic epithelium.

TABLE 6-2. Indications for Endoscopic Mucosal Resection

Esophagus
  Barrett's esophagus ("visible" areas of high grade dysplasia)
    Short Barrett, noncircumferential: complete ablation
    Long Barrett, circumferential: surgery
    Elderly patients and/or comorbidities: EMR ± PDT (circumferential mucosectomy under evaluation)
  Barrett's esophagus ("nonvisible" areas of high grade dysplasia)
    Surgery
    Circumferential mucosectomy (randomized trials needed)
  Early stage carcinoma (m1, m2)
  Granular cell tumor
  Benign lesions
    Adenomatous polyps
Stomach
  Early Gastric Cancer
    Differentiated adenocarcinoma
    Mucosal cancer < 20 mm if lesion elevated
    Mucosal cancer < 10 mm if lesion depressed, well-demarcated borders
  Benign lesions
    Adenomatous polyps
    Hyperplastic polyps
Duodenum
  Ampullary and peri-ampullary adenomas (FAP still controversial)
  Ampullary and peri-ampullary cancer
    Surgery refused or unfit for surgery
  Subepithelial undefined mass lesions
    Stromal cell tumors, neuroendocrine tumors, etc
Colon
  Early stage adenocarcinoma
    Flat or depressed cancer limited to the epithelium
    Flat or depressed cancer (sm1)
    Sessile lesions, including "laterally spreading tumors"
  Subepithelial undefined mass lesions
    Stromal cell tumors, neuroendocrine tumors, etc

EMR = endoscopic mucosal resection; FAP = familial adenomatous polyposis; m = mucosa; PDT = photodynamic therapy; sm = submucosa.

In patients with *long BE segments*, the sequential treatment of EMR to remove the visible areas of HGD, followed by PDT that could destroy the invisible foci of malignancy has been proposed. Buttar and colleagues (2001) treated 17 *nonsurgical patients* with *superficial esophageal cancer*. EMR improved staging in 47% of patients. Strictures occurred in 30% of patients, but the combined treatment was effective in eliminating the superficial cancer (Buttar et al, 2001).

The safety of *circumferential EMR* in patients with nonvisible HGD has been evaluated. Five patients with multifocal HGD and/or intramucosal cancer, and seven with "invisible" HGD were included. During every session, EMR removed 30 to 40 mm in length and three-quarters of the circumference. EMR sessions were scheduled every 3 to 4 weeks until the complete removal of BE. A monofilament polypectomy snare was used, without submucosal injection. No recurrences were observed after a median follow-up of 9 months. Two strictures occurred, but were solved with bougienage (Seewald et al, 2003).

A randomized study comparing two EMR techniques has been carried out by May and colleagues (2003) in patients with *early esophageal cancer*. Fifty EMRs were performed with the "suck-and-ligate" technique, without submucosal injection, and 50 were performed with the EMR cap-assisted (EMR-C) after submucosal injection of diluted epinephrine. No difference was observed between the two techniques. After EMR, 57% of patients had residual neoplasia at the first follow-up (May et al, 2003).

TABLE 6-3. Selected Studies on Endoscopic Mucosal Resection in Barrett's Esophagus

Author	Number of Pts or Lesions	Size of Lesion (mean [cm])	Technique	Histology Pre-EMR	Histology Post-EMR	Change in Diagnosis	Complications (%)	Follow-Up Months (mean)	Recurrence (%)
May et al, 2003	72 pts, 100 lesions	NOS	EUS, VLD, EMR-C, Injection	Invasive AC: 78			BI: 2%	20.7	6/62 (9.7%)
Seewald et al, 2003	12 pts	5 (median)	EUS, Snare	HGD/IMC (visible): 5 IMC (non visible): 7	BE: 2, LGD: 1, HGD: 5, Invasive AC:4	75%	BI: 33, Stricture: 17	−9 (median)	0
Ahmad et al, 2002	19 pts/101	0.5–3	EUS, EMR-C, Snare, Injection	Invasive AC: 6, HGD: 6, NOS: 7	Invasive AC: 8, HGD: 4, LGD: 1, Benign: 6	58%	BI: 11	≥ 24	0
Buttar et al, 2001	17 pts	8.0	EUS, VLD-PDT, Injection	IMC: 7, AC: 10	IMC: 7, AC: 10	47%	BI: 6, Stricture: 30	13	HGD: 1*, LGD: 1, AC: 1
Nijhawan et al, 2000	25 pts	7	EUS, Lift-and-Cut, VLD, Injection	BE: 2, LGD: 8, HGD: 5, AC: 9, Other: 1	BE: 2, LGD: 3, HGD: 5, AC: 13, Other: 2	48%	0	14.6	0

AC = adenocarcinoma; BE = Barrett's esophagus; BI = bleeding; EGJ = esophagogastric junction; EMR = endoscopic mucosal resection; EUS = endoscopic ultrasonography; HGD = high grade dysplasia; IMC = intramucosal carcinoma; LGD = low grade dysplasia; NOS = not otherwise specific; PDT = photodynamic therapy; Pts = patients; VLD = variceal ligator device.
*Persistence of HGD.

Post-EMR Stenosis

Dysphagia has been reported after EMR involving more than two-thirds of the circumference. An esophageal *stenosis* was observed in 13 of 19 (68%) patients who underwent an extended EMR. When the longitudinal length was > 30 mm, stenosis occurred in all patients. Recently, we demonstrated the feasibility of circumferential mucosectomy (3 cm in length) in an animal model. Stenosis was observed in one out of four cases, and it was probably due to an insufficient amount of solution in the submucosa (Conio et al, 2001).

Stomach and Duodenum

EGC

The EMR is now an established treatment for patients with *small EGC*. The outcome of 479 ECGs treated by EMR has been reported. Among patients with intramucosal cancers, 5.7% had recurrence. In the group of 127 patients with incomplete resection, 24 had surgery and 9 had further endoscopic therapy. Among patients with unfavorable prognosis, 18% had a local recurrence, after a median follow-up of 4 months. The perforation rate was 5%. Tanabe and colleagues (2002) performed EMR in 106 patients with EGC. "En bloc" resection was performed in patients with a lesion < 10 mm in diameter, and piecemeal in lesions ranging between 10 to 20 mm. One (1.5%) perforation occurred in the "en-bloc" group and was managed endoscopically. When the lesion was completely resected, no recurrences occurred. Cancer recurred in 3 (2.8%) patients, all with a lesion greater than 15 mm (Tanabe et al, 2002). Unrecognizable submucosal spread is frequently the cause of local recurrence. The analysis of *diffuse-type mucosal gastric cancer* less than 20 mm in diameter macroscopically has been carried out. In patients with *atrophic mucosa*, the distance between macroscopic and microscopic margins was about 10 mm.

Undifferentiated mucosal cancers should *not* be treated by EMR as the risk of metastasis to lymph nodes is about 4.2%, and *gastrectomy* should be advised. Abe and colleagues (2003) removed a 42 × 30 mm malignant lesion of the lesser curvature of the cardia by "en bloc" EMR by using the IT knife. Five weeks later, laparoscopic lymphadenectomy was carried out. Histopathologic evaluation did not detect neoplastic infiltration in the 28 lymph nodes removed (Abe et al, 2003).

If the cancer is located in a position that precludes an adequate endoscopic approach, a combined surgical-endoscopic procedure can be adopted. The use of a 15 mm trocar inserted into the stomach, through which a double channel gastroscope can be placed, has been described to perform EMR of an early cardia cancer.

The efficacy of the IT-knife in performing one piece resection of gastric lesions has been evaluated. "En-bloc" resection rates were 82% for lesions of 10 mm, 75% for those between 11 and 20 mm, and 14% for those greater than 20 mm. No recurrences were observed. However, bleeding and perforation occurred in 22% and 5% of cases, respectively (Ohkuwa et al, 2001).

The use of the ligating device has been reported in the removal of antral lesions of ≤ 10 mm. The maximum diameter resected was 12.8 × 11.0 mm. EMR can be carried out in the duodenum. The main application is represented by SP in familial adenomatous polyposis *(FAP) patients*, even those involving the papilla of Vater.

Colorectum

Some selected studies on EMR in colorectal benign/noninvasive lesions are reported in Table 6-4. The use of EMR-C in the colon is *still controversial*. Tada and colleagues (1996) obtained full thickness resection of the mucosal layer and one third of the submucosal layer. Some authors prefer the standard snare excision technique, as in the case of Bergmann and Beger (2003) who treated 57 patients with SP and early stage carcinoma, ranging from 10 to 50 mm. Complications occurred in two patients, in whom submucosal injection failed to raise the mucosa. Yoshikane and colleagues (1999) performed a successful "en bloc" resection in 15 of 17 colorectal tumors ≤ 40 mm in diameter, whereas "piecemeal" resection was successful in those larger than 40 mm. Recurrence occurred in one patient with a 45 mm lesion. The percentage of bleeding ranges from 1 to 9% in some studies, whereas an increased risk, from 12 to 45%, has been experienced by other authors (see Table 6-4).

We resected 139 SP (86 in the right colon) by either snare polypectomy alone or with EMR-C. The median diameter of the lesions was 20 mm in the right colon and 30 mm in the remaining bowel. Normal saline plus epinephrine solution (50 to 100 cc) was injected into the submucosa. EMR-C was performed in 46 patients (18 in the right colon). Bleeding occurred in 10.8% of the polyps. APC was used adjunctively in 45 patients. Invasive carcinoma was found in 17 SP and surgery was performed in 10 of them. After a median follow-up of 12.3 months, local recurrence was detected in 21.9% of polyps with no invasive cancers, and in none of the patients with invasive carcinoma who did not undergo surgery. The recurrence rate was similar regardless of the use of APC in the completion of EMR.

The *recurrence rate* after EMR of sessile colorectal polyps ranges between 0 to 46%, depending on the polyp size and the period of follow-up. Recurrence may occur in 100% of cases if remnants of adenoma are still in place, and the application of APC can decrease the recurrence to only 50%.

TABLE 6-4. Selected Studies on Colorectal Endoscopic Mucosal Resection

Author	Polyps (sessile/total)	Size (mean [mm])	Technique	Malignancy	Complications	Follow-Up Months	Recurrence*
Doniec et al, 2003	141/186	47	S ± E	HGD: 25% (47/186), Invasive AC: 9% (7/82)	Bl: 18% (26/141), P: 1% (1/141)	40	4% (7/175)
Regula et al, 2003	82/82	29 (median)	S ± APC	Invasive AC: 9% (7/82)	Bl: 12% (10/82), Postcoagulation sdr: 2% (2/82)	37 (mean)	13% (10/78)
Bergmann et al, 2003	non polypoid lesion: 71	25.4	S or EMR-C ± SE	HGD: 21% (15/71), Early AC:11% (8/71), Advanced AC: 3% (2/71)	Bl: 1% (1/71), P: 1% (1/71)	18	3% (2/65)
Dell'Abate et al, 2001	35/104	34	S ± SS	HGD: 23% (24/104), Invasive AC: 26% (9/35)	Bl: 3% (1/35)	34 (median)	25†
Binmoeller et al, 1996	129/176	≥ 30	S + E	HGD: 12% (21/176), Malignant: 8% (15/176)	Bl: 45% (58/129)	20 (median)	Adenoma: 16% (19/117), AC: 28% (2/7)
Walsh et al, 1992	116/116	30	S	HGD: 7% (8/116), AC: 16% (18/116)	Bl: 9% (10/116)	33.6	28% (18/65)

AC = adenocarcinoma; APC = Argon Plasma Coagulation; Bl = bleeding; E = epinephrine; EMR = endoscopic mucosal resection; HGD = high grade dysplasia; NOS = not otherwise specified; P = perforation; S = snare; SS = saline; sdr = syndrome; SE = saline + epinephrine.
*For patients with follow-up.
†Metachronous or recurrent.

Complications

Ulcerated lesions, such as scars following previous ablative attempts, have fibrosis, which seals the submucosa with the muscularis propria, and EMR should *not* be attempted.

The most frequent complication is *bleeding*. Injection of normal saline plus epinephrine is sufficient to stop the bleeding. The placement of *hemoclips* can prevent delayed hemorrhage.

The risk of *perforation* during EMR in the upper digestive tract is 0.06 to 5%. Perforation can be prevented by avoiding the removal of large lesions "en bloc", and repeating the injection when the piecemeal approach is used. Muscular resections have been reported in spite of the injection. A *pinhole perforation* can be managed endoscopically by placing *hemoclips*.

Conclusions

Data from the literature are encouraging and surgery can be avoided in a large number of patients with early gastrointestinal cancers. More training and exposure is required for gastroenterologists and trainees to become conversant with this technique. EMR should be performed by endoscopists, who are able to cope with procedural complications such as bleeding and perforation. EMR is a technique in evolution. However, randomized trials comparing EMR with surgery or other ablative endoscopic techniques are lacking, and EMR remains an unproven therapy.

Supplemental Reading

Abe N, Mori T, Izumisato Y, et al. Successful treatment of an undifferentiated early stage gastric cancer by combined en bloc EMR and laparoscopic regional lymphadenectomy. Gastrointest Endosc 2003;57:972–5.

Ahmad NA, Kochman ML, Long WB, et al. Efficacy, safety and clinical outcomes of endoscopic mucosal resection: a study of 101 cases. Gastrointest Endosc 2002;55:390–6.

Bergmann U, Beger HG. Endoscopic mucosal resection for advanced non-polypoid colorectal adenoma and early stage carcinoma. Surg Endosc 2003;17:475–9.

Binmoeller KF, Bohnacker S, Selfert H, et al. Endoscopic snare excision of "giant" colorectal polyps. Gastrointest Endosc 1996;43:183–8.

Buttar NS, Wang KK, Lutzke LS, et al. Combined endoscopic mucosal resection and photodynamic therapy for esophageal neoplasia within Barrett's esophagus. Gastrointest Endosc 2001;54:682–8.

Conio M, Sorbi D, Batts KP, et al. Endoscopic circumferential esophageal mucosectomy in a porcine model: an assessment of technical feasibility, safety, and outcome. Endoscopy 2001;33:791–4.

Dell'Abate P, Iosca A, Galimberti A, et al. Endoscopic treatment of colorectal benign-appearing lesions 3 cm or larger: techniques and outcome. Dis Colon Rectum 2001;44:112–8.

Doniec JM, Lohnert MS, Schniewind B, et al. Endoscopic removal of large colorectal polyps: prevention of unnecessary surgery? Dis Colon Rectum 2003;46:340–8.

Feitoza AB, Gostout CJ, Burgart LJ, et al. Hydroxypropyl metylcellulose: a better submucosal fluid cushion for endoscopic mucosal resection. Gastrointest Endosc 2003;57:41–7.

Matsuzaki K, Nagao S, Kawaguchi A, et al. Newly designed soft prelooped cap for endoscopic mucosal resection of gastric lesions. Gastrointest Endosc 2003;57:242–6.

May A, Gossner L, Behrena A, et al. A prospective randomized trial of two different endoscopic resection techniques for early stage cancer of the esophagus. Gastrointest Endosc 2003;58:167–75.

Nijhawan PK, Wang KK. Endoscopic mucosal resection for lesions with endoscopic features suggestive of malignancy and high-grade dysplasia within Barrett's esophagus. Gastrointest Endosc 2000;52:328–32.

Ohkuwa M, Hosokawa K, Boku N, et al. New endoscopic treatment for intramucosal gastric tumors using and insulated-tip diathermic knife. Endoscopy 2001;33:221–6.

Regula J, Wronska E, Polkowski M, et al. Argon plasma coagulation after piecemeal polypectomy of sessile colorectal adenomas: long-term follow-up study. Endoscopy 2003;35:212–8.

Seewald S, Akaraviputh T, Sitz U, et al. Circumferential EMR and complete removal of Barrett's epithelium: a new approach to management of Barrett's esophagus containing high-grade intraepithelial neoplasia and intramucosal carcinoma. Gastrointest Endosc 2003;57:854–9.

Shimizu Y, Tsukagoshi H, Fujita M, et al. Long-term outcome after endoscopic mucosal resection in patients with esophageal squamous cell carcinoma invading the muscularis mucosae or deeper. Gastrointest Endosc 2002;56:387–90.

Tada M, Inoue H, Yabata E, et al. Colonic mucosal resection using a transparent cap-fitted endoscope. Gastrointest Endosc 1996;44:63–5.

Tanabe S, Koizumi W, Mitomi H, et al. Clinical outcome of endoscopic aspiration mucosectomy for early gastric cancer. Gastrointest Endosc 2002;56:708–13.

Walsh RM, Ackroyd FW, Shellito PC. Endoscopic resection of large sessile colorectal polyps. Gastrointest Endosc 1992;38:303–9.

Yamamoto H, Kawata H, Sunada K, et al. Success rate of curative endoscopic mucosal resection with circumferential mucosal incision assisted by submucosal injection of sodium hyaluronate. Gastrointest Endosc 2002;56:507–12.

Yoshikane H, Hidano H, Sakakibara A, et al. Endoscopic resection of laterally spreading tumours of the large intestine using a distal attachment. Endoscopy 1999;31:426–30.

CHAPTER 7

ORAL CONSIDERATIONS IN PATIENTS WITH GASTROINTESTINAL DISORDERS

MICHAEL A. SIEGEL, DDS, MS, AND WENDY S. HUPP, DMD

This chapter is intended to assist the attending physician in the diagnosis, management, or referral of oral conditions that might complicate the management and/or control of patients with gastrointestinal (GI) and liver diseases. Dental health care professionals can assist with patients requiring diagnosis of oral manifestations of GI disorders and drug actions and interactions, as well as by providing routine dental maintenance and restorative procedures. Maintaining dental health serves to minimize the risk of secondary infection from an oral source and improve the quality of life for these patients.

The common embryogenesis of the GI tract and oral cavity is occasionally reinforced for the clinician when he or she finds heterotopic gastric mucosal cysts in the tongue or oral mucous membranes. More frequently, oral manifestations of commonly occurring GI disease or the sequelae of indicated medical therapy complicate the management of afflicted patients and warrant attention by both the physician and the dentist.

Inflammatory Bowel Disease

The medical and dental literature abounds with articles describing extra-abdominal, oral signs of inflammatory bowel diseases (IBDs), which include *aphthous-like ulceration, gingivitis, candidiasis, pyostomatitis vegetans, cobblestone appearance* of the oral mucosa, *oral epithelial tags* and folds, persistent *lip swelling, lichenoid mucosal reactions, granulomatous inflammation* of minor salivary gland ducts, and *angular cheilitis*. Current dental literature focuses on the oral status of IBD patients with regard to the potential use of thalidomide against antitumor necrosis factor-α for the treatment of recalcitrant oral granulomatous lesions, caries rate, salivary antimicrobial proteins, and infections of bacterial and fungal origins. Interestingly, oral manifestations of IBD may precede the onset of intestinal radiographic lesions by as long as a year or more. IBD is of interest to both physicians and dentists because of their complicating oral sequelae and their diagnosis and management.

Crohn's Disease

Crohn's disease (CD) is an inflammatory disease of the small or large intestine. The inflammation involves all the layers of the bowel. Oral lesions may be either symptomatic or asymptomatic and affect 6 to 20% of patients afflicted with CD. Most oral manifestation occur in patients with active intestinal disease and their presence frequently correlates with disease activity. *Recurrent aphthous*-like ulcers are the most common oral manifestation of CD. It is uncertain whether the oral manifestations are a true expression of CD, preexisting and/or coincidental findings, a direct result of medical intervention, or a manifestation of an associated problem such as anemia. Certainly, *minor salivary gland duct pathology, cobblestone mucosal architecture*, and *pyostomatitis vegetans* represent granulomatous changes that are characteristic of CD. Biopsies of these small, nonhealing, multiple aphthous-like ulcers reveal *granulomatous inflammation*. Less frequently, CD patients develop *inflammatory hyperplasia* of the oral mucosa with a cobblestone pattern, *diffuse swelling of the lips and face*, *indurated polypoid tissue* tags in the vestibule and retromolar pad area, and persistent *deep linear ulcerations* with hyperplastic margins. *Granulomatous lesions* have also been observed in the salivary glands, where they may cause rupture of the ducts and mucus retention cyst formation.

Various medications have been reported to cause *oral lichenoid* (lichen planus-like) drug reactions, including anti-inflammatory and sulfa-containing preparations, which are commonly used to manage IBD patients. Superinfection with *Candida albicans* may represent a reaction to the bacteriostatic effect of sulfasalazine, a primary manifestation of the disorder, or an impaired ability of neutrophils to kill this granuloma provoking fungus (Curran et al, 1991). This underscores the sometimes subtle intraoral clinical signs and symptoms of CD that may render a dentist invaluable to the physician working up a patient with previously undiagnosed CD.

IBD patients often complain of pain associated with ulcerative lesions in the oral cavity. Palliative sodium bicarbonate mouth rinses (one-half teaspoon of baking soda in eight ounces of water) may be rinsed and expectorated. Moderate potency topical steroid preparations, such as 0.05% *fluocinonide, desoximetasone,* and *triamcinolone,* or ultrapotency preparations such as *clobetasol* and *halobetasol* can be topically applied to the lesions, 4 times daily (not to exceed 2 continuous weeks). Ointments and creams are useful when the lesions are localized and direct topical application is possible. In cases when lesions are disseminated or oropharyngeal in distribution, *dexamethasone elixir* 0.5 mg/5 mL can be used as a rinse or gargle for 1 minute, 4 times daily and expectorated. The patient must be advised that prolonged use of topical steroids will result in mucosal atrophy, systemic steroid absorption (especially with the ultrapotency preparations), and an increased incidence of mucosal candidiasis.

IBD patients appear to be at an increased risk of dental caries as well as bacterial and fungal infections. These are multifactorial in etiology but appear to be related to either the patient's altered immune status or diet (Benvenius, 1988; Malins et al, 1991; Muerman et al, 1994; Rooney, 1984; Sundh and Emilson, 1989; Sundh et al, 1993). Oral manifestations of anemia such as *pallor, angular cheilitis*, and *glossitis* may occur, particularly in undiagnosed or poorly controlled disease has been reported in patients with active ulcerative colitis (UC).

UC

The oral changes that occur in UC are nonspecific and uncommon, with an incidence of < 8%. Major and minor forms of aphthous-like stomatitis has been reported in patients with active UC. There is nothing unique about these lesions and it has been proposed that their appearance is either coincidental or suggestive of a compromised immune system. However, the ulcers in patients with UC may result from blood loss directly related to the UC or to nutritional deficiencies of iron, folic acid, and vitamin B_{12}. In addition, anti-inflammatory medications such as 5-aminosalicylates, the mainstay of UC treatment, are excreted in the saliva and are known to cause aphthous-like ulcers in some individuals. A new crop of oral ulcers often heralds a flare-up of the bowel disease in patients prone to develop oral aphthae. Other nonspecific forms of oral ulceration associated with concomitant skin lesions have been reported. Pyoderma gangrenosum may occur in the form of deep ulcers that sometimes ulcerate through the tonsillar pillar.

Deep tissue vegetative or proliferative lesions that undergo ulceration and then suppuration characterize lesions of pyostomatitis vegetans. It is speculated that pyostomatitis vegetans lesions are due to effects of circulating immune complexes, induced by antigens that are derived from the gut lumen or the damaged colonic mucosa, because these lesions disappear with a total colectomy (Calobrisi et al, 1995). UC patients also can develop hairy leukoplakia, a lesion of the lateral tongue borders most commonly associated with acquired immunodeficiency syndrome (Fluckiger et al, 1994). This lesion probably serves as a marker of severe immunosuppression, and may be exacerbated by corticosteroids or other immunosuppressive agents.

Medical management of UC may necessitate alterations of dental therapy. A number of oral considerations are related to the therapeutic use of corticosteroids. Major oral surgical or periodontal procedures can precipitate adrenal insufficiency if the steroid doses are not adjusted properly. Patients undergoing oral surgery require increased doses of steroids before and after the procedure because their own adrenal response to stress is compromised. Further, patients on immunosuppressive agents, such as azathioprine (AZA), might be expected to have changes in the white and red blood cell counts, so total and differential white blood cell counts should be made available to the consulting dentist or oral surgeon who is contemplating major dental reconstruction or surgery. Routine maintenance dental therapy such as cleanings or simple restorations should be unaffected by steroid or immunosuppressive therapy.

In patients with a history of chronic bleeding, blood studies should be undertaken to rule out the presence of anemia or coagulopathy for any dental patient undergoing periodontal therapy or extractions likely to result in intraoral hemorrhage. Sulfasalazine interferes with folate metabolism, and supplemental folic acid may be needed especially if a macrocytic anemia is revealed in a complete blood count.

Finally, patients taking the immunosuppressive agent such as AZA may also exhibit signs of hepatic suppression. Abnormal liver function tests should be discussed with the attending dentist who might prescribe analgesic or antibiotic medications that are metabolized in the liver.

Peptic Ulcer Disease

Oral manifestations of peptic ulcer disease are rare unless there is anemia from GI bleeding or persistent regurgitation of gastric acid as a result of pyloric stenosis that leads to dental erosion, typically of the palatal aspect of the maxillary teeth. Vascular malformations of the lip have been reported and range from a very small macule to a large venous pool (Guis et al, 1963; Siegel and Jacobson, 1999).

Physicians should advise dentists that aggravation of the peptic ulcer disease might be minimized by avoidance of actions that increase the production of acid. Thus, lengthy dental procedures should be avoided or spread out over shorter appointments to minimize stress. To avoid aspirations patients should not be left in a supine or sub-supine position for lengthy periods during dental appointments. Dentists should be advised to avoid administering drugs that exacerbate ulceration and cause GI distress such as aspirin and other nonsteroidal anti-inflammatory drugs. Instead, acetaminophen products should be recommended. Additionally, because many of the antacids containing calcium, magnesium, and aluminum salts bind antibiotics such as erythromycin and tetracycline, the dentist should be reminded that administration of one of these drugs within 1 hour of antacid therapy may decrease the absorption of the antibiotic as much as 75 to 85%. Consequently, erythromycin and tetracycline should be taken 1 hour before or 2 hours after ingestion of antacids. Patients who exhibit dental phobia may be candidates for oral or intravenous sedation in order to effectively treat them dentally.

Dry mouth (xerostomia) is a common complaint in patients taking anticholinergic drugs. Patients who wear either complete or partial dentures are particularly troubled by xerostomia. Denture adhesives and artificial saliva may aid in the retention of their dental prostheses. Dentate patients are at an increased risk of dental caries if the hyposalivation is prolonged or if the patient places sugar-containing candies or antacids into the mouth in an effort to stimulate saliva flow. In these cases, dental referral is prudent to ensure that appropriate preventive measures are instituted. Medical management of peptic ulcer disease often includes the use of medications that may cause xerostomia. If the patient specifically complains of dry mouth, it may be possible to alter the specific drug type or dosage. Various therapy modalities for dry mouth are available such as artificial saliva, alcohol-free mouth rinses or increased fluid intake. Class V (root) caries are sequelae of dry mouth, even in patients who have been relatively caries free prior to the disease. Commonly used sialogogues, such as pilocarpine or cevimeline, may be contraindicated due to their parasympathomimetic action. If reflux into the oral cavity is present, referral to the dentist for restorative dental therapy is indicated.

Prior to extensive oral surgical or periodontal procedures, physicians should consult with the dentist of record who should be advised of the patient's serology, especially if the patient has had a history of ulcer perforation and subsequent hemorrhage resulting in anemia. Delayed healing and risk of bacterial infection, particularly anaerobic bacterial infection due to tissue hypoxia, and the potentially grave side effects of respiratory depression induced by narcotic analgesics, are examples of such associated oral surgical risks in the chronically anemic GI patient. Cimetidine and rantidine, drugs commonly prescribed for duodenal ulcer patients, have occasionally been associated with thrombocytopenia and may compete with antibiotics or antifungal medications as noted below.

Gastroesophageal Reflux Disease

Gastroesophageal reflux disease (GERD) with or without a *hiatal hernia* is one of the most commonly occurring diseases affecting the upper GI tract. The incidence of GERD is increasing in the developed world; upwards of 10% of the population experience heartburn daily. During gastroesophageal reflux, gastric contents (chyme) passively move up from the stomach into the esophagus. Although this can occur normally, if it is associated with symptoms, it may be attributed to GERD.

Patients who experience GERD complain of dysgeusia (foul taste), dental sensitivity related to hot or cold stimuli, dental erosion, and/or pulpitis. Dental thermal sensitivity is generally due to erosion of enamel by gastric acid. Erosion of enamel leads to exposed dentin and thermal sensitivity. On occasion, if the erosion is severe, irreversible pulpal (nerve) damage may result that requires root canal therapy. Mild baking soda mouth rinses may be swished and expectorated to minimize dysgeusia due to acid reflux. Dental referral should be sought in order to provide *topical fluoride applications* using *custom-made occlusive tray delivery* in order to ensure optimal dental mineralization and reduction of thermal sensitivity. The dentist can restore tooth structure destroyed by gastric acid erosion in order to provide comfort and aesthetics and to minimize further hard tissue damage. It is preferable to institute oral preventive measures at the earliest possible time in order to minimize the need for extensive dental restoration.

Medical therapy can affect the dental management of patients with GERD in a number of ways. Patients taking *cimetidine* (Tagament) or other H_2 receptor antagonists may experience a toxic reaction to *lidocaine* (or other amide local anesthetics) if they are injected intravascularly. Cimetidine also has been shown to inhibit the absorption and, therefore, the blood concentration of azole antifungal drugs such as *ketaconazole* via the potent inhibition of the cytochrome P-450 3A4 enzyme system. Soft tissue changes such as esophageal stricture and fibrosis may complicate intubation if the patient requires general anesthesia for an oral maxillofacial procedure. Oral mucosal changes are minimal, however erythema and mucosal atrophy may be present as a result of chronic exposure of tissues to acid. Mild sodium bicarbonate rinses may again be useful if mild signs of stomatitis are present.

Eating Disorders

The two most common eating disorders are anorexia nervosa and bulimia (Ruff et al, 1992). A variety of specialists, including gastroenterologists, psychiatrists, psychologists, dentists, internists, clinical social workers, nurses, and dietitians, must provide the treatment of eating disorders. There is a separate chapter on this topic (see Chapter 38, "Anorexia Nervosa and Bulimia").

The cardinal oral manifestation of eating disorders is severe erosion of the enamel on the lingual surfaces of the maxillary teeth. Acids from chronic vomiting are the cause (Shaw, 1994; Tylenda et al, 1991). Examination of the patient's fingernails and volar surfaces of the fingers may disclose abnormalities related to using these fingers to initiate purging. Mandibular teeth are not usually affected to the same degree as the maxillary teeth. Parotid enlargement may develop as sequelae of starvation.

Malabsorption Syndrome

Oral manifestations of malabsorption may be seen as mucosal and *gingival pallor, angular cheilitis*, and *atrophic or a beefy-red glossitis*. Additionally, as previously described, oral manifestations of anemia, may occur, particularly in undiagnosed or poorly controlled disease. Nutritional deficiencies are directly related to the section of the bowel affected by the GI disease. Persistent malnutrition is often a problem and the dentist can assist the physician in monitoring compliance with recommended dietary supplementation.

Gardner's Syndrome

Gardner's syndrome consists of intestinal polyposis, which represents premalignant lesions and multiple, *impacted supernumerary (extra) teeth*. This disorder is inherited as an autosomal dominant trait, and few afflicted patients with this syndrome reach the age of 50 years without surgical intervention. In a young patient with a family history of Gardner's syndrome, a dental radiograph such as a *panogram (linear tomogram)* can provide the earliest indication of the presence of this disease process. The at-risk patient should be referred for this radiograph at the earliest possible opportunity.

Plummer-Vinson Syndrome

The Plummer-Vinson syndrome, originally described as "hysterical dysphagia," is noted primarily in women in the fourth and fifth decades of life. Dysphagia is the hallmark of this disorder resulting from esophageal stricture causing many patients to have a fear of choking (Hoffman and Jaffe, 1995). Patients may present with xeroderma and a lemon-tinted cutaneous pallor, spoon-shaped fingernails (koilonychia), and splenomegaly. The oral manifestations are the direct result of an iron deficiency anemia. These include an *atrophic glossitis* with *erythema* or *fissuring, angular cheilitis, thinning* of the vermilion borders of the lips, and *leukoplakia* of the tongue. Inspection of the oral mucous membranes will disclose atrophy and hyperkeratinization. These oral changes are similar to those encountered in the pharynx and esophagus. Carcinoma of the upper alimentary tract has been reported in 10 to 30% of patients (Chen and Chen, 1994). Thorough oral, pharyngeal, and esophageal examination are mandatory to ensure that carcinoma is not present. Artificial salivas may reduce the sensation and, thereby, the fear of choking.

Peutz-Jegher's Syndrome

Multiple intestinal polyps throughout the GI tract, primarily in the small intestines, characterize Peutz-Jegher's syndrome. Malignancies in the GI and elsewhere in the body have been reported in approximately 10% of patients with this syndrome. *Pigmentation* of the face, lips, and oral cavity, present from birth, is a hallmark of this syndrome. Interestingly, the facial pigmentation fades later in life, although the intraoral mucosal pigmentation persists. No specific oral treatment is necessary.

Cowden's Syndrome

Cowden's syndrome (multiple hamartoma and neoplasia syndrome) is an autosomal dominant disease characterized chiefly by facial trichilemmomas, GI polyps, breast and thyroid neoplasms, and oral abnormalities. Cowden's syndrome is considered a cutaneous marker of internal malignancies (Mignogna et al, 1995). *Pebbly, papilloma-like lesions* and multiple fibromas may be found widely distributed throughout the oral cavity (Porter et al, 1996).

Liver Diseases

Oral findings are usually associated with vitamin deficiencies, bleeding, and anemia, including *angular cheilitis, glossitis,* and *mucosal pallor*. Yellow pigmentation may be observed on the oral mucosa and may be accompanied by scleral and cutaneous *jaundice*. Salivary gland dysfunction, secondary to Sjogren's syndrome, may be associated with primary biliary cirrhosis. Pigmentation of oral mucosa is only rarely observed in hemochromatosis.

The physician should advise dental professionals that a dental patient presenting with a history of liver cirrhosis deserves special attention. Patients with cirrhosis may have significant hemostatic defects, because of nutritional deficiency, an inability to synthesize clotting factors, or because of secondary thrombocytopenia. Medical management such as replacement with fresh frozen plasma and platelets can be employed prior to anticipated oral surgical or periodontal procedures. Specifically, a complete blood count, prothrombin time or international normalized ratio, partial thromboplastin time , platelet count, and bleeding time should be obtained and transmitted to the dentist (Glick, 1997). The dentist can assist the physician with regard to dietary counseling deemed necessary to manage nutritional deficiency.

A consulting physician is essential to properly manage the dental patient with liver cirrhosis. In patients with a history of encephalopathy, the dentist should avoid narcotics, sedatives, and tranquilizers. Additionally, there may be an induction of liver enzymes leading to a need for increased dosages of certain medications. The patient with ascites may not be able to fully recline in the dental chair due to increased pressure on abdominal vessels. Liver transplant patients on immunosuppressive therapy should be monitored for systemic infection of oral-pharyngeal origin, oral viral infection (herpes simplex, cytomegalovirus), and oral ulcers of unknown origin. Oral manifestations of acute graft-versus-host disease in the posttransplant patient can present as a mucositis, whereas chronic graft-versus-host disease will resemble oral lichen planus.*

Supplemental Reading

Arendt DM, Frost R, Whitt JC, Palomboro J. Multiple radiopaque masses in the jaws. J Am Dent Assoc 1989;118:349–51.

Benvenius J. Caries risk in patients with Crohn's disease: a pilot study. Oral Surg Oral Med Oral Pathol 1988;65:304–7.

Calobrisi SD, Mutasim DF, McDonald JS. Pyostomatitis vegetans associated with ulcerative colitis: temporary clearance with fluocinonide gel and complete remission after colectomy. Oral Surg Oral Med Oral Pathol Oral Radiol Endod 1995;79:452–4.

Chan SWY, Scully C, Prime SS, et al. Pyostomatitis vegetans: oral manifestation of ulcerative colitis. Oral Surg Oral Med Oral Pathol 1991;72:689–92.

Chen TS, Chen PS. Rise and fall of the Plummer-Vinson syndrome. J Gastroenterol Hepatol 1994;9:654–8.

Curran FT, Youngs DJ, Allan RN. Candidacidal activity of Crohn's disease neutrophils. Gut 1991;32:55–60.

Dhote R, Bergmann JF, Leglise P, et al. Orocecal transit time in humans assessed by sulfapyridine appearance in saliva after sulfasalazine intake. Clin Pharmacol Ther 1995;57:461–70.

Douglas LR, Douglass JB, Sieck JO, Smith PJ. Oral management of the patient with end-stage liver disease and the liver transplant patient. Oral Surg Oral Med Oral Pathol Oral Radiol Endod 1998;86:55–64.

Ficarra G, Cicchi P, Amorosi A, et al. Oral Crohn's disease and pyostomatitis vegetans: an unusual association. Oral Surg Oral Med Oral Pathol 1993;75:220–4.

Fluckiger R, et al. Oral hairy leukoplakia in a patient with ulcerative colitis. Gastroenterol 1994;106:503–8.

Ghandour K, Moneim I. Oral Crohn's disease with late intestinal manifestations. Oral Surg Oral Med Oral Pathol 1991;72:565–7.

Guis JA, Boyle DE, Castle DD, et al. Vascular formations of the lip and peptic ulcer. JAMA 1963;133:725–9.

Glick M. Medical considerations for dental care of patients with alcohol-related liver disease. J Am Dent Assoc 1997;128:61–70.

Gorlin RJ, Jirasek JE. Oral cysts containing gastric or intestinal mucosa: unusual embryologic accident or heterotopia. J Oral Surg 1970;28:9–11.

Halme L, Meurman JH, Laine P, et al. Oral findings in patients with active or inactive Crohn's disease. Oral Surg Oral Med Oral Pathol 1993;76:175–81.

Hansen LS, Silverman S, Daniels TE. The differential diagnosis of pyostomatitis vegetans and its relation to bowel disease. Oral Surg 1983;55:363–73.

Healy CM, Farthing PM, Williams DM, et al. Pyostomatitis vegetans and associated systemic disease: a review and two case reports. Oral Surg Oral Med Oral Pathol 1994;78:323–8.

Hegarty A, Hodgson T, Porter S. Thalidomide for the treatment of recalcitrant oral Crohn's disease and orofacial granulomatosis. Oral Surg Oral Med Oral Pathol 2003;95:576–85.

Hoffman RM, Jaffe PE. Plummer-Vinson syndrome: a case report and literature review. Arch Int Med 1995;155:2008–11.

Kano Y, Shiohara T, Yagita A, et al. Erythema nodosum, lichen planus and lichen nitidus in Crohn's disease: report of a case and analysis of T-cell receptor V gene expression in the cutaneous and intestinal lesions. Dermatology 1995;190:59–63.

Katz JO, Chilvarquer LW, Terezhalmy GT. Gardner's syndrome: report of a case. J Oral Med 1987;42:211–5.

Lipsett J, Sparnon AL, Byard RW, et al. Embryogenesis of enterocystomas-enteric duplication cysts of the tongue. Oral Surg Oral Med Oral Pathol 1993;75:626–30.

Malins TJ, Wilson A, Ward-Booth RP. Recurrent buccal space abscesses: a complication of Crohn's disease. Oral Surg Oral Med Oral Pathol 1991;72:19–21.

Muerman JH, Halme L, Laine P, et al. Gingival and dental status, salivary acidogenic bacteria, and yeast counts of patients with active or inactive Crohn's disease. Oral Surg Oral Med Oral Pathol 1994;77:465–8.

Mignogna MD, Lo Muzio L, Ruocco V, Bucci E. Early diagnosis of multiple hamartoma and neoplasia syndrome (Cowden syndrome): the role of the dentist. Oral Surg Oral Med Oral Pathol Oral Radiol Endod 1995;79:295–9.

Physicians desk reference, 55th ed. Montvale: Medical Economics; 2001.

Plauth M, Jenss J, Meyle J. Oral manifestations of Crohn's disease: an analysis of 79 cases. J Clin Gastroenterol 1991;13:29–37.

Porter S, Cawson R, Scully C, Eveson J. Multiple hamartoma syndrome presenting with oral lesions. Oral Surg Oral Med Oral Pathol Oral Radiol Endod 1996;82:295–301.

Rooney TP. Dental caries prevalence in patients with Crohn's disease. Oral Surg 1984;57:623–4.

Ruff JC, Koch MO, Perkins S. Bulimia: dentomedical complications. Gen Dent 1992;40:22–5.

Schnitt SJ, Antonioli DA, Jaffe B, et al. Granulomatous inflammation of minor salivary gland ducts: a new oral manifestation of Crohn's disease. Hum Pathol 1987;18:405–7.

Shaw BM. Orthodontic/prosthetic treatment of enamel erosion resulting from bulimia: a case report. J Am Dent Assoc 1994;125:188–90.

Siegel MA. Oral manifestations of gastrointestinal disease: diagnosis and treatment. In: Bayless TM, editor. Current therapy in gastroenterology and liver disease-3. Hamilton(ON): BC Decker; 1989. p. 1–5.

Siegel MA, Balciunas BA. Medication can cause severe ulcerations. J Am Dent Assoc 1991;122:75–7.

Siegel MA, Jacobson JJ. Inflammatory bowel diseases and the oral cavity. Oral Surg Oral Med Oral Pathol Oral Radiol Endod 1999;87:12–4.

Siegel MA, Jacobson JJ, Braun RJ. Diseases of the gastrointestinal tract. In: Greenberg MS, Glick M, editors. Burkets oral medicine: diagnosis and treatment. 10th ed. Hamilton (ON): BC Decker; 2003. p. 389–406.

Stege P, Visco-Dangler L, Rye L. Anorexia nervosa: review including oral and dental manifestations. J Am Dent Assoc 1982;104:648–52.

Sundh B, Emilson CG. Salivary and microbial conditions and dental health in patients with Crohn's disease: a 3-year study. Oral Surg Oral Med Oral Pathol 1989;67:286–90.

Sundh B, Johansson I, Emilson GC, et al. Salivary antimicrobial proteins in patients with Crohn's disease. Oral Surg Oral Med Oral Pathol 1993;76:564–9.

---

*Editor's Note: An extensive bibliography is included for the gastroenterologist unfamiliar with some of these topics.

Tylenda CA, Roberts MW, Elin RJ, et al. Bulimia nervosa: its effects on salivary chemistry. J Am Dent Assoc 1991;122:37–41.

Van Dis ML, Parks ET. Prevalence of oral lichen planus in patients with diabetes mellitus. Oral Surg Oral Med Oral Pathol Oral Radiol Endod 1995;79:696–700.

Vincent SD, Fotos PG, Baker KA, Williams TP. Oral lichen planus: the clinical, historical, and therapeutic features of 100 cases. Oral Surg Oral Med Oral Pathol 1990;70:165–71.

Ward CS, Dunphy EP, Jagoe WS, et al. Crohn's disease limited to the mouth and anus. J Clin Gastroenterol 1985;7:516–21.

Wescott WB, Correll RW. Oral and perioral pigmented macules in a patient with gastric and intestinal polyposis. J Am Dent Assoc 1984;108:385–6.

CHAPTER 8

Oropharyngeal Dysphagia

Peter J. Kahrilas, MD, and John E. Pandolfino, MD

Oropharyngeal dysphagia is a common disorder associated with high morbidity and mortality. The prevalence of dysphagia among individuals older than 50 years of age has been estimated to range from 16 to 22%. In addition, up to 13% of hospitalized patients and 50% of nursing home residents have feeding problems of which most are attributed to oropharyngeal dysphagia. The complications of oropharyngeal dysphagia are severe and include dehydration, malnutrition, aspiration, pneumonia, and death. As our population continues to age, oropharyngeal dysphagia will become an increasing problem associated with complex medical and ethical issues.

Mechanics of Swallow

Oropharyngeal swallowing begins with a voluntary oral phase that is then followed by a pharyngeal phase. The oral phase of swallowing is essentially voluntary and highly variable depending upon stimuli such as taste, environment, hunger, and motivation. Disorders of the oral phase of swallowing occur with many conditions characterized by global neurologic dysfunction, such as head trauma, cerebral tumors, or cerebral vascular accident. Once initiated, the pharyngeal phase of swallowing results in a transient reconfiguration from a respiratory to an alimentary pathway by opening the inlet to the esophagus and sealing the inlet to the larynx. Mechanistically, the pharyngeal phase of swallowing is complex and can be subdivided into several closely coordinated actions:

1. Nasopharyngeal closure by elevation and retraction of the soft palate
2. Upper esophageal sphincter (UES) opening
3. Laryngeal closure
4. Tongue loading (ramping)
5. Tongue pulsion
6. Pharyngeal clearance

Precise coordination of these events is crucial, and defects in the biomechanical mechanisms may lead to nasopharyngeal regurgitation, dysphagia, aspiration, and diverticulum formation. Table 8-1 summarizes the mechanical elements of the swallow, along with the manifestation and consequence of dysfunction and the representative conditions in which they are encountered.

Evaluation and Classification of Oropharyngeal Dysphagia

The evaluation of patients with presumed oropharyngeal dysphagia should focus on the following five basic questions:
1. Does the patient describe true dysphagia as opposed to globus sensation?
2. Is dysphagia oropharyngeal or esophageal in origin?
3. Is the dysphagia secondary to a structural or functional neurogenic or myogenic disorder?
4. Is there an underlying causative disorder that can be treated?
5. Should therapy be directed toward the underlying etiology of dysphagia or directed at treating the complications?

TABLE 8-1. Patterns and Manifestations of Oropharyngeal Dysphagia

Mechanical Element	Biomechanical Mechanism	Evidence of Dysfunction	Typical Diseases
Nasopharyngeal closure	Soft palate elevation	Nasopharyngeal regurgitation, nasal voice	Myasthenia gravis
Laryngeal closure	Laryngeal elevation, arytenoid tilt, vocal fold closure	Dysphagia, postswallow residue/aspiration, diverticulum formation	Cricopharyngeal bar, CVA, Parkinson's disease
Tongue loading and bolus propulsion	Lingual sensation and control	Sluggish, misdirected bolus	Parkinson's disease, surgical defects, cerebral palsy
Pharyngeal clearance	Pharyngeal shortening, pharyngeal contraction, epiglottic flip	Postswallow residue/aspiration	Polio, postpolio, oculopharyngeal dystrophy, CVA

Reproduced with permission from Kahrilas, 1999.
The table includes the mechanical elements of normal swallowing along with the manifestations and consequences of dysfunction and the representative conditions in which they are encountered.
CVA = cerebral vascular accident.

50 / Advanced Therapy in Gastroenterology and Liver Disease

These questions can usually be answered with a detailed history and physical exam. However, further diagnostic tests may be needed to determine both the cause of oropharyngeal dysphagia and the proper treatment (Figure 8-1).

History

The patient history is extremely important in the evaluation of oropharyngeal dysphagia, and is usually sufficient to answer the first two questions regarding the

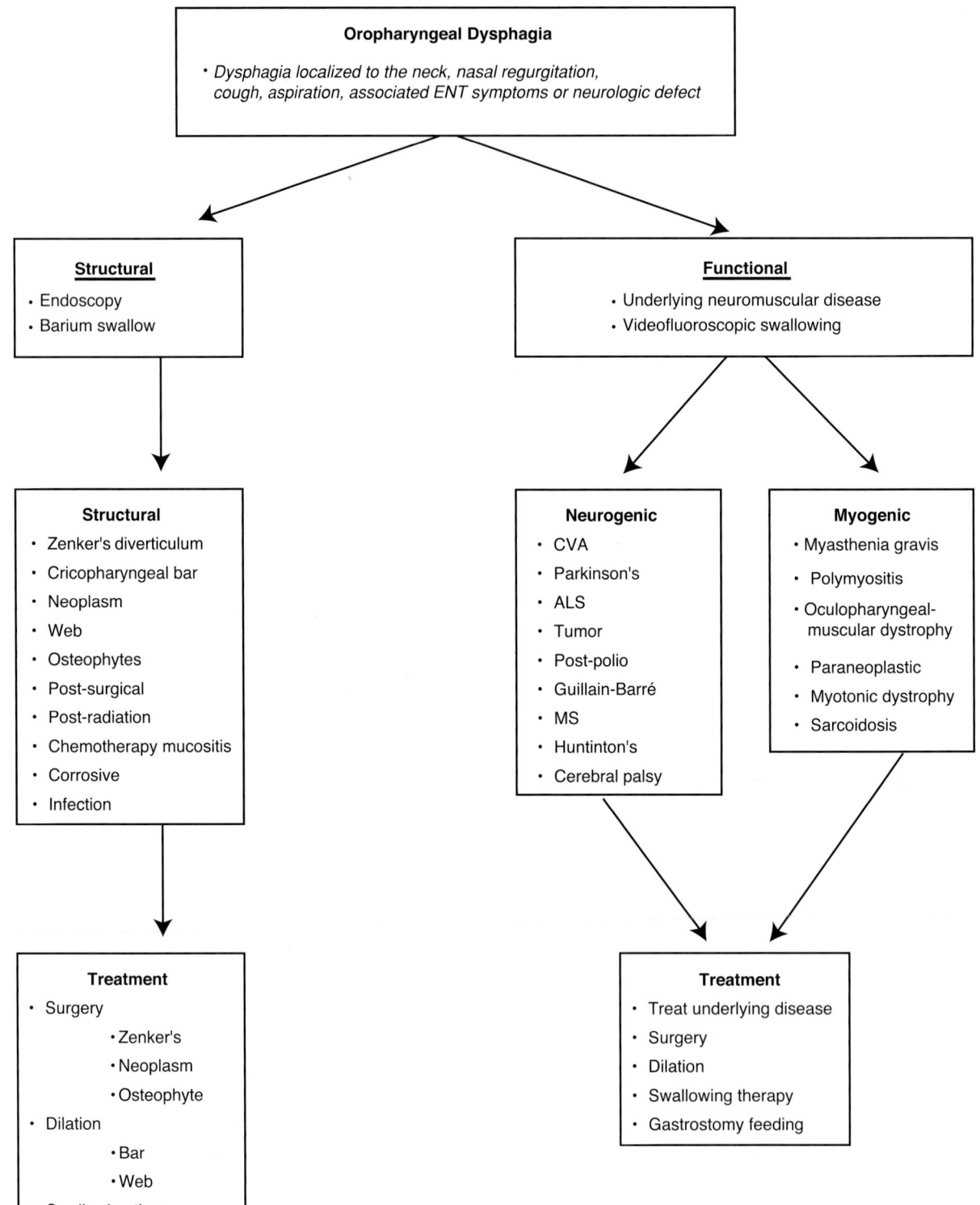

FIGURE 8-1 Management algorithm for oropharyngeal dysphagia. ALS = amyotrophic lateral sclerosis; CVA = cerebral vascular accident; ENT = ear, nose, and throat; MS = multiple sclerosis.

presence and location of dysphagia. Major objectives of the history are to first determine if dysphagia is present and then to differentiate oropharyngeal dysphagia from esophageal dysphagia. In cases of oropharyngeal dysphagia, patients are able to accurately localize bolus hang-up in the neck; however, they mistakenly identify the neck as the locus of bolus hang-up with esophageal dysphagia about 15 to 30% of the time. Therefore, obtaining a history of symptoms such as aspiration, coughing, nasopharyngeal regurgitation, or drooling is of significant value in distinguishing oropharyngeal dysphagia from esophageal dysphagia. Distinguishing oropharyngeal dysphagia from globus sensation may be difficult. Unlike dysphagia, which occurs only during swallowing, globus sensation is a constant sensation of a foreign body present in the throat. If the history is consistent with globus and evaluation with radiographic and endoscopic examinations are negative, most patients with globus respond to explanation and reassurance.

Physical Examination

Physical examination may play a role in (1) diagnosing underlying systemic or metabolic disorders, (2) localizing the neuranatomic level and severity of a causative neurologic lesion when present, and (3) determining the degree that dysphagia is affecting the fluid and nutritional status of the patient. Examination of the oral cavity, head, and neck should include palpation for obstructing masses, lymph nodes, goiter, and a pharyngeal pouch (usually on the left). Neurologic examination is mandatory because findings may indicate cranial nerve dysfunction, neuromuscular disease, cerebellar dysfunction, or an underlying movement disorder. Of note, contrary to popular belief, the gag reflex is not predictive of pharyngeal swallowing efficiency or aspiration risk because it is absent in 20 to 40% of asymptomatic normal adults.

Radiographic–Endoscopic Examinations

If the causative disease of oropharyngeal dysphagia is not apparent after a careful history and physical examination, further diagnostic studies are indicated. The first task is to distinguish between structural and functional abnormalities of intrinsic musculature, peripheral nerves, or central nervous system control mechanisms, because their management implications are very different. Structural abnormalities resulting from trauma, surgery, tumors, caustic injury, congenital anomalies, or acquired deformities are identified by endoscopic and/or radiographic examination. Endoscopy may be performed either transorally or transnasally to identify tumors, webs, or hypopharyngeal diverticula. Barium studies may also define areas of obstruction and are very helpful in diagnosing cricopharyngeal bars and hypopharyngeal diverticula.

VIDEOFLUOROSCOPY

After structural defects have been excluded, *videofluoroscopy* evaluation of swallowing is used for an evaluation of oropharyngeal function. This study has frequently been referred to as a modified barium swallow and various protocols comprised of a series of swallow tasks have been described by Jones and Donner (1991). During the swallowing tasks, images are obtained in a lateral projection, framed to include the oropharynx, palate, proximal esophagus, and proximal airway. The images are then evaluated with respect to the following four categories of oropharyngeal dysfunction:

1. Inability or excessive delay in initiation of pharyngeal swallowing
2. Aspiration
3. Nasopharyngeal regurgitation
4. Residue of the ingestate within the pharyngeal cavity after swallowing

In addition to defining the functional abnormality, this procedure also allows for evaluation of the efficacy of various compensatory dietary modifications, postures, and swallowing maneuvers in improving swallowing dysfunction. *Intraluminal manometry* can complement videofluoroscopy by providing information on the strength of pharyngeal contraction, the completeness of UES relaxation, and the relative timing of these events. This may provide useful information regarding UES dysfunction and may help distinguish impaired UES function from weak pharyngeal contractions.

Treatment

Structural Etiologies

Identification of obstructing lesions that cause dysphagia will lead to specific management in most cases. These lesions are usually localized with endoscopic and radiographic evaluation. Benign lesions, such as *pharyngeal* or *cricopharyngeal strictures* and *cervical webs*, usually respond to simple dilation with semisolid bougies, the endoscope itself, or with balloon inflation. *Tumors* will require surgery, antineoplastic therapy, or some combination of these therapies. *Cervical osteophytes*, if prominent, may also cause significant obstructive symptoms secondary to anterior bulging into the hypopharynx. This entity is correctable by surgical removal of the bony spur.

HYPOPHARYNGEAL DIVERTICULI AND CRICOPHARYNGEAL BAR

The most common structural abnormalities of the hypopharynx associated with dysphagia are hypopharyngeal diverticula and cricopharyngeal bars. Acquired hypopharyngeal diverticula are most common in men after the age of 60 years and typically present with symptoms of dysphagia, halitosis, postswallow regurgitation, or even aspiration of material from the pharyngeal pouch. The most frequent site of herniation is Killian's dehiscence between the oblique fibers of the inferior pharyngeal constrictor and the cricopharyngeus muscle in the midline posteriorly, this being the location of a Zenker's diverticulum. Other locations of acquired pharyngeal diverticula can be found at sites of potential weakness of the muscular lining of the hypopharynx. Hypopharyngeal diverticula have been hypothesized to result from either delayed UES relaxation, failure of relaxation, or premature contraction. However, more current data suggest that the development of these diverticuli is the result of a restrictive myopathy associated with diminished compliance of the cricopharyngeus muscle. The muscle relaxes normally during swallowing, but it cannot distend normally, resulting in the appearance of a cricopharyngeal indentation, or bar, during a barium swallow. The increased stress on the hypopharynx from the increased intrabolus pressure proximal to the bar leads to the formation of hypopharyngeal diverticula.

The treatment of hypopharyngeal diverticula is endoscopic or surgical *cricopharyngeal myotomy with or without a diverticulectomy*. Cricopharyngeal myotomy reduces both the resting sphincter tone and resistance to flow across the UES. Good or excellent results can be expected in 80 to 100% of Zenker's patients treated by *transcervical myotomy* combined with *diverticulectomy* or *diverticulopexy*. In addition, *endoscopic CO_2 laser myotomy* of the cricopharyngeus is safe and effective and has been proposed as an alternative to surgical myotomy in elderly patients with severe comorbidities. A limited procedure may be adequate, but a *definitive* approach to the problem of pulsion diverticula should involve *both* diverticulectomy and myotomy. Diverticulectomy alone risks recurrence because the underlying obstruction at the level of the cricopharyngeus is not relieved. Similarly, myotomy alone does not treat the hypopharyngeal diverticulum and the patient will remain at risk for aspiration and regurgitation. *Small diverticula* may spontaneously disappear following myotomy.

Whether or not a *cricopharyngeal bar* in the absence of a diverticula requires treatment is unclear. Certainly, if dysphagia exists and combined fluoroscopic/manometric analysis demonstrates reduced sphincter opening in conjunction with elevated upstream intrabolus pressure, there is good rationale for treatment. Anecdotal evidence suggests that in this scenario, simple dilation with a *large caliber bougie* may be efficacious and certainly a reasonable initial treatment option. Subjects not responding to dilation should be referred for cricopharyngeal myotomy.

Functional Etiologies

Oropharyngeal dysphagia may be one of the most devastating pathologic consequences of primary neurological or muscular diseases. Management of functional causes of oropharyngeal dysphagia begins with definition of the aberrant physiology described in Table 8-1. This is most easily accomplished with a videofluoroscopic modified barium swallow study. After the patient's swallowing dysfunction has been defined, the following four specific issues pertaining to management of oropharyngeal dysphagia can be addressed:

1. Identification of an underlying disease
2. Characterization of a disorder amenable to surgery or dilation
3. Identification of a specific pattern of dysphagia amenable to swallowing therapy
4. Assessment of aspiration risk

IDENTIFYING UNDERLYING DISEASE

A potential outcome of the swallowing evaluation is the identification of an underlying neuromuscular, neoplastic, or metabolic disorder that will dictate specific management. For example, dysphagia can be the presenting symptom in patients with *myopathy, myasthenia, thyrotoxicosis, motor neuron disease,* or *Parkinson's disease*. In each instance, identification of the underlying disease will result in a specific treatment. Whether treatment of the underlying disorder improves swallowing function depends on both the natural history of the disease and whether or not an effective treatment exists.

DISORDERS AMENABLE TO SURGERY

The efficacy of *myotomy* in *neurogenic dysphagia* is variable with most series evaluating the efficacy of myotomy in neurogenic dysphagia being uncontrolled without specific outcome measures. After combining data from 15 studies examining the efficacy of myotomy on neurogenic dysphagia, an overall favorable response was noted in 63% of subjects with an operative mortality of 1.8% (Cook and Kahrilas, 1999). Determining which patients may respond to myotomy remains unclear, however, it does appear that *pharyngeal propulsion* may be an important factor in predicting outcome.

SPECIFIC PATTERNS OF DYSPHAGIA AMENABLE TO SWALLOWING THERAPY

In addition to providing insight into the underlying etiology of functional oropharyngeal dysphagia, the radiographic evaluation can be used to test selected compensatory or therapeutic treatment strategies. *Compensatory treatments* include *postural changes, modifying food delivery or consistency*, or the use of *prosthetics*. For example, *head turning* can eliminate aspiration or pharyngeal residue by favoring more functional structures in patients with hemiparesis (Logemann, 1998). Similarly, *diet modifications* can reduce the "difficulty" of the swallow. Therapeutic strategies are designed to alter the physiology of the swallow, usually by improving the range of motion of oral or pharyngeal structures using voluntary control of oropharyngeal movement during swallow. A recent study performed by Shaker and colleagues (2002) tested the effect of *suprahyoid muscle strengthening* in restoring swallow function. All patients randomized to the exercise routine had significant improvement in UES opening and were able to resume oral feedings (Shaker et al, 2002). Depending on the severity of the impairment, level of motivation, and global neurologic intactness, defective elements of the swallow can be selectively rehabilitated. For a detailed description of the techniques and limitations of swallow therapy, the reader is referred to treatises on the topic by Cook and Kahrilis (1999) and by Logemann (1998).

Detection of Severe Aspiration

Oropharyngeal dysphagia associated with aspiration is a frequent outcome associated with stroke, occurring in 33% of stroke patients overall and 67% of those with brainstem strokes. Among the subset of stroke patients who develop oropharyngeal dysphagia after the stroke, pneumonia occurs in 43 to 50% of these patients during the first year and has a mortality of 45% (Croghan et al, 1994; Johnson et al, 1993). Videofluoroscopy is believed to be the most sensitive test for detecting aspiration, capable of detecting aspiration not evident by bedside evaluation in 42 to 60% of patients. Despite the logical association between deglutitive aspiration and the subsequent development of pneumonia, this sequence is not inevitable. Available studies suggest that radiographic aspiration has a positive predictive value of only 19 to 68% and a negative predictive value of 55 to 97% for pneumonia. Nonetheless, the evidence does suggest that *detection of aspiration* is a *predictor of pneumonia risk*, and that its *detection dictates intervention*. Strategies to prevent aspiration may take the form of compensatory swallowing strategies, nonoral feeding, or corrective surgery. *Nonoral feeding does not necessarily eliminate* the risk of aspiration. A study by Croghan and colleagues (1994) evaluating the risk of aspiration pneumonia in 22 patients with radiographic aspiration reported that the 15 subjects that had feeding tubes placed had a significantly higher rate of pneumonia and death compared with those without feeding tubes. This finding suggests that *aspiration of oral secretions* may be important in determining pneumonia risk and has led some to consider further measures such as *cuffed tracheostomy* to protect the airway.

Supplemental Reading

Cook IJ. Diagnosis and management of cricopharyngeal achalasia and other upper esophageal sphincter opening disorders. Curr Gastroenterol Rep 2000;2:191–5.

Cook IJ, Gabb M, Panagopoulos V, et al. Pharyngeal (Zenker's) diverticulum is a disorder of upper esophageal sphincter opening. Gastroenterology 1992;103:1229–35.

Cook IJ, Kahrilas PJ. AGA technical review on management of oropharyngeal dysphagia. Gastroenterology 1999;116:455–78.

Croghan JE, Burke EM, Caplan S, Denman S. Pilot study of 12-month outcomes of nursing home patients with aspiration on videoflouroscopy. Dysphagia 1994;9:141–6.

Davies AE, Kidd D, Stone SP, MacMahon J. Pharyngeal sensation and gag reflex in healthy subjects. Lancet 1995;345:487–8.

Goyal RK. Disorders of the cricopharyngeus muscle. Otolaryngol Clin North Am 1984;17:115–30.

Groher M, Bukatman R. The prevalence of swallowing disorders in two teaching hospitals. Dysphagia 1986;1:3.

Horner J, Massey EW, Riski JE, et al. Aspiration following stroke: clinical correlates and outcome. Neurology 1988;38:1359–62.

Johnson ER, McKenzie SW, Sievers A. Aspiration pneumonia in stroke. Arch Phys Med Rehabil 1993;74:973–6.

Jones B, Donner MW. The tailored examination. In: Jones B, Donner MW, editors. Normal and abnormal swallowing. New York: Springer-Verlag; 1991. p. 33–50.

Kahrilas PJ. Motility disorders of the esophagus. In: Yamada T, editor. Textbook of Gastroenterology. Volume One. 3rd ed. Philadelphia: Lippincott Williams and Wilkins; 1999. p. 1199–234.

Logemann J. Evaluation and treatment of swallowing disorders. 2nd ed. Austin (TX): Pro-ed; 1998.

Shaker R, Easterling C, Kern M, et al. Rehabilitation of swallowing by exercise in tube-fed patients with pharyngeal dysphagia secondary to abnormal UES opening. Gastroenterology 2002;122:1314–21.

Walker AE, Robins M, Weinfeld FD. The National Survey of Stroke. Clinical findings. Stroke 1981;12:I13–44.

CHAPTER 9

Gastroesophageal Reflux: Medical Therapy

Radu Tutuian, MD, and Donald O. Castell, MD

The availability of highly effective medications with infrequent side effects for treatment of a condition that affects 40% of the adult US population leads to an almost "knee jerk reflex" answer to the patient's complaint "Doctor, I've got heartburn." Many practitioners will prescribe a proton pump inhibitor (PPI) once daily. Fortunately, this approach is highly successful in most patients despite the inability of PPIs to correct the underlying pathophysiology of gastroesophageal reflux disease (GERD), which is an abnormally relaxing lower esophageal sphincter (LES) with or without an abnormal esophageal motility leading to an abnormal amount of acid gastric material in the esophagus. By decreasing the acidity of the refluxed material, however, PPIs do satisfy the following two major goals of medical therapy in GERD: (1) healing of lesions and (2) alleviation of symptoms. We will discuss the practical, day-to-day approach to the medical treatment of GERD.

Initial Treatment

PPIs

It is our opinion that patients in whom the diagnosis of GERD is suspected based on their clinical presentation should be started on a once daily PPI 15 to 30 minutes before breakfast. This recommendation is supported by the observation that this class of medication has the best available efficacy/side effect profile. Several studies in the late 1980s and early 1990s showed the superiority of PPIs over the then standard-of-care histamine-2 receptor antagonists (H_2RAs) in both the healing of esophagitis and symptom control. Currently five PPIs are commercially available in the United States with the following Food and Drug Administration (FDA)-approved daily doses:
1. Omeprazole 20 mg and 40 mg
2. Lansoprazole 15 mg and 30 mg
3. Rabeprazole 20 mg
4. Pantoprazole 40 mg
5. Esomeprazole 40 mg

Improvement in symptoms can be expected in about 78% of cases (range 62 to 94%) and healing of esophagitis in 83% of cases (range 71 to 96%) (DeVault and Castell, 1999).

Superiority of one PPI over the others is controversial. For each study showing one PPI being superior to another there are others showing the opposite. Overall, based on similar esophagitis healing rates approaching 90% at 8 weeks (Caro et al, 2001) and similar intragastric pH profiles after 7 days of dosing (Tutuian et al, 2000) all first generation PPIs (omeprazole [Prilosec], lansoprazole [Prevacid], rabeprazole [Aciphex], pantoprazolen [Protonix]) can be considered to have equivalent effectiveness (Figure 9-1). Minor differences in pharmacodynamics can be shown, such as earlier onset of action, but these should have little importance in the long-term management of a chronic disease (Horn, 2000). Local differences in price may be an important factor in selection.

The more recent "second generation" PPI, esomeprazole (Nexium), is the active s-isomer in the racemic mixture of omeprazole, a formulation approach that produces longer duration of intragastric acid control than the four original PPIs. Results from a large, double blind study suggest that the advantages of esomeprazole become more clinically important in patients with higher grades of esophagitis (Figure 9-2) (Castell et al, 2002).*

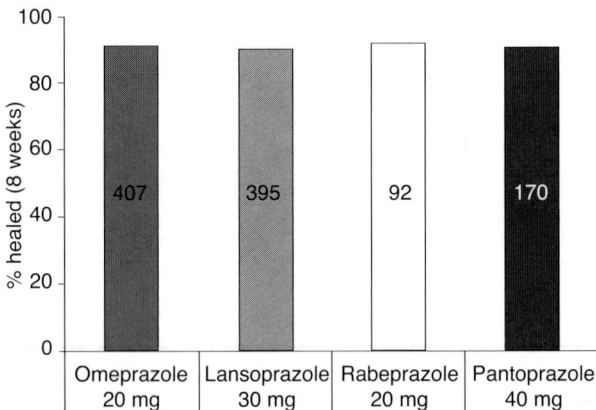

FIGURE 9-1. Comparison of acute healing rates for first-generation proton pump inhibitors. Bars indicate percent healing after 8 weeks of treatment. Numbers indicate patients in respective multicenter prospective studies.

---

*Editor's Note: Who should be esophagoscoped to determine severity?
Author's Reply: We focused primarily on the medical therapy of GERD but would be happy to expand on this issue. We consider that patients with alarm symptoms (eg, dysphagia, weight loss, gastrointestinal bleeding, or anemia) should be endoscoped. Also, patients with long-standing reflux disease (ie, more than 5 years) and over the age of 40 years should consider having a one-time endoscopy to rule out Barrett's esophagus.

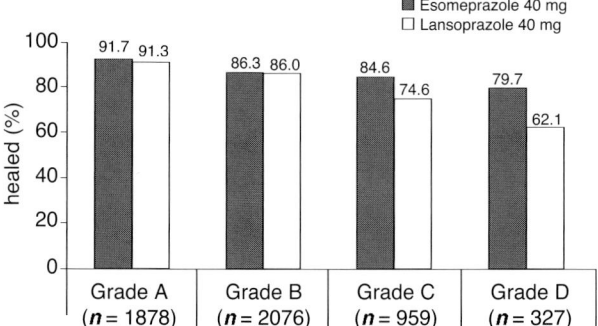

FIGURE 9-2. Comparison of esomeprazole versus lansoprazole in 8-week healing rates of erosive esophagitis by baseline grade of esophagitis. The benefits of esomeprazole are higher in more severe cases of esophagitis. Adapted from Castell et al (2002).

Lifestyle Modifications

We believe that patients with a chronic disorder, such as GERD, should be educated about those lifestyle modifications that they can adopt to assist treatment of their symptoms. Although some would argue that these lifestyle modifications have, in part, lost their importance since acid suppressive therapy became available, the Guidelines of the American College of Gastroenterology recommend them as adjuncts to treatment (DeVault and Castel, 1999). Still, physicians or nurses should discuss the approaches shown in Table 9-1. The next chapter is devoted to lifestyle changes for the GERD patient (see Chapter 10, "Lifestyle Measures for the Treatment of Gastroesophageal Reflux Disease").

H₂RAs

Because PPIs have very few side effects (about 3% of patients may have diarrhea, headache, or allergic reactions), the primary limiting factor in their use is cost. Interpreting the healing rates on H₂RAs (around 50%) versus PPIs (> 80%) from a financial perspective, treating only those patients who failed H₂RAs with PPI is cost saving compared to treating every patient with PPI. However, if one considers that the improved GERD symptom response to PPIs often leads to decreased patient visits, the total costs are likely to be less. An over the counter low dose of PPI or H₂RA can be used for mild intermittent symptoms.

Pregnancy

When it comes to treatment of pregnant patients, PPIs, except lansoprazole (class B), are included among class C drugs (animal studies show adverse fetal effects but there are no controlled human studies or no animal or human studies that weigh possible fetal risk versus maternal benefit). There are no controlled trials evaluating the safety of PPIs in humans, but metanalysis of thousands of patients indicate these drugs to be safe in pregnancy. Still the decision is left to the physician to weigh the risks and benefits of the treatment. Even though it is not as effective, *sucralfate* (Carafate) (healing rates of esophagitis around 40%) is likely to be "safer" because this drug is minimally absorbed systemically.

Promotility Agents

Conceptually promotility agents should be the ideal approach to GERD based on the hypothesis that normalizing underlying dysmotility or augmenting existing motility would decrease reflux and esophageal acid contact time. All available agents have limited efficacy or unacceptable side effects.

Bethanechol is a cholinergic agonist that will increase esophageal peristalsis and LES pressure but also stimulate gastric secretion. Compared to placebo it will improve GERD symptoms but does not have any advantages in healing esophagitis. At the recommended dose for treatment of GERD (25 mg 4 times daily) it may have cholinergic side effects, including diarrhea, abdominal cramping, fatigue, and blurred vision.

Metoclopramide (Reglan) is a smooth muscle stimulant that inhibits dopamine receptors. It enhances gastric emptying and LES pressure but has no effect on esophageal peristalsis. Even though it may improve GERD symptoms it does not show healing rates to justify its side effect profile, which includes galactorrhea, menstrual dysfunction, lethargy, and extrapyramidal motor defects. The most concerning side effect is tardive dyskinesia, which can occur in up to 20% of patients and can be permanent.

Cisapride stimulates acetylcholine release increasing LES pressure and accelerating gastric emptying. Placebo controlled trials have shown significant improvement in GERD symptoms, but because of its cardiovascular side effects (life threatening ventricular tachycardia) it is no longer available.

Tegaserod (Zelnorm), a selective 5-hydroxytryptamine-4 receptor partial agonist, which has promotility activity throughout the gastrointestinal (GI) tract, is also considered

---

TABLE 9-1. Lifestyle Modifications for Gastroesophageal Reflux Disease Symptoms

Eat smaller meals
Avoid high fat meals
Avoid fast eating
Avoid late meals/stay upright for 3 hours postprandially
Avoid saliva stimulating agents (ie, hard candies, chewing gum)
Restrict smoking, alcohol, coffee, chocolate
Weight loss
Sleep with the head of the bed elevated (or sleep on the left side)
Check medication list
Use OTC medications for "breakthrough" symptoms

OTC = Over the counter.

to decrease visceral sensitivity and promote gastric emptying. In GERD patients it has been shown to decrease postprandial esophageal acid exposure suggesting a potential role in treatment of GERD.

Domperidone and *erythromycin* are the other promotility agents currently used for treatment of GERD. Both agents enhance gastric emptying while not having significant effects on esophageal peristalsis. Their side effect profile may also limit their clinical utility.

It is our opinion that promotility agents (metoclopramide, domperidone, erythromycin, and tegaserod) have historically fallen short of expectations. Their inferior healing rates compared to PPIs and unfavorable side effect profiles indicate that these medications should not be used alone in treating GERD.

Treatment of Patients with Persistent Symptoms on Once Daily PPI

Because acid-suppressive therapy is very effective and has few side effects, specialists (gastroenterologists and GI surgeons) are likely to see only the "tip of the iceberg" represented by patients with severe or persistent symptoms not responsive to standard treatment (Bennet and Castell, 1999).

The concept of treatment failure of daily PPI was initially surprising because early literature obtained from parietal cell cultures described these drugs as irreversibly binding to the proton pumps, the hydrogen/potassium ATPases that functions as the final common step in acid secretion. The isolated cell studies showed 1,000-fold accumulation of these drugs in the canaliculi, relating the area under the plasma concentration curve and net plasma concentration to their effect, and indicated that synthesis of proton pumps takes 36 to 96 hours. In contrast, 24-hour intragastric pH studies in healthy volunteers and GERD patients showed that the mean duration of intragastric pH > 4 following a steady state single dose of any of the five PPIs ranges from 10 to 14 hours. This can be explained by a variety of factors, including that, in vivo PPIs bind 70 to 80% of active pumps, not all pumps are active at the same time, synthesis of new pumps is continuous, and the half-life of the PPIs range between 2 to 4 hours.

Several studies indicate that individual patient responses to PPIs vary widely. Therefore, we recommend switching to another PPI as the first step in patients not responding to one PPI. Attention should also be paid to the frequency and severity of symptoms. Patients with occasional breakthrough symptoms should be instructed to take an antacid as needed.

In patients with continuing symptoms, the next step is to increase the dose of the PPI. Divided doses of PPIs work better than simply doubling the morning dose. It is also important to pay attention to the timing of PPI dosing in relation to meals. The ideal window to take the PPI is 15 to 30 minutes before meals. This allows absorption of the medication to provide availability to the proton pumps when they are activated by the meal. PPIs taken before meals provide the best intragastric pH control (Khoury et al, 1999). Inadequate timing is frequently seen clinically, especially when patients are prescribed PPI twice daily without further instructions, as they frequently take the medication in the morning and before bedtime (without a meal). Table 9-2 outlines the "step-up" approach to acid suppression therapy we use for GERD. Going directly to PPI dosing before breakfast and dinner is another "step-up" approach.*

Management of "Refractory" GERD (Persistent Symptoms on PPI Twice Daily)

Patients with persistent symptoms on twice-daily PPI given in ideal dosing before breakfast and before dinner are challenging. At this point we recommend reevaluating their symptoms and further testing because the symptoms might be due to persistent acid reflux, nonacid reflux, or not related to gastroesophageal reflux at all.

Patients with atypical supraesophageal symptoms (ie, laryngitis, hoarseness, chronic cough, asthma) should be treated for at least 4 to 6 months on high dose PPI before declaring their atypical GERD symptoms refractory to therapy. There is a chapter on extraesophageal manifestations of GERD. In patients with predominantly persistent nocturnal symptoms, bedtime H_2RAs should be added in the attempt to control nocturnal acid breakthrough. Studies from our laboratory have indicated that up to 80% of patients receiving PPI twice daily before meals have at least 60 continuous minutes of overnight intragastric pH < 4 (nocturnal acid breakthrough) and addition of bed-

TABLE 9-2. Suggested Approach to Acid-Suppressive Therapy

Step	Medical Regimen
1	Single dose PPI (AM AC)
2	Switch to another PPI
3	PPI AM plus H_2RA at bedtime
4	PPI bid AC
5	PPI bid AC plus H_2RA at bedtime

AC = before meals; AM = morning; bid = twice daily; H_2RA = histamine-2 antagonist; PPI = proton pump inhibitor.

*Editor's Note: How long to continue successful therapy with PPIs is another question. When to taper to once per day? When to go to H_2RAs? When to stop?
Author's Reply: Because GERD is a chronic disease patients with correctly diagnosed GERD should be on acid suppressive therapy indefinitely. Studies indicate that 70 to 80% of patients with healed esophageal lesions will relapse when switched to H_2RAs or daily PPI therapy is discontinued. With the exception of patients with Barrett's esophagus, in whom we recommend high dose PPI twice daily with/without bedtime H_2RA, we discuss with patients the possibilities of tapering down the PPI treatment, switching to H_2RAs based on their symptoms.

time H$_2$RA decreased this proportion to 32%. Despite concerns regarding tolerance to H$_2$RAs, this combination is effective long term in many patients.

Testing patients with persistent symptoms on PPI twice daily or "maximal acid control" (ie, PPI twice daily before meals + H$_2$RA at bedtime) will often clarify which one of the three possible causes account for the symptoms. We recommend combined multichannel intraluminal impedance and pH (MII-pH) testing on therapy as the best currently available technique in detecting gastroesophageal reflux of all types. Because combined MII-pH detects reflux by measuring changes in electrical resistance along the MII-pH probe within the esophageal lumen, it can detect both acid and nonacid reflux. Initial studies with this technique indicate that approximately 20% of patients with persistent symptoms on acid-suppressive therapy with at least twice-daily PPI have their symptoms related to continuing acid reflux. The majority traditionally present a diagnostic dilemma as to whether their symptoms are associated with nonacid reflux or not associated with any type of GERD. Combined MII-pH testing will further clarify this possible association, separating those patients with persistent symptoms due to nonacid reflux from those without temporal association between symptoms and any type of reflux. Therefore, we believe that combined MII-pH on PPI twice-daily before meals should be considered the next step in the diagnostic approach to patients not responding to PPI therapy (Figure 9-3).

In patients with documented persistent acid reflux on PPI bid ± H$_2$RA we recommend testing for hypersecretory status (ie, serum gastrin level and possible secretin stimulation test) and recommend *increasing the dose* of acid suppressive medication or referral for *antireflux procedures*. Patients with *symptomatic nonacid reflux* should be offered antireflux surgery. Endoscopic antireflux procedures should be offered only in centers with experience and adequate follow-up. There are limited pharmacologic options for nonacid reflux. To date, γ-aminobutyric acid *(GABA) B-receptor agonists* (ie, baclofen) have been proposed as medications to decrease the frequency of *transient LES relaxations* and studies indicate that *baclofen* decreases both acid and nonacid reflux (Vela et al, 2003). The side effect profile (dizziness, muscular weakness, fatigue) of these medications is the main limiting factor. In patients in whom symptoms cannot be associated with acid or nonacid reflux episodes, other, nonreflux, causes of their symptoms should be investigated.

Who Should Be Referred for Surgery?

Surgery is an effective therapy for GERD and the surgical option is a reasonable consideration for any patient with documented *persistent acid or nonacid reflux* associated with their symptoms, particularly *young patients* and those with *poor compliance*. On the other hand, patients should be cautioned that surgery is not 100% successful, and that there is also a risk of developing new symptoms, including dysphagia, bloating, inability to belch, and increased flatulence. We do not recommend surgery for patients labeled as "medical failures" by persistent symptoms despite medical therapy unless their symptoms have been documented to be related to reflux, either acid or nonacid. Chapter 12 ("Surgery for Gastroesophageal Reflux Disease") covers surgery for gastroesophageal reflux.

Summary

GERD is a chronic condition requiring long-term treatment. Potent acid-suppressive therapy is currently the most important and successful medical therapy. Step-up medical therapy can be accomplished according to Table 9-2. Although healing of esophagitis is usually achieved with a

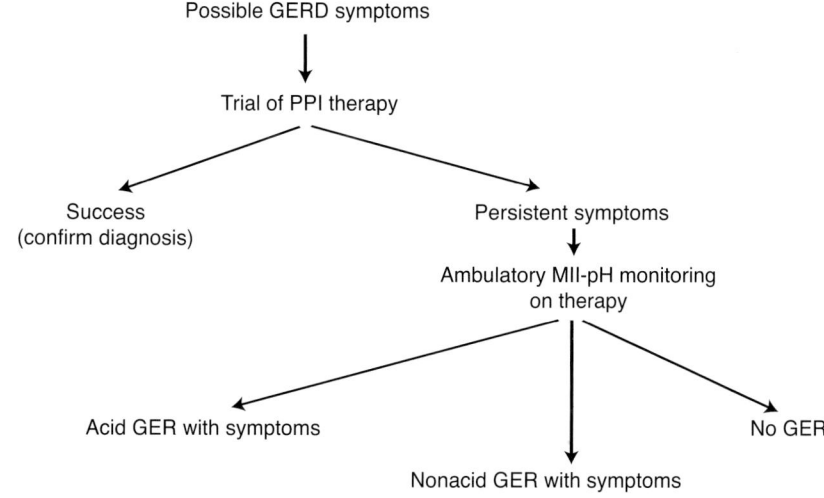

FIGURE 9-3. Suggested diagnostic gastroesophageal reflux disease (GERD) algorithm. GER = gastroesophageal reflux; MII-pH = multichannel intraluminal impedance and pH; PPI = proton pump inhibitor.

single dose of any PPI in over 80% of cases, symptoms are more difficult to control. Patients with persistent symptoms on therapy should be tested (with combined MII-pH or with pH probe) for association of symptoms with acid, nonacid, or no reflux. Long-term follow-up studies indicate that PPIs are effective, tolerable, and safe medications. Promotility agents have shown limited efficacy and their side effect profile often outweighs benefits.

Supplemental Reading

Bennet JR, Castell DO. Overview and symptom assessment. In: Castell DO, Richter JE, editors. The esophagus. 3rd ed. Philadelphia: Lippincott Williams & Wilkins; 1999. p. 33–43.

Caro JJ, Salas M, Ward A. Healing and relapse rates in gastroesophageal reflux disease treated with the newer proton-pump inhibitors lansoprazole, rabeprazole, and pantoprazole compared with omeprazole, ranitidine, and placebo: evidence from randomized clinical trials. Clin Ther 2001;23:998–1017.

Castell DO, Kahrilas PJ, Richter JE, et al. Esomeprazole (40 mg) compared with lansoprazole (30 mg) in the treatment of erosive esophagitis. Am J Gastroenterol 2002;97:575–83.

DeVault KR, Castell DO. Updated guidelines for the diagnosis and treatment of gastroesophageal reflux disease. Am J Gastroenterol 1999;94:1434–42.

Horn J. The proton-pump inhibitors: similarities and differences. Clin Ther 2000;22:266–80.

Khoury RM, Katz PO, Castell DO. Post-prandial ranitidine is superior to post-prandial omeprazole in control of gastric acidity in healthy volunteers. Aliment Pharmacol Ther 1999;13:1211–4.

Tutuian R, Katz PO, Castell DO. A PPI is a PPI is a PPI: lessons from prolonged ambulatory pH monitoring. Gastroenterol 2000;118(Suppl 2):A17.

Vela MF, Tutuian R, Katz PO, Castell DO. Baclofen decreases acid and non-acid post-prandial gastro-oesophageal reflux measured by combined multichannel intraluminal impedance and pH. Aliment Pharmacol Ther 2003;17:243–51.

Chapter 10

Lifestyle Measures for the Treatment of Gastroesophageal Reflux Disease

William C. Orr, PhD

The implementation of lifestyle and behavioral measures in the treatment of gastroesophageal reflux disease (GERD) has been a popular notion in the treatment of this disease. The rationale behind these treatments often relates to simple logic. For example, it would seem logical that elevating the head of the bed would be advantageous to preventing the retrograde flow of gastric contents. Similarly, with obese individuals, the additional intra-abdominal pressure caused by a pendulous abdomen would logically seem to favor the retrograde flow of gastric contents. Empirically, physicians have realized that dietary measures can significantly alter symptom complaints in patients with frequent heartburn. Although there is a dearth of randomized, controlled clinical trials to test these various clinical interventions, a number of studies have been done to test the efficacy of these measures in smaller populations. This review will specifically address the existing empirical data relating to lifestyle measures and the treatment of GERD. It would be prudent to keep in mind the admonition noted in the practice review guidelines published by the American College of Gastroenterology in regard to the treatment of GERD, which notes as follows: "common sense would argue in favor of implementing these procedures even without randomized controlled clinical trials documenting efficacy"(DeVault and Castell, 1999).

Dietary Measures

Enhanced Gastroesophageal Reflux

Typically it has been presumed that there are two mechanisms that provoke heartburn via food intake. First, some foods with a more acidic pH, such as citrus fruits, have been shown to directly irritate the lining of the esophagus and produce heartburn, and, second, some foods have been shown to decrease the lower esophageal sphincter (LES) pressure, thereby predisposing to gastroesophageal (GE) reflux. Data with regard to the effect of a high fat meal are conflicting; however, there appears to be a consensus that chocolate does decrease the LES pressure (Nebel and Castell, 1973; Pehl et al, 1999; Murphy and Castell, 1988). Peppermint, garlic, and onions are food constituents that clinically appear to induce heartburn in many patients. These compounds have a similar derivation and are often categorized as carminatives. In our laboratory, we undertook a study to directly test one of these constituents (ie, raw onions), and its effect on postprandial reflux (Allen et al, 1990). In this study, we had normal individuals eat a hamburger with and without a large raw onion. In the onion condition it was shown that there was a significant postprandial increase in esophageal acid contact. Peppermint has also been shown to induce GE reflux, but this may be confounded by the fact that dissolving a peppermint may have the salubrious effect of enhancing salivation, which will facilitate acid clearance. Chewing gum may also induce increased salvation with similar effects on esophageal acid clearance.

Heartburn and esophageal irritation are common experiences in individuals with an acid sensitive esophagus who ingest citrus fruit juices. A recently published survey showed a significant correlation between the acidity of the citrus juices and heartburn score (Feldman and Barnett, 1994). On this basis, it would seem reasonable to advise patients to avoid *chocolate, citrus fruits,* and *fruit juices,* as well as carminatives, such as *onions* and *garlic*. Data with regard to high fat content on LES pressure are equivocal, but it would seem rational to advise individuals to avoid high fat foods, at least with regard to their effect on delayed gastric emptying and GE reflux. Two studies have been done that address the issue of carbonation and caffeine. Crookes and colleagues (1999), did not find any differences between carbonated water, caffeine-free Pepsi, or regular Pepsi, and concluded that LES changes are due to gas rather than caffeine level or pH. On the other hand, in a study designed to test the difference between regular coffee and decaffeinated coffee, Pehl and colleagues (1997) found that decaffeinated coffee indeed did reduce the percent of acid contact time in the esophagus.

Gastric Distention

An obvious and inexorable effect of eating is gastric distention. Because evidence is now clear that gastric distention does induce transient lower esophageal sphincter relaxations (TLESR), it would seem that food ingestion alone would predispose to reflux via the mechanism of TLESR. Again, although no randomized control trial exists to document the efficacy of this measure, it would seem prudent to advise patients to avoid large volume meals as well as carbonation.*

The Role of Obesity

Weight loss is generally recognized as an important lifestyle measure to observe in the treatment of GERD, and obesity is felt to be a significant risk factor for GERD. Until fairly recently, this approach was based only on the logical assumption that increased girth promotes an increase in intra-abdominal pressure, thereby facilitating the retrograde flow of gastric contents into the esophagus. In more carefully analyzing the relationship between obesity and GERD, the relationship between GE reflux per se and the symptoms of GERD must be taken into account. For example, it is now well-established that 50% or fewer of reflux events are associated with a symptom such as heartburn or regurgitation, and the relationship between 24-hour esophageal pH measures of esophageal acid contact and the presence or absence of esophagitis is relatively poor. Therefore, any indictment of weight loss simply because it does not reduce the absolute percent of esophageal acid contact time is probably not warranted. Further complicating the assessment of these relationships is the fact that there appears to be a significant difference between males and females in the relationship between obesity and GERD. Female susceptibility has been demonstrated in epidemiological studies (Nilsson et al, 2003). Thus, any study with a preponderance of men in the subject population would be most likely not to show any particular relationship between obesity and the presence or absence of GERD symptoms.

An example of the complexity of these relationships can be illustrated in two studies done by the same large group of collaborators (Nilsson et al, 2003; Lagergren et al, 2000). In a study published in 1999, the authors concluded that there was no relationship between body mass and GERD symptoms, and this applied to both severity and duration of reflux symptoms. In a more recent study, published in 2003, the authors reached a very different conclusion. In this study they reported a significant association between body mass and symptoms of GERD. They noted that the association was stronger in women, particularly in premenopausal women, and that the use of hormone therapy appears to strengthen this association. In the discussion of this article, the authors commented on their previous work and suggested that a paucity of males in that particular study biased the results toward negativity. Other epidemiological studies have documented a strong relationship between obesity, GERD symptoms, and the presence of adenocarcinoma (AC) in the distal esophagus (Mayne and Navarro, 2002). Another epidemiological study has shown a significant relationship between increased body mass index, hiatal hernia, and esophagitis (Wilson et al, 1999).

Thus, the preponderance of epidemiological data would suggest a strong association between obesity and GERD symptoms, as well as the well-known complications of GE reflux per se, such as esophagitis and AC of the esophagus. On the basis of these data, it would seem prudent to recommend weight loss in patients with GERD, or preferably the prevention of substantial weight gain to levels that would be significantly beyond the patient's ideal body weight.

Other Factors

Other lifestyle modifications that are commonly recommended to GERD patients include avoiding alcohol intake, cessation of smoking, and altering sleeping position.

Alcohol itself does appear to irritate the lining of the esophagus and to produce heartburn via direct contact with the esophageal mucosa. *Beer* and *wine* both have been shown to induce reflux, but interestingly, this does not appear to be an effect of alcohol content or the pH of the ingested liquid. For wine aficionados, *white wine* does appear to be more problematic than *red wine*, and both appear to be substantially more provocative than tap water (Pehl et al, 1998).

Smoking

Most, but not all, studies show that smoking has a negative effect on LES pressure, and perhaps more importantly, diminishes the concentration of salivary bicarbonate. This latter factor indirectly could be extremely important in view of data that have shown that reducing salivation will markedly retard esophageal acid clearance and, conversely, enhancing salivation will facilitate acid clearance. In view of epidemiological data suggesting a relationship between smoking and AC of the distal esophagus, and the overall negative health consequences of smoking, a strong recommendation to stop smoking would be advisable for GERD patients.

Gravity

It has been axiomatic among primary care physicians, and even gastroenterologists, that *elevation of the head of the bed* for sleeping is a prudent approach to reducing GE reflux. Recent studies have shown this to be a much more complicated issue. For example, it appears that elevating the head of the bed may not actually reduce episodes of GE reflux, but indeed may facilitate acid clearance. Other studies have shown that the subpopulations of GERD patients

---

*Editor's Note: Foods that delay gastric emptying, such as fatty meals, will also contribute to gastric distension and should be limited. Patients often cite meals with tomato sauce, which are possibly multifactorial.

with bipositional reflux and esophagitis benefit with regard to efficacy of elevating the head of the bed. Those with upright reflux without esophagitis did not benefit (Shay and Johnson, 1994). In view of these data, it would seem that a routine recommendation of elevating the head of the bed should be reconsidered, and perhaps should be implemented only in the subpopulation of patients with esophagitis (Meining and Classen, 2000).

Sleeping Position

With regard to sleeping position per se, it appears that the *left lateral position* does actually reduce acid reflux in the esophagus compared to the right lateral position, and it would be sensible to recommend that patients with significant heartburn complaints sleep in the left lateral position. There is a further physiologic basis for this in that the right lateral position does appear to induce a higher frequency of transient LES relaxations.

In summary, regarding sleeping for better control of reflux, it would appear that the best recommendation would be to *sleep in the left lateral decubitus position*, and perhaps only in patients who have *documented esophagitis* would one recommend *elevating the head of the bed*.

A Word About Sleep

It has now been well established that GE reflux is associated with significant sleep complaints, many of which may be referred to primary care physicians, or gastroenterologists who care for patients with GERD (Shaker et al, 2003). It has been noted above that sleeping position does affect reflux, and patients should avoid sleeping in the right lateral position. It is known that disturbed sleep and transient arousals from sleep do tend to be associated with reflux events in GERD patients. Thus, the logical conclusion would be that if these transient arousal responses, and improved sleep, could be accomplished, reflux events during sleep would be reduced. In addition, snoring and obstructive sleep apnea have also been shown to be associated with increased complaints of heartburn and esophageal acid contact time. Furthermore, the majority of GERD patients complain of nighttime heartburn, and awakenings from sleep due to heartburn. In addition, such patients also show a marked decrease in the quality of life. It is important for the clinician to be aware of the fact that sleep complaints may be related to GERD, and even in instances where heartburn does not seem to be a particular problem, "silent" reflux can be contributing to sleep disorders.

It is of interest that the common recommendation of avoiding a meal within 2 hours before going to bed may not be particularly well founded. We have conducted a study in which a late evening meal did not necessarily produce an increase in sleep-related esophageal acid contact time (Orr and Harnish, 1998). In patients with sleep complaints without typical symptoms of heartburn, it is tempting to prescribe a hypnotic drug for temporary relief of the sleep disorder. In general, this is not a good idea unless the clinician is convinced the patient does not have any symptoms of nocturnal heartburn. Depressing the level of consciousness during sleep will almost certainly result in a prolongation of esophageal acid contact time if reflux events do occur, and this would be placing the patient at additional risk for the development of complications of reflux. The most obvious approach to GERD-related sleep complaints is to eliminate GE reflux. There is evidence now that this will indeed improve the sleep in patients with significant heartburn complaints. In short, in patients with concomitant sleep complaints who also have significant complaints of heartburn, the best approach is to effectively ameliorate the reflux symptom. The notion that reflux is not an issue in sleep complaints if patients do not complain particularly of heartburn is probably erroneous. In such patients, without an obvious cause of reflux and sleep disturbance, such as sleep apnea, a trial with an acid suppressing medical therapy, for example, proton pump inhibitor treatment, would be appropriate. Although ingesting a meal 2 hours before bedtime may not bother all patients, it should be recognized that such meals are often high volume meals (ie, eating out), and as noted above this should be avoided.

Conclusions

Although the data to support the overall efficacy of lifestyle measures is modest, on the basis of the available scientific data, it still appears to be a reasonable adjunct approach to the treatment of patients with GERD. It would seem that lifestyle modifications alone have only a very modest effect on reducing symptoms of heartburn and GE reflux, but would add to an overall approach to the treatment of GERD to include over the counter and prescription medication. It also appears that more recent data suggest that *lifestyle measures* will be more effective in certain subpopulations of patients, such as *obese females* and patients with *documented esophagitis*. Implementing lifestyle modifications initially in patients presenting to a primary care physician could be limited primarily to dietary measures, avoiding alcohol and smoking, and avoiding sleep in the right lateral position.

Supplemental Reading

Allen ML, Mellow MH, Robinson MG, et al. The effect of raw onions on acid reflux and reflux symptoms. Am J Gastroenterol 1990;85:377–80.

Crookes PF, Hamoi N, Thiesen J, et al. Response of lower esophageal sphincter to ingestion of carbonated beverages. Gastroenterology 1999;116:A.

DeVault K, Castell D. Updated guidelines for the diagnosis and treatment of gastroesophageal reflux disease. Am J Gastroenterol 1999;94:1434–42.

Feldman M, Barnett C. Relationship between the acidity and osmolality of popular beverages and reported postprandial heartburn. Gastroenterology 1994;108:125–31.

Lagergren J, Bergstrom R, Nyren O. No relation between body mass and gastro-oesophageal reflux symptoms in a Swedish population based study. Gut 2000;47:26–9.

Mayne S, Navarro S. Diet, obesity and reflux in the etiology of adenocarcinomas of the esophagus and gastric cardia in humans. J Nutr 2002;3467S–70S.

Meining A, Classen M. The role of diet and lifestyle measures in the pathogenesis and treatment of gastroesophageal reflux disease. Am J Gastroenterol 2000;95:2692–7.

Murphy DW, Castell, DO. Chocolate and heartburn: evidence of increased esophageal acid exposure after chocolate ingestion. Am J Gastroenterol 1988;83:633-6.

Nebel O, Castell DO. Inhibition of the lower oesophageal sphincter by fat: a mechanism for fatty food intolerance. Gut 1973;134:270–4.

Nilsson M, Johnsen R, Ye W, et al. Obesity and estrogen as risk factors for gastroesophageal reflux symptoms. JAMA 2003;290:66–72.

Orr WC, Harnish MJ. Sleep related gastro-oesophageal reflux: provocation with a late evening meal and treatment with acid suppression. Aliment Pharm & Ther 1998;12:1033–8.

Pehl C, Pfeiffer A, Wendl B, et al. Different effects of white wine and red wine on lower esophageal sphincter pressure and gastroesophageal reflux. Scand J Gastroenterol 1998;33:118–22.

Pehl C, Pfeiffer A, Wendl B, et al. The effect of decaffeination of coffee on gastro-oesophageal reflux in patients with reflux disease. Aliment Pharmocol Ther 1997;11:483–6.

Pehl C, Waizendorfer A, Wendl B, et al. Effect of low and high fat meals on lower esophageal sphincter motility and gastroesophageal reflux in healthy subjects. Am J Gastroenterol 1999;94:1992–6.

Shaker R, Castell, DO, Schoenfeld PS, Spechler SJ. Nighttime heartburn is an under-appreciated clinical problem that impacts sleep and daytime function: the results of a Gallup survey conducted on behalf of the American Gastroenterological Association. Am J Gastroenterol 2003;98:1487–93.

Shay SS, Johnson LF. Upright refluxers without esophagitis differentiated from bipositional refluxers with esophagitis by simultaneous manometry and pH monitoring conducted in two postures before and after a meal. Am J Gastroenterol 1994;89:992–1002.

Wilson L, Wenzhou M, Hirschowitz B. Association of obesity with hiatal hernia and esophagitis. Am J Gastroenterol 1999;94:2840–4.

CHAPTER 11

Management of Extraesophageal Presentations of GERD

Joel E. Richter, MD

It has been suggested that gastroesophageal reflux disease (GERD) may be the cause of a wide spectrum of conditions, including noncardiac chest pain, asthma, chronic cough, posterior laryngitis, recurrent pneumonitis, and even dental erosions (Richter, 2000). If true, these "extraesophageal" manifestations of GERD combined with classic reflux disease may well adversely affect 40 to 50% of the US population at some time in their life.

The Conundrum

Over the last 15 years, I have found the extraesophageal manifestations of GERD the most challenging area to perform good research and to define accurate treatment paradigms for. In fact, over time my enthusiasm has begun to wane about how "common" an important problem this is. Let me explain.

The literature suggests that the majority of patients with extraesophageal GERD do not have the classic symptoms of heartburn or acid regurgitation. For example, reflux symptoms are absent in 40 to 60% of asthmatics, in 57 to 94% of patients with ear, nose, and throat (ENT) complaints, and in 43 to 75% of patients with chronic cough in whom GERD is suspected to be causing their symptoms (Richter, 2000). In contrast, studies find that 80 to 90% of patients with acid reflux-related chest pain have associated classic reflux symptoms (Hewson et al, 1991). Obviously, the "silent reflux" of this syndrome contributes to difficulties in making this diagnosis. If true, physicians must consider GERD in the differential diagnosis of these problems either early, when classic symptoms are present, or when alternative diagnoses have been excluded.

Furthermore, traditional tests for GERD are not extremely helpful in patients with extraesophageal manifestations. The prevalence of endoscopic evidence of esophagitis is low in these patients in the range of 10 to 30%, and, when present, is usually mild. This is in sharp contrast to the 47 to 79% prevalence of esophagitis in patients with typical GERD symptoms. Without classic reflux symptoms and/or esophagitis, physicians often turn to 24-hour esophageal pH testing to help confirm the diagnosis. Unfortunately, esophageal pH testing is not a perfect test, and controversies exist relating to probe placement (pharyngeal vs upper esophagus) and the tendency for false negative tests (20 to 50%). Thus, a negative test may not confidently exclude the diagnosis of GERD-related extraesophageal symptoms. On the other hand, a positive test only confirms the coexistence of GERD with patients' "atypical" symptoms and does not assure a cause-and-effect relationship. The latter can only be proved with confidence when the extraesophageal symptoms or signs markedly improve or resolve with aggressive medical treatment or surgical antireflux therapy.

This conundrum with extraesophageal GERD is summarized by the pyramid shown in Figure 11-1. The presence of erosive esophagitis is the foundation of our treatment strategies for GERD. Esophagitis has excellent specificity for reflux disease and heartburn; therefore, treatment studies, especially those with proton pump inhibitors (PPIs), have response rates usually exceeding 85 to 95%. On the other hand, nonerosive GERD, which is intuitively a milder disease because esophageal damage is not present, only responds in 60 to 80% of cases. Drug efficacy is not the issue; rather, despite the presence of classic reflux symptoms some of these patients have factors other than acid accounting for their complaints. This complex relationship among symptoms, presence of GERD, and causal relationship is further compounded as one goes up the pyramid with the extraesophageal presentations of GERD. Esophageal pH testing does not allow resolution of this issue. Aggressive therapeutic trials, usually with PPIs, must be used instead.

Therapeutic Trials

The use of therapeutic trials to identify patients with true GERD-related extraesophageal complaints is ideal in clinical practice, but it is impractical for large clinical trials of drug efficacy. Reliable predictors of response to therapy are needed; unfortunately, these are not available, and therefore we have little means of "enriching" our study populations with patients who have true GERD-related extraesophageal symptoms. This key issue probably accounts for the variable treatment results seen with both aggressive medical and surgical antireflux regimens, and it makes scientific evidence-based algorithms for treating these patients very difficult. For example, asthma studies with PPIs by Harding and Sontag (2000) have found only

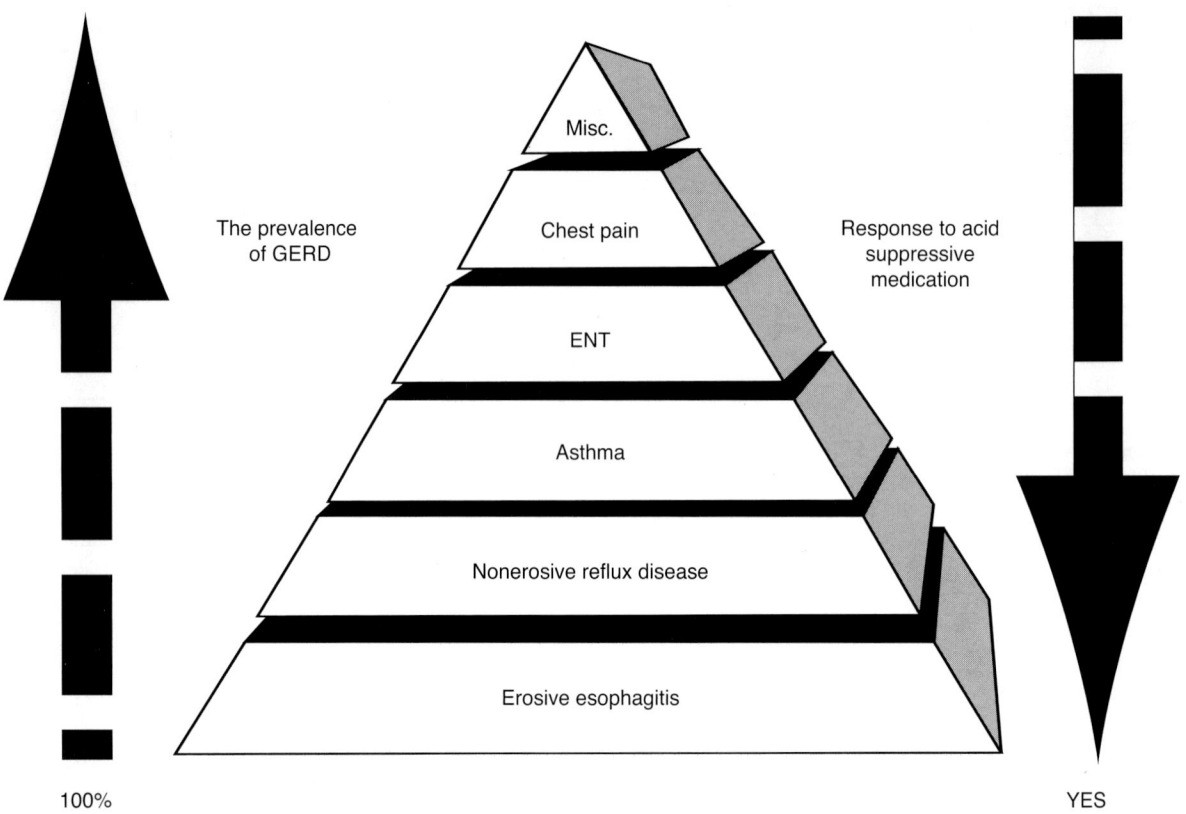

FIGURE 11-1 The Reflux Pyramid. Response to acid suppression and prevalence of gastroesophageal reflux disease (GERD) is best at the base of the pyramid. ENT = ear, nose, and throat; misc = miscellaneous.

inconsistent results in the improvement of asthma after aggressive treatment of GERD. Furthermore, whereas a surgical study by So and colleagues (1998) found that 93% of patients with classic reflux symptoms responded to antireflux surgery, only 56% of patients had relief of their atypical complaints. To complicate this issue further, few placebo-controlled studies are available in this area. In those studies with placebo controls, either the group receiving active treatment did no better than patients on placebo or the response rate in crossover studies was only in the range of 30 to 40%. Here again, the issue is not the effectiveness of available medical or surgical treatments, but rather our current inability to identify with certainty those patients whose extraesophageal complaints are caused by GERD.

General Approach to Extraesophageal Presentation of GERD

Figure 11-2 summarizes my general approach to patients with suspected extraesophageal presentations of GERD. If possible, it is key to exclude other factors that can be leading to these atypical symptoms. If the patient has associated classic reflux symptoms or there is a high suspicion of GERD, especially when other potential etiologies have been excluded, I go directly to an aggressive therapeutic trial with a PPI. As discussed previously, this circumvents problems with pH testing, is more acceptable to the patient, and allows me to define a possible cause-and-effect relationship. No one PPI is superior to another for these trials, although I prefer to be very aggressive, *dosing twice daily, in the morning and before dinner.* As will be discussed in the following sections on individual syndromes, the length of treatment will vary, but these patients usually do not respond as rapidly as classic GERD patients. Marked symptom reduction or improvement is strong clinical evidence that acid reflux is the cause of the patient's complaints. After several months of good symptom relief, I attempt to step down therapy to the minimal dose of PPI, or even H_2 blocker, or lifestyle changes that will control their symptoms. I have little concern about a "placebo" response, because these patients are only looking for relief. Furthermore, stepping all patients down will define those individuals who will relapse, therefore reconfirming the presence of GERD. In patients requiring long-term PPI treatment for relief of extraesophageal reflux symptoms,

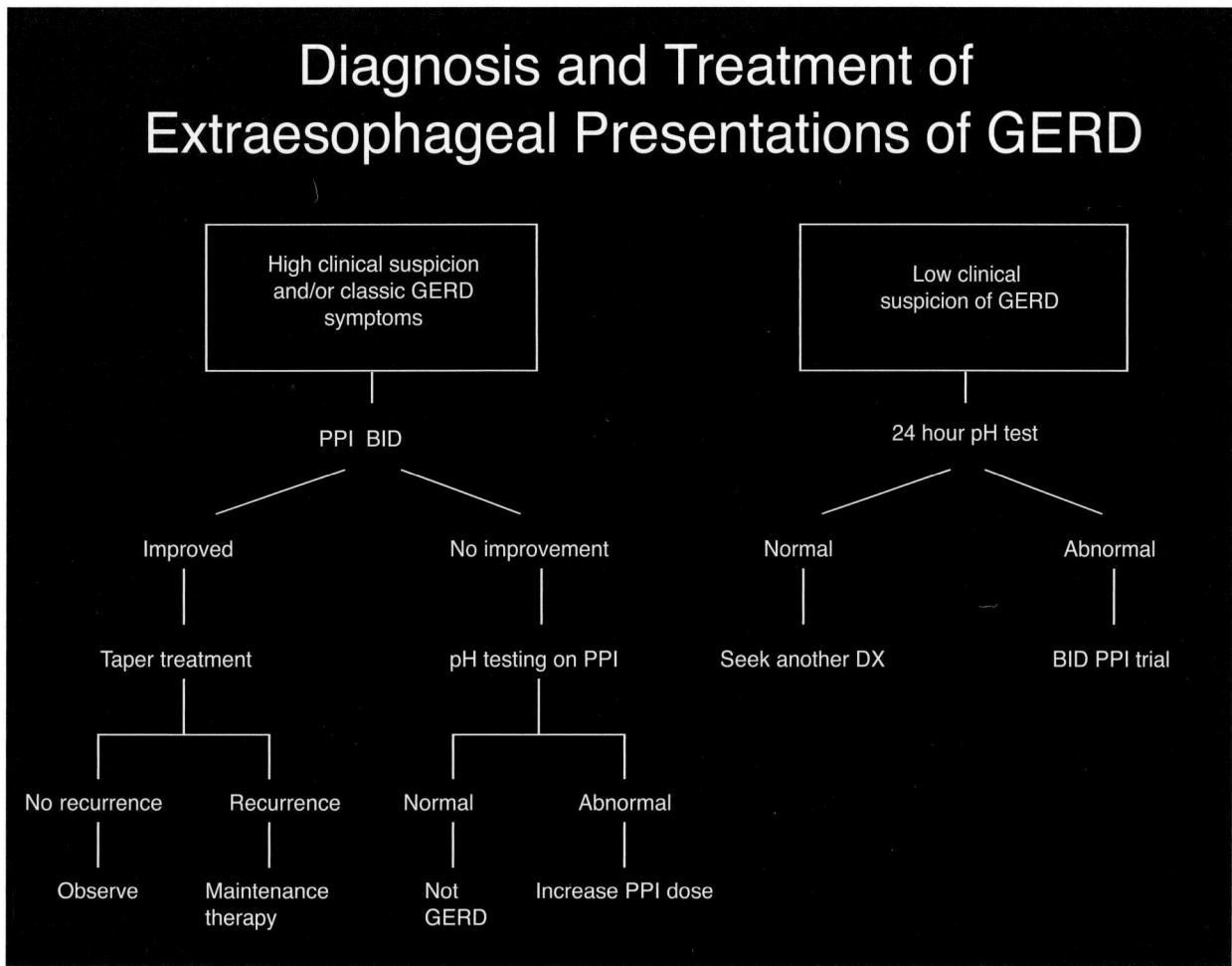

FIGURE 11-2. Algorithm for diagnosis and treatment of extraesophageal presentations of gastroesophageal reflux disease (GERD). PPI = proton pump inhibitor; BID = twice a day; DX = diagnosis.

antireflux surgery is a viable alternative because the response to medical treatment is the best predictor of a good response to surgical treatment (So et al, 1998).

Patients not responding to an aggressive therapeutic trial of a PPI, then undergo 24-hour esophageal pH testing "on" medication. I do not test these patients off medication, because the question is not whether or not they have GERD. Rather, at this point in the clinical dilemma, the issue is whether or not they have had adequate acid control over the last months to improve their possible reflux-related symptoms. The type of pH probe to use is uncertain. Frankly, a single distal probe showing good acid control (< 3 to 4% over 24 hours) should be more than adequate to define this issue. If no acid reflux is defined, then it is like a baseball game—"strike three and you are out"—and I am confident that GERD is not the cause of their symptoms. These patients are then referred back to their primary care physician or specialist for more careful evaluation of other potential etiologies of their complaints.

Possible Nonacidic Reflux

Some authorities, however, suggest that these patients still may be suffering from "nonacidic" reflux. New technology such as impedance combined with pH testing allows the measurement of acid and nonacid reflux high into the esophagus. In our experience with impedance, as well as the older Bilitec technique, which measures bilirubin as a surrogate marker of bile reflux, we found that high doses of PPIs predictably eliminate both acid and nonacid GERD. Rarely, if ever, would I consider antireflux surgery for these patients. Certainly, if they have no symptoms of classic GERD and fail PPIs, with evidence of good control by 24-hour pH testing, the logic for antireflux surgery is only based on the premise of nonacid reflux, which is precarious at best. On the other hand, patients with classic reflux symptoms and atypical complaints may be offered surgery if their heartburn and acid regurgitation symptoms respond well to PPIs, they have appropriate physiology, and they understand the side effects that may be associated with antireflux surgery. The logic here is that these patients have GERD, and surgery offers an appropriate and effective alternative treatment, but no guarantees are made about how their extraesophageal complaints will do.

Low Suspicion of GERD

In patients with *no reflux symptoms* and unusual possible "extraesophageal" complaints (ie, globus, sore throat, burning tongue, or neck pain), I tend to go directly to 24-hour esophageal pH monitoring (see Figure 11-2). A negative test reassures them that acid reflux is not the cause of their complaints and their physicians can begin to look elsewhere. If acid reflux is present, then again a therapeutic trial of a PPI is administered.

Chest Pain

GERD-related chest pain may mimic angina pectoris, even to the point of worsening with exercise. Recent studies by Hewson and colleagues (1991) suggest that about 25 to 50% of patients with noncardiac chest pain have GERD. Multiple placebo-controlled studies now confirm the efficacy and cost savings of a therapeutic trial of a PPI to make the diagnosis and treat this syndrome. In the best study to date, Fass and colleagues (1998) found that a 7-day trial of omeprazole (Prilosec) 40 mg in the morning and 20 mg in the evening had a sensitivity of 78% and specificity of 85% for predicting GERD, when compared with traditional esophageal tests. Additionally, they found a savings of $573 per average patient due to a 59% reduction in the number of diagnostic tests (ie, upper gastrointestinal endoscopy and 24-hour pH tests) performed in these patients. From a practical standpoint, I give the patients a 1-month trial of a PPI taken twice daily, with further testing based on the response at follow-up. There is a separate chapter on esophageal motility disturbances and chest pain (see Chapter 17, "Esophageal Strictures").

Asthma

Studies have suggested that pulmonary disease, especially asthma, may be associated with GERD, based on symptoms or pH testing, in up to 70% of these patients. In reality, studies by Irwin and colleagues (1993) suggest that those patients with difficult to manage asthma (ie, multiple visits to emergency room or hospitalization for asthma exacerbations) are the most likely to have acid reflux as a major cause of their asthma. Other asthmatic groups to consider are nonallergic asthmatics with symptoms beginning in adulthood or asthma patients with classic reflux symptoms, especially regurgitation (Harding and Sontag, 2000).

The results of treatment studies in asthma are inconsistent, but the review by Harding and Sontag (2000) concluded that the medical treatment of GERD-related asthma improved asthma symptoms in over 60% of patients and may reduce the need for asthma medications, but objective improvement of pulmonary function tests was observed in only 25% of patients. Most asthma studies have used omeprazole (Prilosec) or lansoprazole (Prevacid). The dose of omeprazole should be ≥ 20 mg twice daily or the equivalent dose of another PPI given for 3 months or more. This is based on our experience in 30 asthmatics with GERD, of which 27% required more than 20 mg omeprazole for adequate acid suppression documented by serial esophageal pH testing. In the same study, (Harding et al, 1996) we noted that 3 months were required to see maximal symptom improvement.

Cough

GERD is the third most common cause of chronic cough lasting for greater than 3 weeks, following postnasal drip syndromes due to a variety of rhinosinus conditions and asthma. Additionally, 20 to 50% of chronic cough patients have multiple etiologies and the act of coughing can also provoke GERD. Therefore, I believe a careful evaluation for postnasal drip syndromes, asthma, and medications that may provoke coughing (especially angiotensin-converting enzyme inhibitors) needs to be done before indicting GERD as a likely candidate. Postnasal drip can be excluded by a trial of H_1 antagonists and inhaled steroids, as well as by radiographs to exclude sinusitis. Cough variant asthma should be evaluated with a methacholine challenge test, preferably, or a trial of asthma medications.

Treatment trials, which are rarely undertaken with placebo, find that GERD-related cough has a high rate of response to H_2 receptor antagonists, prokinetics, or PPIs over weeks to months of treatment. For example, Poe and Kallay (2003) observed that 75% of their 56 patients improved with a single dose of a PPI, while the remainder responded when metoclopramide (Reglan) or cisapride (Propulsid) was added. The cough was markedly improved or eliminated after 4 weeks in 86% of patients and by 8 weeks in the remaining patients. In the only placebo-controlled PPI study, Ours and colleagues (1999) from my group found that omeprazole (Prilosec) 40 mg twice daily in the morning and at bedtime for 2 weeks was a very reliable method for identifying acid-related cough. Additionally, we found this empirical trial to be three- to five-fold less expensive than manometry and pH testing followed by omeprazole treatment for a positive test. I have now used this approach, most recently substituting esomeprazole (Nexium) 40 mg twice daily for omeprazole (Prilosec) in over 50 patients with cough, in which about 25% responded dramatically and are doing well long term. In the nonresponders, a 24-hour pH test on medication rarely showed evidence of persistent GERD.

Ear, Nose and Throat Disease

GERD may be associated with a number of ENT syndromes, including recurrent hoarseness, throat clearing, sore throat, and globus, and signs, such as laryngitis, vocal cord granulomas, ulcers, leukoplakia, sinusitis, and even laryngeal cancer. These patients are usually diagnosed by our ENT colleagues based upon symptoms and signs of inflammation involving the posterior third of the vocal cords and interarytenoid areas, which are both in close proximity to the upper esophageal sphincter. However, the specificity of these findings has recently been questioned; our study in 100 healthy volunteers without ENT complaints found signs associated with "reflux laryngitis" in 86% of these subjects (Hicks et al, 2002). In these individuals, other causes could usually be found, including smoking, alcohol, excessive voice use, allergies, or asthma.

Case studies without controls suggest that 60 to 90% of patients with suspected acid-related ENT symptoms improve with acid suppression (Wong et al, 2000). Here again, PPIs are more effective than H$_2$ receptor antagonists, and extended treatment for 3 months or more may be required. In our experience with over 60 patients, there was no difference, based on signs and symptoms, between twice daily dosing with omeprazole (Prilosec), lansoprazole (Prevacid), or esomeprazole (Nexium), with 40% of patients responding in 2 months and an additional 20% responding in 4 months. The addition of an H$_2$ receptor antagonist at night was no more effective than twice daily PPI alone. In this area, placebo-controlled studies are particularly lacking. One small study found no efficacy for twice daily lansoprazole for 3 months. Another study randomized 20 patients with signs and symptoms of chronic laryngitis to lansoprazole (Prevacid) 20 mg or placebo twice daily for 3 months. In the PPI group, six patients (50%) achieved a complete symptom response compared with only one patient (10%) in the placebo group, but laryngeal signs generally did not fully resolve. Predictors of response have not been identified in this or other studies, although patients with milder laryngeal signs show better improvement of symptoms.

Summary

The possible extraesophageal symptoms of GERD are a common problem seen by gastroenterologists, internists, and family practitioners. Unfortunately, a strong evidence-based medicine approach for the diagnosis and treatment of these diseases is lacking because the true prevalence and predictors of GERD-related causes have not been identified. Nevertheless, I believe an empirical trial (see Figure 11-2) with twice daily dosing of PPIs (Table 11-1) is the most practical, cost effective, and humane approach for these patients. Symptom resolution or improvement suggests that GERD is causing their complaints, although a placebo response cannot be excluded. However, asymptomatic patients do not really care. Patients should be stepped down to the lowest dose of medication or lifestyle changes that will control their symptoms. Esophageal pH testing is limited to those patients not responding to this aggressive trial and is performed on PPI therapy. If pH testing and a prolonged therapeutic trial are negative, then I believe we have confidently excluded acid-related GERD as a cause of the extraesophageal complaints. I do not believe that nonacid reflux, except for obvious aspiration, causes these complaints and would not send patients for antireflux surgery unless they showed evidence of prior response to medical treatment.

TABLE 11-1. Suggested Treatment Regimens for Extraesophageal Presentations of Gastroesophageal Reflex Disease Based on the Medical Literature

Chest Pain
Omeprazole 40 mg in the am, 20 mg before dinner for 7 days
Any PPI bid × 4 weeks

Asthma
Omeprazole 20 mg bid × 3 months
Lansoprazole 30 mg bid × 3 months
Omeprazole 40 mg in the am × 2 months

Cough
Any PPI in the am × 1–2 months
Omeprazole 40 mg bid × 2 weeks
Esomeprazole 40 mg bid × 2 weeks

ENT syndromes*
Omeprazole 40 mg am or 20 mg bid × 4 months
Lansoprazole 30 mg bid × 4 months
Esomeprazole 40 mg bid × 4 months

bid = twice daily; ENT = ear, nose, and throat; PPI = proton pump inhibitor.
*Adding H$_2$ receptor antagonists at bedtime is no better than bid PPI.

Supplemental Reading

American Thoracic Society. Guidelines for methacholine and exercise challenge testing–1999. Am J Resp Crit Care Med 2000;161:309–29.

Corrao WM, Braman SS, Irwin RS. Chronic cough as the sole presenting manifestation of bronchial asthma. N Engl J Med 1979;300:633–7.

El-Serag HB, Lee P, Buchner A, et al. Lansoprazole treatment of patients with chronic idiopathic laryngitis: a placebo controlled trial. Am J Gastroenterol 2001;96:979–83.

Fass R, Fennerty MB, Hoffman JJ, et al. The clinical and economic value of a short course of omeprazole in patients with noncardiac chest pain. Gastroenterology 1998;115:42–9.

Harding SM, Richter JE, Guzzo MR, et al. Asthma and gastroesophageal reflux: acid suppression therapy improves asthma outcome. Am J Med 1996;100:395–405.

Harding SM, Sontag SJ. Asthma and gastroesophageal reflux. Am J Gastroenterol 2000;95(Suppl):S23–32.

Hewson EG, Sinclair JW, Dalton CB, et al. Twenty-four hour esophageal pH monitoring: the most useful test for evaluating non-cardiac chest pain. Am J Med 1991;65:409–12.

Hicks DM, Ours TM, Abelson TI, et al. The prevalence of hypopharynx findings associated with gastroesophageal reflux in normal volunteers. Voice 2002;16:564–79.

Irwin RS, Carley FJ, French CL. Difficult-to-control asthma: contributing factors and outcome of a systematic protocol. Chest 1993;103:1662–9.

Ours TM, Kavuru MS, Schilz RJ, Richter JE. A prospective evaluation of esophageal testing and a double-blind, randomized study of omeprazole in a diagnostic and therapeutic algorithm for chronic cough. Am J Gastroenterol 1999;94:3131–8.

Poe RH, Kallay MC. Chronic cough and gastroesophageal reflux disease. Experience with specific therapy for diagnosis and treatment. Chest 2003;123:679–84.

Richter JE. Extraesophageal presentations of gastroesophageal reflux disease: an overview. Am J Gastroenterol 2000;95(Suppl):S1–3.

So JBY, Zeitels SM, Rattner DW. Outcome of atypical symptoms attributed to gastroesophageal reflux treated by laparoscopic fundoplication. Surgery 1998;124:28–32.

Wong RKH, Hauson DG, Waring PJ, Shaw G. ENT manifestations of gastroesophageal reflux. Am J Gastroenterol 2000;95(Suppl):S15–22.

CHAPTER 12

Surgery for Gastroesophageal Reflux Disease

J. Andrew Isch, MD, Brant K. Oelschlager, MD, and Carlos A. Pellegrini, MD

Gastroesophageal reflux disease (GERD) is the leading gastrointestinal (GI) disorder in the United States. As such, there are multiple therapies available to treat it. These range from simple lifestyle changes and nonprescription medications to antireflux surgery. With the advent of minimally invasive surgical techniques, the number of operations being performed to treat GERD has increased significantly. This chapter aims to discuss the surgeon's approach to reflux disease and the clinical considerations involved in counseling patients regarding surgical therapies.

Patient Assessment and Perioperative Considerations

Initiating medical therapy usually begins with the recognition of symptoms consistent with GERD, and no formal testing is required. The effects of surgical therapy are not easily reversible, thus the success of an antireflux surgery depends on an accurate diagnosis, quantification of severity, and characterization of anatomic factors associated with GERD. Several diagnostic tests are helpful and often essential to assure a successful operation.

24-hour pH monitoring is the gold standard for confirming and quantifying abnormal reflux. Monitoring is usually done with the distal pH sensor placed 5 cm above the proximal border of the lower esophageal sphincter (LES) while the patient is off all antacid medication. Abnormal reflux is usually defined as a distal esophageal acid exposure (percentage of the time the pH is < 4) > 4% and/or a DeMeester Score (composite score based on study variables) > 14.72. Not only is the amount of reflux important when deciding whether to proceed with an operation, correlation between symptoms and a drop in pH may also be helpful in determining whether a patient's symptoms are due to reflux. If there is more than a 50% correlation between episodes, drops in pH are considered positive. Demonstrating this correlation is helpful in equivocal cases, especially in the face of moderate amounts of reflux.

Manometry is another essential component for examining a patient for a fundoplication, and it serves essentially three functions. First, and perhaps most importantly, it determines the precise location of the LES for subsequent pH probe placement. Second, the LES pressure measurement provides some information about its competency. Finally, manometry allows the surgeon to evaluate esophageal motility. Traditionally this has been used to predict developing dysphagia and if a fundoplication should be tailored to the ability of peristalsis to propel food past it (to be discussed in more detail later).

Upper endoscopy is the third important component of the work-up. It enables the physician to assess for the stigmata of reflux (ie, esophagitis) and to look for other foregut pathologies, including gastric and esophageal ulcers, infections, bile reflux gastritis, peptic strictures, Barrett's esophagus (BE), and upper GI cancers. Biopsies can be obtained, strictures dilated, and other interventions employed as indicated. The presence or absence of foregut abnormalities often has a significant impact on the decision to perform an antireflux procedure.

An *upper gastrointestinal series* (UGI) completes the work-up for the average patient (there are other tests that need to be performed on patients with suspected gastric motility disorders, or laryngeal problems, or others). UGI may detect free reflux or the mucosal changes associated with reflux, but its real value to the surgeon is in determining the anatomy of the gastroesophageal junction. If a hiatal hernia is present on examination, its size, type, and location can be characterized. This will have technical implications at the time of surgery. A large paraesophageal hernia or the presence of a foreshortened esophagus are more demanding operations, and have added technical considerations that must be considered before proceeding with surgical intervention.

Patient Considerations

Antireflux surgery should be considered for patients who have symptoms of GERD, abnormal esophageal acid exposure on objective testing, and who do not suffer from other GI conditions. Those who meet these criteria and desire cessation of medical treatment or better reflux control should be considered for operation. If performed in well-selected patients by surgeons with significant experience with antireflux procedures, surgery provides excellent relief of GERD. Most patients discontinue antacid medical therapy after operation. There is normalization of distal esophageal acid exposure, restoration of LES pressures, and resolution of symptoms in the majority of individuals.

CONFOUNDING CONSIDERATIONS

Antireflux surgery should be approached more cautiously in certain groups of patients. *Obese patients* have a high failure rate with fundoplication; therefore, we recommend obese patients lose weight before proceeding with an operation. The alternative for morbidly obese individuals (body mass index > 40) with GERD is a *Roux-en-Y gastric bypass*. This operation not only aids in weight loss (thus providing other health benefits), but it is an extremely effective antireflux procedure. Patients with multiple comorbidities and previous upper abdominal operations should be approached more cautiously. Patients with severe cardiopulmonary disease may not tolerate general anesthesia or the pneumoperitoneum required to do the operation laparoscopically. Former upper GI or gastric surgery may preclude safe or effective access to the hiatus or make the use of the stomach to construct the wrap more difficult, and sometimes impossible. The most important factor is probably the experience and comfort of the surgeon because multiple technical subtleties encountered at the time of surgery can affect long-term outcome.

Potential Side Effects

Surgery is not without potential side effects, the most common being dysphagia, bloating, diarrhea, and early satiety. Inappropriate geometry of the wrap, tightness of the crural closure, and esophageal peristaltic function are all variables that may lead to *difficulties swallowing* after an operation. The reported incidence varies from 2 to 5% (Anvari and Allen, 2003; Atwood et al, 1992). Although some degree of dysphagia is common immediately after surgery, it generally resolves quickly with expectant management alone. The need for postoperative dilation is unusual, and the need to take down the fundoplication is even less so. *Gas bloating* can occur and is the result of swallowed air that cannot escape by belching secondary to the new wrap. *Early satiety* may result because the gastric volume has been reduced with construction of the wrap. Fortunately, these are also generally short lived and require little or no intervention. *Diarrhea* can occur after surgery and may have several etiologies. In the early postoperative period, infectious (ie, *Clostridium difficile* colitis) and medical causes of diarrhea should be excluded. If diarrhea persists, vagal injury may be the cause. This may be the result of an unrecognized vagotomy or entrapment of the anterior vagus when constructing the wrap. Diarrhea that persists can be treated with dietary manipulation and antidiarrheal medicine.

Outcomes

Outcomes after antireflux surgery are excellent with 85 to 95% of patients experiencing relief of symptoms. These outcomes persist long-term (5 or more years), and can be demonstrated with objective measurements (manometry and pH evaluation) or subjective criteria (Gastrointestinal Quality of Life Index). Failure of the operation to correct reflux and/or recurrent symptoms after a period of apparent success occurs in 5 to 20% of patients within the first 10 years. The etiology of recurrent symptoms can be multiple (technical errors at surgery, disruption of the wrap, poor wound healing, etc) and may require treatment with either medical therapy or re-operation. If a second operation is required, the majority of patients will still have long-term resolution of GERD.

GERD and Airway Disease

Airway manifestations of GERD are now recognized as a significant component of the disease spectrum. Patients with pulmonary or laryngeal disease caused or exacerbated by GERD are much more likely to respond to surgical than medical therapy. Confirming a link between GERD and airway symptoms, such as coughing, sore throat, hoarseness, and asthma with diagnostic testing, however, is difficult. Thus, these patients, as a group, have the highest chance of improvement, and at the same time failure, with surgical therapy. Successful intervention is most likely dependent on picking those patients in whom reflux is the culprit.

One problem is that the exact mechanism by which reflux causes respiratory symptoms is unclear and is likely due to several different mechanisms. Aspiration is one obvious and likely common mechanism of airway injury. Vagal nerve stimulation may induce bronchospasm or potentiate the bronchomotor response to other triggers. Although acidic refluxate likely plays a role in both of these mechanisms, it is possible that neutralized and/or alkaline gastric contents may cause symptoms as well. This may be why medical therapy is often ineffective.

It is therefore not surprising that accurate diagnosis is the most difficult problem in this patient population. The presence of typical symptoms of reflux (heartburn and regurgitation) does not mean that GERD is the cause (because GERD symptoms may be present in up to 40% of the population). Likewise, the absence of heartburn does not exclude GERD as the cause because many patients with clear GERD-induced airway disease never experience heartburn. Because the presence or absence of atypical symptoms is a poor predictor of reflux, more objective measurements are required. Although 24-hour pH monitoring is the gold standard for confirming the diagnosis of GERD, it unfortunately has many shortcomings in patients with predominantly respiratory symptoms. Because GERD is so common, pH monitoring may be abnormal, but in some cases, unrelated to the patient's symptoms. Moreover, respiratory diseases may also cause secondary reflux induced by coughing or due to intrathoracic pressure. Finally, we have noted that a substantial number of these patients have evidence of reflux into their pharynx (and thus likely aspirating), even though their standard esophageal acid exposure is normal.

We have observed that the presence of acid in the pharynx on pH monitoring is a strong predictor of respiratory symptom response to medical and surgical therapy. We have, therefore, used this test liberally and found its positive predictive value to be quite helpful. In patients with laryngeal manifestations (eg, cough, hoarseness) direct laryngoscopy can be of additional value. It can identify erythema, edema, polyps, or other signs of airway irritation or injury. Unfortunately, no individual finding is diagnostic of reflux-induced injury. However, the combination of abnormal laryngoscopy and pharyngeal reflux provides the strongest evidence currently available for reflux-induced airway injury.

Although medical therapy may be effective, it is much less so for respiratory symptoms compared with typical symptoms of GERD. Surgical therapy is more effective in patients with airway symptoms, and this is probably due to the fact that antacid medication cannot adequately control regurgitation and aspiration. In addition to normalizing esophageal acid exposure, surgery eliminates regurgitation and, thus, aspiration potential. This is critical because even small amounts of regurgitation may result in the persistence of airway symptoms (Farrell et al, 1999). Thus, we recommend surgical intervention to patients with atypical symptoms when the evidence suggests that reflux is the etiology.

BE

BE represents a severe form of GERD in which chronic exposure of the esophageal mucosa to gastric contents leads to the development of intestinal metaplasia. The main concern is that BE can subsequently progress to dysplasia and eventually adenocarcinoma (AC). There are two controversial issues that may affect the decision to recommend surgical therapy to patients with BE. The first question to ask is whether an operation will provide long-term control of the patient's symptoms. The second question is whether an operation will affect the natural history of the BE and, thus, reduce the risk of developing cancer.

Control of GERD

Antireflux surgery is effective at controlling GERD. Symptoms are relieved in the vast majority of patients with BE, and this relief has been shown to be durable. There is also objective evidence of superior control of reflux in these patients when pH monitoring is performed, and fewer redevelop esophagitis and stricture after surgery when compared with medical therapy (Atwood et al, 1992). In our own series of 106 BE patients undergoing laparoscopic antireflux surgery between 1994 and 2000 with a mean follow-up of 40 months, 79% had resolution and 93% had improvement in their heartburn. Ninety-four percent had improvement in their regurgitation, and 83% had improvement in their dysphagia. As a group there was a significant increase in the LES pressure (9.0 to 19.2 mm Hg) and a drop in the amount of reflux to normal levels (distal acid exposure from 27.9 to 4.0% and a DeMeester score from 100.6 to 17.1) after surgery. Certainly antireflux procedures in patients with BE can be more difficult (secondary to higher incidence of large hiatal hernias, esophageal inflammation, and shortened esophagus) and require meticulous technique, but good results are attainable.

Regression of BE

The most important aspect of BE is its propensity to progress to dysplasia and AC. Because medical therapy does not seem to decrease this risk, the goals of treating patients with BE have not included modulating this risk. Our group and other authors have recently shown that an effective operation cannot only limit progression, but in some patients it can lead to the regression of BE (Hofstetter et al, 2001). In our own series of 54 patients with short segment BE (< 3 cm), 30 (55%) had complete regression of their disease at a mean follow-up of 43 months after surgery. Other authors have also reported the regression of dysplasia after surgery (DeMeester and DeMeester, 1999; Low et al, 1999).

Continued Surveillance

Although regression of BE is possible after operation, surgery does not alleviate or replace the need for ongoing surveillance of these patients. In our own series, the complete regression of long segment BE (> 3 cm) did not occur, although many patients did have a reduction in total length of disease.

Two factors may be responsible for the superior response of the epithelium to surgical therapy. First, medical therapy titrated to symptom relief usually does not eliminate acid exposure (Dixon et al, 2001). Second, there may be a significant role of alkaline and bile reflux in the pathogenesis of BE progression. Supporting the concept that reflux must be dramatically reduced for regression of BE to occur, we found that regression occurred only when surgical therapy effectively reduced all types of reflux. Thus, antireflux surgery controls symptoms, allows for the discontinuation of medicine, and gives the patient the best chance at regression of the disease. Therefore, laparoscopic antireflux surgery is an excellent option that should be considered and offered to most patients with BE.

Other Considerations

Ineffective Esophageal Motility

There has long been concern about performing a fundoplication in patients with abnormal peristaltic function of the esophagus. For this reason manometry is generally recommended in the preoperative work-up, with surgeons performing a partial fundoplication or "tailoring" the operation when manometric data reveal ineffective esophageal motility. The implication of this is not trivial. Ineffective esophageal motility is more likely in patients with severe GERD, and many studies have demonstrated the inferiority of a partial fundoplication compared with a total fundoplication. There is increasing evidence, however, to suggest that a total fundoplication does not increase the incidence of dysphagia in patients with ineffective peristalsis. Because a full fundoplication provides superior reflux control, it would be preferred if it did not lead to higher incidence of dysphagia.

At the University of Washington, we abandoned the use of a partial (Toupet) fundoplication in 1997 for most patients with impaired peristalsis. We observed that although both procedures were effective at controlling typical symptoms of GERD (heartburn, regurgitation, etc), a total fundoplication was more likely to relieve existing dysphagia than a partial fundoplication. Furthermore, there was essentially no development of new dysphagia, the most feared outcome. It is now our practice to perform a full 360° wrap in all patients, with the exception of those who essentially have aperistalsis of the esophagus.

Paraesophageal Hernia

Paraesophageal hernias are a type of hiatal hernia in which a portion of the stomach (generally fundus) herniates into the mediastinum with the gastroesophageal junction either below the diaphragm (type 2 hernia) or above the diaphragm (type 3 hernia). Traditionally, surgeons considered the presence of a paraesophageal hernia a surgical emergency/urgency. This dogma resulted from two papers published in the late 1960s and early 1970s by Skinner and colleagues (1967) and by Hill (1973). They observed a high incidence of acute gastric volvulus, which carried with it a high operative mortality rate. More experience, a reduction in operative mortality, and recent studies seem to have tempered this finding and approach. Stylopoulos and colleagues (2002) demonstrated that published studies overestimate the mortality of emergency surgery (17% vs 5.4%), and if elective surgery is routinely recommended, it would be more beneficial than observation in less than one in five patients.

Elective repair in this generally elderly patient population carries significant risk. Therefore, we recommend repair through a laparoscopic approach of paraesophageal hernias in younger, healthy patients (no matter what their symptoms) and in those patients whose symptoms seem to justify risk.

Conclusions

Most individuals who suffer from GERD will never require an operation. We believe, however, that certain groups of patients will benefit significantly from surgical therapy. If the goals of the operation are clear, and patients are evaluated and selected appropriately, surgical therapy for GERD can be recommended with the confidence that the disease will be cured and the majority of patients will be satisfied.

Supplemental Reading

Anvari M, Allen C. Five-year comprehensive outcomes evaluation in 181 patients after laparoscopic Nissen fundoplication. J Am Coll Surg 2003;196:51–7.

Atwood SE, Barlow AP, Norris TL, Watson A. Barrett's oesophagus: effect of antireflux surgery on symptom control and development of complications. Br J Surg 1992;79:1050–3.

Bowrey DJ, Peters JH, DeMeester TR. Gastroesophageal reflux disease in asthma: effects of medical and surgical antireflux therapy on asthma control. Ann Surg 2000;231:161–72.

Carlson MA, Frantzides CT. Complications and results of primary minimally invasive antireflux procedures: a review of 10,735 reported cases. J Am Coll Surg 2001;193:428–39.

DeMeester SR, DeMeester TR. The diagnosis and management of Barrett's esophagus. Adv Surg 1999;33:29–68.

Dixon MF, Neville PM, Mapstone NP, et al. Bile reflux gastritis and Barrett's oesophagus: further evidence of a role for duodenogastro-oesophageal reflux? Gut 2001;49:359–63.

Farrell TM, Smith CD, Metreveli RE, et al. Fundoplication provides effective and durable symptom relief in patients with Barrett's esophagus. Am J Surg 1999;178:18–21.

Hill LD. Incarcerated paraesophageal hernia: a surgical emergency. Am J Surg 1973;126:286–91.

Hofstetter WL, Peters JH, DeMeester TR, et al. Long-term outcome of antireflux surgery in patients with Barrett's esophagus. Ann Surg 2001;4:532–9.

Kamolz T, Granderath F, Pointner R. Laparoscopic antireflux surgery. Surg Endosc 2003. [In press]

Katzka DA. Motility abnormalities in gastroesophageal reflux disease. Gastroenterol Clin North Am 1999;28:905–15.

Katzka DA, Castell D. Successful elimination of reflux symptoms does not insure adequate control of acid reflux in patients with Barrett's esophagus. Am J Gastroenterol 1994;89:989–91.

Low DE, Levine DS, Dail DH, Kozarek RA. Histological and anatomic changes in Barrett's esophagus after antireflux surgery. Am J Gastroenterol 1999;94:80–5.

Lund RJ, Wecher GJ, Raiser F, et al. Laparoscopic Toupet fundoplication for gastroesophageal reflux disease with poor esophageal body motility. J Gastointest Surg 1997;1:301–8.

Patti MG, Arcerito M, Feo CV, et al. An analysis of operations for gastroesophageal reflux disease: identifying important technical elements. Arch Surg 1998;133:600–7.

Simpson WG. Gastroesophageal reflux disease and asthma. Diagnosis and management. Arch Intern Med 1995;155:798–803.

Skinner DB, Belsey RH, Russell PS. Surgical management of esophageal reflux and hiatus hernia. Long-term results with 1,030 patients. J Thor Cardio Surg 1967;53:33–54.

Stylopoulos N, Gazelle GS, Rattner DW. Paraesophageal hernias: operation or observation? Ann Surg 2002;236:492–500.

Wetscher GJ, Glaser K, Hinder RA, et al. Respiratory symptoms in patients with gastroesophageal reflux disease following medical therapy and following antireflux surgery. Am J Surg 1997;174:639–43.

CHAPTER 13

Endoscopic Therapies for Gastroesophageal Reflux Disease

Reza Shaker, MD, and Walter J. Hogan, MD

The treatment paradigm for gastroesophageal reflux disease (GERD) disorders was well established at the onset of the second millennium. Potent antacid medications and laparoscopic fundoplication surgery were well-accepted treatment modalities effective for the great majority of GERD sufferers. However, there remained a significant minority of GERD patients unable or unwilling to be aided by these conventional therapies. Some patients were unresponsive or did not tolerate medications; others were noncompliant or adverse to lifelong use. Some patients were volume regurgitators or developed supraesophageal complications of GERD, and operative therapy was often an unwanted alternative therapy.

Recently, the combination of sophisticated technology and instrument design was adapted to endoscopic treatment modalities for GERD. Two of these unique devices were introduced into the medical community 3 years ago following United States Food and Drug Administration (FDA) approval. Since then an estimated 8,000 to 9,000 patients with GERD problems have been treated with endoscopic devices. Two additional perendoscopic treatments have received approval for clinical use in treating GERD and other devices are soon to follow. The introduction of this new unique approach to treating GERD patients raises the important question: Do these endoscopic devices fulfill an unmet need, or is this technology in search of a mission?

This chapter discusses the unique devices and techniques in detail and the potentials and pitfalls associated with the clinical infusion of perendoscopic techniques to treat GERD patients. The future role of this treatment modality for treating GERD patients is in the evolutionary stages and much more information is required before its clinical usefulness is established.

The Gastroesophageal Junction

The focus of perendoscopic treatments to prevent gastric reflux is directed towards the gastroesophageal junction (GEJ). Both the physiologic and anatomic components to the acid reflux barrier occupy this zone (Figure 13-1). Primary factors enhancing gastroesophageal reflux are a hypotensive lower esophageal sphincter (LES) pressure and transient LES relaxations (tLESrs). Structural alterations at the anatomic hiatus enhance the opportunity for orad escape of gastric contents into the esophagus.

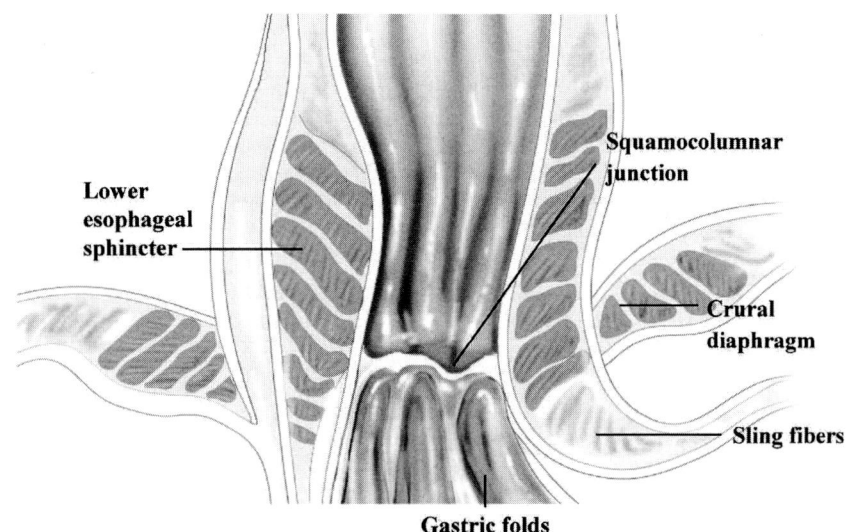

FIGURE 13-1. Schema of gastroesophageal junction (GEJ).

The zone of the LES is approximately 4 cm in length. The proximal 2 cm of the LES is surrounded by the crural diaphragm; the distal portion of the sphincter is intra-abdominal in position. Sling or oblique fibers of the gastric fundus located beneath the LES contribute to the overall antireflux barrier. The sling fibers anatomically form a "C" configuration. (The open side of the "C" is oriented to the lesser curvature of the stomach) (Boyle et al, 1985). A "flap valve" results from this design. Pressure within the gastric fundus accentuates the "flap valve" mechanism, which embraces the distal portion of the esophagus and enhances the LES pressure (Mittal et al, 1995).

tLESr events are a vagovagal reflex and are triggered by gastric distention. The afferent receptive field is located in the gastric cardia and fundus where vagal fibers with specialized terminal endings called intraganglionic laminar endings (IGLEs) exist (Zagorodnyuk et al, 2001). These IGLEs are deformity sensitive neural transducers arranged within the proximal stomach and appear to be responsible for receptive relaxation and tLESr initiation.

The majority of patients with severe esophagitis have an axial hiatus hernia (Jones et al, 1991). Thinning and elongation of the phrenoesophageal membrane leads to herniation of the stomach into the posterior mediastinum. Hiatal hernias may range in size from a type I or "sliding" variety to a type IV that is associated with a large enough hiatal defect to allow other organs to enter the sac (Kahrilas and Pandolfino, 2004). A hiatal hernia may add complicating features to the GERD algorithm by several mechanisms. A hernia may impair acid clearance from the esophagus, or crural contractions can force compartmentalized acid upwards into the distal esophagus. A large hiatal hernia is associated with widening of the esophageal hiatus that impairs the ability of the crural diaphragm to function as a sphincter (Sloan et al, 1992). Finally, hiatal hernias are associated with loss of the flap valve mechanism and the intra-abdominal portion of the esophagus obviating important factors in the prevention of gastroesophageal reflux (Mittal and Balaban, 1997).

Thus, gastroesophageal reflux is multifactorial offering a number of target choices for proponents of perendoscopic therapies.

Perendoscopic GERD Therapies

Several endoscopic devices have been developed and used to treat GERD patients during the past 4 years. The current perendoscopic devices and vendors are listed in Table 13-1. Despite considerable numbers of procedures performed to date, endoscopic treatment modalities for GERD have escaped the scrutiny of carefully designed, randomized, sham studies to critically evaluate their efficacy. Patient treatment groups have been carefully selected to avoid the majority of GERD sufferers with severe problems. Head-to-head studies comparing endoscopic GERD treatment with currently accepted treatment modalities for reflux disease are lacking. Factors to consider in the endoscopic treatment of GERD are shown in Table 13-2. Clinical outcome results of endoscopic GERD treatments have been determined almost exclusively on the basis of short-term, open-label trials. There has been a paucity of peer-reviewed publications. Finally, concerns about the safety, durability and cost-effectiveness of endoscopic GERD therapy have yet to be adequately answered.

Despite these imposing, critical issues, the number of new endoscopic devices introduced as treatment options for GERD is growing. Premarketing guidelines for future devices for GERD therapy are shown in Table 13-3. At present, perendoscopic GERD treatment modalities have been designed to augment the reflux barrier based on one of the

TABLE 13-1. Endoscopic Devices for Gastroesophageal Reflux Disease Therapy

Device	Vendor	Antireflux Mechanism	FDA Approval
Stretta	Curon Medical Inc, Sunnyvale, CA	RF thermal energy	Yes
Endocinch	CR Bard, Inc, Murray Hill, NJ	Sewing/plication	Yes
ESD	Wilson-Cook Med, Inc, Winston-Salem, NC	Sewing/plication	Yes
Enteryx	Boston Scientific, Natick, MA	Injection biopolymer	Yes
Plexiglass	Rohn & Haas, Philadelphia, PA	Injection biopolymer	No
Plicator	NDO Surgical Inc, Mansfield, MA	Plication technique	No
Gatekeeper	Medtronic, Minneapolis, MN	Implantable biopolymer	No

FDA = US Food and Drug Administration; RF = radiofrequency.

TABLE 13-2. Factors in Endoscopic Therapy for Gastroesophageal Reflux Disease

- Esophagus: Vigorous contractions; longitudinal, shortening; GEJ angulation; wall thickness
- Procedure: Large diameter overtubes; blinded balloon inflations/needle deployment; injections/placement of foreign polymers; instrument impaction
- Anesthesia: Increased amount conscious sedation; general infrequently
- Competence: Adequate training and experience with device/technique

GEJ = gastroesophageal junction.

TABLE 13-3. Future Endoscopic Gastroesophageal Reflux Disease Devices Premarketing Guidelines

- Stringent FDA assessment for approval
- Mandatory sham, controlled trials
- Assured safety of device/procedure
- Longevity of therapeutic benefit
- Comparisons to conventional treatments
- Applicability to all GERD patients
- Cost-effectiveness treatment modality

FDA = US Food and Drug Administration; GERD = gastroesophageal reflux disease.

following three general techniques: (1) radiofrequency (RF) thermal energy, (2) sewing or plication, and (3) injectable or implantable biopolymers. A review of these sophisticated technologies and procedures is necessary to gain an appropriate perspective into the current and future role for this approach to GERD management.

RF Thermal Energy Systems

Background

RF ablation techniques are not new to medicine. RF energy has been used over the decades to treat a variety of medical disorders ranging from tumor ablation to accessory A-V pathway disruption in patients with Wolff-Parkinson-White Syndrome. The effects of Stretta RF on the GEJ are incompletely elucidated to date but appear to be a combination of focal tissue remodeling and/or afferent vagal neurolysis.

Earlier studies to determine the effect of RF energy on tissue alteration in the GEJ were performed on porcine and canine models. Histopathic assessment was inconclusive in the pig study whereas the dog model demonstrated marked muscle hypertrophy and fibrosis (Utley et al, 2000). Segments of tissue from the gastric cardia showed a significant increase in thickness after RF energy delivery. However, an endoscopic ultrasonogram (EUS) study in a small group of patients performed prior to and 6 months following RF treatment showed no significant alteration in the wall thickness in the GEJ region (Dibaise et al, 2002).

A second potential mechanism for RF effect may be disruption of the vagal mechanosensory mechanism, which triggers tLESrs (ie, neurolysis). Human studies have shown a significant reduction in the frequency of distention-induced tLESrs at 3 and 6 months in a group of 20 patients following Stretta treatment (Tam et al, 2003). The postprandial tLESr rate diminished from a mean of 6.8 to 5.2 per hour during a 3-hour postmeal recording period. In this study, it should be noted that the RF energy delivery to the cardia was more intense than currently recommended. A most recent preliminary report suggests RF energy may also effect sensory factors in the GEJ zone (Ark et al, 2003). A group of 13 patients were examined before and 3 and 6 months after RF treatment for GERD. The Bernstein acid perfusion test (infusion of 0.1 HCl into the mid-esophagus for 30 minutes) was performed as part of the investigation. Before RF treatment all patients had a positive symptomatic response during the acid infusion test. Six months after RF therapy, 4 patients became insensitive to acid infusion, and the mean time before symptoms were experienced by the patients during acid infusion was prolonged significantly from 9 ± 6 to 17 ± 1 minutes.

Device: Stretta System

Curon Medical Inc (Sunnyvale, CA) received approval from the FDA to market the "Stretta System" for treatment of GERD in April 2000. The Stretta System consists of a 4-channel control module generator for automated modulation of RF energy output while constantly monitoring tissue temperature and the RF delivery catheter. The circuitry is completed by an electrode pad applied to the back and connected to the control module. The catheter RF delivery component consists of a distal inflation balloon covered by 4 electrode strips or sheaths positioned radially at 90° increments. (The catheter system can be continuously irrigated with water during RF energy delivery from ports adjacent to the needle entry sites.) Within each delivery sheath is a curved 5.5 mm needle electrode that is deployed into tissue during balloon distention. During the flow of RF current between the needle and surrounding tissue, thermocouples in the base and tip of the nickel-titanium catheters provide constant feedback information to the control module about the tissue temperatures. The computerized control algorithm continuously ensures optimal target tissue temperature of 85°C at the electrode tip and below 50°C at the mucosa. This provides spherical thermal lesions in the tissue surrounding the tip while the overlying mucosa remains relatively unaffected by RF injury.

Procedure

Anatomic distances from the squamocolumnar junction (SCJ) to the incisor teeth are obtained at initial endoscopic examination. Following placement of a guidewire, the endoscope is removed and the Stretta catheter is inserted over the wire and positioned 1 cm above the SCJ based on the interval markings on the shaft of the instrument relative to the electrode sites. The electrodes are deployed during balloon inflation (2.5 psi) into the muscle of the GEJ. RF energy is delivered for 90 seconds; reduction in the electrode impedance is displayed on the consul screen as the electrodes penetrate into muscle. Following completion of the initial set of lessons, the balloon is deflated, the needles retracted, and the catheter is rotated 45°. A second set of lesions are made in the same axial plane establishing a circular ring of 8 RF thermal burns. Three additional rings are created in a similar manner at 0.5 cm above the SCJ, at the SCJ, and 0.5 cm below. Following this, the catheter is inserted into the stomach, the balloon is inflated to 25 cc and the ensemble is retracted against the hiatus and the electrodes are deployed once again. Two "pull-back" rings of 12 lesions are formed subsequently in the cardia. Optimally, 14 lesion sets (56 RF sites) are delivered during a total of 21 minutes of active RF therapy (Figure 13-2).

In the initial open-label report of 47 patients treated with the Stretta procedure, conscious sedation involved midazolam (mean 6.7 mg; range 2.0 to 13.5) and either fentanyl (mean 13.4 mg; range 75 to 275) or meperidine (mean 114 mg; range 12.5 to 300). Multiple lesion sets were created (mean 13.8 ± 2.5) with a mean total procedure time

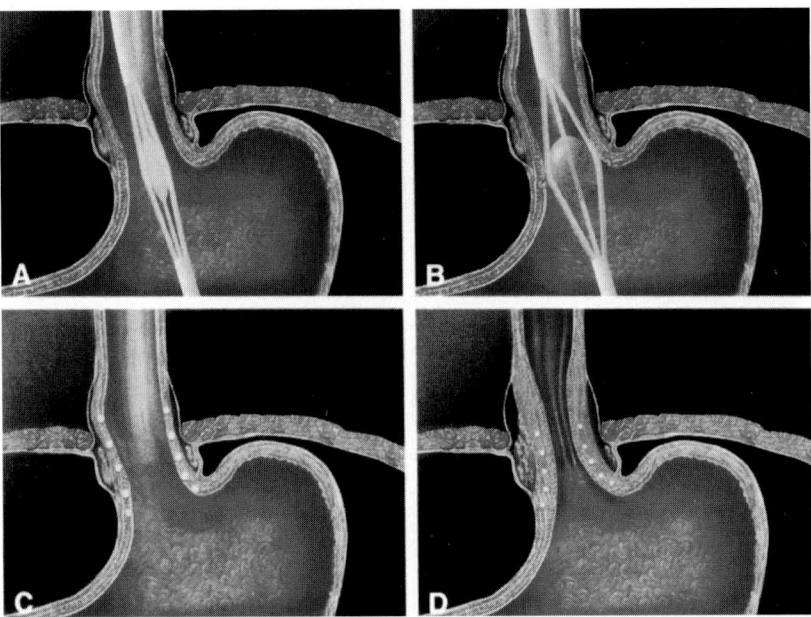

FIGURE 13-2. Stretta System (Curon Medical Inc, Sunnyvale, CA) radiofrequency thermal energy system.

of 69 ± 17 minutes. In this report, the RF energy delivery time was 52 ± 10 minutes (Triadalfilopoulos et al, 2001).

Endoscopic Suturing (Plication)

BACKGROUND

Endoscopic suturing devices developed for gastric fold plication have undergone a series of redesigns and retesting in laboratory animals over the last decade. The initial trial of suturing in humans was published in abstract form in 1994 by Swain and colleagues. Endoscopic suturing of proximal gastric fundic folds (gastroplasty) is designed to alter the anatomy of the GEJ by cinching the cardia along the lesser gastric curvature accentuating the angle of this.

DEVICE: ENDOCINCH SYSTEM

The Bard Interventional Endoscopic Suturing System (EndoCinch) was approved by the US FDA for clinical use as an alternative treatment modality for GERD in May 2000. This system originally included a miniature-sewing capsule attached to an endoscope, a knot pusher, metal-tagged sutures, and suture cutter. The current model has a small ring and peg-cinching tag that obviates the necessity for hand-tying knots, cutting suture ends, and cinching together the tag parts at the surface of the gastric tissue (Swain et al, 2000).

Procedure The EndoCinch procedure requires an overtube and two upper endoscopes. The metal sewing capsule is attached to the tip of the first endoscope; the second endoscope cinches sutures through a catheter device that deploys a ceramic plug and ring through which the sutures are threaded. Only two intubations per procedure are necessary.

A 19.7 mm overtube is inserted over a 15-mm Savary-type dilator and advanced over a guidewire into the stomach. The first endoscope with mounted sewing capsule is passed through the overtube below the GEJ to the desired location. Gastric tissue is aspirated into the hollow end of the sewing capsule for 10 seconds. A handle attached to the biopsy port on the endoscope advances a hollow-core needle, which has been back-loaded with a metal tilt-tag attached to a 3.0 suture through the sectioned tissue. A stiff wire pushed through the hollow needle by the control handle drives the metal tilt-tag forward to be captured into the sewing capsule tip. The suturing system is withdrawn through the overtube along with the tilt-tag attached to the suture. The same tilt-tag suture is reloaded into the hollow core needle and the sewing procedure is repeated. The second stage is optimally placed 1 to 1.5 cm away from the first stitch. Subsequently, the two stitches are pulled together and cinched by the ceramic plug and ring attached to the second endoscope (Figure 13-3).

Effect Two to three plications are formed during the EndoCinch procedure. The plications most commonly are placed circumferentially 1 cm below the GEJ at the 3-6-9 o'clock positions or in linear fashion 1, 2, and 3 cm below the GEJ. The majority of the stitches are placed in the submucosa. The initial multicenter study used a technique that averaged 8 steps per plication (repeated for each additional plication) (Filipi et al, 2001). The mean procedure time took 68 minutes, and 17% of patients required general anesthesia. A more recent publication of experience using the EndoCinch technique reported a mean procedure time of 45 minutes (range

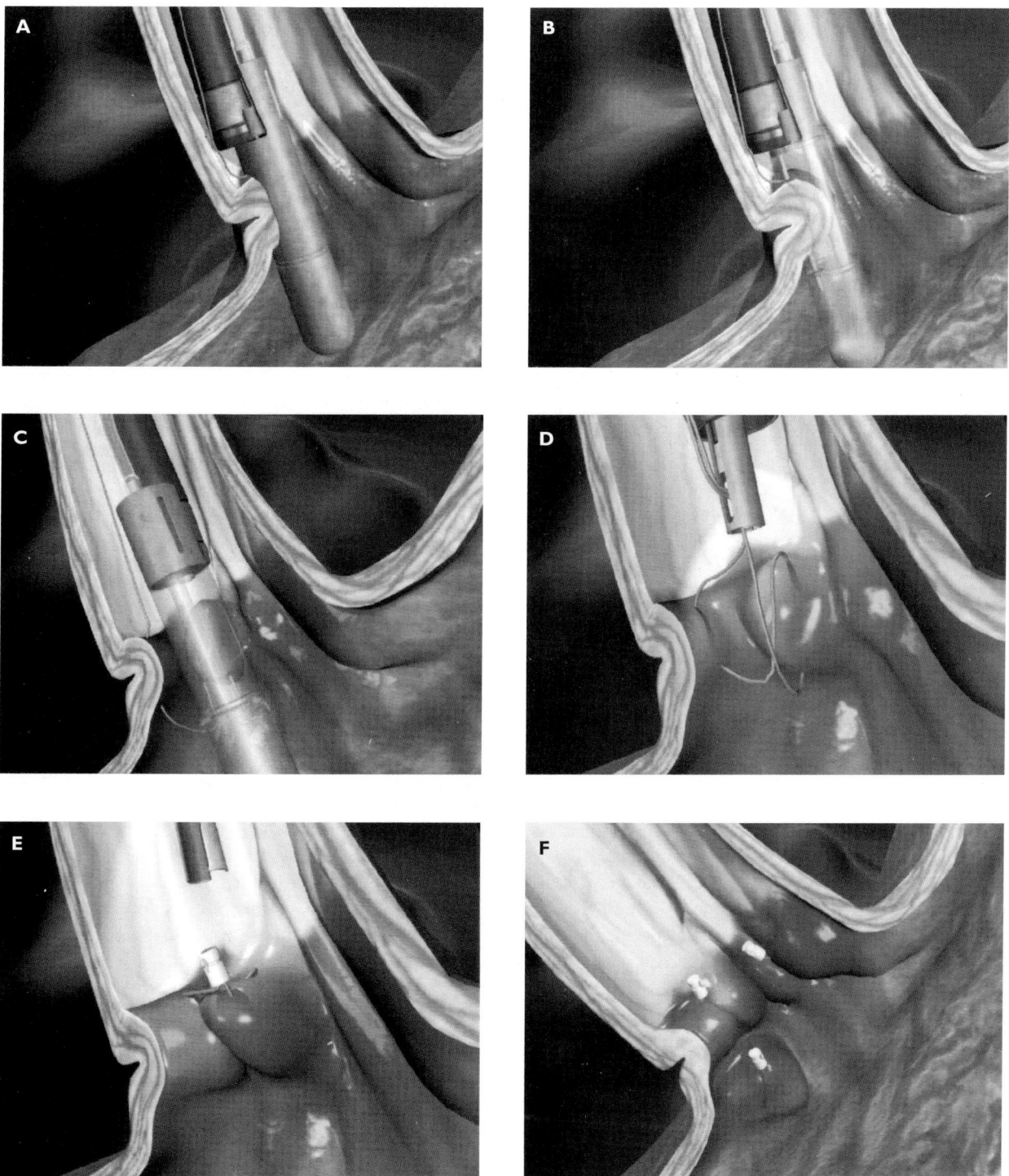

FIGURE 13-3. EndoCinch (Bard Interventional Endoscopic Suturing System, CR Bard Inc, Murray Hill, NJ). Step-wise sequence of application is shown top left to bottom right.

25 to 100 minutes). Conscious sedation included the use of midazolam (mean dose 21 mg [range 8 to 60 mg]) and pethidine (mean dose 108 mg [range 25 to 100 mg]).

The therapeutic effectiveness of the EndoCinch gastroplication procedure to "tighten" the cardiac component of the acid reflux barrier has been compromised by the instability/loss of the submucosal stitches over time. In a recent preliminary report, a gastroplication procedure was performed in 96 patients. A total of 250 sutures were placed. Endoscopic surveillance of suture integrity was performed at three intervals following the procedure. At median of 14 weeks surveillance only 39% of all patients had all plications intact, and at median of 29 weeks only 8% of patients had preserved plication. At the third endoscopy at 62 weeks, none of the sutures were observed intact (Ben-Menachem et al, 2003). In fact, the permanence of the plication sutures has been sufficiently problematic that welding (cautery) of the adjacent gastric folds has been attempted to augment plication security (Lehman et al, 2002).

Device: ESD System

The Wilson-Cook Endoscopic Suturing Device (ESD) received FDA approval in 2003. The device consists of a flexible Sew-Right device with proximal grip handle and Ti-Knot device, external accessory tube attachable to the flexible upper endoscope, suture (braided 2.0 polyester), and a titanium knot-dipping device. This instrument requires only one intubation procedure to form multiple plications because the Sew-Right and Ti-Knot devices can be reloaded through the external accessory tube. The Sew-Right element contains 2 needles controlled by a toggle switch. A continuous single suture is used to stitch adjacent gastric folds beneath the SCJ (Figure 13-4).

Procedure

The external accessory channel is secured to the upper gastrointestinal endoscope. The Sew-Right unit is loaded with suture and a vacuum cap is advanced distally over the sewing device. The ensemble is inserted into the accessory channel and advanced into the stomach where it is visualized by the endoscopist. A needle selector on the toggle switch is oriented to the right. A proximal gastric fold is aspirated into the vacuum cap and suction applied through a port on the handle mechanism. Squeezing and releasing the handle grip extends the first (right) needle outward, securing the suture, and dragging it through the tissue. Subsequently, the needle returns to its former position. Suction is released, the needle selector or the handle is switched to the left and the second needle is advanced in similar sequence.

The sewing unit is removed. The suture ends are back-loaded through the distal end of the Ti-Knot. The Ti-Knot unit is passed through the accessory channel over the two sutures to the surface of the gastric folds. A proximal level on the Ti-Knot is squeezed, which crimps a preloaded titanium knot while simultaneously severing the excess suture.

Effect

Despite FDA clearance for clinical use, there is no information available currently about the effectiveness of gastric plication stitches applied through this mechanism.

Device: Full-Thickness Plication System

The full-thickness endoscopic plication system (NDO Surgical Inc, Mansfield, MA) device consists of a reusable instrument with a control handle, which actuates the distal end of the device, providing retroflexion and opening and closing the instrument arms and deploying a suture-based implant. The instrument contains two channels. A tissue helical retractor, designed to penetrate the gastric fold to the depth of the serosa, is inserted through the first channel. The retractor is made of stainless steel and biocompatible polymers and includes a protective sheath covering, which stabilizes the mucosal surface while securing the gastric wall and pulling it into the outstretched instrument arms. The second channel provides passage of a 5.9 mm pediatric endoscope for direct visualization of the procedure. The implant affixed to the open arms of the plicator consists of pretied 2.0 suture prethreaded onto 2 titanium retention bridges. The suture bolsters are made of soft, flexible expanded polytetrafluoroethylene materials (Figure 13-5).

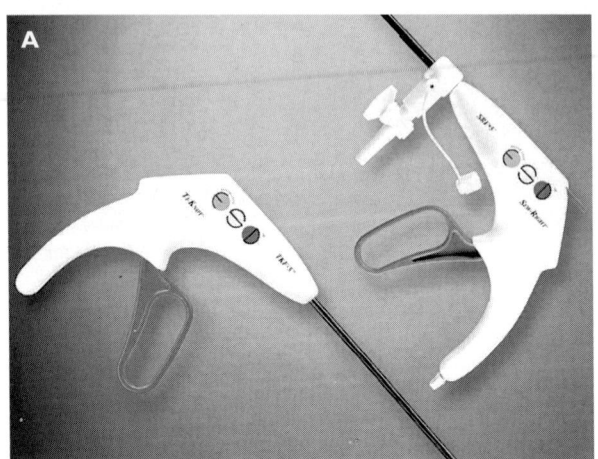
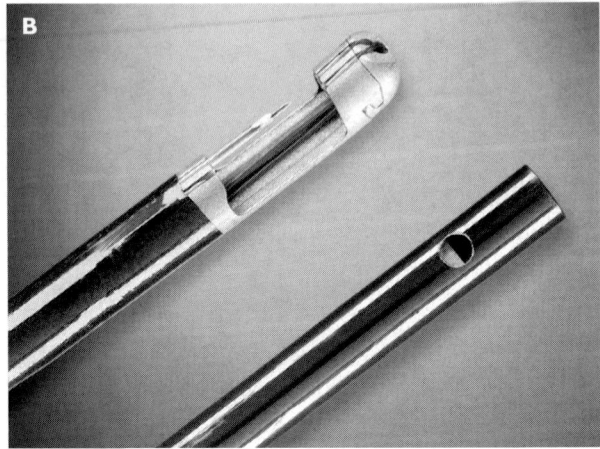

FIGURE 13-4. ESD system (Wilson-Cook Endoscopic Suturing Device, Wilson-Cook Med, Inc, Winston-Salem, NC).

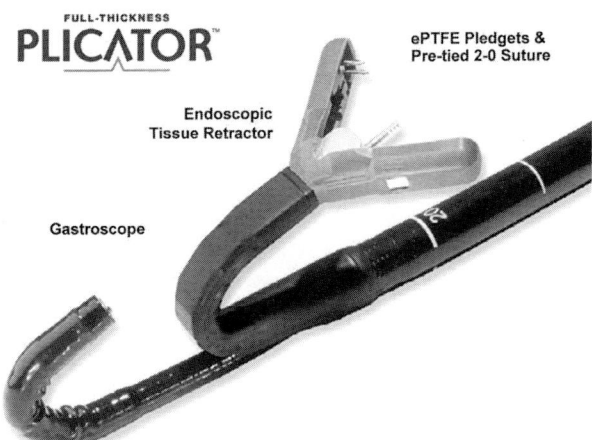

FIGURE 13-5. Plicator (NDO Surgical Inc, Mansfield, MA) full-thickness plication system. ePTFE = polytetrafluoroethylene.

Procedure

A 60 F overtube is inserted over a 54 F Savary dilator, which passed over a guidewire into the stomach (Figure 13-6). The plicator is passed through the overtube 10 to 12 cm below the GEJ. The overtube is subsequently retracted into the esophagus proximal to GEJ (see part 1 of Figure 13-6). The stomach is distended with air and the plicator is retroflexed viewing the anterior side of the cardia (see part 2 of Figure 13-6). Once the plicator is positioned, the arms are opened and the catheter with the corkscrew tip is advanced to penetrate the gastric tissue to the serosa within 1 to 2 cm of the GEJ (see part 3 of Figure 13-6). Following this, the full thickness of the gastric wall is retracted into the span of the open arms (see part 4 of Figure 13-6). The instrument arms are closed (est. 5 cm "bites") and the implant is deployed forming one large plication composed of 2 full-thickness segments of the cardia (see part 5 of Figure 13-6). The device is disengaged from the implant, the arms are closed, and the instrument is straightened and removed together with the endoscope.

Effect

The plicator provides deeper gastric cardia apposition in forming the plication than the other suturing devices. It is anticipated that over a period of time, there will be "fusing" of the opposing serosal sides of the stomach wall with tightening of the cardia providing increased durability of the plication.

In the initial publication, mean procedure time was 21 minutes. Midazolam and meperidine were administered

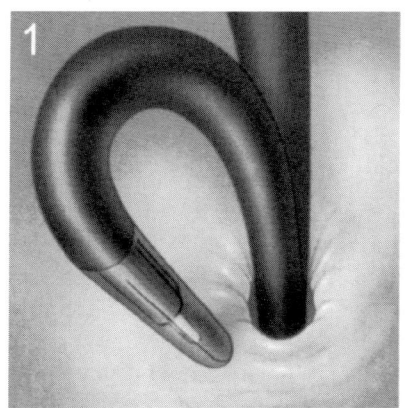
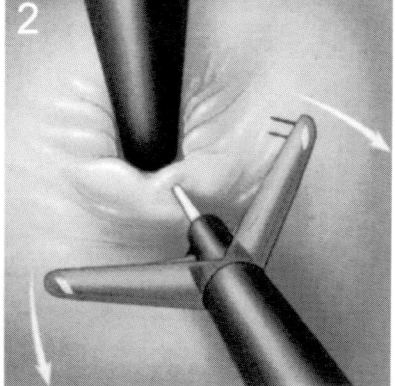
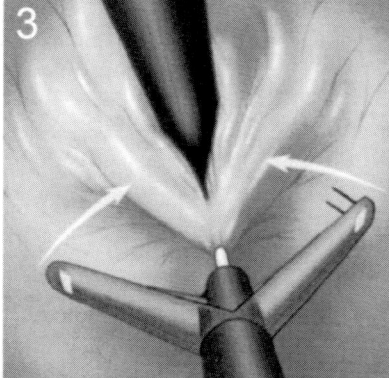
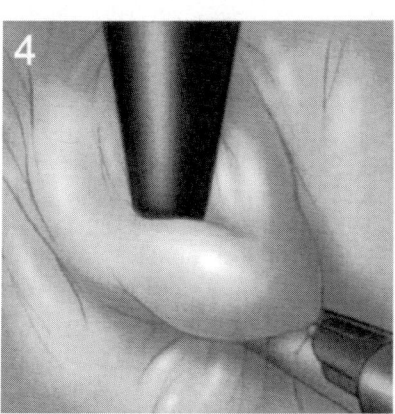
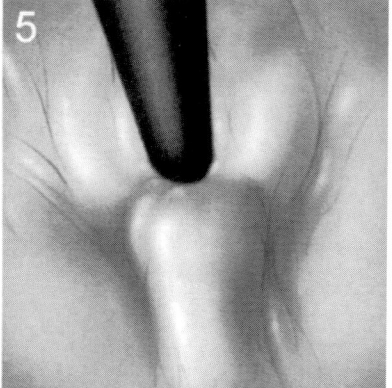

FIGURE 13-6. Stepwise sequence of Plicator system technique.

as conscious sedation, but no dosages were given. This device has not yet received FDA approval for clinical use.

Injection/Implantation of Biopolymers

BACKGROUND

Endoscopic submucosal injection of bovine collagen (O'Connor and Lehman, 1998) or *polytetrafluoroethylene* (Shafik, 1996) into the zone of the EGJ has been attempted in the past with the goal of increasing tissue compliance and altering the dimensions and radial asymmetry of the LES. Clinical improvement was transient because collagen is biodegraded and polytetrafluoroethylene particles migrate from the implantation site.

A biodegradable polymer, *ethylene-vinyl-alcohol copolymer* (*Enteryx*, Boston Scientific, Natich, MA) has been used successfully for embolization of arteriovenous malformations (Terada et al, 1991). Enteryx is a biocompatible polymer (8% weight/volume [w/v] with a radiopaque contrast agent [30% w/v tantalum powder] dissolved in an organic liquid carrier (dimethyl sulfoxide [DMSO]). Upon injection and contact with tissue or body fluids, the DMSO rapidly diffuses into tissue and results in precipitation of the polymer as a spongy mass. The viscosity of Enteryx before tissue contact is quite low. This permits injection through a 23 to 25 gauge needle. The biopolymer is neither biodegradable nor antigenic and migration or shrinkage of the material has not been demonstrated. Biocompatibility tests have been approved by domestic and international standards organizations. Enteryx injection into the minipig model has demonstrated mature, well-delineated fibrous capsules surrounding the implants into muscle at the LES zone after 3 months (Mason et al, 2000).

DEVICE

Enteryx (Boston Scientific, Natich, MA) *Injection Therapy*
The injection therapy requires an upper gastrointestinal endoscope, a 4 mm needle (23 to 25 gauge) injection catheter, a catheter flush unit, and a vial of Enteryx solution (Figure 13-7).

Procedure

Enteryx injection is performed in a unit equipped with fluoroscopy. Prophylactic antibiotics are usually administered. The injection catheter is introduced through the biopsy channel of the endoscope. The needle catheter is flushed with DMSO and filled completely with Enteryx. The tip for the injection catheter was placed at or 1 to 2 mm below the SCJ. The mucosa is punctured and Enteryx solution injected along the muscle layer or deep submucosal layer of the cardia. If the polymer forms an arc, noted fluoroscopically, additional material is injected at the same site. Otherwise, multiple separate 1 to 2 cc injections are performed in a circumferential (4-quadrant) fashion. Six to 8 cc total of Enteryx is injected although ≥ 6 cc is associated with more chest pain. The injection rate is limited to 1 cc/min to allow for polymerization and heat dissipation, the needle remains in situ to avoid backflow of material. A gray surface color with a mass effect bulging into the lumen is indicative of a shallow submucosal injection. If this is observed, injection is stopped and a new injection site is chosen. The average procedure time was 33.8 ± 10 min in one report of 85 patients (Johnson et al, 2003). Total fluoroscopy time was 11.8 ± 7.9 min. Mucosal sloughs occur with submucosal injection causing superficial ulcers, which apparently heal without problems.

Effect

Enteryx injection does not appear to "bulk" the GEJ. Observations at follow-up endoscopy show no luminal narrowing or structural abnormalities. In one report, 9 patients with underlying esophageal disease received Enteryx injection 4 to 5 hours prior to esophagectomy. Subsequently, histologic exam of the resected esophagus demonstrated polymer substance implanted into the deep submocosa contiguous with the circular muscle and within the muscularis propria in all patients with implants occasionally extending into the subserosa (Peters et al, 2003). The primary effect of Enteryx may be alteration of distal esophageal compliance.

DEVICE: PLEXIGLAS IMPLANTATION

Polymethylmethacrylate (PMMA) has been used for dental prosthesis and tissue expansion in plastic surgical operations for decades. The PMMA (100 μm) microspheres have a smooth completely rounded surface that permits injection through a needle. The substance used as a carrier for PMMA is a heated 3.5% bovine spongious encephalitis-free gelatin (1:3 suspension PMMA). Following implantation, the gelatin is phagocytized by macrophages (within 5 months) and replaced by fibroblasts and collagen fibers. The spheres are encapsulated by connective tissue and at

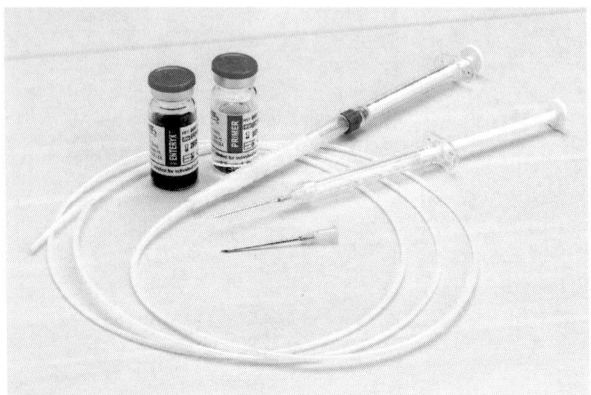

FIGURE 13-7. Enteryx (Boston Scientific, Natick, MA) injection solution and catheter delivery system.

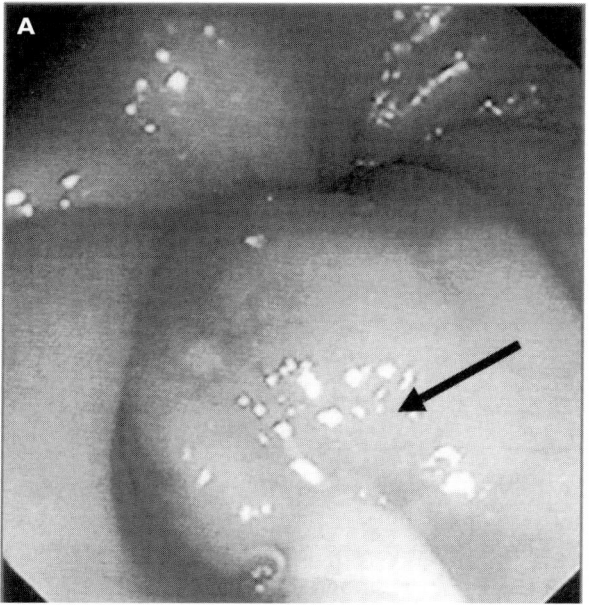 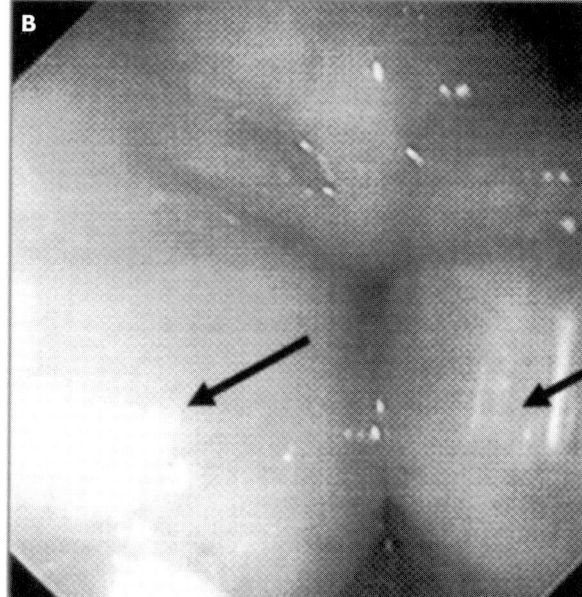

FIGURE 13-8. Plexiglas (PMMA) (Rohn & Hass, Philadelphia, PA) implantation. Appearance of distal esophagus following Plexiglas injections.

least two-thirds of the total volume of the implant remains at the injection site (Lemperle et al, 1995).

Procedure

Skin tests and antibody titers to gelatin are performed because of the large quantities of PMMA used for endoscopic therapy. In the only report to date using this injection therapy, a flexible sigmoidoscope was used (Feretis et al, 2001). The sterilized PMMA implant material is prepared in 3 mL syringes and injected into the submucosa 1 to 2 cm proximal SCJ through a shortened 90-cm catheter with a 4-mm long, 21-gauge retractable needle. Five to six injections were performed in different sites until the swelling of the esophageal folds resulted in their close luminal approximation. The treatment was repeated a second or third time depending on patient's GERD symptoms (Figure 13-8).

Effect

Procedure time averaged between 10 to 30 minutes. Followup EUS demonstrated "continuing presence" of PMMA particle at all sites in the entire group of 10 patients (Feretis et al, 2001). The properties of PMMA implant make it a potential EGJ bulking agent. The product has not received FDA approval. Further publications or follow-up studies on the use of PMMA injection treatment have not appeared since the original report.

DEVICE: EXPANDABLE HYDROGEL PROSTHESIS

The Gatekeeper (Metronics, Minneapolis, MN) technique places miniature expandable hydrogel prosthesis at the GEJ during endoscopic observation. The hydrogel prosthesis expands over 75% volume in 24 hours following tissue placement. The device includes a 16-mm overtube with a distal rigid segment containing a shelf-like structure, a 2.4-mm diameter hydrogel delivery system (needle, dilator, sheath), an injection catheter, and a packet of the hydrogel prosthesis.

Procedure

The upper gastrointestinal endoscope is inserted within the overtube and both devices passed into the distal esophagus over a guidewire to the GEJ. Suction applied from the endoscope retracts esophageal tissue into the bottom shelf of the overtube. Through a second channel in the overtube, a needle injection catheter is inserted. Saline is injected into the submucosa causing a bleb or pocket. The injection catheter is removed and the prosthesis delivery tube passed through the channel to the site of the bleb where a slit is formed. The sheath portion of the delivery system remains within the submucosal opening following removal of the needle/dilator mechanism. A dessicated 1.5-wide, 18-mm long hydrogel prosthesis is inserted into the proximal opening of the sheath and advanced by a push rod through the sheath into the submucosal slit. Following removal of the sheath, the esophageal fold is dislodged from the overtube shelf with air inflation and torque on the tube. Additional prosthesis can be placed simply by rotation of the overtube and repetition of placement technique(Figure 13-9).

Effect

Up to 12 prostheses have been placed at one time, but 6 appear to be the average number. The procedure takes approximately 15 minutes for initial prosthesis placement and 5 minutes for each additional insertion. The hydrogel

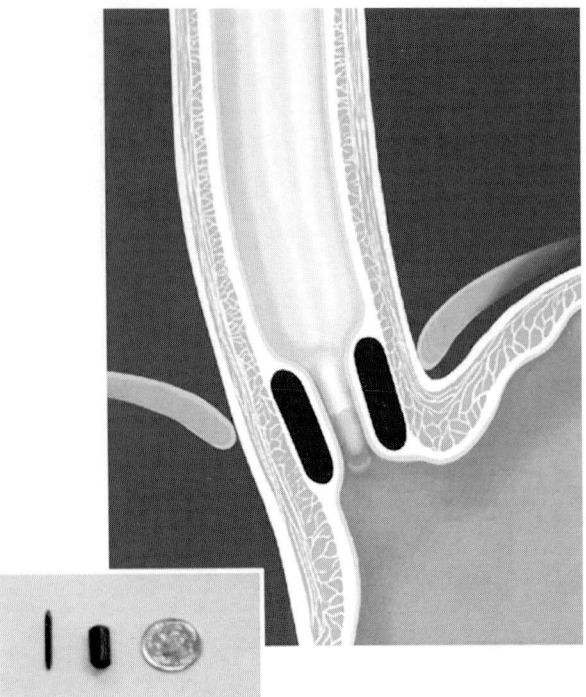

FIGURE 13-9. Gatekeeper (Medtronic, Minneapolis, MN). Expandable hydrogel prosthesis placement.

prothesis will slough if placed superficially, however. In one recent preliminary multicenter report, the Gatekeeper technique was used in a group of 60 patients, 20% of prosthesis were lost in the first week. In 6 months follow-up of one-third of the group, 75% of prosthesis were retained (Fockens et al, 2003). The mechanism of Gatekeeper appears to be a "bulking" or "augmentation" of the LES zone.

Endoscopic GERD Treatment Trials

Overview

The vast majority of clinical studies that have evaluated endoscopic treatment modalities for GERD have been open-label trials or anecdotal reports. Despite the fact that several of these endoscopic technologies were introduced into clinical medicine over 3 years ago and thousands of GERD patients have been treated, only a single randomized sham controlled study has been performed and published (Corley et al, 2003). A number of criticisms therefore are well-directed towards the conclusions drawn by their authors from the results of these other clinical trials. Patients who have been enrolled in these clinical trials all have symptoms of heartburn, regurgitation, and require antacid medication. Ambulatory 24-hr pH results are > 4.0% for total acid exposure. However, patients with a hiatal hernia > 2.0 cm and/or esophagitis > grade 2 LA classification are excluded from study participation. Complications of stricture formation and Barrett's esophagus are also exclusionary factors.

A large group of 474 GERD patients were recently examined in a retrospective study to determine eligibility for endoscopic GERD treatment using the standard restrictive criteria of these trials. Only 88 patients (32%) fulfilled the eligibility criteria (Rhoads et al, 2003). The patient populations included in these endoscopic GERD treatment trials are inadequately detailed in virtually every report. They have a "partial" or "poor" response to proton pump inhibitor (PPI) medication, often despite elevated daily doses.

The primary efficacy outcome is comparison of the use of PPI medications before versus after endoscopic treatment. Standard questionnaires are frequently used to obtain this information. Secondary outcomes are based on quantitation of patient symptoms using heartburn scores, validated GERD-Health Related Quality of Life (GERD-HRQL) questionnaire and quality of life issues measured by the Medical Outcomes Study form, SF-36. Endoscopic assessment of the esophageal mucosa before and after endoscopic treatment is often lacking in many of these reports. There are a myriad of reports concerning the results of endoscopic treatments of GERD. The following were selected as the best examples.

Treatment Trial Results

The most extensive report of endoscopic GERD treatment results is the 6 to 12 months Stretta US open-label trial (Triadafilopoulos et al, 2002). Ninety-four patients from the original 118 patients receiving Stretta RF treatment were examined after 12 months. GERD-HRQL scores improved from a mean of 27 to 9; heartburn scores were reduced 50% in 68% of patients and SF 36 scores improved significantly. There was a significant improvement in distal esophageal acid exposure (10.2 to 6.4%) although this parameter did not normalize in the majority of patients.

Eighty-eight percent of patients required daily PPI therapy at baseline. At 12 months follow-up, only 30% of patients required PPI therapy. (Interestingly, only 15% of patients were using PPI medication at the 6-month period.) Esophagitis grades were not improved although the majority of patients had 0 to grade I mucosal changes at entry into the study.

The only sham controlled study reported to date involved 64 patients from 8 participating centers who were randomized to Stretta RF GERD treatment (35 patients) or a sham procedure (29 patients). At 6 months, interested sham patients crossed over to active treatment. The 6-month assessment showed that the Stretta RF treated group had significantly improved both heartburn symptoms and quality of life scores. These symptom improvements continued at 12 months. However at 6 months, there were no differences in daily medication use between the treatment group and the control population (17 patients [55%] versus 14 patients [61%]). There was no difference in total acid exposure between the two groups to explain the improvement in GERD symptoms in the treatment group.

ENDOCINCH

The initial multicenter study with the Bard EndoCinch suturing device enrolled 64 patients with standard GERD entry criteria (Filipi et al, 2001). Ten patients withdrew from the study before the 6-month evaluation period. Heartburn severity, frequency, and regurgitation improved. The total acid exposure (< 4.0) time was also reduced significantly after EndoCinch therapy, but did not approach normalization.

Two-year open-label follow-up studies from two centers evaluated the results of Bard EndoCinch GERD therapy (Rothstein et al, 2001; Haber et al, 2001) on antacid medication usage. Their results were basically similar following suture plication, 25% of the patients discontinued all PPI medication and slightly > 25% reduced the quantity of medication. However, > 40% of patients continued on full dose medication despite the plication treatment.

In a more recent report on the outcomes of EndoCinch therapy, 22 of 26 patients completed a 1-year follow-up (Mahmood et al, 2003). At 12 months, heartburn symptoms and regurgitation scores improved significantly, whereas PPI medication was reduced by 64%. At the end of a 1-year survey, 14 patients eliminated PPIs completely whereas 8 patients remained on PPIs. Twenty-four hour pH metry monitoring was repeated after 3 months in 21 patients. There was significant improvement in mean DeMeester scores (44.1 versus 33.3) and reduction in percentage of upright acid exposure (13.5 versus 9.8), and number of reflux episodes (177.4 versus 118.2). Nonetheless, supine acid exposure (8.2 versus 7.1) and total esophageal acid exposure time (11.1 versus 9.3) were not significantly altered after EndoCinch treatment.

ENTERYX INJECTION SYSTEM

The Enteryx injection system was evaluated in 85 patients with GERD symptoms responsive to PPI medication in a 6-month follow-up report (Johnson et al, 2003). The use of PPI medication was eliminated in 74% of patients and reduced > 50% in another 10% of patients. HRQL improved from a score of 24 (preimplantation) to 4 at follow-up. Mean total esophageal acid exposure was significantly decreased from 9.5 to 6.7%; (26 of 71 patients [37%] had normalized their total acid exposure time). Interestingly, mean LES length appeared to increase from 2.0 to 3.0 cm following Enteryx therapy.

GATEKEEPER REPAIR SYSTEM

Data on the effectiveness of the Gatekeeper Repair System for treating GERD is inconclusive as of February 2004. A preliminary report from a multicenter study involving 60 patients has yielded some information about this technique (Fockens et al, 2003). As many as six protheses were implanted into the GEJ zone. At 3-month evaluation, the GERD-HRQL scores improved in 31 patients (21 versus 12). The total acid exposure on 24-hr pH metry decreased in 11 patients from 9.2 to 8.3%.

PLICATOR

The Plicator (full thickness plication) was recently evaluated in a multicenter study of 64 GERD patients (Pleskow et al, 2003). GERD-HRQL scores improved from 12.6 to 6.9 in 41 patients at 6-months follow-up. Prior to treatment 92% of patients required daily PPI medication; at 6 months posttherapy only 17% of patients needed daily medication. However, the mean to total acid exposure (pH < 4.0) decreased only 21% at 6 months in 35 patients and normalized in only 31%.

Open-Label Trials: The Caveat

The enthusiasm by investigators involved in current endoscopic GERD treatment trials is prompted by apparent symptom improvement in many patients following application of these devices. Interpretation of results in an open-label trial is suspect. The initial open-label Stretta trial of 47 patients which prompted FDA approval likened the Stretta Device equivalent to fundoplication surgery (Triadofilopoulos et al, 2001). In rebuttal to this "premature judgment," Dr Peter Kahrilas (1996) wrote "with a disease (GERD) that can have a 60% placebo response rate, it is simply not good enough to equate a 60% symptomatic response in an uncontrolled trial to existing data on alternative therapies that utilized different trial design, different clinical end points and very different patients" (Kahrilas, 2003). Schoenfeld and Scheiman (2003) are quite explicit in their concerns about the composition of an appropriately designed treatment trial. Randomization, concealed allocation and double-blinding are the only study design techniques proven to prevent an inflated estimate about the benefits of treatment."

It is worthwhile to point out that the results of the only randomized sham controlled trial (Stretta) (Corley et al, 2003) heartburn severity and associated QOL measures were significantly improved for up to 12 months in the treated group. However acid exposure and antacid requirements were similar in both treatment and sham groups.

Current Status

The therapeutic effectiveness of endoscopic treatments for GERD patients, for the most part, remains unproven.

Safety Issues

Endoscopic devices to treat GERD have been associated with complications. Postmarketing surveillance data was obtained on 1,200 patients undergoing Stretta RF treatment (Zagorodnyuk et al, 2001). A total of 15 significant complications occurred in the first 6 months after FDA approval. These complications included five esophageal perforations and two deaths. The number of complications following Stretta RF procedure may have decreased, but there continues to be morbidity associated with this endoscopic GERD therapy. A 2002 report of 118 patients who were treated with the Stretta procedure recorded 13 patients with chest distress for 2 to 5 days, 7 patients with mild transient unobstructive dysphagia, and 2 patients with delayed bleeding (1 to 3 weeks) who did not require transfusions. The morbidity rate in this study was 1.7% (Noar et al, 2002).

The EndoCinch procedure is also associated with morbidity. In the 1-year EndoCinch study, "minor" adverse effects of sore throat, vomiting, abdominal pain, chest soreness, dysphagia, and bloating, described as "transient" and resolving spontaneously within 72 hours, were reported. Two patients had significant postprocedure bleeding and one of the patients required transfusion. A "gastric mucosal tear" was observed in one patient (Mahmood et al, 2003).

The Enteryx procedure can cause significant morbidity. In the report on 85 patients treated by injection therapy, 92% experienced retrosternal pain (rated as "mild to moderate") that resolved in 2 weeks requiring prescribed analgesics in 70% of patients. Dysphagia occurred in 17 patients and lasted for 2 to 12 weeks. Ten patients experienced low grade fever for 1 to 3 days. Overall, the rate of adverse effects was 34% in this series of Enteryx-treated GERD patients (Johnson et al, 2003).

A pharyngeal perforation related to introduction of the overtube was reported in the Gatekeeper study while chronic nausea prompted the endoscopic removal of the prostheses after 3 weeks (Fockens et al, 2003).

The long term complications associated with the current array of endoscopic devices to treat GERD are unknown.

A complete 46-item bibliography is available from rshaker@mcw.edu

Supplemental Reading

Ark J, VanOlmen A, D'Haens G, et al. Radiofrequency delivery at the gastroesophageal junction in GERD improves acid exposure and symptoms and decreases esophageal sensitivity to acid infusion [abstract]. Gastroenterology 2003;148:A–19.

Ben-Menachem T, Goel S, Zonla M, et al. Endoscopic surveillance of plication after endoluminal gastroplication (ELGP) for GERD [abstract]. Gastrointest Endosc 2003;M1731:AB–1128.

Boyle IT, Altshuler SM, Nixon TE, et al. Role of the diaphragm in the genesis of lower esophageal sphincter pressure in the cat. Gastroenterology 1985;88:723–30.

Chuttani R, Sud R, Sachdev G, et al. A novel endoscopic full-thickness plicator for the treatment of GERD: a pilot study. Gastrointest Endosc 2003;58:770–6.

Corley DA, Katz P, Wo J, et al. Improvement of gastroesophageal reflux symptoms after radiofrequency energy: a randomized sham-controlled trial. Gastroenterology 2003;125:668–76.

Dibaise JK, Brand RE, Quigley EMM. Endoluminal delivery of radiofrequency energy to the gastroesophageal junction in uncomplicated GERD: efficacy and potential mechanism of action. Am J Gastroenterol 2002;97:833–42.

Feretis C, Benakis P, Demopoules C, et al. Microscopic implantation of plexiglas (PMMA) microspheres for treatment of GERD. Gastrointest Endosc 2001;53:423–426.

Filipi C, Lehman G, Rothstein RI, et al. Transoral flexible endoscopic suturing for the treatment of GERD: a multicenter trial. Gastrointest Endosc 2001;53:416–422.

Fockens P, Bruno MJ, Custamayne G, et al. Endoscopic augmentation of the lower esophageal sphincter for treatment of GERD: multicenter study of the Gatekeeper Reflux Repair System [abstract]. Gastrointest Endosc 2003;57:AB–97.

Haber GB, Marcon NE, Kortan P, et al. A 2-year follow-up of 25 patients undergoing endoluminal gastric plication (ELGP) for gastroesophageal reflux disease (GERD) [abstract]. Gastrointest Endosc 2001;53:AB-116.

Jackman WM, Wang XZ, Friday KJ, et al. Catheter ablation of accessory atroventricular pathways (Wolff-Parkinson-White Syndrome) by radiofrequency current. N Engl J Med 1991;324:1605–11.

Johnson DA, Ganz R, Aisenberg J, et al. Endoscopic deep mural implantation of Enteryx for the treatment of GERD: 6-month follow-up of a multicenter trial. Am J Gastroenterol 2003;98:250–8.

Jones MP, Sloan SS, Rabine JC, et al. Hiatal hernia size is the determinant of esophagitis presence and severity in gastroesophageal reflux disease. Am J Gastroenterol 1991;26:921–6.

Kahrilas PJ. Gastroesophageal reflux disease. JAMA 1996;276:983–8.

Kahrilas PJ. Radiofrequency energy treatment of GERD [editorial]. Gastroenterology 2003;125:970–3.

Kahrilas PJ, Pandolfino JE. In: Castell DO, Richter JE, editors. Hiatus hernia in the esophagus: 4th ed. Philadelphia: Lippincott Williams & Wilkins; 2004. p. 389–407.

Kim MS, Holloway R, Dent J, Utley DS. Radiofrequency energy (RFC) delivery to the gastric cardia inhibits triggering of transient lower esophageal sphincter relaxations and gastroesophageal reflux in dogs. Gastrointest Endosc 2003;57:17–22.

Lehman GA, Dunne DP, Hiestenk K, et al. Suturing plication of cardia with EndoCinch device: effect of supplemental cautery- a human prospective randomized trial [abstract]. Gastroenterology 2002:122:4.

Lemperle G, Gautier-Hagan N, Lemperle M. PMMA microspheres for skin tissue augmentation. Part 2: clinical investigation. Plast Reconstr Surg 1995;96:627–34.

LeVeen H, Wapnick S, Piccone V, et al. A tumor eradication by radiofrequency therapy; response in 21 patients. JAMA 1976;153:2198–200.

Mahmood Z, McMahon BP, Arfin Q, et al. Endocinch therapy for gastroesophageal reflux disease: a one-year prospective follow-up. Gut 2003;52:34–9.

Mason RJ, Hughes M, Lehman GA, et al. Endoscopic augmentation at the cardia with a biocompatible injectable polymer in a porcine model [abstract]. J Surg Endosc 2000;14:S166–230.

Mittal RK, Balaban DH. The esophagogastric junction. N Engl J Med 1997;336:924–32.

Mittal RK, Holloway RH, Penagini R, et al. Transient lower esophageal sphincter relaxation. Gastroenterology 1995;109:601–10.

Noar M, Knight S, Bidlack D. Long-term experience with the Stretta procedure in medically refractory GERD patients: the first 14 months [abstract]. Gastroenterology 2002;112:4.

O'Connor MD, Lehman GA. Endoscopic placement of collagen at the lower esophageal sphincter to inhibit gastroesophageal reflux: a pilot study of 10 medically intractable patients. Gastrointest Endosc 1988;34:106–12.

Peters JH, Silverman DE, Stein A. Lower esophageal sphincter injection of a biocompatible polymer accuracy of implantation assessed by esophagectomy. Surg Endosc 2003;17:547–50.

Pleskow D, Rothstein R, Kozarek R, et al. Endoscopic full-thickness plication for GERD; a multicenter study [abstract]. Gastrointest Endosc 2003;57:AB–96

Rhoads S, Goel S, Foegl R, et al. A large proportion of patients with symptomatic reflux disease are ineligible for endoscopic therapy [abstract]. Gastrointest Endosc 2003;S1531;AB–119.

Rothstein RI, Pohl H, Grave M, et al. Endoscopic gastric plication for the treatment of GERD: two-year follow-up results [abstract]. Am J Gastroenterol 2001;S36:A–107

Schoenfeld P, Scheiman J. An evidence-based approach to clinical practice guidelines. Clin Gastroenterol Hepatol 2003;1:57–63.

Shafik A. Intraesophageal polytef injection for the treatment of reflux esophagitis. Surg Endosc 1996;10:329–31.

Sloan S, Kahrilas PJ. Impairment of esophageal emptying with hiatal hernia. Gastroenterology 1991;100:596–605.

Sloan S, Rademaker AW, Kahrilas PJ. Determinants of gastroesophageal junction incompetence: hiatal hernia, lower esophageal sphincter or both? Ann Intern Med 1992;117:977–82.

Swain CP, Kadirk A, Manathan SS, et al. Sewing at flexible endoscopy in human gastrointestinal tract [abstract]. Gastrointest Endosc 1994;40:AB–35.

Swain P, Park PO, Kjellin T, et al. Endogastroplasty for gastroesophageal reflux disease [abstract]. Gastrointest Endosc 2000;51:AB–114.

Tam WCE, Schoeman MN, Zhang Q, et al. Delivery of radiofrequency energy to the lowest oesophageal sphincter and gastric cardia inhibits transient lower oesophageal sphincter relaxations and gastro-oesophageal reflux in patients with reflux disease. Gut 2003;57:479–85.

Terada T, Nakamura Y, Nakai K, et al. Embolization of arteriovenous malformations with peripheral aneurysms using ethylene vinyl alcohol copolymer; report of three cases. J Neurosurg 1991;75:625–60.

Triadafilapoulos G, DiBaise JK, Nostrant TT, et al. Radiofrequency energy delivery to the gastroesophageal junction for the treatment of GERD. Gastrointest Endosc 2001;53:407–15.

Triadofilapoulos G, DiBaise JK, Nostrant TT, et al. The Stretta procedure for the treatment of GERD: 6 and 12 month follow-up of the US open-label trial. Gastrointest Endosc 2002;55:149–56.

US Food and Drug Administration. Center for Devices and Radiological Health. Available at: www.fda.gov/edrh.

Utley DS, Kim M, Vierra MA, Triadafilopoulos G. Augmentation of the lower esophageal sphincter pressure and gastric esophageal junction: a porcine model. Gastrointest Endosc 2000;52:81–6.

Zagorodnyuk VP, Chen BN, Brookes SJ. Intraganglionic laminar endings are mechano-transduction sites of vagal tension receptors in the guinia pig stomach. J Physiol 2001;534:255–68.

CHAPTER 14

Barrett's Esophagus

Richard E. Sampliner, MD

Barrett's esophagus (BE) is a change in the lining of the distal esophagus from the normal squamous epithelium to an intestinal-like mucosa that includes goblet cells. BE is a complication of gastroesophageal reflux disease (GERD), and its importance lies in its potential for the development of adenocarcinoma (AC) of the esophagus and esophagogastric junction. These two simple statements carry a great deal of meaning, which translates into major management issues. The diagnosis of BE is confirmed only when there is an abnormal appearing segment in the distal esophagus at endoscopy and the biopsy documents intestinal metaplasia. Because BE is a complication of reflux, the primary therapy is aimed at controlling GERD. The role of medical and surgical therapy will be discussed in this chapter. The malignant predisposition of BE raises a different and complex issue of preventing the development of AC of the esophagus. The current estimate of the incidence of AC of the esophagus in patients with BE (0.5% per year) is clearly *less* than what was formerly thought (Drewitz et al, 1997; Shaheen et al, 2000). However, this risk remains much greater than that of an individual without BE. In addition, it has become clear that the majority of patients with BE die from causes not related to AC of the esophagus (Conio et al, 2001).

Treating GERD

BE represents the severe end of the spectrum of GERD. Patients typically have prolonged exposure to a pH < 4 in their distal esophagus, which is more acidic than that experienced by other patients with GERD. Appropriate therapy involves proton pump inhibitors (PPIs). The controversy with therapy is not what class of agents to use (the most potent one) but what the *endpoint of therapy* should be. Escalation to twice daily dosing may be necessary to control symptoms in some patients with BE. However, it is clear that even with control of reflux symptoms, patients with BE commonly have ongoing abnormal esophageal acid exposure. A randomized trial demonstrated that PPIs control esophageal acid exposure more effectively than H2 receptor antagonist therapy (Montgomery et al, 2001). There is also a trial showing similar outcomes in relation to dysplasia in patients treated medically with PPIs compared with antireflux surgery (Parilla et al, 2003). Antireflux surgery is usually effective in lessening reflux; it normalizes esophageal acid exposure in the majority of patients. If surgery, which usually prevents reflux of all gastric contents, fails to completely stop neoplastic progression, it would be unexpected for pharmacologic treatment to do so. Currently, in theory, therapy is driven by the pragmatic endpoint of relieving patients' symptoms. Until there is data showing that an intervention that more rigorously controls esophageal acid exposure has an impact on the development of cancer, the standard practice of relieving symptoms will not change.*

Antireflux Surgery

The role of fundoplication in patients with BE has shifted over the decades. The rapid introduction and success of laparoscopic fundoplication has increased the application of this procedure. Antireflux surgery is appropriate in patients with volume reflux (ie, ongoing regurgitation even when their heartburn is controlled) and in patients who prefer a surgical approach to taking daily medications. Theoretically, the mechanical correction provided by antireflux surgery would most effectively prevent the reflux of gastric contents into the esophagus and, therefore, have maximum beneficial effect. There are no large randomized studies of medical versus surgical therapy to document an impact on the incidence of AC of the esophagus. A large meta-analysis from the published literature on therapy of BE by Corey and colleagues (2003), suggests that the incidence of cancer is similar whether the therapy has been medical or surgical (Corey et al, 2003). Surprisingly, one of the experienced surgical groups in the country has a five-year series with antireflux surgery in patients with BE that demonstrates a 20% failure rate in relation to symptoms, recurrence of hiatal hernia, and abnormal 24-hour pH (Hofstetter et al, 2001). Most patients with BE have hiatal hernias, and patients with longer segments of BE tend to have longer hiatal hernias. Antireflux surgery in patients with large hiatal hernias can be more of a technical challenge. There is a separate chapter on antireflux surgery (see Chapter 11, "Management of Extraesophageal Presentations of GERD").

---

*Editor's Note: A flaw in this concept is the observations that patients who develop BE become less symptomatic with acid reflux.

Preventing AC of the Esophagus

There is only one form of therapy that is clinically believed to prevent the development of AC of the esophagus. It is an *esophageal resection,* once high grade dysplasia (HGD) has been documented. This is assuming that the patient has only HGD and, in fact, is not harboring an occult AC that has already spread to regional lymph nodes. In addition, there is emerging data that photodynamic therapy used to endoscopically ablate HGD can reduce the development of AC of the esophagus as described in the next chapter (see Chapter 15, "Ablative Therapy in Esophageal Disease"). In the face of cancer risk, we are left with surveillance endoscopy as a tool of early detection and potential intervention to improve survival. On the horizon is the possibility of chemoprevention as a strategy to decrease the development of AC.

Esophagectomy

Esophagectomy has been the *standard procedure for HGD and early AC* of the esophagus. The operative mortality is sensitive to the volume of procedures performed at an institution, but even at high volume institutions (greater than six procedures per year), the operative mortality remains 3%. The morbidity is 30% and includes primarily cardiopulmonary and anastomotic leaks. The five-year survival for esophagectomy for early AC in recent studies exceeds 80%. These excellent results are due to patient selection, experienced centers, and improved contemporary perioperative management.

Surveillance Endoscopy

Whether the individual is a candidate for endoscopic surveillance is the first issue to address in a patient with BE. Is the patient so debilitated that he cannot undergo periodic endoscopy? Does the patient agree to regular endoscopic surveillance and is he capable of adhering to such a program? Is the patient willing to undergo endoscopic or surgical intervention? We need to inform our patients that even if they follow the recommended schedule of endoscopy, it is possible for a more advanced cancer to be found. The patients need to understand that surveillance endoscopy is an empiric approach that does not guarantee uniform success.

The first step of endoscopy in a patient with BE is to document whether or not the mucosa is regular. A regular mucosa requires systematic quadrantic biopsies every 2 cm. However, if there are marked irregularities in the mucosa, endoscopic mucosal resection (EMR) needs to be considered to adequately stage the patient. There is a separate chapter on EMR (see Chapter 6, "Endoscopic Mucosal Resection"). If the resected specimen demonstrates cancer in the lamina propria, this may be a sufficient intervention. However, if the cancer goes beyond the muscularis mucosa, there is a 25% likelihood of regional lymph node involvement. Such a cancer requires either surgical resection or chemoradiation.

Surveillance endoscopy is performed by the majority of gastroenterologists in the United States. Clinical guidelines published by the American College of Gastroenterology suggest that the frequency of endoscopy should be driven by the grade of dysplasia (Figure 14-1). Interval endoscopy and systematic biopsies are recommended with the interval determined by the severity of dysplasia. If a patient has no dysplasia on quadrantic biopsies every 2 cm of BE appearing mucosa, then a repeat endoscopy should be done in the next 2 years to document the lack of dysplasia. Once this is documented, the patient can undergo endoscopy every 3 years (Sampliner, 2002).[†]

If a patient is found to have low grade dysplasia (LGD), a repeat endoscopy should be performed within the next 6 months to document that this is the highest grade of dysplasia that is present in the esophagus. If LGD is documented on the second endoscopy, then this patient can undergo annual endoscopy with systematic biopsies until no dysplasia is found on two consecutive endoscopies. The *limited information* on the natural history of LGD suggests that the majority of these patients will have no dysplasia during follow-up endoscopy and *10% of patients* will progress to HGD or adenocarcinoma of the esophagus.[‡] If a patient is found to have HGD, a repeat endoscopy within the next 3 months is appropriate to rule out the presence of AC of the esophagus. Then the options of continuing surveillance, endoscopic ablation and resectional surgery remain.

A major controversy in the surveillance for BE is the commitment of necessary resources and the cost effectiveness. The ability to concentrate surveillance on high risk patients would be most advantageous. The last decade has seen an explosion of information on the molecular biology of carcinogenesis in BE. However, no biomarker or panel of markers has been validated as predictive of cancer in multicenter follow-up studies of patients with BE.

The optical detection of dysplasia is another emerging area that could help more effectively risk-stratify patients with BE. If validated, these techniques could recognize dysplasia in the absence of biopsy and allow for endoscopic therapy during the same procedure. Laser-induced fluorescence, light scattering spectroscopy, fluorescence spectroscopy, Ramen spectroscopy, and fluorescence induced with 5-aminolevulinic acid are all being evaluated. None of these techniques is ready for clinical application.

[†]Editor's Note: Getting the recommended number and distributions of surveillance biopsies, as well as having pathology support, is important if using any guidelines.

[‡]Editor's Note: This guarded view of indefinite or LGD in BE is less pessimistic than that commonly held for LGD in the colon in inflammatory bowel disease patients.

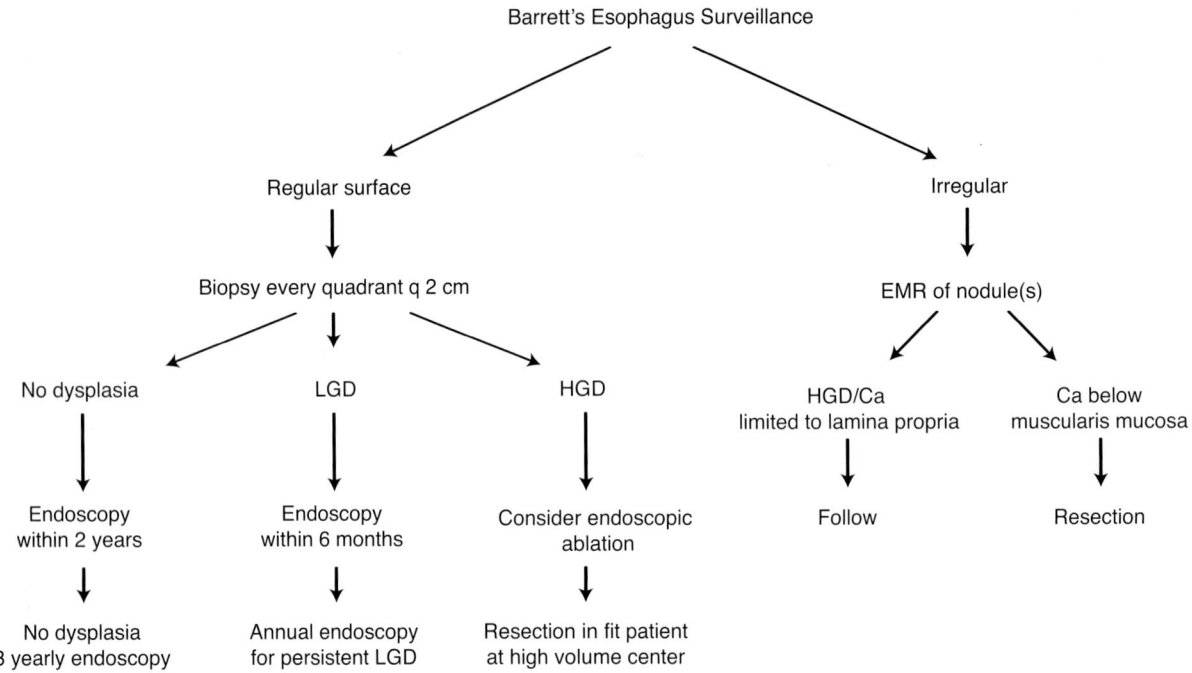

FIGURE 14-1. Barrett's esophagus surveillance. EMR = endoscopic mucosal resection; HGD = high grade dysplasia; LGD = low grade dysplasia.

Endoscopic Ablation

The preliminary data now available from a large multicenter trial, which randomized patients to photodynamic therapy using porfimer sodium with PPI versus PPI alone, suggest that this therapy is ready to enter the clinical arena. This is the largest randomized trial to date on any therapy in patients with BE. With a minimum follow-up of 2 years, there has been a documented decrease in the development of AC of the esophagus in patients undergoing photodynamic therapy. Thus, a therapy less than esophageal resection, may offer the opportunity to reduce the development of AC of the esophagus by 50% while maintaining esophageal function. The immediate potential mortality of esophagectomy is avoided, but the possibility of failure to eliminate the later development of cancer in the in situ esophagus is an additional issue that the patient and physician must face. Other forms of endoscopic ablation therapy are still considered experimental. The widely applied modalities have been thermal, including argon plasma coagulation and multipolar electrocoagulation. The next chapter (see Chapter 15) is about ablation therapy in esophageal disease.

Chemoprevention

There is much epidemiologic case control literature documenting that aspirin and nonsteroidals reduce the likelihood of the development of cancer of the esophagus, including AC by an estimated 43%. Chemoprevention trials are currently being initiated, but there are currently no data to guide clinical practice. Given the widespread use of aspirin for cardiovascular prophylaxis and nonsteroidal anti-inflammatory drugs for musculoskeletal problems in the at risk population (older males), the future use of one of these agents for chemoprevention seems likely. The fact that patients with BE are already treated with PPIs reduces the risk of the GI toxicity of these agents.

Conclusions

Major developments in the medical and surgical therapy of GERD, including PPI therapy and antireflux surgery, have been applied to patients with BE in the last decade. In spite of emerging techniques for the optical recognition of dysplasia and of the profusion of potentially predictive molecular markers of cancer risk, surveillance endoscopy and biopsy remain the cornerstone of efforts to improve survival from AC of the esophagus in patients with BE. Photodynamic therapy for HGD in BE is entering the clinical arena. Esophagectomy performed at a high volume institution remains a procedure with mortality and morbidity issues, but with excellent long term survival in early AC detected during surveillance. Chemoprevention offers a less invasive strategy for the future prevention of AC of the esophagus.

Supplemental Reading

Conio M, Cameron AJ, Romero Y, et al. Secular trends in the epidemiology and outcome of Barrett's oesophagus in Olmsted County, Minnesota. Gut 2001;48:304–9.

Corey KE, Schmitz SM, Shaheen NJ. Does a surgical anti-reflux procedure decrease the incidence of esophageal adenocarcinoma in Barrett's esophagus? A meta-analysis. Am J Gastroenterol 2003:In press.

Corley DA, Kerlikowske K, Verma R, Buffler PA. Protective association of aspirin/NSAIDs and esophageal cancer: a systematic review and meta-analysis. Gastroenterol 2003;124:47–56.

Drewitz DJ, Young MA, Maples MR, Ramirez FC. Esophageal mechanosensitivity in Barrett's esophagus. A prospective study with age matched controls. Gastroenterol 1997;112:A106.

Ell C, May A, Gossner L, et al. Endoscopic mucosal resection of early cancer and high grade dysplasia in Barrett's esophagus. Gastroenterol 2000;118:670–7.

Hofstetter WL, Peters JH, DeMeester T et al. Long-term outcome of antireflux surgery in patients with Barrett's esophagus. Ann Surg 2001;234.

Montgomery E, Goldblum JR, Greenson J, et al. Dysplasia as a predictive marker for invasive carcinoma in Barrett's esophagus: a follow-up study based on 138 cases from a diagnostic variability study. Hum Pathol 2001;32:379–88.

Parilla P, Martinez de Haro L, Ortiz A, et al. Long-term results of a randomized prospective study comparing medical and surgical treatment of Barrett's esophagus. Ann Surg 2003;237:291–8.

Peters FTM, Ganesh S, Kuipers EJ, et al. Endoscopic regression of Barrett's oesophagus during omeprazole treatment: a randomised double blind study. Gut 1999;45:489–94.

Shaheen NJ, Crosby MA, Bozymski EM. Is there publication bias in the reporting of cancer risk of Barrett's esophagus? Gastroenterol 2000;119:333–8.

Sampliner RE, Practice Parameters Committee ACG. Updated guidelines for the diagnosis, surveillance, and therapy of Barrett's esophagus. Am J Gastroenterol 2002;97:1888–95.

CHAPTER 15

Ablative Therapy in Esophageal Disease

Sanjay Jagannath, MD, and Marcia I. Canto, MD, MHS

Barrett's esophagus, defined as the replacement of normal esophageal squamous epithelium with specialized columnar metaplasia characterized by goblet cells (Sampliner, 1998), is a condition that often arises in the setting of chronic gastroesophageal reflux disease. The presence of Barrett's epithelium is clinically important because it represents a premalignant condition that predisposes to the development of esophageal adenocarcinoma (AC). There is a separate chapter on endoscopic ultrasound and fine needle aspiration (see Chapter 5, "Endoscopic Ultrasound and Fine Needle Aspiration").

The incidence of esophageal AC is the highest among all cancers in the United States and Western Europe. The estimated 5-year survival of esophageal cancer (EC) is a dismal 5 to 10%, and, currently, it represents the seventh leading cause of cancer death worldwide. The overall risk of developing EC in the setting of Barrett's epithelium is estimated to be approximately 0.5% per year; however, the relative risk of developing malignancy in Barrett's epithelium is 30 to 125 times greater than that reported in the non-Barrett's epithelium population (Drweitz et al, 1997; Shaheen et al, 2000; Conio et al, 2003; Provenzale et al, 1994). The risk of malignancy is greatest in Barrett's epithelium with advanced dysplasia, where the finding of occult AC in this population is as high as 30%. Prophylactic esophagectomy is generally recommended for patients with known high grade dysplasia, and it can often be performed with low mortality and excellent long term survival in high volume surgical centers (Heitmiller, 2003; Falk et al, 2000; Pellegrini and Pohl, 2000; Tseng et al, 2003). However, recent studies have emphasized the risks associated with surgical resection and thus generated interest in minimally invasive treatment techniques (Berkmeyer et al, 2002).

The question of what to do with patients who are not surgical candidates for an esophagectomy remains. The current recommendation is to perform ablative therapy of the esophagus for patients with dysplastic Barrett's epithelium or early mucosal AC. The goal of Barrett's epithelium ablation is to eliminate or at least downgrade mucosal dysplasia. The premise is that destruction of premalignant Barrett's epithelium followed by normal squamous re-epithelialization in an anacid environment results in curing of Barrett's epithelium and eliminates the risk of esophageal AC.

After the publication of the first case report in 1993, various ablative therapies have been reported, including laser therapy (Nd:YAG), argon plasma coagulator, multipolar or bipolar electrocoagulation, photodynamic therapy (PDT), endoscopic mucosal resection (EMR), and cryotherapy. Despite the paucity of well-designed trials with long term follow-up to support using ablative techniques, there is a general tendency among gastroenterologists to incorporate ablative techniques into their practice. In response to a survey conducted in 2002, only 15% of physicians believed ablation lowered the risk of AC and only 19% believed using ablation was supported by the medical literature; however, 25% of physicians did use ablation at the time of initial survey, and this percentage increased to 36% in the follow-up survey (Gross et al, 2002).

This chapter discusses the various ablative techniques that have been studied in patients and their results. It will not discuss, however, EMR indications or techniques since this is reviewed in a separate chapter dedicated to EMR (see Chapter 6, "Endoscopic Mucosal Resection"). In addition, discussions regarding experimental or possible future techniques (eg, cryotherapy, chemoprevention) will not be discussed, at this time, because there are no published human trials. The goal of successful ablation therapy should be complete ablation of Barrett's epithelium without evidence of recurrence over a long period of follow-up.

An important caveat is to note that there is currently *no indication* for ablative therapy of *nondysplastic Barrett's epithelium* outside of approved clinical trials. The risk of developing AC in the setting of nondysplastic Barrett's epithelium is very low, and these patients should be maintained on a proton pump inhibitor (PPI) and undergo routine endoscopic surveillance. Finally, the authors will discuss how they incorporate ablative techniques in their practice. There is a separate chapter on Barrett's esophagus (see Chapter 14, "Barrett's Esophagus").

Ablation with Thermal Electrocoagulation

Thermal coagulation of the Barrett's mucosa can be accomplished using bipolar and heat probes with an overall success rate of approximately 75%. Sampliner and colleagues

(2001) treated 58 patients with non-dysplastic Barrett's epithelium with up to six sessions of multipolar electrocoagulation. Over a short follow-up period, 78% had endoscopic and histologic reversal of Barrett's epithelium. Similar results were obtained in another study, by Kovacs and colleagues (1999), with 27 patients and 4.5 months of follow-up.

The mucosa is treated until there is a uniform white coagulum, and the treatment is repeated monthly until ablation of the Barrett's mucosa is achieved. The rate of residual or recurrent columnar lined epithelium is approximately 20 to 30%, and the follow-up periods range from 4.5 months to 3 years. Advantages to thermal ablation include its wide availability, inexpensive cost, and relatively few major side effects (Eisen, 2003).

Most published trials demonstrate the efficacy and overall safety of thermal ablation of Barrett's mucosa, but unfortunately, few studies involve patients with dysplastic Barrett's epithelium. Sharma and colleagues (1999) reported long term follow-up in 11 patients (4 of whom had low grade dysplasia), where a mean length of 4.4 cm of Barrett's epithelium was ablated. After mean follow-up period of 3 years, 3 patients had residual intestinal metaplasia, but none had associated dysplasia.

Ablation with Laser Therapy

Two types of lasers have been used to ablate Barrett's epithelium, Nd:YAG (1064 nm; depth of injury 3 to 4 mm), and KTP (532 nm; depth of injury 1 mm) (Eisen, 2003). Table 15-1 summarizes selected studies evaluating the success of laser therapy to achieve complete ablation of Barrett's epithelium. Most trials report eradication rates of approximately 70 to 80% with laser therapy and complication rates of 0 to 17% (Luman et al, 1996; Weston and Sharma, 2002).

Bonavina and colleagues (1999) prospectively evaluated Nd:YAG laser eradication of Barrett's epithelium. They documented eradication in 8 of 12 patients with tongues of Barrett's, 1 of 4 patients with circumferential Barrett's epithelium, and in both patients with short-segment Barrett's epithelium. In addition, 1 patient progressed in a 6-month period to develop AC *underneath* regenerated squamous epithelium. It is apparent that in some patients, although the superficial mucosa regenerates with normal squamous epithelium (also known as "neo-squamous epithelium"), deep mucosal islands of Barrett's epithelium and/or carcinoma may develop. These islands are not endoscopically visible, may occur with any type of ablative therapy, and represent a failure of ablative therapy.

The remaining published studies in Table 15-1 evaluated the success of laser ablation therapy in patients with dysplastic (predominantly high grade) and early AC. Collectively, the complete response rate averaged 80%, with a mean follow-up period of 16.5 months (Salo et al, 1998; Gossner et al, 1998; Weston and Sharma, 2002). The complication rate ranged from 0 to 17.6%, and primarily included stricture formation requiring dilation for management. The most commonly reported side effects included odynophagia, early dysphagia, and chest pain. Laser may be best suited for small areas of dysplastic Barrett's epithelium or cancer, especially if a clinician decides to use a second mode of ablative therapy for residual short segment dysplastic Barrett's epithelium.

Ablation with Argon Plasma Coagulator

The argon plasma coagulator is a device that allows high frequency electric current to be conducted "contact-free" through ionized, electrically conductive argon gas. The optimal distance between the probe and the target tissue is between 2 to 8 mm, and the depth of injury is more superficial than laser or PDT (Eisen, 2003; Grund and Farin, 2000).

Table 15-2 lists the eradication rates for argon plasma coagulator in some published series success (Mork et al, 1998; Van Laethem et al, 1998). Successful or *complete eradication* (CE) is defined as histologic ablation of Barrett's epithelium at the time of follow-up. Identification of Barrett's epithelium underneath the regenerated squamous epithelium ("Barrett's neo-epithelium") is considered a failure of ablation. The majority of studies ablated non-dysplastic Barrett's epithelium with argon plasma coagulator, showing an overall average CE of 73%, a Barrett's neo-epithelium rate of approximately 24%, and an overall major complication rate of 2.7%. Pereira-Lima and colleagues

TABLE 15-1. Ablative Treatment with Lasers

Authors	Patients (N)	Mean Follow-Up (mo)	Mean Laser Tx (N)	CE of Barrett's Epithelium (%)	Complications (%)
Luman et al, 1996	8 ND	6	NR	0	0
Salo et al, 1998	11	26	4	82	NR
Gossner et al, 1999	10	10.6	2.4	80	0
Bonavina et al, 1999	18 ND	14	3	61	11
Weston and Sharma, 2002	14	12.8	NR	78	17

CE = complete eradication at time of follow-up; ND = non-dysplastic Barrett's epithelium; NR = not reported.

TABLE 15-2. Ablative Treatment with Argon Plasma Coagulator

Authors	Patients (N)	Mean Follow-Up (mo)	CE of Barrett's Epithelium (%)	Barrett's Neo-Epithelium (%)	Complications (%)
Mork et al, 1998	15 ND	9	73	6.7	0
Van Laethem et al, 1998	17 ND	12	53	61	12
Grade et al, 1999	9 ND	NR	78	22	0
Schulz et al, 2000	73 ND	12	99	0	4.3
Tigges et al, 2001	22 ND, F	12	91	NR	NR
Basu et al, 2002	50 ND	12	32	44	0
Morino et al, 2003	23 ND, F	31.9	87	9	0
Byrne et al, 1998	30	9	70	30	10
Pereira-Lima et al, 2001	33	10.6	97	NR	12
Kahaleh et al, 2002	39	36	38	NR	NR
May et al, 1999	3 AC	24.3	67	33	0
Van Laethem et al, 2001	17 AC	24	76	NR	NR

AC = adenocarcinoma; CE = complete eradication at time of follow-up; F = fundoplication; ND = non-dysplastic Barrett's epithelium; NR = not reported.

(2001), while using a higher powered argon plasma coagulator (60 Watts), reported a 97% CE rate in ablating non-dysplastic Barrett's epithelium, but also reported major complications including strictures, chest pain lasting up to 10 days, pneumomediastinum, subcutaneous emphysema, high fevers, and pleural effusions.

For patients with dysplastic Barrett's epithelium or intramucosal AC, the average CE rate was 70% and the average Barrett's neo-epithelium rate was 31%; a reminder that *surveillance continues indefinitely despite ablation therapy* (Kahaleh et al, 2002).

One study, which prospectively followed patients for 1 to 4 years after treatment with argon plasma coagulator, found that endoscopic and histologic *recurrence rates* increased with each year of follow-up. The endoscopic and histologic recurrence rates were 10% and 40% respectively at year 1; at 4 years, both rates were 62%. Two patients progressed to cancer. Multivariate analysis revealed that short segment Barrett's epithelium and a normalized pH on PPI were predictors of sustained effects of argon plasma coagulator ablation. The authors, themselves, did not recommend the wide application of argon plasma coagulator for ablation of Barrett's epithelium (Kahaleh et al, 2002).

In general, approximately 2 to 4 argon plasma coagulator sessions performed at weekly intervals are required to ablate Barrett's epithelium. Common side effects include chest pain and odynophagia (as high as 30%). Studies have reported that argon plasma coagulator ablation was less successful in long segment Barrett's epithelium in comparison to short segment Barrett's epithelium (Basu et al, 2002; Kahaleh et al, 2002). In addition, a case report has been published of a 68-year-old man who developed intramucosal AC underneath regenerated squamous epithelium 18 months after argon plasma coagulator ablation of non-dysplastic Barrett's epithelium (Van Laethem et al, 2000). Perhaps, if Barrett's epithelium was never ablated, earlier detection of the AC would have been accomplished with routine surveillance. The overwhelming concern is that residual premalignant glands may remain after ablation therapy, and that the early diagnosis of neoplastic changes may be compromised by the squamous re-epithelialization. The bottom line is that argon plasma coagulator *may be useful in short segment dysplastic Barrett's epithelium,* but probably should *not* be considered an ideal first choice for therapy.

Ablation with PDT

PDT is a nonthermal ablative technique resulting in local tissue ablation. A photosensitive compound (usually porfimer sodium or delta-aminolevulinic acid [ALA]) is administered to the patient prior to activation using endoscopically applied laser light. The laser generates a monochromatic beam, which activates the photosensitive compound and generates cytotoxic singlet oxygen radicals resulting in rapid vascular stasis, hemorrhage, and an acute inflammatory reaction, followed by direct and anoxia-induced tumor cell death (Overholt, 1992).

The localized effect of PDT is based on several factors: the relative specificity of a photosensitizer for malignant tissue, the directed application of light, the transmission depth of the wavelength of light, and the oxygen content of the tissue (Adler and Baron, 2001). The remaining tissue heals with little cumulative or systemic toxicity; therefore PDT can be repeated and does not interfere with or preclude other forms of therapy.

The most common photosensitizers used in Barrett's ablation along with their relevant clinical properties are listed in Table 15-3 (Eisen, 2003; Prosst et al, 2003). Clinical contraindications to PDT include known porphyria (or hypersensitivity to porphyrins), tumor infiltration into the respiratory tract, and the presence of an esophagopulmonary fistula. Relative contraindications may include symptomatic pleural or pericardial effusions and unstable

TABLE 15-3. Characteristics of Photodynamic Therapy Photosensitizers

Photofrin (Porfimer Sodium)	Aminolevulinic Acid
Available in United States	Not available in US
Intravenous administration	Oral administration (5-ALA)
(2 mg/kg)	Topical administration (delta-ALA)
Risk for photosensitivity	Risk of photosensitivity
(4 to 6 weeks)	(1 to 2 weeks)
High selectivity for tumor	Limited depth of penetration (2 mm)

ALA = aminolevulinic acid.

arrythmias (Maier et al, 2001).

Patients may develop transient substernal or epigastric pain, odynophagia, or worsening dysphagia. Fever, leukocytosis, and asymptomatic pleural effusions may be present, and often resolve in several days without intervention. Major complications include perforation, aspiration, fistulas, and stricture formation (Reilly and Fleischer, 1991).

Photosensitivity can occur in approximately 60% of patients treated with PDT (Webber et al, 1999). Photofrin is primarily retained by the reticuloendothelial system of the liver, spleen, and kidney, and redistributed into the skin. Given that the longest half-life of Photofrin is 36 days, skin photosensitivity can occur for up to 3 months. Patients are cautioned to avoid direct sunlight, strong fluorescent or incandescent light, strong residential indoor lights, and radiant heat for at least 30 days. Skin photosensitivity can vary from mild erythema and pruritus, to severe erythema and edema, to blisters with skin desquamation. Topical sunscreens are not beneficial because they block ultraviolet light and not infrared light. Most patients develop at least a tan (Marcon, 1994; Saidi and Marcon 1998)! Different photosensitizers have been tested, including 5-ALA, which carries a lower rate of skin photosensitivity; however, the depth of penetration and efficacy of the ALA compounds may be less than Photofrin.

Table 15-4 lists selected clinical trials showing the efficacy of PDT in dysplastic Barrett's epithelium and early ACs (Barr et al, 1996; Gossner et al, 1998). Overholt and colleagues (2001) in their pioneering trial used a balloon fiber-centering device meant to flatten the esophageal mucosa to theoretically help reduce overtreatment and stricture formation. Subgroup analysis showed an overall mean eradication rate of 90% for dysplastic Barrett's epithelium. One-third of patients in the study developed strictures, and 6% developed Barrett's epithelium under neo-squamous epithelium. Other studies have used PDT without a centering balloon, and found identical stricture rates (Wolfsen et al, 2002). Studies that used 5-ALA appear to report fewer complications likely because the depth of penetration is less when compared to porfimer sodium. Panjehpour and colleagues (2000) designed their study to determine if steroid injection into the esophageal mucosa would reduce stricture formation in patients with PDT. They reported a comparable complication rate of approximately 30% and found that steroid injection did not reduce the risk of stricture development

Recently, the *Food and Drug Administration (FDA) has approved PDT for eradication of Barrett's epithelium with high grade dysplasia* based on the results of the PHO-BAR trial. In an unpublished-to-date randomized, multicenter, international trial, 200 patients with Barrett's epithelium with high grade dysplasia were randomized to receive PDT versus omeprazole alone. At 12 months follow-up, 41% of patients had CE of Barrett's epithelium and 72% had elimination of high grade dysplasia when compared with the control group. The PDT group had a near threefold decrease in the development of AC as compared to the omeprazole group. This has been the basis for FDA approval of PDT for eradication of high grade dysplasia in the United States and Canada (Overholt et al, 2001; Wolfsen, 2002). In the vast majority of PDT studies, a second mode of ablative therapy (argon plasma coagulator, NdYAG laser, or thermal coagulation) is used when residual Barrett's epithelium is found. The future of PDT is promising, but it depends on improving further photosensitizers with improved efficacy and decreased toxicity, improved targeting of dysplastic or neoplastic mucosa, and, hopefully, decreased cost.

Considerations When Choosing Ablative Therapy

Most of the published literature on ablative therapy for Barrett's epithelium lacks control groups and randomization. The primary endpoint is usually absence of Barrett's

TABLE 15-4. Photodynamic Therapy in Dysplastic Barrett's Epithelium and Early Cancer

Authors	Patients (N)	Agent	Mean Follow-Up (mo)	CE of Barrett's Epithelium (%)	Complications (%)
Barr et al, 1996	5	5-ALA	12	60	0
Gossner et al, 1998	32 HC	5-ALA	9.9	88.5	0
Overholt et al, 1999	100 HC	POR	19	77	34
Panjehpour et al, 2000	60 HC	POR	NR	80 to 90	30
Wolfsen et al, 2002	48 HC	POR	18.5	84	0

AC = adenocarcinoma; 5-ALA = 5-aminolevulinic acid; C = adenocarcinoma; CE = complete eradication at time of follow-up; H = high grade dysplasia; NR = not reported; POR = porfimer sodium.

epithelium (or downgrading from dysplastic Barrett's epithelium) or intramucosal carcinoma at the time of follow-up. Without adequate long term follow-up, it is impossible to document answers to critical questions, such as the following: (1) the durability of the neo-epithelium, (2) the decrease in the need for endoscopic surveillance, or (3) the elimination or decrease in cancer/death rates, and (4) the cost-effectiveness of ablative therapy.

Listed below are several important tenets to follow in clinical practice when choosing to perform ablation therapy in the esophagus.
1. Patients with high grade dyplasia/intramucosal cancer should undergo surgical resection at a center with high volume experience in esophagectomies, if they are surgical candidates.
2. Nonsurgical candidates with intramucosal cancer or high grade Barrett's epithelium should be offered ablative treatment. There is a separate chapter on palliative therapy for carcinoma of the esophagus (see Chapter 22, "Palliation of Esophageal Cancer"). There is no role for ablative therapy of non-dysplastic Barrett's epithelium outside of an approved clinical trial.
3. Patients undergoing ablative therapy should receive high-dose acid suppression with a PPI so that squamous epithelial regeneration can occur in an anacid environment.
4. Patients with focal lesions amenable to treatment (eg, a nodule of intramucosal cancer or high grade dysplasia) should be considered for EMR with or without PDT, depending on availability. The authors' preference is to do EMR followed by PDT in 1 to 2 months if residual Barrett's epithelium and high grade dysplasia or cancer persists. If EMR is unavailable, then the authors would choose PDT. There is a separate chapter on EMR (see Chapter 6, "Endoscopic Mucosal Resection").
5. Patients with long segments of dysplastic Barrett's epithelium should be treated with PDT preferentially. Argon plasma coagulation should not be the first choice for ablation in long segment dysplastic Barrett's epithelium. If multiple areas of residual dysplastic lesions persist, then retreatment with PDT should be considered. Other options include using another modality (eg, laser, argon plasma coagulation, thermal coagulation).

Summary

It is evident from reviewing the current literature on ablative therapies for Barrett's epithelium that there is significant promise in these techniques. Mainstays of good clinical practice remain using PPIs and endoscopic surveillance to monitor for progression of Barrett's epithelium, and referral of patients with high grade dysplasia or intramucosal cancer for esophagectomy, if they are surgical candidates. There is no role for ablative therapy of non-dysplastic Barrett's epithelium outside of approved clinical trials. Options for ablative therapy of dysplastic Barrett's epithelium and intramucosal AC include thermal ablation, lasers, argon plasma coagulation, and PDT. The overall eradication rate is approximately 70 to 90%, but long term eradication remains to be proven. Each therapeutic option has associated complications. Understanding the distribution and histology of Barrett's epithelium will help physicians choose appropriate ablative therapies. None of these options preclude continued endoscopic surveillance. A technique that permanently eliminates Barrett's epithelium and intramucosal cancer remains elusive. A complete 53-item bibliography is available at <sjagann1@jhmi.edu>.

Supplemental Reading

Adler DG, Baron TH. Endoscopic palliation of malignant dysphagia. Mayo Clin Proc 2001;76:731–8.

Barr H, Shepard NA, Dix A, et al. Eradication of high-grade dysplasia in columnar-lined (Barrett's) oesophagus by photodynamic therapy with endogenous generated protoporphyrin IX. Lancet 1996;348:584–5.

Basu KK, Pick B, Bale R, et al. Efficacy and one year follow up of argon plasma coagulation therapy for ablation of Barrett's oesophagus: factors determining persistence and recurrence of Barrett's epithelium. Gut 2002;51:776–80.

Berkmeyer JD, Siewars AE, Finlayson EV, et al. Hospital volume and surgical mortality in the United States. N Engl J Med 2002;346:1128–37.

Bonavina L, Ceriani C, Carazzone A, et al. Endoscopic laser ablation of nondysplastic Barrett's epithelium: is it worthwhile? J Gastrointest Surg 1999;3:194–9.

Byrne JP, Armstrong GR, Attwood SE. Restoration of the normal squamous lining in Barrett's esophagus by argon plasma coagulation. Am J Gastroenterol 1998;93:1810–5.

Conio M, Blanchi S, Lapertosa G, et al. Long-term endoscopic surveillance of patients with Barrett's esophagus. Incidence of dysplasia and adenocarcinoma: a prospective study. Am J Gastroenterol 2003;98:1912–3.

Drweitz DJ, Sampliner RE, Garewal HS. The incidence of adenocarcinoma in Barrett's esophagus: a prospective study of 170 patients followed 4.8 years. Am J Gastroenterol 1997;92:193–4.

Eisen GM. Ablation therapy for Barrett's esophagus. Gastrointest Endosc 2003;58:760–9.

Falk GW, Rice TW, Goldblum JR, et al. Jumbo biopsy forceps protocol still misses unsuspected cancer in Barrett's esophagus with high-grade dysplasia. Gastrointest Endosc 2000;52:197–203.

Gossner L, May A, Stolte M, et al. KTP laser destruction of dysplasia and early cancer in columnar lined Barrett's esophagus. Gastrointest Endosc 1999;49:8–12.

Gossner L, Stolte M, Sroka R, et al. Photodynamic ablation of high-grade dysplasia and early cancer in Barrett's esophagus by means of 5-aminolevulinic acid. Gastroenterology 1998;114:448–55.

Grade AJ, Shah IA, Medlin SM, et al. The efficacy and safety of argon plasma coagulation therapy in Barrett's esophagus. Gastrointest Endosc 1999;50:18–22.

Gross CP, Cruz-Correa M, Canto MI, et al. The adoption of ablation therapy for Barrett's esophagus: a cohort study of gastroenterologists. Am J Gastroenterol 2002;97:279–86.

Grund KE, Farin G. Clinical application of argon plasma coagulation in flexible endoscopy. In: Tytgat Guido NJ, Classen M, Waye JD, Nakazawa S, eds. Practice of therapeutic endoscopy. 2nd ed. London: Harcourt Publishers Limited; 2000. p. 87–100.

Heitmiller RF. Prophylactic esophagectomy in Barrett's esophagus with high-grade dysplasia. Langenbecks Arch Surg 2003;388:83–7.

Kahaleh M, Van Laethem JL, Nagy M, et al. Long-term follow-up and factors predictive of recurrence in Barrett's esophagus treated by argon plasma coagulation and acid suppression. Endoscopy 2002;34:950–5.

Kovacs BJ, Chen YK, Lewis TD, et al. Successful reversal of Barrett's esophagus with multipolar electrocoagulation despite inadequate acid suppression. Gastrointest Endosc 1999;49:547–53.

Luman W, Lessels AM, Palmer KR. Failure of Nd-YAG photocoagulation therapy as treatment for Barrett's esophagus—a pilot study. Eur J Gastroenterol Hepatol 1996;8:627–30.

Maier A, Tomaselli F, Matzi V, et al. Does new photosensitizer improve photodynamic therapy in advanced esophageal cancer? Lasers Surg Med 2001;29:323–7.

Marcon N. Photodynamic therapy and cancer of the esophagus. Semin Oncol 1994;21(6Suppl15):20–3.

May A, Gossner L, Gunter E, et al. Local treatment of early cancer in short Barrett's esophagus by means of argon plasma coagulation: initial experience. Endoscopy 1999;31:497–500.

Morino M, Rebecchi F, Giaccone C, et al. Endoscopic ablation of Barrett's esophagus using argon plasma coagulation (APC) following surgical laparoscopic fundoplication. Surg Endosc 2003;17:539–42.

Mork H, Barth T, Kreipe HH, et al. Reconstitution of squamous epithelium in Barrett's oesophagus with endoscopic argon plasma coagulation: a prospective study. Scand J Gastroenterol 1998;33:1130–4.

Overholt BF. Laser and photodynamic therapy of esophageal cancer. Semin Surg Oncol 1992;8:191–203.

Overholt BF, Haggitt RC, Bronner MP, et al. A multicenter, partially blinded randomized study of the efficacy of photodynamic therapy (PDT) using porfimer sodium (POR) for the ablation of high-grade dysplasia (HGD) in Barrett's esophagus (BE): results of 6-month follow-up [abstract]. Gastroenterology 2001;120:A79.

Overholt BF, Panjehpour M, Haydek JM. Photodynamic therapy for Barrett's esophagus: follow-up in 100 patients. Gastrointest Endosc 1999;49:122–5.

Panjehpour M, Overholt BF, Haydek JM, et al. Results of photodynamic therapy for ablation of dysplasia and early cancer in Barrett's esophagus and effect of oral steroids or stricture formation. Am J Gastroenterol 2000;95:2177–84.

Pellegrini CA, Pohl D. High-grade dysplasia in Barrett's esophagus: surveillance or operation? J Gastrointest Surg 2000;4:131–4.

Pereira-Lima JC, Busnello JV, Saul C, et al. High power setting argon plasma coagulation for the eradication of Barrett's esophagus. Am J Gastroenterol 2001;95:1661–8.

Prosst RL, Wolfsen HC, Gahlen J. Photodynamic therapy for esophageal diseases: a clinical update. Endoscopy 2003;35:1059–68.

Provenzale D, Kemp JA, Arora S, et al. A guide for surveillance of patients with Barrett's esophagus. Am J Gastroenterol 1994;89:670–80.

Reilly HF III, Fleischer DE. Palliative treatment of esophageal carcinoma using laser and tumor probe therapy. Gastroenterol Clin North Am 1991;20:731–42.

Saidi RF, Marcon NE. Nonthermal ablation of malignant esophageal strictures: a photodynamic therapy, endoscopic intratumoral injections, and novel modalities. Gastrointest Endosc Clin N Am 1998;8:465–91.

Salo JA, Salminen JT, Kiviluoto TA, et al. Treatment of Barrett's esophagus by endoscopic laser ablation and antireflux surgery. Ann Surg 1998;227:40–4.

Sampliner R, and The Practice Parameters Committee of the American College of Gastroenterology. Practice guidelines on the diagnosis, surveillance, and therapy of Barrett's esophagus. Am J Gastroenterol 1998;93:1028–32.

Sampliner RE, Faigel D, Fennerty MB, et al. Effective and safe endoscopic reversal of nondysplastic Barrett's esophagus with thermal electrocoagulation combined with high-dose acid inhibitition: a multicenter study. Gastrointest Endosc 2001;53:554–8.

Sampliner RE, Hixson LJ, Fennerty MB, et al. Regression of Barrett's esophagus by laser ablation in an anacid environment. Dig Dis Sci 1993;38:365–8.

Schulz H, Miehlke S, Antos D, et al. Ablation of Barrett's epithelium by endoscopic argon plasma coagulation in combination with high-dose omeprazole. Gastrointest Endosc 2000;51:659–63.

Shaheen NJ, Crosby MA, Bozymski EM, et al. Is there a publication bias in the reporting of cancer risk in Barrett's esophagus? Gastroenterology 2000;119:333–8.

Sharma P, Bhattacharyya A, Garewal HS, et al. Durability of new squamous epithelium after endoscopic reversal of Barrett's esophagus. Gastrointest Endosc 1999;50:159–64.

Tigges H, Fuchs KH, Maroske J, et al. Combination of endoscopic argon plasma coagulation and antireflux surgery for treatment of Barrett's esophagus. J Gastrointest Surg 2001;5:251–9.

Tseng EE, Wu TT, Yeo CJ, et al. Barrett's esophagus with high-grade dysplasia: surgical results and long-term outcome—an update. J Gastrointest Surg 2003;7:164–70.

Van Laethem JL, Cremer M, Peny MO, et al. Eradication of Barrett's mucosa with argon plasma coagulation and acid suppression: immediate and mid term results. Gut 1998;43:747–51.

Van Laethem JL, Jagodzinski R, Peny MO, et al. Argon plasma coagulation in the treatment of Barrett's high-grade dysplasia and in situ adenocarcinoma. Endoscopy 2001;33:257–61.

Van Laethem JL, Peny MO, Salmon I, et al. Intramucosal adenocarcinoma arising under squamous re-epithelialisation of Barrett's oesophagus. Gut 2000;46:574–7.

Webber J, Herman M, Kessel D, Fromm D. Current concepts in gastrointestinal photodynamic therapy. Ann Surg 1999;230:12–23.

Weston AP, Sharma P. Neodymium:yttrium-aluminum garnet contact laser ablation of Barrett's high grade dysplasia and early adenocarcinoma. Am J Gastroenterol 2002;97:2998–3006.

Wolfsen HC. Photodynamic therapy for mucosal esophageal adenocarcinoma and dysplastic Barrett's esophagus. Dig Dis 2002;20:5–17.

Wolfsen HC, Woodward TA, Raimonda M. Photodynamic therapy for dysplastic Barrett esophagus and early esophageal adenocarcinoma. Mayo Clin Proc 2002;77:1176–81.

CHAPTER 16

ESOPHAGEAL INFECTIONS

C. MEL WILCOX, MD

Despite advancements in immunosuppressive therapy and antimicrobial prophylaxis for organ transplant patients and the advent of highly active antiretroviral therapy (HAART) for human immunodeficiency virus (HIV) infections, esophageal infections remain an important clinical problem. The likely cause(s) of esophageal infection can often be determined based on the underlying mechanism(s) and degree of immunodeficiency, the clinical presentation including the character and severity of esophageal symptoms, physical findings, and routine laboratory tests. Endoscopic examination is the gold standard for the diagnosis of esophageal infections. Endoscopy is not only diagnostic based on the appearance of the lesions, but directed mucosal biopsy of identified abnormalities can be safely performed for a definitive diagnosis.

With the efficacy of current therapies, treatment of esophageal infections is rewarding for both patients and physicians. Even those patients with the most severe immunodeficiency, such as those with the acquired immunodeficiency syndrome (AIDS), will obtain clinical improvement with appropriate treatment. Despite this efficacy, however, when immunodeficiency persists, true cure of the infection is rare and, thus, necessitates *long term secondary prophylaxis to prevent relapse*. Where possible, removal of predisposing factors will expedite resolution and prevent recurrence. The use of HAART to restore immune function plays a central role in the "treatment" of all immunodeficiency-related complications in AIDS. There is a separate chapter on gastrointestinal (GI) and nutritional complications of HIV infection (see Chapter 46, "Gastrointestinal and Nutritional Complications of HIV Infection"). Recommended treatment regimens for common esophageal infections are summarized in Table 16-1.

Candida and Other Fungi

Candida spp, principally *Candida albicans*, are the most prevalent esophageal pathogens. When *Candida* is found in the normal host, a search for and correction of any predisposing factors plays an important role in both resolving the disease and preventing recurrence. Such factors include antibiotic use, inhaled or ingested corticosteroids, diabetes mellitus, malnutrition, and esophageal motility disturbances.

Therapy is highly effective for *Candida* esophagitis with either oral or intravenous medications. Although species other than *Candida albicans* cause esophagitis (eg, *Candida tropicalis*), speciation is not required as treatment is generally the same, regardless of species. The choice of therapy primarily depends upon the cause, severity, and expected duration of immune dysfunction. If disease is found incidentally at the time of endoscopy and the cause for candidal infection can be easily reversed (see above), no therapy may be necessary. Although *nonabsorbable locally acting treatments,* such as *nystatin* or *clotrimazole troches,* may be the therapy of choice for patients with *disease limited to the oropharynx, systemic therapy* is generally indicated for symptomatic esophageal disease. For patients with mild symptoms, minimal immunocompromise, and readily reversible immunodeficiency, a short course of a systemic agent may be given. When symptoms are more severe, an abbreviated course (7 days) of oral systemic therapy is indicated to provide more rapid symptom resolution. Immunocompromised transplant and AIDS patients

TABLE 16-1. Treatment Regimens for Common Esophageal Disease

Pathogen	Drug	Dosage	Route	Duration	Efficacy
Candida	Ketoconazole	200–400 mg/d	po	7–14 d	< 80%
	Fluconazole	100 mg/d	po/IV	7–14 d	≈ 80%
	Itraconazole	200 mg/d	po/IV	7–14 d	≈ 80%
	Amphotericin B	0.5 mg/kg/d	po/IV	7 d	> 95%
	Caspofungin	50 mg/d	IV	7–14 d	> 90%
CMV	Ganciclovir	5 mg/kg bid	IV	2–4 wks	≈ 75%
	Foscarnet	90 mg/kg bid	IV	2–4 wks	≈ 75%
	Cidofovir	5 mg/kg weekly	IV	2–4 wks	≈ 75%
	Valganciclovir	900 mg bid	po	2–4 wks	–-
HSV	Acyclovir	400 mg 5 times/d	po/IV	14 d	> 90%
	Valacyclovir	1 g tid	po	14 d	> 90%
	Famciclovir	500 mg tid	po	14 d	> 90%
	*Foscarnet	90 mg/kg bid	IV	14 d	> 95%
	*Ganciclovir	5 mg/kg/d	IV	14 d	> 95%
Idiopathic Ulcer	Prednisone	40 mg/d taper	PO	4 wks	> 90%
	Thalidomide	200–300 mg/d	PO	4 wks	> 90%

bid = twice daily; CMV = cytomegalovirus; HSV = herpes simplex virus; IV= intravenous; po = orally; tid = three times daily.
*Same dosage as for CMV.

with *Candida* esophagitis should routinely be treated with systemically acting agents. Patients with granulocytopenia are at risk for disseminated candidal infection, which mandates the use of systemically acting agents as well.

Orally administered systemically active agents include *ketoconazole, fluconazole,* and *itraconazole.* Although all of these agents are effective for the treatment of *Candida* esophagitis, *fluconazole* is the *drug of choice* because of its excellent absorption, prolonged half-life, minimal side effects, and demonstrated superiority over both ketoconazole and itraconazole (Barbari et al, 1996). Suspension formulations of fluconazole and itraconazole are a good option when odynophagia is severe. It should be recognized that ketoconazole has a number of important *drug interactions* (eg, *cyclosporine*). Also, both ketoconazole and itraconazole require an *acid milieu for absorption*, which has relevance for patients with AIDS in whom hypochlorhydria has been observed, as well as for patients receiving proton pump inhibitors. The significantly lower cost of ketoconazole, however, warrants consideration for patients with minimal immunocompromise and minimal or mild symptoms when a short course of a systemically acting agent is preferable. A brief course of *intravenous* therapy (*fluconazole, amphotericin B*) may be required when oral intake is contraindicated or compromised.

Clinical resistance to azole therapy has been observed, and both the cumulative dose of azole and the severity of immunodeficiency have been linked to resistance. Because of the concern for resistance, generally acute treatment of symptomatic episodes should be provided instead of long term maintenance therapy. When standard doses of antifungal therapy are ineffective, drug resistance should be suspected and the *dose of medication should be escalated.* Some patients may require 300 to 400 mg/d or more of fluconazole to control their symptoms. When these high doses are reached, switching from fluconazole to itraconazole should be considered. This is occcasionally helpful, but higher doses of itraconazole will also be necessary. *Flucytosine* has been used in *combination therapy,* but is ineffective as a single agent therapy, and I would not recommend its routine use. *Intravenous amphotericin B* is usually required when high dose (> 400 mg/d fluconazole) treatment fails. An emerging alternative here would be *caspofungin*, which also has to be given intravenously but has minimal toxicity (Arathoon et al, 2002). Immune reconstitution, when associated with improvements in CD4 T lymphocyte count, may be effective for refractory disease and provides effective secondary prophylaxis for patients with AIDS. Indeed, if significant immune reconstitution occurs with HAART, long term prophylaxis can be discontinued.

Other Fungi

Fungal infection of the esophagus with pathogens other than *Candida* is rare. Primary infection and hematogenous dissemination to the esophagus has been described with *Aspergillus, Histoplasma,* and *Blastomyces.* Mediastinal disease with adenopathy leading secondarily to *tracheoesophageal fistula* is a well-documented mechanism of disease from *Histoplasma* and *Blastomyces. Aspergillus* and histoplasmosis should be treated initially with intravenous *amphotericin B* in the immunocompromised patient. Alternatives to amphotericin B for *Histoplasma* include *itraconazole,* if the patient is eating and not using medications which induce P450 enzymes, *caspofungin,* and, in the near future, *voriconazole.* Itraconazole is adequate therapy for histoplasmosis in the normal host. For patients with these fungal infections, consultation with an infectious disease specialist is recommended given the serious nature of these infections and the need for long term treatment.

Empiric Antifungal Therapy

Given the prevalence of *Candida* esophagitis in AIDS, empiric antifungal therapy is widely prescribed for symptomatic patients. A prospective randomized trial comparing endoscopy with *empiric fluconazole* in HIV-infected patients with esophageal symptoms demonstrated a high response rate and substantial cost savings with fluconazole, and no patient failing empiric therapy developed complications before definitive endoscopic examination (Wilcox et al, 1996). Although not critically studied, an empirical approach is commonly employed in other immunocompromised patients. If patients do not improve rapidly following empiric therapy, I do not recommend additional empiric trials, such as with antiviral therapy. Similarly, *immunosuppressed transplant patients* who develop esophageal symptoms while already receiving prophylactic antimicrobial therapy, *warrant endoscopic examination* rather than additional empiric trials or radiological studies. This is particularly true if the patient is receiving *cyclosporine,* given the many drug interactions with this agent.

Viruses

Although viral esophagitis may occur in the "normal" host, a search for underlying immune dysfunction is always warranted. Regardless of immune function, viral esophagitis usually requires therapy. *Long term secondary prophylaxis* may be required when immunodeficiency persists and cannot be reversed.

A wealth of experience in both immunocompetent and immunodeficient patients has shown the efficacy of *acyclovir*, a nucleoside analog, for the treatment of esophageal disease. Even in patients with severe immunodeficiency, such as those with AIDS, a clinical and endoscopic response can be observed in essentially all treated patients. When severe odynophagia hampers oral intake or when there is a question of drug absorption, intravenous administration

(5 mg/kg every 8 hours) should be given. Acyclovir is generally well tolerated and has few side effects. *Valacyclovir*, a prodrug of acyclovir, and *famciclovir* are the newest agents available. These drugs have been more widely tested for genital disease and herpes zoster and demonstrate efficacy and tolerability equivalent to acyclovir. The advantage of these agents is reduced drug dosing, although at higher cost. I generally *recommend* using *acyclovir for 10 to 14 days* given its record of success and lower cost. However, if compliance is an issue, either valacyclovir or famciclovir would be reasonable substitutes. Although rare, resistance should be suspected when there is clinical failure of acyclovir; in this setting, *intravenous foscarnet* is the drug of choice and will lead to clinical cure in most patients.

Until recently, only intravenous therapies were available for *Cytomegalovirus (CMV) disease*, including ganciclovir, foscarnet, and cidofovir. *Ganciclovir* and *foscarnet* are equally effective for the treatment of CMV esophagitis resulting in cure in most transplant patients and symptomatic improvement in approximately 70 to 80% of patients with AIDS (Shafran et al, 1996). *Cidofovir* is an attractive agent given its long half-life, which makes once weekly administration possible. The new formulation of *ganciclovir (valganciclovir)* has excellent *oral* absorption and minimal toxicity. In fact, serum concentrations are equivalent to intravenous administration of ganciclovir. Trials with this agent have shown *equivalency* to intravenous ganciclovir for induction therapy for CMV retinitis in AIDS. To date, there is more limited but favorable experience in the transplant patient for the *prophylaxis* of gastrointestinal disease (Winston et al, 2003). Because of these favorable attributes, *valganciclovir* has become a first line therapy for mild disease and for prophylaxis. Until more data is available, treatment with intravenous ganciclovir should be initiated until there is complete resolution following acute CMV disease in both AIDS and transplant patients. This may be followed by valganciclovir for maintenance therapy until the immunosuppressive regimen is either discontinued (bone marrow transplant) or significantly reduced (solid organ transplant). In patients with AIDS, the diagnosis of *GI CMV disease* necessitates *opthalmologic examination* because 10 to 20% of patients have *coexistent retinitis* necessitating long term therapy. There is a separate chapter (see Chapter 46, "Gastrointestinal and Nutritional Complications of Human Immunodeficiency Virus Infection") on GI and nutritional complications of HIV infections.

The side effect profiles of ganciclovir and foscarnet are different. *Ganciclovir* is associated with *myelosuppression*, which may be severe, especially when other bone marrow suppressive drugs such as azidothymidine are coadministered. Severe granulocytopenia or anemia can be treated successfully despite continued ganciclovir therapy with granulocyte colony-stimulating factor provided other marrow suppressive drugs are discontinued. *Foscarnet* causes reversible renal insufficiency, hypocalcemia, and hypophophatemia. Renal insufficiency may be prevented by vigorous saline hydration before and during drug administration in combination with dose adjustments based on creatinine clearance. *Cidofovir* is also associated with renal insufficiency, which limits it widespread use. Administration of probenecid (2 g) 3 hours before infusion, as well as 1 L of saline 1 hour before drug infusion, will help reduce renal insufficiency. All drugs for herpes viruses only inhibit viral replication; thus, relapse is frequent following therapy if immunodeficiency remains. In patients with AIDS, the *relapse rate of CMV esophagitis* is *approximately 50%* and is *similar for herpes simplex virus*. The relapse rate for transplant patients also remains high until immunosuppressive therapy can be reduced. Fortunately, despite long term administration, CMV resistance to ganciclovir and foscarnet is uncommon.

Bacteria Including Mycobacteria

Bacterial esophagitis is very rare and has been described almost exclusively in patients with *hematologic malignancies* complicated by severe *granulocytopenia*. Single case reports have described *actinomycosis* and *nocardiosis* of the esophagus in patients with AIDS. Given the microbiology of bacterial esophagitis, these mixed infections require *broad spectrum antibiotics* with agents effective for both *oral flora* and *gram-negative enteric pathogens*. A second or third generation *cephalosporin plus vancomycin* is an appropriate initial therapy pending culture results.

Mycobacterial involvement of the esophagus remains uncommon regardless of the cause of immunosuppression, but can rarely also be observed in normal hosts, especially in areas of the world with high prevalence rates of tuberculosis. *Mycobacterium tuberculosis* causes esophageal disease usually through contiguous involvement by infected mediastinal lymph nodes. *Tracheoesophageal fistula* or *traction diverticulum* is often the result. Despite the prevalence of intestinal and systemic disease with *Mycobacterium avium* complex in AIDS, esophageal involvement is still very rare.

Regardless of the cause of immunodeficiency, 9-month multidrug regimens are usually curative for tuberculosis, provided drug resistance is not present. *Closure of tracheoesophageal fistula* has also been documented following *antituberculous therapy alone*. Therefore, before considering surgical repair of a fistula or even endoscopic stenting, a *prolonged trial of medical therapy* should be undertaken. Long-term therapy for *Mycobacterium avium* complex can only be considered suppressive. The most effective agents for this infection are clarithromycin and ethambutol (Wilcox et al, 1996). Use of HAART can also limit the need for long term suppressive therapy.

Protozoa

In developed countries, protozoal infections of the esophagus are extraordinarily rare and occur almost exclusively in patients with AIDS. In such patients, reported esophageal pathogens include *Pneumocystis carinii*, *Cryptosporidium parvum*, and *Leishmania donovani*. Therapy for these agents is generally ineffective except for *trimethoprim-sulfamethoxazle* combination therapy for *Pneumocystis*. Institution of HAART is the primary "therapy." In Central and South America where *Trypanosoma cruzi* is endemic, this organism characteristically involves the myenteric plexus of the esophagus resulting in an *achalasia-like picture* with *megaesophagus* termed *Chaga's disease*. This disorder mimics idiopathic achalasia clinically, radiographically, endoscopically, and manometrically. Treatment with *niftutimox* 8 to 10 mg/kg/d in 4 divided doses may be helpful if the disease is diagnosed early. However, patients who present with end-stage esophageal disease will gain little and should be treated similarly to idiopathic achalasia with surgery or endoscopic therapies.

Idiopathic Esophageal Ulcer

Early on in the AIDS epidemic, large esophageal ulcerations, which lacked a specific etiology despite extensive histopathologic examination of ulcer tissue, were recognized. These ulcers, termed idiopathic esophageal ulcers (IEU) or aphthous ulcers, are very common, having been found in 41% of HIV-infected patients with esophageal ulcer, and are seen in the later stages of immunodeficiency when the CD4 T lymphocyte count is < 100/mm (Wilcox et al, 1995). Because IEU is a diagnosis of exclusion, endoscopy and biopsy are the only definitive diagnostic tests.

IEUs respond rapidly to either prednisone or thalidomide with clinical and endoscopic cure in > 90% of patients. I generally initiate treatment with prednisone at 40 mg/d and taper 10 mg per week. Addition of once weekly fluconazole may be helpful to prevent esophageal candidiasis, which may complicate steroid therapy. Prednisone is inexpensive and very well tolerated. We use thalidomide for patients intolerant or refractory to prednisone. Because of its known sedative effect, we start with 200 mg/d given at bedtime. The most common side effects are rash and neuropathy. Caution must be exercised and patients must be educated if thalidomide is used, given its horrific teratogenic effects.

Supplemental Reading

Arathoon E, Gotuzzo E, Noriega LM, et al. Randomized, double-blind, multicenter study of caspofungin versus amphotericin B for treatment of oropharyngeal and esophageal candidiases. Antimicrob Agents Chemother 2002;46:451–7.

Barbari G, Barbarini G, Calderon W, et al. Fluconazole versus itraconazole for *Candida* esophagitis in acquired immunodeficiency syndrome. Gastroenterol 1996;111:1169–77.

Blanshard C, Benhamou Y, Dohin E, et al. Treatment of AIDS-associated gastrointestinal cytomegalovirus infection with foscarnet and ganciclovir: a randomized comparison. J Infect Dis 1995;172:622–8.

Shafran SD, Singer J, Zarowny DP, et al. A comparision of two regimens for the treatment of *Mycobacterium avium* complex bacteremia in AIDS: rifabutin, ethambutol, and clarithroymcin versus rifampin, ethambutol, clofazimine, and ciprofloxacin. N Engl J Med 1996;335:377–83.

Wilcox CM, Alexander LN, Clark WS, Thompson SE. Fluconazole compared with endoscopy for human immunodeficiency virus-infected patients with esophageal symptoms. Gastroenterol 1996;110:1803–9.

Wilcox CM, Schwartz DA, Clark WS. Esophageal ulceration in human immunodeficiency virus infection: causes, diagnosis, and management. Ann Intern Med 1995;123:143–9.

Winston DJ, Yeager AM, Chandrasekar PH, et al. Valacyclovir Cytomegalovirus Study Group. Randomized comparison of oral valacyclovir and intravenous ganciclovir for prevention of cytomegalovirus disease after allogeneic bone marrow transplantion. Clin Infect Dis 2003:36:749–58.

CHAPTER 17

MANAGEMENT OF ESOPHAGEAL STRICTURES

ASYIA AHMAD, MD, FAULLIN PALETSKY, MD, AND JAMES C. REYNOLDS, MD

Benign esophageal strictures are believed to develop as a result of chronic inflammation causing fibrous tissue formation and collagen deposition (Spechler, 1995). It is estimated that 65 to 70% of all benign strictures are peptic in origin and a result of chronic uncontrolled gastroesophageal reflux (a full list of other etiologies of esophageal strictures is listed in Table 17-1). Strictures become clinically apparent when patients complain of progressive dysphagia to solids. Heartburn, present in 75% of patients with peptic strictures, and chronic cough, regurgitation, and asthma can also be present. Symptoms may be subtle in which the patient slowly changes their eating habits or overt with recurrent food impactions.

Modern esophageal dilatation techniques can effectively eliminate symptoms of dysphagia in nearly all patients without the need for surgical intervention. An effective management strategy of esophageal strictures includes the use of optimal dilatation techniques and the appropriate management of the underlying causes.

Management of Esophageal Strictures

PREDILATATION EVALUATION

A thorough evaluation of the esophagus should be performed prior to esophageal dilatation. An esophagram is helpful in locating diverticula, hiatal hernias and tortuousity that may be less clearly seen during endoscopy. Endoscopy can be used to identify esophageal ulceration and Barrett's esophagus and allow for brushings and biopsy samples to be taken. Both studies are capable of characterizing the stricture, which is essential to the dilatation process. Strictures that are < 2 cm, straight and patent are known as *simple strictures*. Strictures that are > 2 cm, tortuous and not easily traversed by the endoscope are known as *complicated strictures*. During endoscopy, the endoscope or an open biopsy forcep can be used to help approximate the length and width of the stricture.

Prior to dilatation, the patient should be examined for any contraindications to the procedure, including severe coagulopathy, active bleeding, or an ulcerated stricture. It is imperative that the patient is cooperative and capable of being safely sedated. Once the patient is deemed a suitable candidate for esophageal dilatation, they should understand about the risks and benefits of the procedure. They should be told about adhering to a clear liquid diet for 24 to 36 hours before the procedure especially if tight strictures, gastroparesis or esophageal diverticula are present (Devita and Reynolds, 2002).

TECHNICAL CONSIDERATIONS

The selection of the dilator is a key step in the dilatation process. Mechanical dilators and the balloon dilators are two main types of dilators used today (Table 17-2). The *mechanical or push dilator* stretches the stricture by exerting both

TABLE 17-1. Differential Diagnosis of Esophageal Strictures

Benign	Malignant
Peptic*	Primary esophageal neoplasms
Corrosive	Benign
Radiation-induced	Leiomyoma
Sclerotherapy-induced	Granular cell
Pill-induced	Malignant
Epidermolysis bullosa	Squamous cell carcinoma
Infectious	Adenocarcinoma
Graft-vs-host disease	Pseudoachalasia (GE junction tumor)
Crohn's disease	Metastatic disease to the esophagus
Eosinophilic esophagitis	
Postop	
Extrinsic lesions	
Vascular abnormalities	

*Represents 65 to 70% of all strictures.
GE = gastroesophageal.

TABLE 17-2. Main Dilators for Esophageal Dilatation

Mercury Bougies
   Hurst–blunt tip
   Maloney–tapered tip
Wire Guided
   Jackson Plummer–metal olives
   Eder Puestow–metal olives
   Savary Gillard–hollow core polyvinyl
   Celestin–Neoplex stepped diameter
Polyethylene Balloons
   Through-the-scope (TTS)
   Guidewire facilitated (over-the-wire, OTW)
Hybrid TTS-guide wire

radial and axial forces as it traverses the stricture. These dilators can be passed blindly (Maloney or Hurst dilators) or they can be passed with the assistance of a guidewire (Savary-Gilliard, Eder-Puestow, or Celestin dilators). On the other hand, balloon dilators exert only radial forces as they stretch the stricture and are divided into two groups. The *through-the-scope (TTS)* balloons are positioned under direct visual guidance using the endoscope. The *over-the-wire (OTW)* balloons are positioned by fluoroscopic visualization over a guidewire. Although numerous studies have compared the effectiveness of the various dilators, a consistent consensus regarding the superiority of one dilator over the other has not been achieved. (Yamamoto et al, 1992; Cox et al, 1994).

The goals of dilatation are to produce symptomatic relief for the patient in a safe manner and to prevent recurrence of the stricture. Most patients will experience dysphagia when the luminal diameter of the esophagus is < 13 mm. Therefore, the aim of the dilatation procedure is to stretch the stricture in order to achieve a residual diameter of at least 15 mm (Schatzki and Gary, 1953). Strictures are elastic in nature after the procedure is completed. Recurrent dysphagia seen early after the procedure may be secondary to elastic recoil to a size smaller than the largest dilator passed during the procedure. The initial size of the dilator should approximate the width of the stricture that is going to be dilated (Nostrant, 1995). During the dilation session up to three dilators of consecutive sizes can be used. This rule known as Boyce's "rule of threes" is generally followed in order to insure safety although there is no data supporting this approach. A repeat dilatation session can be done approximately 72 hours after the initial session if further stretching of the stricture is required.

Blindly Passed Dilators

The two types of unguided bougies are the Maloney and Hurst dilators. The *Hurst* was the first of these dilators to be developed and consists of a mercury core encased by a rubber shell with a blunt end. The *Maloney* is a modified version of the Hurst, which has a tapered end instead of a blunt end (Figure 17-1). This improved design allows for easier entry into the esophagus with less shearing stress and is therefore the more common of the unguided dilators used today. These dilators used to be known as the mercury filled dilators, but this potentially toxic metal has been removed from all new dilators. Maloney dilators are made in a variety of sizes up to 60 F (20 mm) although dilators < 30 F are rarely used. Success rates between 80 and 98% have been seen using the Maloney dilator (Wesdorp et al, 1982). Morbidity rates of 4% and a perforation rate of up to 0.3% have been documented (Hernandez et al, 2000). The use of dilators without the guidance of a wire or endoscopy should be limited. Clearly, only uncomplicated, relatively wide diameter strictures in an esophagus without diverticula or tortuousity should be considered for such techniques. Historically, Maloney dilators have often been favored because of their low cost, ease of use, relative safety, and because they are easily reusable. Furthermore, dilatations using the Maloney can be performed without sedation or fluoroscopy in a cooperative patient. (Pereira-Lima et al, 1999; McClave et al, 1993). Such an approach was common in the era before proton pump inhibitors (PPIs) were used to treat reflux. The major disadvantages of these dilators are that they have the ability to coil in the esophagus above a narrow stricture, a tumor shelf, or a large hiatal hernia. The use of fluoroscopic guidance in preventing these complications is controversial. It is believed that fluoroscopy is most useful in patients with large hiatal hernias or peptic-induced strictures rather than Schatzi's ring (Tucker, 1992). In addition, fluoroscopy has been shown to improve relief of dysphagia and luminal patency over the blinded techniques.

Technique

A complete endoscopic examination is performed in the standard left lateral position. The patient is then positioned in either an upright position or in a left lateral position at 30 degrees in preparation for the dilatation. The upright position may be awkward in a sedated patient but has been associated with better success rates. The patient's chin should be tilted downward to reduce the angle leading into the laryngeal vestibule and to facilitate passage into the esophagus. The patient's pharynx should be anesthetized with topical spray and the dilator should be lubricated in preparation for the procedure. Two of the endoscopist's fingers (preferably the fellow's fingers) should be used to hold down the tongue in order to guide the dilator away from the hard and soft palate at the appropriate angle. The dilator is rotated both clockwise and counterclockwise while it is maneuvered down the esophagus. The dilator is then removed with a steady, swift movement.

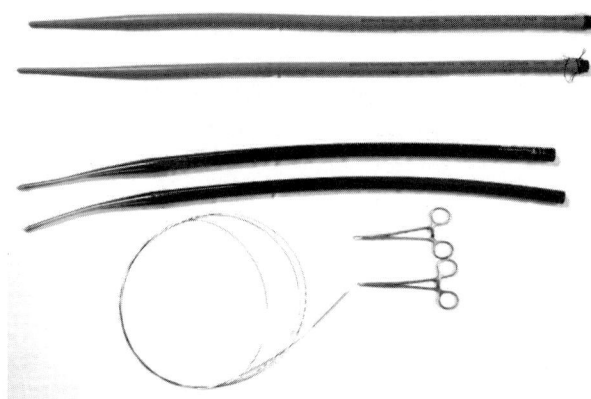

FIGURE 17-1. The top dilators represent tungsten filled Maloney dilators. The bottom two dilators are wire guided Savary dilators. The marked guidewire and hemostats are included.

Wire-guided Polyvinyl Dilators

The *Savary* and *Eder-Puestow* dilators are mechanical dilators passed through strictures over a previously passed guidewire. The Savary has largely replaced the olive-shaped Eder-Puestow dilators, which were developed before flexible endoscopy. The Savary dilators are reusable, noncompressible, gradually tapered dilators (see Figure 17-1). These dilators contain a central opening through which a guidewire can be passed. They also contain radiopaque markers to aid in fluoroscopic detection. A kit of these dilators includes various sizes in 3 F (1 mm) intervals up to a size of 60 F (20 mm). The set also includes replacement guidewires, which is marked at standard lengths. These dilators are strongly recommended over unguided dilators when dealing with narrow, complicated strictures or anatomic abnormalities, such as esophageal diverticula or large hiatal hernias (Kadakia et al, 1991; Anand, 1992). They also are used when unguided dilators are unsuccessfully passed through a stricture. Disadvantages to these dilators are the need for fluoroscopy or endoscopy to properly position the guidewire. In addition, guidewire associated complications can occur. Bends in the wire can lead to point of trauma in either the esophagus or gastric mucosa. Curling of wire can also lead to inadequate passage of the dilator and laceration or hematoma. Despite these potential complications, the morbidity and mortality is low when using these dilators (Marshal et al, 1996).

Technique

The objective in using Savary dilators is to correctly place the guidewire across the stricture and into the antrum of the stomach. Either endoscopic or fluoroscopic assistance can be used to achieve this goal. In the endoscopic method, the endoscope is advanced carefully through the stricture and into the stomach. A guidewire is then passed through the endoscope under direct visualization and advanced into the antrum. In cases in which the endoscope cannot be passed through the stricture, it is prudent to advance the endoscope to the proximal edge of the stricture and then use fluoroscopy to manipulate the guidewire past the stricture and into the stomach (Kadakia et al, 1993). In cases in which the guidewire meets resistance, it is prudent to withdraw a small portion of the wire, change the angle or wiggle the wire and then try to advance again. Some endoscopists have passed the wire through a tight untraversable stricture without the use of fluoroscopy; however, this is neither standard nor advisable. Once the guidewire is placed, the endoscope must be carefully removed without disturbing the position of the wire. This can best be accomplished by the "one to one" method in which an assistant withdraws the endscope as the endoscopist advances the wire in a one to one manner. Using the markings on the guidewire as the sole means for insuring placement has proved inaccurate with wire migration of up to 30 cm. Once the endoscope has been removed, a hemostat should be placed at the mouth to stabilize the wire in position. The dilator should then be passed over the guidewire to the level of the hemostat, and then a second hemostat is placed at the proximal end of the dilator. The hemostat at the mouth is then removed and the dilator is passed through the mouth and esophagus while it is carefully ensured that a constant length of wire remains outside the mouth. The dilator is passed expeditiously, but gently, using a rotating motion. The angle of the dilator should be as straight as possible and the guidewire should remain taut to prevent kinking. Once the dilator is fully inserted it can be removed over the wire. Up to 3 dilators (each 1 or 2 mm larger than the former) can be performed over the same wire at 1 session. If further dilatation is necessary, another session can be performed in 3 days.

Balloon Dilators

Hydrostatic Balloon Dilatation

The OTW and TTS balloon are two types of balloon dilators that have been used for dilatation of esophageal strictures. The OTW uses balloons that are passed over a wire and positioned in the stricture using fluoroscopy. TTS balloons are placed through the working channel of the endoscope and allow direct visualization of the stricture and the balloon during dilatation (Figure 17-2). The main difference between balloon dilators and mechanical dilators is that balloon dilators exert only radial forces and not the shearing forces produced by the mechanical dilators. Another characteristic is that the balloons expand to a set diameter and may rupture if too much force is applied (Graham and Smith, 1985). Although these features appear to enhance safety, no trial has shown a significantly lower complication rate when using these dilators as compared to polyvinyl bougies (Shemesh and Czerniak, 1990; Saeed

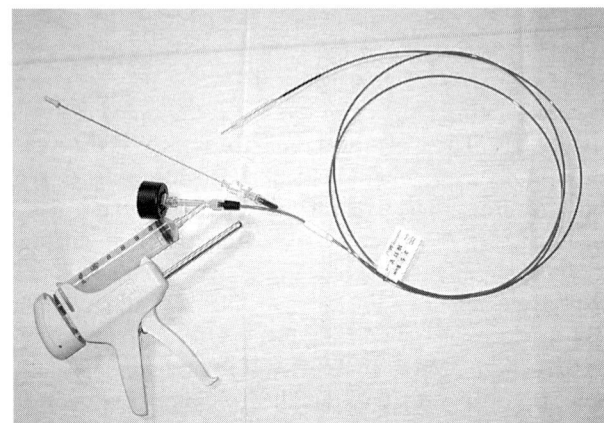

FIGURE 17-2. A through-the-scope (TTS) balloon with pressure gun is represented.

1997). In a national survey, the *overall perforation rate was 0.3%*. This rate may be an overestimate of the true complication rate because a substantial proportion of these patients had either a malignant or tight, eccentric stricture. In this same study, the hemorrhage rate was 2% and was largely secondary to the sharp tip at the end of the balloon catheter. Overall, the balloons are still most advantageous for dilating *narrow, tortuous long strictures*, and the technical success and immediate symptom relief approaches 88% (Kozarek, 1986). There are some disadvantages to the balloons, including loss of tactile sense, low shelf life secondary to balloon rupture, and higher costs.

Technique

An endoscopy is first performed to evaluate the stricture and assess the risk for perforation or laceration of the esophagus. In the case of the TTS balloon, the endoscope is withdrawn just proximal to the stricture. The TTS balloon is then sprayed with a *lubricating silicon spray* in order to aid in its passage through the scope channel and into the lumen. The balloon is passed through the working channel of the scope and into the middle of the stricture and then carefully inflated. The exact balloon diameter to be used depends of the size of the stricture. General recommendations suggest using a 10 mm balloon for strictures with a diameter between 2 and 4 mm, a 12 mm balloon for strictures between 5 and 12 mm, and a 15 mm balloon for strictures > 9 mm in diameter. The balloon is sustained in maximal inflation for 20 to 60 seconds. The balloon is then deflated and the procedure can be repeated an additional time. If necessary, the entire procedure can be repeated during another session in a few days.

The OTW balloon dilators are less frequently used than the TTS balloons. The OTW balloons use guidewire placement and fluoroscopy monitoring during stricture dilatation. The presence of radio-opaque markings at either end of the balloon also helps insure proper placement of the balloon within the stricture. During dilatation, the balloon is held inflated for 20 to 60 seconds and the disappearance of the narrowed portion of the stricture signifies success. The use of hydrostatic dilatation for achalasia is discussed in Chapter 19, "Management of Achalasia".

Special Conditions

Refractory Strictures

Special attention has to be taken in refractory strictures that require multiple, frequent dilatations. The most common cause of refractory strictures is *caustic ingestion, surgery induced (anastomotic), or radiation therapy*. Due to their complex nature, these strictures should be dilated using either polyvinyl or balloon dilators. Fluoroscopy may be necessary in maneuvering through tight, tortuous strictures.

Patients with refractory symptoms may need to undergo surgical correction in order to alleviate their symptoms.

Epidermolysis Bullosa

Epidermolysis bullosa is a heterogenous group of rare disorders causing severe bullous formation on the skin and mucosa membranes. Dystrophic epidermolysis bullosa is a hereditary form of this condition that also includes severe blister formation of the esophagus. These bullous lesions can occur in the proximal or distal esophagus and lead to scarring from minor trauma, including contact with food or acid reflux. Therefore, esophageal dilatation may worsen the preexisting damage already occurring in the esophagus. In this condition, mechanical dilatation is avoided since its shearing forces can lead to further strictures and perforation. If dilatation is necessary, hydrostatic balloons are preferred since only radial forces are applied. Patients may ultimately require esophageal resection in order to achieve sustained relief (McBride, 1989).

Complications of Esophageal Dilatation

Disruption of the esophageal wall and subsequent bacteremia or hemorrhage is an important complication of esophageal dilatation. Esophageal hemorrhage after dilation is consistently < 2% according to a recent AGA review. On the other hand, the rate of esophageal damage during esophageal dilatation differs depending on the method of evaluation. Esophagrams following balloon dilatation have shown extravasations of contrast into the intramural wall in 9% of patients with contrast penetrating through the transmural thickness of the esophagus in an additional 12% (Kang et al, 1998). On the other hand, the rate of clinically relevant perforations requiring aggressive medical or surgical care is lower ranging from < 0.1 to 2% (Kang et al, 1998). The rate of perforation is also dependent on a variety of factors. Bougie dilatation may lead to a higher rate of esophageal disruption than balloon dilators because of the shearing forces it produces. Strictures treated with frequent intervals between dilatation sessions have also been associated with an increased frequency of perforations (Tulman and Boyce, 1981). Corrosive-induced strictures have perforation rates as high as 33%, exceeding the perforation rate for strictures of other benign etiologies (McLean and LeVeen, 1989).

Esophageal Perforation

Patients with significant pain, fever or leukocytosis should be examined for esophageal perforation. An esophagram may display extravasation of contrast into the mediastinum or a chest radiograph may show air in the mediastinum. Patients with mild symptoms and minimal extravasation of contrast into the mediastinum may be treated conservatively with antibiotics, parenteral nutrition (PN), and nasogastric suction. Patients with free perforation and leakage of contrast into the mediastinum, pleural space or abdomen must undergo surgery in addition to receiving antibiotics and PN. In patients who are septic and are poor surgical candidates, an esophageal stent may be temporarily placed to seal the perforation site.

BACTEREMIA

Trauma to a strictured, damaged esophagus during esophageal dilatation may lead to bacteremia. Rates of bacteremia detected by postdilatation blood cultures is 22% by some recent studies in contrast to studies performed in the 1980s that showed rates of 50% or higher (Botoman and Surawicz, 1986). The majority of isolated organisms prove to be *Streptococcus viridans*, refuting earlier beliefs that the source of the bacteremia was the result of incompletely sterilized dilators (Zuccaro et al, 1998). Factors that may predispose to bacteremia during esophageal dilatation include multiple passes with dilators, the use of bougie dilators instead of balloons, and dilatation of malignant strictures or tight strictures that are not easily traversed by the endoscope (Nelson et al, 1998). Bacteremia is highest during the first few minutes following the procedure and drops from 22 to 5% 30 minutes after the procedure. *Antibiotic prophalaxis prior to esophageal dilatation remains controversial.* Current practice is to administer preprocedure antibiotics to patients at high risk. It is still debatable if patients with moderate risk should receive antibiotics. Currently, the American Heart Association advises *prophylaxis* for patients undergoing esophageal dilatation, whereas the American Society for Gastrointestinal Endoscopy has remained neutral on the issue (Dajani et al, 1997). Recommendations are diverse since case reports of bacterial endocarditis or abscess formation as a result of esophageal dilatation are rare. The lack of evidence has led some experts to believe that providing antibiotic prophylaxis is not warranted and lends itself to adverse drug reactions and antimicrobial resistance (Meyer, 1998). There is a separate chapter on endoscopic disinfection (see Chapter 4, "Endoscopic Disinfection").

Recurrence of Esophageal Strictures

The treatment of esophageal strictures with dilatation has had a major impact on relieving symptoms of dysphagia. On the other hand, recurrence of strictures after initial dilatation has proved to be a major problem. *The 1-year recurrence rate for strictures is approximately 60%, with only 40% of patients remaining symptom-free* (Ogilvie et al, 1980; Patterson et al, 1983). Studies have looked at different characteristics that may play a role in subsequent need for repeat dilatations. Factors such as cause of stricture, severity of stricture, presence of esophagitis or initial diameter of dilatation have not consistently correlated with stricture recurrence. Recently it has been shown that weight loss or lack of heartburn correlate with need for repeat dilatation but this has yet to be reconfirmed (Agnew et al, 1996). Other factors, such as nonsteroidal anti-inflammatory drug use, have revealed conflicting data.

ACID SUPPRESSION

One treatment that has consistently shown to reduce the number of stricture dilatations is *acid suppression* therapy. Acid suppression therapy has been shown to reduce the 1-year recurrence rate to 30% (Lundell, 1992). An added effect has been shown with the use of PPIs over histamine receptor antagonists. One randomized prospective study comparing postdilatation use of omeprazole (Prilosec) 20 mg daily to ranitidine (Zantac) 150 mg twice daily revealed a significant lower need for redilatation and improved dysphagia in the omeprazole group at 1 year (Smith et al, 1994). Another study using the same medications showed a significant decrease in stricture recurrence at 10 months as judged by radiologic and endoscopic criteria (Silvis et al, 1996). Therefore, *acid suppression therapy with PPIs is recommended in the treatment of benign* esophageal strictures.

INTRALESIONAL STERIOD INJECTIONS

Intralesional steroid injections may help reduce the number of dilatation sessions needed for patients with refractory benign strictures. This adjuvant therapy has allowed for greater achievable dilator sizes as well as increased symptom-free intervals between dilatation sessions with negligible complications or side effects (Zein et al, 1995; Kirsch et al, 1991). Steroid injections work by suppressing collagen formation and subsequent fibrosis and may be effective without coinciding dilatation. In fact, by decreasing the need for repetitive dilatations, this modality may prove to lower the overall risk of complications behind frequent dilatation sessions. This intervention may be most successful and cost effective among those forms of strictures that are highly relapsing. Studies suggest that placement of the steroid injections in the thickest part of the stricture is optimal. Endoscopic ultrasound guided injection may be the most precise manner in which to insure adequate placement of steroids into the stricture (Bhutani et al, 1997). Although intralesional steroid injections have shown promise, there is no consistent guideline for their use in esophageal strictures.

TEMPORARY STENTS

Temporarily placed *nitinol stents* may increase the interval between esophageal dilatation sessions for recurrent benign strictures. These expandable wire mesh stents are most frequently used in *aggressive strictures*, such as those resulting from *radiation therapy* or *corrosive* substances. Although the optimal duration that these stents should remain in place is not well established, they have been shown to have an excellent safety profile (Song et al, 2000). Presently, a biodegradable stent that maintains its integrity and allows for remodeling of the esophageal stricture without the dangers of a long term foreign body is being developed (Fry and Fleischer, 1997).

Novel Dilatation Techniques/Self Dilatations

Over the past decade, a number of innovative approaches have been devised for the management of complicated or highly relapsing strictures that are poorly amenable to medical or surgical interventions. One method involves dedication from the patients to *dilate their own strictures*. This technique is best reserved for chronic upper to mid-esophageal strictures such as those resulting from corrosive or pill esophagitis (Robinson and Gear, 1991). In this technique, the patient is instructed to swallow a catheter coated with a steroid paste. A balloon at the end of the catheter is inflated allowing the stricture to stretch. The patient then pulls out the apparatus completing the procedure. The patient repeats this dilatation technique frequently over several months until complete relief is achieved.

Combined Approach

Another clever technique that has been designed to safely dilate nearly obstructed or fistulizing esophageal strictures, is the *combined antegrade and retrograde dilatation procedure* (Bueno et al, 2001). In this technique, an endoscope is inserted through a preexisting or newly placed gastrostomy tube, in an effort to pass a guidewire through the distal aspect of the stricture. A guidewire is fluoroscopically passed through the stricture and captured by a peroral endoscope. This is followed by antegrade Savary dilatation of the complicated stricture. Other endoscopists have documented variations of this technique (Lew and Kochman, 2002).

Conclusion

Esophageal dilatation is a safe and effective therapy for the management for esophageal strictures with an overall complication rate of < 2%. It is important to properly assess the characteristics of the stricture in preparation for the dilatation procedure. Blindly passed dilators are suitable only for simple, short and symmetrical strictures with little risk for complications. Polyvinyl and hydrostatic balloon dilators are used for complicated, angulated, and long strictures, as well as refractory strictures. A guidewire and/or fluoroscopy aid in improving the efficacy and safety of the procedure. Peptic stricture recurrence can be markedly reduced by effectively inhibiting acid reflux with the long term use of high dose PPI therapy. A complete 66 item reference list is available at <james.reynolds@drexel.edu>.

Supplemental Reading

Agnew SR, Pandya SP, Reynolds RPE, Preiksaitis HG. Predictors for frequent esophageal dilations of benign peptic strictures. Dig Dis Sci 1996;41:931–6.

American Society for Gastrointestinal Endoscopy. Antibiotic prophylaxis for gastrointestinal endoscopy. Gastrointest Endosc 1995;42:630–5.

Anand BS. Eder-Puestow and Savary dilators. Hepato-Gastroenterol 1992;39:494.

Bhutani MS, Usman N, Shenoy A, et al. Endoscopic ultrasound miniprobe-guided steroid injection for treatment of refractory esophageal strictures. Endoscopy 1997;29:757–9.

Botoman VA, Surawicz CM. Bacteremia with gastrointestinal endoscopic procedures. Gastrointest Endosc 1986;32:342–6.

Boyce HW. Precepts of safe esophageal dilation. Gastrointest Endosc 1977;23:215.

Bueno R, Swanson SJ, Jaklitsch MT, et al. Combined antegrade and retrograde dilation: a new endoscopic technique in the management of complex esophageal obstruction. Gastrointest Endosc 2001;54:368–72.

Cox JG, Winter RK, Maslin SC, et al. Balloon or bougie for dilatation of benign oesophaeal stricture? An interim report of a randomized controlled trial. Gut 1988;29:1741–7.

Cox JG, Winter RK, Maslin SC, et al. Balloon or bougie for dilatation of benign esophageal stricture? Dig Dis Sci 1994;39:776–81.

Dajani AS, Taubert KA, Wilson W, et al. Prevention of bacterial endocarditis: recommendations by the American Heart Association. JAMA 1997;277:1794–801.

DeVita JJ, Reynolds JC. Esophageal dilation techniques. Practical Gastroenterol 2002;16:46–57.

Dooner J, Cleator IGM. Selective management of benign esophageal strictures. Am J Gastroenterol 1982;77:172–7.

Earlam R, Cunha-Melo JR. Benign oesophageal strictures: historical and technical aspects of dilatation. Br J Surg 1981;68:829–36.

Fry SW, Fleischer DE. Management of a refractory benign esophageal stricture with a new biodegradable stent. Gastrointest Endosc 1997;45:179–182.

Glick ME. Clinical course of esophageal stricture managed by Bougienage. Dig Dis Sci 1982;27:884–88.

Graham DY, Smith JL. Balloon dilation of benign esophageal stenoses. Gastrointest Endosc 1985;31:171–4.

Graham DY, Tabibian N, Schwartz JT, Smith JL. Evaluation of the effectiveness of through-the-scope balloons as dilators of benign and malignant gastrointestinal strictures. Gastrointest Endosc 1987;33:432–5.

Hernandez LJ, Jacobson JW, Harris MS. Comparison among the perforation rates of Maloney, balloon and Savary dilation of esophageal strictures. Gastrointest Endosc 2000;5:460–2.

Hine KR, Hawkey CJ, Atkinson M, Holmes GKT. Comparison of the Eder-Puestow and Celestin techniques for dilating benign oesophageal strictures. Gut 1984;25:1100–2.

Ho SB, Cass O, Katsman RJ, et al. Fluoroscopy is not necessary for Maloney dilation of chronic esophageal strictures. Gastrointest Endosc 1994;41:11–4.

Kadakia SC, Cohan CF, Starnes EC. Esophageal dilation with polyvinyl bougies using a guidewire with markings without the aid of fluoroscopy. Gastrointest Endosc 1991;37:183–6.

Kadakia SC, Parker A, Carrougher JG, et al. Esophageal dilation with polyvinyl bougies, using a marked guidewire without the aid of fluoroscopy: an update. Am J Gastroenterol 1993;88:1381–5.

Kang SG, Song HY, Lim MK, et al. Esophageal rupture during balloon dilation of strictures of benign and malignant causes: prevalence and clinical importance. Radiology 1998;209:741–6.

Kirsch M, Blue M, Desai RK, Sivak MV. Intralesional steroid injections for peptic esophageal strictures. Gastrointest Endosc 1991;37:180–2.

Kozarek RA. Hydrostatic balloon dilation of gastrointestinal stenoses: a national survey. Gastrointest Endosc 1986;32:15–9.

Lanza FL, Graham DY. Bougienage is effective therapy for most benign esophageal strictures. JAMA 1978;240:844.

Lee M, Kubik CM, Polhamus CD, et al. Preliminary experience with endoscopic intralesional steroid injection therapy for refractory upper gastrointestinal strictures. Gastrointest Endosc 1995;41:598–600.

Lew RJ, Kochman ML. A review of endoscopic methods of esophageal dilation. J Clin Gastroenterol 2002;35:117–26.

Lundell L. Acid suppression in the long-term treatment of peptic stricture and Barrett's oesophagus. Digestion 1992;51:49–58.

Marks RD, Shula M. Diagnosis and management of peptic esophageal strictures. Gastroenterologist 1996;4:223–7.

Marshal JB, Afridi SA, King PD, et al. Esophagal dilation with polyvinyl (American) dilators over a marked guidewire: practice and safety at one center over a 5-yr period. Am J Gastroenterol 1996;91:1603–6.

Maynar M, Guerra C, Reyes R, et al. Esophageal strictures: balloon dilation. Radiology 1988;167:703–6.

McBride MA, Ergun GA. The endoscopic management of esophageal strictures. Gastrenterol Clinics NA 1994;4:595–620.

McClave SA, Brady PG, et al. Does fluoroscopic guidance for Maloney esophgageal dilation impact on the clinical endpoint of therapy: relief of dysphagia and achievement of lumenal patency. Gastrointest Endosc 1993;43:93–7.

McClave SA, Woolfolk GM. Techniques for dilation of esophageal strictures. Gastrointest Endosc 1999;37:183.

McLean GM, LeVeen RF. Shear stress in the performance of esophageal dilation: comparison of balloon dilation and bougienage. Radiology 1989;172:983–6.

Meyer GW. Endocarditis prophylaxis for esophageal dilation: a confusing issue? Gastrointest Endosc 1998;48:641–3.

Nelson DB, Sanderson SJ, Azar MM. Bacteremia with esophageal dilation. Gastrointest Endosc 1998;48:563–7.

Niv Y, Bat L, Motro M. Bacterial endocarditis after Hurst bougienage in a patient with a benign esophageal stricture and mitral valve prolapse. Gastrointest Endosc 1985;31:265–7.

Nostrant TT. Esophagal dilatation. Dig Dis 1995;13:337–55.

Ogilvie AL, Ferguson R, Atkinson M. Outlook with conservative treatment of peptic oesophageal stricture. Gut 1980;21:23–5.

Patterson DJ, Graham DY, Smith JL, et al. Natural history of benign esophageal stricture treated by dilatation. Gastroenterol 1983;85:346–50.

Pereira-Lima JC, Ramires RP, Zamin I, et al. Endoscopic dilation of benign esophageal strictures: report on 1043 procedures. Am J Gastroenterol 1999;94:1497–501.

Raines DR, Branch WC, Anderson DL, Boyce HW. The occurrence of bacteremia after esophageal dilation. Gastrointest Endosc 1975;22:86–7.

Robinson MHE, Gear MWL. Self-dilation of oesophageal strictures. Gut 1991;32:1076–8.

Saeed ZA. Balloon dilation of benign esophageal stenoses. Hepato-Gastroenterol 1992;39:490.

Saeed, ZA, Ramirez FC, Hepps KS, et al. An objective end point for dilation improves outcome of peptic esophageal strictures: a prospective randomized trial. Gastrointest Endosc 1997;45:354–9.

Saeed ZA, Winchester CB, Ferro PS, et al. Prospective randomized comparison of polyvinyl bougies and through-the-scope balloons for dilation of peptic strictures of the esophagus. Gastrointest Endosc 1995;41:189–94.

Schatzki R, Gary JE. Dysphagia due to a diaphragm-like localized narrowing in the lower esophagus ("lower esophageal ring"). Am J Roentgenol 1953;70:911–22.

Schlitt M, Mitchem L, Zorn G, et al. Brain abscess after esophageal dilation for caustic stricture: report of three cases. Neurosurgery 1985;17:947–51.

Shemesh E, Czerniak A. Comparison between Savary-Gilliard and balloon dilatation of benign esophageal strictures. World J Surg 1990;14:518–22.

Silvis SE, Farahmand M, Johnson JA, et al. A Randomized blinded comparison of omeprazole and ranitidine in the treatment of chronic esophageal stricture secondary to acid peptic esophagitis. Gastrointest Endosc 1996;43:216–20.

Silvis SE, Nebel O, Rogers G, et al. Endoscopic complications. Results of the 1974 American Society for Gastrointestinal Endoscopy survey. JAMA 1976;235:928–30.

Smith PM, Kerr GD, Cockel R, et al. A comparison of omeprazole and ranitidine in the prevention of recurrence of benign esophageal stricture. Gastroenterol 1994:107:1312–8.

Song HY, Jung HY, Park SH, et al. Covered retrievable expandable nitinol stents in patients with benign esophageal stricture: initial experience. Radiology 2000;217:551–7.

Spechler SJ. Complications of gastroesophageal reflx disease. In: Castell DO, editor. The esophagus, 2nd ed. Boston: Little, Brown; 1995. p. 533–44.

Stephenson PM, Dorrington L, Harris OD, Rao A. Bacteremia following esophageal dilation and esophago-gastroscopy. Aust N Z J Med 1977;7:32–5.

Stoddard CJ, Simms JM. Dilation of benign oesophageal strictures in the outpatient department. Br J Surg 1984;71:752.

Tucker LE. The importance of fluoroscopic guidance for Maloney dilation. Am J Gastroenterol 1992;87:1709–11.

Tulman AB, Boyce HW. Complications of esophageal dilation and guidelines for their prevention. Gastrointest Endosc 1981;27:229–34.

Wesdorp ICE, Bartelsman JFWM, Hartog Jager FCA, et al. Results of conservative treatment of benign esophageal strictures: a follow-up study in 100 patients. Gastroenterol 1982;82:487–93.

Yamamoto H, Hughes RW, Schroeder KW, et al. Treatment of benign esophageal stricture by Eder-Puestow or balloon dilators: a comparison between randomized and prospective nonrandomized trials. Mayo Clin Proc 1992;67:228–36.

Yin TP, Dellipiani AW. Bacterial endocarditis after Hurst bougienage in a patient with a benign oesophageal stricture. Endoscopy 1983;15:27–8.

Zein NN, Greseth JM, Perrault J. Endoscopic intralesional steroid injections in the management of refractory esophageal strictures. Gastrointest Endosc 1995;41:596–7.

Zuccaro G, Richter JE, Rice TW, et al. Viridans streptococcal bacteremia after esophageal stricture dilation. Gastrointest Endosc 1998;48:568–73.

Chapter 18

Esophageal Motor Disorders and Chest Pain

Ray E. Clouse, MD.

The swallowing process begins in the oropharyngeal phase. Oropharyngeal motor dysfunction results primarily from central nervous system (CNS), cranial nerve, and striated muscle disease, and motility disorders are common causes of oropharyngeal dysphagia. Control of motor activity shifts largely to the intramural nerve plexus once peristalsis passes the first several centimeters of esophagus, correlating with transition from striated to smooth muscle in the esophageal wall. Motor dysfunction in these distal regions is an important cause of esophageal symptoms, but unlike oropharyngeal dysphagia, structural lesions are more common causes of esophageal dysphagia. The subject of this chapter is the management of motility disorders involving the smooth-muscle region and chest pain related to motor dysfunction in that region.

Types of Esophageal Motor Dysfunction

The terminology used in describing esophageal motility disorders is not fully standardized. At Washington University we classify dysmotility using a simple scheme representing the two principal types of motor dysfunction (Figure 18-1). The first leads to impaired contraction in the esophageal body and/or lower esophageal sphincter (LES). Resultant *hypomotility* predisposes the patient to gastroesophageal reflux disease (GERD), either by increasing reflux events or delaying clearance of refluxate. The second type of motor dysfunction reflects inadequate or failed inhibition of contraction in these same regions or an imbalance between contraction and inhibition. Neural inhibitory effects are required for the correct timing of contraction in the esophageal body and for appropriate relaxation of the LES. The resultant

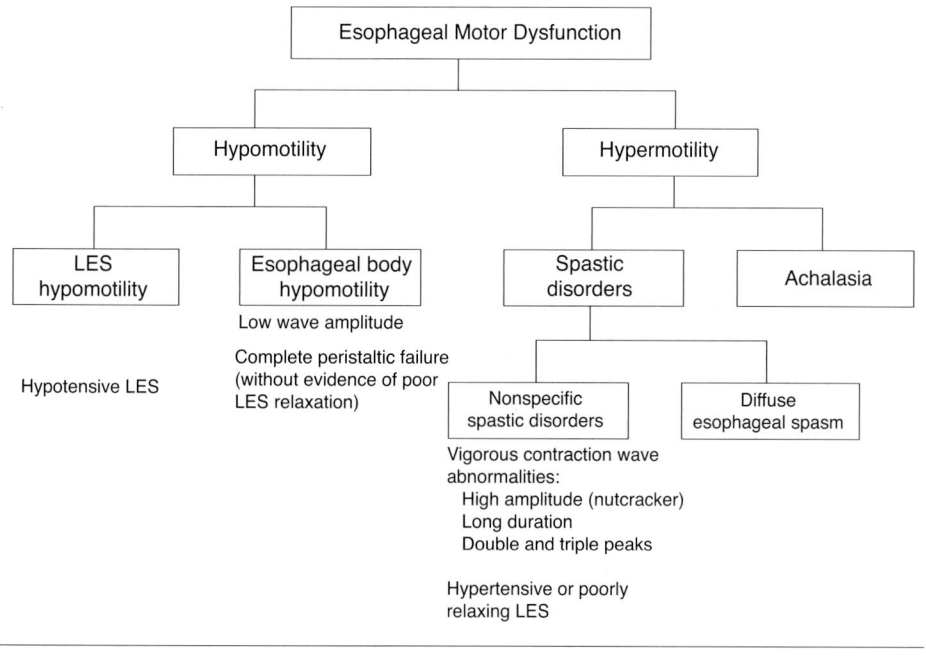

FIGURE 18-1. A method for categorizing motor disorders of the distal esophagus and lower esophageal sphincter (LES) based on principal type of motor dysfunction. Some patients have a mixture of hypomotility and hypermotility features and cannot be classified solely into one branch. Hypermotility typically is associated with hypersensitivity to endogenous, intraluminal, and chemical stimuli, whereas hypomotility is associated with hyposensitivity. From Clouse (1997).

hypermotility manifests as rapid propagation or nonperistaltic contraction in the esophageal body, exaggerated contraction response of high amplitude or broad duration, hypertension of the LES, and inadequate or incomplete LES relaxation. Advanced manifestations of hypermotility (no normal peristalsis and incomplete LES relaxation) typify achalasia. Less developed patterns of hypermotility that display intermittently normal peristalsis and LES relaxation are classified as spastic disorders. Some overlap occurs between spastic disorders and achalasia that cannot be fully differentiated manometrically.

One often-overlooked management aspect is concurrent esophageal sensory dysfunction. A variety of conditions associated with hypomotility also are associated with *hyposensitivity* to intraluminal stimuli, such as acid or distention. In contrast, conditions associated with hypermotility, particularly the spastic disorders, also are associated with increased sensation and symptom reproduction with such stimuli (*hypersensitivity*). Although these relationships are incomplete, co-occurrence of sensory and motility alterations is sufficiently common that the relationship should be considered in management.

Causes of Esophageal Chest Pain

The location and radiation patterns of esophageal chest pain often mimic cardiac angina, mandating a thorough investigative approach. Pain is produced by diseases involving the mucosa and esophageal wall as well as by noxious luminal stimuli. GERD is the most commonly identified etiology of discrete esophageal pain episodes that are differentiated from heartburn. At least 40% of patients with otherwise unexplained chest pain will have evidence of pathologic reflux, either as esophagitis at endoscopy or elevated acid exposure time on ambulatory pH monitoring. Of the remainder, at least one-third will have close association of chest pain episodes with acid reflux events, although their responsiveness to acid suppressant therapy is reduced compared with those having pathologic reflux.

If no objective measure of GERD is present in patients with otherwise unexplained chest pain, the patient is diagnosed with functional chest pain, even if the pain seems acid provoked (Clouse et al, 1999). Studies using acid, balloon distension and electrical stimulation of the esophagus as sensory stimulants, and symptoms or direct physiologic measures of brain activity as the response, demonstrate that the primary abnormality is a misinterpretation of stimulus significance in the CNS. These observations may help explain the high prevalence of anxiety and affective disorders in patients with unexplained chest pain, disorders that can influence central perception of somatic signals and pain reporting. Either the distorted processing of esophageal sensory information or the comorbid psychiatric disturbances may be responsible for autonomic reactivity that also appears a part of the syndrome. This discussion is germane to understanding the relationship of unexplained chest pain to esophageal motility disorders, as a certain degree of motor dysfunction, especially hypermotility, may be produced by this pathophysiology. Figure 18-2 illustrates these relationships and provides a conceptual framework for the treatment strategies outlined in this chapter, particularly for the spastic disorders.

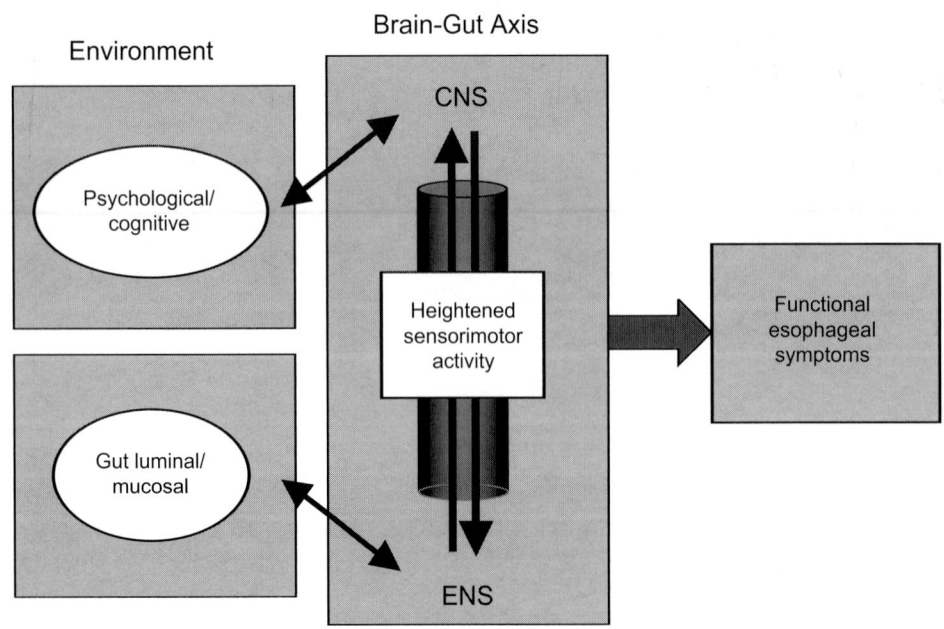

FIGURE 18-2. A model of the pathophysiologic elements involved in functional chest pain and other functional esophageal symptoms. Heightened sensory and motor activity, reflecting underlying errors in central signal processing and possibly exaggerated autonomic response to these processing errors, are the core abnormalities. These features are provoked by luminal stimuli (such as acid and distention) at the level of the enteric nervous system (ENS) and by psychological and cognitive influences at the level of the central nervous system (CNS). Each box represents a potential treatment target.

Management of Hypomotility Disorders

Hypomotility often is discovered incidentally during the investigation of GERD, during preoperative evaluations preceding antireflux surgery, and when clarifying the nature of dysmotility found on barium radiographs. Sometimes hypomotility is sought to support a diagnosis of connective tissue disease (eg, scleroderma or related illnesses). With the exception of its participation in the production of GERD, hypomotility rarely is symptomatic. One might expect dysphagia from severe hypomotility of the esophageal body, but dysphagia should not be attributed to this finding until intrinsic and extrinsic structural lesions as well as nonobstructive GERD have been excluded.

Management of the patient with dysphagia and esophageal hypomotility begins with thorough exclusion of obstructive processes, even to the point of empiric dilatation when no explanation is identified during endoscopy. Dietary modification toward soft foods, avoidance of foods that exacerbate esophageal dysphagia (meat, bread), and positioning to facilitate gravitational effects on postprandial emptying should be recommended. A therapeutic trial of a proton pump inhibitor (PPI) is indicated even with normal endoscopy to exclude a contribution from nonobstructive reflux disease. Medications that promote esophageal motility are of limited availability. Cisapride enhances contraction in the mid-esophagus and can promote esophageal clearance. Preliminary information indicates that it has some effect in mild to moderate hypomotility. Whether tegaserod, another 5-hydroxytryptamine-4 agonist, has similar properties is presently unknown, and other agents have not been tested.

Management of Hypermotility Disorders

Achalasia

Achalasia is the hallmark hypermotility disorder, wherein dysmotility results from death of intramural inhibitory neurons. The presentation typically includes dysphagia, with regurgitation and chest pain being reported by large subsets of patients. Management is palliative, as no treatment can reverse the neural loss (Dunaway and Wong, 2001). The neural defect leads to both aperistalsis and obstruction at the level of the nonrelaxing LES. Reversing obstruction is key to treatment, as aperistalsis is less relevant to the symptomatic presentation—just as in severe hypomotility.

Treatments are divided into those producing muscle relaxation and those producing muscle disruption. There is a separate chapter on achalasia management (see Chapter 19, "Management of Achalasia"). Relaxation of the LES can be accomplished independent of inhibitory nerves with calcium channel blockers and nitrates (Hoogerwerf and Pasricha, 2001). *Nifedipine* 10 mg orally or *isosorbide dinitrite* 5 mg sublingually immediately before meals will transiently reduce LES pressure and improve esophageal symptoms in 70% of patients. Benefits per dose are brief; sustained responses over time occur in a minority of achalasia patients. Side effects of headache and orthostasis interfere with use of these medications. Consequently, smooth-muscle relaxants typically are used for short term gains while planning a more durable management approach.

Botulinum toxin injection, 80 to 100 units at the level of the LES, produces sphincteric relaxation by interfering with cholinergic innervation (Hoogerwerf and Pasricha, 2001; Gui et al, 2003). Initial symptomatic improvement occurs in > 80% of patients, but duration of response to a single injection averages < 8 months. As-needed injection for symptomatic relapses can keep nearly 60% of patients satisfied for up to 2 years, but 1 to 3 injections per year may be required to achieve this outcome. Neither smooth-muscle relaxants nor botulinum toxin injection improve emptying of the esophagus as much as they improve symptoms. Good esophageal emptying may be needed to prevent long term complications associated with achalasia (aspiration pneumonia, carcinoma). Consequently, botulinum toxin also has been reserved for patients in whom more durable treatments are unacceptable or in whom its short term gains would be satisfactory.

Pneumatic dilatation with a 30 to 40 mm diameter balloon positioned across the LES remains the most common treatment worldwide for achalasia. A step-wise dilatation program beginning with the 30 mm balloon and progressing to larger balloons as needed for unsatisfactory outcome has become popular (Kadakia and Wong, 2001). This approach may reduce the risk of perforation, which approximates 3%. Perforation caused by pneumatic dilatation can be managed nonoperatively in selected cases, but thoracotomy is required in the majority. Surgical myotomy often can be performed at the time of thoracotomy. On average, two-thirds of achalasia patients can be managed with pneumatic dilatation, but an objective test of emptying as well as symptoms may be required to establish adequacy of treatment effect (Vaezi, 2001). Risk of perforation and subsequent thoracotomy remains the largest deterrent to this approach both by physicians and by patients and has helped shift the emphasis toward minimally invasive surgery in centers where the expertise is available.

Laparoscopic myotomy is now the preferred primary surgical treatment (Balaji and Peters, 2002). A fundoplication is performed at the time of the myotomy. Results 5 years following this procedure suggest that its outcome parallels that from the transthoracic approach. Nearly 90% of patients report at least a very good outcome; recurring dysphagia and the occurrence of new reflux symptoms remain the most important contributors to deterioration in long term gains. Anatomical distortion in the distal esophagus can persist following myotomy or worsen as the esophagus dilates over time. Emptying can progressively worsen such that nothing short of esophagectomy will produce the desired outcome. Results from esophagectomy for advanced achalasia are very good.

Achalasia does not mandate intervention for the patient with limited symptoms or in whom the diagnosis is made incidentally during investigation of unrelated complaints. Progressive dilatation of the esophageal body, however, can place the patient at risk for pulmonary complications and possibly the development of esophageal squamous cell carcinoma. Monitoring for progressive dilatation is recommended with barium studies initially at one- to two-year intervals if observation is the opted approach. Chest pain in achalasia may not respond to interventions directed at reducing LES pressure, improving emptying, and decreasing symptoms more directly related to impaired transit (dysphagia, regurgitation). A trial of PPIs can be offered to patients with persisting chest pain after an otherwise adequate intervention has been accomplished. Exclusion of *Candida* esophagitis is recommended. Preliminary data indicate that low dose tricyclic antidepressant (TCA) regimens, as used for spastic disorders and unexplained chest pain, also are beneficial for chest pain management in achalasia.

Spastic Disorders

The term spastic disorders is applied to a wide spectrum of dysmotility (see Figure 18-1). These disorders are identified from patterns of hypermotility on manometric tracings or presence of tertiary or uncoordinated contractions during barium fluoroscopy. Unlike achalasia, where inhibitory nerve death results in regular evidence of motor dysfunction, the findings in spastic disorder are intermittent, vary in severity from swallow to swallow, and are intermixed with normal findings. The anatomic location of neural dysfunction is uncertain in spastic disorders, and no consistent pathologic abnormality has been detected. Abnormal modulation of motility through central mechanisms may be responsible in some cases.

Spastic disorders typically are discovered during the investigation of esophageal complaints when no structural explanation is present. Appropriate management must take several important facts into consideration (Clouse, 1997; Kahrilas, 2000). First, the manometric or radiologic findings are sufficiently nonspecific for symptoms that careful exclusion of other explanations, esophageal (eg, GERD) and nonesophageal (eg, cardiac), is still required. Second, concurrent abnormalities in esophageal sensation may be as important as motility abnormalities in producing symptoms. Despite the wide variety of spastic disorders (including diffuse esophageal spasm, nutcracker esophagus, and other nonspecific spastic disorders), there presently is no evidence that one should be managed different from another.

Once the spastic disorder is detected and alternative symptom explanations are excluded, management proceeds according to the algorithm shown in Figure 18-3. If the principal symptoms reflect disturbed transit (viz dysphagia or regurgitation), then the spectrum of treatments used for achalasia can be considered (Gui et al, 2003; Balaji and Peters, 2002). Because dysphagia also can be a symptom of altered sensation in these disorders, that is, a sense of disturbed transit without conspicuous obstruction to bolus movement, management approaches used for chest pain sometimes are appropriate. Before considering the more morbid procedures, including pneumatic dilatation or myotomy, it is essential that a relationship of symptoms to impaired transit be demonstrated. This can be accomplished by offering a radio-opaque pill at the time of a fluoroscopic barium swallow to see if symptoms are reproduced with lodging of the pill—usually at the level of the LES.

At my institution, PPIs and antidepressants, either alone or in combination, prove to be the most important management tools for these patients. A PPI trial, either empiric or as directed by findings on 24-hour pH monitoring, is the first step. Patients with refractory symptoms will receive a low dose TCA along with the PPI if there was a symptomatic response, if pathologic reflux has been demonstrated either by endoscopy or pH monitoring, if there was an association of symptoms with reflux events during the pH study, or in place of antireflux therapy if none of these features were present. TCAs appear superior in clinical practice to contemporary antidepressants (Clouse, 1994). I begin with nortriptyline 25 mg at bedtime with an escalation to 50 to 125 mg daily until symptomatic response occurs or side effects prevent further dose increment. In

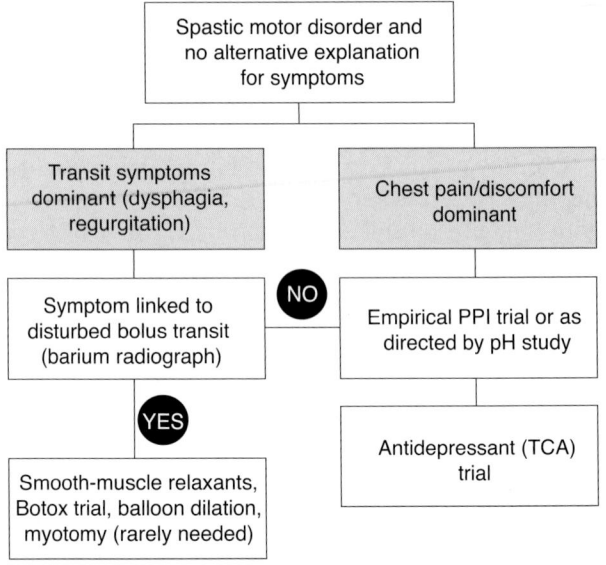

FIGURE 18-3. Management algorithm for patients with otherwise unexplained esophageal symptoms and spastic motor disorders. PPI = proton pump inhibitor; TCA = tricyclic antidepressant.

patients with many somatic symptoms or unexplained syndromes, I start with 10 mg at bedtime. Nortriptyline and desipramine, metabolites of amitriptyline and imipramine, respectively, are better-tolerated TCAs because of their fewer side effects. Treatment for 6 to 24 months is typical in symptomatic responders before withdrawal is attempted. Patients with objective evidence of reflux disease need continuous antireflux therapy; "stepping down" to intermittent antireflux treatment should be tried for other subjects.

Rarely is surgery used in patients with spastic disorders. (Balaji and Peters, 2002). Chest pain is a poor indication, just as chest pain is the least responsive symptom to surgery for achalasia. Most patients with spastic disorders have stable patterns over time and symptoms wax and wane. Long esophageal myotomy is the surgical procedure of choice when esophageal body abnormalities are present; if poor LES relaxation is the dominant finding, a shorter myotomy as for achalasia is performed. Surgery typically is reserved for subjects with advanced spastic motor abnormalities that overlap with achalasia (sometime called "achalasia variants") in whom incomplete LES relaxation is well demonstrated and transit disturbances during radiography correlate well with symptoms.

Management of Unexplained Chest Pain

The most common explanation for recurring substernal chest pain following negative cardiac evaluation is GERD (Fang and Bjorkman, 2001). Approximately 15% of patients will have esophagitis at endoscopy and up to 40% of patients will have elevated acid exposure time during 24-hour pH monitoring. The remaining large subset has no evidence of pathologic reflux. About one-third of these will have a significant association of symptoms with acid reflux events, but as a group, all subjects without pathologic reflux respond less well to antireflux therapy. Twenty-five to 50% of patients with no pathologic reflux will have a spastic motor disorder on manometry, the wide variation in prevalence relating to different thresholds in assigning these diagnoses. Although the therapeutic approach is similar for all patients without pathologic reflux, some options are restricted to those with spastic motor disorders. The treatment algorithm for this group is reflected in Figure 18-3.

Not all patients undergo ambulatory pH monitoring in the primary phase of investigation, making therapeutic trials with PPIs important in the initial aspects of management. A short term (1-week) trial of 40 mg of omeprazole in the morning and 20 mg at night (or an equivalent regimen with an alternative PPI) is sensitive to 80 to 85% of subjects with pathologic reflux. Because the results of therapeutic trials often are ambiguous, nearly all patients with unexplained chest pain will continue such therapy for the early management period. As for pain in presence of spastic motor disorders, TCAs play an important role in rescuing subjects who fail to respond to antireflux therapy alone. Twenty-four-hour pH monitoring may help direct the need to continue antireflux therapy concurrent with antidepressant trials.

Management is challenging for those who respond poorly to these initial approaches. A common error is failure to increase the TCA to a satisfactory dosage, and full psychiatric dosing is required in some subjects (Clouse, 1994). Intolerance to TCA can prompt a trial of a contemporary antidepressant (such as a selective serotonin reuptake inhibitor) in usual psychiatric dosing. The response with regard to chest pain reporting in general has been less satisfactory. I have used other pain modulating agents on occasion, including carbamazepine and gabapentin, but have reserved these medications for refractory and debilitating symptoms or for pain with sharp or lancinating characteristics. Calcium channel blockers also have been used with anecdotal success.

Nonpharmacologic approaches can be useful in unexplained chest pain, just as in other functional gastrointestinal disorders. Cognitive behavioral psychotherapy, deep muscle relaxation, biofeedback, and other stress reduction techniques, are beneficial for some patients. Transcutaneous electrical nerve stimulation, acupuncture, and other alternative approaches, have had anecdotal success, but the best advice is to learn to maximize the use of antidepressants, particularly TCAs, in this patient group.

Supplemental Reading

Balaji NS, Peters JH. Minimally invasive surgery for esophageal motility disorders. Surg Clin North Am 2002;82:763–82.

Clouse RE. Spastic disorders of the esophagus. Gastroenterologist 1997;5:112–27.

Clouse RE. Antidepressants for functional gastrointestinal disorders. Dig Dis Sci 1994;39:2352–63.

Clouse RE, Richter JE, Heading RC, et al. Functional esophageal disorders. Gut 1999;45(Suppl 2):II31–6.

Dunaway PM, Wong RK. Achalasia. Curr Treat Options Gastroenterol 2001;4:89–100.

Fang J, Bjorkman D. A critical approach to noncardiac chest pain: pathophysiology, diagnosis, and treatment. Am J Gastroenterol 2001;96:958–68.

Gui D, Rossi S, Runfola M, Magalini SC. Review article: botulinum toxin in the therapy of gastrointestinal motility disorders. Aliment Pharmacol Ther 2003;18:1–16.

Hoogerwerf WA, Pasricha PJ. Pharmacologic therapy in treating achalasia. Gastrointest Endosc Clin N Am 2001;11:311–24.

Kadakia SC, Wong RK. Pneumatic balloon dilation for esophageal achalasia. Gastrointest Endosc Clin N Am 2001;11:325–46.

Kahrilas PJ. Esophageal motility disorders: current concepts of pathogenesis and treatment. Can J Gastroenterol 2000;14:221–31.

Vaezi MF. Quantitative methods to determine efficacy of treatment in achalasia. Gastrointest Endosc Clin N Am 2001;11:409–24.

CHAPTER 19

Management of Achalasia

William J. Ravich, MD

Achalasia is a disorder of esophageal motility that results from neural damage within the myenteric ganglion cells within the esophageal wall. As a consequence of this injury, the esophageal body cannot generate a progressive peristaltic wave and the lower esophageal sphincter (LES) is unable to relax normally in response to swallowing. The end result is resistance to flow through the (EG) junction.

Presentation

Virtually all patients with achalasia complain of dysphagia and most complain of regurgitation. The dysphagia is typically for both liquids and solids. A small percentage, however, have dysphagia for solids only. Dysphagia is most often localized to the chest, although some point to the neck as the level at which they feel that food sticks. Although regurgitation may occur during or immediately after eating, it commonly occurs after a substantial delay. Delayed regurgitation of recognizable food that occurs hours after eating suggests only a limited set of diagnostic options. Aside from achalasia, hypopharyngeal (Zenker's) or esophageal diverticula are the most likely alternative diagnoses. Less often, regurgitation due to gastroesophageal reflux in the presence of hypochlorhydria may present in a similar manner. Other presentations include weight loss, nighttime cough, and aspiration pneumonia.

Diagnosis

The diagnosis of achalasia is strongly suggested by the findings on a barium esophagram. A dilated esophagus, a column of barium with an air-fluid level, and a tapered narrowing at the EG junction, are highly suggestive of achalasia. The major diagnostic alternatives for this radiograph appearance are a benign or malignant stricture. However, unlike a stricture, the EG junction usually opens intermittently to a few millimeters allowing small spurts of barium to pass into the stomach. Also with a stricture, dysphagia for liquids and solids usually develops only after a long period of dysphagia for solids only, and esophageal dilatation rarely progresses to the extent typically seen in achalasia. In long-standing achalasia, the esophageal lumen may distend to dramatic proportions and take on a tortuous configuration referred to as a "sigmoid esophagus."

Esophageal manometry typically demonstrates complete absence of progressive peristalsis, a high-normal or high resting lower esophageal pressure, and failure of LES relaxation after swallowing. Although LES relaxation is usually < 50% to the intragastric baseline, in a minority of patients, relaxation to the intragastric baseline has been described. However the appearance of this apparently complete relaxation is unusual, demonstrating a much more rapid fall and rise than that seen in normal individuals. This finding corresponds to the minimal distension of the EG junction commonly seen during videoradiographic studies.

In classic achalasia, there is also an absence of contractions in the esophageal body. Although small simultaneous elevations of pressure may follow each swallow, these pressure changes tend to occur earlier than in normal individuals and are of very low amplitude (usually < 30 mm Hg). They represent the effect of pharyngeal contraction—the "pharyngeal squirt"—increasing pressure in the dilatated esophagus, rather than intrinsic esophageal muscular activity. In a variant of achalasia, referred to as *"vigorous achalasia,"* swallowing generates more substantial, but nonetheless simultaneous and, occasionally, multiphasic increases of esophageal pressure that do represent intrinsic esophageal motor activity. Whether vigorous achalasia is an early phase in the evolution of classic achalasia or is a separate condition with a different pathogenesis is unknown.

Patients with radiographic studies compatible with achalasia who are subsequently found to have a malignancy involving the EG junction may meet the manometric criteria for achalasia (referred to as "pseudoachalasia" or "secondary achalasia"). Therefore, manometry cannot be relied on to distinguish between true achalasia and a malignant stricture. Because some patients with achalasia develop carcinoma of the esophagus, this can be an important differential diagnosis.

Endoscopy is sometimes used by gastroenterologists as the first test in the evaluation of dysphagia, on the grounds that the procedure will ultimately be required in the examination of patients presenting with this symptom. This may be a tactical mistake. Although it is true that endoscopy in patients with dysphagia may make radiographic examination unnecessary, barium studies are more helpful, providing information on both motor function and structural disease. The endoscopic findings of achalasia, especially before distension of the esophageal lumen becomes pronounced, may be subtle and easily misinterpreted as normal or a stricture. Nonetheless, it is true that in the face of a barium esophagram compatible with achalasia, endoscopic examination is required to rule out a benign or malignant stricture.

The diagnosis is confirmed when a tight EG junction that does not distend with air insufflation is covered by normal-looking overlying mucosa and allows the endoscope to pass through with little resistance. A retroflexed view of the cardia and fundus should be performed routinely as a double check for possible malignancy. Although there may be some resistance to intubation of the EG junction in achalasia, it is usually minimal with the endoscope passing through with a slight popping sensation. Patients with achalasia are prone to candidial esophagitis due to esophageal stasis. However focal erosive or ulcerative disease in the areas of the EG junction should raise concerns about an alternative diagnosis. A nodular mass is inconsistent with achalasia and suggests a malignancy. Malignancy masquerading as achalasia on barium studies is often infiltrating and may not involve the mucosa on either the esophageal or cardial side of the SC junction. Therefore biopsies and brushings may confirm a malignancy, but cannot rule one out. Excessive resistance to intubation should also suggest the presence of a malignancy, even in the absence of an obvious tumor. Nonetheless, pseudoachalasia is a relatively rare condition and the vast majority of patients with radiographic findings suggesting achalasia have achalasia.

Many authorities insist that all three of the tests mentioned above are required for the diagnosis of achalasia. However, I have rarely seen manometry change a diagnosis of achalasia based on the combination of barium and endoscopic findings. On the rare occasions in which the manometry appears to dictate against achalasia, the discrepancy is almost invariably due to technical problems in the performance or interpretation of the manometric study. I do not feel that manometry is a necessary test for the diagnosis of achalasia.

Treatment Options

Treatment options include *observation, smooth muscle relaxants, intrasphincteric botulinum toxin injection, large diameter balloon dilatation* ("pneumostatic dilation"), or *surgical myotomy* (Table 19-1).

Observation

In clinical practice, patients generally have had symptoms for a long time before they seek medical attention. The symptoms usually progress so slowly in early stages that patients have already exhausted the option of observation without intervention by the time they present to the gastroenterologist. Nonetheless rare patients have sufficiently mild symptoms to allow a delay in treatment. Episodes of *aspiration pneumonia* and *profound weight loss* are clear indications at the earliest practical opportunity. *Nighttime regurgitation* increases the risk of aspiration pneumonia and also warrants intervention, even if the patient would otherwise prefer to delay treatment.

Carbonated Beverages

Pending definitive treatment, *carbonated beverages* increase esophageal emptying by radionuclide study in a large majority of achalasia patients. I therefore often suggest a trial of carbonated beverage during or at the end of a meal, and at bedtime. The mechanism of this response appears to be through stimulating spastic activity in the esophageal body, thereby increasing intra-esophageal pressure sufficiently to overcome resistance from the LES. However this pressure may also cause discomfort or regurgitation in its own right, and only about 50% of patients feel the overall effect to be beneficial, whereas others find that it increases symptoms. We therefore let the patient decide whether to continue with these carbonated beverage chasers.

Smooth Muscle Relaxants

After the introduction of calcium channel blockers to medical practice it was discovered that sublingual administration of these drugs decreases LES resting pressure transiently. Although some patients do seem to respond symptomatically to smooth muscle relaxant therapy, the benefit is usually partial in degree and often diminishes over time. Also high doses may be required to obtain a substantial symptomatic response, and patient tolerance for the vasodilatory effect of these drugs, even in standard doses, may be limited. Ironically, there is evidence that the older long acting nitrates may have more profound effects on the esophageal muscle function than do calcium channel blockers.

TABLE 19-1. Therapeutic Options in Achalasia

- Observation*
- Oral or sublingual smooth muscle relaxants*
- Intrasphincteric botulinum toxin injection
- Large-caliber balloon dilatation
- Surgical myotomy

*Usually not feasible as long term treatment.

Intrasphincteric Botulinum Toxin Injection

The concept of injecting botulinum toxin into the LES of achalasia patients was suggested by Pankaj Pasricha, as a gastrointestinal fellow at Johns Hopkins. After a series of animal studies confirmed its effect on LES pressure and it did not appear to cause significant histologic injury, we began to study its effect in achalasia patients with gratifying results. These results have been confirmed in controlled trials at Hopkins and elsewhere.

Observations based on these studies and on subsequent clinical experience, include the following:

1. Treatment is remarkably safe. Complications are, for the most part, the same and no more frequent than those associated with diagnostic upper endoscopy in achalasia patients. Occasional patients (perhaps 10 to 20%) do have transient and usually mild chest pain. Very rarely, patients have some reflux symptoms that are generally short lived.
2. Older patients respond better than younger patients
3. Patients with vigorous achalasia respond better than those with classic achalasia
4. The mean duration of response exceeds 1 year in some series, but is substantially shorter in others. The reason for these reported differences is unclear.
5. Virtually all patients ultimately relapse symptomatically and require retreatment. Although patients who initially respond usually respond to reinjection, there is a drop off in the response rate with repeat injections. Conversely, if a patient does not respond initially to two injections, they are unlikely to respond to additional injections.

Balloon Dilatation

Dilatation for achalasia dates back to the seventeenth century when Thomas Willis described the successful use of periodic dilatation with whalebone of various sizes in a patient who in retrospect is thought to have had achalasia. Unfortunately serial dilatation for achalasia usually results in only a temporary and partial symptomatic response. A better response can be obtained with the use of *large diameter balloon dilatators* (≥ 30 mm) placed across the EG junction and distended rapidly to obliterate the waist produced by the contracted LES.

A variety of balloon dilatators have been used for this purpose. Overtime, a consensus has been reached that a low compliance balloon that could be blown up with sufficient pressure to a predetermined maximum diameter, and could not be further distended once that diameter was reached, had the best effect–complication profile. Traditionally, at least in the United States, a 35 mm balloon was used in adults and a 30 mm balloon was used for the occasional child with achalasia. Earlier reinforced latex balloons were replaced by polyethylene balloons, largely due to concerns about disinfection of reusable balloon dilatators.

In the United States, commercially available polyethylene balloons with central channels for placement over a guide wire are available with outer diameters of 30, 35 and 40 mm when fully distended; outside the United States, dilatators with diameters up to 50 mm are available. To minimize the risk of perforation, reported to range between 1 and 5% in recent series, there has been a tendency among endoscopists to start with the 30 mm balloon, reserving the 35 mm balloon for patients in whom the initial treatment fails. Some endoscopists will go on to dilatate with a 40 mm balloon if the 35 mm balloon does not achieve an adequate result. However others feel that the increased risk associated with these larger balloons favors moving toward other options, especially surgery.

The usual approach is to perform the dilatation as part of an upper endoscopy. The guide wire is positioned in the distal stomach. The scope is withdrawn and the dilatator is passed under fluoroscopic control until it straddles the EG junction. The balloon is then inflated by a rapid, stepwise sequence of increments until the waist is obliterated as observed under fluoroscopy. The balloon is then deflated, to a sigh of relief from the patient who generally experiences at least moderate pain during the period of full inflation. There is considerable variation in technique described in the medical literature concerning the duration of time for which balloon distension is maintained, ranging from 15 seconds to 2 minutes, and there are no objective studies to favor one recommendation over another.

Traditionally, the pressure required to achieve full distension is noted and is determined again at the end of the procedure; a drop in the pressure required that distends the EG junction ≥ 3 pounds per square inch suggests good response. However, the real effect of treatment is based on the patient's symptomatic response, generally augmented by other postprocedural objective studies. It is common to see some streaks of blood on the deflated balloon after it is removed, suggesting that a mucosal tear has occurred. The clinical response presumably reflects traumatic injury to the sphincter muscle. The literature suggests that a good long term response can be obtained in 60 to 90% of patients, with clinically significant postdilatation reflux disease being uncommon. A major advantage over surgery is that the patients can generally return to their regular daily regimen the next day.

Surgery

The choice between surgery and dilatation as the primary mode of treatment is often determined by local referral patterns. When gastroenterologists with an interest in the esophagus are the first line of referral, dilatation is most often performed. When patients are referred directly to surgeons, surgery is more likely to be performed as the initial therapeutic intervention. Which group dominates in a particular locale appears to be passed down through generations of physicians and is based more on tradition than evidence. Studies suggest a good to excellent result from surgical myotomy in 70 to 90% of patients. Overall, a 10% better response rate with surgery over dilatation is supported in the literature. However, outcomes may be more operator dependent with myotomy than with dilatation.

This better response rate for myotomy, however, comes with some baggage. Although some surgeons claim excellent results without postoperative reflux problems, others have found clinically significant gastroesophageal reflux occurs in a large proportion of patients. For that reason, myotomy is often combined with an antireflux procedure. However, in the face of absent peristalsis, fundoplication can interpose an obstructive element, therefore, at least conceptually, counteracting the primary goal of surgery. For this reason, when antireflux surgery is included, a partial fundoplication is usually preferred. Myotomy can be performed through either a thoracic or abdominal approach. It is my impression that abdominal surgeons tend to favor the addition of an antireflux component, whereas thoracic surgeons do not.

Aside from reflux, postoperative problems include early or late recurrence of obstructive symptoms. Early recurrence may be due to inadequate myotomy or obstruction by the wrap. Late recurrence may also be due to an inadequate myotomy, but is more likely to occur from a reflux-induced inflammation and stricture formation. It is often difficult to distinguish between these alternative causes.

Recently there has been a trend towards thoracoscopic or laparoscopic approach to myotomy. The benefits of minimally invasive surgery are primarily in terms of faster postoperative recovery and less patient discomfort. Although these benefits are real and often sufficient to make a patient favor a surgical option that they might otherwise refuse, it is unlikely that minimally invasive surgery is in fact superior to its open variant in terms of long term results. Nonetheless, the introduction of laparoscopic and thoracoscopic myotomy has created a more balanced playing field, in which surgery and dilatation are increasingly seen as valid initial treatment options.

Personal Approach

I virtually always begin evaluation of unexplained dysphagia with barium studies (Figure 19-1). More mistakes are made by leaping directly to endoscopy than for any other reason. Once the diagnosis of achalasia is suggested by barium esophagram, assuming an endoscopy has not already been performed, I perform an endoscopy to rule out benign or malignant stricture. Clues to an alternative diagnosis include an obvious fungating mass lesion obstructing the lumen, significant erosive disease, inability or excessive resistance to intubate the EG junction, and a mass on retroflexed view of the gastric cardia and fundus.

In the face of a consistent barium esophagram and in absence of any of these suspicious findings, the diagnosis of achalasia is virtually assured. As based on currently available sutides, neither LES pressure nor the category of achalasia would be likely to change my therapeutic decisions; manometry is of interest, but is not essential before treatment. Although the distinction between vigorous and classic achalasia have prognostic significance, my treatment approach is not dramatically altered by the category of achalasia. If there is doubt after endoscopy, a computed tomography scan and endoscopic ultrasound (EUS) are

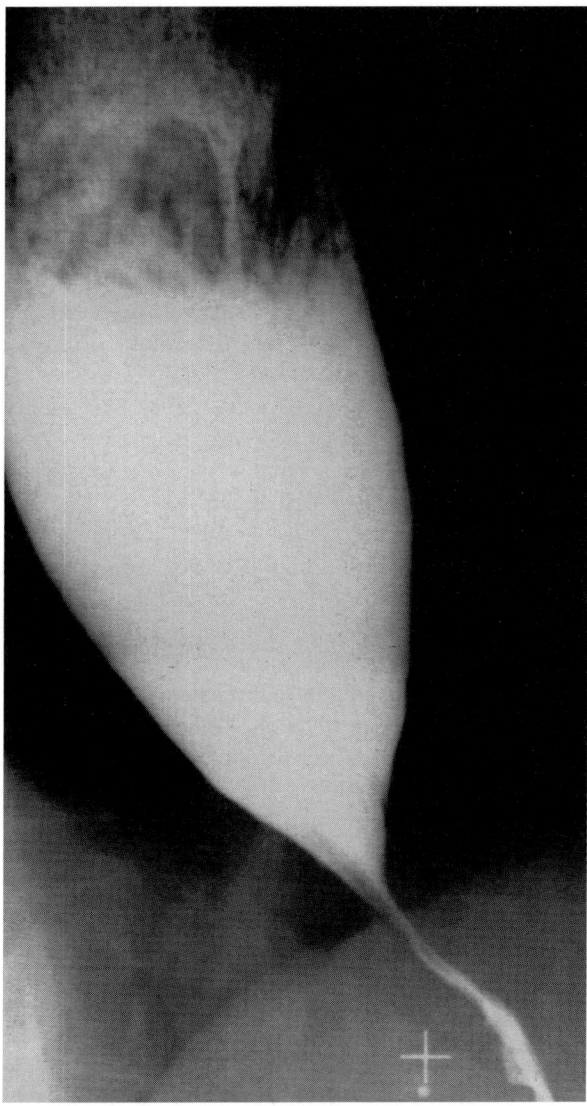

FIGURE 19-1. The barium study shows a dilatated esophagus with a column of barium mixed with retained food and an air-fluid level at the top, extending up from a smooth tapered stenotic EG junction.

more likely to help in the diagnosis of a cancer posing as achalasia than is manometry.

As mentioned, continued observation is rarely an option. Nonetheless the urgency of treatment is increased by a history suggesting a high aspiration risk and by the degree of weight loss. I often suggest an empirical trial of carbonated beverage with meals or just before bedtime to see if I can improve the patient's symptoms pending arrangement for treatment. If nighttime coughing is a problem, the patient should avoid lying down within a few hours of eating and should elevate the head of the bed. I may use a *short acting sublingual nitroglycerin* for the patient who has intermittent chest pain or a *longer acting sublinqual nitrate* for temporary alleviation of symptoms if other interventions must be delayed. However, given the limited response and frequent side effects, I do not generally recommend the long term use of smooth muscle relaxants unless the patient refuses alternative treatment options.

Botulinum Toxin

Although I believe that botulinum toxin should be discussed, the relatively short duration of effect favors the use of other treatment options unless the patient is a poor operative risk or extremely risk adverse. Multiple studies have confirmed that the *elderly* are substantially more likely to respond to botulinum toxin than are the young. Therefore botulinum toxin seems a better choice for the elderly patient with significant comorbidities. The need for multiple treatments that would presumably continue indefinitely should be adequate explanation to all but the most risk adverse young to seriously consider other options.

The original studies of intrasphincteric botulinum toxin used a 20 units/mL solution of botulinum toxin type A, injecting 1 mL into each of 4 sites around the circumference of the LES achalasia with a sclerotherapy catheter. Because of the increased pressure in the LES and the dilatation of the esophageal lumen above, the sphincter muscle stands out, making it easy to inject directly into the belly of the muscle. In those early studies we used a modified injection technique, pushing the needle deeply into the muscle for the first half of each injection and then relaxing the pressure and pulling back slightly on the injection catheter. The concept was to give some of the bolus relatively deeply and then relatively superficially. Others have suggested injecting the toxin from the gastric side during scope retroflexion, but targeting the injection sites would seem to be more difficult with this approach. I have not tried it.

The total dose that we used was somewhat serendipitous. The original animal studies were performed with a total of 40 units for arbitrary reasons. The 80-unit dose in humans was simply extrapolated based on the difference in body weight between the pigs used in the animal studies and average sized humans. Subsequent studies have not shown any obvious benefit to higher doses, but it seems wasteful to throw out 20 units from the standard 100-unit vial. I currently use a 25 unit/mL solution and inject it in 0.5 mL aliquots in 8 separate sites scattered around the EG junction.

A few caveats about botulinum toxin are in order. First, although EUS-guided injection has been described, it increases the complexity and cost of the procedure. I do not think there is evidence that EUS offers any therapeutic advantage over visually directed injection. Second, the toxin is inactivated by preservatives, so nonbacteriostatic saline should be used to reconstitute the toxin. Third, the toxin is also inactivated by agitation. This would include the agitation that results from the rapid introduction of the diluting solution that occurs when the syringe is introduced into the vacuum-sealed vial. I therefore purposely break the seal with an unattached needle before injecting the solution into the vial to prepare the solution. Fourth, laboratory technicians who work with botulinum toxin often develop antibodies to the toxin, presumably from skin contact. Although it is unclear that this poses a significant health risk, it seems best to avoid antibody development. Endoscopy personnel should be taught to use gloves routinely when reconstituting and using the toxin, if only to assure that they will be candidates for botulinum toxin therapy if and when they need it.

Balloon Dilatation

I still favor balloon dilatation over surgery for achalasia as my first approach. The costs, overall complication rate, and recovery time is shorter for dilatation than for surgery, my perforation rate is below 1%, most perforations that do occur are confined and can be treated without surgery, and finally most patients who do perforate ultimately have a satisfactory response to the dilatation (albeit only after a period of anxiety and discomfort resulting from the resulting hospitalization). Although the percentage with a very good to excellent response may be slightly lower with dilatation than with surgery, the benefits seen in my analysis offset this advantage. Surgery is like the "girl with the curl"—the results are often very good, but they can on occasion be horrid. The often rosy reports from the surgical literature do not accurately reflect the general results seen in patients referred to me in my outpatient clinic. I prefer the slightly decreased rate of response to dilatation to the irrevocable step of surgery.

My approach to dilatation is as follows. I make sure the endoscopy assistant is at the ready with suction device in hand at initial endoscopic intubation. After evacuation of as much liquid esophageal contents as possible, I turn the patient supine and mark the chest with a metal marker (a paper clip serves quite well) at the level of the EG junction by means of the fluoroscope to detect the scope tip positioned at the proximal end of the LES. For the first dilatation, I always use a 30 mm achalasia balloon dilatator. The balloon is then positioned across the EG junction. Although traditionally dilatation is performed with air inflation ("pneumostatic dilatation"), I find that with the currently available balloon dilatators, it is sometimes difficult to confirm the position of the inflated balloon. As accurate balloon positioning is of paramount importance, I inflate the balloon with a one-fourth strength contrast solution to improve visualization of the balloon during distention. I gradually distend the balloon to make sure the waist created by the LES remains in the middle one-third of the balloon. During inflation, the balloon may tend to migrate up or down, squeezed out by the sphincter pressure, a pressure that is obvious to the person holding the balloon catheter. I ask an assistant to resist this axial pressure. Should the waist position be suboptimal, the balloon must be completely deflated prior to repositioning, otherwise the LES will be displaced and may be difficult to locate fluoroscopically. Finally, when the position of the partially inflated balloon is satisfactory, the balloon is inflated through a series of a rapid series of 5 cc increments until the waist is totally obliterated. Because the sphingomanometer that comes with the currently available achalasia balloons is poorly designed for the use of hydrostatic inflation, I use one of the pumps designed for the type of balloons used for strictures. Although there is a slightly greater risk of perforation reported with increasing distention pressure, it is not clear that there is a maximum pressure at which the attempt should be aborted, short of the bursting pressure of the balloon.

Surgery

Patients who choose surgery as their initial intervention, or who fail dilatation, should be referred to a surgeon with substantial experience in the field of esophageal surgery. Both the length of the myotomy and the performance of the fundoplication seem to be more of an art than a science. Experience and past results are very important for outcomes. Because of the shorter recovery times, I generally send patients to someone experienced in *minimally invasive surgery* for achalasia. At our institution, this has been a laparoscopic surgeon. In others, thoracoscopic surgeons appear to dominate. I do not think there is convincing evidence in favor of one over the other. Should a follow-up surgery be required because of bad results, we have tended to favor an open procedure on the grounds that the second surgery should have the best exposure possible in what may be the last good chance at surgical correction. However minimally invasive surgery for failed myotomies have been described.

Follow-Up

Should the initial botulinum treatment be unsuccessful or result in a response of limited duration, I will generally perform a second injection of the same dose of toxin before deciding to move onto an alternative approach. We have found that if the second injection fails, additional attempts are fruitless. Should the first dilatation fail, I will perform a second, this time with a 35 mm achalasia balloon. I feel that dilatation with larger balloons is associated with *a significant escalation in the risk of perforation,* and I only use the available 40 mm balloon under unusual circumstances and usually only if the patient wants to avoid other options at all costs.

After treatment, I primarily follow the patient's clinical response, using objective studies to provide new baselines and to correlate with symptoms. Of the available tests, the post-treatment LES pressure appears to be the best indicator of long term response after both botulinum toxin injection and dilatation. However, manometry is fairly noxious for the patient. I offer, but do not insist, that the patient go through with this procedure just to obtain this prognostic information. The change in other objective findings is variable, and often correlates poorly with symptoms. Under study conditions, although there are usually statistical improvements in objective studies in the study population as a whole, it is not uncommon to find dramatic discrepancies between the symptomatic and objective responses, and between different objective measures of response. I find it difficult to justify a repeat intervention on the basis of objective response alone if the patient is doing well clinically. More typically, I will obtain a follow-up barium esophagram after the initial series of treatment are completed, either to document esophageal emptying and the diameter of the esophageal lumen after a clinical response is achieved, or to reassess in preparation for alternative therapies if the patient's symptoms do not improve adequately.

After successful treatment, I will generally suggest that I see the patient in clinic on a yearly basis and do some form of objective testing—either barium esophagram or solid-phase radionuclide study—for the first few years. I will consider retreatment if symptoms recur or if there is evidence of progressive dilatation of the esophagus. In general when symptoms do recur, I will go through the various options again and help the patient decide, in light of the adequacy and duration of the previous response, whether to repeat the last treatment option or move onto an alternative choice.

Supplemental Reading

Annese V, Basciani M, Borrelli O, et al. Intrasphincteric injection of botulinum toxin is effective in long-term treatment of esophageal achalasia. Muscle Nerve 1998;21:1540–2.

Annese V, Basciani M, Perri F, et al. Controlled trial of botulinum toxin injection versus placebo and pneumatic dilation in achalasia. Gastroenterol 1996;111:1418–24.

Annese V, Bassotti G, Coccia G. A multicentre randomised study of intrasphincteric botulinum toxin in patients with oesophageal achalasia. GISMAD Achalasia Study Group. Gut 2000;46:597–600.

Bonavina L, Incarbone R, Antoniazzi L, Peracchia A. Does previous endoscopic treatment affect the outcome of laparascopic heller myotomy? Ann Chir 2000;125:45–9.

Csendes A, Braghetto I, Henriquez A, Cortes C. Late results of a prospective randomised study comparing forceful dilatation and oesophagomyotomy in patients with achalasia. Gut 1989;30:299–304.

Eckardt VF, Aignherr C, Bernhard G. Predictors of outcome in patients with achalasia treated by pneumatic dilation. Gastroenterol 1992;103:1732–8.

Ellis FH Jr, Watkins E Jr, Gibb SP, Heatley GJ. Ten to 20-year clinical results after short esophagomyotomy without an antireflux procedure (modified Heller operation) for esophageal achalasia. Eur J Cardiothorac Surg 1992;6:86–9.

Gelfond M, Rozen P, Gilat T. Isosorbide dinitrate and nifedipine treatment of achalasia: a clinical, manometric and radionuclide evaluation. Gastroenterol 1982;83:963–9.

Howard PJ, Maher L, Pryde A, et al. Five year prospective study of the incidence, clinical features, and diagnosis of achalasia in Edinburgh. Gut 1992; 33:1011–5.

Hunter JG, Trus TL, Branum GD, Waring JP. Laparoscopic Heller myotomy and fundoplication for achalasia. Ann Surg 1997;225:655–64.

Imperiale TF, O'Connor JB, Vaezi MF, Richter JE. A cost-minimization analysis of alternative treatment strategies for achalasia. Am J Gastroenterol 2000;95:2737–45.

Kadakia SC, Wong RK. Graded pneumatic dilation using Rigiflex achalasia dilators in patients with primary esophageal achalasia. Am J Gastroenterol 1993;88:34–8.

Katz PO, Gilbert J, Castell DO. Pneumatic dilatation is effective long-term treatment for achalasia. Dig Dis Sci 1998;43:1973–7.

Malthaner RA, Todd TR, Miller L, Pearson FG. Long-term results in surgically managed esophageal achalasia. Ann Thorac Surg 1994;58:1343–6.

Nair LA, Reynolds JC, Parkman HP, et al. Complications during pneumatic dilation for achalasia or diffuse esophageal spasm. Analysis of risk factors, early clinical characteristics, and outcome. Dig Dis Sci 1993;38:1893–904.

Okike N, Payne WS, Neufeld DM, et al. Esophagomyotomy versus forceful dilation for achalasia of the esophagus: results in 899 patients. Ann Thorac Surg 1979;28:119–25.

Panaccione R, Gregor JC, Reynolds RP, Preiksaitis HG. Intrasphincteric botulinum toxin versus pneumatic dilatation for achalasia: a cost minimization analysis. Gastrointest Endosc 1999;50:492–8.

Pasricha PJ, Rai R, Ravich WJ, et al. Botulinum toxin for achalasia: long-term outcome and predictors of response. Gastroenterol 1996;110:1410–5.

Pasricha PJ, Ravich WJ, Hendrix TR, et al. Intrasphincteric botulinum toxin for the treatment of achalasia. N Engl J Med 1995;332:774–8.

Patti MG, Feo CV, Arcerito M, et al. Effects of previous treatment on results of laparoscopic Heller myotomy for achalasia. Dig Dis Sci 1999;44:2270–6.

Ponce J, Garrigues V, Pertejo V, et al. Individual prediction of response to pneumatic dilation in patients with achalasia. Dig Dis Sci 1996;41:2135–41.

Prakash C, Freedland KE, Chan MF, Clouse RE. Botulinum toxin injections for achalasia symptoms can approximate the short term efficacy of a single pneumatic dilation: a survival analysis approach. Am J Gastroenterol 1999;94:328–33.

Streitz JM Jr, Ellis FH Jr, Williamson WA, et al. Objective assessment of gastroesophageal reflux after short esophagomyotomy for achalasia with the use of manometry and pH monitoring. J Thorac Cardiovasc Surg 1996;111:107–12.

Urbach DR, Hansen PD, Khajanchee YS, Swanstrom LL. A decision analysis of the optimal initial approach to achalasia: laparoscopic Heller myotomy with partial fundoplication, thoracoscopic Heller myotomy, pneumatic dilatation, or botulinum toxin injection. J Gastrointest Surg 2001;5:192–205.

Vaezi MF, Richter JE, Wilcox CM, et al. Botulinum toxin versus pneumatic dilatation in the treatment of achalasia: a randomised trial. Gut 1999;44:231–9.

CHAPTER 20

Management of Acute Variceal Bleeding

Paul J. Thuluvath, MBBS, MD, FRCP

Gastroesophageal variceal bleeding is an unpredictable complication of cirrhosis with an associated mortality of 15 to 30% with each bleeding episode, and about one-third of all deaths in patients with cirrhosis could be directly attributed to acute variceal bleeding. *Prevention of first bleeding (primary prophylaxis)* is therefore as important as *treatment of acute bleeding* and *secondary prophylaxis*. Patients with large varices or red signs, and those with an elevated hepatic venous wedge pressure gradient (> 12 mm Hg), should be treated with *nonselective β-blockers* to prevent the first bleed. Those who present with acute bleeding should be managed in an optimal fashion to reduce early mortality. The past decade has seen tremendous progress in the management of acute variceal bleeding. A large number of randomized, controlled studies have been published on this topic comparing various treatment options, but these studies have uniformly lacked the sample size to show an improvement in survival. However, careful observations based on these studies, as well many meta-analyses performed on these studies, have made it possible for the clinicians to devise better strategies to manage these patients (Figure 20-1).

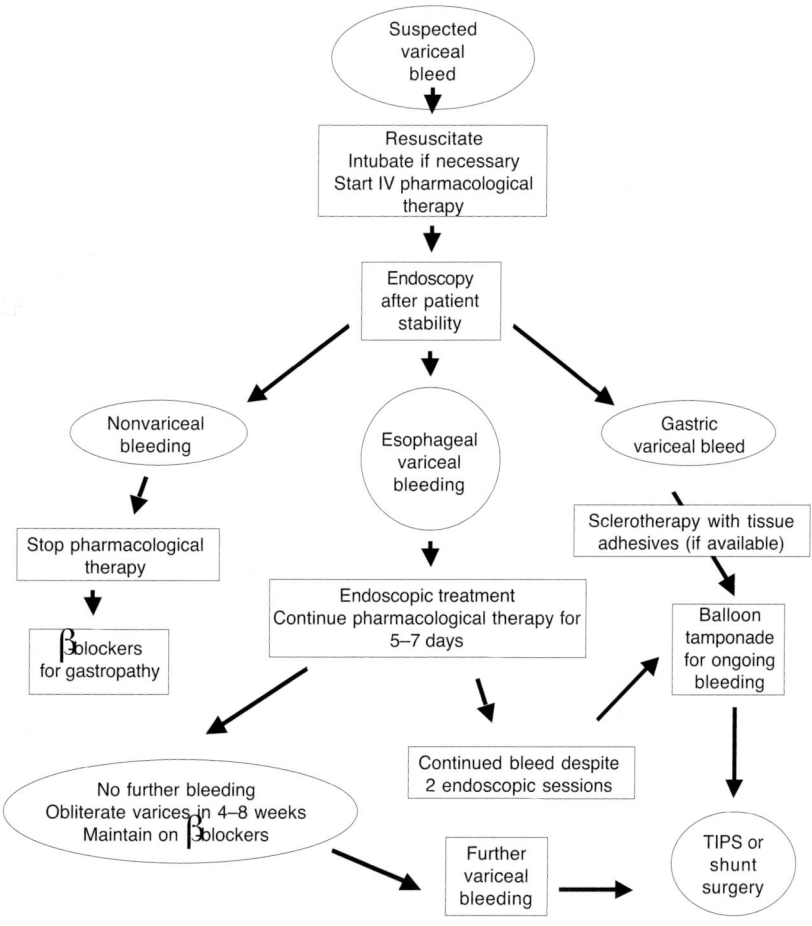

FIGURE 20-1. IV = intravenous; TIPS = transjugular intrahepatic portosystemic shunting.

Resuscitative Measures

Management of acute variceal bleeding includes *general resuscitative* measures and *specific treatment* aimed at arresting the variceal bleeding. It is important to protect airways in an encephalopathic patient, particularly during endoscopic procedures and balloon tamponade, since aspiration pneumonia is a major cause of morbidity and mortality in these patients. Measurement of central venous pressure is a sensitive guide to the blood volume status but caution should be exercised in the presence of tense ascites because diaphragmatic compression of the right atrium by the ascites may lead to an overestimation of the readings. *Pulmonary capillary wedge pressure* is the most accurate guide to control blood volume and may be invaluable in the presence of major ongoing bleeding. Blood volume restitution should be prompt and as accurate as possible to protect vital organs, particularly renal function. The ideal replacement fluid is *blood* and colloid is reserved for immediate infusion until blood becomes available. Isovolemic replacement should be the aim with care taken to avoid major overexpansion of the circulation that may precipitate further bleeding due to the associated increase in portal pressure. There is increasing evidence to support routine prophylactic antibiotics in those with ascites and in those with active bleeding. Control of bleeding is slower in patients with bacterial infection. It is therefore important to detect and treat complications, such as aspiration pneumonia and spontaneous bacterial peritonitis, at the earliest opportunity.

Because bleeding from a nonvariceal source is common in chronic liver disease, endoscopy should be performed when patient is stabilized. This may also be the ideal time to perform a therapeutic procedure to stop bleeding or prevent early rebleeding. If variceal bleeding is suspected, pharmacological treatment should be initiated while the patient is resuscitated before endoscopic confirmation of gastroesophageal variceal bleeding. Early pharmacologic treatment may improve the efficacy of endoscopic treatment as well as the survival.

Pharmacologic Treatment

The major benefit of *pharmacologic therapy* is that it can be given without any specialized training, even to the unstable patient. The safety margin and efficacy of some of the vasoconstrictor drugs used for this purpose has been less than desirable, but there have been major improvements in this area recently.

Vasopressin

Vasopressin, a peptide hormone, causes splanchnic arterial vasoconstriction, thereby reducing portal blood flow and portal pressure. The main side effects of vasopressin are secondary to nonselective arterial vasoconstriction. These include ischemia of the myocardium, abdominal viscera and lower limbs, left heart failure, hypertension, and arrhythmia. In randomized, controlled studies, between 30 to 60% experienced one or more complications and about 25% of patients were withdrawn because of a major complication. A combination of vasopressin and nitroglycerine has been shown to reduce the hemodynamic side effects of vasopressin without attenuating the effect on portal inflow. The transdermal route may be preferred because of ease of administration. The reported efficacy of vasopressin is around 50 to 60% compared with 40% with placebo. Because of the poor safety profile and the availability of safer alternatives, vasopressin is not recommended for the management of acute variceal bleeding. However, if it was used because of its low costs, it should be used in combination with nitroglycerine.

Terlipressin (or glypressin) (triglycyl lysine vasopressin), currently not available in the United States, is a prodrug that is converted to lysine vasopressin in vivo. Terlipressin (glypressin) has properties similar to those of vasopressin, and unlike vasopressin, it can be given as bolus doses through a peripheral line. For unexplained reasons, terlipressin does appear to offer enhanced control of bleeding (efficacy around 80%), with fewer side effects compared to vasopressin when used with or without nitroglycerin. Repeated administration of terlipressin has been found to be as effective as sclerotherapy to control acute bleeding and to prevent early rebleeding.

Somatostatin and Octreotide

Somatostatin and *octreotide*, a cyclic octopeptide analogue of somatostatin, cause splanchnic vasoconstriction by a direct effect on vascular smooth muscle and possibly by inhibiting the release of vasodilatory peptides such as glucagon. Continuous infusion of somatostatin has been found to produce a sustained decrease in HVWPG and blunt the rise in HVWPG in response to test meal and blood transfusion. However, to obtain optimal results, both these drugs need to be given as *repeated bolus doses* in *addition to a continuous infusion*. Although the standard dose of somatostatin is 250 µg bolus followed by 250 µg/hr, a higher dose (500 µg/hr) may benefit those who demonstrate active bleeding during emergency endoscopy.

A number of studies have compared somatostatin and octreotide with placebo, endoscopic treatment, or tamponade. These studies have clearly shown that both drugs are free of any major side effects, even when these were used as continuous infusion over 5 to 7 days. These studies also have shown a significant trend favoring somatostatin and

---

Editor's Note: Vasopressin has been found to be superior to epinephrine for cardiac asystole and vasopressin following epinephrine may be more effective than epinephrine alone for refractory cardiac arrest (Wenzel et al, 2004).

octreotide compared with either placebo or vasopressin. Infusion of somatostatin or octreotide has been shown to be comparable to balloon tamponade or endoscopic treatment. Meta-analyses of controlled trials have shown that *octreotide* is *superior* to *vasopressin/terlipressin*, and *comparable to sclerotherapy*. The side effect profile of octreotide is similar to placebo and significantly better than vasopressin/terlipressin. The excellent safety margin of these drugs allows their use in the emergency department while the patient is resuscitated and also over the first few days after the bleeding to prevent early rebleeding.

Endoscopic Therapy

ENDOSCOPIC SCLEROTHERAPY

Endoscopic sclerotherapy has an efficacy rate of 75 to 90%. Endoscopic band ligation is an alternative to sclerotherapy. Meta-analytical studies have shown that hemostasis rates with band ligation are comparable to sclerotherapy in patients with active variceal bleeding. However, no specific benefits have been shown for this technique over injection sclerotherapy during active bleeding. Band ligation has been found to be safe in children with acute variceal bleeding. Although endoscopic treatment may be marginally better than somatostatin/octreotide in some meta-analytical studies, many carefully performed studies and a recent meta-analysis have failed to show any significant advantage for either form of treatment when used alone. Moreover, sclerotherapy was associated with more adverse events than somatostatin/ octreotide.

BAND LIGATION, TISSUE ADHESIVES

About 15 to 20% of patients treated with endoscopic sclerotherapy develop complications such as bleeding postsclerotherapy ulcers, esophageal stenosis, or perforation of esophagus. It is likely that the complication rates are lower with *band ligation*. *Tissue adhesives* such as *n-butyl-2-cyaoacrylate* have also been used by intravariceal injection to obliterate varices. Tissue adhesives are not approved for intravariceal injection in the United States, but studies from elsewhere have claimed control of bleeding in approximately 90% of cases. The specific role for this treatment may be to obliterate fundal varices that respond unreliably to intravariceal injection of sclerosant or band ligation. *Cerebral toxicity* has been reported with the use of intravariceal injection of tissue adhesives. Currently there is no convincing evidence to recommend routine use of tissue adhesives for esophageal variceal obliteration.

Combination of Endoscopic and Pharmacologic Treatment

A combination of continuous infusion of *octreotide for 5 days along* with either *sclerotherapy* or *band ligation* has been shown to be superior to either sclerotherapy or band ligation alone in reducing early rebleeding and mortality. The combination treatment appears to particularly benefit those patients with shock and ongoing bleeding. In addition, continuous infusion of octreotide also has been shown to be very effective in reducing bleeding from postsclerotherapy esophageal ulceration. Other combination treatments, such as addition of isosorbide mononitrate to somatostatin, have not been shown to have any advantage over somatostatin alone. The current evidence favors the use of a *combination of endoscopic treatment* with *either octreotide or somatostatin*. These drugs should be started prior to endoscopy and continued for *5 to 7 days* after the bleeding episode.

Until recently, it was generally accepted that immediate endoscopic treatment is the optimum treatment for active variceal bleeding, but is critically dependent upon available expertise to attain these high success rates and to minimize complications. The optimum timing of endoscopic treatment with respect to the bleeding episode remains unanswered. The options are immediate treatment with the associated technical difficulties, or delayed treatment after temporary hemostasis is achieved using vasoconstrictive drugs. Because the efficacy of somatostatin, octreotide or terlipressin is comparable to endoscopic treatment, it is reasonable to postpone endoscopy for treatment, as well as to confirm the diagnosis, until the patient is stabilized with pharmcologic intervention. Immediate endoscopic treatment could be reserved for nonresponders to pharmacologic intervention. To reduce early rebleeding, it is advisable to continue vasoconstrictors, such as somatostatin or octreotide (or terlipressin), for the first 5 to 7 days after the bleeding episode.

Predictors of Failure to Control Acute Variceal Bleeding

A reliable model that could predict the failure of hemostasis after an acute bleeding episode will be very useful for risk stratification, management, and research purposes. Many studies have been done, but small sample size, retrospective nature of the study, the heterogeneity of offered therapy and different patient characteristics make it difficult to draw any definite conclusions. However, *active bleeding* at the *time of endoscopy* has been shown to independently predict failure to control bleeding as well as early (30 day) mortality in many studies. Other factors include *higher HVWPG, encephalopathy, low platelet counts, history of alcoholism, shorter interval to admission, and bacterial infections.*

Patients who continue to bleed despite adequate endoscopic and pharmacologic treatment should be managed by *balloon tamponade* followed by *transjugular intrahepatic portosystemic shunting* (TIPS) or surgery.

Balloon Tamponade

Balloon tamponade is a highly effective method of controlling active variceal bleeding. In experienced hands, it is equivalent to endoscopic treatment for the immediate control of bleeding, but efficacy extends only to the period of application. In inexperienced hands, the morbidity and mortality of balloon tamponade may be unacceptably high. Balloon tamponade is best reserved for the management of life threatening bleeding when a risk of exsanguination exists and endoscopic intervention is unlikely to be feasible, or when a combination of endoscopic and pharmacologic treatment has failed to control bleeding. Balloon tamponade should be followed by more definitive treatment within 24 hours. Depending on the situation, the definitive treatment may include endoscopic ligation or sclerotherapy (only in those who had no effective endoscopic treatment prior to balloon tamponade), surgery, and TIPS.

Surgery and TIPS

Although endoscopic therapy at the time of diagnostic endoscopy probably is the optimum approach to an episode of variceal bleeding, TIPS or surgical intervention (shunt or nonshunt procedure) has an important role, particularly in patients who *continue to bleed despite a combination of endoscopic and pharmacologic therapy*. It is reasonable to *repeat endoscopic therapy on a second occasion* before considering it to have failed. However, the decision to progress to TIPS or surgery should not be further delayed in order to prevent the inevitable escalation of operative risks in a deteriorating patient. Patients with ongoing variceal bleeding should be stabilized with *balloon tamponade* prior to TIPS or surgery. The choice between TIPS or surgery depends on the local expertise, and the severity of the liver disease. Patients with *mild disease* (Child A) may be better candidates for *surgical shunt*.

TIPS has evolved as the major "rescue" procedure for the management of acute variceal bleeding in most centers in the United States. TIPS has been increasingly used in the United States as a rescue procedure because of the relative inexperience with emergency shunt surgery in many centers. The morbidity and mortality with TIPS in patients with advanced cirrhosis and ongoing bleeding is similar to that of surgical procedures. In patients with ongoing bleeding and very advanced liver disease (Child-Pugh C), the mortality with TIPS is close to 50% and this is more of a reflection of the severity of liver disease.

If surgery was preferred, the type of surgical shunt chosen should be based on local expertise. *Selective distal splenorenal* shunt requires more operating time compared to either *mesocaval or portocaval* shunt, which makes it generally unsuitable as an emergency procedure. Shunt surgery does not preclude subsequent transplantation, but could be associated with hepatic encephalopathy in a significant number of patients. The most commonly used nonshunting surgery is *esophageal transection* with varying degrees of devascularization, and it is rarely used in the Western hemisphere. The only major concern that arises from the use of devascularization procedures is the adverse effect on liver transplantation because of extensive scar tissue and adhesions. In controlled trials that have compared sclerotherapy with esophageal transection or portocaval shunting, the survival rates were not different between the groups. However, this procedure is rarely done these days in the Western countries because of better alternatives.

Secondary Prophylaxis

Rebleeding is common after the first bleed; 50 to 80% of those who survive the first bleed rebleed within 2 years and most rebleed within 6 weeks after the first bleed. A number of options are available to prevent recurrent bleeding, including *endoscopic treatment, nonselective β-blockers, shunt or nonshunt surgery, TIPS, and liver transplantation*. This area will be discussed in more detail in Chapter 117, "Portal Hypertension."

Recent trials comparing *propranolol/nadolol* with *sclerotherapy/band ligation* have confirmed that both forms of treatment are similar in efficacy. Although it may appear logical to perform long term follow-up endoscopic treatment, there is no convincing evidence to suggest that long term follow-up treatment is superior to short term treatment aimed at obliteration of varices, especially if patients are maintained on β-blockers. Based on the limited data, it appears that addition of *β-blockers to short term endoscopic therapy* may be superior to either treatment alone. This was to be expected since a number of patients on β-blockers do not attain a significant reduction in HVWP. Combination treatment may be useful especially in patients who are less likely to comply with medical treatment or in those who cannot tolerate maximal medical treatment. Currently, *shunt surgery* (preferably *mesocaval shunt or distal splenorenal* shunt) is reserved for patients with good synthetic function (Child A) and recurrent variceal bleeding who fail endoscopic and pharmacologic treatment. *TIPS* is very effective in preventing recurrent rebleeding, but it is associated with very high rates of shunt stenosis and occlusion. The current indication for TIPS is as a bridge to transplantation in patients with advanced cirrhosis (Child B or C) who present with recurrent rebleeding despite variceal obliteration and pharmacologic therapy. The mortality after variceal bleeding and the long term survival following the index bleed are directly related to the severity of liver disease. It is difficult to imagine that the various treatment options discussed here are likely to improve liver function and, hence, survival. *Liver transplantation*, with 5-year survival rate reaching 85 to 90% percent, is the treatment of choice for patients with advanced liver disease.

Gastric Varices

The incidence of *gastric varices* in published reports varies from 6 to 16%, and the incidence appears to increase after esophageal variceal obliteration. Gastric varices are usually seen in association with esophageal varices or, rarely, in isolation as in splenic vein thrombosis (segmental portal hypertension). The overall *mortality* from bleeding gastric varices is *over 50%*. Although the management of gastric varices is similar to that of esophageal varices, endoscopic sclerotherapy using sclerosant should be reserved only for lesser curve varices or varices within a hiatus hernia. *Tissue adhesives*, as discussed earlier, may be used to inject fundal varices during active bleeding or preferably after the initial bleeding has stopped. It is technically difficult to inject fundal varices when there is active bleeding. If balloon tamponade is unsuccessful in patients with bleeding fundal varices, one should proceed immediately to TIPS or shunt surgery. Splenectomy is curative when isolated fundal varices are seen in association with splenic vein thrombosis.

Ectopic Varices

Bleeding from nongastroesophageal sites varies from 1.6 to 5% in the large reported series. The common ectopic sites, usually seen in association with esophageal varices, are *duodenum, colon, anorectum, and enterostomy*. Rarely these varices may be localized, especially in the colon, and result from superior or inferior vein thrombosis, tumor infiltration, adhesions, or congenital malformation. The management of the bleeding depends on the site of bleeding, the severity of liver disease, and the local expertise. Because there are no controlled studies, it is difficult to recommend any special strategy. Shunt surgery may be the best line of management for bleeding varices in the duodenum, jejunum, ileum, and enterostomy. If portal vein is patent and the expertise for TIPS is readily available, TIPS should be considered as the first line of management before other forms of shunt surgery. Anecdotal reports suggest that duodenal varices and ileostomy varices can be managed successfully by sclerotherapy or feeding vessel embolization, but one has to consider carefully the postsclerotherapy complications, such as duodenal perforation and stoma dysfunction, and the high recurrence rate after embolization. Tissue adhesives may be used in selected cases. Colonic varices are usually localized and can be managed by local resection. When colonic varices are seen in association with esophageal varices, TIPS may be a safer alternative. Anorectal varices can be safely treated with sclerotherapy or by underrunning with an absorbable suture.

Recommendations

Nonselective β-blockers should be used for primary prophylaxis in patients with advanced liver disease and large varices. Optimal resuscitation in a timely fashion is crucial for a better outcome in patients with acute variceal bleeding. Pharmacologic intervention while the patient is resuscitated is safe and beneficial, and pharmacologic treatment should be continued for 5 to 7 days to prevent early rebleeding. Endoscopic diagnosis and therapy should be performed when patient is adequately resuscitated and stabilized. TIPS or shunt surgery should be reserved for nonresponders to a combination of pharmacologic and endoscopic therapy, and should not be delayed when endoscopic therapy has failed on two separate occasions. Bleeding fundal varices are managed by either early surgery or TIPS, and balloon tamponade should be used to control active bleeding. If tissue adhesives are available, endoscopic treatment with these agents may be an alternate option for bleeding gastric or ectopic varices before considering surgery or TIPS. A combination of β-blockers (± nitrates) and endoscopic treatment (preferably banding) may be a logical approach for secondary prophylaxis. TIPS or shunt surgery should be reserved for patients who rebleed despite a combination of endoscopic and pharmacologic therapy. Liver transplantation is the treatment of choice for patients with advanced liver disease and recurrent variceal bleeding.

Supplemental Reading

Avgernos A, Nevens F, Raptis S, Fevery J. Early administration of somatostatin and efficacy of sclerotherapy in acute esophageal variceal bleeds: the European Acute Bleeding Esophageal Variceal Episodes (ABOVE) randomized trial. Lancet 1997;350:1495–9.

Banares R, Albillos A, Rincon D, et al. Endoscopic treatment versus endoscopic plus pharmacologic treatment for acute variceal bleeding: a meta-analysis. Hepatology 2002;35:609–15.

Ben-Ari Z, Cardin F, McCormick AP, et al. A predictive model for failure to control bleeding during acute variceal hemorrhage. J Hepatol 1999;31:443–50.

Besson I, Ingrad P, Person B, et al. Sclerotherapy with or without octreotide for acute variceal bleeding. N Engl J Med 1995;333:555–60.

Cales P, Masliah C, Bernard B, et al. Early administration of vapreotide for variceal bleeding in patients with cirrhosis. French Club for the Study of Portal Hypertension. N Engl J Med 2001;344:23–8.

Corley DA, Cello JP, Adkisson W, et al. Octreotide for acute esophageal variceal bleeding: a meta-analysis. Gastroenterology 2001;120:946–54.

D'Amico G, Pagliaro L, Bosch J. The treatment of portal hypertension: a meta-analytic review. Hepatology 1995;22:332–54.

D'Amico G, Pietrossi G, Tsrantino I, Pagliaro L. Emergency sclerotherapy versus vasoactive drugs for variceal bleeding in cirrhosis: a Cochrane meta-analysis. Gastroenterol 2003;124:127–91.

Escorsell A, Ruiz del Arbol L, Planas R, et al. Multicenter randomized controlled trial of terlipressin versus sclerotherapy in the treatment of acute variceal bleeding: the TEST study. Hepatology 2000;32:471–6.

Imperiale TF, Carlos Teran J, McCullough AJ. A meta-analysis of somatostatin versus vasopressin in the management of acute esophageal variceal hemorrhage. Gastroenterology 1995;109:1289–94.

Levacher S, Letoumelin P, Pateron D, et al. Early administration of terlipressin plus glyceryl trinitrate to control active upper gastrointestinal bleeding in cirrhotic patients. Lancet 1995;346;865–8.

Lo GH, Lai KH, Cheng JS, et al. A prospective, randomized trial of butyl cyanoacrylate injection versus band ligation in the management of bleeding gastric varices. Hepatology 2001;33:1060–4.

Moitinho E, Escorsell A, Bandi JC, et al. Prognostic value of early measurements of portal pressure in acute variceal bleeding. Gastroenterology 1999;117:626–31.

Planas R, Quer JQ, Boix J, et al. A prospective randomized trial comparing somatostatin and sclerotherapy in the treatment of acute variceal bleeding. Hepatology 1994;20:370–5.

Sung JJY, Chung SCS, Lai CW, et al. Octreotide infusion or emergency sclerotherapy for variceal haemorrhage. Lancet 1993;342:637–41.

Sung JJY, Chung SCS, Yung MY, et al. Prospective randomised study of effect of octreotide on rebleeding from oesophageal varices after endoscopic ligation. Lancet 1995;346:1666–9.

Thuluvath PH, Krishnan A. Primary prophylaxis of variceal bleeding. Gastrointest Endosc 2003;58:558–67.

Tripathi D, Therapondos G, Jackson E, et al. The role of transjugular intrahepatic portosystemic stent shunt (TIPSS) in the management of bleeding gastric varices: clinical and hemodynamic correlations. Gut 2002;51:270–4.

Wenzel V, Krisner AC, Arntz HR, et al. A comparison of vasopressin and epinephrine for out-of-hospital cardiopulmonary resuscitation. N Engl J Med 2004;350:105–13.

CHAPTER 21

Cancer of the Esophagus

Michael K. Gibson, MD, and Arlene A. Forastiere, MD

Treatment of esophageal cancer (EC) remains a challenging endeavor that is best approached by a multidisciplinary team. Furthermore, significant controversy exists regarding the standard of care for this group of complex patients. Although this aggressive cancer remains difficult to treat and even more difficult to cure, recent advances in screening, diagnosis, treatment, and supportive care are resulting in progress (Polednak, 2003). The goal of this chapter is to provide up-to-date and concise guidance to the health care providers working together to better the outlook for patients with EC. After a brief review of epidemiology, the primary focus will be on treatment, be it with palliative or curative intent. Although supportive care is an integral part of treatment, another full chapter in this text is devoted to palliative care (see Chapter 22, "Palliation of Esophageal Cancer").

The chapter will be presented in the same sequential manner that clinicians use when they approach a referred patient who is already diagnosed. A review of initial broad considerations will be followed by more detailed discussions of staging—with particular emphasis on categorizing patients as either curable or not. Specifics of treatment will be stratified by the presenting stage, with the majority of discussion involving the controversial area of locally advanced (curable) disease. The chapter concludes with a few words about follow-up and recurrent disease.

Epidemiology

Although the overall number of cases of EC in the United States continues to rise—estimated at 13,900 cases in 2003—the change in epidemiology is more striking. Squamous cell cancer (SCC) used to be the most common histology; however, due to a steady increase in adenocarcinoma (AC) over the past several decades, this histology currently makes up the majority of new diagnoses. Most of these cases are thought to arise from *Barrett's esophagus (BE)*, a premalignant condition that results from chronic gastroesophageal reflux that is likely exacerbated by obesity and hiatal hernia.

Concurrent with the emergence of two distinct histologic types is the necessity of considering the differences between these two entities when initially assessing a patient. Although the treatment approach typically does not vary greatly by histologic type of EC, differences in epidemiology, pathophysiology, and tumor behavior may impact management. *SCC* is more common in patients with a history of alcohol and tobacco use, is stable in incidence in the United States, tends to be located in the upper and middle esophagus, and has a greater tendency to recur locally. Locoregional nodes occur in the upper mediastinum, and mestastatic disease is more commonly found in the supraclavicular nodes and lung parenchyma. *AC* is related to gastroesophageal reflux and BE, is increasing in incidence, occurs usually in the distal esophagus and gastroesophageal junction, and is more likely to recur in abdominal nodes and distant organ sites. Locoregional nodal spread is via the retroperitoneum to include the celiac and gastrohepatic regions, whereas metastases typically are found in the liver and occasionally on the peritoneum. Finally, *differentiating distal esophageal AC from primary gastric cancer* is also critical, as treatment of these two cancers differs.

Initial Considerations

Staging

The initial overview of a patient with EC is a multidisciplinary effort that addresses a number of factors, including tumor histology, staging, and overall health status. An experienced team approach will enable choice of appropriate treatment. The team should include the following:

1. A medical oncologist
2. A radiation oncologist
3. A thoracic surgeon skilled at esophagectomy
4. A gastroenterologist with experience performing endoscopic ultrasound (EUS)
5. A nutrionist familiar with parenteral nutrition
6. Nurses, intensivists and anesthesiologists skilled at caring for these complex patients

Familiarity with these procedures and patients is critical—several studies demonstrate that outcome correlates with surgical volume, expertise of the ultrasonographer, and adequacy of nutritional support (Nozoe et al, 2002; Schlick et al, 1999; Dimick et al, 2003).

Perhaps the single most important factor in the evaluation is staging. It determines whether the patient will be treated with curative or palliative intent. Because tissue is obtained most often by endoscopic biopsy, new referrals will have a general description of the endoluminal tumor, including appearance, location within the esophagus (cervical, mid, distal, gastroesophageal junction [GEJ]), and extent of luminal obstruction. Following biopsy confirmation, EUS is now the standard modality for determining T and local N stage, the factors most highly correlated with prognosis in patients with locally advanced disease.

EUS

For the primary tumor, EUS provides reliable information about the extent of tumor penetration into, and possibly through, the esophageal wall. Depth of penetration, defined as T stage, correlates with both the extent of lymph node involvement as well as resectability. This directly impacts treatment and prognosis—T_4 lesions that invade adjacent structures such as the aorta, vena cava or pericardium are unresectable—and lymph node status correlates with survival. Supplementing information about tumor depth is the ability to image local (periesophageal and celiac) lymph nodes, with the added benefit of endoscopic biopsy if desired for confirmation. For lesions in the distal esophagus or involving the GEJ, EUS also provides information about extension of tumor into the gastric cardia and celiac lymph nodes. Retroflexing the endoscope to detect tumors that emanate primarily from the cardia is essential. In this situation, biopsy of the fundus is important, because these lesions that extend into the body of the stomach are treated as primary gastric tumors. Involvement of celiac nodes (M_{1a}) in disease that straddles the GEJ is still considered locally advanced and thus curable EC. There is an earlier chapter (see Chapter 5, "Endoscopic Ultrasound and Fine Needle Aspiration") on endoscopic ultrasound and fine needle aspiration.

COMPUTED TOMOGRAPHY AND POSITRON EMISSION TOMOGRAPHY SCANS

Computed tomography (CT) and *positron emission tomography (PET)* are then used to assess for distant metastases (M stage). Until the advent of routinely available PET, CT was the imaging approach of choice for detecting distant lymph nodes and solid organ metastases. CT is still used to stage every patient and to follow each patient for response to therapy. Recent studies by Flamen and colleagues (2000), however, suggest a powerful role of PET in detecting distant disease that is missed by CT. The current approach is to obtain a PET (or PET/CT) scan on every patient considered for curative therapy. In those with PET-detected lesions not seen on CT, the finding should be *confirmed* with biopsy or additional imaging before denying potential curative treatment. A small fraction of patients with distal lesions will also have *occult peritoneal metastases* that are too small for detection on PET. However, because all patients slated for curative therapy undergo *jejunostomy tube placement*, the peritoneum is visualized directly prior to initiation of treatment.

Performance Status

As with other tumor types, the overall health status of the patient prior to treatment correlates with how well treatment is tolerated. Studies continue to demonstrate that this variable—*performance status*—remains the *single most important predictor of outcome* in cancer patients. Patients with EC most commonly present with dysphagia, weight loss, and pain, all factors that contribute to decreased performance status. These combined with the aggressive—and often toxic—nature of treatment, especially for the 50% of patients who present with potentially curable disease, can create a significant management challenge. As such, performance status is paramount as both a *factor to be treated primarily* and a factor that *significantly impacts the therapeutic approach* to the cancer.

TREATING PERFORMANCE STATUS

Regarding performance status as a factor to be treated, the initial therapy often involves an intervention designed to improve performance status. *Pain* is assessed and treated at the initial visit. *Nutritional deficiency*, usually related to dysphagia, is also addressed. Each patient is introduced to a nutritionist who helps to jointly determine the best way to supplement nutrition in order to mitigate weight loss and hopefully achieve weight gain. For patients with metastatic disease, oral intake can often be restored with an *esophageal stent*. If this is inadequate or not possible, a *percutaneous gastrostomy (PEG)* or *surgical jejunostomy tube* is placed. For patients triaged to undergo *curative therapy, stents are avoided*. There is some concern for esophageal perforation when a stent is present in the radiation field. If neoadjuvant therapy followed by esophagectomy is planned, a *surgically placed jejunostomy* tube is preferable to a PEG so as not to violate the gastric wall.

DETERMINING TREATMENT AGGRESSIVENESS

Determining appropriate level of treatment aggressiveness in the setting of performance status may be challenging even to the most experienced clinician. In this case, consideration includes the above as well as medical comorbidities relating to fitness for surgery, aggressive chemoradiotherapy, or cytotoxic drugs. As a general rule, *combined modality approaches (chemoradiotherapy ± surgery)* are *reserved* for the *healthiest* patients with *curable* disease. For those *less healthy* but still curable, surgical colleagues may consider *primary esophagectomy*. However, esophagectomy, even in the absence of preoperative treatment, is a major procedure with significant morbidity and mortality.

Concomitant chemoradiotherapy without surgery may be as difficult to tolerate as esophagectomy, especially given issues of *mucositis* and *cytopenias*. Therefore, in those patients with curative disease but poor performance status, the same palliative approaches that are usually reserved for those with metastatic disease are often pursued. For both curable patients with poor performance status as well as in those with primary metastatic disease, the palliative modality and regimen again must be tailored to the patient's performance status. Further discussion of this follows in the section of palliative chemotherapy.

Therapy of Locally Advanced Disease

Although the best management of curable EC remains controversial, several approaches are available and can be tailored based on the condition of the patient, location of tumor within the esophagus, and T stage. The three major treatment modalities of chemotherapy, radiotherapy and surgery can be combined in a number of ways, and within each modality there are further choices of types and schedules of drugs, dose and schedule of radiotherapy and approach to esophagectomy. Although the options are broad, certainties do exist. There are two generally accepted standards of care that can be offered to patients with locally advanced disease—*primary surgery* and *primary chemoradiotherapy*. Two special cases, however, are worth reviewing. Because of the difficulty of resecting *cervical esophageal lesions*, these are treated with *primary chemoradiotherapy*, not surgery. The same approach is taken with unresectable T₄ lesions.

Primary Esophagectomy

One accepted standard of care for curable disease is primary esophagectomy. The results obtained with surgery alone in two randomized trials of surgery versus chemotherapy followed by surgery show a surgical cure rate of approximately 25% at 3 years of follow-up (Kelsen et al, 1998; Medical Research Council Oesophageal Cancer Working Group, 2002). Patients with an R0 resection (complete resection with negative margins) did better than those without, but this was achieved in only 50 to 60% of patients. *Adjuvant local radiotherapy* reduces local recurrence in patients with *positive surgical margins*, and this is the sole indication. It is unclear whether adjuvant chemotherapy or chemoradiotherapy is beneficial.

Concomitant Chemoradiotherapy

A *second standard of care*, which is *at least equivalent to surgery*, is *primary concomitant chemoradiotherapy (CRT)*. The benchmark is the Intergroup (RTOG 85-01) study first published in 1992 (Herskovic et al, 1992) then with further follow-up in 1999 (Cooper et al, 1999). Five-year survival was 27% in the CRT group and 0% in the radiation alone group. *This study established chemoradiotherapy as a curative option, provided an approach for patients who could not or did not want to have surgery, and confirmed that radiation alone was not curative.*

Preoperative Chemotherapy

Another approach of recent interest and active study but *not yet standard of care* is *chemotherapy alone followed by surgery*. Two large, published, randomized trials provide *conflicting* results. The US study led by Kelsen and colleagues (1998) evaluated three cycles of 5-fluorouracil (5-FU) and cisplatin followed by surgery and found no difference in survival. The UK Medical Research Council study led by McDonald evaluated two cycles of 5-FU and cisplatin followed by surgery and found a survival benefit to preoperative chemotherapy. Given the difficulty in resolving these opposing results, further trials are awaited, and *preoperative chemotherapy alone should be used only in the setting of a clinical trial.*

Trimodality Approach

Our preference for patients with *good performance status* and *resectable lesions* is to use *preoperative (neoadjuvant) concomitant CRT* followed by *transhiatal esophagectomy*. The *tri-modality approach* evolved from the observation that current standards still result in significant failures. Patients who undergo primary surgery often recur with distant metastases, whereas a substantial proportion of those undergoing definitive CRT recur locally. There are theoretical advantages of combining CRT with surgery. Micrometastatic systemic disease is treated with chemotherapy, the primary tumor is downstaged with chemoradiation (taking advantage of the radiosensitizing properties of cytotoxics), and residual macro or micrometastatic disease is resected.

There are at least four *randomized trials of preoperative CRT versus surgery alone*. The trials by Urba and colleagues (2001) and Walsh and colleagues (1996) showed benefit whereas the two by LePrise and colleagues (1994) and Bosset and colleagues (1997) did not. The results are summarized in Table 21-1. Although the results are conflicting, no trial is considered definitive or without fault. In addition, comparing the studies is difficult because of differences in factors that include sequencing of chemotherapy and radiation; doses, types and schedules of chemotherapy; and radiation and surgical outcome. Although the results of these trials and other phase II studies have led to adoption of preoperative CRT as *accepted treatment within community practice, the results are mixed. This approach cannot be considered standard of care and is best used in the confines of a clinical trial.*

TABLE 21-1. Combined Modality Therapy Options For Locally Advanced Disease

Resectable
 Primary surgery
 Chemotherapy followed by surgery (Kelsen et al, 1998; Medical Research Council Oesophageal Cancer Working Group, 2002)
 *Chemoradiotherapy (neoadjuvant) followed by surgery (Bossett et al, 1997; Le Prise et al, 1994; Urba et al, 2001; Walsh et al, 1996)
Unresectable
 Radiotherapy
 *Concomitant chemoradiotherapy (Herskovic et al, 1992)

	R0 Resection Surgery Only Arm	3-Year Survival, Surgery	3-Year Survival, CMT*	Median Follow-up for Survivors	Histology	Schedule
Preoperative Chemoradiotherapy						
Le Prise	Not available (total n = 86)	47%[†]	47%[†]	Not available	Squamous	Sequential to 20 Gy
Bosset	69% (94/137)	34%	36%	55.2 months	Squamous	Sequential, Interrupted (no 5-FU) to 37 Gy
Urba	88% (44/50)	16%	30%	8.2 years	Both	Concurrent to 45 Gy
Walsh	Not available (total n = 113)	6%	32%	> 5 years	Adeno	Concurrent to 40 Gy
Preoperative Chemotherapy						
Kelsen	59% (135/227)	26%	23%	46.5 months	Both	N/A
MRC	54% (215/402)	25%	32%	37.9 months	Both	N/A
Primary Chemoradiotherapy, 5-year Survival						
Herskovic	N/A	CRT 27%	R only 0%	12.5 months	Both	CRT, 64 Gy R, 50 Gy

CMT = combined modality therapy; CRT = chemoradiotherapy; 5-FU = 5-fluorouracil.
*Approach preferred by authors.
[†]Survival at 1 year (3 year results not available).

INSTITUTIONAL EXPERIENCE

Nevertheless, our group continues to have success with this approach. Our most recent series of 92 patients documented a *5-year survival of 40%* in patients treated with *5-FU and cisplatin* based regimens followed by *transhiatal esophagectomy* (Kleinberg et al, 2003). Currently, each potentially curable patient undergoes an *extensive examination* by our multidisciplinary team. Each patient is *staged* with EUS and PET/CT to rule out unresectable and/or metastatic disease. If still eligible based on the staging and evaluation of performance status, the patient is then *examined by a radiation oncologist and thoracic surgeon skilled in esophagectomy*. All patients then have a *staging laparoscopy* and *jejunostomy* tube placed and undergo a comprehensive nutritional examination. Once these pretreatment steps are completed, patients are then treated with *5-FU and cisplatin concomitant with daily radiotherapy to 45 Gy* followed by *transhiatal esophagectomy* or a clinical trial. Surgery is carried out between *4 to 8 weeks after conclusion of CRT*. Patients who obtain a *pathologic complete response (~30%)* to preoperative therapy have a markedly *better survival* than those who do not.

Metastatic Disease

Metastatic disease is incurable, so the goal is to maximize the quality of life while prolonging life. Palliation remains a major concern and in general follows the approaches outlined in the previous section. Although *chemotherapy is effective in approximately 50%* of patients, approaches to *pain management* and *nutrition* succeed in almost everyone. Pain is treated with combinations of short and long acting narcotics as well as local radiotherapy if needed. Again, swallowing may be restored with stent placement, and nutrition can always be provided through a PEG or jejunostomy tube. There is another chapter (Chapter 22 "Palliation of Esophageal Cancer") that is devoted to palliation of esophageal carcinoma.

Chemotherapy is given in *doublets* and chosen based on projected efficacy, patient performance status/medical comorbidities, and the side effect profile of the agents used. Increasing the number of drugs beyond two does not seem to increase efficacy. There is significant experience with combinations of *cisplatinum* and *5-FU*. More recently published regimens were developed in phase II clinical trials, often at single institutions. Some remain in abstract form.

For those patients with good performance status, several regimens are available. Our *preference* is to enroll this group in *clinical trials*. The National Cancer Institute provides a Web site (<www.cancer.gov>) that includes a database of trials that is searchable by state and type of trial (phase I, II, or III). Although *infusional 5-FU and cisplatin may be considered* the standard of care, it is *inconvenient* and can be associated with *significant mucositis*. Doublets containing newer agents can be given, often weekly, in the outpatient setting without a central venous catheter (Enzinger et al, 1999). One approach is the doublet of weekly *cisplatin* and *irinotecan* developed by Ilson and colleagues (1999). *Paclitaxel* is also active and continues to be studied by our group, including in combination with *cisplatin, carboplatin,* or *irinotecan* (Ilson et al, 2000). More recent trials are evaluating the role of alternatives to 5-FU and paclitaxel, such as *capecitabine* and *docetaxel*. Biologically targeted agents such as *tyrosine kinase inhibitors* will likely have a role in the future but are currently investigational in EC.

In patients with a *lower performance status*, one must consider regimens with a more favorable side effect profile or give reduced doses of previously mentioned combinations. Although carboplatin as a single agent has no activity in AC, it may be substituted for cisplatin in a doublet for patients with SCC and preexisting neuropathy or renal dysfunction. Similarly, paclitaxel may be replaced by docetaxel in patients with poorer overall health status or preexisting neuropathy. The potential for *irinotecan to produce diarrhea* must be considered in patients with marginal fluid or nutrition status. If diarrhea is projected to cause a problem, either reduce the dose or choose a regimen that does not contain irinotecan. Another option is *single agent capecitabine*, which is an *oral prodrug* that provides an alternative to infusional 5-FU.

Follow-Up/Recurrent Disease

Patients who undergo complete resection after preoperative CRT are examined with CT scan every 4 to 6 months. Biopsies are performed on masses from suspicious lesions. The role of PET in monitoring for postoperative recurrence

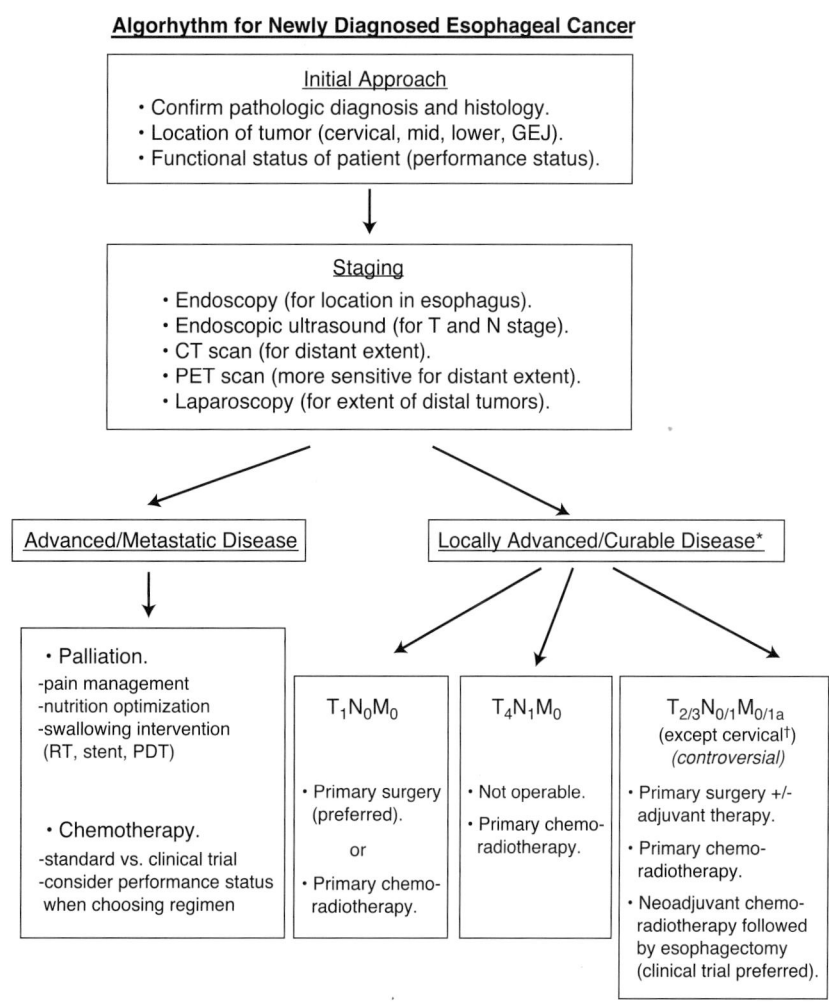

FIGURE 21-1. Algorithm for newly diagnosed esophageal cancer. CT = computed tomography; GEJ = gastroesophageal junction; PET = positron emmision tomography.
*Includes M_{1a} for distal lesions.
†Primary chemoradiotherapy

remains investigational. Patients with recurrent disease are treated similarly to those with primary metastatic disease, with particular attention placed on *performance status* and *ability to tolerate additional chemotherapy*. The small subgroup of patients who have tumor progression during preoperative treatment (< 5% in our experience) are offered similar palliative interventions.

Summary

EC remains a disease for which much progress is needed. We hope that if providers follow this multidisciplinary approach in a thorough and measured manner, outcomes for this group of complex patients will continue to improve.

Supplemental Reading

Bosset JF, Gignoux M, Triboulet JP, et al. Chemoradiotherapy followed by surgery compared with surgery alone in squamous-cell cancer of the esophagus. N Engl J Med 1997;337:161–7.

Cooper JS, Guo MD, Herskovic A, et al. Chemoradiotherapy of locally advanced esophageal cancer: long-term follow-up of a prospective randomized trial (RTOG 85–01). Radiation Therapy Oncology Group. JAMA 1999;281:1623–7.

Dimick JB, Pronovost PJ, Cowan JA, et al. Surgical volume and quality of care for esophageal resection: do high-volume hospitals have fewer complications? Ann Thorac Surg 2003;75:337–41.

Enzinger PC, Ilson DH, Kelsen DP. Chemotherapy in esophageal cancer. Semin Oncol 1999;26:12–20.

Flamen P, Lerut A, Van Cutsem E, et al. Utility of positron emission tomography for the staging of patients with potentially operable esophageal carcinoma. J Clin Oncol 2000;18:3202–10.

Herskovic A, Martz K, al-Sarraf M, et al. Combined chemotherapy and radiotherapy compared with radiotherapy alone in patients with cancer of the esophagus. N Engl J Med 1992;326:1593–8.

Ilson DH, Forastiere A, Arquette M, et al. A phase II trial of paclitaxel and cisplatin in patients with advanced carcinoma of the esophagus. Cancer J 2000;6:316–23.

Ilson DH, Saltz L, Enzinger P, et al. Phase II trial of weekly irinotecan plus cisplatin in advanced esophageal cancer. J Clin Oncol 1999;17:3270–5.

Jemal A, Murray T, Samuels A, et al. Cancer statistics, 2003. CA Cancer J Clin 2003;53:5–26.

Kelsen DP, Ginsberg R, Pajak TF, et al. Chemotherapy followed by surgery compared with surgery alone for localized esophageal cancer. N Engl J Med 1998;339:1979–84.

Kleinberg L, Knisely JP, Heitmiller R, et al. Mature survival results with preoperative cisplatin, protracted infusion 5-fluorouracil, and 44-Gy radiotherapy for esophageal cancer. Int J Radiat Oncol Biol Phys 2003;56:328–34.

Le Prise E, Etienne PL, Meunier B, et al. A randomized study of chemotherapy, radiation therapy, and surgery versus surgery for localized squamous cell carcinoma of the esophagus. Cancer 1994;73:1779–84.

Lukanich JM. Section I: epidemiological review. Semin Thorac Cardiovasc Surg (Epidemiology) 2003;15:158–66.

Medical Research Council Oesophageal Cancer Working Party. Surgical resection with or without preoperative chemotherapy in oesophageal cancer: a randomized controlled trial. Lancet 2002;359:1727–33.

Nozoe T, Kimura Y, Ishida M, et al. Correlation of pre-operative nutritional condition with post-operative complications in surgical treatment for oesophageal carcinoma. Eur J Surg Oncol 2002;28:396–400.

Polednak AP. Trends in survival for both histologic types of esophageal cancer in US surveillance, epidemiology and end results areas. Int J Cancer 2003;105:98–100.

Schlick T, Heintz A, Junginger T. The examiner's learning effect and its influence on the quality of endoscopic ultrasonography in carcinoma of the esophagus and gastric cardia. Surg Endosc 1999;13:894–8.

Urba SG, Orringer MB, Turrisi A, et al. Randomized trial of preoperative chemoradiation versus surgery alone in patients with locoregional esophageal carcinoma. J Clin Oncol 2001;19:305–13.

Walsh TN, Noonan N, Hollywood D, et al. A comparison of multimodal therapy and surgery for esophageal adenocarcinoma. N Engl J Med 1996;335:462–7.

CHAPTER 22

Palliation of Esophageal Cancer

Shou-jiang Tang, MD, and Norman E. Marcon, MD

Although esophageal cancer (EC) accounts for 1% of all cancers, it surprisingly represents 12% of all cancer deaths and is the seventh leading cause of cancer death worldwide. The treatment of EC is tailored to the stage of the disease. For mucosal dysplasia, such as high grade dysplasia of intramucosal cancer, curative endoluminal therapy is now a reality. However, EC is frequently not resectable at the time of diagnosis due to local invasion or metastasis. The prognosis is very poor once the tumor has extended beyond the esophageal wall, with 5-year survival rates of 5 to 10%. It is not known why patients with EC carry such a poor prognosis compared to patients with gastric cardiac cancer, whose 5-year survival rate is around 45%. The difference in lymphatic drainage and local lymphocytic infiltration may play a role. Because of the usually grim prognosis of EC at diagnosis, and because many patients have significant comorbidities that make them unlikely candidates for curable esophagectomy, palliation of dysphagia and nutritional support become the primary goals of therapy. The management of EC should be multidisciplinary involving gastroenterologists, oncologists, radiation oncologists, surgeons, and a palliative care team (Best, 2001; Weigel et al, 2002; Hujala et al, 2002).

Chemoradiation therapy may be provided as palliative therapy to relieve dysphagia for patients with good functional status. Dysphagia can be alleviated by external bean with or without endoluminal brachytherapy radiation therapy in patients with poor functional status (Hujala et al, 2002). Chemoradiation or radiation therapy alone can be complicated by radiation-induced esophagitis, esophageal strictures, and tracheoesophageal fistulas (TEF).

For locally advanced cancer, surgery is appropriate. The results so far have been disappointing for staging EC after chemoradiation therapy in hopes to carry out resection. In some centers, radiation and chemotherapy is given if dysphagia persists despite endoscopic stent placement. For gastroenterologists, the traditional role is to provide endoscopic palliation of dysphagia and nutritional support. Endoscopic measures include (1) debulking tumor tissue using electrocoagulation, laser therapy, argon plasma coagulation (APC), photodynamic therapy (PDT), and injection therapy and (2) maintaining lumenal patency with dilatation, esophageal endoprostheses, and feeding tubes placement.

Palliation of EC is related to the available endoscopic skills, local expertise, and socioeconomic factors. No patient wants to die from disease. Hopefully in the future, we can better and truly palliate/control this cancer as new biological treatments become available.

Nutrition

For patients with EC, oral nutrition is ideally provided after esophageal stent placement. However, in some patients, oral nutrition may be supplemented with feeding gastrostomy. Feeding gastrostomy tubes can be placed percutaneously under endoscopic or radiological guidance or assistance before radiation and chemotherapy. If the tumor responded well to radiation and chemotherapy, the feeding gastrostomy tube may be removed eventually. Some patients prefer to keep gastrostomy tube patency as a safety measure if tumor recurs.

Debulking Modalities

Electrocoagulation

Monopolar, bipolar, and heater probes work by coagulating malignant tissue. Although all techniques have been reported as being successful in the elimination of tumor-associated dysphagia, limited data is available comparing these modalities. Until more comparative data is available, selection is dictated more by resource availability and the provider's expertise. Complications include transient chest pain, fever, leucocytosis, worsening of dysphagia from the resultant edema, and, occasionally, perforation.

Laser Therapy

Endoscopic laser treatment usually with Nd:YAG is best suited in debulking short, noncircumferential lesions in the mid- to distal esophagus. The laser probe is introduced through the endoscopic channel and treatment begun in a caudal to rostral direction. The effective depth of destruction can be as much as 4 to 6 mm. The procedure may be performed in several sessions for long or bulky tumors. Treatment response is usually related to tumor length, circular extend, and relationship to the esophageal sphincters. Short segments in the distal esophagus are easier to treat. Laser treatment of proximal segments may be better tolerated and easier with general anesthesia. Laser treatment can restore luminal patency in up to 90% of patients, with improvement in dysphagia in 70 to 85% of cases. For longer and severe circumferential cancer, relief of dysphagia is usually short-lived and repeat sessions are required. Complications include all those associated with thermal therapies, including transient dysphagia, chest pain, pleural effusions, fever, and perforation (1 to 15%). The major disadvantages of this modality include the high equipment costs, difficulty in using the laser in angulated areas (cricopharyngeus and lower esophagus), and the not uncommon requirement for several sessions before desired results are achieved. Types of lasers available for endoscopic usage include Nd:YAG and diode lasers. Nd:YAG coagulates vessels and tissues at lower power and vaporizes tissues at high power. Although palliation of dysphagia is now mainly performed with endoscopic prostheses, for asymmetrical or noncircumferential lesions, thermal debulking is still appreciated. Some studies have revealed a prolonged dysphagia improvement period by debulking with Nd:YAG laser followed by external bean radiation and intraluminal brachytherapy.

APC

APC is a noncontact thermal technique that limits the maximal coagulation depth to less than 2 to 3 mm (Figures 22-1 and 22-2). The existence of both side and forward viewing APC probes permits more precise targeting of the malignant tissue. The major disadvantage is its limited depth of penetration requiring several sessions. Due to the limited depth of thermal effect, bulky tumors cannot be effectively treated by APC. APC is effective in ablating residual tissues and achieving hemostasis with low risk of perforation (0.5%). In one study on advanced ECs, APC in conjunction with endoscopic balloon dilatation achieved a success rate of 84% within 2 treatment sessions in the palliation of dysphagia (Heindorff et al, 1998). The perforation rate in this study was 8%, which is comparable to laser therapy. The relative high perforation rate is likely due to the adjunctive use of balloon dilatation. In addition, APC is particularly useful in managing malignant and hyperplastic tissue overgrowth/ingrowth associated with the use of an esophageal stent. Compared to Nd:YAG laser therapy, which may destroy the metal meshes, APC generally does not damage the stent. However, there are reports using APC endoluminally to cut the nitinol stents. The major advantages of APC over laser therapy include relatively low equipment costs and tangential delivery of thermal energy.

PDT

PDT is a unique debulking nonthermal technology with the clever use of a photosensitizing drug and the activating red laser beam. Laser light activates the drug to generate singlet oxygen. Singlet oxygen released locally is highly toxic to the microvasculature of the tumor leading to ischemic necro-

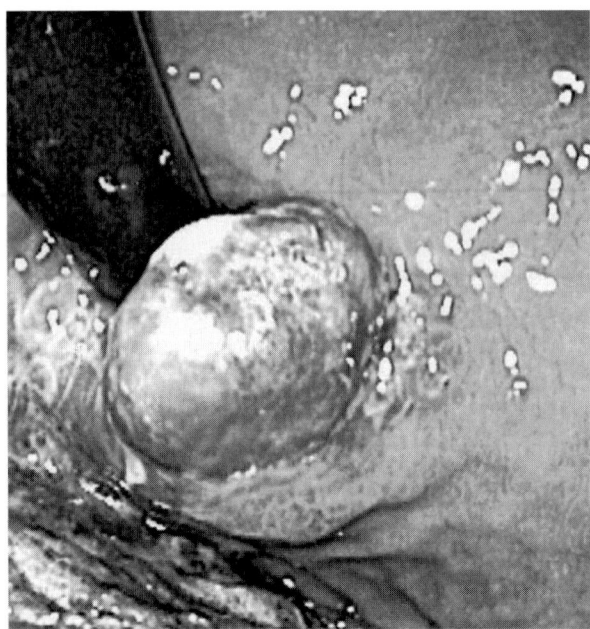

FIGURE 22-1. Endoscopic view of a recurrent esophageal adenocarcinoma before argon plasma coagulation treatment for palliation.

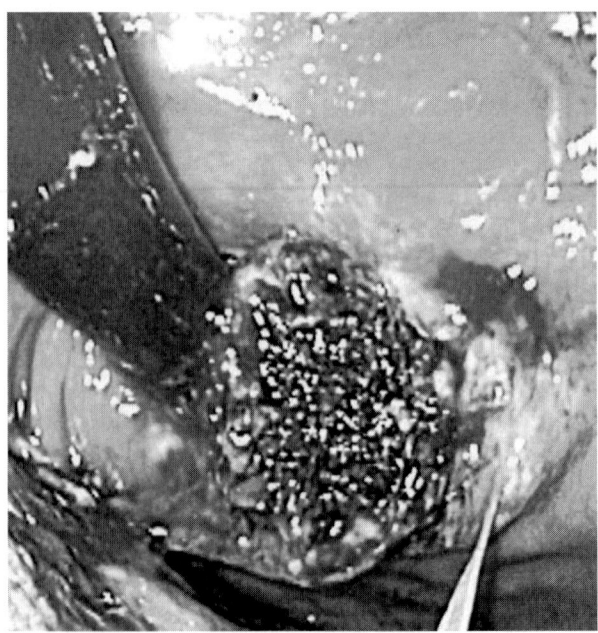

FIGURE 22-2. Endoscopic view of the residual esophageal adenocarcinoma after argon plasma coagulation therapy.

sis. There may also be an immunological effect as well as a local apoptotic effect. PDT involves drugs, light sources, and light delivery systems. The light for PDT can be delivered endoluminally by microlens fibers, cylindrical diffusers, or inflatable balloon applicators. Drug and light dosimetry and tissue oxygenation determine the treatment effects. PDT can be employed in curative and palliative management of EC (Figures 22-3 and 22-4) (Lightdale, 2000). A randomized study compared PDT (Photofrin) with Nd:YAG laser for palliation of advanced EC (Lightdale et al, 1995). Improvement in dysphagia was equivalent between the two treatment arms. Objective tumor response was significantly higher with PDT at 1 month (32% versus 20%, $p < .05$). There was no survival difference between the two treatment arms. In this study, the PDT arm had a better tumor response for certain tumor subtypes, including tumors longer than 10 cm, tumors located within the upper third of the esophagus, and tumors located within the angulated portion of the lower esophagus.

PDT is carried out with greater ease and is associated with fewer acute perforations than Nd:YAG laser therapy. In addition, PDT can be used to obliterate tumor ingrowth associated with the use of endoprostheses, but the experience is limited. The main disadvantages associated with PDT include the high drug and equipment costs, as well as the photosensitivity that occurs from the residual drug in the skin. The one major limitation of PDT is for large tumor masses where the light penetration is limited. A light guide is placed "free hand" in the center of the tumor. For bulky tumors, intratumoral insertion of short diffuser (1 to 2 cm) can lead to more destruction. PDT treatment can be repeated. However, the high cost of repeated drug infusion makes esophageal prostheses a better option. Complications resulting from the use of PDT include esophageal strictures occurring in 10 to 50% of patients, transient fever, and pleural effusion. Fistulas and perforations are rare. M-Tetra (hydroxyphenyl)chlorine (Foscan) is an experimental photosensitizer that provides more destruction but with a higher incidence of bleeding and perforation.

Injection Therapy

A more established, but now less commonly used technique in the palliation of malignant dysphagia is endoscopic injection therapy. The procedure involves the direct injection of a cytotoxic agent into the tumor tissue using an injection catheter. Although 100% ethanol is the most commonly used agent, the successful use of other agents has been reported (eg, 3% polidocanol, 2.5% sodium morrhuate/5-fluorouracil mixture, and cisplatin/epinephrine mixture). In one randomized trial comparing injection with laser ablation, dysphagia improved in 78% of subjects treated with ethanol, and no significant differences in efficacy or complications were found between the two groups (Carazzone el al, 1999). Complications of alcohol injection include mediastinitis and TEF formation. The extent of resultant tissue necrosis with injection is less predictable than the necrosis associated with the incremental thermal ablative therapies, and many patients require further treatment sessions to sustain symptom relief. Although advantages of the technique include its universal availability and low equipment costs, lack of standardization of the technique and its relatively short efficacy have limited its utility in recent years.

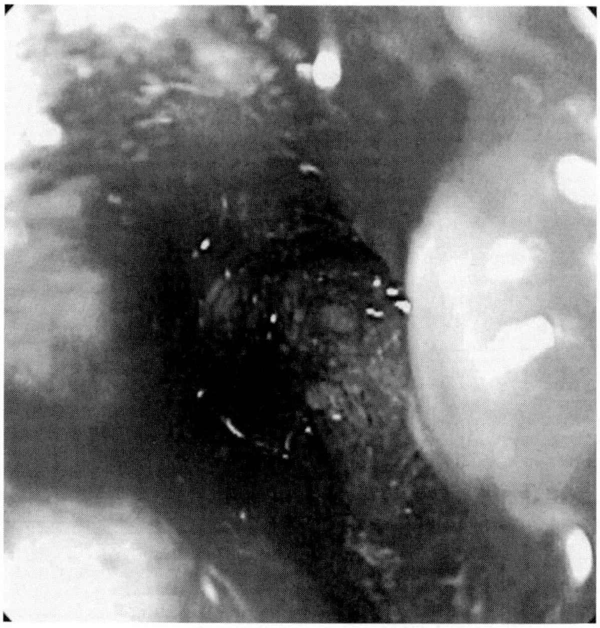

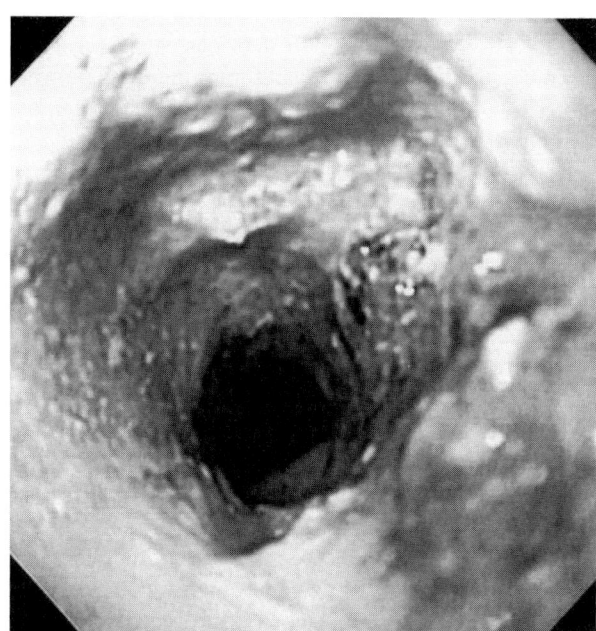

FIGURE 22-3. Endoscopic view of an inoperable esophageal adenocarcinoma before photodynamic therapy for palliation.

FIGURE 22-4. Forty-eight hours after the photodynamic therapy, the luminal diameter is much increased resulting from tumoral necrosis.

Endoscopic Dilatation

The efficacy of endoscopic dilatation for palliation of dysphagia is short term, but occasionally the effects are prolonged. More importantly, esophageal dilatation allows a more comprehensive evaluation of a malignant lesion where the distal margin cannot be assessed because the tumor is impassable even using miniscopes. Endoscopic dilatation can also be used for radiation-induced esophageal strictures, anastomotic strictures, and anastomotic tumor recurrence. In addition, dilatation is often used in conjunction with other palliative modalities, such as endoscopic injection, APC, laser ablation, and stent placement. Dilatation can be performed either with Savary-Gilliard dilators over a stiff wire or with balloon dilators introduced over a wire through the scope under direct endoscopic vision. The use of fluoroscopy is recommended to ensure safe passage of the Savary wire in each technique. In some very tight strictures that cannot be maneuvered by miniscopes, guide wires with a hydrophilic coating (Terumo type) may be used, usually under fluoroscopic guidance. Complications associated with dilatation include perforation risk (around 4%), chest pain, bleeding, and bacteremia. The risk of perforation is slightly increased when dilatation is used in conjunction with other endoscopic palliative measures.

Esophageal Endoprostheses

The insertion of esophageal endoprostheses or stents is a common approach to the palliative management of dysphagia (Baron, 2001; Siersema et al, 2003). Stent placement should only be undertaken after very careful scrutiny of the clinical situation (eg, tumor stage, length, position, and expected prognosis of the patient). Because of the potential complications associated with stent placement (eg, stent migration, perforation, and stent tumor ingrowth or overgrowth), consideration of these factors is especially important before stent placement. A stent should be considered permanent after deployment and is the ultimate form of palliation before the patient dies. The risk of stent-associated complications is increased if patients subsequently undergo chemoradiation or radiation therapy. To minimize the risks associated with stent placement, tumors that can be adequately treated with thermal or PDT ablative therapies should first be treated in that fashion for as long as possible before stent placement is contemplated. If the stent is patent and the patient still complains of dysphagia, the patient needs to be considered for radiation and chemotherapy, although it is unlikely that radiation or chemotherapy will prolong either survival or quality of life. Before stent placement, endoscopic examination of the tumor should be carried out to measure the lesional length, location, and the distance from the lesion to the upper or lower esophageal sphincters. Generally, the stent should be 4 to 6 cm longer than the tumor, allowing 2 cm above and below the lesion. During stent placement, under fluoroscopic guidance, the metal markers can be placed as external skin markers to mark the proximal and distal ends of the tumor. Repositioning of the stent can be achieved by withdrawal and/or reconstraining (Wallstent) the partially deployed stents.

Different options in stent selection include plastic or metal, coated or uncoated, and the various designs offer different degrees of tensile strength, memory, and expansive radial forces. The use of rigid plastic stents has fallen significantly since the introduction of self-expandable metallic stents (SEMS), partly because of their higher complication rates (associated with preplacement dilatation), and partly because metallic stents are easier to use and deploy and tend to cause less pain. In one randomized study comparing plastic stents to SEMS, there was no significant difference in complications or mortality rate between the two groups (O'Donnell et al, 2002). The SEMS demonstrated advantages in terms of quality of life, survival, and cost effectiveness after 4 weeks. If a patient's expected survival is relatively short and the cost of the stent is an issue, a covered plastic stent, such as a Polyflex esophageal stent (Willy Rüsch, Kernen, Germany) (Figure 22-5), should be considered over the SEMS in the palliation of EC.

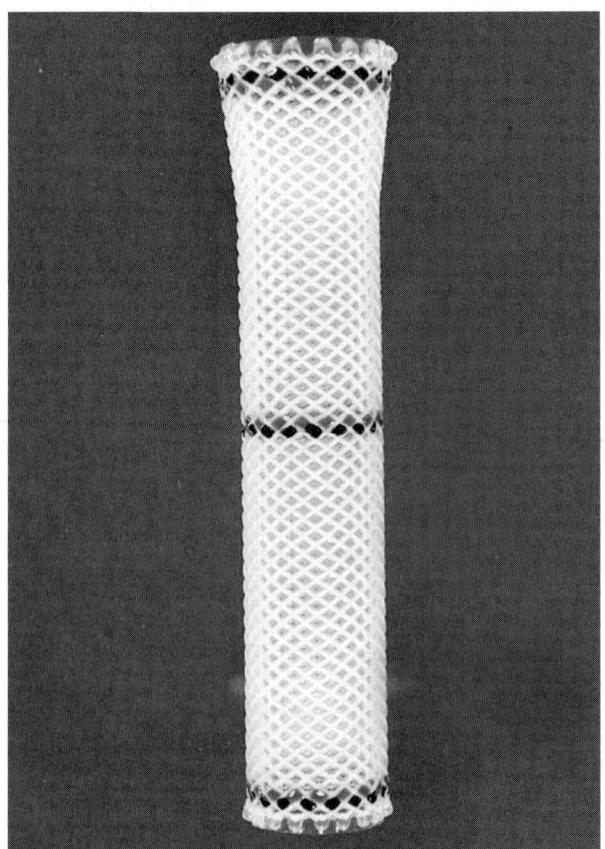

FIGURE 22-5. Polyflex covered plastic stent.

Most available data on SEMS is retrospective and uncontrolled. The immediate palliation of malignant dysphagia with SEMS is 78 to 96%, with a stent migration rate of 4 to 9%, a tumor ingrowth of 3 to 37%, a need for subsequent intervention rate of 3 to 78%, and a major complications (ie, bleeding, perforation, aspiration, and fistula) rate of 3 to 17%. Most metal stents are safe if patients undergo magnetic resonance imaging (Table 22-1).

There are four commonly used covered metal stents for esophageal stenting: Ultraflex stent (Microvasive/Boston Scientific, Natick, Massachusetts), Wallstent II (Boston Scientific), Flamingo Wallstent (Boston Scientific, available only in Europe), and Gianturco-Z stent (Wilson-Cook Medical, Winston-Salem, North Carolina) (see Table 22-1 and Figures 22-6 to 22-8). In one randomized trial, there was no difference in rates of dysphagia improvement, subsequent recurrence of dysphagia (24 to 36%), or complication (18 to 36%) between the Ultraflex stent, the Flamingo Wallstent, or the Z stent (Siersema et al, 2001). In another study comparing covered with uncovered SEMS, there was a higher tumor ingrowth rate in the uncovered SEMS arm (30 versus 3%) leading to a significantly higher endoscopic reintervention rate (27 versus 0%). However, there was no difference in patient survival or quality of life measures between the two arms. Data comparing the SEMS to other therapeutic modalities available for palliation of EC is limited. One randomized trial compared SEMS with combination therapy of endoscopic laser therapy/external beam radiotherapy in patients with cancer that was not resectable. It found no difference in rates of dysphagia improvement or survival advantage between the two palliation arms. However, there was a lower incidence of restenosis and major complications in the SEMS arm. Stenting was also demonstrated to be more cost effective.

TABLE 22-1. Specifics of US Food and Drug Administration-Approved Expandable Metal Stents for Esophageal Use in North America

	Ultraflex	Wallstent II	Z Stent
Material	Nitinol	Elgiloy	Stainless steel
Covering	Yes	Yes	Yes
Design	Mesh	Mesh	Zigzag
Radial Force	+	+++	++
Lumen diagmeter (mm) (flanges/shaft)	23–28/17–22	28/20	21–25/18–22
Covered length (cm)	7–12	8, 13	8–14
Degree of foreshortening*	up to 30%	≈ 20%	0%
MRI-friendly	Yes	Yes	No

MRI = magnetic resonance imaging.
* Stent foreshortening generally will not affect stent deployment. The Ultraflex has postdeployment radiopaque markers that indicate exactly where the stent will reside after deployment.
†The foreshortening is variable depending on the nature of the stricture and compression of the stent within that stricture.

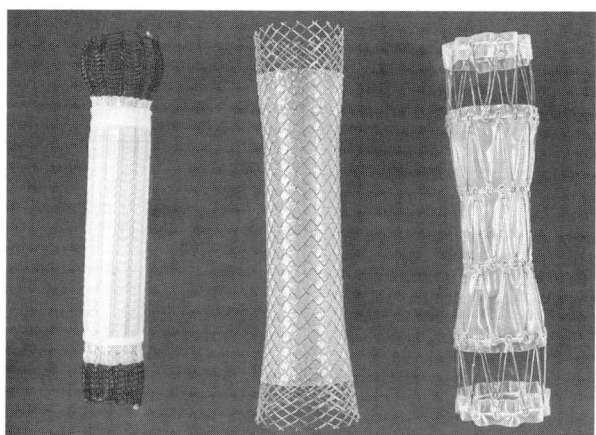

FIGURE 22-6. US Food and Drug Administration-approved covered expandable metal stents for esophageal use in North America, from the left to the right: Ultraflex stent, Wallstent II, and Z stent.

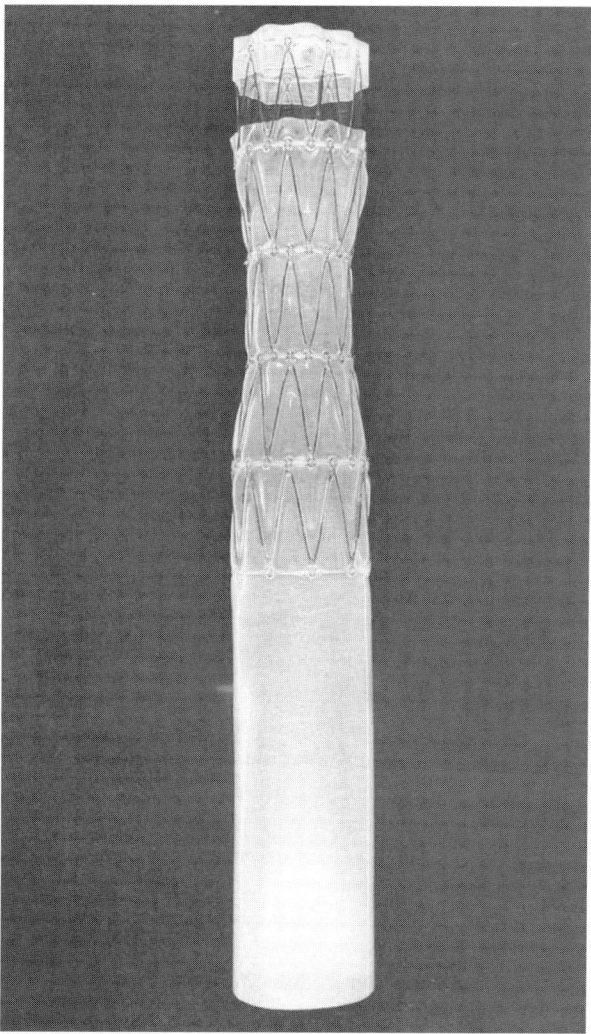

FIGURE 22-7. Z stent with antireflux valve.

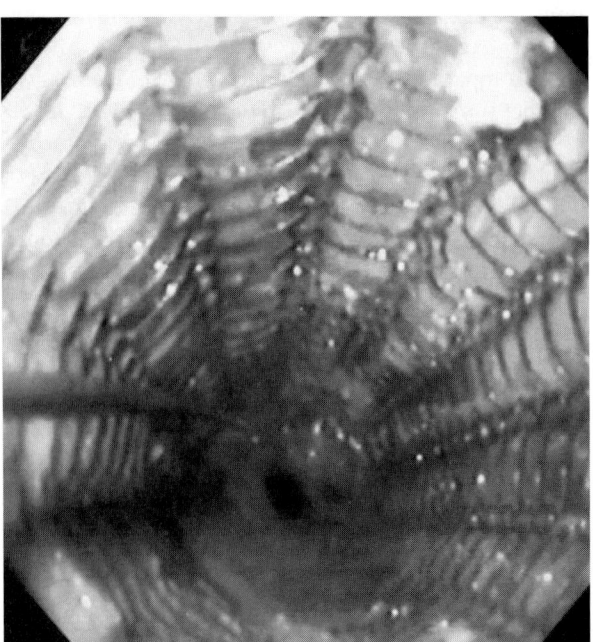

FIGURE 22-8. Endoscopic view of an Ultraflex stent deployed in the esophagus.

There are several special situations concerning esophageal stent placement. For malignant intraluminal cancers located near the upper sphincter, if the tumor is within 2 to 3 cm of the upper sphincter, SEMS can be placed; however, careful positioning with metallic markers and maintenance of the patient in a supine position is usually needed during stent placement. The more difficult situation is when the tumor invades the upper sphincter. In these situations, thermal therapy or PDT could be tried. The issues are tracheal compression or foreign body sensation after stent deployment. A small caliber plastic tube could be used in connection with a feeding gastrostomy. There have been reports using Montgomery salivary bypass tubes (Boston Scientific, Natick, Massachusetts), latex rubber tubes (Celestin, Medoc Ltd, Atlanta, Georgia.) or Tygon polyvinyl endoprostheses for palliation in the cervical esophagus (Weigel et al, 2002). In cases of extrinsic compression and infiltration of the esophagus from metastatic, pulmonary or lymphatic malignancies without a shelf in the esophagus, dilatation followed by placement of stent with wide flange can be tried. To minimize stent migration, in some instances, endoscopically placed clips may be used to prevent stent migration, especially in patients where the stricture is extrinsic and/or not overly tight. Another way is to anchor the stent with an umbilical thread passed transnasally and overhung around the ear (Hujala et al, 2002). The availability of covered SEMS has significantly changed the management of TEF, esophageal fistulas, or perforation resulting from other palliative measures.

Untreated TEF carries a very poor prognosis primarily from aspiration pneumonia and the covered SEMS has become the first line of treatment. Closure of the fistula is achieved in 70 to 100% of patients with SEMS. For persistent TEF despite stent placement, placement of an airway stent should be considered to close the fistula. It should be noted that placement of an SEMS does not prevent further subsequent enlargement of the existing fistula or development of further fistulas (Heindorff et al, 1998).

Aspiration precautions, such as elevation of the head of the bed and aggressive acid suppression with proton pump inhibitors, are needed to prevent aspiration and reflux if a stent without an antireflux mechanism is placed across the gastroesophageal (GE) junction. An esophageal stent with an antireflux device may be of value under such circumstances.

Stent occlusion and migration are the most significant complications occurring in long term cancer survivors. Stent occlusion is caused by tumor overgrowth and by reactive tissue hyperplasia/granulation tissue. APC, Nd:YAG laser, PDT, or placement of a second overlapping stent can be considered to relieve the occlusion. For very long and large tumors, placement of two overlapping stents can minimize tumor overgrowth. Dietary precautions should be practiced by all patients, such as adherence to a mechanical soft or pureed diet to prevent food impaction within or above the stent. Stents tend to migrate more commonly distally than proximally. Long circumferential tumors minimize stent migration. The approach to migration depends on the type of stent, extent of migration, and whether any complications have occurred as a consequence of migration. Chemoradiation or radiation therapy predisposes the pre-placed stent to migrate due to tumor shrinkage. The migration rate may be affected by stent diameter with larger caliber stents being less likely to migrate, but this finding has to be balanced by the possibility that larger caliber stents may increase the rate of complication from stent erosion through the esophageal wall. Finally partially covered stents with wider distal flanges may prove useful in reducing the rate of stent migration, although this is not proven by the available data. Ongoing advances in endoprostheses material and design aim to reduce tissue overgrowth, stent migration, and acid reflux in cases where the stent traverses the GE junction. For cases where the stent has migrated into the stomach, controversy exists over whether to adopt a "watchful waiting approach" or whether to try to remove the stent immediately. If the migrated stent in the stomach interferes with gastric emptying and the patient's functional status is good, the stent could be removed either endoscopically or by laparotomy.

Based on current data, no particular type of SEMS can be recommended to be ideal for all causes of malignant dysphagia. Local resource availability, technical expertise and familiarity, and other factors need to be considered during the decision-making process.

Perspective

The increasing use of endoscopic screening and surveillance programs, advanced imaging techniques, such as high frequency endoscopic ultrasound and optical coherence tomography, and new endoscopic interventions, such as endoscopic mucosal resection, may lead to early detection and better treatment of esophageal mucosal dysplasia and cancer. Early intervention could lead to better prognosis or cure. There has been a technological expansion of resources available for dealing with both early and advanced EC. Advances in biotechnology offer hope for patients with advanced cancer, such as gene-based therapy and molecular-targeted drugs. Coated chemotherapeutics and radiation emitting metal stents may decrease the stent occlusion rates. These endeavors may ultimately lead to a greater success in reducing the mortality associated with EC and in prolonging quality of life with malignant cellular stabilization.

Supplemental Reading

Baron TH. Expandable metal stents for the treatment of cancerous obstruction of the gastrointestinal tract [review]. N Engl J Med 2001;344:1681–7.

Carazzone A, Bonavina L, Segalin A, et al. Endoscopic palliation of oesophageal cancer: results of a prospective comparison of Nd:YAG laser and ethanol injection. Eur J Surg 1999;165:351–6.

Frenken M. Best palliation in esophageal cancer: surgery, stenting, radiation, or what? [review]. Dis Esophagus 2001;14:120–3.

Heindorff H, Wojdemann M, Bisgaard T, Svendsen LB. Endoscopic palliation of inoperable cancer of the oesophagus or cardia by argon electrocoagulation. Scand J Gastroenterol 1998;33:21–3.

Hujala K, Sipila J, Minn H, et al. Combined external and intraluminal radiotherapy in the treatment of advanced oesophageal cancer. Radiotherapy Oncol 2002;64:41–5.

Lightdale CJ. Role of photodynamic therapy in the management of advanced esophageal cancer [review]. Gastrointest Endosc Clin N Am 2000;10:397–408.

Lightdale CJ, Heier SK, Marcon NE, et al. Photodynamic therapy with porfimer sodium versus thermal ablation therapy with Nd:YAG laser for palliation of esophageal cancer: a multicenter randomized trial. Gastrointest Endosc 1995;42:507–12.

O'Donnell CA, Fullarton GM, Watt E, et al. Randomized clinical trial comparing self-expanding metallic stents with plastic endoprostheses in the palliation of oesophageal cancer. Br J Surg 2002;89:985–92.

Siersema PD, Hop WC, van Blankenstein M, et al. A comparison of 3 types of covered metal stents for the palliation of patients with dysphagia caused by esophagogastric carcinoma: a prospective, randomized study. Gastrointest Endosc 2001;54:145–53.

Siersema PD, Marcon NE, Vakil N. Metal stents for tumors of the distal esophagus and gastric cardia [review]. Endoscopy 2003;35:79–85.

Weigel TL, Frumiento C, Gaumintz E. Endoluminal palliation for dysphagia secondary to esophageal carcinoma [review]. Surg Clin North Am 2002;82:747–61.

Chapter 23

Helicobacter pylori and Gastroduodenal Disease

Mae F. Go, MD

Helicobacter pylori infection is associated with multiple gastroduodenal disorders, including *gastritis, peptic ulcer disease (PUD), gastric adenocarcinoma (AC),* and *gastric mucosa-associated lymphoid tissue (MALT) lymphoma.* H. pylori infection can be detected in half the world's population. Virtually everyone infected develops chronic active gastritis. Chronic infection is linked to a higher risk of peptic ulcer and a small but increased risk for gastric malignancy, particularly in those individuals who are genetically susceptible. Prevalence of the infection in the general US population is about 20 to 30%, with higher prevalence in some population subgroups, such as those living in crowded and poor socioeconomic conditions. Prevalence of the infection is more common in the older population and in those who have immigrated to the United States from a country with a high endemic prevalence of the infection. It is postulated that prevalence of the infection will continue to decline because of improved health and socioeconomic conditions in addition to eradication of the infection.

Diagnosing *H. pylori* Infection

Tests to detect *H. pylori* infection can be divided into nonendoscopic and endoscopic tests (Table 23-1). If a patient is undergoing *endoscopy, gastric biopsy,* samples can be obtained for the *rapid urease test (RUT) or histology;* the accuracy of both these techniques is 90 to 95%. If *H. pylori* status is sought, the RUT is a cost effective test. If there is concern about malignancy, gastric tissue for histology should be obtained. Most pathologists can identify *H. pylori* on hematoxylin and eosin stain and special stains. Accurate nonendoscopic tests include the *urea breath test (UBT)* and the *H. pylori stool antigen test (HpSA).* Both these tests are useful for *initial diagnosis* and also for *confirmation of eradication.* Because of the increasingly high rate of false-positive results, *blood antibody tests are less useful,* unless it is clear that the patient has not been previously exposed to *H. pylori* eradication therapy. Immunoglobulin G antibodies to *H. pylori* can remain present for years after successful eradication.

Tests that detect "active" infection include the endoscopic biopsy tests, the UBT, and the HpSA. If possible, these tests should be performed while the patient is not taking proton pump inhibitors (PPIs), high dose histamine-2 receptor antagonists, or antibiotics. These agents can decrease accuracy of the biopsy-based tests (RUT, histology), the UBT, and the HpSA by as much as 15 to 25%. Because it is not practical to stop acid-suppressing drugs before patient examination, if endoscopy is being performed, two biopsies (one from antrum and another from body of the stomach) may increase yield of the RUT in the patient on a PPI.

Peptic Ulcer Disease

It is estimated that one in six people with chronic *H. pylori* infection will have a peptic ulcer sometime in his or her lifetime. Initial studies indicated that > 90% of peptic ulcers were caused by *H. pylori* infection. More recent examination of clinical trials in the United States showed that 60 to 70% of duodenal ulcers are causally related to this infection (Laine et al, 1998). Numerous studies from around the world have confirmed that eradication of the infection significantly decreases recurrent PUD. It is now generally accepted that *all patients presenting with a peptic ulcer should be tested for H. pylori infection.* If positive, the patient should receive appropriate *H. pylori* eradication treatment. Most authorities feel that once the infection is eradicated, acid suppression for ulcer prophylaxis is unnecessary as long as the patient is not on other "ulcerogenic" agents, such as nonsteroidal anti-inflammatory drugs (NSAIDs) (Liu et al, 2003). The increasing use of NSAIDs and acetylsalicylic acid (ASA) is likely to "shift" the balance of ulcer etiology from *H. pylori* to *NSAIDs, ASA,* and cyclooxygenase-2 (COX-2)

TABLE 23-1. Tests to Detect *Helicobacter pylori* Infection

	Sensitivity	Specificity
Nonendoscopic		
Blood Antibody Test[†]	85%	70 to 80%
Urea Breath Test (C-13, C-14)*	95%	95%
Stool Antigen Test*	90 to 95%	85 to 90%
Endoscopic		
Rapid Urease Test*	90 to 95%	90 to 95%
Histology*	90 to 95%	90 to 95%
Culture*	50%	100%

*Tests with decreased accuracy if patient is on proton pump inhibitors, high dose histamine-2 receptor antagonists, or antibiotics.
[†]May obtain false-positive result if patient has received prior *Helicobacter pylori* eradication treatment.

inhibitors (*coxibs*) in the coming years. This trend makes testing for *H. pylori* in an ulcer patient even more important in order to identify potential cause(s) of the ulcer.

Should one *confirm eradication* of the infection in the peptic ulcer patient? There is general agreement that eradication should be confirmed in all patients *presenting with a complicated ulcer*. A recent prospective study by Arkkila and colleagues (2003) is one of many studies demonstrating that eradication of *H. pylori* in the complicated ulcer patient significantly reduces recurrent ulcer unless other inciting agents are present. After healing of their bleeding peptic ulcer, 223 *H. pylori*-positive patients were randomized to eradication treatment or to PPI treatment with placebo. The 1-year follow-up with endoscopic evaluation showed that only 2% of patients with successful *H. pylori* eradication had suffered a recurrent ulcer compared with 38% of those with *H. pylori* infection. There is less agreement about confirming eradication in the patient with an uncomplicated ulcer, but this has been largely based on costs of testing. The decreased costs of *H. pylori* diagnostic tests and their widespread availability now make it reasonable to consider confirming eradication in individuals who have undergone *H. pylori* eradication treatment.

H. pylori and NSAIDs

The meta-analysis from Huang and colleagues (2002) showed that *H. pylori* infection and NSAID use were independent risk factors for PUD; together they contribute at least an additive increased risk for ulcer development. Both factors also increased the risk of ulcer bleeding but NSAIDs appeared to be a more frequent cause of bleeding than *H. pylori* infection. These conclusions were confirmed by the above-mentioned study from Arkkila and colleagues (2003). Eradication of *H. pylori* resulted in a significantly decreased ulcer recurrence at the 1-year follow-up in patients initially presenting with a bleeding peptic ulcer. In those patients using ASA or NSAIDs, only 4% of patients with successful *H. pylori* eradication developed ulcer relapse compared with 58% of those who were *H. pylori*-positive. The use of both ASA and NSAIDs increased ulcer rates to 75% in those with *H. pylori* infection compared with only 6% of those without *H. pylori* infection. This study suggested that *H. pylori* infection might be a more significant risk factor for recurrent ulcer disease than use of NSAIDs and/or ASA, because there were significantly fewer ulcer relapses in those with *H. pylori* eradication even though they used NSAIDs and/or ASA.

Because NSAIDs and ASA are important causes of ulcer disease, should patients on NSAIDs be tested for *H. pylori* infection to exclude this ulcer risk factor? This issue remains controversial. Studies from Asia suggest that eradication of *H. pylori* prior to chronic NSAID use will significantly reduce endoscopic gastroduodenal lesions (Chan et al, 1997). By contrast, there appears to be no significant benefit of immediate eradication of *H. pylori* infection in patients who develop ulcer disease while on chronic NSAID therapy. Studies from the United Kingdom suggest that healing of a peptic ulcer is enhanced if *H. pylori* infection is present in patients who have been on long term NSAIDs (Yeomans et al, 1998). A prospective study from Hong Kong suggested that maintenance therapy with a PPI was more effective than *H. pylori* eradication to reduce recurrent ulcer bleeding in patients taking chronic NSAIDs (Chan et al, 2001). In this same patient population there was no difference between *H. pylori* eradication and PPI maintenance therapy in the patient who developed an ulcer while taking ASA. This remains a controversial area but management by a "risk stratification" strategy may be helpful in decision making.

If patients are beginning chronic NSAID use and have a prior history of ulcer disease, there is a clear indication for testing for *H. pylori* infection; eradication treatment should be offered to the patient if a positive test result is obtained. If there is no prior history of peptic ulcer but the patient has other risk factors such as older age (> 65 or 70 years of age) and is using other "ulcerogenic" agents, such as steroids, testing for *H. pylori* infection is reasonable. If the patient is young without other comorbidities, benefits of testing for *H. pylori* infection will be less useful. If the patient has been on chronic NSAIDs and develops a peptic ulcer, *H. pylori* eradication therapy could be "held" until after the ulcer(s) has healed.

H. pylori and Gastric Malignancy

H. pylori infection was designated a definite carcinogen by the Interagency on Cancer Research arm of the World Health Organization. The Eurogast Study showed that chronic *H. pylori* infection increased risk of gastric AC by four- to sixfold. Uemura and colleagues (2001) showed that *H. pylori* infection was a significant risk factor for developing gastric cancer (GC) in a Japanese population. However, screening for *H. pylori* infection to prevent GC has not been shown to be cost effective in modeling studies of the general US population. Parsonnet and colleagues (1996) postulated that this might be *cost effective only* in those *individuals of Japanese origin*. However, many authorities agree that first-degree relatives of patients with GC should be screened for *H. pylori* infection because these individuals are at greater risk for GC development. Recent studies indicate that individuals with certain polymorphisms in interleukin-1β and other "proinflammatory cytokines" may be at greater risk for developing gastric AC, but these types of markers are not readily available and additional factors may be important (El-Omer et al, 2003).

MALT Lymphoma

H. pylori infection will be detected in 85 to 90% of low grade gastric MALT cases, so *H. pylori* infection should be sought and eradicated. Partial to complete remission will be observed in as many as 75% of patients with successful *H. pylori* eradication (Steinbach et al, 1999). Relapses have occurred with *H. pylori* reinfection. If high-grade disease is present, eradication alone will be insufficient. Chemotherapy, radiation, and surgery are options to consider. There is a separate chapter on gastric lymphoma (see Chapter 33, "Primary Gastric Lymphoma")

Chronic Gastritis

The patient with *intestinal metaplasia and atrophy* on gastric biopsies presents another type of patient for whom there are no follow-up management guidelines. If the patient has *H. pylori* infection, the infection should be eradicated. Unless the patient has additional risk factors, such as first-degree relative with GC, or has a Japanese background, the vast majority of patients with gastric intestinal metaplasia and atrophy are unlikely to develop GC. In general, interval endoscopic surveillance is not performed.

H. pylori and Nonulcer Dyspepsia

H. pylori prevalence is higher in patients with nonulcer dyspepsia (NUD) compared to the general population, but it is unclear whether infection causes dyspepsia. Disparate results have been obtained from the many prospective studies assessing long term (1 year) symptom improvement in NUD patients randomized to *H. pylori* eradication versus placebo (or PPI) (Laine et al, 2001). The most recent Cochrane systematic review update by Moayyedi and colleagues (2003) shows a small but statistically significant benefit for eradication of *H. pylori* infection in the patient with NUD with a number needed to treat of 15. Similar findings were described in the prospective German multicenter ELAN study in which the therapeutic gain was only 10% in NUD patients with successful *H. pylori* eradication (Malfertheiner et al, 2003).

Although these studies support intervention (*H. pylori* eradication) in the NUD patient, one should also identify the numerous potential factors contributing to the patient's dyspepsia. Many patients will have symptom improvement immediately after successful *H. pylori* eradication only to develop recurrence of their dyspepsia shortly thereafter. The provider must be prepared for this "refractory" dyspepsia. Psychosocial factors are often important issues to explore in many patients with NUD.*

Treatment

H. pylori Eradication Treatment

Effective US Food and Drug Administration (FDA)-approved eradication regimens are now available. "PPI-

*Editor's Note: This concept is discussed in the excellent chapter nonulcer dyspepsia (see Chapter 30, "Management of Nonulcer Dyspepsia").

based triple" regimens are the first line therapies in the United States. These regimens consist of *amoxicillin and clarithromycin* in addition to a *PPI* (Table 23-2). FDA-approved treatment durations are *10 or 14 days*, except for rabeprazole-based triple therapy, which has been approved for *7-day treatment*. Another eradication regimen is the quadruple regimen, which includes *Pepto Bismol, metronidazole, tetracycline*, and a *PPI*; this regimen should be prescribed for *14 days*. Per protocol eradication rates are about 85 to 90% for all these eradication regimens. If penicillin allergy exists, *metronidazole* can be substituted for amoxicillin in the PPI-triple therapy or the quadruple therapy can be used. Selection of initial eradication therapy should include general assessment of prior exposure to the antibiotics in the eradication therapy. If the patient has been exposed to *metronidazole*, then the quadruple regimen should not be used initially, but rather the PPI-based triple. If the patient has been previously treated with *clarithromycin*, then quadruple therapy may be more appropriate initial treatment. If the patient has failed one eradication therapy, then the other regimen should be used (Howden and Hunt, 1998).

Summary

H. pylori infection is causally linked to gastritis, PUD, and gastric malignancy. Understanding the role of this microorganism in gastroduodenal disorders continues at a rapid pace because of the tremendous number of investigations in progress around the world. Good management guidelines are available for PUD, but controversy remains about screening for *H. pylori* in the patient beginning NSAIDs or in the patient who has been on NSAIDs. Although this

TABLE 23-2. FDA-Approved Eradication Regimens for *Helicobacter pylori* Infection

Bismuth-Metronidazole-Tetracycline (Helidac) therapy for 14 days
Pepto Bismol 2 tabs po qid
Metronidazole 250 mg po qid
Tetracycline 500 mg po qid
Plus H$_2$RA for 8 weeks or PPI for 4 to 6 weeks
PPI-bid triple therapy for 10 or 14 days
Omeprazole (Prilosec) 20 mg or Lansoprazole (Prevacid) 30 mg po bid (Prevpac)
Amoxicillin (Amoxic) 1 g po bid
Clarithromycin (Biaxin) 500 mg bid
PPI bid triple therapy for 7 days
Rabeprazole (Aciphex) 20 mg po bid
Amoxicillin (Amoxic) 1 g po bid
Clarithromycin (Biaxin) 500 mg bid
PPI qd triple therapy for 10 days
Esomeprazole (Nexium) 40 mg qd
Amoxicillin (Amoxic) 1 g po bid
Clarithromycin (Biaxin) 500 mg bid

bid = twice daily; FDA = US Food and Drug Administrtion; H$_2$RA = histamine-2 receptor antagonist; po = by mouth; PPI = proton pump inhibitor; qd = every day; qid = four times daily.

infection has been labeled as a definite carcinogen, screening for this ubiquitous infection does not appear to be cost effective in the general US population. Benefit of eradication in the NUD patient continues to be uncertain, but recent studies indicate a small therapeutic gain for sustained symptom improvement in these patients. *H. pylori* infection and associated clinical disorders remains a complex and controversial subject. Disparate conclusions are often based on differences in population demographics and study designs. Management strategies have been based on guidelines from consensus conferences, but these strategies must remain flexible as new study findings become available.

Supplemental Reading

The EUROGAST Study Group. An international association between *Helicobacter pylori* infection and gastric cancer. Lancet 1993;341:1359–62.

Arkkila PET, Seppala K, Kosunen TU, et al. Eradication of *Helicobacter pylori* improves the healing rate and reduces the relapse rate of nonbleeding ulcers in patients with bleeding peptic ulcer. Am J Gastroenterol 2003;98:2149–56.

Chan FK, Chung SC, Suen BY, et al. Preventing recurrent upper gastrointestinal bleeding in patients with *Helicobacter pylori* infection who are taking low-dose aspirin or naproxen. N Engl J Med 2001;344:967–73.

Chan FK, Sung JJ, Chung SC, et al. Randomised trial of eradication of *Helicobacter pylori* before non-steroidal anti-inflammatory drug therapy to prevent peptic ulcers. Lancet 1997;350:975–9.

El-Omar EM, Rabkin CS, Gammon MD, et al. Increased risk of noncardia gastric cancer associated with proinflammatory cytokine gene polymorphisms. Gastroenterology 2003;124:1193–201.

Howden CW, Hunt RH. Guidelines for the management of *Helicobacter pylori* infection. Ad Hoc Committee on Practice Parameters of the American College of Gastroenterology. Am J Gastroenterol 1998;93:2330–8.

Huang JQ, Sridhar S, Hunt RH. Role of *Helicobacter pylori* infection and non-steroidal anti-inflammatory drugs in peptic-ulcer disease: a meta-analysis. Lancet 2002;359:14–22.

Laine L, Hopkins RJ, Girardi LS. Has the impact of *Helicobacter pylori* therapy on ulcer recurrence in the United States been overstated? A meta-analysis of rigorously designed trials. Am J Gastroenterol 1998;93:1409–15.

Laine L, Schoenfeld P, Fennerty MB. Therapy for *Helicobacter pylori* in patients with nonulcer dyspepsia. A meta-analysis of randomized, controlled trials. Ann Intern Med 2001;134:361–9.

Liu C-C, Lee C-L, Chan C-C, et al. Maintenance treatment is not necessary after *Helicobacter pylori* eradication and healing of bleeding peptic ulcer. Arch Intern Med 2003;163:2020–4.

Malfertheiner P, Muessner J, Fischback W, et al. *Helicobacter pylori* eradication is beneficial in the treatment of functional dyspepsia. Aliment Pharmacol Ther 2003;18:615–25.

Moayyedi P, Deeks J, Talley NJ, et al. An update of the Cochrane Systematic review of *Helicobacter pylori* eradication therapy in nonulcer dyspepsia: resolving the discrepancy between systematic reviews. Am J Gastroenterol 2003;98:2621–6.

Parsonnet J, Harris RA, Hack HM, Owens DK. Modelling cost-effectiveness of *Helicobacter pylori* screening to prevent gastric cancer: a mandate for clinical trials. Lancet 1996;348:150–4.

Steinbach G, Ford R, Glober G, et al. Antibiotic treatment of gastric lymphoma of mucosa-associated lymphoid tissue. An uncontrolled trial. Ann Intern Med 1999;131:88–95.

Uemura N, Okamoto S, Yamamoto S, et al. *Helicobacter pylori* infection and the development of gastric cancer. N Engl J Med 2001;345:784–9.

Yeomans ND, Tulassay Z, Juhasz L, et al. A comparison of omeprazole with ranitidine for ulcers associated with nonsteroidal antiinflammatory drugs. Acid Suppression Trial: Ranitidine versus Omeprazole for NSAID-Associated Ulcer Treatment (ASTRONAUT) Study Group. N Engl J Med 1998;338:719–26.

CHAPTER 24

NONSTEROIDAL ANTI-INFLAMMATORY DRUGS AND GASTROINTESTINAL COMPLICATIONS

Francis K. L. Chan, MD, and David Y. Graham, MD

Nonsteroidal anti-inflammatory drugs (NSAIDs) are among the most widely used medications in the world. For example, there were more than 111 million NSAID prescriptions written in 2000 in the United States. NSAID use is associated with an increase in the risk of clinical upper gastrointestinal (UGI) events including symptomatic ulcer and ulcer complications (ie, bleeding, perforation, and gastric outlet obstruction). The individual risk of UGI complications in average risk NSAID users is estimated to be between 2 to 4% per year (or 2 to 4 per 100 patient years). Despite this relatively low frequency of untoward events, the high volume of use results in an estimated 16,500 deaths annually among arthritis patients from the gastrointestinal (GI) toxicity of NSAIDs.

In addition to serious complications, up to 50% of NSAID users experience dyspepsia. The presence of dyspepsia has little or no correlation with the presence of gastroduodenal ulcers and the presence of dyspepsia is, at most, very weakly associated with the presence of NSAID-induced ulcers. NSAID-associated UGI complications frequently occur without antecedent symptoms such that the absence of symptoms cannot be equated with the absence of risk. NSAID-associated dyspepsia tends to occur in two types: one that is *responsive to antisecretory drug therapy* and *one that is not*. It is likely that antisecretory drug responsive dyspepsia is related to NSAID-associated damage to the *esophagus*. It has been recognized that chronic blood loss and hypoalbuminemia are poorly related to visible NSAID damage to the upper GI tract. There is also increasing evidence of small bowel injury among chronic NSAID users. It is unknown what proportion of antisecretory drug unresponsive dyspepsia originates in the small intestine. There is a separate chapter on NSAID-induced injury to the small and large intestine (see Chapter 60 "Nonsteroidal Anti-Inflammatory Drug-Induced Small and Large Intestinal Injury").

Ulcerogenic Potential of NSAIDs

Although all NSAIDs can cause GI injury, some NSAIDs are more ulcerogenic than others. In general, the ulcerogenic potential of an NSAID correlates with its anti-inflammatory activity. NSAIDs with a *high analgesic effect at doses with low anti-inflammatory* activity, such as *ibuprofen*, are *less ulcerogenic* than NSAIDs that achieve acceptable analgesic effects only at doses with *high anti-inflammatory activity* (eg, *piroxicam*). Clinically, the ulcer risk observed with various NSAIDs is in part a reflection of prescribing behavior. For example, ibuprofen is frequently used at analgesic doses (1.2 g or less per day) for noninflammatory pain conditions. When full anti-inflammatory doses are given (eg, 2.4 g/d), it is not possible to distinguish ibuprofen from other NSAIDs.

The primary mechanism for NSAID damage to the gastric mucosa is related to suppression of prostaglandin synthesis. Thus, administration of NSAIDs parenterally or rectally does not reduce the risk of ulcers or ulcer complications. The same argument applies regarding use of enteric-coated or delayed release formulations, which have no advantages over the parent NSAIDs in terms of the risk for UGI complications (Graham, 1996).

Risk Estimation

The choice of NSAID and the strategy for prevention of risk both relate to the known risk factors for NSAID-induced UGI complications (Table 24-1). In clinical practice, patients who require NSAIDs should be stratified according to the nature and number of risk factors, as follows: (1) low risk (absence of risk factors), (2) moderate risk (one to two risk factors), and (3) high risk (prior ulcer complications, concomitant low dose aspirin, or three risk

TABLE 24-1. Risk Factors for Nonsteroidal Anti-Inflammatory Drug-Induced Ulcer Complication

History of peptic ulcer disease (especially prior ulcer complications)
Old age (> 60 years)
High dose NSAID use
Use of multiple NSAIDs
Recent institution of NSAIDs (within 30 days)
Cardiovascular diseases
Concomitant use of low dose aspirin
Concomitant use of anticoagulants
Concomitant use of steroids

NSAID = nonsteroidal anti-inflammatory drug

factors or more) (Table 24-2). A history of an ulcer complication is the single most important factor that predicts UGI complications with NSAID use. In fact, a history of prior UGI complications is also the most ominous predictive factor for *Helicobacter pylori* ulcers. With *H. pylori* ulcers, eradication of the *H. pylori* infection essentially eliminates the risk of future untoward events. In contrast, the natural history of patients with complicated NSAID ulcers is largely unknown except in the short term (ie, 6 months to 1 year). Understanding this natural history is among the most important questions remaining to be answered in ulcer disease. For example, does the risk decrease with time, and, if so, what amount of time off NSAIDs is required to return to baseline risk? Patients with a history of a complicated UGI event associated with low dose aspirin should also be treated as high risk (Weisman, 2002). Concomitant use of NSAID and low dose aspirin substantially increases the risk of ulcer complication compared with NSAID use alone. The exact mechanism is uncertain. Low dose aspirin probably also provokes bleeding from mucosal ulcerations induced by NSAIDs.

Risk Reduction

The presence of an active *H. pylori* infection increases the risk of a UGI complication two to fourfold. We therefore recommend that all patients scheduled for chronic aspirin or NSAID therapy be tested for *H. pylori* and that the infection be eradicated if present (Huang et al, 2002). An additional advantage of *H. pylori* eradication is prevention of chronic antisecretory drug therapy-associated worsening of *H. pylori*-associated corpus gastritis.

The best method of risk reduction is to avoid NSAIDs particularly in high risk individuals. This is often not practical when treating an inflammatory condition. However, patients with degenerative arthritis or other noninflammatory pain conditions should receive non-NSAID analgesics as their first line therapy. If NSAIDs are required for analgesia, one should prescribe an NSAID with a *high analgesic effect and low anti-inflammatory action* (eg, ibuprofen [Advil]) and the lowest effective dose should be used. Cyclooxygenase-2-inhibitors (COX-2) are a reasonable alternative and can provide good analgesia with increased safety but at greater expense. One of the acknowledged risk factors is use of *multiple NSAIDs,* and many patients will take both prescription NSAIDs and nonprescription NSAIDs without their doctors being aware (eg, prescription ibuprofen for arthritis and over-the-counter naproxen for a headache). Use of multiple NSAIDs compounds the risk of complications (ie, moves the patient into a higher risk category), and the patient should be warned to avoid this behavior. For patients who require NSAIDs for inflammatory conditions, current evidence indicates that COX-2 inhibitors (eg, celecoxib [Celebrex] or rofecoxib [Vioxx]) are preferred over even the least ulcerogenic conventional NSAID (ibuprofen) in terms of UGI toxicity. The question remains as to whether the use of a COX-2 inhibitor and combined treatment with a low toxicity conventional NSAID and an antisecretory drug or misoprostol are equal in terms of safety and efficacy. This issue is discussed in Chapter 2, "Decision Analysis in the Management of Digestive Diseases."

TABLE 24-2. Number of Risk Factors and the Estimated Incidence of Nonsteroidal Anti-Inflammatory Drug-Induced Ulcer Complications

Number of Risk Factors*	Annualized Incidence of NSAID-Induced Ulcer Complications
0	0.8%
1	2%
2	7.6 to 8.6%
3	18%

NSAID = nonsteroidal anti-inflammatory drug.
*A history of ulcer complications is the single most important risk factor that outweighs the combined effects of other risk factors. It should be noted that this study was done before the importance of *H. pylori* was accepted and it is not taken into account. Adapted from Silverstein et al, 1995.

Cardiovascular Diseases and Renal Failure

Patients with cardiovascular diseases or renal insufficiency and inflammatory arthritis pose special management problems because both NSAIDs and COX-2 inhibitors aggravate cardiovascular and renal diseases by inducing fluid retention, hypertension, and renal impairment. These renal adverse events are common in patients with decompensated heart failure, preexisting renal impairment, and those who receive angiotensin-converting enzyme inhibitors. Importantly, COX-2 inhibitors offer no advantage over conventional NSAIDs in terms of renal adverse events, and both should be avoided if possible in these high risk patients. The question regarding whether the COX-2 inhibitor, rofecoxib, is associated with an *increase in the risk* of acute myocardial infarction remains unresolved. COX-2 inhibitors lack an antiplatelet activity, such that patients with coronary heart disease should continue prophylactic treatment with low dose aspirin despite the use of COX-2 inhibitors.

Given the better gastrointestinal (GI) safety profile of COX-2 inhibitors over conventional NSAIDs, COX-2 inhibitors are the preferred anti-inflammatory drugs for moderate to high risk patients (Table 24-3) who receive concomitant low dose aspirin. Unfortunately, low dose aspirin itself is associated with a substantial risk of UGI complications. Current data suggest concomitant low dose aspirin partially or completely negates the beneficial safety effects of COX-2 inhibitors. Thus, patients on *low dose aspirin who require anti-inflammatory therapy,* regardless of NSAIDs or COX-2 inhibitors, should receive cotherapy with an *anti-*

TABLE 24-3. Risk Stratification and Strategies to Prevent Nonsteroidal Anti-Inflammatory Drug-Induced Upper Gastrointestinal Complications

	Low Risk*	Moderate Risk†	High Risk‡
Asymptomatic	1. Least ulcerogenic NSAID at the lowest effective dose for analgesia 2. COX-2 inhibitors for inflammatory arthritis	1. COX-2 inhibitor 2. NSAID + PPI NSAID + PPI	COX-2 inhibitor + PPI or misoprostol Endoscopy
Dyspepsia	1. Consider switching to another NSAID 2. NSAID + H₂RA		
Concomitant aspirin	NSAID + H₂RA, PPI or misoprostol	COX-2 inhibitor + PPI or misoprostol	COX-2 inhibitor + PPI or misoprostol

COX-2 = Cyclooxygenase-2-inhibitors; H₂RA = H₂ receptor antagonist; NSAID = nonsteroidal anti-inflammatory drug; PPI = proton pump inhibitor.
*Low risk = no risk factor; †Moderate risk = two risk factors or less (excluding a history of ulcer complications or concomitant use of low dose aspirin); ‡High risk = a history of ulcer complications or three risk factors or more.

secretory drug (an H₂ receptor antagonist [H₂RA] or proton pump inhibitor [PPI] or misoprostol) (see Table 24-3).

Concomitant Steroids or Anticoagulant Therapy

Concomitant steroids or anticoagulant therapy substantially increases the risk of UGI complications in patients receiving NSAIDs. Current evidence indicates that concomitant steroid use does not increase the risk of clinical UGI events in patients receiving COX-2 inhibitors compared with patients receiving a traditional NSAID, such as *naproxen*. Thus, the use of a COX-2 inhibitor is a good alternative to combined treatment with a gastroprotective agent and a conventional NSAID for patients receiving steroid therapy.

Although experimental studies suggest there is no interaction between COX-2 inhibitors and anticoagulants, this has not yet been confirmed by actual clinical outcome studies. Since patients who receive anticoagulant therapy usually have serious medical conditions, such as prosthetic heart valve replacement, and deep vein thrombosis and the consequence of GI bleeding or withholding anticoagulants is potentially disastrous, we recommend the use of steroids instead of NSAIDs or COX-2 inhibitors for acute, short term inflammatory conditions, such as an attack of gouty arthritis. Alternatively, we recommend the combination of *a COX-2 inhibitor* and *misoprostol*. Misoprostol is preferred because anticoagulants can provoke bleeding from preexisting mucosal ulcerations anywhere in the GI tract and antisecretory drugs only protect the proximal GI tract. Theoretically, the combination of a COX-2 inhibitor and misoprostol reduces the risk of both upper and lower GI bleeding. This hypothesis has not been tested clinically.

Gastroprotective Agents

There are many clinical studies using "endoscopic ulcers" as an endpoint. There are far fewer using clinically important outcomes such as a UGI complication. In addition, most of the "endoscopic ulcer" studies did not separate *H. pylori* infected patients (which would include a variable number with *H. pylori* ulcers) from *H. pylori* negative patients. It has become evident that the prevention of endoscopic ulcers differs between those with and without *H. pylori* infection. For example, the PPI omeprazole (Prilosec) was superior to low dose *ranitidine* (Zantac) (150 mg twice daily) or low dose *misoprostol* (Cytotec) (200 μg twice daily) among those with *H. pylori* infection. In contrast, omeprazole was less effective and not significantly different from ranitidine among those without *H. pylori* infection and was actually inferior to low dose misoprostol. Low dose misoprostol was even superior to omeprazole for healing of "endoscopic" gastric ulcers among those without *H. pylori* infection (Graham, 2002; Silverstein, 1995). Head-to-head outcome studies using clinically important end points are clearly needed. At the present time it is impossible to determine which combination (H₂RAs, PPIs, or misoprostol) is best. It has been suggested that the *combination* of an *antisecretory drug* (either an H₂RA or PPI) and low dose *misoprostol* (200 μg twice daily) may provide the best overall protection. The only large scale study showing partial protection used misoprostol, but patients were not stratified in relation to their *H. pylori* status. It is currently impossible to make recommendations based on data. *PPIs* are superior to H₂RAs for suppression of acid secretion and are *generally preferred* because they are better tolerated than misoprostol and require only a single daily dose.

Management of NSAID-Associated Dypepsia, Ulcers, and Their Complications

NSAID-Associated Dyspepsia

Although dyspepsia does not predict the development of symptomatic ulcer or ulcer complications with NSAID therapy, it is a common problem that often leads to discontinuation of treatment, repeated endoscopic examinations, and frequent use of gastroprotective agents. Because it is impractical to endoscope every patient with NSAID-associated dyspepsia, we recommend empirical treatment with gastroprotective agents for low to moderate risk patients and endoscopic evaluation for high risk patients (see Table 24-3). For low risk patients, switching to another NSAID or cotherapy with an H$_2$RA often relieves dyspeptic symptoms (see Table 24-3). Antisecretory drugs are useful in patients with reflux-like or ulcer-like dyspepsia. For moderate risk patients, PPIs are preferred to H$_2$RAs because they are more potent, which theoretically should make them more effective (see Table 24-3). However, there are limited comparative data in NSAID users without *H. pylori* infection, and the data that are available show more similarities with PPIs than differences. Nonetheless, unless cost is a critical issue PPIs are preferred for all but those with minimal risk. If cost is the critical issue, we recommend double dose H$_2$RAs or single dose plus low dose misoprostol.

Although COX-2 inhibitors cause less dyspepsia than conventional NSAIDs, there is no evidence regarding whether substitution for a COX-2 inhibitor can resolve NSAID-associated dyspepsia. Management of dyspepsia in high risk patients (ie, a history of ulcer complication or multiple risk factors) remains difficult and there are remarkably little data to guide the physician. We recommend use of a COX-2 inhibitor and a PPI. If symptoms persist despite receiving combination therapy, we recommend endoscopy to exclude conditions like erosive esophagitis, penetrating ulcers, gastric outlet obstruction, or gastric malignancy (see Table 24-3).

Ulcers and Their Complications

While symptomatic gastroduodenal ulcers may develop during NSAID therapy, one can never be confident that the ulcer is actually benign. If endoscopy is done, a biopsy should be performed on any gastric ulcer to exclude malignancy. It is recommended that a definite ulcer should be followed until complete healing. This is especially important with large ulcers (≥ 2 cm). Biopsies of the normal appearing mucosa should also be taken to confirm that *H. pylori* is not present. NSAIDs should be withheld. If *H. pylori* infection is present, it should be eradicated as it is impossible to determine whether the ulcer was caused by NSAIDs, *H. pylori* infection, or both. Curing the infection removes one of the most important causes of recurrent ulcer disease. The choice of diagnostic test for *H. pylori* during the early phase is complicated because many factors may be present that may lead to *false negative diagnostic* tests, such as the presence of *blood* in the stomach or recent use of *antibiotics, bismuth*, or *PPIs*. All of the tests for active infection including rapid urease tests, urea breath tests, stool antigen tests, histology, and culture are affected with *false negative results* in the range of 20 to 50% of the cases. Nonetheless, a positive test for active infection indicates *H. pylori* infection. The issue is what to do if the tests are negative. A gastric biopsy for histological confirmation of *H. pylori* is often best as it can be performed at the time of endoscopy. It is important to obtain both antral and corpus biopsies to reduce the chance of a negative biopsy resulting from suppression of the infection by antibiotics, bismuth, or PPIs. There is no urgent need to treat an *H. pylori* infection, and when in doubt, we generally use a urea breath test after ulcer healing. Whichever test for active infection is used, it is important that the *PPI be discontinued for at least 2 weeks* before testing. One can use an H$_2$RA without a negative influence on testing. Although serology can always be used, we believe that a positive *H. pylori* serology test should always be followed-up with a test for active infection before starting therapy. The *recommended* H. pylori *eradication regimens* include *a PPI or ranitidine, bismuth citrate* plus *amoxicillin*, and *clarithromycin* for a minimum of at least 1 week. The antimicrobial therapy may be given before or after a course of PPI for ulcer healing. Commencing antibiotics after a course of PPI has the advantage of enhancing the efficacy of PPI for ulcer healing in the presence of *H. pylori* infection. However, one has to wait for 4 weeks posteradication to confirm successful cure of the infection. Starting antimicrobial therapy before a course of PPI may modestly reduce the efficacy of PPI, but one only needs to wait for 2 weeks after stopping PPI to check ulcer healing and the final *H. pylori* status. Again, we substitute an H$_2$RA for the PPI until we are confident that the *H. pylori* infection has been eradicated. The preceding chapter (see Chapter 23, "*Helicobacter pylori* and Gastroduodenal Disease") is on *H. pylori* infection.

Anti-Inflammatory Therapy in the Presence of Active Ulcers

As a general rule, one should substitute non-NSAID analgesics for NSAIDs in the presence of active ulcers. Most NSAID ulcers will heal spontaneously after stopping NSAID therapy but healing is accelerated with antisecretory drug therapy. NSAID ulcers will heal with standard doses of PPIs despite continued NSAID use but the time to complete healing may be prolonged. Thus, patients with active ulcers who cannot discontinue anti-inflammatory therapy should receive the least ulcerogenic NSAID at the lowest effective dose plus cotherapy with a gastroprotective agent, preferably a PPI.

Patients who presented with active bleeding from NSAID ulcers are at high risk of early rebleeding after initial endoscopic hemostasis. We recommend a bolus of 80 mg of a PPI intravenously followed by a continuous PPI infusion at 8 mg/h for the first 72 hours as this provides the best control of intragastric pH. Intravenous therapy is then followed by high dose oral PPI (eg, omeprazole 40 mg twice or three times daily, or its equivalent). *A short course of steroid therapy* often controls the inflammatory arthritis and is *preferred* over continuing NSAIDs in this dangerous period.

Refractory NSAID Ulcers

The most common cause of refractory NSAID ulcer is continued NSAID use. A detailed history, repeated questioning, or interviewing family members often provides a clue to surreptitious use of NSAIDs. Serum salicylates levels are helpful to identify surreptitious aspirin users. Patients with unhealed NSAID ulcers should be treated with a prolonged course of high dose PPI (eg, omeprazole 40 mg twice daily) until the ulcer is healed. Based on the authors' experience, combined treatment with high dose PPI and misoprostol is probably best but this has not been studied prospectively. These chronic, difficult to heal, ulcers recur rapidly when NSAIDs or aspirin are restarted. It is unclear whether switching to a COX-2 inhibitor after ulcer healing would reduce the rate of ulcer recurrence. Substitution of a COX-2 for a traditional NSAID is not thought to have an advantage over conventional NSAIDs with regard to ulcer healing. There is experimental evidence in animals that COX-2 inhibitors actually impair gastric ulcer healing, but the affects in humans are unknown. Thus, we do not recommend switching from a conventional NSAID to a COX-2 inhibitor in the management of refractory NSAID ulcer. Cessation of NSAID use is often the only effective measure to promote ulcer healing.

Very High Risk Patients

Patients with prior ulcer complications are in the highest risk group. Those who have a recent history of ulcer complications (eg, within 6 months) are at much higher risk than those with a remote history of complicated ulcers. The risk of rebleeding from *H. pylori* ulcers without *H. pylori* eradication ranges from 1 to 3% per month. The early studies did not separate *H. pylori* from NSAID ulcers such that it was impossible to discern whether one was studying the natural history of *H. pylori* ulcers in NSAID users, or NSAID ulcers in those with *H. pylori* infection, or some combination. Recent data suggest that the natural history of complicated NSAID ulcers is similar to that of *H. pylori* ulcers with approximately the same or higher risks of rebleeding if they continue to use NSAIDs. Because ulcers tend to recur at previous ulcer sites, the high incidence of recurrent bleeding in patients with recent complicated ulcers is probably due to the breakdown of immature scar tissue.

Current evidence indicates that combined treatment with a PPI plus a conventional NSAID and treatment with a COX-2 inhibitor without a gastroprotective are comparable but equally disappointing in eliminating the risk of ulcer complication in very high risk patients (Graham, 2002). The lack of a control group or a group in whom no NSAIDs were given precludes determining whether either approach actually reduced the risk of recurrent ulcer bleeding. The rebleeding rate with either was approximately 10 per 100 patient years (ie, 10% per year) and, as such, was unacceptably high. Thus, we recommend that these patients avoid NSAIDs. If this is impossible, we recommend the combination of a COX-2 inhibitor and a PPI and/or misoprostol. For frail elderly patients, the combination of a COX-2 inhibitor, a PPI, and misoprostol should be considered.*

Supplemental Reading

Chan FK, Sung JJ. Role of acid suppressants in prophylaxis of NSAID damage. Best Pract Res Clin Gastroenterol 2001;15:433–45.

Graham DY. Critical effect of *Helicobacter pylori* infection on the effectiveness of omeprazole or prevention of gastric or duodenal ulcers among chronic NSAID users. Helicobacter 2002;7:1–8.

Graham DY. Nonsteroidal anti-inflammatory drugs, *Helicobacter pylori*, and ulcers: where we stand. Am J Gastroenterol 1996;91:2080–6.

Graham DY. NSAIDs, *Helicobacter pylori*, and Pandora's Box. N Engl J Med 2002;347:2162–4.

Huang JQ, Sridhar S, Hunt RH. Role of *Helicobacter pylori* infection and non-steroidal anti-inflammatory drugs in peptic-ulcer disease: a meta-analysis. Lancet 2002;359:14–22.

Silverstein FE, Graham DY, Senior JR, et al. Misoprostol reduces serious gastrointestinal complications in patients with rheumatoid arthritis receiving nonsteroidal anti-inflammatory drugs. A randomized, double-blind, placebo-controlled trial. Ann Intern Med 1995;123:241–9.

Weisman SM, Graham DY. Evaluation of the benefits and risks of low-dose aspirin in the secondary prevention of cardiovascular and cerebrovascular events. Arch Intern Med 2002;162:2197–202.

---

*Editor's Note: Thanks for calling, take two plus two and call the office in the morning.

CHAPTER 25

Peptic Ulcer Disease

Joseph R. Pisegna, MD

The stomach plays a central role in the digestive tract owing in large part to the fact that it is the initial site for gastrointestinal (GI) digestion and that, through the release of peptide mediators, it regulates both secretion and motility. In the twentieth century, key discoveries were made in understanding the hormonal regulation of acid secretion with the discovery of gastrin, secretin, and cholecystokinin (CCK), as well as their receptors. The description of a syndrome linked to the gastric hormone gastrin, Zollinger Ellison (ZE) syndrome, showed a direct cause and effect relationship between this hormone and the development of uncontrolled gastric acid. The discovery of the organism, *Helicobacter pylori*, and its role in the genesis of peptic ulcerations, came to light late in the twentieth century and has provided new insights into the role of this organism and gastric mucosal host defense mechanisms. Similarly, with the increasing use of nonsteroidal anti-inflammatory drugs (NSAIDs) for the treatment of rheumatologic conditions, the role of these iatrogenic agents in the genesis of peptic ulcer disease (PUD) was appreciated. More recently new developments in the field of inhibition of gastric acid secretion and PUD treatment have improved our ability to cure peptic ulcers. However, despite two centuries of investigations, as well as improved treatments and prevention, PUD has not been completely cured and continues to account for a significant morbidity and mortality. There are separate chapters on *H. pylori* (see Chapter 23, "*Helicobacter pylori* and Gastroduodenal Disease"), NSAIDs (see Chapter 24, "Nonsteroidal Anti-Inflammatory Drugs and Gastrointestinal Complications"), and gastrinomas (see Chapter 26, "Gastrinoma"). Peptic ulcer therapy is also discussed in the first two chapters on evidence (see Chapter 1, "Using Evidence-Based Medicine in Patient Care") and on analyses (Chapter 2, "Decision Analysis in the Management of Digestive Diseases").

Epidemiology

Despite efforts to reduce the level of gastric acid secretion, there remain a substantial number of patients admitted each year with PUD. In a recent study in US veterans it was shown that, although there has been an appreciable reduction in hospitalizations for both gastric and duodenal ulcer disease over the past three to four decades, the level has reached a plateau (El-Serag and Sonnenberg, 1998). Furthermore, there appears to be > 1 million cases of PUD recurrences in the United States each year (Munnangi and Sonnenberg, 1997). The major complication resulting from PUD is the risk for the development of upper GI bleeding. GI bleeding remains a major cause of morbidity and mortality despite newer endoscopic approaches because there remains an approximately 15 to 20% risk of re-bleeding following successful hemostasis. There is a separate chapter on GI Bleeding (see Chapter 28, "Upper Gastrointestinal Bleeding").

It is speculated that factors such as advanced age, medical comorbidities, use of NSAIDS, use of antiplatelet agents, warfarin derivatives, and infection with *H. pylori*, either alone or in combination, explain the high morbidity and mortality associated with complicated PUD. Genetic factors were once thought to be important in predisposing some individuals to the development of PUD, however, to date, there have been no direct links made with the exception of patients with *ZE syndrome* and *multiple endocrine neoplasia type I*. *Cigarette smoking* is known to be a risk factor in PUD. It is postulated that cigarette smoking reduces the levels of gastric mucosal prostaglandins and, hence, impairs gastric mucosal defensive factors (Cryer et al, 1992). The association between alcohol and PUD is less clear given that some studies have been unable to demonstrate a strong association between modest alcohol consumption and the development of PUD in the noncirrhotic patient (Stern et al, 1984). Similarly, there is no known association between dietary factors and the development of PUD. It had been purported that certain types of foods could predispose to the development of PUD, such as spicy foods, caffeine, and alcohol, but these factors have been disputed. The relationship between emotional states and the development of PUD has not been firmly resolved. As discussed below, acid secretion is dependant upon the release of neurohormonal mediators and there has been recent evidence showing that these mediators link the brain and GI tract. In animal models, stress results in the release of corticotrophin-releasing factor (CRF) and activation of the CRF receptor that mediates visceral hypersensitivity and intestinal motility (Million et al, 2003). However, to date, there has not been a definitive link between emotional stress and the development of PUD.

Stress-Related Erosive Syndrome

The development of stress-related PUD represents a special case and is recognized as being increasingly more important, especially in the hospitalized patient. These types of ulcerations occur in the critically ill patient, and the ulcerations can be generally characterized as being superficial with only 1.5 to 3.5% presenting with clinically significant bleeding (Mutlu et al, 2001). In these critically ill patients, however, bleeding from stress ulcers is exacerbated by coexistent coagulopathy and in these cases there is a significant increase in mortality and increased costs related to the length of intensive care unit (ICU) stay. The development of stress-ulcer bleeding can be thought of as one of the factors related to mortality in these patients, and should be considered a marker of overall severity of critical illness (Lewis et al, 2000). There is a chapter on stress-related erosive syndrome (see Chapter 27, "Management of Stress-Related Erosive Syndrome").

Physiology of Gastric Acid Secretion

The secretion of gastric acid is the principle role of the gastric oxyntic gland apparatus and is regulated by a complex neurohormonal process. Interplay between neurocrine, paracrine, and endocrine regulation occurs via acetylcholine, histamine, and gastrin, respectively for each of these processes. The parietal cell is primarily responsible for the synthesis and release of acid; however other cellular components of the oxyntic gland include the gastric D cells and enterchromaffin-like (ECL) cells. In general, acid secretion can be divided into the following two phases: (1) the cephalic phase and (2) the peripheral phase (Zeng et al, 1999).

The major neural regulator of acid secretion is through the vagus nerve. Stimulation by the vagus nerve results in cholinergic stimulation of the muscarinic receptor on the parietal cell (Wolfe and Soll, 1988). Our understanding of the mechanisms involved in the cephalic phase of acid secretion have been improved by the observation that enteric neurons in the gastric mucosa contain the neuropeptide, pituitary adenylate cyclase activating polypeptide (PACAP) which has been shown to stimulate release of histamine from the ECL cell (Zeng et al, 1999). Presumably, higher cortical perceptions of food activate the cephalic phase of acid secretion.

The peripheral phase of gastric acid secretion occurs once food comes into contact with the gastric mucosa. Ingested proteins stimulate the release of gastrin from gastric G cells. The receptor-mediated pathway for this process is still largely unknown. Gastrin released from the G cell stimulates the CCK-2 or gastrin receptor that is expressed on the gastric ECL cell. Gastrin, like PACAP, stimulates the release of histamine from the ECL cell. Histamine acts at the histamine-2 (H_2) receptor expressed on the parietal cell to stimulate hydrogen/potassium ATPase (H^+/K^+-ATPase).

Acid Secretion and Pathophysiologic Consequences

GASTRIC MUCOSAL DEFENSE

The gastric mucosa is exposed to acid pH and to large volumes of gastric acid secretion. To prevent the development of mucosal damage, mechanisms have evolved to afford the mucosal lining *protection (gastric mucosal defense)*. These normal defense mechanisms can be disrupted in various pathophysiologic situations, such as mucosal stress that is caused by NSAIDs or *H. pylori*, and in patients that are being treated in the ICU.

In the hospital setting, medical and surgical patients develop the risk of peptic ulcerations because of the development of gastric mucosal hypoxia with consequent disruption to the tight junctions that inherently prevent the back-diffusion of gastric acid as well as from the release of inflammatory mediators (Cook et al, 1994). Patients that are at particular risk for the development of stress PUD include those with severe sepsis, those requiring mechanical ventilation or coagulopathy, and burn and neurosurgical patients. The risk of GI bleeding is the greatest in those patients with *respiratory failure* and *coagulopathy*. Importantly, patients in the ICU that undergo enteral feedings may fare better than those patients who are maintained without feeding by mouth (NPO).

Stress ulceration results from a combination of reduced blood flow to the gastric mucosa as well as disturbances in acid–base balance. During periods of stress there is constriction of splanchnic blood vessels resulting in local gastric mucosal hypoxia with consequent acidemia. One hypothesis is that cytokines released during periods of respiratory compromise result in the release of catecholamine that occurs in the ICU setting. Stress ulcerations are perhaps the most common manifestation of PUD in the hospitalized patient. Our current thinking is that the release of albeit small levels of gastric acid in these patients, in combination with the release of pepsinogen and bile salt reflux, act as injurious agents to the mucosa that is compromised by hypoperfusion. Increased bleeding occurs in those patients with diminished clotting factors or with platelet dysfunction.

Clinical Presentations of PUD

The history should include a review of medications especially NSAIDS and acetylsalicylic acid (ASA). Family history should focus on a history of PUDs. Although there is no genetic link identified, patients with multiple endocrine neoplasia (MEN) type I can provide a history of ulcer disease. Similarly, a review of family history for the presence of *H. pylori* may be useful. In many cases the patient is asymptomatic, whereas in others the symptoms include abdominal pain, hematemesis, or melena. In patients with ZE syndrome the most common presentation of uncontrolled gastric acid hypersecretion is diarrhea, abdominal pain, and, occasionally, upper GI bleeding from postbulbar ulcerations. Classically, patients presenting with PUD will experience a burning or gnawing pain in the epigastrium, or occasionally the hypogastrium, that occurs several hours after meals and typically improves with food ingestion. Presumably acid secretion that is stimulated by meals leads to the pain symptom and the ingestion of food results in buffering of gastric acidity. The pain will be similarly alleviated by the ingestion of antacids or histamine-2 receptor antagonists (H$_2$RAs). Pain related to PUD can be frequently confused with the characteristic pain related to gastroesophageal reflux disease (GERD). In the latter, however, the patients are more likely to report that there is movement of the pain from the epigastrium into the esophagus. The pain related with both PUD and GERD may be improved with meal ingestion, antacids, or H$_2$RAs. A careful history should include whether the patient obtains relief of the pain with various maneuvers. Occasionally, patients with PUD may report radiation of pain to the right upper quadrant which can be confused with pain related to biliary colic, and if the patient has a posterior duodenal ulcer, the pain may radiate to the back and be confused with the pain related to pancreatic diseases. It is often difficult to distinguish functional dyspepsia from true PUD without a diagnostic test. Clearly PUD remains in the differential diagnosis for patients diagnosed with dyspepsia. Last, an endoscopic approach with biopsy is needed to distinguish benign gastric ulcers related to PUD from gastric cancer.

Role of *H. pylori* and NSAIDs

There is a very strong epidemiologic link between *H. pylori* infection and the development of PUD. The proof that this association exists has been described following the observation that a significant proportion of patients with PUD have co-infection coupled with the observation that eradication strategies result in a significantly lowered risk for the development of PUD. Controversies exist as to whether *H. pylori* should be eradicated in patients who test positive for infection as a means of preventing the development of PUD. There is a greater likelihood for the development of PUD in patients who have coexistent *H. pylori* and NSAID usage. The treatment of *H. pylori* infection and the management of NSAID-induced ulcers are described in Chapter 23 "*Helicobacter pylori* and Gastroduodenal Disease"; Chapter 24 "Nonsteroidal Anti-Inflammatory Drugs and Gastrointestinal Complications"; Chapter 29, "Chronic Gastritis"; and Chapter 33, "Primary Gastric Lymphoma."

Role of ZE Syndrome

The *ZE syndrome* results from the development of a *gastrinoma* tumor-releasing gastrin (see Chapter 26, "Gastrinoma"). Gastrin, a potent activator of parietal cell release of gastric acid stimulates gastric hypersecretion in these patients. Gastrinomas belong to a larger group of neuroendocrine tumors (NETs) of the GI tract. The most common of these tumors in the GI tract are gastrinomas. With regards to their overall prevalence, NETs are relatively rare and account for < 1% of malignant tumors of the GI tract and an overall population prevalence of only 1 per 100,000 persons (Pisegna, 2002). Patients with ZE syndrome can be generally divided into either sporadic or those that are MEN I-associated. Thus far, genetic testing has failed to identify a genetic link in patients with sporadic ZE syndrome, whereas a genetic locus has been identified in those patients who have MEN I associated disease. Natural history studies have identified that patients with the sporadic ZE syndrome are more likely to have pancreatic tumors that are larger at the time of surgery and have a greater predisposition for the development of metastatic disease compared to patients with MEN I syndrome. In general, patients with sporadic ZE syndrome can be cured of disease if the gastrinoma tumors can be identified and surgically extirpated, whereas in those patients with MEN I Syndrome, the surgical cure rate is low (Pisegna and Sawicki, 1998).

DIAGNOSIS

Given that nearly one-third of ZE syndrome patients may also have the MEN I syndrome, serum measurements of parathyroid hormone and calcium are recommended. The diagnosis of ZE syndrome is usually established by hypergastrinemia (ie, > 100 pg/mL) in combination with gastric acid hypersecretion (ie, > 15 mEq/h). Histologic proof of the presence of gastrinomas is often difficult because of the small tumor size, especially if the gastrinoma occurs in the duodenum. A *secretin test* is sometimes clinically useful if there are equivocal findings on the gastrin level or gastric acid output. Patients with gastrinoma generally will have a serum gastrin measurement > 500 pg/mL. A gastrin measurement of > 1000 pg/mL is nearly diagnostic of ZE syndrome. False positives can occur with the use of proton pump inhibitors (PPIs) due to the inhibition of gastric acid secretion and the consequent feedback stimulation of antral G cells. In practice, the PPI should be discontinued for at least 1 week prior to the reassessment of serum gastrin and for gastric acid secretary studies. The secretin stimulation test (Figure 25-1) can be used if the results are equivocal. Synthetic secretin is now available. The sensitivity is approximately 90% for the diagnosis of ZE syndrome. A basal gastrin level administration of secretin (2 units/kg) intravenously is followed by measurements of serum gastrin. A positive test is an increase in serum gastrin of over 200 pg/mL within 10 to 15 minutes.

GASTRIC ANALYSIS

Gastric analysis can be easily performed with the placement of a nasogastric (NG) tube in the dependant portion of the

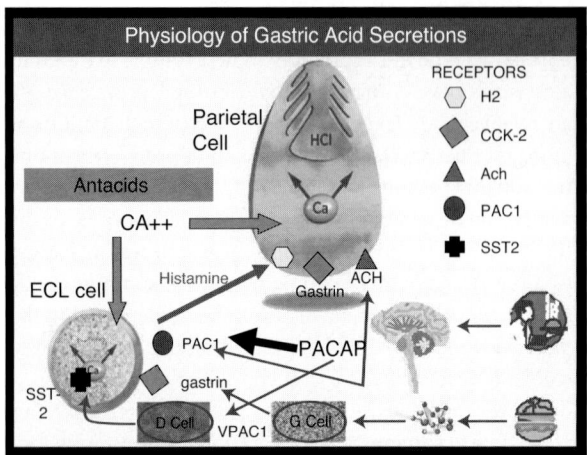

FIGURE 25-1. Physiology of gastric acid secretion. Adapted from Zeng et al (1999). Ca++ = calcium ion ; CCK = cholecystokinin; ECL = enterchromaffin-like; H₂ = histamine-2.

stomach and aspiration of gastrin contents over a 1-hour period and is a reflection of the basal level of acid secretion. This is generally measured as four 15-minute collections. To calculate the level of acid output, concentration of acid is measured using a titration method wherein sodium hydroxide (NaOH) is used to titrate the sample of gastric juice to pH 7.0 and the concentration of hydrogen ion is determined by the amount of NaOH required to titrate the sample to pH 7.0. Output of acid is then determined by multiplying the titratable acidity and the volume of gastric juice collected. The maximal acid output, which is a reflection of the parietal cell mass, can be similarly determined following the administration of pentagastrin subcutaneously (Pisegna, 2002).

Natural History of Upper GI Bleeding From PUD

When examining a patient for PUD, it is important to determine which subgroup of patients has an increased risk for the development of upper GI bleeding. Of the possible causes of upper GI bleeding, PUD remains the most frequent. If a patient required a blood transfusion with a previous PUD GI bleed, there is a more significant risk for re-bleeding. ASA or NSAIDs use and *H. pylori* presence suggest a PUD-related cause for the GI bleeding. The use of anticoagulation is particularly important because anticoagulation and antiplatelet agents generally increase the amount of bleeding and dictate changes in therapy to include reversal of anticoagulation and the timing for an endoscopic therapy. Patients in an ICU have other coexistent medical problems that increase their overall morbidity and mortality in the setting of an upper GI bleed. Patients with ZE syndrome who present with upper GI bleeding generally will have uncontrolled gastric acid secretion. Close attention to fluid imbalances as a result of the gastric acid hypersecretion (ie, up to 4 L/day of losses) will need to be addressed as well as volume losses from GI bleeding (Oh and Pisegna, 2003). High doses of intravenous (IV) proton pump inhibition are usually necessary in these patients.

Management of Upper GI Bleeding

There is a balance between offensive agents and gastric defensive protective factors that help to protect the gastric mucosa from injury. The gastric mucosa is protected by epidermal growth factor, an intact microcirculation, an alkaline mucosal barrier, and prostaglandins. Factors predisposing to an increased risk for bleeding in PUD include (1) ischemia, (2) bile reflux, and (3) a reduced pH. The majority of cases of upper GI bleeding can be controlled without the requirement of exploratory abdominal surgery by using endoscopy combined with hemostasis and the use of potent antisecretory medications, such as the PPIs. Upper endoscopy permits both the location and cause of upper GI bleeding as well as the determination of risk of re-bleeding based upon the morphology and size of the ulcer. A clean-based peptic ulcer would have < 5% risk of re-bleeding, whereas an actively bleeding ulcer would have an approximately 90% risk of bleeding. Ulcers with either an overlying clot or stigmata of recent bleeding would have an intermediate risk for re-bleeding. In patients admitted with upper GI bleeding secondary to PUD most re-bleeding occurs within the first 3 days of hospitalization (see Chapter 28, "Upper Gastrointestinal Bleeding").

ENDOSCOPIC MANAGEMENTS

Upper GI bleeding can be managed endoscopically in one of several manners (Figure 25-2). Using either a heater probe, Bicap electrocautery, injection with either 0.9% saline or absolute 100% ethanol, or a combination of these techniques, adequate hemostasis of a bleeding vessel can be achieved (Laine and Estrada, 2002). Alternative methods that have been used include laser photoablation. In one study the re-bleeding rate was only 6.5% in the combination group, whereas treatment with epinephrine alone resulted in a 22.2% risk of re-bleeding (Chung et al, 1997). At our medical center, we typically inject the ulcer perimeter with a dilute epinephrine solution (1:10,000) and subsequently apply electrocautery to the base of the ulcer to permit coaptation of the vessels underlying the ulcer. Upper endoscopy permits a "second-look" at the source of ulcer bleed. In one study from our medical center, a "second-look" endoscopy was shown to be cost effective at preventing re-bleeding (Spiegel et al, 2003). In addition, for patients presenting with gastric ulcers, upper endoscopy is performed 8 weeks or so following the presentation of upper GI bleeding to ensure complete ulcer healing and exclude the possibility of gastric malignancy.

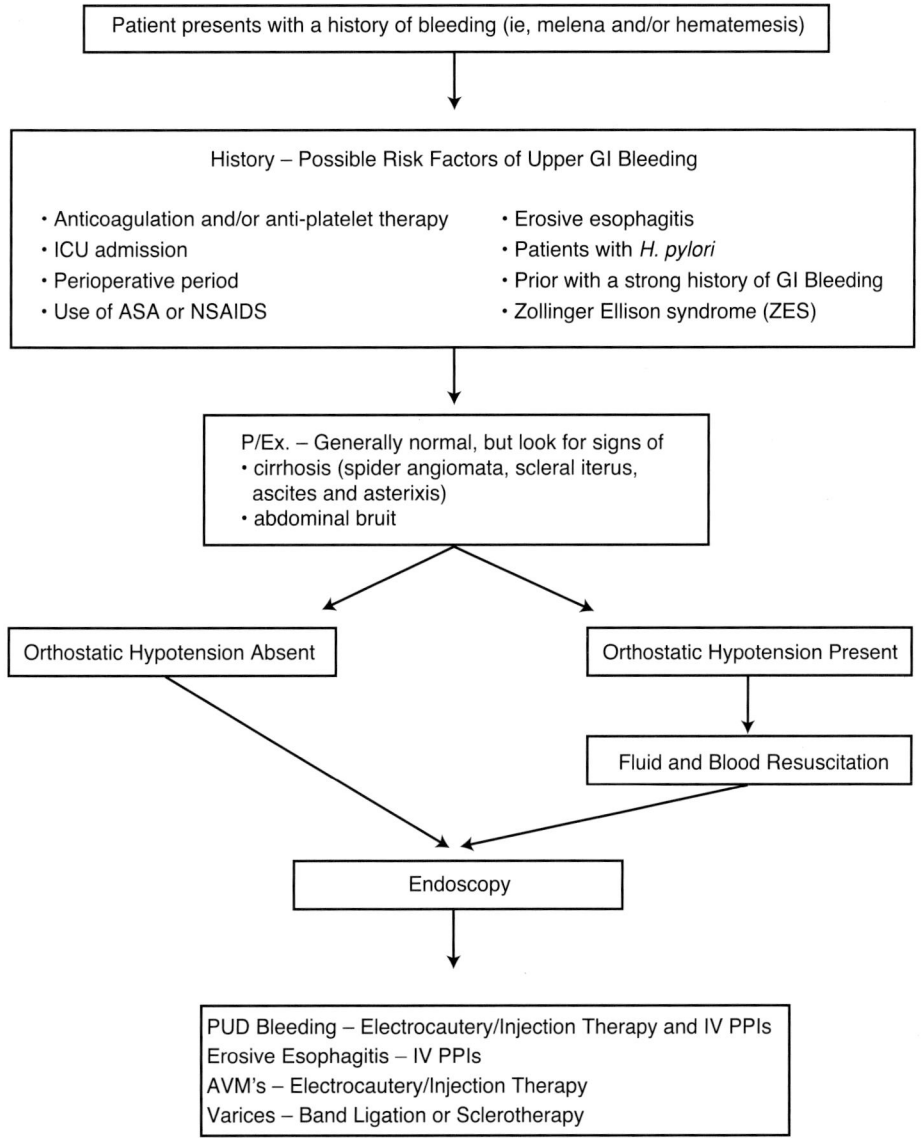

FIGURE 25-2. Algorithm for the management of upper gastrointestinal bleeding. Adapted from Zeng et al, 1999. ASA = acetylsalicylic acid; GI = gastrointestinal; ICU = intensive care unit; IV = intravenous; NSAIDs = nonsteroidal anti-inflammatory drugs; PPI = proton pump inhibitor; ZE = Zollinger Ellison.

Pharmaco-Physiology of PPIs' Actions

PPIs as a group have a similar mechanism of action and a similar chemical composition, possessing a substituted benzimidazole. Unlike the H₂RAs, which are receptor antagonists, the PPIs are "prodrugs" that require an activation step to exhibit efficacy. As "prodrugs" these agents require a protonation step that occurs in the cannalicular space of the parietal cell. There are subtle differences amongst the PPIs with respect to the rapidity at which this occurs. All of the available PPIs are enterically coated allowing for their passage from the stomach to the duodenum. Within the duodenum the enteric coating dissolves exposing the prodrug for absorption and circulating in the bloodstream for approximately 45 minutes during which time there is concentration of the drug within the parietal cell cannalicular space. Given that the cannalicular space has a pH of approximately 1.0, there is rapid activation of the PPI that thereby permits the "activated" PPI to bind to cysteine sites within the H^+/K^+-ATPase. Any condition which impairs the movement of the enterically coated PPI from arriving to the duodenum, such as a gastric emptying disorder, diabetic gastroparesis or a pyloric stricture will reduce the absorption and hence bioavailability of the PPI. In patients with prior Billroth anastamosis the effect of continued bile reflux has an uncertain effect on the absorption and bioavailability of PPIs.

Unlike with H₂RAs, PPIs inactivate only "activated" H^+/K^+-ATPase. The acid pump exists as either an inactive pump within the cytoplasm or an active pump that is embedded into the cannalicular space. Given that PPIs concentrate within the cannalicular space and are activated within this acidic space, PPIs can only block those pumps that are present within this space. Therefore, to attain a maximal effect from the administration of PPIs, one would need to dose these agents at a time in which the pumps are most active. As discussed earlier in the physiology of gastric acid secretion, the pumps are most active following the ingestion of a protein meal. Dosing of the PPI should therefore be done approximately 30 to 60 minutes before ingestion of a protein meal. It is our practice to administer these agents approximately 30 to 60 minutes before breakfast in the morning and if a nighttime dose is required to do so again, 30 to 60 minutes before dinner.*

Pharmacologic Management of PUD

We shall focus on the use of PPI therapy (see Table 25-1) for the treatment of PUD because studies have shown their superiority over H₂RAs (Yeomans et al, 1998). Similarly, when one looks at maintenance data, PPIs remain the dominant treatment modality (Agrawal et al, 2000). In patients who are coinfected with *H. pylori* specific antibiotic therapy is indicated (see Chapter 23, "*Helicobacter Pylori* and Gastroduodenal Disease"). In those patients who are ingesting NSAIDS, the goal of therapy is to discontinue the use of the offending agent and to continue to treat with PPI therapy. The majority of ulcers (*H. pylori*-and NSAID-associated) will heal within 8 weeks of therapy (Walan et al, 1989). For those patients in whom NSAIDs cannot be discontinued some studies have suggested that the use of BID PPI therapy may permit judicious use of NSAIDs in selected cases (Langman et al, 1991). To improve the healing of NSAID-associated ulcers, some have advocated that the patient should discontinue the use of NSAIDS altogether if this can be done safely. If not, one should consider using the lowest possible dose of NSAID coupled with PPI therapy. Some NSAIDs, such as nonaceylated salicylates, have a lower ulcerogenic potential and should be tried. Last, the use of a cyclooxygenase-2 selective agent, such as rofecoxib or celecoxib, should be employed either alone or with a protective agent, such as misoprostol (Laine, 2001).

In patients who fail to show a response after 8 to 12 weeks of ulcer therapy, one should consider these patients to have refractory PUD. In many cases the issue surrounding this is related to compliance. As noted earlier, for PPIs to have a maximal efficacy for inhibiting gastric acid secretion they should be taken 30 to 60 minutes before protein meal ingestion. If a patient has a problem in gastric emptying (ie, diabetic gastroparesis), the PPI will not be able to achieve maximal absorption and consideration should be given in these patients to treatment with an H₂RA. If *H. pylori* infection has not been considered up to this point in time a serum or breath test investigation should be undertaken. Similarly, concomitant use of NSAIDs may lead to a refractory ulcer (Lanas et al, 2000). In a patient with duodenal postbulbar ulcerations, consideration should be given to a diagnosis of ZE syndrome by measuring a serum gastrin and performing a gastric analysis. Last, if the ulcer is a gastric ulcer, serious consideration should be given to exclude gastric adenocarcinoma or an

TABLE 25-1. Food and Drug Administration Approved Antisectretory Medications

Agent	Dose	Route
H₂ Receptor Antagonists		
Ranitidine (Zantac)	300 mg	po, IV
Famotidine (Pepcid)	40 mg	po, IV
Nizatadine (Axid)	300 mg	po
Cimetidine (Tagamet)	800 mg	po, IV
Proton Pump Inhibitors		
Omeprazole (Prilosec)	20 to 40 mg	po
Lansoprazole (Prevacid)	15 to 30 mg	po
Pantoprazole (Protonix)	40 to 80 mg	po, IV
Rabeprazole (Aciphex)	20 to 40 mg	po
Esomeprazole (Nexium)	20 to 40 mg	po

IV = intravenous; po = by mouth.

---
* Editor's Note: Please note that the esophagologists writing in earlier chapters said 15 minutes before breakfast and dinner, although the stomach doctors prefer a longer lag time.

infectious etiology such as cytomegalovirus or *H. simplex*.

Pharmacologic Management of Upper GI Bleeding

In the past few decades we have witnessed major changes in the pharmacologic management of PUD, upper GI bleeding, and GERD. The advent of PPIs has transformed our ability to manage acid secretory conditions. Although there is still a role for H2RAs for the occasional heartburn sufferer and in pregnancy, there is really no place for this therapy for PUD (Ruigomez et al, 1999). Historically, the treatment of excess gastric acid secretion relied upon the use of antacids and H2RAs. Currently, there are the following four US Food and Drug Administration (FDA)-approved H2RAs (see Table 25-1): *(1) cimetidine (Tagamet), (2) ranitidine (Zantac), (3) famotidine (Pepcid)*, and *(4) nizatadine (Axid)*. None of these agents have an indication for the prevention of re-bleeding secondary to PUD, and therefore, their efficacy is limited in PUD. H2RAs have been used for the past several decades and they have a long track record for safety. They are available in both oral and parenteral forms (Levine et al, 2002). With continued usage H2RAs result in *tachyphylaxis*, with diminished efficacy over time. With IV treatment this generally occurs after approximately *24 hours of use*. To date, there are no controlled studies that have shown efficacy for their use in the prevention of PUD re-bleeding. This is probably accounted for by the tachyphylaxis, which occurs with continued usage. Another limiting factor with the use of the H2RAs in the prevention of re-bleeding following ulcer hemostasis is their inability to raise the intragastric pH above a threshold level of approximately 6 (Pisegna, 2002).

Unlike the H2RAs, PPIs as a group have a different mechanism of action, which permits a greater amount of inactivation of parietal cell secretory function. PPIs have now been used for over two decades and have been used in a multitude of clinical investigations, which have demonstrated their safety and efficacy. PPIs currently approved by the FDA include *(1) omeprazole (Prilosec), (2) lansoprazole (Prevacid), (3) pantoprazole (Protonix), (4) rabeprazole (Aciphex)*, and *(5) esomeprazole (Nexium)*. Each has a similar mechanism of action although they are formulated differently. Only pantoprazole is available in both oral and IV formulations, although clinical studies are underway in the United States for the development of IV lansoprazole and esomeprazole formulations. Pantoprazole has been approved by the FDA for the inpatient management of erosive esophagitis, as well as conditions associated with gastric acid hypersecretion, including ZE syndrome (Metz et al, 2001). Each of these agents can be administered *orally* as slurry by suspending the tablet or capsule with sodium bicarbonate to permit NG infusion. Although this approach may have some merits in the chronic suppression of PUD they have major limitations because of absorption in the acute PUD setting, in which case an IV administration would be a preferable route of administration.

As a group, the PPIs act by inhibiting H^+/K^+-ATPase, the final step in the synthesis of gastric acid. Studies have shown that to achieve the optimal reduction in ulcer rebleeding rate, *the intragastric pH should be suppressed to a pH value ≥ 6 or greater*. Given that PPIs act by blocking the final step in the synthesis of gastric acid they are as a group more effective than H2RAs. *Therefore, they are the preferred method of managing the patient with PUD except perhaps in pregnancy* (Li et al, 2000; Yacyshyn and Thomson, 2000).

In the setting of a patient with upper GI bleeding, the goal of antisecretory therapy is to *increase the intragastric pH above 6* during the period preceding and following endoscopic hemostasis. The rationale for achieving this intragastric pH is to improve platelet function and the coagulation cascade to stabilize the clot formation (Barkun et al, 1999). This is facilitated with the development of IV formulations of PPIs, such as pantoprazole, omeprazole, and lansoprazole. The use of IV PPIs reduces the rate of ulcer rebleeding (Lau et al, 2000). The dose of IV *omeprazole (Prilosec)* that was shown to effectively reduce rebleeding was an 80 mg loading dose followed by a continual infusion of 8 mg/h (Lau et al, 2000). Furthermore, the use of IV PPIs in the setting of acute PUD bleeding was shown to be cost effective for the more serious ulcer bleeds (Spiegel et al, 2003). In another study, IV *pantoprazole*

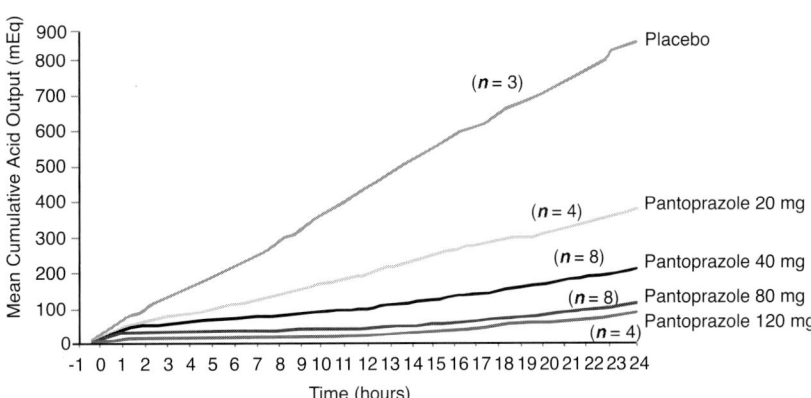

FIGURE 25-3. Dose-dependent inhibition of gastric acid secretion.

(Protonix) was able to dose-dependently (Figure 25-3) inhibit gastric acid secretion in a pentagastrin-stimulated model of ZE syndrome as well as in a cohort of ZE syndrome patients. The optimal dose of pantoprazole in each study was 80 mg administered twice daily. Gastric acid was inhibited rapidly (ie, within 1 hour) and the duration of effect was nearly 20 hours.*

Supplemental Reading

Agrawal NM, Campbell DR, Safdi MA, et al. Superiority of lansoprazole versus ranitidine in healing nonsteroidal antiinflammatory drug-associated gastric ulcers: results of a double-blind, randomized, multicenter study. NSAID-Associated Gastric Ulcer Study Group. Arch Intern Med 2000;160:1455–61.

Barkun AN, Cockeram AW, Plourde V, Fedorak RN. Review article: acid suppression in non-variceal acute upper gastrointestinal bleeding. Aliment Pharmacol Ther 1999;13:1565–84.

Chernow B, Soldano S, Cook D, et al. Positive end-expiratory pressure increases plasma catecholamine levels in non-volume loaded dogs. Anaesth Intensive Care 1986;14:421–5.

Chung SS, Lau JY, Sung JJ, et al. Randomized comparison between adrenaline injection alone and adrenaline injection plus heat probe treatment for actively bleeding ulcers. BMJ 1997;314:1307–11.

Cook DJ, Fuller HD, Guyatt GH, et al. Risk factors for gastrointestinal bleeding in critically ill patients. Canadian Critical Care Trials Group. N Engl J Med 1994;330:377–81.

Cryer B, Lee E, Feldman M. Factors influencing gastroduodenal mucosal prostagalandin concentrations: roles of smoking and aging. Ann Intern Med 1992;116:636–40.

Diebel L, Kozol R, Wilson RF, et al. Gastric intramucosal acidosis in patients with chronic kidney failure. Surgery 1993;113:520–6.

Dubois A. Control of gastric acid secretion. In: Brandt LJ, editor. Clinical practice of gastroenterology. Philadelphia: Current Medicine, Inc; 1999. p. 180–8.

El-Serag HB, Sonnenberg A. Opposing time trends of peptic ulcer and reflux disease. Gut 1998;43:327–33.

Feldman M. Gastric secretion: normal and abnormal. In: Feldman M, Scharschmidt BF, Sleisenger MH, editors. Gastrointestinal and liver disease. Philadelphia: WB Saunders Company; 1998. p. 587–603.

Green FW Jr, Kaplan MM, Curtis LE, Levine PH. Effect of acid and pepsin on blood coagulation and platelet aggregation: a possible contributor to prolonged gastroduodenal mucosal hemorrhage. Gastroenterology 1978;74:38–43.

Konturek SJ. Prostaglandins in pathophysiology of peptic ulcer disease. Dig Dis Sci 1985;30(11 Suppl):105–8S.

Laine L. Approaches to nonsteroidal anti-inflammatory drug use in the high-risk patient. Gastroenterology 2001;120:594–606.

Laine L, Estrada R. Randomized trial of normal saline solution injection versus bipolar electrocoagulation for treatment of patients with high-risk bleeding ulcers: is local tamponade enough? Gastrointest Endosc 2002;55:6–10.

Lanas A, Remacha B, Sainz R, Hirschowitz BI. Study of outcome after targeted intervention for peptic ulcer resistant to acid suppression therapy. Am J Gastroenterol 2000;95:513–9.

Langman MJ, Brooks P, Hawkey CJ, et al. Nonsteroidal antiinflammatory drug associated ulcer: epidemiology, causation, and treatment. J Gastroenterol Hepatol 1991;6:442–9.

Lau JY, Sung JJ, Lee KK, et al. Effect of intravenous omeprazole on recurrent bleeding after endoscopic treatment of bleeding peptic ulcers. N Engl J Med 2000;343:310–6.

Levine JE, Leontiadis GI, Sharma VK, Howdens CW. Meta-analysis: the efficacy of intravenous H2-receptor antagonists in bleeding peptic ulcer. Aliment Pharmacol Ther 2002;16:1137–42.

Lew EA, Pisegna JR, Starr JA, et al. Intravenous pantoprazole rapidly controls gastric acid hypersecretion in patients with Zollinger-Ellison Syndrome. Gastroenterology 2000;118:696–704.

Lewis JD, Shin EJ, Metz DC. Characterization of gastrointestinal bleeding in severely ill hospitalized patients. Crit Care Med 2000;28:46–50.

Li Y, Sha W, Nie Y, et al. Effect of intragastric pH on control of peptic ulcer bleeding. J Gastroenterol Hepatol 2000;15:148–54.

Malledant Y, Tanguy M, Saint-Marc C. Digestive stress hemorrhage. physiopathology and prevention. Ann Fr Anesth Reanim 1989;8:334–46.

Merki HS, Wilder-Smith CH. Do continuous infusions of omeprazole and ranitidine retain their effect with prolonged dosing? Gastroenterology 1994;106:60–4.

Metz DC, Ferron GM, Paul J, et al. Proton pump activation in stimulated parietal cells is regulated by gastric acid secretory capacity: a human study. J Clin Pharmacol 2002;42:512–9.

Metz DC, Forsmark C, Lew EA, et al. Replacement of oral proton pump inhibitors with intravenous pantoprazole to effectively control gastric acid hypersecretion in patients with Zollinger-Ellison syndrome. Am J Gastroenterol 2001;96:3274–80.

Million M, Grigoriadis DE, Sullivan S, et al. A novel water-soluble selective CRF 1receptor antagonist, NBI 35965, blunts stress-induced visceral hypersensitivity and colonic motor function in rats. Brain Research 2003;985:32–42.

Munnangi S, Sonnenberg A. Time trends of physician visits and treatment patters of peptic ulcer disease in the United States Arch. Int Med 1997;157:1489–94.

Mutlu GM, Mutlu EA, Factor P. GI complications in patients receiving mechanical ventilation. Chest 2001;119:1222–41.

O'Laughlin JC, Silvoso GK, Ivey KJ. Resistance to medical therapy of gastric ulcers in rheumatic disease patients taking aspirin: a double blind study with cimetidine and follow-up. Dig Dis Sci 1982;27:976–80.

Oh DS, Pisegna JR. Pharmacologic treatment of upper gastrointestinal bleeding. Curr Treat Options Gastroenterol 2003;6:157–62.

Pisegna JR. Chapter 41: Zollinger-Ellison Syndrome and other hypersecretory states. In: Feldman M, Friedman LS, Sleisenger MH, editors. Sleisenger & Fordtran's gastrointestinal and liver disease: pathophysiology/diagnosis/management. 7th ed. Philadelphia: Saunders; 2002.

Pisegna JR. New ideas about managing gastrointestinal haemostatic complications in surgical patients. Surg Rounds 2002;25(Suppl):19.

---

*Editor's Note: A complete 49-item bibliography can be obtained at <jpisegna@ucla.edu>.

Pisegna JR. Pharmacology of acid suppression in the hospital setting: focus on proton pump inhibition. Crit Care Med 2002;30(6 Suppl):S356–61.

Pisegna JR, Martin P, McKeand WM, et al. Inhibition of pentagastrin-induced gastric acid secretion by intravenous pantoprazole: a dose response study. Am J Gastroenterol 1999;94:2874–80.

Pisegna JR, Sawicki M. Chapter 70: multiple endocrine neoplasias. In: Haskell CM, editor. Cancer treatment. 5th ed. New York: WB Saunders Co; 1998.

Ritchie WP Jr. Acute gastric mucosal damage induced by bile salts, acid, and ischemia. Gastroenterology 1975;68:699–707.

Ruigomez A, Garcia Rodriguez LA, Cattaruzzi C, et al. Use of cimetidine, omeprazole, and ranitidine in pregnant women and pregnancy outcomes. Am J Epidemiol 1999;150:476–81.

Sarosiek J, Jensen RT, Maton PM, et al. Salivary and gastric epidermal growth factor in patients with Zollinger-Ellison syndrome: its protective potential. Am J Gastroenterol 2000;95:1158–66.

Silen W. The prevention and management of stress ulcers. Hosp Pract 1980;15:93–100.

Spiegel BM, Ofman JJ, Woods K, Vakil NB. Minimizing recurrent peptic ulcer hemorrhage after endoscopic hemostasis: the cost-effectiveness of competing strategies. Am J Gastroenterol 2003;98:86–97.

Stern AI, Hogan DL, Isenberg JI. A new method for quantitation of ion fluxes across in vivo human gastric mucosa: effect of aspirin, acetaminophen, ethanol and hyperosmolar solutions. Gastroenterology 1984;86:60–70.

Tremblay L, Valenza F, Ribeiro SP, et al. Injurious ventilatory strategies increase cytokines and c-fos m-RNA expression in an isolated rat lung model. J Clin Invest 1997;99:944–52.

von Bethmann AN, Brasch F, Nusing R, et al. Hyperventilation induces release of cytokines from perfused mouse lung. Am J Respir Crit Care Med 1998;157:263–72.

Walan A, Bader JP, Classen M, et al. Effect of omeprazole and ranitidine on ulcer healing and relapse rates in patients with benign gastric ulcer. N Engl J Med 1989;320:69–75.

Wank SA. PACAP upsets stomach theory. J Clin Invest 1999;104:1341–42.

Wolfe MM, Soll AH. The physiology of gastric acid secretion. N Engl J Med 1988;319:1707–15.

Yacyshyn BR, Thomson AB. Critical review of acid suppression in nonvariceal, acute, and upper gastrointestinal bleeding. Dig Dis 2000;18:117–28.

Yeomans ND, Tulassay Z, Juhasz L, et al. A comparison of omeprazole with ranitidine for ulcers associated with nonsteroidal antiinflammatory drugs. Acid Suppression Trial: Ranitidine Versus Omeprazole for NSAID-Associated Ulcer Treatment (ASTRONAUT) Study Group. N Engl J Med 1998;338:719–26.

Zapata-Sirvent RL, Greenleaf G, Hansbrough JF, Steinsapir E. Burn injury results in decreased gastric acid production in the acute shock period. J Burn Care Rehab 1995;16:622–6.

Zeng T, Athmann C, Kang H, et al. PACAP type I receptor activation regulates ECL cells and gastric acid secretion. J. Clinical Investigation 1999;104:1383–91.

CHAPTER 26

GASTRINOMA

CHANDRA ARE, MD, FRCS, AND CHARLES J. YEO, MD, FACS

Gastrinomas

The incidence of gastrinoma is 0.2 to 1 per million or ≤ 0.1% of all patients with duodenal ulcer disease. The majority of these patients have hepatic or nodal involvement (60%) at the time of presentation. In the absence of hepatic involvement, long term survival is possible. Resection of gastrinoma is associated with a biochemical cure in up to 30% of sporadic forms, whereas the same is difficult to accomplish in MEN I patients. MEN I–related patients have multiple tumors, exhibit different tumor behavior, and are essentially impossible to cure compared to patients with sporadic gastrinomas.

Site

Gastrinomas present either in association with multiple endocrine neoplasia (30%) or sporadically (70%) in the remaining patients. Differences exist between the two types in terms of presentation, associated findings, and the ability to achieve biochemical and clinical cure. *Duodenal gastrinoma* is the most common location for both types, although some series have shown that MEN I is associated with a higher incidence of duodenal primaries. Although *pancreatic adenomas* (of any type) are more common in MEN I, *pancreatic gastrinomas* are more frequent in the sporadic form. Primary duodenal gastrinomas are also known to be a more frequent cause of Zollinger-Ellison (ZE) syndrome than previously thought. They are usually < 1 cm in size (smaller than pancreatic gastrinomas), located predominantly in the proximal portion of the duodenum (80%), and metastasize to regional lymph nodes in two-thirds of the patients.

Clinical Presentation

Certain clinical scenarios should arouse the suspicion of gastrinoma. They include *multiple peptic ulcers, persistence or recurrence of ulcer disease* despite adequate medical or surgical treatment, ulcers in *unusual locations* (such as beyond the first portion of the duodenum), and younger age at presentation. Patients with persistent *diarrhea and ulcer disease, spontaneous jejunal perforation*, or *severe esophagitis*, also need to be investigated to rule out gastrinoma. Patients with *multiple endocrine neoplasia* can present with ulcer disease in conjunction with hypercalcemia or nephrolithiasis. One-third of patients with MEN I–related gastrinoma may have no evidence of other endocrinopathy. Thus, even patients with "sporadic" gastrinoma should undergo periodic screening to rule out MEN I, and be considered for genetic testing.

Duodenal gastrinomas usually tend to be smaller than pancreatic gastrinomas; 80% of duodenal gastrinomas are < 1 cm in size compared to pancreatic gastrinomas, which are usually > 3 cm in size. Gastrinomas frequently metastasize to regional lymph nodes and the liver. Lymph node metastases are seen in > 50 % of patients in both groups, whereas liver metastases are more frequently seen in pancreatic (32 to 54%) than in duodenal gastrinomas (5 to 14%). Pancreatic gastrinomas tend to be more aggressive and are associated with a worse prognosis than duodenal gastrinomas (10 year survival of 50% versus 94%). Metastasis to the liver seems to be related to the size of the primary lesion. Lesions located to the left side of the superior mesenteric artery in the pancreas tend to be larger in size.

It appears that there may be two forms of gastrinoma, *aggressive* and *nonaggressive types*. The aggressive type is usually present in females, comprises 25% of the cases, is associated with a short disease duration, larger tumors, pancreatic location, a higher incidence of liver metastasis, and a poorer prognosis.

Diagnosis

The majority of patients with gastrinoma will present with symptoms and signs of peptic ulcer disease at some stage. The diagnosis is established based upon a battery of tests. A basal gastric output of > 15 mEq/h (> 5 mEq/h if the patient had any prior acid reducing surgery) is helpful in diagnosis, but gastric acid analysis is a test that is rarely performed. Serum gastrin levels are used to diagnose gastrinoma (Maton, 1994). Fasting serum gastrin levels of > 200 pg/mL (> 100 pg/mL prior to 1994) and an incremental increase by > 200 pg/mL after secretin stimulation is performed to confirm the diagnosis of gastrinoma. After withdrawing all acid inhibiting medications, secretin is injected as a bolus (2 U/kg). Serum gastrin levels are measured at 2, 5, 10, and 20 minutes after injection, and an incremental rise in the gastrin of > 200 pg/mL (95.4 pmol/L) is considered positive. It should also be noted that increased gastrin can be found in conditions other than ZE syndrome (Table 26-1). Use of proton pump inhibitors (PPIs) is the most common of these conditions.

It is not common to perform formal gastric acid analysis today. However, it is important to document that a patient suspected of harboring a gastrinoma makes acid. Thus, at endoscopy, measurement of gastric pH should be performed. A common error in diagnosis is to consider gastrinoma in the differential diagnosis of a patient with dyspeptic symptoms and an elevated serum gastrin, only to discover that the patient is achlorhydric (makes no acid) with a diagnosis of atrophic gastritis or pernicious anemia.

PREOPERATIVE LOCALIZATION

The majority of gastrinomas arise in the duodenum, pancreas, and the peripancreatic lymph nodes. In < 5% of the patients, they can be found in unusual locations such as the heart, kidney, liver, bile ducts, lung, mesentery, or bone. The modalities available to detect gastrinomas preoperatively are *ultrasonography* (US) (*transabdominal and endoscopic*), *computed tomography* (*CT*) *scan, magnetic resonance imaging* (*MRI*) *scan, portal venous sampling* (rarely done), *secretin angiography*, and *somatostatin receptor scintigraphy* (SRS) (Modlin et al, 2000) (Table 26-2). Using a combination of CT, angiography and portal venous hormone sampling (Yeo, 2000; Cho and Mittleman, 2000), > 90% of pancreatic islet cell tumors can be localized preoperatively (Y. CT, US, and MRI can help localize gastrinomas preoperatively

TABLE 26-1. Differential Diagnosis of Hypergastrinemia

Increased Gastrin, Increased Acid	Increased Gastrin, Normal to Reduced Acid
Zollinger-Ellison syndrome	Proton pump inhibitor
Retained excluded antrum	Atrophic gastritis
Antral G cell hyperplasia	Perinicous anemia
Gastric outlet obstruction	Postvagotomy state
	Renal failure
	Short gut syndrome

TABLE 26-2. Diagnostic Modalities to Localize Gastrinoma

Modality	Sensitivity
Abdominal ultrasonography	20 to 30%
Endoscopic ultrasonography	80 to 85%
Intraoperative ultrasonography	90%
CT scan	50 to 60%
MRI	25 to 40%
Somatostatin receptor scintigraphy	90%
Portal venous sampling (rarely performed)	70 to 90%

CT = computed tomography; MRI = magnetic resonance imaging.

in 60%, 25%, and 20% of patients, respectively (Zogakis et al, 2003). Nearly all gastrinomas overexpress somatostatin receptor subtypes 2 and 5, and, therefore, most have an affinity for *radiolabelled somatostatin analogues*. SRS can therefore be used to locate the *primary lesion*, as well as any *metastases*, if present. In addition, SRS can help *locate* gastrinomas present at unusual locations. Single photon emission computed tomography (*SPECT*) *imaging* is used with SRS to help identify the lesions and to differentiate them from nearby organs. SRS is most sensitive in detecting metastases related to gastrinoma. Unfortunately, SRS can *miss small lesions* (< 1 cm), *cannot delineate* the exact location in areas containing many organs, and does not give an accurate estimate of the size of the lesion. Therefore, *CT scan* and *MRI* are still performed to increase the accuracy of preoperative localization.

SRS

Nonetheless, the most accurate method of preoperative localization is SRS, which has a sensitivity based on size (< 1 cm: 30%, 1 to 2 cm: 64%, and > 2 cm: 96%). SRS can also help detect metastatic disease in liver, lung, or bone, the presence of which will affect operative decision making. In one study, SRS was helpful in detecting hepatic metastases in 54% of patients that were not detected by other means (Yeo, 1994). Combining SRS and endoscopic US (EUS) has been shown to increase the overall sensitivity.

EUS

Recently, preoperative EUS has been used to help localize the lesion. EUS can help localize the lesion to a particular organ and can be linked to fine needle aspiration to achieve a tissue diagnosis. In skilled hands EUS has a better sensitivity than MRI, CT, or US. EUS has a high sensitivity in localizing lesions in the pancreas, in comparison to a lesion located in the duodenum or other areas. Unfortunately, the sensitivity of EUS is operator dependent, and it often does not provide accurate information about the presence of gastrinoma in unusual locations or widespread metastatic disease.

Management

One algorithm for management of gastrinoma is outlined in Figure 26-1. Once the diagnosis of gastrinoma is made, therapy with PPIs is initiated to control symptoms. After this, the workup is designed to localize and stage the lesion. If the patient has unresectable disease due to extensive liver metastases, biopsy is performed to obtain a tissue diagnosis and surgery is typically not indicated. If there is no evidence of unresectable disease, abdominal exploration is performed. The results of the preoperative localization studies guide the operative exploration. However, patients

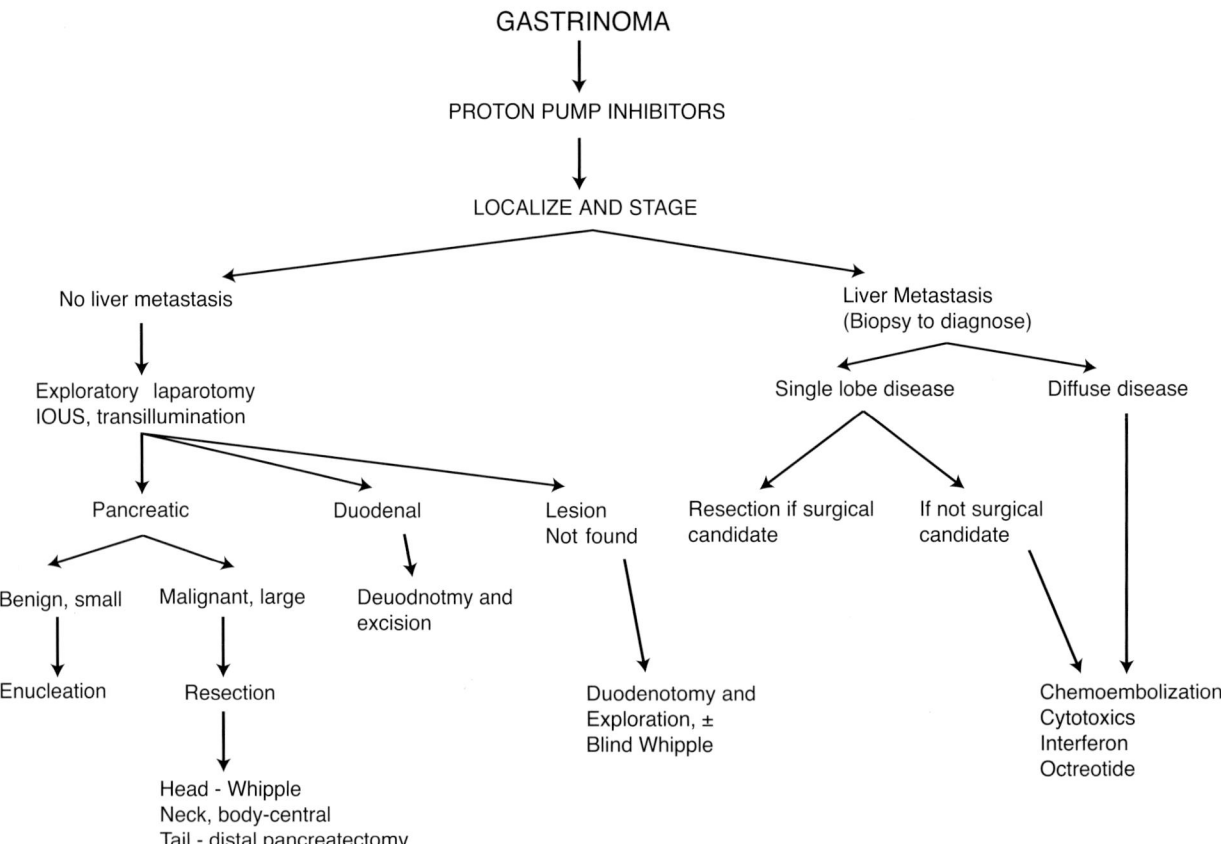

FIGURE 26-1. Algorithm for management of gastrinoma. IOUS = intraoperative ultrasonography.

with biochemically proven sporadic gastrinoma should undergo exploration even if localization tests fail to identify a tumor.

Tumor Removal

The focus of the surgical approach to gastrinomas is to prevent the development of metastatic disease in both types (sporadic and MEN I–related) and to achieve a biochemical cure in patients with sporadic gastrinoma. Even after resection, it is rarely possible to achieve biochemical cure in patients with MEN I. In patients with MEN I, the hypercalcemia is initially dealt with using parathyroidectomy, followed by surgery for gastrinoma. Following parathyroidectomy, a decrease in basal and postsecretin stimulation gastrin levels is noted. Even when a curative resection is not possible for MEN I–associated gastrinoma, a debulking procedure can be considered. Debulking reduces the hormone producing cell mass and improves symptoms, enables more predictable medical management, and decreases tumor mass for cytotoxic therapy. Although controversial, one typical option involves enucleation of duodenal lesions and partial pancreatectomy or pancreatic enucleation. Some recommend this approach only if preoperative localization tests identify a lesion ≥ 2 to 3 cm in size.

The treatment of ZE syndrome due to sporadic gastrinoma in the era of 1950 to 1980 often consisted of palliative gastrectomy to prevent life threatening bleeding and other complications of intractable peptic ulcer disease. Currently, PPIs can control acid related problems in almost all patients and therefore there is virtually no role for palliative surgery. Surgical intervention now consists of locating and excising the primary tumor with lymph node dissection and resection of metastases, if present. Ten-year disease-free survival and eugastrinemia can be obtained in about one-third of patients with sporadic gastrinoma.

Abdominal Exploration

Although preoperative studies have helped in tumor localization, the technique of abdominal exploration for gastrinoma is standardized. A generous Kocher maneuver is performed, to allow proper bimanual palpation of the duodenum and the pancreatic head. Complete palpation of the body and tail of pancreas requires entering the lesser sac and may include medial mobilization of the spleen and tail of the pancreas. Thorough palpation should be combined with intraoperative ultrasonography (IOUS), with consideration given to transillumination of the duodenum and a duodenotomy. IOUS can help detect pancreatic lesions that are not palpable and also detect previously undetected liver metastases. Seventy to 90% of gastrinomas are found in the gastrinoma triangle. This lies to the right of the superior mesenteric artery and therefore more attention should be focused on this area (the head of pancreas and duodenum). The gastrinoma triangle is bound by the junction of the cystic and common hepatic duct superiorly, the junction of the second and third portions of the duodenum inferiorly, and the junction of the neck and body of the pancreas medially.

Duodenal gastrinomas are found in decreasing order of frequency from the first (71%) to the second (21%) to the third portion (8%). Accurate preoperative or intraoperative localization helps in deciding the location and extent of duodenotomy. In the absence of preoperative localization, IOUS and intraoperative endoscopy with transillumination can help decide the location of duodenotomy. If all measures fail, a generous laterally-placed duodenotomy in the second portion of the duodenum is performed. Lesions on the lateral duodenal wall are excised with full-thickness 2 to 3 mm margins, whereas lesions on the medial wall are excised submucosally.

Pancreatic head gastrinomas can often be treated with enucleation. Pancreaticoduodenectomy may be required when enucleation or local resection is not possible (Udelsman et al, 1993; Phan et al, 1997; Phan et al, 1998). Distal pancreatic lesions can be treated with enucleation or distal pancreatic resection. For lesions in the neck of the pancreas, enucleation or central pancreatectomy are performed.

Unresectable Metastic Gastrinoma

Patients with *unresectable metastatic gastrinoma* can be treated via various methods, including (1) chemotherapy (cytotoxics), (2) hormonal therapy with octreotide, (3) hepatic artery embolization, (4) chemoembolization, or (5) interferon. The overall response rate with multiple drug regimens such as 5-*fluorouracil*, *doxorubicin* and *streptozocin* is < 50%. Hormonal therapy with *octreotide* has been reported to ameliorate symptoms due to hypergastrinemia. As most of the symptoms can now be controlled with *PPIs*, the role of octreotide is questionable. Hepatic artery embolization or chemoembolization for unresectable liver metastases may help with the symptoms by reducing tumor load. This is due to the fact that these lesions are hypervascular and derive most of their blood supply from hepatic artery radicles. *Interferon* has been used with biochemical response rates of 40% and tumor reduction by up to 10%. Interferon functions by reducing tumor peptide production and as an antitumor agent. None of these therapies appear to be associated with reproducible survival benefits, although no large studies have investigated this issue.

Prognosis

Long term biochemical cure is difficult or impossible to achieve in patients with MEN I–associated gastrinoma. Almost all patients with MEN I will have recurrent disease and 10-year biochemical cures rarely occur. In contrast, 50% and 35% of sporadic gastrinoma patients undergoing surgical resection may be disease free at 5- and 10-year follow-up, respectively. Up to 93% of patients with MEN I–gastrinoma are alive 15 years after diagnosis, provided appropriate medical therapy is maintained. This, combined with the difficulty in achieving biochemical cure in MEN I has led some to conclude that aggressive surgical management should be reserved for the sporadic form.

Controversies Associated with Surgical Treatment of Gastrinomas

Surgery or Not?

Surgical treatment of gastrinoma depends on whether the lesion is sporadic or a part of the MEN I syndrome. Several studies have shown that the long-term cure rates after surgery for patients with gastrinoma associated with MEN I are very low (< 10%) (Table 26-3). Most authorities currently recommend that surgery not be performed for lesions < 2 to 2.5 cm in patients with gastrinoma and MEN I. Lesions > 2.5 cm are to be excised, as they are associated with a higher risk of liver metastases. Surgery in this group is performed not for biochemical cure, but for prevention of disease progression.

In contrast, sporadic gastrinoma is associated with postoperative eugastrinemia rates of 60% (immediate postoperative), 50% (5 years), and 35% (10 years). In addition, exploration for sporadic gastrinoma identifies the lesion in almost 90% of the patients, even if the preoperative localization studies fail. Therefore, routine surgical exploration is recommended for all patients with sporadic gastrinoma, except for those patients with clearly unresectable metastatic disease.

TABLE 26-3. Cure Rates for MEN 1 Gastrinoma

Study	Number of Patients	Cure Rate (%)
Farley (1992)	15	0
Melvin (1993)	18	5
Norton (1999)	28	6
Norton (2001)	48	0

Routine Removal of Lymph Nodes

Although rare, lymph node primary gastrinomas do exist and some patients are cured by lymph node excision only. As a part of most operations for gastrinoma, lymph nodes in the peripancreatic and periduodenal regions are excised, even if they are benign in appearance.

Role of Parietal Cell Vagotomy

Between 60 and 70% of patients undergoing exploration for sporadic gastrinoma continue to require acid reducing medications after surgery. Because of the expense of long-term PPI use and the risk of noncompliance, parietal cell vagotomy should be considered at the time of exploratory surgery, particularly if the primary lesion is not resected, or if dissemination is identified.

Summary

Gastrinomas are rare tumors and can occur sporadically or in association with the MEN I syndrome. Patients with the sporadic form are more likely to be cured by surgical resection. Due to the low cure rates with MEN I, only select patients with MEN I are typically subjected to surgery. Long-term survival is common in the absence of metastatic disease in both the sporadic and MEN I forms of gastrinoma. The most important prognostic factor is the presence of liver metastases, which adversely affect survival. PPIs can reduce acid production and greatly reduce complications related to the overproduction of acid.

Supplemental Reading

Cho K, Mittleman M. Portal vein sampling. In: Savader, Trerotola, editors. Venous interventional radiology with clinical perspectives, 2nd ed. New York: Thieme Medical Publishers; 2000. p. 569–80.

Maton P. Zollinger-Ellison syndrome. In: Bayless TM, editor. Current therapy in gastroenterology and liver disease. 4th ed. St. Louis: Mosby; 1994. p.127–31.

Modlin IM, Schmid SW, Tang LH, et al. Endocrine tumors of the pancreas. In: Dervenis C, Bassi C, editors. Pancreatic tumors: achievement and prospective. Stuttgart: Thieme-Verlag; 2000. p. 332–54.

Phan GQ, Yeo CJ, Cameron JL, et al. Pancreaticoduodenectomy for selected periampullary neuroendocrine tumors: fifty patients. Surgery 1997;122:989–97.

Phan GQ, Yeo CJ, Hruban RH, et al. Surgical experience with pancreatic and peripancreatic neuroendocrine tumors: review of 125 patients. J Gastrointest Surg 1998;2:473–82.

Udelsman R, Yeo CJ, Hruban RH, et al. Pancreaticoduodenectomy for selected pancreatic endocrine tumors. Surg Gynecol Obstet 1993:177:269–78.

Yeo CJ. A surgeon's perspective on portal venous sampling (and selective arterial provocative testing) for islet cell tumors. In: Savader, Trerotola, editors. Venous interventional radiology with clinical perspectives, 2nd ed. New York: Thieme Medical Publishers; 2000. p. 581–90.

Yeo CJ. Endocrine tumors of the pancreas. In: Bayless TM, editor. Current therapy in gastroenterology and liver disease. 4th ed. St. Louis: Mosby; 1994. p. 664–70.

Zogakis T, Gibril F, Libutti S, et al. Management and outcome of patients with sporadic gastrinoma arising in the duodenum. Ann Surg 2003;238:42–8.

Chapter 27

Management of Stress-Related Erosive Syndrome

Jaime A. Oviedo, MD and M. Michael Wolfe, MD

The clinical features of stress-related erosive syndrome (SRES) have been well characterized since the initial endoscopic description by Lucas and colleagues in 1971 (Lucas et al, 1971). Stress-related lesions in the stomach and duodenum can be detected endoscopically within several hours of a critical illness, trauma, or surgery as multiple punctate subepithelial hemorrhages, erosions, or superficial ulcerations (Schuman et al, 1987). Mucosal injury may be identified in 70 to 100% of critically ill patients admitted to an intensive care unit (ICU), and the risk of developing these lesions appears to be directly correlated with the severity of the underlying illness (Schuster et al, 1984). The presence of endoscopic mucosal damage does not necessarily imply that clinically significant SRES hemorrhage will ensue, however, when documented, the presence of diffuse shallow mucosal injury is the landmark feature in the diagnosis SRES.

Many terms have been used to describe this entity, including *stress ulcer syndrome, stress gastritis, stress-related mucosal disease,* and *stress related syndrome* (Goldin and Peura, 1996). The principal feature of SRES is its relationship to serious systemic disease, such as *sepsis, massive burn injury, head injury associated with increased intracranial pressure, severe trauma,* and *multiple system organ failure.*

Epidemiology

The incidence of overt SRES hemorrhage appears to be declining (Ben-Menachem et al, 1996). This decrease is likely due to significant advances in the ICU monitoring and support of the critically ill patient, including optimization of hemodynamic status, tissue oxygenation, and treatment of sepsis. Estimates of the incidence of SRES are also affected by the criteria used to define the problem. The definition may incorporate clinical or endoscopic criteria or be a combination of both. When microscopic blood loss is adopted as the sole clinical criterion, SRES occurs in virtually 100% of ICU patients (Maier et al, 1994). *SRES-related overt hemorrhage* is defined as hematemesis, bloody gastric aspirate, melena, or hematochezia. *Clinically significant SRES hemorrhage* is, in turn, defined as overt hemorrhage in combination with either orthostatic changes in pulse and blood pressure, a 2 g/dL drop in hemoglobin or 2 unit blood transfusion requirement within a 24-hour period. When this definition is adopted, SRES-related hemorrhage occurs in *up to 30% of ICU patients.*

Once bleeding of any etiology occurs in the ICU, mortality rates increase five fold (Cook et al, 1999). Overt gastrointestinal (GI) bleeding from SRES is felt to contribute to or cause death in up to *30 to 80% of critically ill patients,* in contrast to the 10 to 25% mortality rate in ICU patients without GI hemorrhage. The vast majority of these deaths are not directly attributable to the upper GI hemorrhage itself, but rather reflect the nature and severity of the underlying illness.

Pathophysiology

Although the pathophysiology of SRES is not fully understood, gastric acid and pepsin appear to play a dominant role in the development of the gastroduodenal lesions characteristic of this entity. Both increased stress and head injury are associated with increased gastrin-mediated acid production (Beejay and Wolfe, 2000). As with other acid-related disorders, SRES appears to result from an imbalance between aggressive and defensive factors. Normal mechanisms of gastric mucosal integrity depend on an intact microcirculation, which ensures an adequate supply of nutrients to the mucosa and, in conjunction with the mucous layer, neutralizes hydrogen ions and other locally noxious agents. Mucosal ischemia appears to be the critical factor in the pathogenesis of SRES. Critical illness is commonly associated with hypovolemia, the release of pro-inflammatory cytokines, and increased catecholamines production, which in turn lead to *splanchnic hypoperfusion* (Fisher et al, 1995). Reductions in mucosal blood flow promote intracellular acidosis, the release of nitric oxide, the production of oxygen-derived free radicals, increased cell permeability, a decrease in the synthesis of prostaglandins, and diminished acid buffering capacity. In addition, *mucosal ischemia* leads to decreased mucus and bicarbonate secretion and defects in epithelial cell restitution after injury, all of which contribute to the back-diffusion of hydrogen ions into the gastroduodenal mucosa. *Back-diffusion of acid* is thought to play a central role in the disruption of the surface epithelial barrier, which may later progress to erosive lesions resulting in clinically significant hemorrhage. Small amounts of luminal acid may be sufficient to induce gastroduodenal damage, and SRES can occur even when gastric acid secretion is diminished.

Risk Factors

Most patients in an ICU are at risk for SRES, and those most susceptible to gastroduodenal mucosal injury are patients with severe systemic disease. *Mechanical ventilation for at least 48 hours* and *coagulopathy* (platelet count of < 50,000, a partial thromboplastin time of more than twice that of control subjects, or an International Normalized Ratio of prothrombin time of > 1.5) have been identified as the two single most important risk factors (Cook et al, 1994). Other risk factors include *shock, sepsis, multiple or severe trauma, extensive burns* (greater than 35% of body surface area), *central nervous system (CNS) lesions* (ie, intracranial hypertension), *renal failure, liver dysfunction, multiple system organ failure, aspiration pneumonia, postsurgical states, acute coronary syndromes*, and *length of ICU stay* (Cook et al, 1999). The probability of SRES hemorrhage clearly increases proportionally to the number of risk factors present.

Natural History

Although most individuals with stress-related mucosal injury remain asymptomatic, *10 to 20%* of those who do *not* receive prophylactic therapy experience *GI bleeding* of an occult or overt nature. The lesions of SRES differ from those of "classic" peptic ulcers in that they tend to be shallower and more diffuse in location. The initial lesions are almost invariably found in the acid secreting areas of the stomach, the fundus and the body, and occur *within hours of systemic insult*. The lesions consist of multiple, shallow, punctate, subepithelial defects, usually associated with little or no surrounding inflammatory reaction, which tend to ooze rather than bleed massively. If risk factors persist or worsen, the erosions and subepithelial petechial hemorrhages may worsen both in depth and extent, so that extensive *ulceration* can occur in extended areas of the upper GI tract (distal esophagus, gastric antrum, and duodenum) approximately 4 to 5 days after the initial injury. In a small proportion of cases, penetration into the muscularis mucosa and perforation has been described. Both *profound hypoperfusion* and *sepsis* result in deeper SRES lesions, which tend to bleed profusely. Despite approximately 50% of early mucosal lesions having endoscopic evidence of recent or ongoing hemorrhage, the bleeding in these circumstances is typically self-limited, and the majority of patients do well once the underlying illness is resolved.

Therapy

General Measures

As stated above, the risk of overt GI hemorrhage and subsequent death due to SRES are closely related to the underlying disease. Therapy must therefore be directed at treating the cause of physiologic stress. Hypovolemia and shock should be corrected with adequate and aggressive volume resuscitation. Sepsis must be treated aggressively with appropriate antimicrobial therapy, metabolic abnormalities corrected, ventilatory support optimized, and adequate nutrition instituted. Specific medical therapy emphasizes pharmacologic prophylaxis rather than treatment of active bleeding. Interventional therapy encompasses endoscopic, angiographic, and surgical approaches to control overt and clinically significant SRES-related hemorrhage.

Prophylactic Therapy

Although prophylactic therapy has dramatically *reduced* the *incidence* of bleeding in SRES, a *reduction in mortality* due to bleeding *has not been demonstrated*. The inhibition of gastric acid secretion with H_2 receptor antagonists (H_2RAs) or proton pump inhibitors (PPIs) is the method used most extensively. The rationale for this approach stems from in vitro studies where an increase of intragastric pH to 3.5 to 4.0 is associated with decreased conversion of pepsinogen to pepsin and reduced proteolytic activity in the stomach. Moreover, when intragastric pH approaches 7.0, pepsinogen is irreversibly denatured and clotting factors become operable, enabling activation of the coagulation cascade. Finally, platelet aggregation, which occurs only at a pH > 5.9, also contributes to successful hemostasis and prevention of bleeding due to SRES. Although it has been postulated that optimal prophylaxis would require maintenance of intragastric pH at 7.0 or higher, most studies have demonstrated that an *intragastric pH > 3.5 to 4.0 is associated with a reduction of gastroduodenal hemorrhage* (Wolfe and Sachs, 2000).

Other approaches used to prevent GI bleeding due to SRES include the neutralization of gastric acid with antacids, the use of mucosal protective agents such as sucralfate or prostaglandins, and nonpharmacologic measures, such as the administration of enteral nutrition.

ANTACIDS

Antacids effectively neutralize intraluminal gastric acid and inhibit pepsin activity by increasing gastric pH. Antacids significantly reduce the frequency of overt and clinically significant GI bleeding from SRES by 15 to 20%. The goal of acid neutralization therapy is to *increase the intragastric pH to ≥ 4* to inhibit the conversion of pepsinogen to active pepsin and thereby reduce proteolytic activity.

The administration of antacids in the ICU requires close *monitoring of intragastric pH* and *individual titration* to maintain the *pH > 4*. *Gastric residual* should also be assessed to avoid the possibility of distention and subsequent tracheopulmonary aspiration. Antacids may also impair the systemic absorption of drugs, including antibiotics. Other shortcomings of antacids include the increased incidence of diarrhea caused by the high magnesium concentration found in many antacid preparations, the need for frequent administration (every 1 to 2 hours) usually via nasogastric tube, increased nursing time, and elevated cost. Aluminum-based antacids may cause hypophosphatemia, constipation, and metabolic alkalosis, as well as potentially toxic plasma aluminum levels in patients with renal insufficiency. Because antacids are cumbersome to administer and the dose required to maintain intragastric pH near 4.0 is significant, these agents are *no longer the drug of choice* for SERS prophylaxis.

Histamine H2RAs

H2RAs inhibit acid secretion by competitively binding to histamine type 2 receptors located on the basolateral membrane of the gastric parietal cell. Numerous placebo-controlled trials have established the efficacy of H2RAs in preventing overt and clinically significant SRES hemorrhage. A meta-analysis of 16 studies, including 2,133 patients, showed no significant difference in efficacy between antacids and H2RAs in the prevention of clinically significant SRES hemorrhage. Moreover, both regimens were shown to be superior to placebo and were tolerated equally well (Shuman et al, 1987). A more recent meta-analysis suggested that H2RAs may be more effective than antacids in SRES (Tryba and Cook, 1997).

Only *cimetidine* (Tagamet) administered as a continuous intravenous (IV) infusion has Food and Drug Administration (FDA) approved labeling for the prevention of bleeding in critically ill patients. Other H2RAs given in equipotent doses appear to provide equivalent prophylactic efficacy. Cimetidine is typically administered intravenously by continuous infusion at doses of 37.5 to 100 mg/h, while ranitidine (Zantac) is dosed at 6.25 to 12.5 mg/h and famotidine (Pepcid) at 1.7 to 2.1 mg/h; all can be administered with or without a loading dose. Although no randomized controlled trials of adequate sample size have compared dosing regimens (intermittent versus continuous IV infusion) or routes (oral versus IV) using clinically significant bleeding as study endpoint, continuous H2RA infusion appears to provide more stable acid suppression than intermittent therapy (Baghaie, 1995). Continuous infusion administration of H2RAs for more than 48 hours has been associated with tolerance and intragastric pH variability, likely due in part to enhanced gastrin-induced histamine production and competition with H2RAs at the H2 receptor (Baghaie, 1995). A randomized controlled study of 1,200 patients requiring mechanical ventilation compared *IV ranitidine* with *sucralfate* in the prevention of upper GI bleeding. The rate of clinically significant bleeding in the ranitidine group was 1.7% compared with 3.8% for the sucralfate group; the difference was statistically significant ($p = .02$) (Cook et al, 1998).

Although H2RAs are considered to be very safe agents, they do possess both class specific and individual side effect profiles. The most prominent class specific effect is *CNS toxicity*, which appears to be *idiosyncratic* rather than dose-related and occurs more frequently in *elderly patients* and usually *within the first 2 weeks* of therapy. Dose adjustments are necessary in individuals with *impaired renal function*. In addition, *cimetidine* and *ranitidine*, unlike famotidine and nizatidine, *inhibit the clearance of drugs* by the cytochrome P450 system and thereby interfere with the clearance of a wide variety of drugs.

Because of their efficacy, excellent safety profile, and ease of administration, *H2RAs are generally preferred over antacids and PPIs* in the *prevention* of SRES-related GI hemorrhage.

PPIs

PPIs are substituted benzimidazoles that work by irreversibly blocking hydrogen/potassium-ATPase (H^+/K^+-ATPase), the enzyme mediating the final common pathway involved in the secretion of acid. The following PPIs are currently available: (1) *omeprazole* (Prilosec), (2) lansoprazole (Prevacid), (3) rabeprazole (Aciphex), (4) pantoprazole (Protonix), and (5) esomeprazole (Nexium). All PPIs are available as oral agents, and pantoprazole (Protonix) as an IV preparation. PPIs are prodrugs, which are normally activated after systemic absorption in the highly acidic milieu of the secretory canaliculus of *activated* parietal cells. Activation occurs principally after a meal, and because patients at risk for the development of SRES are generally fasting, these drugs would be *significantly less effective unless* administered in a manner that maintains a plasma level exceeding that generally achieved by oral dosing (ie, IV) (Wolfe and Sachs, 2000).

Despite a prolonged biological half-life, the plasma half-life of PPIs is short (1 to 2 hours) and, if administered intermittently, several doses would be required to achieve adequate inhibition of H^+/K^+-ATPase. Tolerance to PPIs has not been reported.

The use of PPIs in SRES prophylaxis is controversial. Although a few small studies have suggested a beneficial effect, no large randomized trials have been performed to date to evaluate the benefit of these agents in the prophylaxis of SRES-associated GI bleeding. Difficulties in the oral administration of omeprazole and lansoprazole to mechanically ventilated ICU patients have not been resolved despite the recent development of suspensions that are somewhat effective in keeping gastric pH > 4. Two studies in mechanically ventilated ICU patients suggested that a *simplified omeprazole suspension* might not only prevent clinically significant SRES-related hemorrhage, but is also safe and cost effective (Phillips et al, 1996; Lasky et al, 1998). However, the studies were small, open label, and nonrandomized. Omeprazole and lansoprazole are acid labile prodrugs that have been formulated as *granules* with an enteric coating designed to dissolve at pH 5.5. Thus, with the bicarbonate suspension the protective enteric coating is dissolved.

Although the drug is purportedly protected from the acidic environment in the gastric lumen by the bicarbonate, many other factors may influence acid exposure, including the amount of bicarbonate, as well as the pH and volume of the solution used to flush the suspension through a nasogastric tube. It is thus possible that the PPI released from the granules undergoes acid-catalyzed conversion to the reactive species, a thiophilic sulfenamide, with inactivation of the drug before arrival at its intended target site (Wolfe et al, 2001).

Although IV pantoprazole (Protonix) is currently approved by the FDA only for patients with gastroesophageal reflux disease (GERD) who are unable to receive oral PPIs, this agent has shown to be beneficial in the prevention of recurrent hemorrhage due to ulcers, and is quite likely to be useful for other indications, including SRES prophylaxis. Studies comparing the ability of IV administrations of H2RAs and PPIs to raise and maintain intragastric pH suggest that, although both can raise the pH to > 4, PPIs are much more likely to maintain this pH. Unlike H2RAs, PPIs can elevate and maintain the intragastric pH at > 6, and unlike H2RAs, tolerance does not develop with IV preparations. Preliminary findings from clinical trials conducted within an ICU setting have shown that intermittent administration of IV pantoprazole is as effective in raising intragastric pH on the first day as a continuous infusion of an H2RA. These data suggest that *intermittent or continuous infusion with an IV PPI may be an alternative to high dose continuous infusions of an H2RA*. If continuous IV infusion is used, the recommended dose of pantoprazole is an *80 mg loading dose, followed by an infusion of 8 mg/h* (Wolfe and Sachs, 2000).

Mucosal Protective Agents

Sucralfate

Sucralfate is a basic nonabsorbable aluminum salt of sucrose octasulfate. Despite weak antacid properties, the protective effect of sucralfate is not mediated by acid suppression or neutralization, but by a mucosal protective effect on the gastric mucosa. The mucosal protection afforded by sucralfate is mediated by several mechanisms, including formation of a protective barrier, stimulation of gastric mucosal blood flow, prostaglandin-mediated increase in mucus and bicarbonate secretion, and by the stimulation of a variety of growth factors that have been implicated in ulcer healing.

Despite this theoretical benefit, the role of *sucralfate* in the prophylaxis of clinically significant SRES hemorrhage is *controversial*. Although some studies suggest that sucralfate is an effective prophylactic agent with a benign side effect profile that possibly includes a lower incidence of nosocomial pneumonia, in many of the studies reviewed, sucralfate was not statistically superior to the control group in preventing SRES hemorrhage. In a large study by Cook and colleagues (1998), including 1,200 mechanically ventilated patients, sucralfate was inferior to ranitidine in the prevention of upper GI bleeding, and there was no significant differences in the rates of ventilator-associated pneumonia between the two agents (Cook et al, 1998). Sucralfate (Carafate) is available as tablets or as liquid slurry that is administered 1 g orally or by nasogastric tube every 4 to 6 hours. Although usually well tolerated, constipation occurs in 2 to 4% of patients receiving sucralfate, and aluminum toxicity has occurred in patients with chronic renal failure.

Despite some theoretical advantages of sucralfate, including its ease of use, lack of need for monitoring, lack of need for supplemental antacid therapy, and cost effectiveness, this agent *cannot* be recommended as the drug of choice in SRES because of discordant study results.

Prostaglandin Analogues

Despite the promise demonstrated in earlier trials, synthetic prostaglandin derivatives, such as *misoprostol* (Cytotec) have not been shown to be effective in the prophylaxis of SRES. Synthetic prostaglandin analogues exert a cytoprotective effect at low doses and have been demonstrated to protect the gastric mucosa from a variety of agents. Given the relatively high cost and major side effects associated with their use, it is unlikely that any large scale randomized clinical trial will be performed to investigate the role of prostaglandin analogues in SRES hemorrhage; therefore, the use of these agents in the prophylaxis of SERS *cannot* be recommended.

Enteral Nutrition

Experimentally, enteral nutrition reduces stress ulceration, preserves gastric mucosal integrity by neutralizing acid, and stimulates mucosal blood flow. Early administration of nutrition to patients with multiple traumas may also reduce the occurrence of septic complications and multiple organ dysfunction syndrome. These findings have led to some small, retrospective clinical trials that suggest a clinically meaningful effect from the administration of enteral nutrition (Pingleton and Hadzima, 1983; Raff et al, 1997; Gurman et al, 1990). Enteral feeding was, however, found to be a significant risk factor for bleeding in a multicenter study (Cook et al, 1994). This discrepancy may be due to differences in location of nutrient delivery. Tubes placed in the stomach may alkalinize stomach contents, whereas jejunal-feeding tubes may stimulate gastric acid secretion. Although it is widely believed that nutrition is of value in preventing SRES, *no large scale, randomized clinical trials* have compared enteral nutrition to pharmacologic therapy in SRES. Therefore, enteral nutrition *cannot presently be recommended* as an effective method in the prophylaxis of SRES.

Medical Therapy of Actively Bleeding SRES

Although cessation of active hemorrhage due to SRES with the use of antacids, H2RAs, PPIs, and sucralfate has been reported, large, controlled trials evaluating their true efficacy have not been performed. Case reports suggest the efficacy of prostaglandins, somatostatin, and IV vasopressin, but none of these agents can be regarded as more than investigational at this point.

INTERVENTIONAL THERAPY

More aggressive forms of therapy are indicated when prophylactic therapy fails and clinically significant SRES hemorrhage persists.

Esophagogastroduodenoscopy (EGD) accurately identifies the site of bleeding in over 95% cases of GI hemorrhage, and not only provides prognostic information about the risk of rebleeding, but also offers a therapeutic potential. If single lesions with active bleeding or stigmata of recent hemorrhage are identified, control of hemorrhage by several means, including *mucosal epinephrine injection, thermal coagulation, multipolar electrocoagulation*, and *clipping*, is successful in over 90% of cases. *Angiography with intraarterial embolization* is useful when bleeding persists despite endoscopic treatment.

SRES hemorrhage *ceases spontaneously* in up to 95% of patients treated conservatively, and only *approximately 5%* will experience *massive SRES hemorrhage*. Even among those patients with major hemorrhage, up to 90% will be controlled by a combination of pharmacotherapy, therapeutic EGD, and interventional angiography. *Surgery* is reserved for cases of severe hemorrhage uncontrolled by other modalities.

Complications of SRES

NOSOCOMIAL PNEUMONIA

The increase in gastric pH that follows the use of acid suppression therapy can permit *gram-negative bacterial overgrowth*, which is believed to be associated with an increased risk of nosocomial pneumonia. Unlike antacids and H$_2$RAs, sucralfate does not significantly elevate gastric pH and is accordingly associated with less gastric bacterial overgrowth. Moreover, an antibacterial mode of action for sucralfate has been suggested. A meta-analysis of trials by Cook and colleagues (1996) examined the drug class specific rates of nosocomial pneumonia and concluded that *sucralfate causes significantly less nosocomial pneumonia*. However, the results of various studies evaluating the risk of nosocomial pneumonia are widely inconsistent. This is perhaps explained by differing definitions of pneumonia, small samples evaluated, and lack of blinding. As previously stated, a large study comparing sucralfate and ranitidine for the prevention of SRES-related bleeding in 1,200 patients requiring mechanical ventilation showed no significant differences in the rates of nosocomial pneumonia between the two groups. Taking all these issues into consideration, it appears that the *positive attributes* of H$_2$RAs outweigh the possible *risk* of nosocomial pneumonia associated with their use. *IV administration of* H$_2$RAs (or possibly PPIs) may *obviate the need for a nasogastric tube*, which may also serve as a conduit for migration of bacteria from the stomach to the pharynx. Further outcome studies will be necessary before definite clinical conclusions can be drawn regarding any comparisons of sucralfate with antisecretory therapies.

Summary and Recommendations

SERS prophylaxis is recommended for the following groups: (1) patients with *coagulopathy*, (2) patients requiring *mechanical ventilation for more than 48 hours*, (3) patients with a history of GI *ulceration* or *bleeding within the last year*, and (4) patients with *any two* of the other known *risk factors* (Table 27-1) (Wolfe et al, 2001). Antacids, H$_2$RAs, and sucralfate have all been shown to be effective in *preventing* clinically significant bleeding due to SRES, particularly if the intragastric pH is *maintained > 4*. Although no studies evaluating IV PPIs in the prophylaxis of SRES have been reported, available data suggest that intermittent or continuous IV administration of *pantoprazole* can maintain gastric pH > 4 in the fasting ICU patient at high risk for bleeding, similar to *cimetidine continuous infusion*. Moreover, acid suppression with IV pantoprazole increases over time, whereas the inhibitory effects of H$_2$RAs are reduced by the second day of therapy. Oral administration of PPIs cannot be recommended for SERS prophylaxis due to suboptimal bioavailability and uncertain efficacy of these agents when administered via nasogastric tube to fasting individuals.

Although the drug of choice depends to some extent on local preferences, until well-designed, randomized, controlled trials are performed, *H$_2$RAs by continuous IV infusion may represent the best option. Intermittent IV dosing or continuous infusion* of a *PPI* might be expected not only to adequately inhibit acid secretion, but also to allow a smooth transition to oral PPI therapy, especially in patients who may

TABLE 27-1. Risk Factors for Stress-Related Erosive Syndrome

Respiratory failure requiring mechanical ventilation
Coagulopathy
Hypotension and shock
Sepsis
Multiple or severe trauma
Extensive burns
Severe central nervous system injury
Hepatic failure
Renal failure
Acute coronary syndromes
Multiple system organ failure
Aspiration pneumonia
Postorgan transplant
Major surgery and postsurgical states
Long ICU stay

Adapted from Wolfe et al, 2001.
ICU = intensive care unit.

require chronic maintenance therapy for other acid-related conditions, such as GERD. None of the pharmacologic therapies reviewed is of proven value once hemorrhage begins; however, the *interventional techniques* at our disposal are very effective in controlling acute bleeding.

Supplemental Reading

ASHP Therapeutic Guidelines on Stress Ulcer Prophylaxis. ASHP Commission on Therapeutics and approved by the ASHP Board of Directors on November 14, 1998. Am J Health Syst Pharm 1999;56:347–79.

Baghaie AA, Mojtahedzadeh M, Levine RL, et al. Comparison of the effect of intermittent administration and continuous infusion of famotidine on gastric pH in critically ill patients: results of a prospective, randomized, crossover study. Crit Care Med 1995;23:687–91.

Beejay U, Wolfe MM. Acute gastrointestinal bleeding in the intensive care unit. The gastroenterologist's perspective. Gastroenterol Clin North Am 2000;29:309–36.

Ben-Menachem T, Fogel R, Patel RV, et al. Prophylaxis for stress-related gastric hemorrhage in the medical intensive care unit. A randomized, controlled, single blind study. Ann Intern Med 1994;121:568–75.

Ben-Menachem T, McCarthy BD, Fogel R, et al. Prophylaxis for stress-related gastrointestinal hemorrhage: a cost effectiveness analysis. Crit Care Med 1996;24:338–45.

Cook DJ, Fuller HD, Guyatt GH, et al. Risk factors for gastrointestinal bleeding in critically ill patients. Canadian Critical Care Trials Group. N Engl J Med 1994;330:377–81.

Cook D, Guyatt G, Marshall J, et al. A comparison of sucralfate and ranitidine for the prevention of upper gastrointestinal bleeding in patients requiring mechanical ventilation. Canadian Critical Care Trials Group. N Engl J Med 1998;338:791–7.

Cook D, Heyland D, Griffith L, et al. Risk factors for clinically important upper gastrointestinal bleeding in patients requiring mechanical ventilation. Canadian Critical Care Trials Group. Crit Care Med 1999;27:2812–7.

Cook DJ, Reeve BK, Guyatt GH, et al. Stress ulcer prophylaxis in critically ill patients. Resolving discordant meta-analyses. JAMA 1996;275:308–14.

Czaja AJ, McAlhany JC, Pruitt BA Jr. Acute gastroduodenal disease after thermal injury. An endoscopic evaluation of incidence and natural history. N Engl J Med 1974;291:925–9.

Fisher RL, Pipkin GA, Wood JR. Stress-related mucosal disease. Pathophysiology, prevention, and treatment. Crit Care Clin 1995;11:323–45.

Goldin GF, Peura DA. Stress-related mucosal damage. What to do or not to do. Gastrointest Endosc Clin N Am 1996;6:505–26.

Gurman G, Samri M, Sarov B, et al. The rate of gastrointestinal bleeding in a general ICU population: a retrospective study. Intensive Care Med 1990;16:44–9.

Haglund U. Stress ulcers. Scand J Gastroenterol Suppl 1990; 175:27–33.

Lasky MR, Metzler MH, Phillips JO. A prospective study of omeprazole suspension to prevent clinically significant gastrointestinal bleeding from stress ulcers in mechanically ventilated trauma patients. J Trauma 1998;44:527–33.

Lewis JD, Shin EJ, Metz DC. Characterization of gastrointestinal bleeding in severely ill hospitalized patients. Crit Care Med 2000;28:46–50.

Lucas CE, Sugawa C, Riddle J, et al. Natural history and surgical dilemma of "stress" gastric bleeding. Arch Surg 1971;102:266–73.

Maier RV, Mitchell D, Gentilello L. Optimal therapy for stress gastritis. Ann Surg 1994;220:353–60.

Marrone GC, Silen W. Pathogenesis, diagnosis and treatment of acute gastric mucosal lesions. Clin Gastroenterol 1984;13:635–50.

Navab F, Steingrub J. Stress ulcer: is routine prophylaxis necessary? Am J Gastroenterol 1995;90:708–12.

Phillips JO, Metzler MH, Palmieri MT, et al. A prospective study of simplified omeprazole suspension for the prophylaxis of stress-related mucosal damage. Crit Care Med 1996;24:1793–800.

Pingleton SK, Hadzima SK. Enteral alimentation and gastrointestinal bleeding in mechanically ventilated patients. Crit Care Med 1983;11:13–6.

Raff T, Germann G, Hartmann B. The value of early enteral nutrition in the prophylaxis of stress ulceration in the severely burned patient. Burns 1997;23:313–8.

Schuster DP, Rowley H, Feinstein S, et al. Prospective evaluation of the risk of upper gastrointestinal bleeding after admission to a medical intensive care unit. Am J Med 1984;76:623–30.

Shuman RB, Schuster DP, Zuckerman GR. Prophylactic therapy for stress ulcer bleeding: a reappraisal. Ann Intern Med 1987;106:562–7.

Tryba M. Sucralfate versus antacids or H2-antagonists for stress ulcer prophylaxis: a meta-analysis on efficacy and pneumonia rate. Crit Care Med 1991;19:942–9.

Tryba M, Cook D. Current guidelines on stress ulcer prophylaxis. Drugs 1997;54:581–96.

Wolfe MM, Sachs G. Acid suppression: optimizing therapy for gastroduodenal ulcer healing, gastroesophageal reflux disease, and stress-related erosive syndrome. Gastroenterology 2000;118(2 Suppl 1):S9–31.

Wolfe MM, Welage LS, Sachs G. Proton pump inhibitors and gastric acid secretion. Am J Gastroenterol 2001;96:3467–8.

CHAPTER 28

UPPER GASTROINTESTINAL BLEEDING

GREGORY J. MONKEWICH, MD, FRCPC, AND GREGORY B. HABER, MD, FRCPC

Acute nonvariceal upper gastrointestinal bleeding (NVUGIB) is associated with substantial rates of morbidity and mortality despite the remarkable advances in endoscopic therapies over the last 30 years. The largest British epidemiologic study of acute upper gastrointestinal (UGI) bleeding reported an overall mortality rate of 14% (11% in emergency admissions and 33% in inpatients), similar to rates published in earlier studies (Rockall et al, 1995). However, the age-standardized mortality was unchanged, likely because of an increased proportion of elderly patients and their attendant higher risks of death. Thus, it appears that our efforts are not in vain. This chapter provides the gastroenterologist with an evidence-based approach to acute NVUGIB with emphasis on the available therapeutic endoscopic modalities.

Patient Resuscitation and Timing of Endoscopy

Patients with acute NVUGIB should undergo endoscopy soon after presentation. Most authors suggest endoscopy within 12 to 24 hours (Spiegel et al, 2001), although randomized controlled outcome data are lacking. The largest randomized trial ($N = 124$) demonstrated that early endoscopy (< 12 hours) is safe and effective, decreases transfusion requirements compared to delayed endoscopy (12 to 24 hours), but does not decrease mortality (Lin et al, 1996). Resource utilization (hence costs) appears to be reduced with early endoscopy via a decrease in the length of stay and the number of postdischarge physician visits (Lee et al, 1999).

Patients with hemodynamic instability or suspected severe bleeding should undergo more urgent endoscopy following an initial resuscitation. Facilities for urgent after-hours endoscopy must be available. The ideal settings for resuscitation and endoscopy in this scenario are the emergency department, intensive care unit, or endoscopy suite with the support of experienced nurses. Prior to the endoscopy, one should consider (1) airway protection via endotracheal intubation, (2) central venous access, (3) correction of coagulopathy with plasma, (4) consultation with an anesthesiologist (propofol sedation), and (5) consultation with a general surgeon and intensivist.

It is preferable to start blood transfusion before endoscopy unless the severity of the bleeding demands earlier assessment.

Preparation for Endoscopic Therapy

Intravenous Erythromycin

Residual blood and clot in the stomach limits visibility and hinders therapeutic intervention. *Erythromycin* is a motilin agonist that induces gastric emptying. Frossard and colleagues (2002) suggested that infusion of erythromycin before endoscopy in patients with recent hematemesis makes endoscopy shorter and easier and reduces the need for a repeat procedure. Patients admitted within 12 hours of hematemesis ($n = 105$) were randomly assigned to intravenous (IV) erythromycin (250 mg) or placebo administered 20 minutes before endoscopy. A clear stomach was found more often in the erythromycin group (82% vs. 33%; $p < .001$). Erythromycin shortened the procedure (13.7 vs 16.4 minutes; $p = .036$) and reduced the need for second-look endoscopy (6 vs 17 cases; $p = .018$). The length of stay and the transfusion requirement did not differ significantly between the 2 groups and no complications were noted.

Another study randomized 41 patients to either erythromycin (3 mg/kg IV over 30 minutes) or no treatment (Coffin et al, 2002). Endoscopy was performed 30 to 90 minutes after the infusion (unblinded) and the quality of the examination was assessed on a subjective scale. The need to perform a second diagnostic endoscopy was also assessed. The qualities of the endoscopic examinations were significantly better in the erythromycin group (score 2.5 vs 1.5; $p = .02$), but the difference in the number of patients who required a second diagnostic endoscopy was not statistically significant (3 vs 10; $p = .089$), although there was a trend in that direction. Erythromycin did not interfere with the endoscopy and no adverse events were observed.

Nasogastric Aspirate

The nasogastric aspirate (NGA) may have diagnostic merit, but it cannot be recommended as a standard for the triage of patients with NVUGIB. A retrospective study of whether NGA can predict findings at endoscopy reported that a bloody NGA was associated with the presence of a high risk lesion (HRL) at endoscopy (Aljebreen et al, 2004). However, patients from the same database without a NGA had the same rate of HRL and the same rate of endoscopic therapy, suggesting that diagnoses and treatments were not modified by the results of NGA.

Some suggest that NGA carries prognostic value whereby fresh blood is predictive of adverse outcomes (Corley et al, 1998). Further randomized trials are needed to determine whether NGA may improve preendoscopic risk stratification of patients with NVUGIB. The role of NGA in monitoring patients after primary endoscopic hemostasis has yet to be determined.

Multidisciplinary Teams for GI Bleeding

Multidisciplinary clinical care protocols may improve the efficiency of caring for patients with acute GI bleeding. Podila and colleagues (2001) created a multidisciplinary team who developed by consensus an evidence-based GI bleeding clinical care protocol for the management of acute nonvariceal upper and lower GI bleeding. Outcomes measured in the first 8 months of protocol implementation were compared with those measured during the two preceding years. The number of admissions for protocol patients younger than 65 years of age was significantly lower than that of the preprotocol patients. The length of stay for protocol inpatients was reduced (mean 3.5 days) with no significant difference in the 30-day rates of recurrent bleeding, mortality, or hospital readmission. Further research is warranted.

Choice of Equipment

Therapeutic endoscopy suites should have available a selection of endoscopes for the management of NVUGIB. For most cases, the ideal endoscope is a two-channel therapeutic gastroscope with an irrigation pump that allows irrigation and suctioning through one channel and therapeutic instrumentation through the other. The Olympus GIF-2T160 gastroscope is 12 mm in diameter and has 2.8 mm- and 3.7 mm-diameter channels. Instruments are passed through the 2.8 mm channel, whereas the 3.7 mm channel is used for the irrigation and suction. Endoscopes with a specific high volume dedicated injection channel, now incorporated into many of the standard endoscopes, serve a similar purpose. These work with a foot pedal controlled infusion pump. In difficult to reach areas, a regular gastroscope may be better with the advantage of allowing bending at a smaller radius than the larger therapeutic gastroscopes. A side-viewing duodenoscope is often necessary for the treatment of lesions at the junction of the first and second parts of the duodenum or on the lesser curvature of the stomach. A new generation of endoscopes incorporating a second and opposite bending section may allow "en face" access to all areas of the upper gastrointestinal tract (eg, the "M-scope", Olympus GIF-2T240M, Olympus Optical, Tokyo, Japan).

Gastroscopes with large diameter working channels ("clot-busters"), such as the Olympus GIF-XTQ160 (6 mm channel), are useful when large amounts of blood and clot obscure visibility. Alternatively, a large-bore (≥ 34 French) orogastric tube may be used to lavage the stomach (Peterson, 1981).

Which Lesions to Treat

Peptic ulcers are the most common cause of acute NVUGIB accounting for 37 to 44% of all cases. Endoscopic therapy reduces the rates of recurrent bleeding, emergency surgery, and blood transfusion (Gralnek et al, 1998). The modified Forrest classification (Laine and Peterson, 1994) is widely used to describe the appearance of an ulcer base and predict the likelihood of recurrent bleeding (Table 28-1). The generalizability to clinical practice of this scheme for risk stratification is hampered by interobserver variability in interpreting stigmata of hemorrhage, because estimates have suggested major disparities (Laine et al, 1994; Lau et al, 1997; Mondardini et al, 1998). (For example, what is the risk of recurrent bleeding for the duodenal ulcer illustrated in Figure 28-1) Clean-based ulcers have a very low risk of recurrent bleeding (5%) and should not receive endoscopic

TABLE 28-1. Prevalence and Recurrent Bleeding Risks of Bleeding Peptic Ulcer

Endoscopic Appearance	Forrest Class	Prevalence (%)	Risk of Recurrent Bleeding (%)
Clean base	III	42	5
Flat spot	II c	20	10
Adherent clot	II b	17	22
Nonbleeding visible vessel	II a	17	43
Active bleeding	I	18	55

Adapted from Laine L, et al 1994.

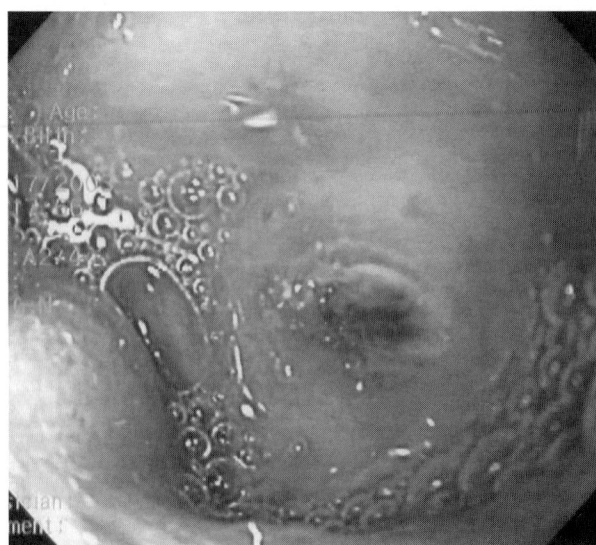

FIGURE 28-1. What is the risk of recurrent bleeding for this duodenal ulcer?

therapy. Oozing, spurting, and visible vessels should receive endoscopic therapy, whereas the management of adherent clot is controversial. Conservative management of tightly adherent clots has a good outcome with a recurrent bleeding rate of only 8% (Laine et al, 1996). However, a body of evidence supports the attempt to remove adherent clot and the subsequent treatment of uncovered vessels. The routine practice in our unit is to pre-inject around the ulcer base with 2 to 5 mL of epinephrine (1:10,000 dilution), followed by an attempt to remove the clot with vigorous washing. If necessary, we snare the clot peripherally and then centrally to assess how secure it is. When a vessel is identified we employ thermocoagulation (MPEC/HP) and/or hemoclipping. Spraying the ulcer base with 3% hydrogen peroxide may improve visualization of the vessel (Kalloo et al, 1999; Wu et al, 1999).

Doppler Ultrasound

A potential refinement to the Forrest risk stratification of bleeding ulcers is the use of *Doppler ultrasound* at the ulcer base to objectively determine whether a vessel is present. A prospective randomized study compared the therapeutic outcomes using a "Doppler" classification and the modified Forrest classification (Kohler et al, 1997). A "Doppler-positive" ulcer base was determined if the Doppler probe identified a vessel within 1 mm of the base of the ulcer. There was less recurrent bleeding in the Doppler group as well as lower emergency surgery and mortality rates.

A prospective nonrandomized trial by Wong and colleagues (2000) evaluated the risk of recurrent bleeding in 52 patients with bleeding peptic ulcers by measuring Doppler signals before and immediately following endoscopic therapy. Of the 23 lesions that received endoscopic therapy, 12 were Doppler signal-positive before treatment. The 30-day recurrent bleeding rate was 11% (1 of 9) in the posttreatment signal-negative ulcers compared to 100% (3 of 3) in the posttreatment signal-positive ulcers ($p = .03$). The early obstacles to this novel approach will be its cost and technical complexities, but further research is warranted.

Other Lesions

Dieulafoy's lesions account for 0.3 to 6.8% of acute upper GI bleeds. In a series of 40 Dieulafoy lesions, 80% were located in the stomach and 17.5% in the duodenum (Schmulewitz and Baillie, 2001). Combination therapy (injection therapy plus thermocoagulation) was successful in 36 patients (90%). Mallory-Weiss tears account for 4.5 to 11% of cases of NVUGIB. Most stop bleeding spontaneously; however 14 to 30% have needed surgery or other therapies which now have been supplanted by endoscopic therapy. Cameron's lesions are usually associated with iron deficiency anemia but may present as acute NVUGIB in up to 33% of cases. Neoplasms and postpolypectomy bleeds are other common causes. The endoscopist must maintain a broad differential diagnosis to appropriately manage bleeding lesions. Figure 28-2 illustrates a sentinel bleed from an aneurysm of the gastroduodenal artery that would have been inadequately managed with just a hemoclip.

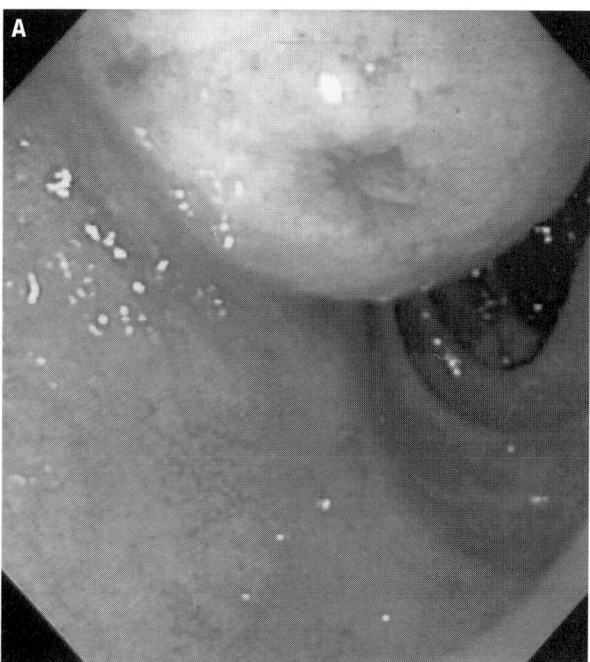

FIGURE 28-2A. Sentinel bleed from an aneurysm of the gastroduodenal artery protruding into the duodenal cap.

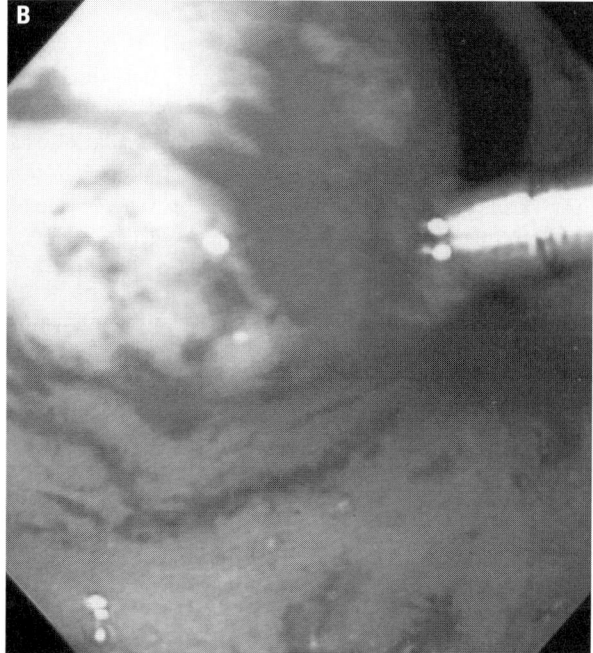

FIGURE 28-2B. A single hemoclip applied to the lesion shown in Figure 28-2A.

Injection Therapy

The agents available for injection therapy include the following: (1) *epinephrine, (2)* sclerosants (*polidocanol, ethanolamine, cyanoacrylate, sodium tetradecyl, and absolute ethanol*), and (3) clot-inducing substances (*thrombin and fibrin glue*).

Injection therapy initiates hemostasis by any of several mechanisms depending on the agent used. Although epinephrine causes vasoconstriction and alters platelet function, local tissue tamponade is probably the most important contributor to its hemostatic effect. Sclerosants such as polidocanol cause tissue necrosis, secondary inflammation, and venous and arterial thrombosis. Absolute ethanol causes profound tissue dehydration, secondary inflammation, and necrosis. Clot-inducing substances induce thrombosis without tissue injury.

A meta-analysis of trials of patients with high risk bleeding ulcers confirmed the effectiveness of injection therapy by showing significant reductions in recurrent bleeding and emergency surgery rates (Cook et al, 1992) Reduced mortality was not shown with injection therapy alone but did exist with combination therapy (discussed below).

Epinephrine

Epinephrine for the treatment of bleeding peptic ulcer was pioneered by Chung and colleagues (1988). We prefer epinephrine as the initial agent to stop active bleeding and give a clear view of the vessel. A four-quadrant injection of epinephrine 0.1 mg/mL (1:10,000 dilution) using a 23 gauge needle (Marcon-Haber, Wilson Cook) requires approximately 10 mL. We follow this with direct injection into the responsible vessel. Nonbleeding visible-vessels are managed the same way. Resistance to injection occurs commonly in chronic peptic ulcers with fibrotic bases and may require a metallic needle (NM-1K, Olympus). Epinephrine does not cause tissue damage, and cardiovascular effects are rare due to its extensive first pass metabolism in the liver. Despite adequately delivered epinephrine, the rate of recurrent bleeding from ulcers remains 15 to 20%. Thus, as discussed below, *combining epinephrine* with *other hemostatic modalities* has been studied extensively.

Sclerosants

The available sclerosants and their dosing regimens are summarized in Table 28-2. The benefit of injecting a sclerosant following epinephrine is controversial. Some studies have shown a benefit, especially in those with spurting hemorrhage (Lin et al, 1993), whereas others have not. Because of the risk of gastric necrosis and the lack of added benefit to epinephrine, we do not recommend adding sclerosants after epinephrine injection. Several studies have shown good results for endoscopic injection of ethanol, but possibly with a higher risk of local complications and perforation.

Thrombin

Church and colleagues (2003) randomized 247 patients presenting with severe peptic ulcer bleeding to heater probe (HP) plus thrombin injection or to HP plus placebo injection. Successful primary hemostasis was achieved in 97% of the patients. Recurrent bleeding developed in 15% of both groups. There was no difference in emergency surgery and mortality rates and there were no adverse events.

Kubba and colleagues (1996) randomized 140 patients to injection with epinephrine alone versus epinephrine combined with large doses of human thrombin (600 to 1000 IU). Only 4.5% of patients in the thrombin group experienced recurrent bleeding compared with 20% in the epinephrine group. Thus, thrombin had a significant benefit in arresting peptic ulcer bleeding.

Fibrin Glue

In a large European multicenter trial of 854 patients (Rutgeerts et al, 1997) the recurrent bleeding rates were 15% in the group treated with repeated injection of fibrin glue (fibrinogen and thrombin) plus epinephrine, 19% in

TABLE 28-2. Sclerosants Available for Injection Therapy

Sclerosant	Dose	Method	Brand, Manufacturer
Polidocanol	0.5 to 2%	0.5 to 1.0 mL aliquots, 4 quadrant (max 5 mL of 1% solution)	Aethoxysklerol; Kreussler Pharma GmbH, Wiesbaden, Germany
Ethanolamine oleate	5%	Needle primed with Lipiodol 0.5 mL + 0.5 mL Lipiodol	Histoacryl; Braun Melsungen, Germany
N-butyl-2-cyanoacrylate			Lipiodol; Byk Gulden, Konstanz, Germany
Sodium tetradecyl sulfate	3%		
Absolute ethanol	98%	0.2 to 0.4 mL aliquots using a tuberculin syringe (maximum 2 mL)	

the group treated with a single injection of fibrin glue plus epinephrine, and 23% in the group treated with injection of polidocanol plus epinephrine. The difference between the repeated injection of fibrin glue and polidocanol was statistically significant and there was a tendency towards less recurrent bleeding with repeated injection compared with single injection.

In Canada and the United States, fibrin glue kits are approved for surgery only and may not be used for injection into tissues or blood vessels due to the theoretical risk of thromboembolism. Other potential risks include anaphylaxis and transmission of viral infections. The latter may be eliminated in the future with recombinant fibrinogen and thrombin. A proposed advantage of fibrin glue in NVUGIB is less potential to injure tissues despite repeated use, although this has yet to be proved.

Commercially prepared fibrin glue kits include Beriplast P fibrin sealant (Centeon Pharma GmbH, Marburg, Germany [not available in Canada, USA]), Hemaseel (Hemacure, FL), and Tisseel Kit VH (Baxter, CA). The Tisseel Kit VH supplies human fibrinogen (made from pooled fresh frozen plasma) and bovine thrombin in separate vials. The fibrinogen is a freeze-dried powder that must be reconstituted by mixing it with a solution containing a fibrinolysis inhibitor (bovine aprotinin). The thrombin is also freeze-dried and must be reconstituted using a calcium chloride solution. The two reconstituted solutions are drawn into separate syringes.

To ensure that clot formation occurs only at the injection site Rutgeerts and colleagues (1997) used a special dual-lumen injector needle (eg, Endo-Flex GmbH, Voerde, Germany) to simultaneously apply the separate thrombin and fibrinogen solutions. Alternatively, the solutions may be delivered sequentially through a standard single lumen injector needle.

The US Food and Drug Administration restrictions and the aforementioned risks notwithstanding, widespread applicability of fibrin glue in the setting of acute UGI bleeding is open to question: the kits require refrigeration (2° to 8°C); the vials must be preheated to 37°C for approximately 10 minutes; mixing the solutions takes at least another 5 minutes; and the special dual-lumen injector needle ideally should be available for simultaneous application of the two solutions. The reconstituted solutions can be kept in their vials or syringes for up to 4 hours.

Thermocoagulation

The principle of *thermocoagulation* is the generation of heat on the bleeding vessel such that edema develops, tissue proteins coagulate, and the vessel contracts. Contact devices allow coaptation of the responsible vessel, which likely contributes to the hemostatic effect. Tissue coagulation requires a temperature of approximately 70°C.

Four classes of thermal coagulation devices are available as follows: (1) *heater probe* (HP), (2) *multi-polar/bipolar electrocautery* (MPEC/BPEC), (3) *argon plasma coagulation* (APC), and (4) *laser thermocoagulation*. The first two are contact devices and employ coaptation in addition to heat to initiate hemostasis. The latter two are non-contact devices.

HP

The HP delivers heat directly at a constant temperature via a heating coil inside the aluminum cylinder at its tip. The delivered energy is selected on the heater probe unit (HPU, Olympus) (range 5 to 30 Joules in 5-Joule increments). We usually select the highest output, namely 30 Joules. The HP is applied to the vessel with coaptive pressure and the foot pedal is pressed and held until the pre-set energy delivery stops spontaneously. The duration of activation of the HP varies directly with the energy setting. Some authors suggest repetitive delivery of the energy (2–3 times) before removing the probe (Chung et al, 1997). The tip of the HP is Teflon-coated to reduce tissue adhesion and the water port permits irrigation of the thermocoagulation site when the right foot pedal is pressed. Two probe sizes are available (2.8 mm and 3.7 mm diameter). We use the 3.7 mm probe as it provides better coaptation than the 2.8 mm probe which often slips off the vessel.

MPEC/BPEC

MPEC probes deliver thermal energy by completion of an electrical circuit between two electrodes on the tip of the probe through nondesiccated tissue. The circuit is completed locally and electrical grounding is not required. As the targeted tissue desiccates, conductivity diminishes, limiting the maximum temperature (~100°C) and the depth and breadth of tissue injury. A foot pedal controls irrigation via a port at the probe tip; alternatively, water may be flushed manually using a syringe. Both the thermal and coaptative components can be applied either tangentially or en face to the targeted vessel. Repeated application often results in a build-up of coagulum at the tip which impedes conduction and necessitates removal and cleaning of the probe.

APC

The principle of APC is the conduction of high frequency monopolar alternating current to target tissues through ionized argon plasma. Electrons flow through a channel of electrically activated ionized argon gas from the probe electrode to the targeted tissue causing thermal coagulation at the interface. As the tissue surface loses its electrical conductivity because of desiccation, the plasma stream shifts to adjacent nondesiccated (conductive) tissue.

The APC probe is a flexible Teflon tube with a tungsten electrode contained in a ceramic nozzle at its tip.

Coagulation depth is dependent on the generator power setting, the duration of application, and the distance from the probe tip to the target tissue. The operative distance between the probe and the tissue ranges from 2 to 8 mm. The argon arc contacts the tissue closest to the electrode allowing for direct or tangential coagulation. Probes are available that direct the plasma parallel (end-firing) or perpendicular (side-firing) to the axis of the catheter.

We prefer the end-firing probes. Pulsed APC delivery modes may offer a more precise application of the argon beam. Cipolletta and colleagues (1998) compared APC with HP in a small group of patients ($n = 41$) with bleeding peptic ulcers. Initial hemostasis, recurrent bleeding, and emergency surgery rates were comparable in both groups. Chau and colleagues (2003) in a larger trial, compared APC with HP plus injection therapy for bleeding peptic ulcers. Although a statistically significant difference was not observed, the sample size was not large enough to demonstrate a significant benefit over standard therapy.

APC has also been compared with epinephrine (1:10,000) plus polidocanol (1%) injection. Recurrent bleeding and mortality rates were similar in both groups; however, this study was also limited by its small sample size ($n = 80$).

Laser Thermocoagulation

Although laser thermocoagulation was one of the earliest modalities used to treat bleeding peptic ulcers, today it is seldom used due to its expense and technical complexity. A randomized study compared the efficacy of Nd:YAG laser, HP, and MPEC in the treatment of active bleeding from peptic ulcers (Hui et al, 1991). Ninety-one patients were randomized to receive laser, HP, or MPEC. There was no significant difference between the groups in the rate of recurrent bleeding, the duration of hospital stay, and the proportion requiring emergency surgery. However, the cost per patient was higher with laser compared to HP and MPEC.

Combination Therapy (Injection Therapy + Thermocoagulation)

Many centers combine injection therapy and thermocoagulation for the endoscopic control of bleeding peptic ulcers. Injection therapy is carried out first followed by thermocoagulation. Supportive evidence includes the study by Lin and colleagues (1999) in which 96 patients with active peptic ulcer bleeding or nonbleeding visible vessels were randomized to receive either epinephrine, BPEC, or combination therapy. Recurrent bleeding episodes were fewer and the volume of blood transfused was less in the combination therapy group compared to the other two groups. No differences were observed in the rates of emergency surgery and mortality among the three groups.

High risk patients with arterial spurting may receive a greater benefit from combination therapy. A study by Chung and colleagues (1997) randomized 276 patients with actively bleeding ulcers to either epinephrine injection or epinephrine plus HP. Overall, there were no differences in the rates of initial hemostasis, recurrent bleeding, mortality, and blood transfusion. However, the subgroup of patients with arterial spurting had shorter hospital stays (4 d vs 6 d, $p = .01$) and less need for emergency surgery (6.5% vs 29.6%, $p = .03$).

Endoscopic Hemoclipping

Endoscopic hemoclipping (HC) was introduced in 1975 by Hayashi and colleagues, but its initial applicability was limited by technical complexities. Its renaissance in the late 1980s as a third endoscopic hemostatic modality was largely due to improved instruments and was encouraged by its theoretic safety advantages over injection and thermal therapies. Hemoclips may achieve immediate hemostasis without tissue injury.

Most studies have used the manually-loaded Olympus rotatable clipping devices. Several clip sizes are available with jaw-angles measuring 90° or 135°. Disposable preloaded clipping devices include QuickClip (Olympus) and Tri-Clip (Wilson-Cook).

Bleeding Peptic Ulcers

Early studies lacking control groups demonstrated the safety and efficacy of hemoclips for the treatment of high risk bleeding peptic ulcers (Binmoeller et al, 1993). Randomized studies are available comparing HC to the other hemostatic modalities for bleeding peptic ulcers (Cipolletta et al, 2001) randomized 113 patients to either HP (10 F) or HC (Olympus MH-858 long clips) in the treatment of severe ulcer bleeding. HC was safe and effective and was reported superior to HP for the prevention of early recurrent bleeding. Endoscopic therapy was not technically feasible in eight HP patients and six HC patients. Contrary results were published by Lin and colleagues (2002) who randomized 80 patients to either HC or HP and found that the initial hemostasis rates were better with HP as was the total number achieving ultimate hemostasis. In difficult to access areas, the rate of hemostasis was better with HP.

Comparisons of HC to injection therapy are available: Chou and colleagues (2003) found HC to be superior to injection with distilled water. Chung and colleagues (1999) randomized 82 patients to either HC, injection with hypertonic saline epinephrine (HSE), or combined treatment. HC was as effective as HSE and combined treatment did not provide a significant advantage. Complications did not occur with HC. The study by Gevers and colleagues (2002), which randomized 101 patients to HC, injection therapy (epinephrine + polidocanol), or combined treatment,

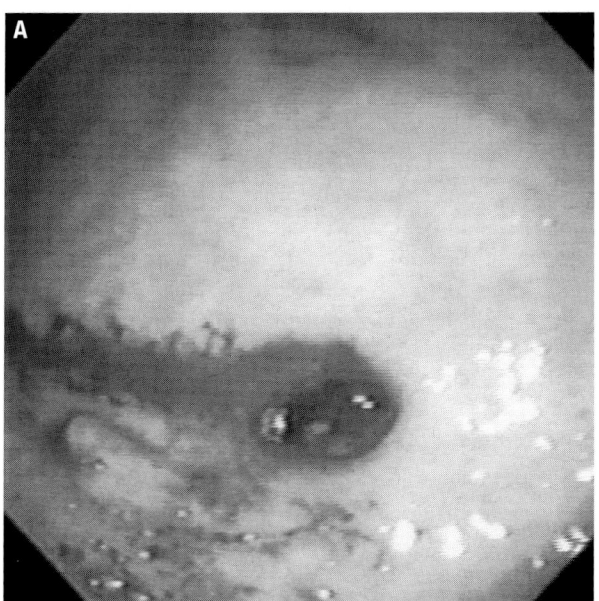

FIGURE 28-3A. Gastric Dieulafoy lesion located on the lesser curvature.

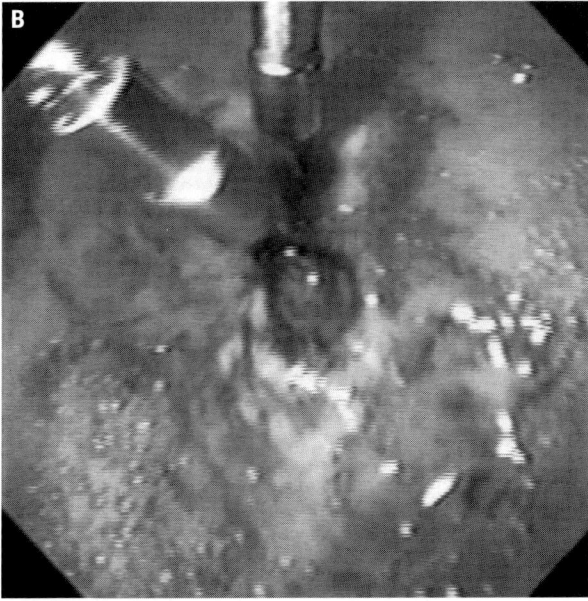

FIGURE 28-3B. Successful hemoclipping of the gastric Dieulafoy lesion shown in Figure 28-3A.

demonstrated that HC was inferior overall to injection therapy. Although their data is retrospective, Nishiaki and colleagues (2000) compared hemoclips to ethanol injection in bleeding peptic ulcers and found no significant difference in the hemostatic effect between these two methods.

It is our practice to start with injection therapy followed by HP/MPEC. When feasible we have placed clips to appose the edges of the ulcer. Theoretically, adding HC after combination therapy may reduce the rate of recurrent bleeding, however, there are no studies that have examined this approach. To be effective, lesions must be accessible for HC deployment. This is difficult at the proximal posterior gastric wall or at the junction of the first and second parts of the duodenum. We prefer the manually-loaded devices over the disposable preloaded clips because clip deployment is more reliable. The 90° jaw-angle clips also seem to hold better than the 135° jaw-angle clips.

Dieulafoy's Lesions

Figure 28-3 illustrates a gastric Dieulafoy lesion located on the lesser curvature. Permanent hemostasis was achieved with two hemoclips. Yamaguchi and colleagues (2003) prospectively examined the short and long term outcomes of HC application for primary hemostatic treatment of Dieulafoy's lesions. Of the 34 patients, 79.4% of the patients had active bleeding. Initial hemostasis was achieved with HC in 94.1% and the rate of recurrent bleeding was 9.3%. There was one death from unrelated causes and the remaining patients were followed for a mean of 53.8 months (range 19 to 90 months). Another Dieulafoy's lesion developed in one patient during follow-up, but in a different location compared with the index lesion.

Chung and colleagues (2000) divided 24 patients into mechanical (9 hemoclipping, 3 band ligation) and injection groups. The average number of endoscopic sessions needed to achieve permanent hemostasis for the mechanical and injection groups were 1.17 and 1.67, respectively. Initial hemostasis was achieved in 91.7% of patients undergoing mechanical therapy and 75% of those undergoing injection therapy, with none in the former group needing subsequent surgery in comparison to 17% of the latter group. The rate of recurrent bleeding in the mechanical therapy group was significantly lower in comparison to that of the injection therapy group (8.3% versus 33.3%, $p < .05$). Higher efficacy in terms of initial hemostasis and less recurrent bleeding was achieved by mechanical hemostatic therapy with hemoclip and band ligation compared with injection therapy.

Mallory-Weiss Tears

Huang and colleagues (2002) randomized 35 patients with Mallory-Weiss tears (MWT) (oozing or spurting vessels) to either HC (mean 2.5 clips) or injection therapy (epinephrine, mean volume 7.9 mL). Primary hemostasis was achieved in every patient. In each group there was one case of recurrent bleeding, which was managed by repeating the treatments to which they had been previously randomized. There were no *second* episodes of recurrent bleeding, no procedure-related complications, and surgery was avoided in all patients.

MWT with active bleeding (spurting, streaming or oozing), visible vessels or fresh adhesive clots received HC in a study by Yamaguchi and colleagues (2001). Follow-up endoscopy was performed within 24 hours, after 5 days and at 1 to 2 months. Of the 58 patients with MWT, HC was performed in 26 and was technically successful in each. The average number of hemoclips used was 2.8 (range 1 to 8). No complications, recurrent bleeding episodes or deaths resulted. Follow-up endoscopy showed no evidence of hemoclip-induced tissue injury.

Endoscopic Band Ligation

Several small case series of endoscopic band ligation (EBL) for the treatment of Dieulafoy's lesions have demonstrated its safety and efficacy. No complications have been reported. In one study, 22 of 23 patients with NVUGIB (locations: stomach 10; Billroth II anastomosis 10; duodenum 2; jejunum 1) were treated successfully with no recurrent bleeding (Nikolaidis et al, 2001).

A recently published retrospective comparison of EBL versus bipolar electrocoagulation demonstrated comparable efficacy in the treatment of Dieulafoy's lesions, Mallory-Weiss tears, gastric angiodysplasias, and postpolypectomy gastric ulcer bleeds (Matsui et al, 2002).

Salvage Therapy

Surgery

The timing of surgical intervention in NVUGIB is controversial. The issue is that early surgery can prevent recurrent bleeding that may be fatal, whereas, on the other hand, a high operative rate will include patients whose bleeding may not have recurred, some of whom will die as a direct result of postoperative complications. There are very few randomized trials on the topic of the timing of surgery in ulcer bleeding and the likelihood of additional trials is lessening given the decrease in volume of ulcer operations as a result of progress in endoscopic management and *Helicobacter pylori* eradication.

In general, salvage therapy with surgery is recommended if the site of bleeding cannot be identified at endoscopy or if arterial spurting is not controlled by endoscopic methods. When the bleeding is so severe that the patient is in hypovolemic shock, then early surgery is advisable. In younger, more resilient patients, the mortality is less which allows for a more conservative approach.

Endovascular Intervention

Arterial embolization may be used as an alternative to surgery if bleeding is not controlled by endoscopic therapy. The goal of arterial embolization is to decrease the blood pressure at the bleeding site thereby facilitating the formation of an effective clot (Hamlin et al, 1997) Superselective catheterization and the use of resorbable agents avoid tissue ischemia. There is a separate chapter on GI bleeding (see Chapter 102, "Gastrointestinal Bleeding: Therapeutic Radiologic Approaches").

Gelatin (*Gelfoam*, Upjohn Corp) is a widely used resorbable agent. When large particles are used, vessel recanalization typically occurs 1 to 3 weeks following resorption. Gastric and bowel infarction is rare, but the risk is increased in patients with prior abdominal surgeries or those with variant vascular anatomy. Therefore, both the celiac and superior mesenteric arterial distributions must be completely visualized prior to embolization to avoid possible gastric and bowel infarctions (Hamlin et al, 1997).

Nonresorbable materials such as coils are used for large bleeding vessels, chronic ulcers, and neoplasms. These materials are necessary to prevent recanalization of the embolized vessel and recurrent bleeding. Coils placed in bleeding vessels may facilitate their identification at surgery (by palpation or under fluoroscopy) should this be necessary.

The *left gastric artery* supplies the fundus and gastroesophageal junction, whereas the *gastroduodenal artery* supplies the duodenum, pylorus, and greater curvature. In patients with gastric bleeding, the left gastric artery usually supplies the bleeding vessel and may be embolized safely. Gastric ischemia is rare due to its collateral blood supply and rich submucosal vascular network. In addition to bleeding ulcers, gastric Dieulafoy's lesions have been embolized successfully.

In patients with duodenal bleeding, the gastroduodenal artery or one of its branches is often responsible. The *inferior pancreaticoduodenal arteries* contribute to the dual vascular supply in the duodenum. Superselective catheterization and embolization of the gastroduodenal artery often reduces perfusion pressure sufficiently to initiate hemostasis.

Medical Therapy

Acid Suppression in Bleeding Peptic Ulcers

A proton pump inhibitor (PPI) should be administered once the endoscopic diagnosis of a bleeding peptic ulcer is made as this will reduce the risk of recurrent bleeding and the need for surgery (Bustamante and Stollman, 2000). The optimal dosing regimen, route of administration, and subset of patients that are most likely to benefit have yet to be determined. We initiate an 80 mg bolus of *pantoprazole* (Protonix) (the only parenteral PPI available at our institutions) and follow it with an 8 mg/hr infusion for 72 hours.

PPI therapy is commonly initiated by emergency and other physicians prior to consultation with a gastroenterologist. It has been shown through a hypothetical cohort and decision analysis that this scenario is likely to be cost effective (Enns et al, 2003).

Studies of acid suppression have not shown a reduction in mortality. *Recognition and treatment of comorbid illnesses* is likely a more important strategy to reduce mortality.

Somatostatin/Octreotide

Available evidence does *not* support the routine use of somatostatin or octreotide in acute NVUGIB. A subgroup analysis of investigator-blinded trials (eight studies) within a meta-analysis demonstrated that the efficacy of somatostatin for the prevention of recurrent bleeding was modest and was limited to peptic ulcer bleeding (Imperiale and Birgisson, 1997). The need for surgery did not differ significantly between the somatostatin group and the control group, nor did the difference in the blood transfusion requirements. Other studies (Lin et al, 1995; Coraggio et al, 1998) have shown similar efficacy compared to H_2-receptor antagonists and less efficacy compared to endoscopic therapy (Barkun et al, 2003).

Recurrent Bleeding

Although initial hemostasis rates following endoscopic treatment in patients with severe bleeding ulcers exceed 94%, the rate of recurrent bleeding is substantial (15 to 20%). The patients at highest risk of recurrent bleeding are those whose bleeding *developed during hospitalization* for another reason, and those with *large or deep ulcers, hypotension at presentation, comorbid illness, and severe coagulopathy*.

Recurrent bleeding may be managed by endoscopic retreatment or emergency surgery. Recurrent bleeding from small ulcers is often the result of inadequate initial thermocoagulation and endoscopic retreatment is worthwhile in these circumstances.

Lau and colleagues (1999) compared emergency surgery to endoscopic retreatment for recurrent bleeding after initial endoscopic hemostasis using epinephrine plus HP. Forty-eight patients were randomized to endoscopic retreatment and 44 were randomized to surgery. The recurrent bleeding rate was 8.7%, which is lower than the rates (15 to 25%) reported in other studies. Although the long term hemostasis rate was lower with endoscopic retreatment (73% vs 93%), the complication rate was significantly higher in the surgical group (36.4 % vs 14.6%), despite the higher rate of ulcer perforation observed with endoscopic retreatment over initial treatment. Hospital length of stay, transfusion requirements, and 30-day mortality did not differ between the groups.

Further randomized trials are needed to determine whether other modalities such as hemoclipping can increase the rate of long term endoscopic hemostasis. In addition, the role of preemptive elective surgery following endoscopic retreatment in patients at high risk of recurrent bleeding should be evaluated.

Second-Look Endoscopy

Scheduled endoscopic retreatment and surveillance "second-look" endoscopy are controversial approaches to bleeding peptic ulcer management. Although some studies have shown lower recurrent bleeding rates with repeated treatments, most studies have shown no benefit. The caveats of repeated endoscopy are at least twofold. Firstly, the delay of a definitive surgical intervention may be deleterious, particularly if the patient's clinical status deteriorates during that time (Olejnik et al, 2003). Secondly, endoscopic retreatment may increase the risk to the gastric or duodenal tissues, including necrosis which could lead to perforation. Most studies suggest that the number needed to treat (NNT) to prevent one episode of recurrent bleeding is too high to recommend routine second-look endoscopy. Selection of high risk patients based on clinical and endoscopic parameters may make the NNT smaller.

Future Endoscopic Therapies

Endoscopic Suturing

Endoscopic suturing devices are available and new devices are being developed. A system developed from laparoscopic instruments, the flexible ESD system (Sew-Right and Ti-Knot, Wilson-Cook), is approved for soft tissue approximation. The device has been used primarily for the antireflux indication. Future instruments with a longer reach may allow suturing and apposition of the edges of gastric or duodenal ulcers.

Conclusion

The evidence presented applies to specific parameters as determined by the criteria for inclusion in the trials cited or the accuracy and objectivity of the retrospectively gathered data. How this applies to the individual case presenting to the physician is impacted by further considerations, especially the expertise of the endoscopist, the availability of materials and equipment, and the timing of the intervention in relationship to the bleeding event. This review is a guide to the various modalities useful to the endoscopist, with a perspective on the relative value of the agents and accessories and their appropriate application. Some basic concepts are worthy of emphasis.

In bleeding lesions of the upper GI tract the elasticity and suppleness of the tissues, the size and contractility of the vessels, and the presence of comorbid conditions especially coagulopathy or portal hypertension, all impact in an unquantifiable way on the outcome of the bleeding event. Perhaps the most important issue not addressed in these trials is the certainty of having identified the bleeding site, especially if there are multiple lesions or a non-bleeding lesion assumed to be the site. An example of this might be a major bleeding event due to a Dieulafoy lesion not actively bleeding at the time of the endoscopy, but with an associated small erosion in the antrum wrongly assumed to be the bleeding site. Identification of a visible vessel or the distinction of a red spot versus a clot is not always an easy task. The efficacy of the intervention must be weighed against these less well-defined variables. Principles worth emphasis are as follows:

1. Injectable agents depend on the diffusion of the substance around and to the bleeding vessel, and in that sense the need to precisely pinpoint the bleeding site is less critical. However, epinephrine and other agents eventually are reabsorbed and metabolized and their effect is time limited.
2. Thermal contact devices are more demanding and depend on the ability to access the bleeding point with the device, which may be challenging in certain areas of the upper GI tract. In these situations, the skill and experience of the endoscopist comes into play.
3. Mechanical devices work best when the tissue is supple allowing suction or compression of the gut wall layers and are more difficult to apply with chronic fibrosis. The combination of modalities has become more the norm today, taking into account the need for immediate cessation of bleeding and to sustain this effect so as to prevent recurrent bleeding.

Assembling all these variables into a final and successful treatment algorithm is the challenge and the reward of our work.

Editor's Note: To me, this is the ideal chapter for readers of this book. Well organized, objective data, clear principles of management and then useful comments as to what the authors do day-to-day.

Supplemental Reading

Aljebreen A, Fallone C, Barkun A. Nasogastric aspirate predicts high-risk endoscopic lesions in patients with acute upper-GI bleeding. Gastrointest Endosc 2004;59:172–8.

Barkun A, Bardou M, Marshall JK. Consensus recommendations for managing patients with nonvariceal upper gastrointestinal bleeding. Ann Intern Med 2003;139:843–57.

Binmoeller KF, Thonke F, Soehendra N. Endoscopic hemoclip treatment for gastrointestinal bleeding. Endoscopy 1993; 25:167–70.

Bustamante M, Stollman N. The efficacy of proton-pump inhibitors in acute ulcer bleeding: a qualitative review. [review] J of Clin Gastroenterol 2000;30:7–13.

Chau CH, Siu WT, Law BK, et al. Randomized controlled trial comparing epinephrine injection plus heat probe coagulation versus epinephrine injection plus argon plasma coagulation for bleeding peptic ulcers. Gastrointest Endosc 2003;57:455–61.

Chou YC, Hsu PI, Lai KH, et al. A prospective, randomized trial of endoscopic hemoclip placement and distilled water injection for treatment of high-risk bleeding ulcers. Gastrointest Endosc 2003;57:324–28.

Chung IK, Ham JS, Kim HS, et al. Comparison of the hemostatic efficacy of the endoscopic hemoclip method with hypertonic saline-epinephrine injection and a combination of the two for the management of bleeding peptic ulcers. Gastrointest Endosc 1999;49:13–8.

Chung IK, Kim EJ, Lee MS, et al. Bleeding Dieulafoy's lesions and the choice of endoscopic method: comparing the hemostatic efficacy of mechanical and injection methods. Gastrointest Endosc 2000;52:721–4.

Chung SS, Lau JY, Sung JJ, et al. Randomised comparison between adrenaline injection alone and adrenaline injection plus heat probe treatment for actively bleeding ulcers. BMJ 1997;314:1307–11.

Chung SC, Leung JW, Steele RJ, et al. Endoscopic injection of adrenaline for actively bleeding ulcers: a randomised trial. BMJ Clin Res Ed 1988;296:1631–3.

Church NI, Dallal HJ, Masson J, et al. A randomized trial comparing heater probe plus thrombin with heater probe plus placebo for bleeding peptic ulcer. Gastroenterology 2003; 125:396–403.

Cipolletta L, Bianco MA, Marmo R, et al. Endoclips versus heater probe in preventing early recurrent bleeding from peptic ulcer: a prospective and randomized trial. Gastrointest Endosc 2001;53:147–51.

Cipolletta L, Bianco MA, Rotondano G, et al. Prospective comparison of argon plasma coagulator and heater probe in the endoscopic treatment of major peptic ulcer bleeding. Gastrointest Endosc 1998;48:191–5.

Coffin B, Pocard M, Panis Y, et al. Erythromycin improves the quality of EGD in patients with acute upper GI bleeding: a randomized controlled study. Gastrointest Endosc 2002;56:174–9.

Cook DJ, Guyatt GH, Salena BJ, Laine LA. Endoscopic therapy for acute nonvariceal upper gastrointestinal hemorrhage - a metaanalysis. Gastroenterology 1992;102:139–48.

Coraggio F, Rotondano G, Marmo R, et al. Somatostatin in the prevention of recurrent bleeding after endoscopic haemostasis of peptic ulcer haemorrhage: a preliminary report. Europ J Gastroenterol Hepatol 1998;10:673–6.

Corley DA, Stefan AM, Wolf M, et al. Early indicators of prognosis in upper gastrointestinal hemorrhage. Am JGastroenterol 1998;93:336–40.

Enns RA, Gagnon YM, Rioux KP, Levy AR. Cost-effectiveness in Canada of intravenous proton pump inhibitors for all patients presenting with acute upper gastrointestinal bleeding. Aliment Pharmacol Therapeut 2003;17:225–33.

Forrest JA, Finlayson ND, Shearman DJ. Endoscopy in gastrointestinal bleeding. Lancet 1974;2:394–7.

Frossard JL, Spahr L, Queneau PE, et al. Erythromycin intravenous bolus infusion in acute upper gastrointestinal bleeding: a randomized, controlled, double-blind trial. Gastroenterology 2002;123:17–23.

Gevers AM, De Goede E, Simoens M, et al. A randomized trial comparing injection therapy with hemoclip and with injection combined with hemoclip for bleeding ulcers. Gastrointest Endosc 2002;55:466–9.

Gralnek IM, Jensen DM, Gornbein J, et al. Clinical and economic outcomes of individuals with severe peptic ulcer hemorrhage and nonbleeding visible vessel: an analysis of two prospective clinical trials. Am J Gastroenterol 1998; 93:2047–56.

Hamlin JA, Petersen B, Keller FS, Rosch J. Angiographic evaluation and management of nonvariceal upper gastrointestinal bleeding. Gastrointest Endosc Clin N Am 1997;7:703–16.

Hayashi T, Yonezawa M, Kuwabara T, Kudoh I. The study on staunch clip for the treatment by endoscopy. Gastroenterol Endosc 1975;17:92–101.

Huang SP, Wang HP, Lee YC, et al. Endoscopic hemoclip placement and epinephrine injection for Mallory-Weiss syndrome with active bleeding. Gastrointest Endosc 2002;55:842–6.

Hui WM, Ng MMT, Lok ASF, et al. A randomized comparative study of laser photocoagulation, heater probe, and bipolar electrocoagulation in the treatment of actively bleeding ulcers. Gastrointest Endosc 1991;37:299–304.

Imperiale TF, Birgisson S. Somatostatin or octreotide compared with H2 antagonists and placebo in the management of acute nonvariceal upper gastrointestinal hemorrhage: a meta-analysis. Ann Intern Med 1997;127:1062–71.

Jensen DM. Management of severe ulcer rebleeding. N Engl J Med 1999;340:799–801.

Kalloo AN, Canto MI, Wadwa KS, et al. Clinical usefulness of 3% hydrogen peroxide in acute upper GI bleeding: a pilot study. Gastrointest Endosc 1999;49(4:Pt1):t1–21.

Kohler B, Maier M, Benz C, Riemann JF. Acute ulcer bleeding. A prospective randomized trial to compare Doppler and Forrest classifications in endoscopic diagnosis and therapy. Dig Dis& Sci 1997;42:1370–4.

Kubba AK, Murphy W, Palmer KR. Endoscopic injection for bleeding peptic ulcer: a comparison of adrenaline alone with adrenaline plus human thrombin. Gastroenterology 1996;111:623–8.

Laine L, Freeman M, Cohen H. Lack of uniformity in evaluation of endoscopic prognostic features of bleeding ulcers. Gastrointest Endosc 1994;40:411–7.

Laine L, Peterson WL. Bleeding peptic ulcer [review]. N Engl J Med 1994;331:717–27.

Laine L, Stein C, Sharma V. A prospective outcome study of patients with clot in an ulcer and the effect of irrigation. Gastrointest Endosc 1996;43(2:Pt1):t1–10.

Lau JY, Sung JJ, Chan AC, et al. Stigmata of hemorrhage in bleeding peptic ulcers: an interobserver agreement study among international experts. Gastrointest Endosc 1997;46:33–6.

Lau JY, Sung JJ, Lam YH, et al. Endoscopic retreatment compared with surgery in patients with recurrent bleeding after initial endoscopic control of bleeding ulcers. N Engl J Med 1999;340:751–6.

Lee JG, Turnipseed S, Romano PS, et al. Endoscopy-based triage significantly reduces hospitalization rates and costs of treating upper GI bleeding: a randomized controlled trial. Gastrointest Endosc 1999;50:755–61.

Lin HJ, Hsieh YH, Tseng GY, et al. A prospective, randomized trial of endoscopic hemoclip versus heater probe thermocoagulation for peptic ulcer bleeding. Am J Gastroenterol 2002;97:2250–4.

Lin HJ, Perng CL, Lee SD. Is sclerosant injection mandatory after an epinephrine injection for arrest of peptic ulcer haemorrhage? A prospective, randomised, comparative study. Gut 1993;34:1182–5.

Lin HJ, Tseng GY, Perng CL, et al. Comparison of adrenaline injecttion and bipolar electrocoagulation for the arrest of peptic ulcer bleeding. Gut 1999;44:715–9.

Lin HJ, Wang K, Perng CL, et al. Early or delayed endoscopy for patients with peptic ulcer bleeding: a prospective randomized study. J Clin Gastroenterol 1996;22:267–71.

Lin HJ, Wang K, Perng CL, et al. Octreotide and heater probe thermocoagulation for arrest of peptic ulcer hemorrhage: a prospective, randomized, controlled trial. J Clin Gastroenterol 1995;21:95–8.

Matsui S, Kamisako T, Kudo M, Inoue R. Endoscopic band ligation for control of nonvariceal upper GI hemorrhage: comparison with bipolar electrocoagulation. Gastrointest Endosc 2002;55:214–8.

Mondardini A, Barletti C, Rocca G, et al. Non-variceal upper gastrointestinal bleeding and Forrest's classification: diagnostic agreement between endoscopists from the same area. Endoscopy 1998;30:508–12.

Nikolaidis N, Zezos P, Giouleme O, et al. Endoscopic band ligation of Dieulafoy-like lesions in the upper gastrointestinal tract. Endoscopy 2001;33:754–60.

Nishiaki M, Tada M, Yanai H, et al. Endoscopic hemostasis for bleeding peptic ulcer using a hemostatic clip or pure ethanol injection. Hepato-Gastroenterology 2000;47:1042–4.

Olejnik J, Labas P, Zahradnik V. Possible risks in combining endoscopic and surgical therapy of bleeding peptic ulcers. Hepato-Gastroenterology 2003;50:1169–72.

Peterson WL. Evaluation and initial management of patients with upper gastrointestinal bleeding. J Clin Gastroenterol 1981;(3Suppl2):2–84.

Podila PV, Ben Menachem T, Batra SK, et al. Managing patients with acute, nonvariceal gastrointestinal hemorrhage: development and effectiveness of a clinical care pathway. Am J Gastroenterol 2001;96:208–19.

Rockall TA, Logan RFA, Devlin HB, Northfield TC. Incidence of and mortality from acute upper gastrointestinal haemorrhage in the United Kingdom. BMJ 1995;311:222–6.

Rutgeerts P, Rauws E, Wara P, et al. Randomised trial of single and repeated fibrin glue compared with injection of polidocanol in treatment of bleeding peptic ulcer. Lancet 1997; 350:692–6.

Schmulewitz N, Baillie J. Dieulafoy lesions: a review of 6 years of experience at a tertiary referral center. Am J Gastroenterol 2001;96:1688–94.

Spiegel BM, Vakil NB, Ofman JJ. Endoscopy for acute nonvariceal upper gastrointestinal tract hemorrhage: is sooner better? A systematic review [review]. Arch Intern Med 2001;161:1393–404.

Wong RC, Chak A, Kobayashi K, et al. Role of Doppler US in acute peptic ulcer hemorrhage: can it predict failure of endoscopic therapy? Gastrointestinal Endoscopy 2000; 52:315–21.

Wu DC, Lu CY, Lu CH, et al. Endoscopic hydrogen peroxide spray may facilitate localization of the bleeding site in acute upper gastrointestinal bleeding. Endoscopy 1999;31:237–41.

Yamaguchi Y, Yamato T, Katsumi N, et al. Endoscopic hemoclipping for upper GI bleeding due to Mallory-Weiss syndrome. Gastrointest Endosc 2001;53:427–30.

Yamaguchi Y, Yamato T, Katsumi N, et al. Short-term and long-term benefits of endoscopic hemoclip application for Dieulafoy's lesion in the upper GI tract. Gastrointest Endosc 2003;57:653–6.

CHAPTER 29

Chronic Gastritis

WILFRED M. WEINSTEIN, MD

This chapter deals mainly with those aspects of *chronic gastritis* that carry an *increased risk of carcinoma* at the population level (ie, *intestinal metaplasia [IM]*), or those that arise from the "soil" of chronic gastritis, such as *hyperplastic polyps, adenomas, and nonadenomatous or endoscopically invisible dysplasia*. These are virtually all triggered by *Helicobacter pylori*. Two other conditions associated with different types of mucosal injury will be discussed, including (1) *Ménétrier's disease*, a hypertrophic gastropathy and (2) the *postoperative stomach*, a reactive gastropathy. Both carry an increased risk of cancer. *Gastropathy* is a pattern of mucosal injury in which inflammatory infiltrates may be present but are not the signature feature. In the case of Ménétrier's type of hypertrophic gastropathy the main change is a *"growth disorder"* with expansion of gastric pits to replace the oxyntic acid-secreting glands. *Reactive gastropathy* is a form of mucosal injury with highly reactive epithelial cells and some foveolar hyperplasia and minimal to no inflammation.

IM of the gastric cardia (gastroesophageal junction [GEJ]) is more related to the spectrum of gastroesophageal reflux disease (GERD). Its management will be discussed briefly at the end of this chapter.

What is IM?

IM distal to the gastric cardia is largely a consequence of *H. pylori* infection but other types of injury such as drugs may also result in IM. IM refers to the replacement of normal epithelium by *intestinal-type mucosa*. It parallels the severity of the associated gastritis in terms of its distribution. It may be more dominant in either antrum, body/fundus (oxyntic: acid-secreting mucosa) or the GEJ. Sometimes it may affect all three zones as a pangastritis. IM is associated with an increased risk of the intestinal type of gastric cancer (GC) epidemiologically. This type of cancer accounts for approximately half of all cases. Diffuse cancer of the stomach accounts for the remainder. The diffuse type of GC, although also associated with *H. pylori*, does *not* have associated IM or dysplasia.

The sequence for the development of the intestinal type of GC is given below. Atrophic gastritis refers to a loss of gastric glands. Atrophic gastritis is present when IM replaces most of the gastric glands in a given biopsy down to the muscularis mucosae.

H. pylori → Gastritis → Atrophic Gastritis with IM → Dysplasia → Cancer.

Gastric Biopsy in Clinical Practice

WHENEVER GASTRIC BIOPSIES ARE TAKEN FOR ANY REASON

Whenever gastric biopsies are taken for any reason, I take two biopsies from the distal antrum and two from the mid-body greater curve to size up the terrain (Lunn and Weinstein, 2000). This provides a quick sampling of the two main gland zones of the stomach and potential information regarding two important clinical implications. One is whether there is *concomitant H. pylori infection*. Apart from other issues related to *H. pylori* eradication, it does makes some hyperplastic polyps disappear or diminish in size (this is discussed subsequently). Secondly mid-body greater curve biopsies determine whether there is *concomitant atrophic gastritis*, not uncommonly associated with hyperplastic polyps and adenomas of the stomach. Its finding should prompt the obtaining of *serum B_{12} levels* at the time and, if necessary, periodically in the future to watch for the development of *pernicious anemia (PA)*.

BIOPSY MAPPING OF THE STOMACH

In some instances, biopsy mapping of the stomach is worthwhile. The technique I use is to divide the stomach into five zones, including the fundus body-lesser and greater curves, respectively, and the antrum greater and lesser curves respectively. I generally take two biopsies from the fundus. Then for each zone equidistant biopsies "by eye", I take four from the antrum greater curve, two or three from the antrum lesser curve, four from the body lesser curve and five to six from the body greater curve. In taking random biopsy samples from the stomach and presupposing that target lesions have had samples taken first, one can speed up the process. It is best accomplished by taking the samples by estimated site and not bother getting up close and cleaning each site of blood, mucous, bile, etc. There are other ways that one can speed up biopsy surveillance that are beyond the scope of this topic (Weinstein, 2000).

Management of IM Distal to the Gastric Cardia

Because IM of the stomach is associated epidemiologically with one of the two main types of GC, the *intestinal type*, when we find that, while taking biopsy samples, we worry that we are *"sitting on"* a GC or that one is imminent.

Incidental Finding of IM

In broad brush strokes, the presence of IM is associated with an increased risk of GC. However the finding is such a common reaction pattern to injury that no one recommends endoscopic biopsy surveillance on the basis of the finding of IM alone.

If gastric body biopsies show extensive IM with atrophic gastritis, then the main value of this finding is to indicate that we should do further testing to rule out a *PA-type stomach functionally* (serum gastrin, intrinsic factor antibodies, and serum B_{12}). If there is no apparent B_{12} deficiency in this setting then *annual B_{12} determinations* should be done.

Documented PA-Type Stomach with End-Stage Atrophic Body-Predominant Gastritis with IM

In many *PA stomachs* there is extensive IM. In some others there is less prominent IM but still extensive atrophy of the oxyntic glands, with their replacement by mucous glands (pseudopyloric metaplasia). The approach is the same for all. When this diagnosis is first made it is useful to carefully examine the stomach for polyps and carcinoids. Biopsy mapping for IM and/or dysplasia is not warranted. In a low GC country (Brown and Devesa, 2002) like the United States (only as it refers to Caucasians) there is a question as to whether any follow-up examinations should be done if the first is negative. At follow-up the most significant lesions to be found, if any, are tiny carcinoids (< 5 mm) that do not warrant removal (Lahner et al, 2001). If tiny pinpoint carcinoids are found at the first examination, I repeat the examination in 3 years, and if no change with just tiny carcinoids, then I recheck in 3 years again. Beyond that, the surveillance intervals are tempered by the age of the patient, the absence of new findings, such as larger carcinoids ≥ 5 mm, or other lesions, such as adenomas. If there are no carcinoids at the outset, I still recheck once in 5 years. Carcinoids associated with atrophic gastritis are much more indolent and less aggressive than in the other two settings for gastric carcinoids, namely sporadic, and part of an MEN picture.

If *adenomas* are found, they represent an investigative alarm and the management, as discussed subsequently, is much more proactive.

IM at the Edges of a Gastric Ulcer

If the ulcer looks otherwise benign, rebiopsy of samples can await the usual time for the healing-test. On rebiopsy, the ulcer scar and adjacent (0.5 to 1 cm) mucosa can be biopsied in a 4-quadrant fashion. At that same healing-test endoscopy, it is worthwhile looking around carefully to be sure that there is not an early neoplasm that might be arising in a field of extensive IM.

IM at the Edges of a Suspicious Lesion

Suspicious refers to an irregular shallow ulcer or an area of focal nodularity with or without depressed areas within. If biopsies only reveal IM, I would repeat the endoscopy, take more samples, and even consider mapping the stomach with multiple biopsies (Lunn and Weinstein, 2000). Here the intensity of biopsy is dependent upon the endoscopist's opinion regarding how ominous the lesion appears.

Should *H. pylori* Eradication Therapy be Used to Reverse IM?

One of the best analyses of the issue of whether atrophy and IM regress with *H. pylori* eradication is given in an editorial by Dixon (2001). The *H. pylori* eradication data is a bit more convincing for some reversal of gland atrophy than for IM. At present there is no indication to employ *H. pylori* eradication as a rationale for reversing atrophic gastritis and/or IM of the stomach. However, if samples have been taken and *H. pylori* is present, then I will treat with *H. pylori* eradication in general terms. Others might advocate not taking gastric biopsy samples at all for *H. pylori* (*don't ask, don't tell*) so that the issue does not arise. There is a separate chapter on *H. pylori* (see Chapter 23, "Helicobacter Pylori and Gastroduodenal Disease").

Family History of GC

This is one of the most difficult value judgement calls. There are families with the intestinal type of GC, more so in countries with higher GC risks (Caldas et al, 1999). Familial intestinal type of GC has been defined as (1) at least 2 first- or second-degree relatives affected, with 1 diagnosed before the age of 50 years or (2) 3 or more relatives with intestinal type of GC at any age. Concern arises even if the strict definition is not met (eg, when two first-degree relatives have had GC).

There are no studies that address the question of how often to do endoscopies looking for GC in the family members. I would do one endoscopy with a careful look for any suspicious raised or depressed lesions. Antral and body biopsies as discussed above would give an overview of whether there is extensive IM. Thereafter I would do periodic endoscopy every 3 to 5 years.

Adenomas and Dysplasia Associated with Other Lesions or Endoscopically Invisible (Flat) in the Setting of Chronic Gastritis

Gastric dysplasia is not common, and, therefore, it is useful to get a second opinion from another pathologist to verify that it is present and to verify its grade.

The finding of an adenoma (a visible mass of dysplastic epithelium) is usually in a setting of chronic gastritis, commonly featuring IM (Borch et al, 2003; Kapadia, 2003). One should not be lulled into the parallel with tiny benign adenomas of the colon. The management of these is simple: every adenoma of the stomach should be removed, preferably with endoscopic mucosal resection. In fact any area of dysplasia, and any grade of it, whether in a polyp form or other visible lesion should be excised to exclude cancer beneath (Weinstein and Goldstein, 1994). In this regard endoscopic ultrasonography before resection provides reassurance that there is no deep extension of the adenomatous lesion. Prior to its removal, I repeat an endoscopy in a patient well sedated with antecedent anticholinergic for a drier field and look for synchronous lesions, found not infrequently. And finally I also do a *gastric biopsy mapping* to ensure that there are no areas of endoscopically invisible dysplasia that might change the management from a localized removal of a single visible lesion to having to consider a wider excision or more intense biopsy followup. And again, as it is for hyperplastic polyps, the setting may be atrophic gastritis of the oxyntic mucosa with a- or hypochlorhydria. After removal of gastric adenomas the serial follow-up at 2 to 3 yearly intervals should be done as if the patient had a GC removed. At the first follow-up examination I would do gastric biopsy mapping. If there were no dysplasia identified on biopsy then subsequent examinations might not include detailed biopsy mapping. Of course if there is a strong history of GC in the family and if the patient is younger, biopsy mapping might be incorporated into any subsequent endoscopic examinations.

The other indication for gastric biopsy mapping looking for endoscopically invisible dysplasia (flat dysplasia) is when an adenoma or tumor is going to be resected surgically. In that instance the objective is to examine carefully, and do multiple biopsies, in the part of the stomach that will be left behind. The purpose is to avoid missing synchronous dysplasia away from the resection margins that the pathologist conventionally examines.

If dysplasia is found accidentally at the edges of a gastric ulcer or area of gastric irregularity, the whole lesion should be managed to rule out cancer and synchronous lesions, and it should be removed. The grade of dysplasia for this setting and in adenomas is immaterial. Gastric dysplasia of any grade in a visible lesion should be considered to potentially represent malignancy. This is equivalent conceptually to the DALM lesion in ulcerative colitis.

Gastric Biopsy Mapping after Partial Gastrectomy for GC

If the tumor was the intestinal type of GC, there is likely residual atrophic gastritis and IM. There are no guidelines for follow-up endoscopic surveillance with or without biopsy. Assuming the gastric mucosa was biopsy mapped preoperatively, I would reexamine the gastric remnant in 1 year with multiple biopsies, and if no dysplastic lesions were found, would repeat the examinations every 3 years. If invisible (flat) dysplasia were found in multiple sites, the dilemma of total gastrectomy versus waiting to see if carcinoma develops has to be individualized based upon the frailty of the patient.

Hyperplastic Polyps in the Setting of Chronic Gastritis

These consist of inflammatory change and an increase in the normal epithelial elements, especially the foveolae, similar to the hyperplastic polyp of the colon. Their appearance often qualifies them for the designation descriptively as hyperplastic/inflammatory polyps. They may often be the first sign that there is severe atrophic gastritis of the gastric body mucosa and commonly are associated with *H. pylori* (Borch et al, 2003). If the reader is unconvinced by the suggestion to take antral and gastric body biopsies whenever gastric biopsies are taken for any reason, the setting of hyperplastic polyps is definitely one setting where biopsy of the nonpolyp mucosa will have clinical implications.

They used to be the most common polyp in the stomach and are usually associated with *H. pylori*. Their movement into second place in countries with lower prevalences of *H. pylori* may reflect the fact that, in the overdeveloped world, the disappearance of *H. pylori* brings instead the fundic gland polyp.

H. pylori eradication may cause hyperplastic polyps to shrink or disappear and thus should be done if one is contemplating polypectomy or repeated long term follow up on their account alone (Ljubicic et al, 1999).

One major clinical implication of these is the same as for adenomas. Namely hyperplastic polyps commonly are the herald clue that atrophic gastritis of the gastric body is the associated condition (Borch et al, 2003; Abraham et al, 2001). Its recognition should trigger periodic testing of serum vitamin B_{12} levels to preempt the development of overt PA.

Hyperplastic polyps have traditionally been classified in the category of non-neoplastic polyps. However, it is now clear that they have malignant potential (Nogueira et al, 1999; Ginsberg et al, 1996). For that reason when they reach 5 mm, I agree with the recommendation (Ginsberg et al, 1996) to remove them either with large cup ("jumbo") forceps, ordinary snare polypectomy, or with endoscopic mucosal resection, saline assisted polypectomy (EMR). When they cluster as localized hypertrophy, removal is a much larger undertaking and one has to decide whether to do extensive EMR or to follow with periodic biopsy looking for the development of dysplasia (adenomatous change). If the latter course is followed, then dysplasia of any grade is a mandate for removal, endoscopically or otherwise.

The Postoperative Stomach

There is an increased risk of cancer after partial gastrectomy especially after 20 years. The gastric mucosa after gastric surgery is not that of extensive chronic gastritis with inflammation. Rather it is a reactive gastropathy with prominent surface and foveolar reactive cellular change and foveolar hyperplasia (corkscrew pits). Beginning between *15 and 20 years after the gastric resection,* I would do endoscopy and biopsy screening for dysplasia or overt cancer. I take 4-quadrant biopsies from the region of the stoma (Billroth II) or the gastric side of the gastroduodenal junction (Billroth I). Then biopsy mapping is done by taking multiple biopsies from the lesser and greater curves of the gastric remnant and from the gastric fundus. If endoscopically invisible high grade dysplasia is found and is multifocal, the patient's overall frailty may dictate choosing follow up to cancer rather than removal of the remainder of the stomach. This is one exception to the idea that there is little merit to the follow-up versus removal of low grade dysplasia if identified focally (Weinstein and Goldstein, 1994). In this setting if only low grade dysplasia were discovered on biopsy, I would just continue annual follow-up because the alternative is total gastrectomy.

Ménétrier's Disease

Ménétrier's disease is extremely rare, characterized by a *"growth disorder"* in which the gastric pits (foveolae) become elongated, cystic, and replace oxyntic glands—a hypertrophic gastropathy with variable amounts of inflammatory infiltrate. Ménétrier's carries an increased risk of cancer (Vandenborre et al, 1998). Admonitions are generally given in case reports of these cancers to do periodic surveillance. This is easier said than done because the mucosa consists of a forest of thick polypoid folds in the gastric body. When first encountered, I look carefully for any lesions that stand out in terms of size or color. Then I biopsy map the gastric body and fundus. Thereafter I repeat this practice yearly, recognizing that finding early cancer amongst polypoid folds is a great challenge. The condition is so rare that it is not likely that evidence-based guidelines will be forthcoming to help guide the practice of surveillance for cancer.

IM of the Cardia/GEJ

The interest in the gastric cardia/GEJ is because cardia cancer is increasing at about the same rate as Barrett's associated cancer and also dominates in white males and is inversely related to *H. pylori* infection. The question is whether IM of the cardia could be a precursor warning for a risk of cardia/GEJ cancer.

IM of the cardia is common in GERD patients (approximately 30%), without Barrett's esophagus (BE), and may occur as part of *H. pylori* gastritis. IM of the GEJ may also occur in the general population as a wear-and-tear phenomenon as a result of chronic exposure of the GEJ to gastric contents (Katzka et al, 1998; Fletcher et al, 2001).

There is no indication to routinely biopsy the GEJ in GERD or to otherwise to look for IM of the cardia or GEJ. If one is compelled to look for IM, the question to the pathologist should be framed as *"rule out IM of the cardia/GEJ"*. That question should alert the pathologist that you did not identify Barrett's and thus is designed to avoid its mention in the pathology report. Calling such patients *"ultrashort Barrett's"* is guaranteed to (1) lead to needless worry on the part of the patient and (2) lead to difficulty with obtaining insurance, or having higher payments for life, health, and disability insurance.

In IM of the cardia/GEJ without visible BE, there is no need to do biopsy surveillance to look for dysplasia in advance of cardia cancer. The reason is that IM is extremely common in GERD without BE, and crosses gender and racial lines much more than BE (Hirota, 1999). Women and black patients therefore may commonly have IM of the cardia in GERD yet their risk of cardia cancer is much less. This indicates that there have to be post-IM factors leading to malignancy, just as there are post-IM factors leading to GC in a tiny subset of those millions in the world with IM of the stomach. Also it is theoretically possible that cancer of the GEJ arises in a similar enigmatic fashion as diffuse cancer of the stomach with little in the way of advance-notice "footprints."

Summary

The main implication of finding IM of the stomach or other consequences of chronic gastritis, such as hyperplastic and adenomatous polyps, is to alert the endoscopist to be on the lookout for any synchronous lesions that might also be neoplastic, and to quick-map the stomach for signs of atrophic gastritis, especially of the gastric body. Additionally, suggestions have been given for scenarios when more extensive gastric biopsy mapping is useful. If severe atrophic oxyntic gland gastritis is found in the gastric body, then the main implication for patients is that they are at risk for having or developing vitamin B_{12} deficiency.

Supplemental Reading

Abraham SC, Singh VK, Yardley JH, Wu TT. Hyperplastic polyps of the stomach. Associations with histologic patterns of gastritis and gastric atrophy. Am J Surg Pathol 2001;25:500–7.

Borch K, Skarsgard J, Franzen L, et al. Benign gastric polyps: morphological and functional origin. Dig Dis Sci 2003;48:1292–7.

Brown LM, Devesa SS. Epidemiologic trends in esophageal and gastric cancer in the United States. Surg Oncol Clin N Am 2002;11:235–56.

Caldas C, Carneiro F, Lynch HT, et al. Familial gastric cancer: overview and guidelines for management. J Med Genet 1999; 36:873–80.

Dixon MF. Prospects for intervention in gastric carcinogenesis: reversibility of gastric atrophy and intestinal metaplasia. Gut 2001;49:2–4.

Fletcher J, Wirz A, Young J, et al. Unbuffered highly acidic gastric juice exists at the gastroesophageal junction after a meal. Gastroenterol 2001;121:775–83.

Ginsberg GG, al-Kawas FH, Fleischer DE, et al. Gastric polyps: relationship of size and histology to cancer risk. Am J Gastroenterol 1996;91:714–7.

Hirota WK. Specialized intestinal metaplasia, dysplasia, and cancer of the esophagus and esophagogastric junction: prevalence and clinical data. Gastroenterol 1999;116:277–85.

Kapadia CR. Gastric atrophy, metaplasia, and dysplasia: a clinical perspective. J Clin Gastroenterol 2003;36:S29–36.

Katzka DA, Gideon RM, Castell DO. Normal patterns of acid exposure at the gastric cardia: a functional midpoint between the esophagus and stomach. Am J Gastroenterol 1998;93:1236–42.

Lahner E, Caruana P, D'Ambra G, et al. First endoscopic-histologic follow-up in patients with body-predominant atrophic gastritis: when should it be done? Gastrointest Endosc 2001;53:443–8.

Ljubicic N, Banic M, Kujundzic M, et al. The effect of eradicating *Helicobacter pylori* infection on the course of adenomatous and hyperplastic gastric polyps. Eur J Gastroenterol Hepatol 1999;11:727–30.

Lunn JA, Weinstein WM. Gastric biopsy [In Process Citation]. Gastrointest Endosc Clin N Am 2000;10:723–38, vii.

Nogueira AMMF, Carneiro F, Seruca R, et al. Microsatellite instability in hyperplastic and adenomatous polyps of the stomach. Cancer 1999;86:1649–56.

Vandenborre KM, Ghillebert GL, Rutgeerts LJ, et al. Hypertrophic lymphocytic gastritis with a gastric carcinoma. Eur J Gastroenterol Hepatol 1998;10:797–801.

Weinstein WM. Carditis and cardia intestinal metaplasia are *Helicobacter pylori* related. In: Hunt RH, Tytgat GNJ, editors. *Helicobacter pylori*: basic mechanisms to clinical cure. Dordecht/Boston/London: Kluwer Academic Publishers; 2000. p. 299–307.

Weinstein WM. Mucosal biopsy techniques and interaction with the pathologist [In Process Citation]. Gastrointest Endosc Clin N Am 2000;10:555–72, v.

Weinstein WM, Goldstein NS. Gastric dysplasia and its management. Gastroenterol 1994;107:1543–5.

Zivny J, Wang TC, Yantiss R, et al. Role of therapy or monitoring in preventing progression to gastric cancer. J Clin Gastroenterol 2003;36:S50–60.

CHAPTER 30

THE MANAGEMENT OF NONULCER DYSPEPSIA

MICHAEL P. JONES, MD, FACP, FACG

Dyspepsia is one of the most common problems encountered in gastroenterology practice, and it accounts for 2 to 5% of primary care visits (Switz, 1976; Knill-Jones,1991). Prevalence estimates for dyspepsia range from 12 to 45%, with an average estimate of about 25% (Westbrook et al, 2000; Dominitz and Provenzale, 1999). Although there is turnover in the dyspeptic population with time, many patients experience chronic symptoms (Jones and Lydeard, 1992; Talley et al, 1992). Dyspepsia is associated with diminished quality of life, diminished productivity, and high use of health care resources.

Defining Dyspepsia

Dyspepsia is a symptom and not a diagnosis. It can be broadly defined as pain or discomfort centered in the upper abdomen. "Centered" refers to symptoms chiefly in or around the midline and not the left or right upper quadrants. "Discomfort" refers to unpleasant feelings that stop short of being painful, including upper abdominal fullness, early satiety, bloating, nausea, and retching or vomiting. Importantly, dyspeptic symptoms are not associated with altered bowel habits, but it is recognized that dyspepsia and irritable bowel syndrome (IBS) frequently coexist.

Investigated and Uninvestigated Dyspepsia

An important distinction should be drawn between patients with dyspeptic symptoms that have not been examined (uninvestigated dyspepsia) and those who have been. Investigated dyspeptics can be divided into two groups: those with an identified cause for their symptoms and those whose symptoms have either no obvious cause or a related finding of uncertain clinical significance. Examples of the former category include peptic ulcer disease, gastroesophageal reflux disease (GERD), or pancreaticobiliary disease. Examples of the latter include such things as delayed gastric emptying and visceral hypersensitivity.

Functional Dyspepsia

Dyspeptic patients with no clear structural or biochemical explanation for their symptoms are considered to have functional dyspepsia. Functional dyspepsia is synonymous with the terms *nonulcer* and *idiopathic dyspepsia*. It is broadly defined as persistent pain or discomfort centered in the upper abdomen without organic explanation and not associated with bowel pattern (Talley et al, 1999). Rome II criteria specify that symptoms be present for 12 weeks in the preceding 12 months. Although this rigidity is not required in clinical practice, chronicity is an important feature of functional dyspepsia.

Functional dyspepsia is a heterogenous disorder, and currently favored mechanisms are shown in Table 30-1. Attempts to elicit meaningful etiologies have resulted in the creation of subgroups defined using various symptom criteria (Talley et al, 1999; Colin-Jones et al, 1988; Bytzer et al, 1997). The utility of classifying functional dyspeptics, whether based on symptom clusters or dominant symptoms, remains controversial, because evidence supporting improved clinical outcomes using such an approach is lacking. Perhaps the most relevant change is that the reflux-like subgroup has been abandoned. These patients should be regarded as having GERD until proven otherwise. It is worth noting that a subset of patients with GERD may present with upper abdominal pain or discomfort in the absence of classic heartburn. Currently, three functional dyspepsia subgroups are recognized according to Rome II criteria (Talley et al, 1999). *Ulcer-like dyspepsia* has pain as the predominant symptom. *Dysmotility-like dyspepsia* has an unpleasant nonpainful sensation, such as fullness, bloating, early satiety, or nausea as the predominant symptom. Finally, patients with *unspecified dyspepsia* do not fulfill criteria for either ulcer-like or dysmotility-like dyspepsia.

TABLE 30-1. Potential Etiologies in Functional Dyspepsia

Visceral hypersensitivity
    Impaired gastric emptying
    Impaired postprandial fundic relaxation
    Antral hypomotility
    Gastric dysrhythmias
    Small bowel dysmotility
    Vagal neuropathy
    Duodenal acid hypersensitivity
    Psychosocial disturbances

Approach to the Patient with Functional Dyspepsia

Only 20 to 25% of people with dyspeptic symptoms will seek care. Importantly, symptoms do not appear to discriminate *dyspeptic consulters* from *nonconsulters*. Dyspeptics who consult are characterized by greater worry over serious illness or cancer, heightened levels of anxiety, depression, and illness behavior, as well as recent traumatic life events. Additionally, they tend to employ more *confrontative* rather than social coping styles (Cheng, 2000). In short, although physicians focus most of their efforts on the patient's symptoms, it is not necessarily the symptoms that lead people to consult. To be effective in the examination and management of these patients, clinicians must pay attention to the patients as well as to the patients' digestive tracts.

Consultation

Consultation with a patient with nonulcer dyspepsia should address several important issues, including the following:

1. *Determine the patient's agenda.* Understand why they are seeking care at this time. Address any concerns or fears that they may have regarding their symptoms.
2. *Identify triggering or exacerbating factors.* These include foods, medicines, situations, and life events. If possible, define the events surrounding symptom origination. Functional symptoms often begin or recur at times of significant psychosocial stress (Henningsen et al, 2003; Herschbach et al, 1999).
3. *Evaluate just enough.* The evaluation should address relevant clinical issues and provide diagnostic certainty. It should also, within reason, address any particular concerns the patient might have. Repetitive studies done for persistent symptoms are rarely helpful. In fact, a never-ending diagnostic evaluation only adds uncertainty to the situation and promotes the "sick role."
4. *Formulate a treatment plan in which the patient takes an active role in planning and implementation.* A critical determinant of successful outcomes is that the patient understands and accepts the diagnosis and treatment. This also ensures that educational and patient issues are effectively addressed. The quality of the physician-patient relationship remains a key determinant of clinical success in the treatment of functional digestive disorders (Koloski et al, 2003; Owens et al, 1995).
5. *Follow-up is essential.* Seeing the patient back facilitates the physician-patient relationship and provides an opportunity to gather more information about the patient and their illness. It also allows the physician and patient to review and modify the treatment plan as needed. Very often subsequent visits are more rewarding in eliciting crucial psychosocial information as the patient and physician become more trusting and open with one another.
6. *Take a psychosocial history and examine for psychiatric illness.* Taking a psychosocial history is not something that is emphasized or even routinely discussed in most gastroenterology training programs. It is, however, an important diagnostic and therapeutic tool (Owens et al, 1995). Commonly helpful questions concerning psychosocial issues are shown in Table 30-3.

TABLE 30-2. Diagnostic Measures in Functional Dysplasia

Diagnostic Measures	Utility
History and examination	Critical. Determines symptom etiologies, triggers and associations. Identifies patient agenda and concerns. Assesses psychosocial issues. Establishes therapeutic relationship.
Upper endoscopy	Ideally done during a symptomatic period off medications.
Helicobacter pylori testing	Routinely done but eradication of little value in nonulcer dyspepsia.
Ultrasonography	Routinely done but the finding of cholelithiasis in the setting of dyspepsia may raise more questions than it answers.
Psychometric testing	Rarely done in practice. Often useful in refractory patients.
Gastric emptying study	Clinical utility not defined. Abnormal study does predict response to prokinetics.
Electrogastrogram	Clinical utility not defined.
Gastroduodenal manometry	Rarely helpful unless pseudo-obstruction or partial small bowel obstruction suggested on clinical grounds.
Gastroduodenal sensory testing	Clinical utility not defined. Hypersensitivity versus hypervigilance needs to be clarified.

TABLE 30-3. Useful Questions Regarding Psychosocial Factors in a Patient's Illness

1. Is the patient's illness acute or chronic? *Chronic illness has a greater potential for psychosocial concomitants.*
2. What is the patient's illness history? *A history of multiple vague complaints, multiple procedures, and poor responses to treatment should raise suspicion that psychosocial factors are contributing.*
3. Why is the patient presenting now? *Psychosocial factors often influence care seeking.*
4. Is there a psychiatric diagnosis? *Identifying such a diagnosis that is amenable to treatment can improve outcomes.*
5. Is there a history of abuse? *Abusive experiences are associated with poorer outcomes and are often undisclosed unless sought in a supportive, empathetic fashion.*
6. Is there evidence of unhelpful illness behavior or coping style? *Examples include overly demanding requests for care and unrealistic expectations to find organic disease or a cure.*
7. What are the family dynamics around the illness? *Are there counterproductive family interactions, such as marital power struggles and separation issues with parents and children, that may manifest through illness?*
8. What are the patient's supports? *Strong social support is important for clinical improvement.*

Adapted from Drossman, 1997; and Budavari and Olden, 2003.

Specific Investigations in Nonulcer Dyspepsia

Esophagogastroduodenoscopy and *Helicobacter pylori*

Although most dyspepsia in clinical practice is functional, the diagnosis of functional dyspepsia is a diagnosis of exclusion. A search for organic etiologies should be undertaken, because therapy for many organic causes is more satisfying than therapies for functional disorders. Age, symptoms and practical concerns of the patient and physician should guide investigation of the patient's symptoms. Endoscopy is essential in making the diagnosis of nonulcer dyspepsia. In a gastroenterology practice, essentially all patients referred for evaluation of dyspepsia will have already been tested and treated for *Helicobacter pylori*. Empiric determination of *H. pylori* status in patients with uninvestigated dyspepsia is an arguable strategy that is heavily dependent upon the prevalence of *H. pylori* infection and peptic ulcer disease in the population being served (Jones, 2003). Although opinions remain divided, eradication of *H. pylori* in patients with nonulcer dyspepsia offers a net therapeutic gain of about 9% beyond placebo (Moayyedi et al, 2000).

Other Testing

Other modalities used in the evaluation of functional dyspepsia are listed in Table 30-2. *Ultrasonography* is commonly employed in the evaluation of dyspepsia. In general, pancreaticobiliary disease can be distinguished clinically from dyspepsia. Findings need to be carefully weighed against symptoms prior to undertaking further diagnostic or therapeutic interventions that often have associated morbidity and mortality. *Scintigraphic measures of gastric emptying* are also commonly performed but of limited value. An abnormal gastric emptying test is neither diagnostic nor predictive of a response to prokinetic agents. A similar and even more robust case can be made for *electrogastrography*. *Gastroduodenal manometry* is generally helpful only if pseudo-obstruction or a partial small bowel obstruction is clinically suspected. Finally, gastric sensory testing does not yet have an established clinical role and the concept of visceral hypersensitivity has not fully distinguished itself from hypervigilence (Whitehead and Palsson, 1998).

Psychometric Testing

Although not generally regarded as the realm of the gastroenterologist, *psychometric testing* is often clinically rewarding as it provides an objective, nonjudgemental measurement of certain behaviors and attitudes. From a practical standpoint, in the patient with refractory dyspeptic symptoms and an extensive negative evaluation, more diagnostic information will be obtained by ascertaining the patient's tendency towards somatization or their illness behavior than will be gained by performing more invasive and obscure tests of digestive anatomy or function. Several simple self-administered measures are available in this setting. Perhaps the most widely used instrument is the *Symptom Checklist-90-R* (SCL-90-R). The SCL-90-R is a self-reporting, clinical symptom rating scale consisting of 90 questions (Derogatis and Covi, 1973).

Responses indicate symptoms associated with nine psychiatric constructs. These constructs are somatization, obsessive-compulsive behavior, feelings of inadequacy or inferiority (interpersonal sensitivity), depression, anxiety, hostility, phobic anxiety, paranoid ideation, and psychoticism. SCL-90-R scores for a group of 73 controls and 92 patients with nonulcer dyspepsia are shown in Figure 30-1. There are significant differences for all scales and profound differences for the *somatization* and *depression*. It should be kept in mind that these measures are not diagnostic of any psychiatric disorder and responses must be considered within the context of the clinical scenario and psychosocial history.

Specific Therapies For Nonulcer Dyspepsia

A wide variety of agents have been used to treat nonulcer dyspepsia. Therapeutic efficacy for most agents is limited and biomarkers to predict responses to specific agents are largely lacking. There are however some useful observations that may improve clinical outcomes.

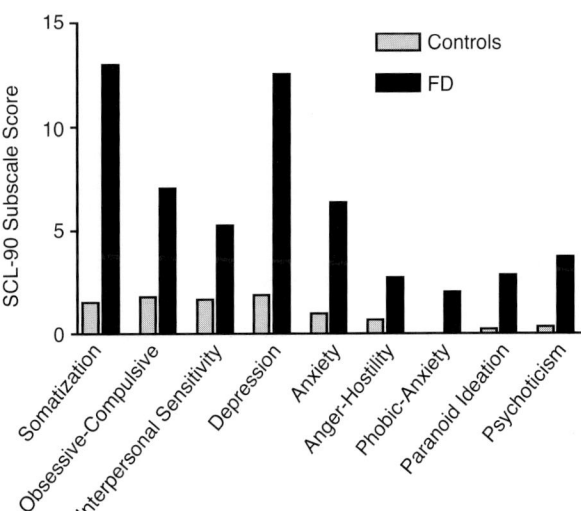

FIGURE 30-1. Symptom Checklist-90-R subscale scores in controls and patients with nonulcer dyspepsia. Significant differences are seen for all scales with the most profound differences occurring on the somatization and depression scales. FD = patients with nonulcer dyspepsia. From Jones et al (2003).

Acid Suppression

Antisecretory medications are the most widely used agents in the treatment of nonulcer dyspepsia. A number of studies have evaluated the efficacy of H$_2$ receptor antagonists (H$_2$RAs) and several meta-analyses have analyzed these trials. Many of the studies with H$_2$RAs have methodological flaws in either study design or enrollment criteria. Epigastric pain and postprandial fullness are the symptoms that are the most relieved (Redstone et al, 2001; Moayyedi et al, 2003). H$_2$RAs provide a modest benefit over placebo with a relative symptom reduction of about 22%. Comparisons of H$_2$RAs with prokinetics or proton pump inhibitors (PPIs) have not shown much advantage for one therapeutic class over the other. Given the low cost and safety of H$_2$RAs, these agents remain reasonable therapeutic agents in the treatment of nonulcer dyspepsia.

There are actually fewer data supporting the use of PPIs in the treatment of functional dyspepsia. Omeprazole has been compared with placebo in a combined analysis of two large trials (Talley et al, 1998). Both 10 mg and 20 mg doses of omeprazole were superior to placebo in patients with reflux-like and ulcer-like dyspepsia. Omeprazole provided a net therapeutic gain of about 8% beyond placebo. Omeprazole was not better than placebo in patients with dysmotility-like symptoms. Another large trial compared lansoprazole (Prevacid) in 15 mg and 30 mg doses with placebo and failed to find significant benefit in any dyspepsia subgroup.

CURRENT USE

Acid suppressive therapy may be of benefit in patients with functional dyspepsia and the benefit appears greatest in patients with *ulcer-like symptoms*. A 2 to 4 week trial of antisecretory therapy at standard doses is reasonable. Therapy should be discontinued if there is no response. Despite a lack of support from existing literature, most gastroenterologists would *empirically use PPIs* rather than H$_2$RAs. Because empiric acid suppression is used to treat both *GERD* presenting as dyspepsia as well as true *nonulcer dyspepsia*, this approach is reasonable.

H. pylori Eradication

A recent meta-analysis reported that eradicating *H. pylori* offers a net therapeutic gain of about 9% beyond placebo (Moayyedi et al, 2000). A second meta-analysis did not find significant improvement in symptoms following eradication (Laine et al, 2001). The disparate results stem from the numbers of trials included. Unfortunately, there do not appear to be any clinical predictors of response to *H. pylori* eradication. The decision to test patients with nonulcer dyspepsia for *H. pylori* infection remains somewhat controversial. If a patient is found to be infected, treatment should be offered but the likelihood of clinical improvement is small.

Prokinetics

The most widely studied prokinetic in the treatment of nonulcer dyspepsia is *cisapride*, but it is currently available in the United States only through an onerous limited access protocol. Although cisapride appeared significantly better than placebo in reducing dyspeptic symptoms, many of the available trials were small in size and publication bias may have influenced results. Comparisons of cisapride with metoclopramide or domperidone or metoclopramide with domperidone have not demonstrated the superiority of one agent over another (Fumagalli and Hammer, 1994; Halter et al, 1997; Van Outryve et al, 1993). *Motilin agonists* have not been well studied, but a recent trial with ABT-229 found it to actually be inferior to placebo in providing symptom relief. *Domperidone* can be obtained from non–US-based pharmacies, often without a prescription. It may also be obtained from compounding pharmacies in the United States with a prescription, but it tends to be much more expensive. Because domperidone has both antiemetic and prokinetic effects without central nervous system toxicity, it is often helpful in patients with dysmotility-like dyspepsia. The starting dose is 10 mg before meals and at bedtime. Although *metoclopramide* (Reglan) remains our first line prokinetic because of availability and expense, domperidone is used in patients who either do not respond to or do not tolerate metoclopramide. To date, there are no published trials of the partial 5-HT$_4$ agonist *tegaserod* in the treatment of nonulcer dyspepsia, but this agent may have efficacy in a subset of patients.

Antidepressants

Antidepressants are commonly used in the treatment of functional digestive disorders and appear to be beneficial (Jackson et al, 2000). In a small trial of seven patients, Mertz and colleagues (1998) showed that 50 mg of *amitriptyline* at bedtime significantly reduced symptoms of nonulcer dyspepsia. Similar results have been seen by Tanum and Malt (1996) with the tetracyclic agent *mianserin*. Interestingly, a response to this agent is *predicted* by both results of a *fenfluramine challenge* and certain *personality constructs*. These personality traits include *low levels of neuroticism*, as well *as low levels of hidden aggression*. Thus, in contrast to acid suppression, *H. pylori* eradication, and prokinetics, there are *biomarkers* that *predict* a *response to antidepressants*. At present, there are no published data for selective serotonin reuptake inhibitors in nonulcer dyspepsia, although studies are underway. *Paroxitene (Paxil)* has been shown to enhance *meal-induced relaxation of the fundus*, but sertraline (Zoloft) exerts no effect on gastric compliance or sensitivity (Ladabaum and Glidden, 2002; Tack et al, 2003).

Anxiolytics

Anxiolytics are *generally avoided* in the management of nonulcer dyspepsia because of the potential for habituation and abuse. There are, however, two scenarios in which these agents appear helpful. The first is in the management of patients with *anxiety* or *panic disorders* who have *prominent dyspeptic features* (Henningsen et al, 2003). Anxiety and panic may be associated with both symptom generation and enhanced symptom perception and decreased symptom tolerance. Additionally, a subset of patients with *panic disorders* may present with digestive symptoms (most often *nausea*) in the *absence* of more classic anxiety symptoms. The SCL-90-R is useful in identifying these patients, as are two other instruments, the Beck Anxiety Index and Spielberger State-Trait Anxiety Index. The second group that may benefit from anxiolytics is made up of patients with *persistent nausea* and *vomiting*. Nausea is an easily conditioned behavior, as has been repeatedly seen in patients with chemotherapy-induced nausea and vomiting. *Lorazepam (Ativan)* is often effective in treating these patients because of its antiemetic and anxiolytic properties.

Buspirone (BuSpar) is an anxiolytic that has fallen from favor in psychiatry but has gained favor in gastroenterology. It is a 5-HT$_{1A}$ agonist that causes *fundal relaxation* (Coulie et al, 1997). In healthy controls it has been shown to significantly decrease postprandial symptom scores. Although therapeutic trials are needed, our anecdotal experience with this agent in upper abdominal bloating and early satiety has been quite positive. Other fundal relaxants include *sumatriptan (Imitrex), tegaserod (Zelnorm), paroxitene (Paxil),* and *citalopram (Celexa)*. All require clinical evaluation.

Psychological Interventions

Psychological interventions in patients with IBS have been evaluated, and a recent systematic analysis supports their efficacy (Spanier et al, 2003). *Hypnotherapy* and *cognitive behavioral therapy* are the modalities best studied. A recent study showed that *hypnotherapy* was *superior* to supportive and medical therapies at both 16 and 56 weeks (Calvert et al, 2002). The results were quite striking with *net therapeutic gains* over medical therapy of 30% for symptoms and 24% for quality of life. It seems likely that psychological interventions will prove to be highly effective in functional digestive disorders, and we have incorporated both behavioral therapy and hypnotherapy into our practice. More rigorous study is needed particularly in the setting of nonulcer dyspepsia. The clinical utility of this intervention will also be highly dependent on the *availability* of *behavioral health specialists* to provide the service and *third party payers* to *reimburse* for what can be a costly treatment.*

---

*Editor's Note: Because of the diffuse nature of nonulcer dyspepsia and the conflicting literature, we have included a larger number of references than with other chapters. I found this a most useful chapter. (TMB)

Supplemental Reading

Agreus L, Svardsudd K, Nyren O, Tibblin G. Irritable bowel syndrome and dyspepsia in the general population: overlap and lack of stability over time. Gastroenterology 1995;109:671–80.

Blum AL, Arnold R, Stolte M, et al. Short course acid suppressive treatment for patients with functional dyspepsia: results depend on *Helicobacter pylori* status. The Frosch Study Group. Gut 2000;47:473–80.

Bortolotti M, Bolondi L, Santi V, et al. Patterns of gastric emptying in dysmotility-like dyspepsia. Scand J Gastroenterol 1995;30:408–10.

Brown C, Rees WD. Dyspepsia in general practice. BMJ 1990;300:829–3.

Budavari AI, Olden KW. Psychosocial aspects of functional gastrointestinal disorders. Gastroenterol Clin North Am 2003;32:477–506.

Bytzer P, Hansen JM, Schaffalitzky de Muckadell OB, Malchow-Moller A. Predicting endoscopic diagnosis in the dyspeptic patient. The value of predictive score models. Scand J Gastroenterol 1997;32:118–25.

Calvert EL, Houghton LA, Cooper P, et al. Long-term improvement in functional dyspepsia using hypnotherapy. Gastroenterology 2002;123:1778–85.

Carvalhinhos A, Fidalgo P, Freire A, Matos L. Cisapride compared with ranitidine in the treatment of functional dyspepsia. Eur J Gastroenterol Hepatol 1995;7:411–7.

Cheng C. Seeking medical consultation: perceptual and behavioral characteristics distinguishing consulters and nonconsulters with functional dyspepsia. Psychosom Med 2000;62:844–52.

Cheng C, Hui WM, Lam SK. Coping style of individuals with functional dyspepsia. Psychosom Med 1999;61:789–95.

Colin-Jones DG, Bloom B, Bodemar G. Management of dyspepsia. Report of a working party. Lancet 1988;1(8585):576–9.

Coulie B, Tack J, Janssens J. Influence of buspirone-induced fundus relaxation on the perception of gastric distention in man. Gastroenterology 1997;112:A715.

Creed F, Craig T, Farmer R. Functional abdominal pain, psychiatric illness, and life events. Gut 1988;29:235–42.

Derogatis LR, Covi L. SCL-90: An outpatient psychiatric rating scale—preliminary report. Psychopharm Bull 1973;9:13–28.

Dobrilla G, Comberlato M, Steel A, Vallaperta P. Drug treatment of functional dyspepsia. A meta-analysis of randomized controlled clinical trials. J Clin Gastroenterol 1989;11:169–77.

Dominitz JA, Provenzale D. Prevalence of dyspepsia, heartburn, and peptic ulcer disease in veterans. Am J Gastroenterol 1999;94:2086–93.

Drossman DA. Irritable bowel syndrome and sexual/physical abuse history. Eur J Gastroenterol Hepatol 1997;9:327–30.

Finney JS, Kinnersley N, Hughes M, et al. Meta-analysis of antisecretory and gastrokinetic compounds in functional dyspepsia. J Clin Gastroenterol 1998;26:312–20.

Fumagalli I, Hammer B. Cisapride versus metoclopramide in the treatment of functional dyspepsia. A double-blind comparative trial. Scand J Gastroenterol 1994;29:33–7.

Halter F, Staub P, Hammer B, et al. Study with two prokinetics in functional dyspepsia and GORD: domperidone vs. cisapride. J Physiol Pharmacol 1997;48:185–92.

Hansen JM, Bytzer P, Schaffalitzky de Muckadell OB. Placebo-controlled trial of cisapride and nizatidine in unselected patients with functional dyspepsia. Am J Gastroenterol 1998;93:368–74.

Henningsen P, Zimmermann T, Sattel H. Medically unexplained physical symptoms, anxiety, and depression: a meta-analytic review. Psychosom Med 2003;65:528–33.

Herschbach P, Henrich G, von Rad M. Psychological factors in functional gastrointestinal disorders: characteristics of the disorder or of the illness behavior? Psychosom Med 1999;61:148–53.

Jackson JL, O'Malley PG, Tomkins G, et al. Treatment of functional gastrointestinal disorders with antidepressant medications: a meta-analysis. Am J Med 2000;108:65–72.

Jian R, Ducrot F, Ruskone A, et al. Symptomatic, radionuclide and therapeutic assessment of chronic idiopathic dyspepsia. A double-blind placebo-controlled evaluation of cisapride. Dig Dis Sci 1989;34:657–64.

Jones MP. Evaluation and treatment of dyspepsia. Postgrad Med J 2003;79:25–9.

Jones MP, Hoffman S, Shah D, et al. The water load test: observations from healthy controls and patients with functional dyspepsia. Am J Physiol Gastrointest Liver Physiol 2003;284:G896–904.

Jones R, Lydeard S. Dyspepsia in the community: a follow-up study. Br J Clin Pract 1992;46:95–7.

Knill-Jones RP. Geographical differences in the prevalence of dyspepsia. Scand J Gastroenterol Suppl 1991;182:17–24.

Koloski NA, Talley NJ, Huskic SS, Boyce PM. Predictors of conventional and alternative health care seeking for irritable bowel syndrome and functional dyspepsia. Aliment Pharmacol Ther 2003;17:841–51.

Ladabaum U, Glidden D. Effect of the selective serotonin reuptake inhibitor sertraline on gastric sensitivity and compliance in healthy humans. Neurogastroenterol Motil 2002;14:395–402.

Laine L, Schoenfeld P, Fennerty MB. Therapy for *Helicobacter pylori* in patients with nonulcer dyspepsia. A meta-analysis of randomized, controlled trials. Ann Intern Med 2001;134:361–9.

Locke GR III. Prevalence, incidence and natural history of dyspepsia and functional dyspepsia. Baillieres Clin Gastroenterol 1998;12:435–42.

Logan R, Delaney B. ABC of the upper gastrointestinal tract: implications of dyspepsia for the NHS. BMJ 2001;323:675–7.

Lyday WD II, DiBaise JK. Metoclopramide-stimulated gastric emptying scintigraphy: does it predict symptom response to prokinetic therapy in chronic gastroparesis? Am J Gastroenterol 2002;97:2474–6.

Lydeard S, Jones R. Factors affecting the decision to consult with dyspepsia: comparison of consulters and non-consulters. J R Coll Gen Pract 1989;39:495–8.

Management of dyspepsia: report of a working party. Lancet 1988;1:576–9.

Mertz H, Fass R, Kodner A, et al. Effect of amitriptyline on symptoms, sleep, and visceral perception in patients with functional dyspepsia. Am J Gastroenterol 1998;93:160–5.

Moayyedi P, Soo S, Deeks J, et al. Systematic review and economic evaluation of *Helicobacter pylori* eradication treatment for non-ulcer dyspepsia. Dyspepsia Review Group. BMJ 2000;321:659–64.

Moayyedi P, Soo S, Deeks J, et al. Systematic review: antacids, H2-receptor antagonists, prokinetics, bismuth and sucralfate therapy for non-ulcer dyspepsia. Aliment Pharmacol Ther 2003;17:1215–27.

Owens DM, Nelson DK, Talley NJ. The irritable bowel syndrome: long-term prognosis and the physician-patient interaction. Ann Intern Med 1995;122:107–12.

Redstone HA, Barrowman N, Veldhuyzen Van Zanten SJ. H2-receptor antagonists in the treatment of functional (nonulcer) dyspepsia: a meta-analysis of randomized controlled clinical trials. Aliment Pharmacol Ther 2001;15:1291–9.

Ricci DA, Saltzman MB, Meyer C, et al. Effect of metoclopramide in diabetic gastroparesis. J Clin Gastroenterol 1985;7:25–32.

Spanier JA, Howden CW, Jones MP. A systematic review of alternative therapies in the irritable bowel syndrome. Arch Intern Med 2003;163:265–74.

Switz DM. What the gastroenterologist does all day. A survey of a state society's practice. Gastroenterology 1976;70:1048–50.

Tack J, Broekaert D, Coulie B, et al. Influence of the selective serotonin re-uptake inhibitor, paroxetine, on gastric sensorimotor function in humans. Aliment Pharmacol Ther. 2003;17:603-8.

Talley NJ. Update on the role of drug therapy in non-ulcer dyspepsia. Rev Gastroenterol Disord 2003;3:25–30.

Talley NJ, Meineche-Schmidt V, Pare P, et al. Efficacy of omeprazole in functional dyspepsia: double-blind, randomized, placebo-controlled trials (the Bond and Opera studies). Aliment Pharmacol Ther 1998;12:1055–65.

Talley NJ, Stanghellini V, Heading RC, et al. Functional gastroduodenal disorders. Gut 1999;45(Suppl 2):II37–42.

Talley NJ, Verlinden M, Snape W, et al. Failure of a motilin receptor agonist (ABT-229) to relieve the symptoms of functional dyspepsia in patients with and without delayed gastric emptying: a randomized double-blind placebo-controlled trial. Aliment Pharmacol Ther 2000;14:1653–61.

Talley NJ, Weaver AL, Tesmer DL, et al. Lack of discriminant value of dyspepsia subgroups in patients referred for upper endoscopy. Gastroenterology 1993;105:1378–86.

Talley NJ, Weaver AL, Zinsmeister AR, Melton LJ III. Onset and disappearance of gastrointestinal symptoms and functional gastrointestinal disorders. Am J Epidemiol 1992;136:165–77.

Tanum L, Bratviet-Johansen K, Malt UF. Fenfluramine challenge test predicts outcome in pharmacological treatment of patients with functional gastrointestinal disorder. J Psychosom Res 1999;47:525–35.

Tanum L, Malt UF. A new pharmacologic treatment of functional gastrointestinal disorder. A double-blind placebo-controlled study with mianserin. Scand J Gastroenterol 1996;31:318–25.

Tanum L, Malt UF. Personality traits predict treatment outcome with an antidepressant in patients with functional gastrointestinal disorder. Scand J Gastroenterol 2000;35:935–41.

Van Outryve M, De Nutte N, Van Eeghem P, Gooris JP. Efficacy of cisapride in functional dyspepsia resistant to domperidone or metoclopramide: a double-blind placebo-controlled study. Scand J Gastroenterol Suppl 1993;195:47–52.

Westbrook JI, McIntosh JH, Talley NJ. The impact of dyspepsia definition on prevalence estimates: considerations for future researchers. Scand J Gastroenterol 2000;35:227–33.

Westbrook JI, Talley NJ. Empiric clustering of dyspepsia into symptom subgroups: a population-based study. Scand J Gastroenterol 2002;37:917–23.

Whitehead WE, Crowell MD, Robinson JC, et al. Effects of stressful life events on bowel symptoms: subjects with irritable bowel syndrome compared with subjects without bowel dysfunction. Gut 1992;33:825–30.

Whitehead WE, Palsson OS. Is rectal pain sensitivity a biological marker for irritable bowel syndrome: psychological influences on pain perception. Gastroenterologyl 1998;115:1263–71.

Wong WM, Wong BC, Hung WK, et al. Double blind, randomised, placebo controlled study of four weeks of lansoprazole for the treatment of functional dyspepsia in Chinese patients. Gut 2002;51:502–6.

CHAPTER 31

GASTROPARESIS

DANIEL C. BUCKLES, MD, AND RICHARD W. MCCALLUM, MD

The diagnosis of gastroparesis should be firmly established by ruling out mechanical obstruction with endoscopy and barium studies and demonstrating delayed gastric emptying by nuclear scintigraphy. Once this is accomplished, the clinician's attention should immediately focus on (1) *restoring nutritional status*, (2) *providing symptomatic relief from nausea and vomiting*, and (3) *improving gastric motility*. These three tasks should be undertaken simultaneously and aggressively with constant reassessment and modification. Any abrupt change in clinical status should prompt diagnostic re-evaluation to rule out causes for symptomatology besides gastroparesis. Figure 31-1 depicts a treatment algorithm that approximates our general approach to treating delayed gastric emptying. *Combination therapy* is the rule rather than the exception, and most patients require *multiple prokinetic* and *antiemetic modalities* for adequate symptom relief. This chapter highlights the following primary goals of treatment in gastroparesis:

1. *Restoration of nutrition*
2. *Prokinetic therapy*
3. *Antiemetic therapy*
4. Incorporating the evolving role of *gastric electrical stimulation* (GES).

Restoration of Nutrition

Many patients with gastroparesis are nutritionally impaired by the time the diagnosis is firmly established. Even if the reduction in body mass index (BMI) is modest, dietary measures are usually tried first. A low fat, low fiber, soft diet with frequent small meals should be initiated and high caloric liquid supplements are often needed to maintain weight. Sometimes patients may have already adapted to their condition by adopting a mostly liquid diet. This can result in less vomiting than a normal diet would and cause the clinician to underestimate the severity of the disorder. If BMI continues to decline despite dietary measures with adequate medical therapy, the patient is having recurrent hospital admissions, not functioning outside the home, or is unable to maintain hydration, a jejunal feeding tube (jejunostomy or J-tube) may be required. These can be placed surgically, endoscopically, or radiologically, depending upon local expertise. J-tubes allow for nocturnal enteral feedings that permit daytime working and functioning. Medications can also be delivered by J-tubes and are absorbed despite intermittent vomiting. Over time, a button device can replace the less cosmetically acceptable tube apparatus. There is a separate chapter on percutaneously placed gastric tubes (PEGs) and percutaneously placed jejunostomies (PEJs) (see Chapter 32, "Percutaneous Endoscopic Gastrostomy"). In general, PEG or combination PEG/PEJ tubes have limited roles in the treatment of gastroparesis. A PEG for gastric decompression should only be considered in the setting of dilated small bowel, such as is found with intestinal pseudo-obstruction. Direct instillation of nutrition into the stomach does not bypass the primary motility problem in gastroparesis, and jejunostomy tubes placed through the pylorus are frequently expelled back into the stomach from the distal duodenum or proximal jejunum with vomiting. Recommending drainage and suction from gastric tubes is not appropriate, as it can lead to potassium depletion and interfere with refeeding goals because of "gastric atrophy." We also do not employ chronic parenteral feeding through central venous lines, as the lines are prone to frequent infection and thrombosis and the expense is not defendable.

Prokinetic Therapy

Dopamine Antagonists

Metoclopramide (Reglan) is the most commonly used prokinetic drug and the agent that we employ as first line therapy. It is a central and peripheral dopamine receptor (D_2) antagonist and a powerful antiemetic at the chemoreceptor trigger zone level while also being effective in improving gastric emptying by increasing antral contractions and decreasing receptive relaxation of the proximal stomach. However, as many as 40% of patients cannot tolerate metoclopramide because of central nervous system (CNS) side effects. If tolerated orally, the usual dose is 10 to 20 mg 30 minutes before meals and bedtime. One strategy for patients who do tolerate this agent orally is to also use it subcutaneously (sc) during periods of worse nausea or vomiting. Metoclopramide sc can be given by the patient (2 mL [10 mg] 2 or 3 times daily) with oral medication during and after hospitalizations while stepping down to

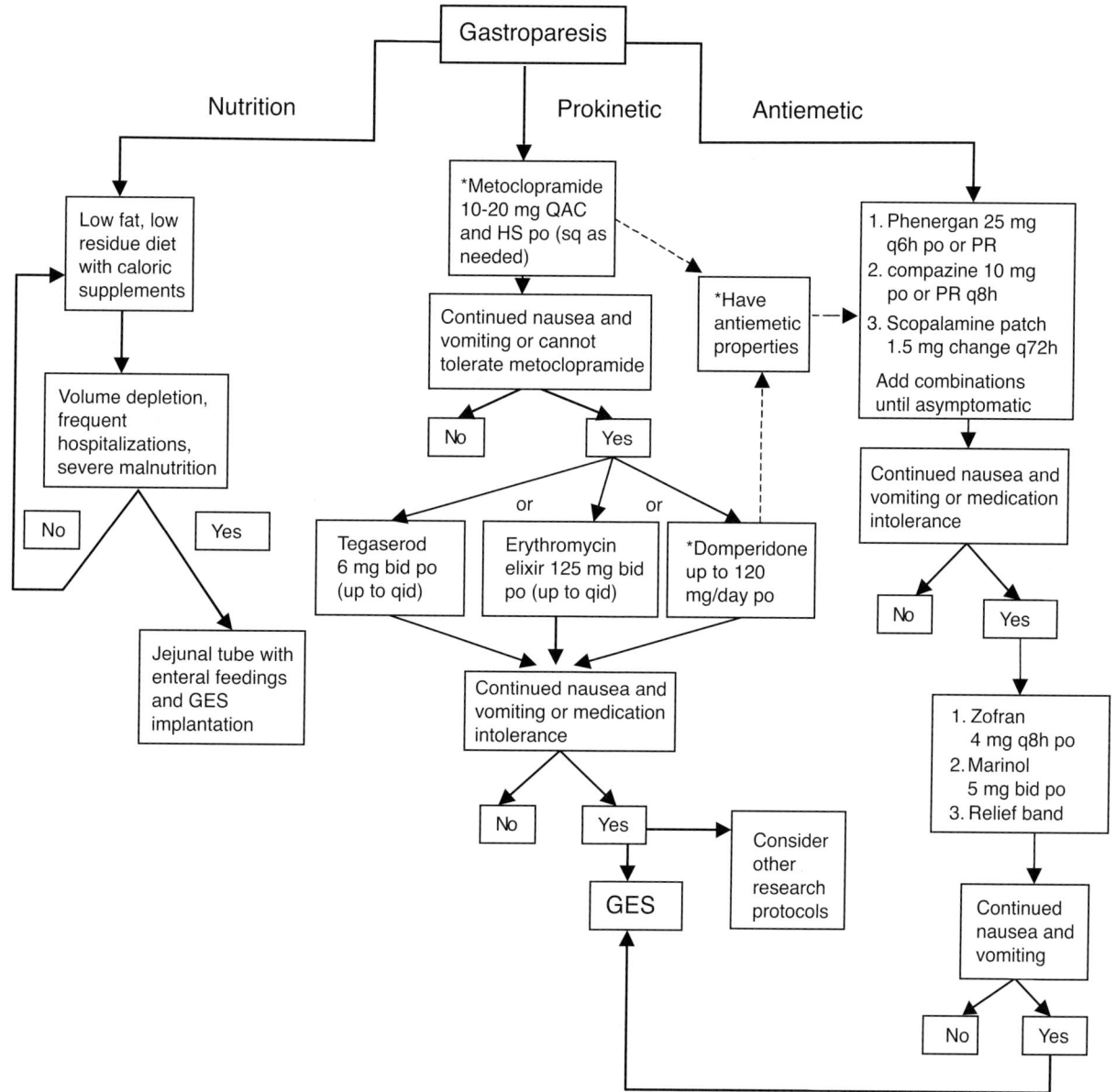

FIGURE 31-1. Gastroparesis treatment algorithm. bid = twice daily; GES = gastric electrical stimulation; po = by mouth; qid = 4 times daily; q8h = every 8 hours.

oral therapy alone or as a bolus supplement at home to control intermittent breakthrough nausea.

For patients that have intolerable side effects on metoclopramide or continued symptomatology, other agents can be used. We frequently substitute *Domperidone* (*Motilium*) for metoclopramide. It is a very effective dopamine-2 antagonist, like metoclopramide, and shares its effect on upper gastrointestinal (GI) motility. It is a potent antiemetic at the chemoreceptor trigger zone but does not cross the blood-brain barrier and, therefore, has no CNS side effects. Unfortunately, however, it is not available in the United States despite the fact that its effectiveness and safety have been established in clinical trials.

Domperidone can be obtained from some compounding pharmacies in the United States and from pharmacies in other countries but is not usually covered by health insurance providers. Domperidone, at doses from 10 mg to 30 mg by mouth (po) 4 times daily (qid) (also given 30 minutes before meals and bedtime), has been shown to significantly reduce GI symptoms and hospitalizations from gastroparesis, enhance quality of life, and accelerate gastric emptying of a solid meal. Domperidone does cause increased serum prolactin levels, and the most commonly reported side effects are gynecomastia in men and breast enlargement and lactation in women. These events occur in approximately 5% of treated patients.

Motilin Agonists

Erythromycin is a useful adjunctive therapy that can be added to metoclopramide or domperidone if nausea and vomiting persist despite maximal tolerated doses of these agents. It attaches to the motilin receptor and stimulates enteric contractility. It is *not* an antiemetic and concomitant agents to address nausea must also be initiated with this agent. Both intravenous and oral forms have been shown to improve gastric emptying rates, but this therapy can be complicated by cramping and abdominal pain. Low doses in a liquid (syrup) form are best to treat gastroparesis (eg, 125 mg 2 or 3 times daily). A potential concern with this agent is that it loses effectiveness over time due to down regulation of the motilin receptor.

5-Hydroxytryptamine Agonists

Cisapride (Propulsid) is the original agent in this class and works by stimulating the stomach via 5-hydroxytryptamine (5-HT4) receptors. It is relatively free of CNS side effects and has been shown to improve gastric emptying of solids and liquids. Unfortunately, the unacceptably high rate of potentially fatal cardiac arrhythmias seen with this drug prompted the US Food and Drug Administration to restrict its use. Consequently, we rarely use this drug outside of special circumstances.

Tegaserod (Zelnorm) (Novartis Pharmaceutical Company) is the most recently approved prokinetic agent. It has recently been FDA-approved for treatment of women with constipation-predominant irritable bowel syndrome (IBS). It is a partial and selective 5-HT$_4$ receptor agonist that possesses GI stimulatory effects from the esophagus to the rectum. Animal and human studies have shown stimulatory motor effects throughout the digestive tract, and it has been shown by Prather and colleagues (2000) to accelerate orocecal transit in patients with IBS. There are data showing improved gastric emptying times in patients with gastroparesis and clinical trials in this subgroup of patients are ongoing. Dosing is recommended as 6 mg po twice daily but in our experience dosing up to 4 times daily is well tolerated without loose stools. We will especially consider introducing this therapy for patients who complain of constipation in addition to their symptoms of gastroparesis. Tegaserod does not have antiemetic properties, and, therefore, would need to be given in combination with standard antiemetics.

Other Agents

Somatostatin (Octreotide) is used for patients with concomitant small bowel motility problems (eg, diarrhea and bacterial overgrowth). Somatostatin works by initiating a migration motor complex beginning in the small bowel, which agitates the gut, moving the bacteria further downstream and helps to sterilize the small intestine. It should be given as 50 to 100 µg sc at night before bed. However, metronidazole or other antibiotics should be given during the day to further address bacterial overgrowth. Somatostatin actually inhibits gastric emptying and hence daytime use would require concomitant prokinetics and administration should not directly precede meals. It can be very effective for treating *dumping syndrome* when given preprandially in this specific clinical setting usually observed postvagotomy or gastric surgery. There is no chapter on peptic ulcer surgery in this edition.

Evolving Therapies

Some reports have shown that diabetic patients with *gastroparesis* have *abnormally high pyloric sphincter pressures*. This has lead to the concept of "pyloric spasm" and the idea that therapies aimed at relaxing the pyloric sphincter could improve gastric emptying. The use of *sildenafil* and local *botulinum toxin A injections* have been proposed to address this particular pathophysiology. Preliminary reports suggest that 100 to 200 Units of *botulinum toxin* injected directly into the pylorus endoscopically is effective in temporarily relieving symptoms in idiopathic and diabetic gastroparesis, although further study is needed (Ezzeddine et al, 2002). It would seem best suited to the setting of an accidental vagal nerve injury accompanying fundoplication or esophageal surgery. Here it would simulate the effects of a pyloroplasty without the necessity for surgery. Since repeated administration will be required, formulation and administration issues may preclude its use as a first line therapy. Sildenafil (Viagra) is a phosphodiesterase inhibitor that leads to increased levels of nitric oxide in the pylorus and hence relaxation. It has been shown to increase gastric emptying in animal models. Its use for gastroparesis in humans is under investigation. A long-acting form with once daily dosing is also being introduced.

GM-611 (Mitemcinal, Chugai Pharmaceutical Company) is a macrolide that, like erythromycin, binds to the motilin receptor and stimulates enteric contractility, but does not have antimicrobial properties. It is currently in phase II trials and has been shown to increase gastric motility and gastric emptying in animal models as well as patients with diabetic gastroparesis. Results of these treatment trials on gastroparesis will be available in the near future.

Mosapride (Takeda Pharmaceutical Company) is an investigational agent and is a 5-HT$_4$ agonist. It has been shown to have stimulatory effects throughout the human GI tract and has less potential for cardiac arrhythmia than its predecessor, Propulsid. It may become a useful agent in the treatment of gastroparetic patients and gastroesophageal reflux and these trials are currently being conducted.

Additional Factors

It is important to alleviate any factors that tend to precipitate or exacerbate nausea and vomiting in patients with gastroparesis. W*omen* appear to be disproportionately susceptible to gastroparesis of any cause. One theory suggests that because progesterone inhibits smooth muscle function, then any insult to gastric smooth muscle control is accentuated in women, who have naturally higher levels of this hormone. Therefore, premenopausal women with gastroparesis sometimes have worse symptoms perimenstrually. Often blocking menses with the gonadotropin-releasing hormone agonist *leuprolide acetate* injections can alleviate these premenstrual problems. Monthly injections of 3.75 mg intramuscularly is the long-acting form. *Migraine headaches* can also cause nausea and vomiting in gastroparetic patients, as in normal individuals. If they are occurring frequently, prophylactic migraine therapy may be warranted. In *diabetic gastroparesis*, glucose control is very important in contributing to nausea and vomiting exacerbations. Glucose levels above 180 mg/dL have been shown to induce gastric dysrhythmias that impair gastric motility, as well as having a direct emetic effect on central control mechanisms. Every effort should be made to address glucose control by identifying underlying infections and addressing insulin use and dietary issues.

Antiemetic Therapy

It is important to remember that nausea will often persist for some time after the initiation of prokinetic therapy that is aimed at restoring gastric motility. The patient's perception of symptom relief starts with nausea and vomiting and this must be immediately addressed while the prokinetics are started. Prokinetics coordinate the motility of the stomach and proximal gut and this effect requires a little longer to work and decrease symptoms than antiemetics which can be effective almost immediately. We recommend aggressive *concurrent antiemetic therapy*, making symptomatic improvement the main goal of medical therapy. Antiemetics should be used liberally and prophylactically to prevent nausea and vomiting rather than treating it after onset. Preventing nausea and vomiting is particularly important for diabetic gastroparesis because nausea can quickly lead to vomiting which can become refractory and evolve to ketoacidosis, emergency room visits, and hospitalizations.

First line agents usually consist of scheduled *promethazine (Phenergan)* at doses of 25 mg po every 6 hours or *prochlorperazine (Compazine)* 10 mg every 8 hours. These agents can also be given in *suppository* form if vomiting is too severe to allow for absorption of orally administered medications. They act centrally on the chemoreceptor trigger zone in the brain affecting cholinergic and dopaminergic receptors to inhibit nausea and vomiting. These medications are relatively effective and inexpensive. However, compazine can cause extrapyramidal side effects and phenergan can cause excessive sedation that may limit their usefulness on a chronic basis.

For patients that have breakthrough nausea despite scheduled therapy with these agents or frequent vomiting that could limit oral absorption, we add a *scopolamine patch*. Patches with 1.5 mg of scopolamine placed behind the ear and changed every 72 hours can provide relief of some nausea. This anticholinergic agent does, however, cause dry mouth, sedation, and blurred vision. Usually these side effects become less pronounced with time, but occasionally, patients are unable to tolerate its use. The patch can also be cut in half to minimize side effects.

Odansetron (Zofran), *granisetron (Kytril)*, and *dolasetron (Anzemet)* are medications that antagonize 5-HT$_3$ receptors and prevent emesis by blocking conduction of vagal afferents up to the chemoreceptor trigger zone, the area postrema of the brain. *Zofran*, the most commonly used medication in this class, is probably the most effective antiemetic medication currently available and is given in oral doses starting at 4 mg every 8 hours. Many patients referred to us are on this therapy for refractory symptoms, but due to the extremely high cost of this medication (about $20.00 [US] per dose), we usually attempt to wean them to more economically viable therapies if chronic use is being contemplated. However, for patients with refractory, severe nausea and vomiting, use of this medication can often be justified.

Dronabinol (Marinol) is an FDA-approved cannabinoid. It works presumably through its effects on cannabinoid receptors in the CNS. It is very effective in preventing nausea, especially when combined with prochlorperazine in patients with chemotherapy-induced nausea. It is fairly expensive, and has the potential for CNS-related side effects, such as euphoria, somnolence, and confusion, but has been tried in patients with refractory symptoms from gastroparesis and can also be used to stimulate food intake.

Low dose tricyclic antidepressants (nortriptyline or amitriptyline) at doses from 10 to 50 mg at night have gained support in the setting of nausea not fully suppressed by the above agents or where "intolerance" or side effects limit dosing. It is thought that symptoms of gastroparesis may be lessened by addressing gastric "visceral hypersensitivity" by reducing postprandial epigastric discomfort, fullness, and bloating and/or raising thresholds to nausea perception in the CNS.

A nonpharmacologic therapy that can be employed in patients with refractory symptoms is the ReliefBand (Woodside Biomedical). It is a Class II medical device that is worn on the wrist of the nondominant hand. It works by transcutaneous acustimulation (ie, it emits a small electrical charge that stimulates the P6 accupressure point on the wrist.) It has been shown to reduce nausea from pregnancy and chemotherapy. It is available for about $90.00 (US) and can be used long term by simply replacing batteries.

GES

For patients who continue to be plagued by disabling nausea and vomiting despite use of the prokinetic and antiemetic therapies outlined above and where there are frequent hospitalizations, poor quality of life, inability to work and worsening nutritional parameters, we next consider implantation of a gastric electrical stimulator (see Figure 31-1). The only currently FDA-approved device is manufactured by Medtronic under the trade name Enterra. At our Center for the Study of Gastrointestinal Nerve and Muscle Function, approximately 50% of patients being referred for gastroparesis are receiving this modality. It is about the size of a cardiac pacemaker and is implanted sc in the abdominal wall at the time of laparoscopy or laparotomy when two electrodes are placed in the smooth muscle about 9.5 to 10.5 cm from the pylorus along the greater curvature of the antrum. The two electrodes are placed 1 cm apart, tangentially, deep in the muscularis propria and connected to the pulse generator in the subcutaneous pocket. Intraoperative endoscopy is performed at the time of implantation to ensure that the leads are not accidentally pushed into the lumen of the stomach and are positioned appropriately in the muscularis propria of the stomach wall.

The pulse generator delivers electrical stimuli to the stomach wall with a higher frequency (12 cpm) than the intrinsic gastric slow wave (2.0 to 4.0 cpm), but uses low energy levels (300 μsec pulse width and 4 to 5 mA). The most commonly seen complication has been pacemaker hardware infection requiring device removal. This has been observed in about 5% of patients, most of whom have been diabetics. The battery life for the device is about 8 years.*

However in recent publications, GES has been shown to significantly reduce nausea and vomiting from gastroparesis in both a double-blind trial and in open-label settings with follow up for as long as 5 years (Abell et al, 2003; Forster et al, 2003). Additionally, a new well controlled study is currently underway to help advance understanding of its clinical efficacy.

The patients studied thus far have diabetic, idiopathic, and postgastric surgery (vagotomy) related gastroparesis. There has been a predictable average response of greater than 50% reduction in nausea and vomiting and other gastroparetic symptoms in approximately 75% of patients. Additionally, in long term follow up studies, improved nutritional parameters, improved diabetic control in patients with diabetic gastroparesis, based on reduced hemoglobin A₁C level, enhanced quality of life, decreased hospitalizations, and decreased health care costs have all been reported with use of this Enterra therapy.

In general, the effect of high frequency–low energy pacing on gastric contractility is unclear, as is the mechanism of action in decreasing symptomatology. Accelerations in gastric emptying times have been noted in some patients (about 20%), however, this response is unpredictable and the majority of treated patients continue to have unchanged and abnormal gastric emptying times after implantation. Furthermore, there has been poor correlation between the changes in symptoms and gastric emptying. Hence there is a need for small volume meals and backup prokinetic therapy to address postprandial fullness and bloating in patients after receiving GES.

It has been hypothesized that the symptomatic improvement that has been observed is caused by modulation of enteric or afferent neural activity that influences symptom perception or influences a central nausea and vomiting control mechanism. Other possible explanations for the efficacy of GES therapy include changes in various electroencephalogram parameters, fundic relaxation, the autonomic nervous system, and perhaps GI peptide mediators.

We currently recommend GES therapy for patients that have had gastroparetic symptoms for over 1 year and are refractory to standard medical management and have abnormal gastric retention (at 2 hours over 60% and 4 hours over 10% using the standardized low fat meal) (see Figure 31-1). Patients with an organic obstruction or pseudo-obstruction, a primary eating or swallowing disorder, chemical dependency, or current pregnancy are not considered as candidates for GES implantation. In view of the minimal effects on gastric emptying, other chronic nausea and vomiting states could be indications in the future for this device (eg, cyclic vomiting syndrome, renal failure, and chronic idiopathic nausea and vomiting). Gastroparetic patients who are being considered for enteral or parenteral nutritional support, have nausea and vomiting despite continuing medical therapy with multiple admissions or are unable to function cannot tolerate medical therapy (see Figure 31-1), diabetic patients being listed for pancreatic and/or renal transplantation who must be maintained on oral immunosuppressants are also candidates for this therapy. In summary, gastric electrical stimulation should be considered at a low threshold, particularly in diabetics, where there is a homogenous pathophysiology resulting in a predictable positive outcome with an accompanying low potential for adverse effects. It has been a major advance in the treatment algorithm (see Figure 31-1) by returning symptomatic gastroparesis patients to functional lifestyles and good quality of life, thus, giving them hope that was not previously present.

---

*Editor's Note: The initial report to the United States Food and Drug Administration in 2000 on the Medtronic device did not show a significant decrease in the median rate of vomiting with the instrument turned on or off.

Supplemental Reading

Abell TR, McCallum RW, Hocking M, et al. Gastric electrical stimulation for medically refractory gastroparesis. Gastroenterology 2003;125:421–8.

Albibi R, McCallum RW. Metoclopramide: pharmacology and clinical application. Ann Intern Med 1983;98:86–95.

Endo J, Nomura M, Morishita S, et al. Influence of mosapride citrate on gastric motility and autonomic nervous function: evaluation by spectral analyses of heart rate and blood pressure variabilities, and by electrogastrography. J Gastroenterol 2002;37:888–95.

Ezzeddine D, Jit R, Katz N, et al. Pyloric injections of botulinum toxin for treatment of diabetic gastroparesis. Gastrointest Endosc 2002:55;920–3.

Forster J, Sarosiek I, McCallum RW, et al. Further experience with gastric stimulation to treat drug refractory gastroparesis. Am J Surg 2003;186:690–5.

Forster J, Sarosiek I, McCallum R, et al. Gastric pacing is a new surgical treatment for gastroparesis. Am J Surg 2001;182:676–81.

Hornbuckle K, Barnett JL. The diagnosis and work up of the patient with gastroparesis. J Clin Gastroenterol 2000;30:117–24.

Lane M, Vogel CL, Ferguson J, et al. Dronabinol and prochlorperazine in combination for treatment of cancer chemotherapy-induced nausea and vomiting. J Pain Symptom Manage 1991;6:352–9.

McCallum RW, Valenzuela G, Spyker D, et al. Subcutaneous metoclopramide in the treatment of symptomatic gastroparesis: clinical efficacy and pharmacokinetics. J Pharmacol Exp Ther 1991;258:136–42.

Peeters TL. GM-611 (Chugai Pharmaceutical). Curr Opin Investig Drugs 2001;2:555–7.

Prather CM, Camilleri M, Zinsmeister AR, et al. Tegaserod accelerates orocecal transit in patients with constipation-predominant irritable bowel syndrome. Gastroenterology 2000;118:463–8.

Richards RD, Davenport K, McCallum RW. The treatment of idiopathic and diabetic gastroparesis with acute intravenous and chronic oral erythromycin. Am J Gastroenterol 1993;88:203–7.

Silvers D, Kipnes M, McCallum RW, et al. Domperidone in the management of symptoms of diabetic gastroparesis: efficacy, tolerability, and quality-of-life outcomes in a multicenter controlled trial. Clin Ther 1998;20:438–53.

Soykan I, Sarosiek I, McCallum R. The effect of chronic oral domperidone therapy on the gastrointestinal symptoms, gastric emptying, and quality of life in patients with gastroparesis. Am J Gastroenterol 1997;92:976–80.

Walsh JW, Hasler WL, Nugent CE, et al. Progesterone and estrogen are potential mediators of gastric slow wave dysrhythmias in nausea of pregnancy. Am J Physiol Gastrointest Liver Physiol 1996;270:G506–14.

CHAPTER 32

Percutaneous Endoscopic Gastrostomy

Abdul Jabbar, MD, Craig J. McClain, MD, and Stephen McClave, MD

Since its initial introduction by Ponsky and colleagues in 1980, percutaneous endoscopic gastrostomy (PEG) has gained wide acceptance as a safe and efficient method of providing enteral alimentation in patients who have functionally intact gastrointestinal (GI) tracts but are unable to swallow or maintain sufficient volitional intake due to a variety of medical conditions. This procedure has been adopted by most centers and is performed in both adults and children with excellent results. Some modifications in technique have been developed, and PEG has replaced surgical gastrostomy in most settings. PEG tube placement is technically easier, less expensive, and performed more rapidly with only local anesthetics and intravenous (IV) conscious sedation, whereas surgical gastrostomy frequently requires general anesthesia. PEG placement numbers are steadily increasing; statistics indicate that PEG placements doubled over the 8 years from 1988 to 1995. In general, PEG tube placement should be considered for patients who require long term enteral feeding for > 4 weeks. For short term nutritional requirements, nasogastric (NG) tubes or nasoenteric tubes are preferred. We will review the indications, complications, nutritional benefits, and ethical issues related to PEG placement.

Indications

The initial indication for PEG placement was to provide long term enteral feeding for patients who were unable to swallow. Other indications have been added as the procedure has continued to evolve (Safadi et al, 1998). PEG tube indications can be divided into two main categories, nutritional and nonnutritional.

Nutritional Indications

The prerequisites for this procedure are a functionally intact GI tract and meaningful longevity of the patient. Nutritional support for patients suffering from cerebrovascular accidents, senile dementia, brain tumors, amyotrophic lateral sclerosis, trauma, and sequelae of extensive neurologic surgery, are the most common nutritional indications for PEG placement. Other appropriate indications include tumors of the oral cavity, head and neck tumors, and severe facial trauma leading to alteration or obstruction of the aerodigestive tract. PEG has been used for nutritional supplementation in patients with inflammatory bowel disease (IBD), short gut syndrome, and malabsorption syndrome. It has also been used in patients with normal swallowing, but inadequate oral intake, to improve their nutritional status. Examples include patients suffering from extensive burns, acquired immunodeficiency syndrome (AIDS) wasting syndrome, anorexia after bone marrow transplantation, and chronic illnesses, such as cystic fibrosis and congenital heart disease. However, the role of enteral feeding in AIDS wasting syndrome is controversial.

Nonnutritional Indications

Nonnutritional indications represent relatively newer applications of PEG. These include chronic enteral administration of unpalatable medications or diets as well as gastric decompression in patients with gastroparesis, abdominal/peritoneal carcinomatosis, or malignant intestinal obstruction. PEG has also been used for GI diversion in radiation enteritis and enterocutaneous fistulas. Other novel uses include nonsurgical therapy for "gas-bloat syndrome" after Nissen-fundoplication, facilitated dilation, and stenting of obstructing esophageal neoplasms, and fixation of the stomach in patients with recurrent gastric volvulus.

Contraindications

Absolute contraindications to PEG placement are the failure or inability to advance the gastroscope through the esophagus or a limited expected life span of a patient. Obstruction of the intestine is considered as a contraindication for PEG placement unless the PEG tube is used for *decompression*. Relative contraindications are massive ascites, peritoneal dialysis, coagulapathy, gastric and esophageal varices, portal hypertensive gastropathy, morbid obesity, prior subtotal gastrectomy, and neoplastic or infiltrative disease of the gastric wall. Cancer patients with ascites are at increased risk for complications and death directly related to PEG placement. Previous abdominal surgery is not an absolute contraindication, and PEG tubes can be safely placed with careful attention to the details of technique and by using "safe tract" technique. PEG tubes can also be placed in patients with a ventriculoperitoneal shunt as long as the site of the shunt can be carefully avoided. A recent retrospective study suggests that PEG tubes can be safely placed within a month after acute myocardial infarction if urgently needed.

Techniques

Since the first description of PEG placement, many commercial kits have been introduced. A few variations of the technique have evolved which include the Ponsky "Pull," the Sachs-Vine "Push," the Russel "Introducer," and primary button methods. Generally, the patient is kept NPO for 6 to 8 hours before the procedure. A single *prophylactic dose* of an *antibiotic* (usually a *cephalosporin*) is used 30 minutes before the procedure. However, selection, duration and timing of antibiotics are controversial. Most studies have shown a benefit with a single dose in reducing risk of infection. One study suggested that if patients are already on broad spectrum antibiotics, they do not need additional antibiotic coverage to provide prophylaxis (Gossner et al, 1999). Before PEG placement, a thorough diagnostic esophagogastroduodenoscopy should be performed because significant pathology may be found in some patients, which may alter the decision for PEG placement.

Pull Technique

The original method described in 1980 by Ponsky and colleagues was a "Pull" technique for PEG placement (Safadi et al, 1998). In this method (after placing the patient in a supine position and starting IV sedation) the endoscope is advanced to complete the upper examination (esophagus, stomach, and duodenum). The stomach is fully inflated. The gastric inflation not only brings the gastric wall closer to the anterior abdominal wall but also helps to displace the left lobe of the liver in cephalad direction and the colon towards the pelvis. Transillumination and movement of the stomach wall during ballottement ensures that the gastric wall will be in close proximity to the anterior abdominal wall and that there are no intervening viscera. A fluid filled syringe is then advanced through the abdominal wall at the spot selected for PEG placement; any air aspirated prior to reaching the stomach suggests interposing bowel and an alternative site should be chosen. The skin is anesthetized with lidocaine and a 1 cm horizontal incision is made. The puncturing cannula is inserted through the abdominal wall into the stomach. A guidewire is passed through the cannula and grasped with a snare. The endoscope is then pulled out along with the snare. Subsequently, the dilating part of the PEG tube is attached to the wire and pulled from the abdominal wall, hence it is called the Pull technique. After several inches are extended, a gastroscope is reintroduced to check the position of the bolster inside the stomach wall. On the outer tube, a crossbar is applied to prevent migration of the tube.

Push Method

The "Push" method is a modification described by Sachs and Vine. The technique is exactly the same as the pull method except that the guidewire, once pulled out of the stomach, is held taut and the feeding tube is pushed over the wire through the mouth, esophagus, stomach, and abdominal wall, and is secured in a similar fashion (Hogan et al, 1986).

Introduce Method

The third method of placing a feeding tube is the *Russel "Introducer"* method. Using the same basic principal as previously described, the stomach is insufflated following endoscope introduction, a needle is thrust into the stomach under endoscopic visualization, a short J shaped guidewire is passed through the needle, and the needle is removed. An introducer with an outer sheath is passed over the wire with a twisting motion until the sheath is clearly visible within the stomach. The introducer is withdrawn leaving only the sheath in the stomach, the gastrostomy tube with a balloon tip is then advanced through the sheath. The gastrostomy tube balloon is inflated under direct endoscopic visualization and the sheath is pealed away. The modification of this procedure is the use of T-fasteners (Versa) to avoid pneumoperitoneum, prevent loss of gastric insufflation and to facilitate the entire procedure. The Russel technique is valuable in patients with esophageal stenosis or larger esophageal tumors. Technically, it is *more difficult* compared to the push or pull methods and has a *higher* incidence of life threatening complications.

Other Methods

Skin level gastrostomy tubes (button type) have been used both as a PEG replacement device, and as a one step technique for initial placement. Radiologic gastrostomy can be considered when an esophageal obstruction is present.

Complications

Several large prospective trials of PEG placement have evaluated the efficacy and safety of the procedure. The frequency of complications observed in the various reports depends upon the definitions used and the population studied. Overall, minor complications were found in 4 to 13% (mean 7%), whereas major complications were found in 1 to 4% (mean 3%). Although major complications are uncommon, mortality associated with major complications was reported at 25% (Foutch et al, 1992). Aspiration and peritonitis were the most common causes for procedure-related mortality

Major complications include aspiration pneumonia, peritonitis, premature removal of the gastrostomy tube, tube migration through the gastric wall, perforation, gastrocolocutaneous fistula, hemorrhage, necrotizing fasciitis, and tumor implantation at the PEG site.

Minor complications include wound infection, inflammation, leakage around the gastrostomy tube, formation of granulation tissue, tube blockage, and fragmentation.

Major Complications

Aspiration can occur during the procedure or later during gastric feeding. It occurs more commonly in neurologically impaired patients. The mortality related to aspiration can be as high as 60%. The best way to prevent these complications is to pay meticulous attention to procedural detail. The patient's stomach should be completely suctioned and overdistension should be avoided to prevent aspiration of gastric contents. Oversedation should also be avoided. The head of the bed should be elevated up 30° to 45° during feeding and continued for 1 hour after. Intermittent or continuous feeding is associated with less aspiration compared to rapid bolus feeding (McClave and Chang, 2003).

Peritonitis after PEG placement occurs in up to 1.2% of patients. Peritonitis can result from several factors such as premature removal or displacement of the tube before tract maturation, internal leakage around the exit stoma, and viscous perforation. Abdominal pain, fever, leukocytosis, and peritoneal findings on physical examination, may herald early peritonitis. If a leak into the peritoneal cavity can be documented on contrast study, early *surgical intervention* may be required. In cases where the tube is pulled out prematurely and there is no sign of peritonitis, the patient can be managed conservatively with IV antibiotics and NG tube decompression.

Buried bumper syndrome occurs in about 22% of cases. In this condition, the internal bumper erodes through the stomach mucosa leading to ulceration. With time, this passage becomes re-epithelialized, covering the bumper, hence the name "buried bumper syndrome." The condition is due to excessive traction or pressure between the internal and external bolster of the tube leading to mucosal ischemia. By designing newer, softer, cup-shaped bumpers and decreasing excessive pressure between the bolster, the incidence has decreased. Typical findings include abdominal pain during feeding, swelling around the stoma, peritubal leaks, and difficulty advancing, pulling or rotating the feeding tube. This syndrome may also present as a local abscess or necrotizing tissue infection. Several techniques for management of this complication have been described. It is important to determine which will be less traumatic to the PEG site, pulling the tube through the abdominal wall, or back into the stomach (McClave and Chang, 2003).

Hemorrhage is a rare complication of PEG placement occurring in 0 to 2.5% of cases. It can result from direct *puncture* of the *vessels* in the gastric wall and can usually be managed by applying tamponade pressure to the internal bumper. Once the bleeding is controlled, the bumper should be loosened to avoid mucosal ischemia. Bleeding at time of procedure can also occur from *mucosal tears* in the esophagus or stomach.

Gastrocolocutaneous fistula is a widely described complication of PEG placement. This complication results either from inadvertent puncture of the intervening colon due to poor gastric insufflation or from migration and erosion of the tube through the colon. It may remain undetected for some time after the procedure. The patient usually presents with severe diarrhea or with stool seeping out around the PEG tube. It can also present in an earlier phase with signs of peritonitis if there is leakage into the peritoneal cavity. Occasionally, this problem may be discovered only when the old PEG tube is replaced with a new tube. In most cases, it can be managed conservatively by removing the gastrostomy tube and allowing the tract and fistula to close.

Necrotizing fasciitis is a rare but potentially lethal complication of PEG placement. Clinical features include localized abdominal pain, edema, erythema, and ecchymoses, with progression to bullae formation and eventually septic shock. Broad spectrum antibiotics with wide surgical debridement are necessary.

PEG site metastasis of head and neck tumors is a rare complication. So far nine cases have been reported. The median time for development of this complication is 8 months post-PEG placement. The exact mechanism of implantation is not known, although direct seeding of the tract by the tumor cells during the procedure is considered to a play major role. Some degree of hematogenous spread has also been speculated. Usually no specific treatment is necessary. Management by local radiation or wide excision have been described.

Minor Complications

One of the most common minor complications of PEG placement is *wound infection*. It can result from several factors. Patient-related factors include diabetes, obesity, malnutrition, chronic treatment with steroids and failure to provide prophylactic antibiotics. Technique-related factors include the fact that push or pull techniques are more likely to lead to wound infection than the introducer technique. The majority of infections are minor. Treatment of local wound infection includes wound care and IV antibiotics administration. Most wound infections will respond to first generation cephalosporin or quinolone. Major infections requiring surgical intervention are relatively rare (Lin et al, 2001).

Excessive drainage around the tube and enlargement of the gastrostomy site may occur for several different reasons. Lateral torsion against the sides of the PEG tract or excess tension applied to the PEG tube can result in localized ischemia and ulceration leading to tract enlargement and excessive drainage. Excessive leakage around the tube can occur from other factors, such as the use of corrosive agents and continuous use of hydrogen peroxide around the stoma and cutaneous fungal infection. The development of exophytic granulation tissue around the stoma can also result in excessive leakage. Stomal enlargement can be managed either by using a skin level device or a clipping device to hold the tube, which will reduce the pivoting action or side torsion of the tube. Local infections should be treated with appropriate antifungal agents or zinc oxide. In some cases, PEG tubes will need to be fully removed and placed at a different location. For exophytic granulation, silver nitrate sticks may be used to cauterize the granulation tissue.

Skin maceration or fungal infection around the stoma may be due to a wet environment caused by occlusive dressings. Usually, no dressing is required. Daily cleaning of the stoma and exposure to air will prevent fungal infection. Antifungal cream may be required to treat the infection.

Pneumoperitoneum is common post-PEG placement. It results from leakage of air into the peritoneal cavity during procedure. In the absence of peritonitis, it has no consequence and should not preclude feeding.

Clogging of the *feeding tube* from medication or the enteral formula is a common problem. Flushing the tube with a declogging agent composed of a viokase tablet and 650 mg of sodium bicarbonate tablet crushed in 10 mL of warm water can usually open the tube. If this fails, a PEG tube brush can be used.

Some patients develop nausea and vomiting after PEG placement, which may be due to transient gastroparesis. In rare cases, ileus may develop with or without significant gastric distension. Decompression of stomach by opening the PEG tube, followed by careful initiation of tube feeding and gradual advancement as tolerated should be sufficient in resolving the ileus.

Diarrhea is a common, albeit poorly defined, complication of enteral feeding that has many potential causes. Antibiotics, sorbitol-containing products, altered bacterial flora, formula composition, and hypoalbuminemia are some of the potential causes. Careful attention should also be paid to fluid and electrolyte management to minimize metabolic complications related to enteral feeding.

PEG-J or Direct-PEJ Tube

Patients intolerant to intragastric feeds need to have a postpyloric feeding tube. This is often due to a combination of gastroesophageal reflux, poor gastric motility, recurrent vomiting, and/or concern for pulmonary aspiration. One advantage of jejunal feeding includes reduction in the risk of aspiration, it is more beneficial for critically ill patients as nearly 15 to 60% of these patients are likely to have gastric feed intolerance (Heyland et al, 2001). In case of acute pancreatitis, jejunal feeding minimizes the stimulation of exocrine pancreatic secretions and helps to speed recovery and reduce overall complications.

The main disadvantage of a PEJ tube is difficulty in initial placement and subsequent proximal displacement. Some patients experience intolerance to feeding from rapid delivery of formula into the jejunum causing symptoms similar to that of dumping syndrome.

PEG-J and direct PEJ can be placed either endoscopically or surgically. The complications from PEG-J are the same as those of PEG. The most unique complication related to PEG-J is migration of the jejunal tube from the small bowel (SB) back into the stomach. Another complication is intermittent SB obstruction caused by the large balloon type internal bolster.

Benefits of Enteral Nutrition

Feeding the gut has several advantages over parenteral nutrition (PN), especially in critically ill patients. Enteral nutrition (EN) helps preserve the structural and functional integrity of the gut. Structural integrity of the gut is maintained by increasing mucosal mass, stimulating epithelial proliferation, and by maintaining villus height. Functional integrity is supported by the EN through its effects on maintaining tight junctions between the cells and therefore preventing translocation of bacteria. Enteral feeding stimulates the blood flow to the gut and also helps in production of a variety of endogenous agents like cholecystokinin, bombesin, and gastrin, all of which have trophic effects on the epithelial cells. Feeding also stimulates immunoglobulin A, which coats bacteria and prevents their adherence to the mucosa, which, in turn, prevents the initiation of the inflammatory cascade. In the setting of major trauma or insult, alimentary exclusion may impair the functional and structural integrity of the gut and can result in bacterial translocation and hence significant systemic infection.

Critically ill patients and patients with major trauma benefit the most from EN. In the critically injured patient, increasing evidence suggest that enteral feeding is important in reducing septic complications such as pneumonia and intra-abdominal abscess. A meta-analysis of eight prospective studies of trauma patients and general surgery patients has concluded that septic complications occurred less commonly in patients with enteral feeding compared to those receiving PN support (Kudsk, 2002).

Nutrition is an important adjuvant therapy for IBD patients to help improve malnutrition. More recent data suggest a role for nutrition as a therapeutic agent using *enteral formula* fortified with *antiinflammatory cytokines* such as *transforming growth factor-β*. There is a separate chapter on PN and EN (see Chapter 54, "Enteral and Parenteral Nutrition").

Timing of EN appears to be important. Instituting enteral feeding within 24 to 48 hours after severe trauma has beneficial effects, whereas delaying 4 to 5 days may be too late to gain these benefits. It is our usual practice to begin tube feeding into the stomach or SB in intensive care unit patients within 24 to 48 hours of admission. Many patients will ultimately recover and eat normally. Patients with problems such as serious head injury, however, may ultimately need to have a PEG placed for long term nutritional support.

The Harris-Benedict formula or a simplistic equation (such as 25 kcal/kg/d) is useful to estimate the amount of calories needed. Once the goal rate has been reached, evaluation with nitrogen balance or indirect calorimetry can help to achieve optimal feeding rate. In general, stressed patients should receive 1.5 to 2 g protein/kg/d with 30 to 35 nonprotein kcal/kg/d, whereas nonstressed patients should receive 1.0 to 1.5 g protein/kg/d and 25 to 30 nonprotein kcal/kg/d.

Several specialized enteral formulas are now available to meet the needs of a variety of patients. Different formulas contain varying degrees of protein, carbohydrate, and fat, depending on the patient's underlying disease process and requirements. Standard formulas contain 50 to 55% carbohydrates, 15 to 20% protein, and 30% fat, the caloric density is ≥ 1 kcal/mL, and the osmolality is close to isotonic (between 280 and 350 mOsm/L). Carbohydrates are in the form of oligosacchrides and polysaccharides. Most of enteral formulas do not contain lactose, avoiding the most common disaccharidase deficiency. Proteins are derived from whey, meat, soy isolates, and various caseinates. Fats are usually supplied by vegetable oils and medium chain triglycerides. Numerous other lipids such as fish oils, borage oil, and structured lipids may be substituted. Fiber is added to some formulas for avoidance of diarrhea. Elemental diets and semi-elemental small peptide formulas may be useful in selected patients with poor SB nutrient absorption. As mentioned, there is a chapter devoted to PN and EN (see Chapter 54).

Ethical Issues with PEG Tube and Artificial Nutritional Support

Obtaining enteral access and feeding patients with a perceived poor quality of life raise a number of medicolegal considerations and ethical issues. This is especially true for the PEG procedure where the endoscopist often serves only as a technician for enteral access, not knowing the patient or family prior to PEG evaluation and without a major role in the subsequent nutritional therapy or follow-up care. Even though PEG placement is a safe procedure with very low mortality, PEG tube outcome can be disappointing in some patients (usually due to the underlying disease process). In determining which patients should receive supplemental feeding through PEG tubes, perceived changes in quality of life, anticipated outcome, and cultural, personal, and religious beliefs, are all factors that have to be taken into consideration (Angus and Burakoff, 2003).

Patients with neurologic injury and dysphagia with increased chance for recovery are excellent candidates for PEG placement. On the other hand, patients with advanced dementia or incurable metastatic cancer may not be good candidates. The benefit of PEG placement in this later group is not as clear, the physician and the patient's family should not have unrealistic expectations, and the ultimate decision for PEG placement may not be made on firm scientific data alone.

Although PEG placement should not be expected to affect aspiration of contaminated oropharyngeal secretions, diverting the level of feeding from the mouth to a lower level in GI tract probably does decrease risk of gastroesophageal reflux and ultimately aspiration pneumonia. PEG placement to help heal pressure sores is more controversial. Empiric sense and previous literature would suggest that improving nutritional status should improve wound healing. However, in the population at risk for decubitus pressure sores, PEG placement is often accompanied by increased use of restraints. Also, PEG placement does not guarantee that nutritional requirements will be met. As a result of these factors, there is often imperceivable improvement in the healing of pressure sores. In dementia, PEG placement probably does not improve quality of life for the patients. However, care of the patient is probably more manageable, and often, families and caregivers report improved quality of life as a result of PEG placement. Most studies confirm that mortality and morbidity associated with PEG placement is not any worse in the population of patients with dementia. Mortality is related to the underlying disease process. Nonetheless, again physicians and families should not have unrealistic expectations about prolonged survival as a result of PEG placement.

Unfortunately, regulations and requirements for nursing home placement often necessitate PEG placement. Ultimately, the physician should be knowledgeable of the issues, participate in informed consent, describe realistic expectations for the procedure, and then support the wishes of the family and the concept of patient autonomy in the final decision for PEG placement.

Supplemental Reading

Angus F, Burakoff R. The percutaneous endoscopic gastrostomy tube: medical and ethical issues in placement. Gastroenterol 2003;98:272–7.

Foutch PG, VanSonnenberg E, Tolbert GA. Complications of endoscopic percutaneous gastrostomy and jejunostomy: recognition, prevention and treatment. Gastrointest Endosc Clin N Am 1992;2:231–9.

Gossner L, Keymling J, Hahn EG. Antibiotic prophylaxis in percutaneous endoscopic gastrostomy(PEG): a prospective randomized clinical trial. Endoscopy 1999;31:119–24.

Heyland DK, Drover JW, McDonald S, et al. Effects of postpyloric feeding on gastroesophageal regurgitation and pulmonary microaspiration: result of randomized controlled trial. Critical Care Med 2001;29:1495–501.

Hogan RB, DeMarco DC, Hamilton JK et al. Percutaneous endoscopic gastrostomy—to pull or push? A prospective randomized trial. Gastrointes Endosc 1986;32:253–8.

Kudsk KA. Current aspects of mucosal of mucosal immunology and its influence by nutrition. Am J Surg 2002;183:390–439.

Lin HS, Ibrahim HZ, Kheng W, et al. Percutaneous endoscopic gastrostomy: strategies for prevention and management of complications. The Laryngoscope 2001;111:1847–52.

McClave SA, Chang WK. Complications of enteral access. Gastrointest Endosc 2003;58:739–51.

Russel TR, Brotman M, Norris F. Percutaneous gastrostomy. A new simplified and cost effective tecnique. Am J Surg 1984;148:132–7.

Safadi BY, Marks JM, Ponskey JL. Percutaneous endoscopic gastrostomy. Gastrointestinal Endos Clinic N Am 1998;8:551–68.

CHAPTER 33

PRIMARY GASTRIC LYMPHOMA

LUIS A. HERRERA, PHD, YINKA DAVIS, MD, AND JULIE PARSONNET, MD

Definition and Epidemiological Data

Primary gastric lymphoma (PGL) belongs to the group of non–Hodgkin's lymphomas that are malignant clonal diseases of the lymphatic system. Gastric lymphomas are considered primary when the stomach is predominantly involved and the intra-abdominal lymphadenopathy, if present, corresponds to the expected lymphatic drainage of the stomach. Patients with palpable subcutaneous nodes, mediastinal lymphadenopathy, or abnormal leukocytes on peripheral blood smear or bone marrow aspirates are not categorized as having PGL. The criteria also exclude those with splenic or liver involvement. These strict criteria exclude many advanced cases, which can result in an underestimate of the frequency of the disease. Most PGL are B-cell in origin, although occasional cases of T-cell and Hodgkin's lymphoma are seen. Although there are several clinico-pathological entities of PGL (eg, *mantle cell lymphoma, lymphocytic lymphoma* [chronic lymphocytic leukemia], and *follicular lymphoma*), a significant proportion of PGL is of low grade histology and arises from *mucosal-associated lymphoid tissue (MALT)*. Normal stomachs do not contain this type of organized lymphoid tissue.

PGL is a rare malignancy occurring in only 1 in 30,000 to 1 in 80,000 of the US population per year. This malignancy represents approximately 2 to 7% of primary gastric tumors and 20% of all primary extranodal lymphomas according to the End Results Groups Cancer Registries in the United States (Aisenberg, 1995). Some recent, well-structured, epidemiological studies have found that the incidence of PGL has increased during the last two decades worldwide. An analysis performed in demographically comparable communities of the United Kingdom and Italy revealed a higher incidence of PGL in northeastern Italy than in the corresponding UK communities, suggesting the existence of geographic variations in the incidence of PGL (Doglioni et al, 1992). Gastric lymphomas occur predominantly in individuals over 50 years of age, with a peak in the seventh decade, but the disease can occur at any age. The male to female ratio is approximately 1.7:1. Because MALT lymphomas are by large the most common pathological entity among all PGLs, this chapter will focus on them.

Histopathology

Low grade MALT lymphomas, recently reclassified as *"extranodal marginal zone lymphomas of MALT-type,"* usually have a very favorable clinical course (Harris et al, 1999). Some MALT tumors may undergo high grade transformation. High grade diffuse large B-cell lymphomas may also arise de novo. Histologically, MALT lymphoma cells infiltrate reactive follicles in the region corresponding to the follicle's marginal zone, spreading diffusely into surrounding mucosa. The tumor cells may resemble germinal center centrocytes or small lymphocytes, or they may assume a monocyte-like appearance. An important feature of MALT lymphomas is the presence of lymphoepithelial lesions formed by invasion of individual glands by aggregates of lymphoma cells (Figures 33-1 and 33-2). The presence of scattered transformed blasts, plasma cell differentiation (which is maximal beneath the surface epithelium), and follicular colonization are characteristics of MALT lymphomas that indicate the cells of low grade gastric MALT lymphoma may be participating in an immune response. MALT lymphoma cells typically sur-

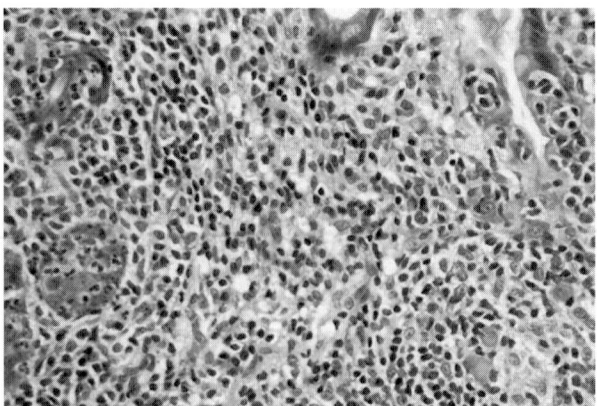

FIGURE 33-1. Active *Helicobacter pylori* gastritis complicated by a low grade extranodal marginal zone B-cell lymphoma (Mucosal-Associated Lymphoid Tissue [MALT] lymphoma). Note the neutrophils in the glands to the left and the atypical lymphocytes infiltrating and destroying the gland in the upper right hand corner (lymphoepithelial lesion). Figure donated by Professor Roger A. Warnke of the School of Medicine at Stanford University.

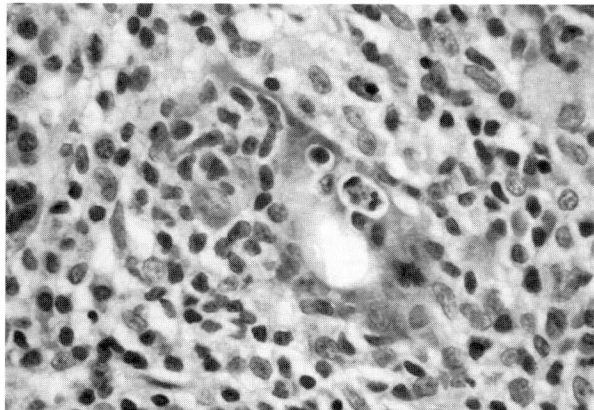

FIGURE 33-2. High magnification of a lymphoepithelial lesion. The gland in the center is being destroyed by the lymphoma cells. One of the epithelial cells is in mitosis. The surrounding lymphomatous infiltrate is composed of round and angulated lymphocytes together with occasional large lymphocytes, histiocytes, and plasma cells. Figure donated by Professor Roger A. Warnke of the School of Medicine at Stanford University.

round reactive B-cell follicles in the distribution of the marginal zone and show a tendency to involve this zone when they disseminate to the lymph nodes and spleen. The B-cells of MALT lymphoma share the cytological features and immunophenotypes of marginal zone B-cells (CD20$^+$, CD21$^+$, CD35$^+$, immunoglobulin [Ig]M$^+$, and IgD$^-$).

The primary lesion is submucosal and originates from the lymphoid tissue in the lamina propria. The invasion occurs outward though the serosa, invading the mucosa during the latter part of the disease process. The most commonly affected site is the *antrum* with the pylorus spared. The entire stomach or multifocal sites may be involved in 5 to 23% of cases. Grossly, the appearance of MALT lymphomas varies from small mucosal ulcerations to large fungating polypoidal masses. Lesions tend to be large with 30% of lymphoma lesions being > 10 cm. The tumor can occasionally take on the characteristics of a diffuse infiltrative process resembling linitis plastica.

Involvement of lymph nodes usually precedes distant metastases. The involvement of adjacent organ ranges from 7 to 29%, with the most common sites being the pancreas, omentum, and spleen. The colon can be occasionally involved with the development of a gastrocolic fistula as a secondary complication of PGL. It has been suggested that dissemination of MALT lymphoma is fostered by the mucosal homing receptor integrin, which is strongly expressed by secondary MALT lymphomas but not by the primary gastric lesion. High levels of integrin expression can also be induced in gastric lymphoma cells following activation by a *Helicobacter pylori* generated T-cell response. The ligand for integrin is the mucosal addressin cell adhesion molecule that is expressed both in the gastric mucosal and splenic marginal zones (Dogan et al, 1997).

Pathogenesis

H. pylori and PGL

It was recognized in 1988 that the cause of acquired gastric MALT is a chronic infection associated with the antigenic *H. pylori*. The first epidemiological studies, in the early 1990s, demonstrated that seropositivity to *H. pylori* was associated with a six-fold increased risk of subsequent gastric lymphoma; an increasing body of evidence has accumulated to strongly support this association (Parsonnet et al, 1994). Other studies validated the dependence of the incidence of MALT lymphoma on the *H. pylori* infection rate. Surgical specimens of gastric MALT lymphoma demonstrated *H. pylori* gastritis in > 90% of the cases. Most strikingly, cure of *H. pylori* infection results in rapid regression and possible cure of most early MALT tumors and even some higher grade tumors.

Molecular Events

The molecular events fundamental for MALT lymphoma pathogenesis have been partially dissected. One of the first steps along this pathway is the acquisition of organized lymphoid tissue after a chronic antigenic stimulation by *H. pylori*. During the prolonged period of lymphoid tissue reactive proliferation, an abnormal B-cell clone arises and replaces the normal population. MALT lymphoma then develops through a series of genetic lesions underlying the progression from a *H. pylori*-dependent lymphoma—with the presence of *H. pylori* strain specific T cells necessary for the growth of lymphoma cells—to a *H. pylori*-independent lesion (Cavalli et al, 2001; Bertoni et al, 2002).

Thirty to 50% of low grade MALT lymphomas carry the t(11;18)(q21;q21) translocation, which is not detected in any other lymphomas, even in MALT lymphomas with large cell components and primary gastric diffuse large B-cell lymphomas. The translocation results in the expression of a chimeric transcript that fuses the apoptosis inhibitor-2 (API2) gene on chromosome 11 to a gene on chromosome 18 called MALT lymphoma translocation (MLT). The normal function of the protein encoded by API2 is to arrest apoptosis. The three domains necessary to suppress apoptosis are always conserved in the chimeric transcript, while its zinc finger domain, which may act as a negative regulator of the apoptosis inhibition, is consistently absent. The function of MLT is still unknown, but it appears to play a role in sub-cellular localization of the chimeric product, which in turn is likely to increase the antiapoptotic effect of API2. The encoded protein contains two immunoglobulin-like C2-type domains, a region homologous with laminin 5α3β, and a domain similar to the mouse immunoglobulin chain VDJ4 sequence. The proportion of MLT that is fused in the expressed transcript is highly variable, due to the varied breakpoints on chromosome 18q.

The t(11;18) appears to be associated with more aggressive clinical behavior. The *translocation* was present in only 3 of 29 gastric MALT lymphomas confined to the gastric wall but in most of those that disseminated beyond the stomach. Moreover, there is some evidence that it might *predict* the *therapeutic response* of gastric MALT lymphoma to *H. pylori* eradication. In one study, this translocation was absent in all gastric MALT lymphomas that showed complete regression, but it was detected in most of nonresponsive tumors, including cases with the disease confined to the gastric wall.

The other recurring chromosomal translocation is t(1;14)(p22;q32) with involvement of BCL-10 on chromosome 1 and the immunoglobulin heavy chain gene on chromosome 14. Wild type BCL-10 is an apoptotic regulatory molecule and acts as a tumor suppressor gene. Aberrant BCL-10 expression occurs frequently without the t(1;14). The combination of t(11;18) and nuclear BCL-10 expression has been reported in advanced gastric MALT lymphomas.

Clinical Presentation and Management

Diagnosis of PGL is often difficult because symptoms are typically vague and nonspecific. The most common presenting symptom is dyspepsia and epigastric pain (Frazee and Roberts, 1992). Nausea, vomiting, perforation, bleeding, and obstruction are uncommon. Thirty percent to 50% of patients with lymphoma that extends to the small bowel initially present with an abdominal emergency (Stephens and Smith, 1998). Lymphadenopathy is rare. Erythema, erosions and ulcers are commonly visualized upon endoscopy, usually in the location of the antrum, and, less frequently, multifocal disease can also be present.

Clinical Staging

Grading of malignancy and staging of disease are the decisive factors that influence the therapeutic modalities in PGL. Staging of gastric lymphomas should include computed tomography (CT) scans of the chest abdomen and pelvis, which demonstrate the extent of the lesion and rule out metastatic disease from a nongastric primary site. Localized GI lymphoma frequently displaces, rather than invades, associated vascular structures. The limitations of CT are the difficulties in differentiating between metastatic lymphadenopathy and reactive lymphoid hyperplasia. A bone marrow biopsy and routine blood test to include lactate dehydrogenase (LDH) should be included in the initial evaluation. Small bowel radiography series demonstrates a potentially malignant lesion in approximately 75% of cases, with the most common finding being enlarged configured gastric folds (Stephens and Smith, 1998). Endoscopy and colonoscopy should also be included in the initial examination. The endoscopic findings are generally a diffuse infiltrative process with thick, rigid folds that do not distend with the aid of insufflation (Nakamura et al, 1995).

The Ann Arbor staging criteria are widely accepted by most clinicians. However, controversy remains; some clinicians believe that the Lugano staging system is more optimal. The Ann Arbor staging was challenged at the Fifth International Conference on Malignant Lymphoma in 1993 and a new proposal was subsequently recommended (see Table 33-1).

Endoscopic ultrasound (EUS) is by far the best modality for the assessment of the vertical extension of gastric lymphomas, thus defining stages I and II (Fischbach et al, 2002). It is accurate in determining the depth of invasion and the presence of perigastric lymphadenopathy. This technique allows for prognostic information on the probability that a histological remission may be obtained after the eradication of *H. pylori*. EUS is not a sensitive technique to diagnose multifocality and horizontal extension of gastric lymphomas (Caletti et al, 1998). The role of EUS in follow up is yet to be determined.

TABLE 33-1. Staging Classification from the Fifth International Conference on Malignant Lymphoma

Stage	Definition
I	Tumor confined to gastrointestinal tract
II	Tumor extending into abdomen from primary site
II1	Local nodal involvement (perigastric/mesenteric)
II2	Distal nodal involvement (para–aortic/paraclaval)
IIE	Penetration of serosa to involve adjacent structures
IV	Disseminated disease or subdiaphragmatic nodal involvement

From Rohatiner et al, 1994.

Therapy

H. pylori Eradication Therapy

H. pylori testing is essential in treating early MALT lymphomas. Testing can be done with a biopsy and histology (with a biopsy preferably obtained from a site without malignancy), breath test, or serology. In infected patients, the first line treatment in all but patients with the largest and most aggressive tumors should be *H. pylori eradication therapy*. Studies have demonstrated a complete remission in about 80% of cases of low grade lymphoma, with a 5% recurrence rate per year (Bayerdörffer et al, 1995). Reports suggest that high grade MALT lymphomas of the salivary glands, duodenum, small intestine, and rectum may also regress with *H. pylori* eradication (Roggero et al, 1995; Wotherspoon et al, 1992). Moreover, some investigators have observed that gastric large cell lymphomas can successfully respond to *H. pylori* eradication therapy and have recommended that treatment with chemotherapy and radiation should be withheld from the initial treatment plan. Of importance is the depth of the lymphoma. Lymphomas infiltrating the mucosa and submucosa are typically treatable with eradication of *H. pylori*. Those infiltrating the deeper layers of the wall have been more refractory to antibiotic therapy. Currently, there is no consensus on the treatment of gastric lymphomas that do not respond to *H. pylori* eradication. Chemotherapy, surgical resection and radiotherapy are some of the treatment modalities that have been used either alone or in combination.

Surgical Therapy

Surgical resection has historically been the mainstay of treatment. Surgery provides the most accurate means of both staging and grading disease. Stage I and stage II disease are more amenable to curative resection with a 52 to 76% success rate in all patients regardless of their staging (De Jong et al, 1999). Failure of resection is usually due to metastatic disease or coexistent morbid conditions. The goal of surgery is to resect the entire tumor with negative margins; the benefit of this must be balanced against the morbidity of the operation and the quality of life expected postsurgery. With the increased use of *H. pylori* treatments, adjuvant therapy, and better understanding of tumor biology, procedures other than surgery are now becoming more widely accepted. Several studies have demonstrated no decrease in survival for patients with involved margins if adjuvant radiation or chemotherapy was given (De Jong et al, 1999).

Chemotherapy and Radiation

Currently, there is much debate about whether chemotherapy and/or radiotherapy should replace surgical resection as the primary treatment modality in tumors that do not respond to antibiotic therapy (Bozzetti et al, 1993). Surgical advocates argue that resection is vital for accurate staging and histological classification, and that having an entire specimen allows the pathologist to adequately evaluate the specimen. With the advances in obtaining biopsies endoscopically and in immunohistopathology, however, these arguments for surgery are becoming less powerful. The main arguments against nonsurgical treatment is that chemotherapy and radiotherapy can lead to *necrosis of the tumor*, resulting in gastric perforation or bleeding. Late complications of radiotherapy, particularly involving the abdominal and retroperitoneal viscera, are also concerns that must be considered. These complications include visceral and ureteric stricture, cystitis, enteritis, anal sphincter dysfunction, and the risk of tumor formation (Brooks and Enterline, 1983).

If disseminated lymphoma involving multiple organs is encountered, surgical cure is unrealistic. The indications for surgery at this stage would be to obtain tissue for diagnosis, repair and visceral perforations and to possibly divert the enteric bowel. Such cases should be directed to chemotherapy and/or radiation.

Palliation

It is often difficult to determine which treatment is best from a review of the recent literature. Results are often comparable in many of the therapeutic regimens. Treatment options should involve the patients, and therapy should be tailored to each individual's needs and preferences. Overall, patients with a diagnosis of *early stage gastric lymphoma* identified on an endoscopic biopsy should be considered for surgical *resection*. This provides local control, which may not be covered by chemotherapy, and allows for correction of possible errors in preoperative staging. Adjuvant chemotherapy plays a role in early stage disease, given that most failures of surgical therapy are extrabdominal. In those patients with evidence of invasion and a definitive biopsy diagnosis, chemotherapy should be considered the mainstay of treatment, with either surgery or radiation providing local control. In patients with nondiagnostic biopsies, surgical exploration and resection need to be considered.

Supplemental Reading

Aisenberg AC. Coherent view of non–Hodgkin's lymphoma. J Clin Oncol 1995;13:2656–75.

Bayerdörffer E, Neubauer A, Rudolph B, et al. Regression of primary gastric lymphoma of mucosa–associated lymphoid tissue type after cure of *Helicobacter pylori* infection. Lancet 1995;1345:1591–4.

Bertoni F, Cavalli F, Cotter FE, Zucca E. Genetic alterations underlying the pathogenesis of MALT lymphoma. Hematol J 2002;3:10–3.

Bozzetti F, Audisio RA, Giardini R, et al. Role of surgery in patients with primary non–Hodgkin's lymphoma of the stomach: an old problem revisted. Br J Surg 1993;80:1101–6.

Brooks, JJ, Enterline HT. Primary gastric lymphomas: a clincopathologic study of 58 cases with long-term follow-up and literature review. Cancer 1983;51:701–11.

Caletti G, Fusaroli P, Bocus P. Endoscopic ultrasonography. Digestion 1998;59:509–29.

Cavalli F, Isaacson PG, Gascoyne RD, et al. MALT Lymphomas. Hematology (Am Soc Hematol Educ Program) 2001;241–58.

De Jong D, Aleman BMP, Taal BG, et al. Controversies and consensus in the diagnosis, work-up and treatment of gastric lymphoma: an international survey. Ann Oncol 1999;10:275–80.

Dogan A, Du M, Koulis A, et al. Expression of lymphocyte homing receptors and vascular addressins in low–grade gastric B-cell lymphomas of mucosa–associated lymphoid tissue. Am J Pathol 1997;151:1361–9.

Doglioni C, Wotherspoon AC, Moschini A, et al. High incidence of primary gastric lymphoma in northeastern Italy. Lancet 1992;339:834–5.

Fischbach W, Goebeler–Kolve ME, Greiner A. Diagnostic accuracy of EUS in the local staging of primary gastric lymphoma: result of a prospective, multicenter study comparing EUS with histopathologic stage. Gastrointest Endosc 2002;56:696–700.

Frazee RC, Roberts J. Gastric lymphoma treatment: medical versus surgical. Surg Clin North Am 1992;72:423–31.

Harris NL, Jaffe ES, Diebold J, et al. The World Health Organization classification of neoplastic diseases of the hematopoietic and lymphoid tissues. Report of the Clinical Advisory Committee meeting, Airlie House, Virginia, November, 1997. Ann Oncol 1999;10:1419–32.

Nakamura S, Akazawa K, Yao T, et al. A clinicopathologic study of 233 cases with special reference to evaluation with MIB–1 index. Cancer 1995;76:1313–24.

Parsonnet J, Hansen S, Rodriguez L, et al. *Helicobacter pylori* infection and gastric lymphoma. N Engl J Med 1994;330:1267–71.

Roggero E, Zucca E, Pinotti G, et al. Eradication of *Helicobacter pylori* infection in primary low–grade gastric lymphoma of mucosa–associated lymphoid tissue. Ann Intern Med 1995;122:767–9.

Rohatiner A, d'Amore F, Coiffier B, et al. Report on a workshop convened to discuss the pathological and staging classifications of gastrointestinal tract lymphoma. Ann Oncol 1994;5:397–400.

Stephens J, Smith J. Treatment of primary gastric lymphoma and gastric mucosa–associated tissue lymphoma. J Am Coll Surg 1998;197:312–20.

Wotherspoon AC, Doglioni C, Diss TC, et al. Regression of primary low–grade B–cell gastric lymphoma of mucosa associated lymphoid tissue type after eradication of *Helicobacter pylori*. Lancet 1992;342:575–77.

CHAPTER 34

Gastric Cancer

Daniel M. Labow, MD, and Murray F. Brennan, MD

Gastric cancer (GC) is an international health problem with an incidence approaching 800,000 people per year. Although uncommon in North America (25,000 cases per year), GC carries a poor prognosis, with more than 12,000 deaths estimated in 2002 (Jemal et al, 2002). This poor outcome is attributed to advanced stage at diagnosis, which precludes a curative resection. However, in the United States patients are being diagnosed at an earlier stage. Gastric adenocarcinoma (AC) is the predominant histology (~95%), followed by leiomyosarcoma/gastrointestinal stomal tumors, lymphoma, and carcinoid. The incidence of gastroesophageal (GE) junction malignancy has risen steadily over the past decade. The treatment and behavior of this disease differs from "true" GC and, thus, for the purposes of this chapter, we will focus on the management of primary gastric AC. There are separate chapters on Barrett's esophagus (Chapter 14, "Barret's Esophagus") esophageal cancer (Chapter 22, "Palliation of Esophageal Cancer"), and on gastric lymphoma (Chapter 33, "Primary Gastric Lymphoma").

Risk Factors

Advanced age, a diet low in fresh fruits and vegetables, alcohol and tobacco consumption, and chronic gastritis with or without associated *Helicobacter pylori* infection are all associated with an increased risk of developing GC. A familial predisposition for developing GC, termed hereditary diffuse gastric cancer (HDGC), has been identified and linked to a mutation in the E-cadherin (*CDH1*) gene. HDGC is characterized by autosomal dominant inheritance, diffuse or multifocal spread, and early age of onset, with cases reported in patients as young as 16 years. This has prompted the controversial recommendation for early, prophylactic gastrectomy for at risk family members (Lewis et al, 2001).

Diagnosis

An important factor in diagnosing GC is a high index of suspicion. Attention to signs and symptoms of gastric pathology, including dyspepsia, gastritis, ulcer disease, early satiety, and weight loss, is important. GC is rarely diagnosed on physical examination, except with widely metastatic disease. Upper endoscopy is the standard for establishing the diagnosis, and clinicians should have a low threshold to recommend endoscopy to patients with suspicious symptoms or from high risk populations. At endoscopy, any suspicious lesions, including ulcers, inflamed areas or masses, should be carefully examined and biopsies should be performed in multiple areas. Special attention to the stomach's shape, mucosal appearance, and distensibility is essential to pick up the more occult, diffuse-type GC, which may be confined to the submucosa and missed on endoscopy.

A number of serum markers have been described in GC, including CEA, CA19–9, and CA72–4 (Marrelli et al, 1999), though none have proven to be sensitive or specific enough to warrant routine use. Gene microarray analysis has implicated a number of gene products, including *TP53* mutations, cell cycle regulators, and ribosomal and mitochondrial proteins, but are currently of research interest only. If the patient is young or has a significant family history, genetic counseling and testing for the *CDH1* gene mutation should be considered.

After the histologic diagnosis of GC has been established, accurate staging of the patient is necessary to make appropriate treatment recommendations and provide definitive therapy.

Preoperative Work-up

After confirmation of the diagnosis of gastric AC, an accurate preoperative work-up is needed to guide the patient down the appropriate treatment algorithm (Figure 34-1). Endoscopic ultrasound (EUS) is the most accurate mode to determine T-stage. Additionally, perigastric lymph nodes and adjacent organ and vascular involvement can be assessed. A computed tomography (CT) scan of the abdomen provides information regarding extragastric disease, which most commonly occurs in the peritoneal cavity or liver. If the lesion was excised at endoscopy and found to be an early T1 or T2 cancer, EUS and CT scans are not necessary, and the patient can be prepared for definitive treatment. For T3 and T4 lesions, a staging laparoscopy should be performed due to the increased chance of metastatic or locally, advanced disease. If metastases are seen on

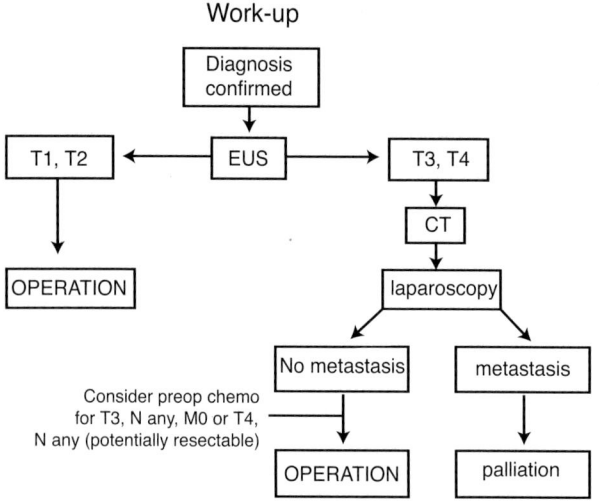

FIGURE 34-1. Treatment algorithm for patients with gastric cancer. CT = computed tomography; EUS = endoscopic ultrasound.

laparoscopy, then a biopsy should be taken and the patient should be referred for palliative chemotherapy. If no metastases are seen, then preoperative chemotherapy in the context of a clinical trial should be considered before definitive surgical therapy. The use of positron emission tomography scans as part of the preoperative work-up is investigational and should be evaluated in the setting of a protocol.

Surgical Management

In patients with early or localized GC, surgical resection remains the only effective therapy for cure. Controversy exists as to the extent of gastric resection and lymphadenectomy, and the value of adjacent organ resection.

Our surgical approach is summarized in Table 34-1. For very early GC (Tis or T1, N0), tailoring the extent of resection to minimize morbidity can be considered. Endoscopic mucosal resection (EMR) has been advocated, particularly in patients with significant comorbidity. This technique is relatively poorly developed in North America and applied more frequently in Asia. There is a separate chapter on EMR (Chapter 6). The endoscopic technique involves injecting saline submucosally to separate the mucosal lesion from the underlying muscularis propria and serosa of the stomach. The lesion is then removed with a 1 cm margin. An alternative is a minimally invasive or laparoscopic approach. Both of these techniques require accurate preoperative localization of the lesion and checking the specimen intraoperatively to ensure complete resection. No long term data exist regarding the survival and local recurrence rates of GC after a "limited" resection.

For patients with *T3, N any or T4, N any (potentially resectable)* disease, *laparoscopy* should be considered to rule out metastatic disease and the patient should be *considered* for *investigational preoperative chemotherapy*. If there is no evidence of metastatic disease on laparoscopy, then a *definitive resection* is performed. Location and size of the lesion determine the extent of resection. Traditionally, *5 to 6 cm* is considered the minimum *acceptable margin*.

Extent of Gastric Resection

Controversy exists as to the appropriate *extent* of gastric resection. There are three choices: (1) *total gastrectomy*, (2) *distal subtotal gastrectomy*, or (3) *proximal subtotal gastrectomy*. A number of prospective trials have examined the extent of gastric resection comparing total gastrectomy with distal subtotal gastrectomy (Gouzi et al, 1989; Bozzetti et al, 1999). None of these studies showed an improved survival based on the extent of gastric resection, though there was increased morbidity with total gastrectomy. For *proximal* lesions, *total gastrectomy* is the traditional choice, although a *proximal gastrectomy* is reasonable if anatomy allows a tension-free, well-perfused gastric remnant. At Memorial Sloan-Kettering Cancer Center (MSKCC), a retrospective review of a prospectively maintained database comparing proximal subtotal with total gastrectomy for cardia and fundus GCs revealed no difference in survival or morbidity between the two groups (Harrison et al, 1998). For larger lesions or those occupying the entire body of the stomach, *total gastrectomy* is necessary. For distal body and/or antral lesions, a *distal, subtotal gastrectomy* is performed.

Extent of Lymph Node Dissection

The extent of lymph node dissection for GC has generated much debate over the past few decades. The extent of lymphadenectomy ranges from limited (D0, D1) to extensive (D3, D4). A D1 dissection involves removal of the perigastric nodes along the lesser and greater curvature of the stomach. A D0 dissection is any removal of lymph nodes

TABLE 34-1. Surgical Management

Preoperative Stage	Laparoscopy?	Neo-adjuvant Therapy?	Extent of Gastric Resection		Nodal Dissection
T$_{1-2}$, N$_0$, M$_0$	No	No	Laparoscopic Local resection		None
			EMR		None
			Open (limited)		D0/D1
T$_3$, N$_{any}$, M$_0$	Yes	Consider	SITE		
			Proximal	TG	D2
T$_4$, N$_{any}$, M$_0$ (potentially resectable disease)	Yes Entire body	Consider TG		PG	
			D2		
			Distal body Antrum	DST	D2

DST = distal, subtotal gastrectomy; EMR = endoscopic mucosal resection; PG = proximal gastrectomy; TG = total gastrectomy.

less than a D1. A D2 dissection involves a D1 dissection plus nodes along the left gastric, common hepatic, splenic arteries, and celiac trunk. D3 adds dissection of lymph nodes along the hepatoduodenal ligament and root of the mesentery, and D4 adds paraaortic and paracolic nodes.

The debate on how extensive a lymphadenectomy is necessary has generated interest in sentinel lymph node biopsy. Proponents of this technique argue that the variable gastric lymphatic anatomy occasionally accounts for lymph node metastases in areas outside the traditional area of lymphadenectomy and, thus, might alert the surgeon to remove nodes that would not otherwise be resected. Currently, this should be considered experimental.

A number of retrospective studies have reported an improved survival in patients who undergo an extended lymph node dissection. These studies have led to extended lymphadenectomy as the standard of care in the majority of Asian centers. Prospective trials have failed to support these findings. Both the Dutch Gastric Cancer Group and the Medical Research Council studies were prospective randomized, multicenter trials designed to examine the benefit of extended of lymph node dissection for gastric AC (Bonenkamp et al, 1999; Cuschieri et al, 1999). Both studies showed equivalent survival between the two groups but significantly increased morbidity, particularly in patients who underwent pancreaticosplenectomy. Recent analysis suggests a small survival benefit for patients with T3 lesions in the Dutch trial. At MSKCC, we have shown equivalent morbidity when comparing D1 and D2 lymphadenectomy. To ensure an adequate number of lymph nodes sampled and with the understanding that improved survival has been shown to be associated with greater than 15 lymph nodes removed, it *is our practice* to perform a *D2 lymphadenectomy without pancreaticosplenectomy for all T3 or greater lesions. For T1 or T2 lesions, a D0 or D1 lymph node dissection* is adequate.

Regardless of the type of gastric resection or lymphadenectomy, the postoperative management is similar. A feeding jejunostomy is not routine. When the patient is passing flatus an oral diet is started. We encourage the patient to eat whatever he can tolerate and do not recommend restrictive "postgastrectomy" diets. Frequent small, high caloric meals work best to prevent significant weight loss and for rapid postoperative recovery.

Adjuvant Therapy

For patients with T1 or T2, N0 disease, surgical resection alone provides definitive treatment. For T3, N any or T4, N any (potentially resectable) disease, laparoscopy should be performed before resection and *investigational neoadjuvant therapy* should be considered if no metastatic disease is found. If the postoperative pathology reveals a T3 or T4, N any lesion, *adjuvant therapy* should be given. Table 34-2 summarizes our approach for adjuvant therapy. The recent

TABLE 34-2. Adjuvant Therapy

Stage	Preop Chemo/XRT?	Postop Chemo/XRT?
T_{1-2}, N_0, M_0	No	No
T_3, N_{any}, M_0	Consider	Yes (clinical trial)
T_4, N_{any}, M_0	Consider (if resectable)	Yes (clinical trial, if resectable)

*T_4, N_{any}, M_0 = unresectable; T_{any}, N_{any}, M_1 = palliative chemotherapy only.

Intergroup 0116 trial included patients with Stage 1B to Stage IV, M0 who were randomized to surgery alone versus surgery plus 4500 cGy and 5–FU, leucovorin (Macdonald et al, 2001). This was the first multicenter trial to demonstrate a *survival advantage* for GC patients after receiving adjuvant therapy (3-year survival of 50% versus 41%, $p < .05$). *Lack of surgical quality control* was the greatest drawback of the trial; more than half of the patients had less than a D1 lymph node dissection. Based on this trial, adjuvant therapy has been adopted in most institutions as the standard of care for patients who undergo curative resection for GC. *However, as all previous adjuvant trials were negative, the use of adjuvant therapy, whenever possible, should be studied in the setting of a clinical trial.* At our institution, we recommend adjuvant therapy for patients who have undergone complete resection with final pathology of T3-4, N any disease. More evidence is needed to improve our understanding of the benefit of adjuvant therapy for GC.

Neoadjuvant Therapy

Because many GC patients are significantly debilitated postoperatively, neoadjuvant therapy has gained attention as a possible approach for patients with advanced GC. One potential benefit is that patients are more likely to tolerate an aggressive chemoradiotherapy regimen preoperatively. The in situ tumor can be used as an in vivo control to assess response to treatment, downstage the tumor, and to allow resection that was not possible before treatment. These benefits are balanced by the increased operative morbidity that is more likely to occur in a previously irradiated field and the potential for over treatment of patients who will not benefit from this regimen. Trials evaluating both neoadjuvant protocols and adjuvant approaches (intraperitoneal, immunotherapy) are currently ongoing.

Outcome and Follow-up

The tendency for GC to present at advanced stages has led to an overall 5-year survival of 24%, whereas in those patients who undergo a curative resection, overall survival improves to 50%, according to our prospectively maintained GC database. Figures 34-2 and 34-3 show the overall survival rates of resected patients stratified by T-stage and N-stage, respectively. Close follow-up is important in patients with GC, although no standard guidelines exist. Weight maintenance is essential and the importance of adequate postoperative nutrition cannot be overemphasized. A thorough history and physical examination, with attention to signs and symptoms of a possible recurrence (such as ongoing weight loss, dysphagia, abdominal pain, and abdominal masses), should prompt immediate investigation. Because most recurrences occur in the first 2 years postoperatively, we recommend follow-up every 4 months for the first 2 years, then every 6 months for the next 3 years, and yearly thereafter. We usually obtain routine blood work every 4 to 6 months for the first 2 years and then yearly. Repeat endoscopy either annually or biannually is performed, depending on the initial extent of disease. Abdominal CT scans are obtained yearly for 5 years, though no established guidelines exist for this practice. All follow-up regimens should be altered according to patient symptoms and tumor characteristics. It is important to remember vitamin B_{12} injections and folate replacement in all patients who have undergone a total or proximal gastrectomy. If any symptoms develop between postoperative visits, thorough and timely investigation with blood work, radiologic imaging, or endoscopy is warranted.

Recurrent GC/Palliative Care

GC recurrence can be both locoregional (anastomotic, in the gastric resection bed, and in the remaining lymph nodes) or distant (liver, lung, and peritoneal carcinomatosis). *Most* patients *recur in the first 2 years* postoperatively. The patients at highest risk of recurrence are those with *advanced stage* at initial operation (ie, T3/T4 and/or any nodal disease). In a select patient population, *reexploration for locally recurrent GC* is warranted. Patients with a long disease-free interval or initial early stage cancer are the subgroups most likely to benefit from re-resection. In general, operation is rarely indicated for locoregional recurrence and virtually never appropriate for distant recurrence.

Palliative procedures for primary, unresectable or recurrent GCs should be tailored to the symptoms the patient defines as the most debilitating. Bleeding and obstruction are the most common. For gastric outlet obstruction, *endoscopically-placed metallic stents* can spare the patient a laparotomy and are effective at restoring gastrointestinal continuity. Unfortunately, this approach only works for lesions in the proximal stomach, GE junction, or antral lesions. Blood loss is usually chronic and periodic blood transfusions often suffice to support the patient. *Palliative chemotherapy and/or radiation therapy* have roles and have been reported to improve quality of life in some patients. A frank discussion between the patient, the patient's family, and the physician is essential for effective palliation of each individual patient's symptoms.

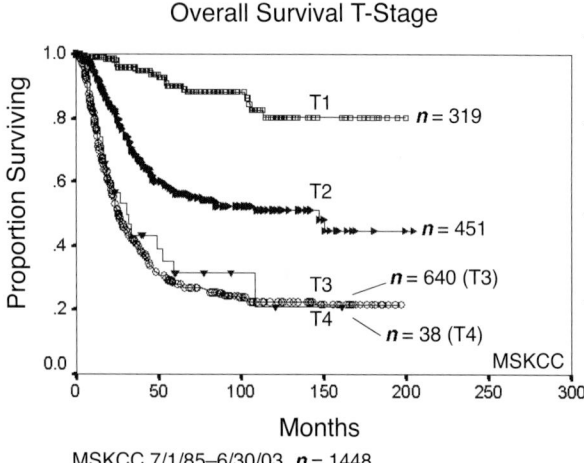

FIGURE 34-2. Kaplan-Meier survival curve for resected patients, stratified by T-stage.

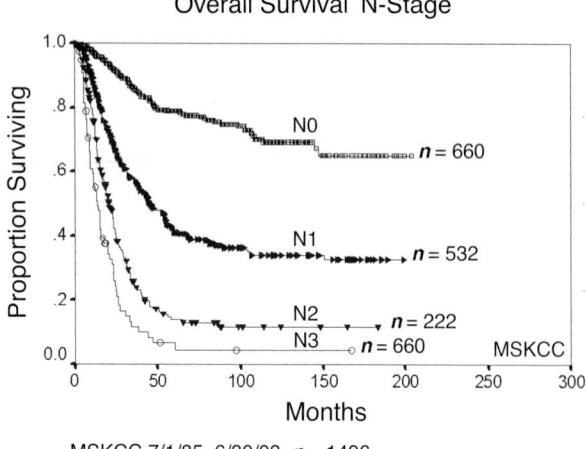

FIGURE 34-3. Kaplan-Meier survival curve for resected patients, stratified by N-stage.

Conclusions

GC is a common disease worldwide, although it is uncommon in North America. Overall survival is poor but improving, with the majority of patients presenting with advanced disease. Surgery is the best treatment for localized disease with recent studies supporting the role of adjuvant chemoradiotherapy to improve survival and decrease local recurrence. Future clinical trials are needed to better our understanding and improve our treatment of this disease.

Supplemental Reading

Bonenkamp JJ, Hermans J, Sasako M, van de Velde CJ. Extended lymph node dissection for gastric cancer. N Engl J Med 1999;340:908–14.

Bozzetti F, Marubini E, Bonfanti G, et al. Subtotal versus total gastrectomy for gastric cancer: five–year survival rates in a multicenter randomized Italian trial. Ann Surg 1999;230:170–8.

Cuschieri A, Weeden S, Fielding J, et al. Patient survival after D1 and D2 resections for gastric cancer: long–term results of the MRC Randomized Surgical Trial. Br J Cancer 1999;79:1522–30.

Gouzi JL, Huguier M, Fagniez PL, et al. Total versus subtotal gastrectomy for adenocarcinoma of the gastric antrum: a French prospective controlled study. Ann Surg 1989;209:162–6.

Harrison LE, Karpeh MS, Brennan MF. Total gastrectomy is not necessary for proximal gastric cancer. Surgery 1998;123:127–30.

Jemal A, Thomas A, Murray T, et al. Cancer statistics, 2002. CA Cancer J Clin 2002;52:23–47.

Lewis FR, Mellinger JD, Hayashi A, et al. Prophylactic total gastrectomy for familial gastric cancer. Surgery 2001;130:612–6.

Macdonald JS, Smalley SR, Benedetti J, et al. Chemoradiotherapy after surgery compared with surgery alone for adenocarcinoma of the stomach or gastroesophageal junction. N Engl J Med 2001;345:725–30.

Marrelli D, Roviello F, De Stefano A, et al. Prognostic significance of CEA, CA19–9, and CA 72–4 preoperative serum levels in gastric carcinoma. Oncology 1999;19:464–9.

CHAPTER 35

OBESITY

LAWRENCE J. CHESKIN, MD

Epidemiology

Obesity has reached epidemic proportions in the United States. In the past generation, the prevalence of obesity has nearly doubled; Sixty-four percent of American adults are now overweight or obese. The recent increase in prevalence is even more dramatic among children and the severely obese, which does not bode well for the future. Indications are that even developing nations are seeing an increase in obesity, in part because of an adoption of Western diet and exercise patterns.

From where does this epidemic come? In the United States, although the percent of kilocalories from fat is decreasing (from a high of 40% to about 33% today), total daily caloric intake is increasing. Coupled with increasing numbers of adults and even children who are sedentary (one-fourth of adults engage in virtually no physical activity aside from activities of daily living). Despite recent discoveries in the molecular genetics of obesity, a major role for genetic influences is not a likely explanation for the rapid recent changes in the prevalence of obesity.

Medical Risks

Obesity is a close second to cigarette smoking as the most important modifiable medical risk factor. It is a significant risk factor for diseases involving essentially every organ system, and even certain cancers (Table 35-1). Obesity is the most important risk factor in the development of type 2 diabetes. The risk of complicating medical conditions increases with the degree of obesity, although for some complications, notably coronary artery disease, type 2 diabetes, and stroke, the risk correlates best with the regional distribution of fat. Central deposition of fat (the "apple-shape" pattern), seen more commonly in men, increases risk, whereas excess fat in the thighs, hips and buttocks, seen more commonly in women (the "pear-shape" pattern), is associated with a lower risk of such conditions.

Obesity also increases overall mortality, and has recently been shown in Framingham and other populations to shorten life expectancy by perhaps 6 years. In addition to the medical risks, and often more motivating for many people seeking to lose weight, are the unfortunate psychosocial consequences of obesity. There is widespread prejudice against obese individuals, even detectable in the opinions of young children. The resulting social and job discrimination contributes to low self-esteem and the high rate of depression among the obese who have sought treatment. Notable also is the greater social stigma borne by obese women compared with obese men in our society, and the higher prevalence of obesity among those of low socioeconomic status, Blacks, and Native Americans.

Definitions

We all know obesity when we see it, but a simple medical definition remains elusive. Obesity is technically defined as an *excess of body fat* (> 25% of body weight for men and > 30% for women) rather than an excess of body weight per se. However, the measurement of percent body fat is difficult and not as intuitive as body weight. Thus, relative weight is a reasonable surrogate measure for the less readily obtained measure of adiposity (percent of body weight constituted by fat).

Weight adjusted for height, or *body mass index* (BMI), defined as weight in kilograms divided by the square of the height in meters, is very useful for defining and grading the severity of obesity and attendant risks. BMI is now the standard measure of relative weight, though it may be a poor reflector of actual degree of adiposity in very muscular individuals (eg, certain types of athletes and laborers). A BMI of 25 to 30 kg/m^2 is defined as overweight, 30 to 40 kg/m^2 as obese, and 40 kg/m^2 as severely/morbidly obese. It is probably best to steer patients away from height-weight tables derived from life insurance data and to *encourage weight loss for medical reasons only*, especially if the patient is young,

TABLE 35-1. Major Health Risks of Obesity

Type 2 diabetes mellitus	Hypertension
Coronary artery disease	Dyslipidemias
Strokes	Carcinoma (especially endometrial, colorectal, esophageal, breast)
Sleep apnea	Gastroesophageal reflux disease
Gallbladder disease	Osteoarthritis
Nonalcoholic fatty liver disease	Infertility
Gout	Thromboembolism

already suffers from complicating medical conditions, or has a strong family history of diabetes or cardiovascular or cerebrovascular disease. For those with *trivial obesity*, the benefits (and motivators) for successful weight loss are perhaps more *psychosocial* than medical. These patients should be encouraged to focus on a healthier *(low refined carbohydrate, low fat, high fiber) diet* and *increased physical fitness* rather than just the number on the scale.

In the case of *abdominal fat deposition*, however, *even mild excess adiposity* may pose a medical problem. A waist circumference of more than 40 inches for men and 35 for women suggests the diagnosis of abdominal obesity and can be easily measured with a tape rule around the narrowest point above the umbilicus. Fortunately, this metabolically active abdominal fat is usually the first to go with weight loss. The pear shape is both safer and more durable than the apple, as many women who attempt to lose weight have learned. From an evolutionary perspective, lower body obesity may have conferred a selective advantage by helping to ensure survival through times of food shortage and being easily mobilized only under the hormonal influences of pregnancy and breastfeeding.

Despite the inescapable fact that *genetic* influences exist (witness adopted twin studies and the increasing number of genetic markers being discovered), genetics does not appear to account for the majority of variability in BMI seen in the population, nor is it an insurmountable barrier in most of those who were fortunate (or unfortunate) enough to draw the genes leading to metabolic efficiency in the lottery of conception. Part of the reason lies in the *learned behaviors*, which are supremely important as modifiers of genetic predisposition and are *good places to focus treatment*.

Treatment

Perhaps no other field of medicine today is as subject to the fads, hype, and unreasonable expectations as the treatment of obesity. There is also the inherent difficulty of reconciling a society whose main fuels are fatty food and ethanol with an ideal body form typified by the Barbie doll. Given that our profession is unlikely to have any say in what body form people are striving for, the next best approach is to lobby for reasonable goal weights for our own patients, encourage those who really need to lose weight to do so, and steer them toward safe, comprehensive treatment.

Realistic Overview

Five components of a comprehensive approach to weight loss are listed in Table 35-2. The omission of any of these items is likely to adversely affect long-term results. The *long-term success rate*, defined as losing weight and keeping most of it off *for 5 years*, is low, perhaps *5 to 15%* in the few studies available. Although this rate is clearly poor, it must be viewed in context and compared with our similarly *poor success in treating other chronic conditions and addictions* (ie, cigarette smoking and drug abuse). In fact, if one views the chronic pleasurable overconsumption of food energy as a kind of addiction, an instructive distinction between food and other reinforcing substances appears. The cigarette smoker need never smoke again; the obese person, however, must learn to coexist with the offending substances in order to live. In this light, the treatment of obesity should be likened not to the cure of an infectious disease but to the *control of a chronic condition*. As such, we *cannot expect many complete cures* and will need to be constantly on the *alert for relapses* in those who appear to be in remission.

Medical Assessment

The first step in treating the obese patient is the medical assessment. The patient may desire weight loss or may be reluctant. By all means encourage the reluctant patient with medical complications of obesity to lose weight, but recognize that any attempt at weight loss will be almost certain to fail, even in the short run, if the patient is not self-motivated to change and does not believes that this change is attainable (self-efficacy).

Begin with a thorough history and physical. The weight history may be of value in identifying precipitants of weight gain and suggesting fruitful avenues for treatment. For example, a change in job leading to a reduction in physical activity may be detected. Also of interest is whether the onset of obesity was in childhood or later in life. Although only about *one-fifth of obese adults* were obese children, *about four-fifths of obese children become obese adults*. Obesity in childhood often results in only an *increase in average cell size, not number*. Treatment of the hyperplastic form of obesity is said to be more difficult because weight reduction does not greatly reduce the number of fat cells, only their average size.

Other information that can be gleaned from the weight history include *postpartum* weight gain (the average woman weighs about 10 lb more 2 years postpartum compared with prepregnancy, but the amount is extremely variable), weight gain after *smoking cessation* (average gain of about 6 lb, again highly variable, and the most common

Table 35-2. Components of Comprehensive Weight Control Programs

1. Medical assessment and monitoring
2. Behavioral assessment and modification
3. Dietary assessment and modification
4. Physical activity assessment and modification
5. Long-term maintenance support

excuse women give for not wanting to quit), and evidence of *yo-yo dieting* and disorders such as *binge eating* (consuming inordinately large amounts of food within a specified period 3 times a week or more in private for over 1 year with loss of control and negative emotional sequelae) or *bulimia nervosa* (binging plus purging, either by vomiting, use of diuretics, or excessive exercise). When an eating disorder is suspected, referral to a center experienced in the treatment of these problems is recommended. There is a separate chapter on anorexia and bulimia (see Chapter 38, "Anorexia Nervosa and Bulimia").

The history should also include questions to help rule out endocrine causes of obesity, such as *hypothyroidism, hyperadrenalism*, and *neuroendocrine tumors*, though in adults even the most common of these, hypothyroidism, is rarely a significant factor in causing obesity. Also inquire about *drugs* that may be associated with weight gain, such as sulfonylureas, insulin, steroids, most psychotropics, and antiseizure medications. Also assess for symptoms suggestive of diseases that often complicate obesity, such as *type 2 diabetes, coronary artery disease, hypertension*, and *sleep apnea*. Symptoms and signs of *depression* should also be sought, as depression is a common accompaniment of severe obesity and may require additional treatment. Childhood or later *sexual* or *physical abuse* is also common, and is usually not volunteered, so it needs to be specifically elicited after rapport has been established. Individual or group counseling may be helpful when sexual or other abuse is detected. The *family history* is of particular interest for endocrine disorders, obesity, and its complications.

The physical examination may be somewhat limited when the patient is morbidly obese, but it can yield evidence of endocrine causes and detect complicating conditions. It is necessary to obtain not only an accurate *weight* and *height* for calculation of the BMI but also the simple tape measurement of the *waist circumference*, an important modifier of the risk in obesity, as previously noted. Laboratory evaluations should serve to screen for the complications of obesity. Blood chemistries should include, in particular, counts of fasting serum *glucose, cholesterol,* and *triglycerides* and *liver function tests*. A *thyroid stimulating hormone* level should be obtained, as well as other endocrine and metabolic tests if a problem is suspected.

Behavioral Assessment

It is critical to gain a sense of the behavioral, as well as the medical aspects, of the patient's situation. This can be accomplished by referral to an appropriately skilled behavioral psychologist and/or through your own discussions with the patient. First, it is important to assess not only specific behaviors, but also the impact of these behaviors and the obesity itself, on the patient's level of functioning and quality of life. It may only emerge with inquiry that the patient has withdrawn from all unnecessary social interactions, or is no longer able to enjoy certain activities or interests because of weight gain, or has suffered job discrimination, to name a few examples.

Also related to quality of life are the patient's expectations about what changes will occur with successful weight control. Although it may be motivating for the patient to believe that life will improve with weight loss, disappointment may follow unless the changes likely to occur have been placed in proper perspective. Medical benefits can certainly be expected with weight loss in the obese suffering from medical complications. For example, patients with type 2 diabetes can often discontinue insulin or oral agents, antihypertensive medications may become unnecessary, sleep apnea usually disappears with as little as a 10 to 15% loss of initial weight, and gastroesophageal reflux disease can improve with weight loss. On another level, however, although self-assurance often increases, the wallflower does not become the life of the party and the competent worker does not get a promotion upon losing weight. Encourage obese patients toward a balanced view by reminding them that societal prejudices about body weight and character are in no way based on fact, and that they are the same good and worthy people whether they weight 300 or 150 lbs. In exploring specific behaviors, it is useful to assist the patient in identifying various *eating cues*. These cues are situations or feelings that lead to eating, often in an inappropriate way. It is axiomatic in our society that physical hunger is rarely a significant part of life, even for the poorest among us. In fact, physical hunger is not an important eating cue for many people, in part because they rarely let themselves get to the point of true hunger. Instead, they may eat in response to a whole host of other cues, most of which are inappropriate. The most common eating cues cited are as follows:

1. Habit ("It's 12:30 so I guess I'll have lunch" or "I have a jelly doughnut and coffee in the car on the way to work")
2. Stress ("I've got to finish this paper, and eating while I work helps me concentrate")
3. Boredom ("There's nothing else to do; a subcategory is watching television and eating at the same time)
4. Emotions ("I eat when I'm depressed or upset")
5. Food as a reward ("After a hard day, I deserve a rich dessert").

Underlying some of these cues is the association of food with love, care, and comfort, which may have its antecedents in early childhood but persists into adult life and, indeed, pervades our culture. The patient should be helped to recognize that using food to deal with stress, boredom, and emotions is, at best, ineffective. The stressful situation, for example, does not resolve with eating. In fact, eating may worsen the problem by distracting a person from dealing directly with the situation while adding the stresses of obesity and its sequelae.

Suggestions

Simply telling a patient not to eat when under stress is useless, of course. Instead, use the following three-step approach. *First*, recommend a period of *observation* and *recording* to enable the patient to recognize the cue. For instance, one can ask the patient to wear his or her watch upside down as a reminder to ask "Why am I reaching for the food at this time?" If the patient is not physically hungry, one of the possibly inappropriate eating cues is most likely in play, and its nature should be guessed at and recorded. *Second*, suggest the *substitution* of other responses for inappropriate eating. For stress, this might be writing down what the stress is, formulating a plan for doing something about it, doing something (besides eating) to relieve the stress on the spot, or, at the very least, substituting a walk around the block or a call to a friend for the bag of potato chips. The third step is *repetition*, that is, to keep making appropriate responses to the problematic cue and to reap the rewards of the new behavior, which include the positive responses of others to the change in approach, not just to eating, but to life, that the patient makes.

Although some degree of change is necessary and beneficial, not every maladaptive behavior must be completely eliminated nor must every rich food be replaced by celery sticks without dip. Although losing a large amount of weight in a reasonable amount of time does require a fairly aggressive diet program, maintaining a new lower weight does not. If the patient can learn to control even partially a few of the more important inappropriate eating behaviors and to shift to a diet somewhat lower in calories than baseline, that is often sufficient to maintain weight in the new, lower range. This is easy to see and difficult to do, but impossible if behaviors are not addressed as part of a comprehensive approach to the treatment of obesity.

Another behavior of interest in obesity is *restraint*. One can simplistically categorize patients as restrained or unrestrained eaters. Restrained eaters believe that they must exercise a good deal of control over their eating—they are always conscious of what they can and cannot eat. Unrestrained eaters do not control their eating to any great extent. Restrained eating may lead to some paradoxical results; once restraint is relaxed, an exaggerated response may ensue (all-or-nothing behavior). Such patients may be superb dieters, but are equally superb at overeating once the diet has been "broken." The issue of restraint is one of too much of a good thing. Although a certain amount of control and monitoring is necessary for maintaining weight loss, high levels of restraint may be more problematic than low ones in the long run. One solution is to *couple* the *teaching of ways* to *control inappropriate eating* cues *with dietary changes* that emphasize *foods lower in fat and calories*, and *higher in fiber* and *water content*, so that lower restraint is required to maintain a given intake. Skipping meals when the patient is physically hungry should be discouraged, and a low calorie, nutritious breakfast encouraged rather than skipping it in the false belief that this will aid weight control.

Dietary Assessment

Although most aspects of diet are more properly characterized as behaviors, the need remains to understand patients' tastes and the macronutrient composition of their usual array of food choices. This information is a tool for suggesting behavioral changes that will comport with the patient's preferences and lifestyle. Although the physician can and should get some idea of these things in talking with the patient, a formal dietary assessment is best done by a dietitian using either a prospective or retrospective food diary.

The results of a *food diary* must be interpreted with caution, as both retrospective underreporting and prospective restrained eating are common. Despite these shortcomings, the information gathered can be very useful. For example, the macronutrient composition of a patient's diet will often be weighted towards fats, simple carbohydrates, and protein. By *cutting fat* and *increasing intake* of *complex carbohydrates*, especially *vegetables* and *fruit*, such patients can considerably increase the volume of food they consume as they attempt to reach and maintain a lower weight.

A helpful tool in altering the composition of the patient's diet is the technique of *gradual change*. For example, a patient reluctant to switch from whole milk to skim milk could first try 2% milk (which is actually 35% fat), get used to this for a month or two, then move on to 1% fat milk for another month. At this point, the patient should notice something interesting: the once-favored whole milk will now taste too oily. At some later date, the final step to skim milk can be made with few or no feelings of deprivation, demonstrating that taste preferences are acquired and eminently changeable even in later life.

Recommend scouring the supermarket aisles (at a time when the patient is not hungry) for *tasty, low fat, or fat-free alternatives* to favored foods. Encourage the patient to explore the wide variety of foods now available and to focus on the good taste of the new choice rather than comparing it with the "real thing." The presentation of nutritional information on food labels is becoming more and more useful, listing not just g of fat, for example, but also the percentage of the daily dietary fat allotment those g represent. The patient should be taught (usually by the dietitian) to read labels and to stay within the fat and calorie "budget."

This is also a good time to *improve the dietary habits* of the *patient's family*, something that is particularly easy to do when the patient is the primary cook and food shopper. Including the family in this process not only improves their diet but also makes it easier for the patient if at least the house can be a temptation-free zone. Even if other members of the family must have junk food, they can be instructed to partake outside the home or to put only individually packaged items in the cupboard. Small-size purchases of rich deserts and the like are desirable in general; the smaller the dietary indiscretion, the less severe the consequences. Unfortunately, portions have risen greatly in the

United States in recent years, especially in meals consumed outside the home. Specific recommendation of types of diets is listed under "Types of Diets."

Exercise Assessment

Exercise alone is, unfortunately, *not* a terribly effective method for losing weight. It is difficult for the untrained person to do enough of it, and most if not all of the expended energy is compensated by increased caloric intake. Exercise is, however, a *superb way to maintain a lower weight after weight loss*, enabling a person to eat somewhat more than a nonexerciser and maintain the same given weight. Regular aerobic exercise and strength training will also improve cardiovascular fitness, trim inches, and promote growth of metabolically more active muscle tissue.

An exercise assessment should include a record of the usual degree of physical activity, any limiting factors such as joint disease or previous injuries, types of activity the patient finds enjoyable, and a measurement by an exercise physiologist of the current fitness level. A formal stress test is not required unless cardiovascular disease is suspected.

A rule of thumb in devising an exercise regimen that will be followed is the *phased-in approach*. Most obese patients start out with a limited capacity to exercise. Rather than suggesting a type of level of activity that is unlikely to inspire adherence, make sure that the plan fits into the patient's schedule and lifestyle.

Lifestyle

The *first* phase consists of increasing the amount of everyday physical activity, so-called "lifestyle" activity, without introducing a formal exercise regimen. Lifestyle activities include taking the stairs in gradually increasing increments, parking the car farther away from the mall entrance, walking to the mailbox, and the like. This step alone may double the level of physical activity in a very sedentary person.

Walking

The *second* phase is a walking plan. People are most likely to comply with such a plan if the walk is scheduled during a break or lunchtime at work, and/or when the daily energy level is the highest (for example, early morning). Having a companion to walk with and a place to walk indoors are also helpful in increasing compliance. *One half hour* is minimum amount of time a patient should make available for each session of exercise. An *hour* is *best* for weight control. The intensity of the exercise is not critical to the burning of calories; walking at a leisurely pace for one hour is roughly equal to walking briskly for half an hour. Allow the patient to set the pace. Initially, it may be quite slow, but in the absence of severe pulmonary, cardiovascular, or joint disease, most patients soon find the going easier and faster. *Goal setting* can strengthen this reinforcement. Have the patient *keep a log* of the time spent walking and the distance covered after each session. The patient can then see the progress being made and set the goal a bit higher from time to time.

Aerobic Exercise

Next, the types of activities performed should be *broadened*. Walking or jogging can and should remain an ingredient at this stage, but with the addition of other forms of *aerobic exercise*. Recommend aerobics classes, stationary or outdoor bicycling, swimming, a cross-country skiing machine, or just about anything else that will burn calories and be enjoyable to the patient. Team or racquet sports and golf can be suggested to provide social interaction as well as to increase energy expenditure. Again, the most important criterion for a good exercise plan is that it be one that the patient is likely to follow and be comfortable with as a *lifelong habit*.

Types of Diets

It is best to start by instilling in your obese patients a degree of skepticism about commercially advertised weight control measures. Many are based on very limited menus, the rationale being that monotony helps curb consumption. Others involve diuretic agents. In fact, any reduced-calorie diet will initially cause diuresis, which will be regained as soon as the period of severe caloric restriction ends.

After the diuretic phase, the amount of weight loss to be expected on any diet obeys a simple formula. Lipolysis of one pound of adipose tissue yields about 3,500 kilocalories; it is therefore *necessary to restrict energy intake and/or increase energy output by about 500 kilocalories per day to lose one pound of fat per week*. Because some muscle may also be lost and muscle is poorer in energy than fat, the rate of weight loss may be somewhat higher than predicted. However, two countervailing factors are at work. First, with sustained moderate-to-severe caloric restriction, a modest reduction in metabolic rate occurs. This decrease makes weight loss somewhat more difficult to achieve, but caloric requirement, corrected for the new, lower weight, fortunately appears to return the prediet level within a few months of resuming a balanced diet. Second, because lower weight means reduced caloric need, the same caloric intake will represent less of a deficit as the patient loses weight. A regular program of physical activity, especially one that includes some resistance exercises, can partially compensate for both these factors by helping to blunt the decrease in metabolic rate and by building muscle mass, which is more metabolically active and therefore has a higher caloric requirement, even at rest, than an equal weight of adipose tissue.

How much of a caloric deficit should be recommended, and in what form should the calories be taken? The answer depends on the degree of obesity, the presence or absence of comorbidities such as type 2 diabetes and hypertension, the results of the behavioral assessment, and, to some extent, the patient's preferences. In any case, it is important to remind the patient that the diet is only part of the overall plan and will fail in the long term unless accompanied by changes in behavior. Use of fat replacers, such as olestra, and sugar substitutes, such as aspartame, may be helpful in reducing overall caloric intake.

Overweight or Moderately Obese

For patients who are overweight or moderately obese (BMI 25 to 32), I recommend a *caloric deficit of 500 to 750 kilocalories per day to achieve 1 to 1.5 pounds of weight loss per week*. The dietitian can design a low calorie, food-based diet that is either balanced-deficit (reducing total number of calories while keeping proportions from carbohydrate, fat, and protein roughly the same as before), or fat-deficit, with most of the caloric reduction resulting from restriction of fat intake. The latter approach is preferable in light of the typical American diet that is too high in fat, especially saturated fat. Also, a greater volume of food can be eaten on a diet that emphasizes complex and vegetable-source carbohydrates and reduces fat to < 30% of calories consumed.

Obese

Patients with a BMI of 33 to 40 will also benefit from a fat-and-calorie reduced diet. It is important however, to recognize that at this level of caloric restriction it will take more than a year to attain a weight loss of 50 to 70 pounds. Few patients can sustain this degree of restriction for that long; therefore, for a limited period a *very low calorie diet* (VLCD) (*fewer than 800 kilocalories per day*) may be needed. The VLCD is justified particularly if the patient already suffers from comorbidities that are likely to be alleviated with significant weight loss. VLCDs can consist of food, commercially available liquid supplements, or a combination of both. With full compliance, the amount of weight lost on a VLCD *ranges from 2.5 to 4 pounds per week*, depending on body mass and level of physical activity. The *initial diuretic phase* may be pronounced and accompanied by (usually transient) lightheadedness, headache, or fatigue. Later symptoms may include constipation and intolerance of cold. Electrolyte abnormalities are rare, but serum should be monitored occasionally and more frequently if the patient may be prone to electrolyte problems because of renal insufficiency or diuretic use. Because of the greater stress on the body and greater need for monitoring of true VLCDs, I prefer to keep the caloric intake *above 800 to 1000 kilocalories per day*.

Gallstones may arise or become symptomatic, probably due to gallbladder stasis, and a decrease in bile acids, which occurs during or immediately after any severely restricted (especially fat-restricted) diet. To prevent stasis, the patient can add to the diet a tablespoon of a fat (preferably an unsaturated fat such as canola or olive oil) taken in one daily dose, which will allow the gallbladder to contract.

A VLCD should be administered only under a physician's supervision and with full attention to the behavioral changes necessary to sustain the weight loss that this regimen will produce.

Severe Obesity

In severe ("morbid") obesity, corresponding to a BMI of 40 kg/m^2 or more, the only practical diet for most patients is a VLCD or other highly restricted diet with careful medical monitoring and long-term follow-up. It should be noted, however, that even a modest weight loss can yield substantial health benefits for morbidly obese patients. Sleep apnea often disappears with as little as a 10% loss in weight, and hypertension, diabetes, and gastroesophogeal reflux may also improve significantly. I do *not* view, nor let my patients view, modest weight loss as a failure or a waste of time. The same is true for patients with lesser degrees of obesity.

Drugs and Surgery

Adjunctive anorectic medications may be useful for the obese patient, either from the start, to enhance compliance with the diet or later, or when compliance begins to waver or hunger becomes an issue. There is little doubt that such medications significantly increase weight loss during the period in which they are used, and may help with maintaining some weight loss (though there tends to be regain even with continued use). Commonly used anorectic drugs are *phentermine* and *sibutramine*. One reasonably effective agent, *ephedrine*, is available over the counter, but may soon be restricted because it has been associated with adverse cardiovascular events. The true amphetamines, diuretics, and thyroid medications should not be prescribed for weight loss. An agent that holds some appeal to me as a gastroenterologist is *orlistat*. This is the only nonsystemically acting prescription medication as yet available. It acts in the lumen of the small bowel by binding to lipases, and thus causes malabsorption of about 30% of ingested fat. It also blocks fat-soluble vitamin and cholesterol absorption. This has two consequences, as follows: (1) a *multivitamin supplement* must be taken at a time when the orlistat is not being taken to prevent deficiencies and (2) there seems to be a greater degree of reduction in cholesterol levels for a given amount of weight loss compared with weight loss resulting from diet alone. Although orlistat has no appetite-curbing effects, it may have an *"Antabuse-like effect"* in that consumption of more than a moderate amount of fat at a sitting will result in unpleasant gastrointestinal consequences. I thus view it as more suitable for patients who are having difficulty avoiding junk food and fats than for patients with increased physical hunger. Whether obesity should be considered a chronic disease and treated on a long-term basis with anorectic or other drugs is in part a philosophical issue. I use these agents only after attempts at dieting have failed in patients who are severely obese and/or who suffer from comorbid conditions.

The surgical treatment of morbid obesity has improved considerably since the days of the jejunoileal bypass and jaw wiring. The next chapter (Chapter 36, "Bariatric Operations") is on obesity surgery. Generally, patients are referred for surgery only if they have a BMI ≥ 40, preferably along with obesity-related health conditions, and have failed to lose or maintain weight loss with a comprehensive, nonsurgical approach. Probably the best procedure currently available is the *gastric bypass*, preferably done *laparoscopically*. This procedure combines *stapling* of the stomach to make a small-capacity proximal gastric pouch with a short-segment bypass of the proximal small bowel created by a *Roux-en-Y loop*. Results are quite good in the short term. Long-term results, as with all methods of weight loss, depend largely on the patient's ability to make behavioral changes. Therefore, aside from access to a hospital with adequate experience in this procedure, the best chance of long term success will come with referring the patient to a center that offers and insists upon extensive preoperative examination and maintenance therapy of long duration consisting of regular sessions in dietary management and behavioral modification. Do not make the mistake of viewing surgery as a treatment that does not require the patient's active involvement; an unmotivated or unguided patient can and will defeat the procedure.

Maintenance

The physician and the patient should both know that the long term results of attempts at weight loss are often poor. It is therefore important to expose that patient, at the beginning of treatment, to the attitudes and behaviors that are likely to foster long-term maintenance of weight loss. These may be summarized as follows:

1. *Readiness*—Correct timing for change is vital. It is folly for your patient to begin a diet when he or she is not yet convinced of the need to do so or is in the midst of a stressful life event such as divorce.
2. *Setting reasonable goals*—Aiming for attainable rather than an "ideal" body weight is advisable. A reasonable long-term goal might be the lowest weight the patient has successfully maintained for 1 year or more during the previous 10 years.
3. *Reliable support systems*—Obtaining helpful assistance aids in both weight loss and maintenance. This usually involves seeking out a friend or relative who knows how to listen and not just give advice.
4. *Building in maintenance*—Planning and executing behavioral changes from day 1 is essential.
5. *Becoming invested in one's goals*—Learning how to talk to oneself in a positive way in order to enhance commitment to self-set objectives is a useful technique.
6. *Making gradual changes*—Modifying food choices and level of physical activity reduces the sense of deprivation and may make the process of change easier and the changes themselves more likely to be permanent.
7. *Keeping records*—Recording weight, foods eaten, exercise, and precipitants of inappropriate eating is an excellent way to identify problem areas and to spot a relapse before it gets out of hand, thereby improving the chances of long term success.
8. *Making it enjoyable*—This is self-explanatory. It is much easier to comply with the new behaviors if they can be enjoyed. If your patient cannot stand to exercise, do not tell him or her to do it anyway. Instead, suggest taking a child to the park or walking around the mall to people watch. The achievement of a *positive change in lifestyle* is, by itself, very reinforcing and should not be discounted as a source of satisfaction and enjoyment.
9. *Being flexible*—This applies to both the physician and the patient. If an approach that has been given a fair trial is not working, or if the patient's circumstances change (eg, a new job), the weight loss plan may need to change, too.

In closing, it should be obvious that helping patients lose weight and keep it off requires a comprehensive and sustained effort. Although it is true that only the patient can do it, this is one area where the diligent and caring physician can make a real difference.

Supplemental Reading

Cheskin LJ. Losing weight for good. Baltimore (MD): Johns Hopkins University Press; 1997.

Folsom AR, Kaye SA, Sellers TA, et al. Body fat distribution and risk for death in older women. JAMA 1993;269;483–7.

Garrow JS. Treatment of obesity. Lancet 1992;340;409–13.

Kayman S, Bruvold W, Stern JS. Maintenance and relapse after weight loss in women—behavioral aspects. Am J Clin Nutr 1990;52:800–7.

Must A, Jacques SD, Dallal GE, et al. Long-term morbidity and mortality of overweight adolescents. N Engl J Med 1992;327;1350–5.

There is an excellent guideline published by the National Heart Lung and Blood Institute:

Clinical guidelines on the identification, evaluation, and treatment of overweight and obesity in adults—the evidence report. Obes Res 1998;6 Suppl 2:51S–209S.

CHAPTER 36

BARIATRIC OPERATIONS

MICHAEL G. SARR, MD, MICHEL M. MURR, MD, AND MICHAEL L. KENDRICK, MD

Once the decision to perform bariatric surgery has been made, the surgeon and, to some extent, the patient, must agree on the type of bariatric operation to be undertaken. This decision is important, because the history of bariatric surgery is a rather dark one. Many different types of operations have been designed and tried, often in clinical settings that did not allow adequate follow-up study of the patients to determine clinical outcomes. One need only remember the ignominious, but appropriate fate of the jejunoileal bypass (JIB) (see below), also called the small intestinal bypass, to fully acknowledge the need to study both short and long term outcomes of even the most theoretically appealing "new" bariatric operations. The indications for surgery are discussed in the preceding chapter (see Chapter 35, "Obesity"), along with the need for continuing medical follow-up.

This chapter will briefly review the history of the different bariatric operations since their birth in the mid 1950s; understanding just a bit of the historical evolution is important in our current understanding of bariatric complications (Balsiger et al, 2000). We will then describe the currently accepted bariatric operations and their expected outcomes, focusing the discussion on the role of the gastroenterologist. The preceding chapter deals with the overall management of obesity. The current chapter will finish with a description of the as yet unproven procedures being evaluated.

History of Bariatric Operations

Basically, operations for weight loss fall under the following three categories: (1) complete malabsorption, (2) gastric restriction (volume reduction of the stomach), and (3) selective malabsorption. Some operations incorporate elements of both gastric restriction and selective malabsorption.

Complete Malabsorption

The first operation designed in the mid 1950s was the jejunocolic bypass. The jejunum was transected 200 cm distal to the ligament of Treitz, the distal end of jejunum was oversewn, and the proximal transected end was sewn to the transverse colon, thereby bypassing the remainder of the jejunoileum. Weight loss was impressive, but bypass of all of the ileum led to severe diarrhea (a combination of a bile salt-induced secretory component as well as steatorrhea). These unacceptable results rapidly spurred the modification termed the jejunoileal bypass (or JIB). This operation, carried out from the early 1960s until the mid to late 1970s, involved transecting the jejunum 14 inches (approximately 36 cm) distal to ligament of Treitz and the ileum 4 inches (approximately 10 cm) proximal to ileocecal junction; gastrointestinal (GI) continuity was restored by anastomosing the proximal jejunum to the distal ileum. The "bypassed" small bowel, about 90% of the jejunoileum, was oversewn proximally and the distal end of the ileum was sewn into the colon (Figure 36-1A). Although theoretically very attractive, it took about 20 years to acknowledge the unacceptable side effects of this operation, which were not infrequent. These included acute hepatic failure, late insidious cirrhosis, oxalate urolithiasis and, occasionally, irreversible oxalate nephropathy, an immune complex arthritis, protein, calorie, vitamin and mineral nutritional deficiencies, and multiple mechanical and bacterial overgrowth sequelae in the "bypassed" segment. Although this operation is no longer performed, there are occasional patients with this anatomy that present clinically today. These patients often present with oxalate nephropathy or metabolic problems that require reversal of the anatomy or are asymptomatic but require close nutritional surveillance (Hassan et al, 2001).

Gastric Restriction

This concept involves decreasing the size of the gastric reservoir into which the ingested food initially resides. The first gastric restrictive procedures, or "gastroplasties" (changing the shape of the stomach), were facilitated by introduction of mechanical surgical staplers and were rapidly dubbed "stomach staplings." Using a stapler, the stomach was separated or "partitioned" into a small upper "pouch" of cardia and fundus (with a 30 to 50 mL volume) that communicated with the rest of the stomach by a narrow 1 cm channel or "stoma" (Figure 36-1B). These operations were attractive in theory (ie, no anastomoses, no anatomic bypass, and, thus, no "malabsorption"), because this "restrictive" anatomy should prevent the patient from overeating at any one meal; moreover, operative mortality and serious morbidity were low. Unfortunately, results

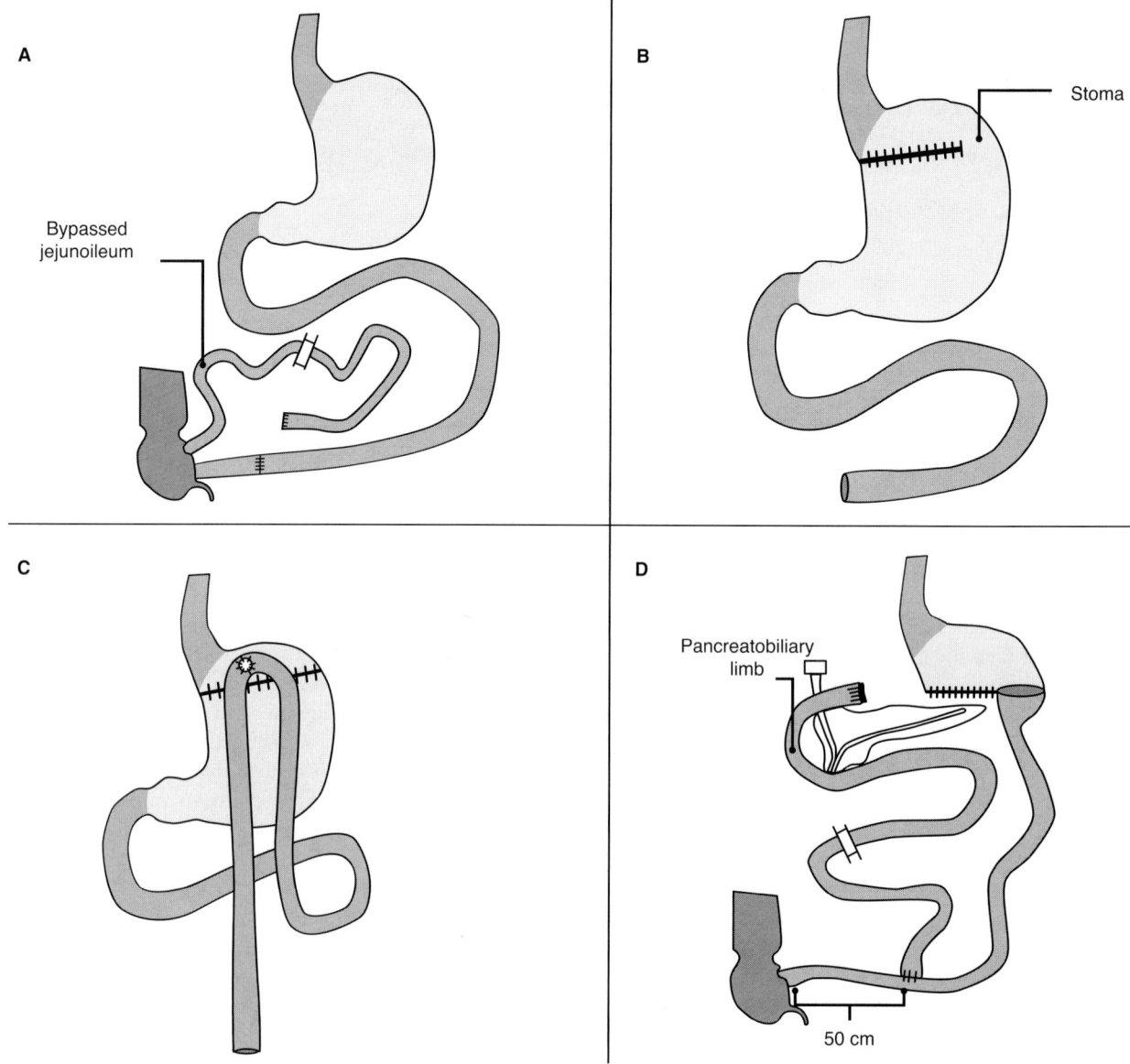

FIGURE 36-1. Previous bariatric procedures no longer performed. Small bowel bypass (A). Gastroplasty (stomach stapling) (B). Loop gastric bypass (C). Scopinaro procedure (partial biliopancreatic diversion) (D).

proved unsatisfactory in > 50% of patients because of eventual staple line disruption or stomal dilatation that abolished the restrictive physiology. Currently performed gastroplasties incorporate multiple applications of a stapler to minimize staple line breakdown and an external band or ring to prevent stomal dilatation. Far too many of these stomach staplings were carried out without detailed follow-up; many of those patients are still seen today with complications of the stomach stapling or insufficient weight loss.

Selective Malabsorption

These procedures are designed to establish a more selective type of malabsorption and to incorporate gastric restriction as well. The first type was the gastric bypass (Figure 36-1C). This operation partitioned the stomach (by a row of staples) into a small upper pouch completely discontinous with the distal stomach. A loop of jejunum was then anastomosed to the proximal pouch. This procedure worked in two ways—first, by its gastric restriction of oral intake and second, by setting up a dumping physiology for high calorie sweets. The vast majority of the stomach and all of the duodenum were bypassed. However, this procedure was complicated by bile reflux esophagitis in over 30% of patients, guiding a modification of the loop anatomy to a Roux limb as currently used today (see below).

The second selective malabsorptive procedure was the partial biliopancreatic diversion designed by Scopinaro and colleagues (1996) in Italy. This operation involves an 80% distal gastrectomy (the restrictive component) and transection of the ileum 250 cm proximal to the ileocecal junction; the distal ileum is sewn to the stomach, while the proximal ileum (the pancreatobiliary limb) is re-anastomosed to the Roux limb of ileum 50 cm proximal to the ileocecal junction (Figure 36-1D). This diversion of the biliopancreatic secretions to the distal ileum leads to bile salt loss into the colon with a subsequent selective maldigestion and thus malabsorption of fats (and fat soluble vitamins). This procedure has not become popular in the United States because of a high incidence of protein/calorie malnutrition and rather severe steatorrhea, but it has spured the current concept of biliopancreatic diversion (BPD).

Currently Accepted Bariatric Operations

The 1991 NIH Consensus Conference on Bariatric Surgery effectively condoned the success of bariatric surgery in appropriate patients. At that time, two operations were recognized as being effective: *vertical banded (Ring) gastroplasty* (VBG) and *Roux-en-Y gastric bypass (RYGB)*. Since then, two others have become "accepted" in current practice: *gastric banding* and *duodenal switch with BPD*.

VBG

This form of gastric restrictive procedure involves a "vertical" line of staples to partition the stomach into a small volume (< 30 mL) pouch along the lesser curvature that communicates with the rest of the stomach through a stoma of 1.1 cm that is banded or ringed externally (with a polypropylene or Silicone prosthesis), which prevents stomal dilatation (Figure 36-2A). VBG was first described in 1980 and was rapidly accepted; many tens of thousands of these procedures were performed after they were "sanctioned" by the 1991 NIH Consensus Conference, and VBG is still performed in some centers. The operative mortality is low (< 1%) and serious morbidity is < 5%; thus, it is a safe operative procedure.

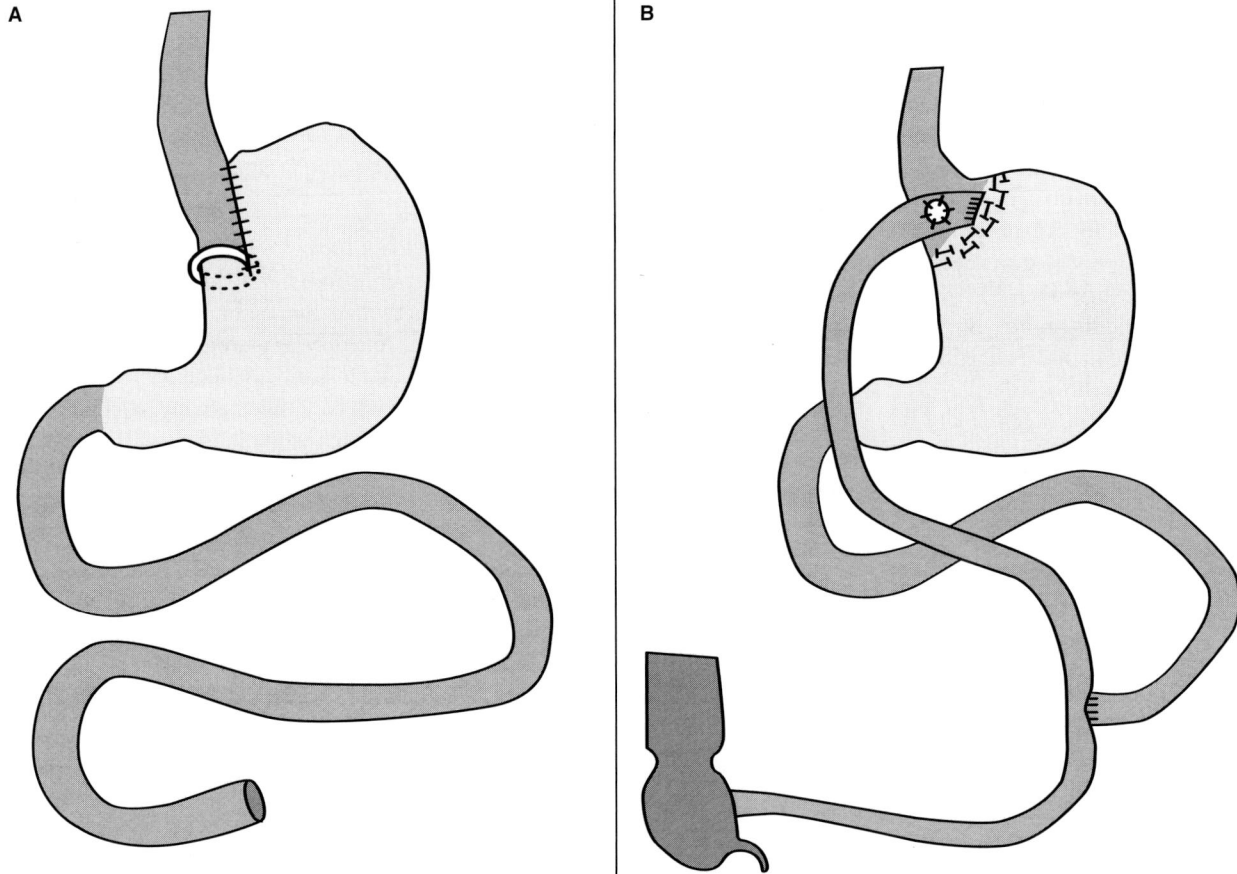

FIGURE 36-2. Current procedures. Vertical banded gastroplasty (VBG) (A). Roux-en-Y gastric bypass (RYGB) (B).

Early success, as measured by weight loss, is quite good, with the majority of patients losing 20 to 35 kg in the first 6 months postoperatively. Unfortunately, in most centers, the long term results after 2 years have been very disappointing for several reasons. First, the incidence of significant staple line breakdown approaches 50%. Also, and possibly more importantly, many patients find that eating solids is difficult, which "encourages" many to alter their diet to the softer solids and liquids. Unfortunately, the poorly restrictive nature of this anatomy that allows ready ingestion of high calorie liquids (milkshakes, ice cream, etc) is counterproductive in maintaining weight loss. Indeed, long term maintenance of weight loss is often poor at 3 years (< 40%) and even worse at 10 years postoperatively (approximately 20%) (Balsiger et al, 2000). For this and other reasons (see below), many groups have abandoned this operation. It had a short-lived rebirth with the description of a minimal access laparoscopic approach, but RYGB has largely replaced this isolated gastric restrictive procedure.

RYGB

RYGB represents the current gold standard bariatric procedure in the United States (Figure 36-2B). This procedure again completely separates the gastric cardia from the remainder of the stomach either by one or more rows of staples or by complete anatomic transection of the proximal stomach. The proximal jejunum is then transected, and the end of a 75 to 150 cm Roux-en-Y limb of jejunum is brought up and anastomosed to the proximal gastric pouch. The proximal jejunum is then anastomosed to the mid jejunum, restoring enteric continuity. This is not a true malabsorptive procedure, because only the stomach, duodenum, and first 40 to 60 cm of jejunum are "bypassed." There should be no malabsorption of ingested nutrients (ie, fat, protein, or carbohydrates) or most vitamins after RYGB; there is, however, a decreased absorption of *iron* and probably *calcium*, much of which is absorbed in the duodenum, and *vitamin B_{12}* because of discoordination of acid breakdown of the cyanocobalamin-pteryl complex with binding of free cyanocobalamin with R Factor and intrinsic factor.

Results with RYGB serve as the benchmark against which newer procedures should be judged (Balsiger et al, 2000). In experienced hands, operative mortality and significant morbidity should be less than 1% and 5 to 8%, respectively. RYGB can also be performed laparoscopically in a large percentage (approximately 70%) of patients, provided they are not too short (< 5 feet or 150 cm tall), too heavy (body mass index [BMI] > 55), or have had previous gastric or significant intra-abdominal surgery (Schauer et al, 2000). Weight loss is superior to VBG, with *average weight loss of about 70% of excess body weight* and 66% of patients *maintaining* a *weight loss of at least 50% of their excess body weight at 5 years.*

Duodenal Switch with BPD

This form of selective malabsorptive operation involves a modified gastric restriction by tubularizing the lesser curvature of the stomach via a greater curvature gastrectomy (Figure 36-3), and a diversion of biliopancreatic secretions to the distal ileum. The latter is accomplished by transecting the duodenum proximal to the ampulla of Vater (Figure 36-3, site A/B), oversewing the distal end of the duodenum (site B), transecting the proximal ileum 250 cm proximal to the ileocecal valve (site C/D), anastomosing the distal end of ileum (site D) to the proximal duodenum (site A), and reimplanting the proximal ileum (site C) into the distal ileum 100 cm proximal to the ileocecal junction (site E). This is a newer operation that is more in vogue on the West Coast of the United States. Although this operation lacks a broad experience across many centers, the operative morbidity and mortality appears to be similar to RYGB. Weight loss, however, appears to be somewhat better than RYGB; however, with the potential for fat malabsorption (via the 100 cm common channel of distal ileum where all digestion/absorption occurs), many bariatric surgeons reserve this procedure for the superobese (BMI > 55).

Gastric Banding (Laparoscopic)

Laparoscopic gastric banding, often referred to as the "lap band", is the new kid on the block (O'Brien et al, 1999). In concept, this as yet unproven bariatric procedure is again theoretically attractive. A silicone band that contains an eccentrically placed "balloon" is placed around the gastric cardia and is connected to a subcutaneous port. As fluid is inserted via the port, the balloon externally "occludes" the lumen of the cardia. The resultant "stoma" diameter is "adjustable" by insertion/removal of fluid from the balloon in the band. This procedure is purely a gastric restrictive operation. It is attractive, in concept, because (1) it is laparoscopic (hospital stay is 1 to 2 days), (2) it is "adjustable," and (3) there is no gut bypass, anastomosis, or malabsorption.

Laparoscopic gastric banding is very commonly performed in Europe and Australia. It has not (yet) been embraced by most bariatric surgeons in the United States, because a preliminary, randomized, prospective trial in US patients showed poor outcomes and was very discouraging (DeMaria et al, 2001). Good long term results are few, and definitive data regarding both its efficacy and potential morbidity are lacking. Without the malabsorptive component, this procedure likely will not equal the RYGB in efficiency and may share the fate of the other restrictive procedures (eg, VBG).

---

*Editor's Note: The preceding chapter (Chapter 35) on obesity points out the need for continued medical involvement after surgery.

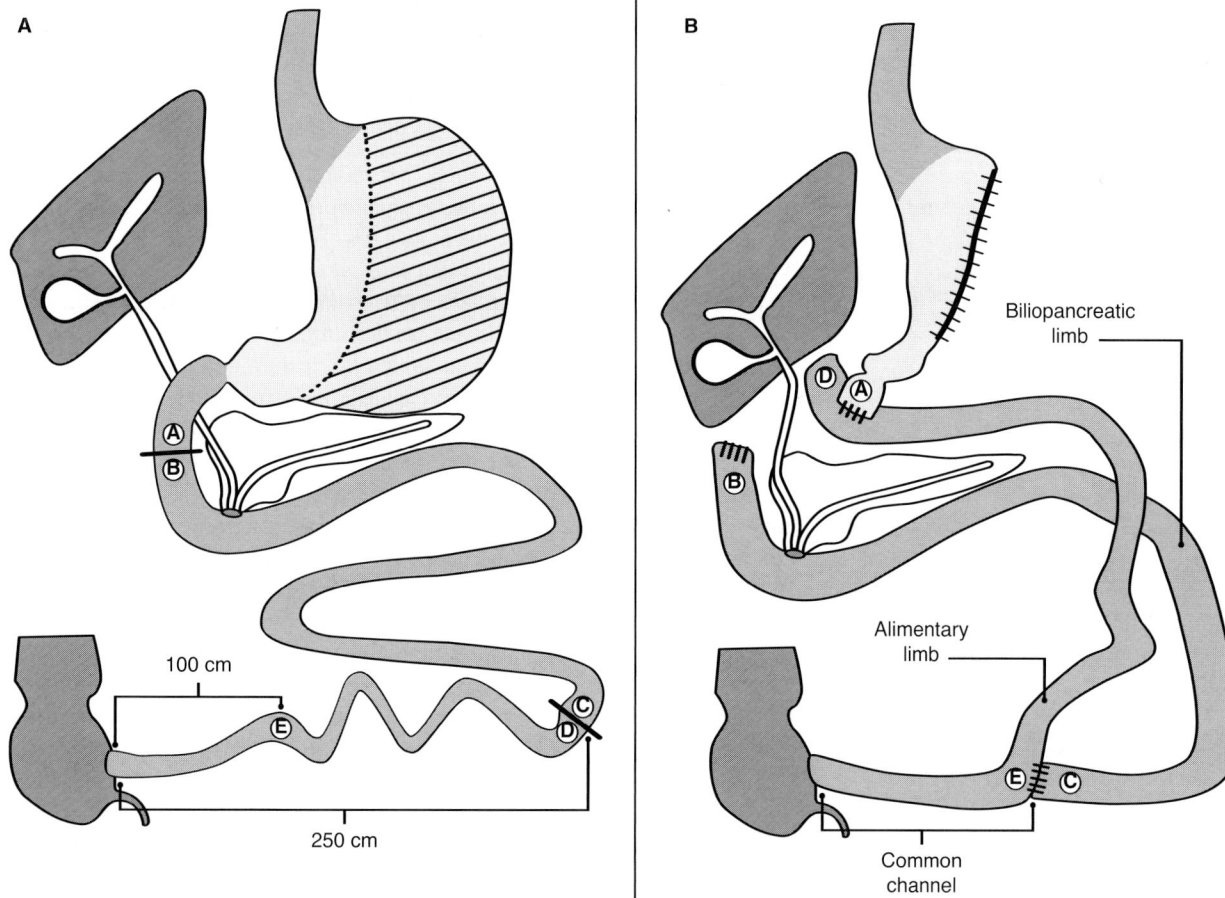

FIGURE 36-3. Duodenal switch with biliopancreatic diversion (BPD).

Gastroenterologic Complications of Bariatric Surgery

Although there are numerous potential metabolic sequelae, the GI complications of bariatric surgery consist primarily of "stomal" problems, GI bleeding, gastroesophageal reflux symptoms/disease, intestinal obstruction, and malabsorption. Each will be discussed separately.

Stomal Problems

Stomal complications involve either obstruction/stricture, bleeding, perforation, or maladaptive eating, and are pertinent to VBG, RYGB, and gastric banding. These narrow stomas can become *acutely obstructed* by incompletely chewed foodstuffs (especially meat) and, on occasion, require endoscopic removal of the obstructing food bolus. These stomas also can become *strictured*, either from ulceration or secondary to enteric erosion by an external band or prosthesis, each of which causes a mechanical obstruction similar in clinical presentation to an esophageal stricture. The former is treated by endoscopic dilatation (effective approximately 50% of the time), while the latter usually requires reoperation. Stomal *ulceration* may cause unrelenting pain and, if unresponsive to acid suppression, may require operative intervention. Stomal *bleeding* is usually from external band erosion or, in patients after RYGB, from acid exposure to the gastrojejunostomy. The latter may occur from staple line breakdown and reflux of acid from the distal "bypassed" stomach into the proximal pouch or from too big a proximal pouch that thus secretes acid. In both situations, the "unprotected" jejunal mucosa of the Roux limb, which no longer has alkaline pancreatobiliary secretions flowing through it, is at high risk for stomal ulceration if gastric acid bathes the gastrojejunostomy. Stomal *perforation* is extremely rare and has a similar pathogenesis to stomal ulceration. Finally, the so-called "maladaptive eating disorder" is related to a functional "obstruction" to the emptying of solid ingested foods from the proximal pouch. This "obstruction" causes the patient to change their diet to primarily liquids and often high calorie foods (milkshakes, ice cream, etc), and their weight often increases. In severe and protracted situations, the patient may become nutritionally challenged. This "maladaptive eating disorder" may be associated with gastroesophageal reflux disease (GERD).

GI Bleeding

GI bleeding can occur early postoperatively (within 2 weeks postoperatively) or in a delayed fashion. *Early postoperative* GI bleeding is usually from the staple line closure of the stomach or from the gastrojejunostomy. When bleeding occurs from the "bypassed" stomach after RYGB, diagnosis is difficult because it cannot be accessed or visualized endoscopically in patients after RYGB. *Later* GI bleeding can be secondary to an *ulcer* at the stoma (after VBG) or at the gastrojejunostomy after RYGB, a classic duodenal ulcer, or, rarely, from a poorly understood *distal antral gastritis* that occurs in the bypassed stomach in about 80% of patients after RYGB. Again, the latter two sources cannot be visualized endoscopically after RYGB; when they are persistent or recurrent, both of these causes may require reoperation and resection of the bypassed stomach. After RYGB, one must not "assume" that an iron deficiency anemia is secondary to blood loss because the anatomy predisposes to *iron malabsorption* and, thus, one should confirm a GI source with an hemoccult test of the stool.

GERD

GERD-like symptoms are quite common after the gastric restrictive procedures (VBG, gastric banding). Symptoms may occur from distal esophageal loading or true reflux of acidic peptic juice from the distal stomach; some investigators believe that emptying of the proximal pouch is disrupted by the gastric restriction, thus permitting esophageal reflux.

After RYGB, symptoms of GERD should not occur. When done correctly, RYGB should be one of, if not the best, antireflux operations because: (1)) there is no acid in the proximal pouch of cardia and (2) the Roux limb anatomy should prevent any alkaline or acid/bile reflux from getting into the esophagus. Thus, symptoms of GERD after RYGB suggest either that the proximal pouch is too big and includes some element of acid-producing parietal cell mass, dehiscence of the staple line separating the proximal gastric pouch from the bypassed stomach (which does make acid that can reflux into the proximal pouch and esophagus), or bile reflux into the esophagus, either from staple line dehiscence or reflux up a Roux limb that is too short, even if the surgeon claimed the Roux limb to be 75 cm long. Endoscopic examination that shows bile in the proximal pouch confirms one of these possibilities. A less common cause can be from an older "loop" gastric bypass (see Figure 36-1C), the precursor to the RYGB, or from what has been dubbed the "mini-gastric bypass," a short-lived "reintroduction" of the loop gastric bypass performed with a short minilaparotomy. GERD from these procedures requires reoperation with relatively simple conversion from the loop anatomy to a Roux anatomy (see Figure 36-2B).

Intestinal Obstruction

As with any intra-abdominal operation, these patients are subject to adhesive small bowel obstruction or incarcerated incisional hernias. However, the "replumbing" of the anatomy also can lead to several variations of localized obstruction. After RYGB or the duodenal switch with BPD, selective obstruction of the biliopancreatic limb can lead to a form of "closed loop obstruction" (similar to an "afferent limb syndrome") characterized by marked postprandial fullness (duodenal distention and, with RYGB, also gastric distention), nausea and nonproductive vomiting (dry heaves), and, on rare occasion, acute pancreatitis or jaundice allegedly related to high pressure duodenopancreatic reflux. This diagnosis is difficult and requires (1) clinical suspicion and (2) confirmation of duodenal and, after RYGB, gastric distention best imaged by computed tomography. Lack of any reflux of contrast into the pancreaticoduodenal limb on oral contrast study is suggestive but not sensitive. Treatment involves reexploration and either adhesiolysis or internal bypass or short-circuiting of bile from the duodenum to the distal jejunum; percutaneous gastrostomy or duodenostomy via radiologic approach will decompress the distention, but the more distal obstruction may not resolve. The other form of intestinal obstruction involves an internal hernia through incompletely closed mesenteric defects created by the "surgical replumbing."

Malabsorption

Global malabsorption of all nutrients (ie, protein, fat, and carbohydrate), which complicated the old JIB (see Figure 36-1A), should no longer occur; any form of "malabsorption" should not occur after a purely gastric restrictive procedure such as VBG (see Figure 36-2A) or gastric banding (Figure 36-4). However, selective malabsorption is not uncommon after RYGB (see Figure 36-2B) or duodenal switch with BPD (see Figure 36-3). These latter procedures bypass the duodenum where much of the iron and calcium is absorbed. Iron malabsorption is usually only symptomatic in menstruating women; treatment may require intravenous iron dextran if oral iron supplementation proves inadequate. Vitamin B_{12} from the diet is also malabsorbed after RYGB because of lack of acid contact and discoordination of binding with R Factor and intrinsic factor.

Fat malabsorption with clinical steatorrhea can also occur. After a duodenal switch with BPD, the common channel (see Figure 36-3) may not be long enough to fully reabsorb bile salts, leading to bile salt wasting, bile salt-induced secretory diarrhea, depletion of the total body bile salt pool, and a subsequent fat malabsorption. Correction may require reoper-

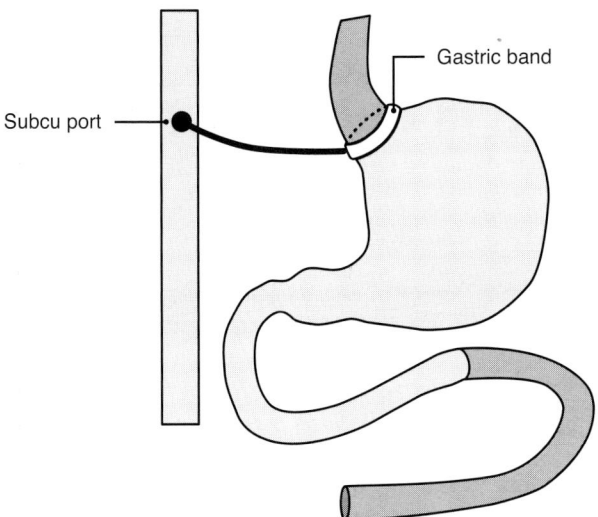

FIGURE 36-4. Gastric banding (usually laparoscopic). Note subcutaneous reservoir, which permits adjustment of the tightness of the band.

ation with moving of the biliopancreatic limb more proximally. Similarly, both BPD and RYGB may on occasion allow a bacterial overgrowth to occur in the bypassed segment, causing diarrhea and steatorrhea. This complication, however, is uncommon and differs from all the problems that occurred after the old JIB surgery in which the "bypassed" jejunoileum did not have pancreatobiliary secretions (trophic secretions) flowing through the bypassed segment.

Weight Regain

Finally, the gastroenterologist may be called upon to help define potentially correctable causes of weight regain. Most patients who are initially successful postoperatively and later regain significant weight are usually "*grazers*" who have changed their diet and eat "all the time." However, the restricting staple line disrupts occasionally after VBG or RYGB, thereby abolishing any gastric restrictive component and allowing unlimited oral intake. Endoscopic examination should show such a staple line disruption clearly.

Additional Approaches

Currently, some investigators are exploring whether electrical gastric stimulation (often incorrectly termed gastric "pacing") will induce early satiety. The justifying "preliminary data" is scanty and early results are equally questionable. This concept is "attractive" because the "pacing" electrodes can be placed laparoscopically; time will tell, however, of its efficacy. There is a separate chapter on gastric stimulation in gastroparesis (see Chapter 30, "The Management of Nonulcer Dyspepsia").

Summary

Until a truly effective pharmacologic therapy for obesity becomes available, bariatric surgery is here to stay. Gastroenterologists will be called upon to treat these patients, even if their local surgical community does not perform bariatric surgery. However, most communities are now either doing bariatric surgery or starting a program. Thus, a rudimentary knowledge of the anatomy and potential complications is imperative for the gastroenterologist and surgeon alike.

Supplemental Reading

Balsiger BM, Kennedy FP, Abu-Lebdeh HS, et al. Prospective evaluation of Roux-en-Y gastric bypass as primary operation for morbid obesity. Mayo Clin Proc 2000;75:673–80.

Balsiger BM, Murr MM, Poggio JL, Sarr MG. Bariatric surgery: surgery for weight control in patients with morbid obesity. Med Clin N Am 2000;84:477–89.

Balsiger BM, Poggio JL, Mai J, et al. Ten and more years after vertical banded gastroplasty as primary operation for morbid obesity. J Gastrointest Surg 2000;4:598–605.

Consensus Development Conference Panel. Gastrointestinal surgery for severe obesity. Ann Int Med 1991;115:956–61.

DeMaria EJ, Sugerman HJ, Meador JG, et al. High failure rate after laparoscopic adjustable silicone gastric banding for treatment of morbid obesity. Ann Surg 2001;233:809–18.

Hassan I, Juncos LA, Milliner DS, et al. Chronic renal failure secondary to oxalate nephropathy: a preventable complication after jejunoileal bypass. Mayo Clin Proc 2001;76:758–60.

O'Brien PE, Brown WA, Smith A, et al. Prospective study of a laparoscopically placed adjustable gastric band in the treatment of morbid obesity. Br J Surg 1999;86:113–8.

Schauer PR, Ikramuddin S, Gourash W, et al. Outcomes after laparoscopic Roux-en-Y gastric bypass for morbid obesity. Ann Surg 2000;232:515–29.

Scopinaro N, Gianetta E, Adami GF, et al. Biliopancreatic diversion for obesity at eighteen years. Surgery 1996;119:261–8.

CHAPTER 37

ALCOHOLISM AND ASSOCIATED DISORDERS

MACK C. MITCHELL JR, MD

Consumption of alcoholic beverages is widely accepted as a normal practice in most Western societies. Consumption of moderate amounts of alcohol does not appear to be harmful, except during pregnancy and in those individuals with a history of alcohol-associated problems or liver diseases, such as chronic viral hepatitis. On the other hand, excessive consumption of alcoholic beverages can lead to serious medical and behavioral consequences. This chapter will cover an approach to the recognition of harmful drinking patterns, definitions of alcoholism and alcohol abuse, and the approach to treatment of both alcoholism and its medical consequences.

Definitions of Alcoholism, Alcohol Abuse, and Hazardous Drinking

In the last decade many professional organizations have established guidelines or limits for safe consumption of alcoholic beverages. The majority of guidelines have defined a standard drink to contain 12 g of absolute ethanol. This is the amount contained, on average, in 12 ounces of beer, 5 ounces of wine, or 1.5 ounces of 80 proof distilled spirits. Although there is some variability in the amount of alcohol considered to be safe or nonhazardous, most guidelines recommend a limit of 2 standard drinks per day or 14 drinks per week for men and half this amount for women. The rationale for the lower limit in women is based on the lower body mass and the observation that women have reduced first pass metabolism of ethanol by the gastric mucosa, leading to a higher amount of ethanol reaching the portal circulation and the liver.

Alcoholism is a complex disorder with both behavioral and medical components, the cause of which is likely to be multifactorial. Many studies have highlighted the importance of *genetic risk factors* in the development of alcoholism and alcohol-related problems, although specific genes for alcoholism have not yet been identified. Definitions of alcoholism reflect the relapsing nature of alcoholism as well as the existence of physical dependence and tolerance to alcohol, lack of control of consumption, and continued use despite the development of problems or harmful consequences.

Definitions

Both the *Diagnostic and Statistical Manual of Mental Disorders* (DSM) and the *International Statistical Classification of Diseases* (ICD) separate alcohol-related problems into two broad categories, alcoholism and alcohol abuse disorders. The primary distinction between alcohol abuse and alcoholism in both the DSM and ICD is the requirement for physical dependence to establish a diagnosis of alcoholism. Furthermore, the ICD definition states that evidence of physical dependence must occur for at least 1 month or must occur repeatedly over 12 months, whereas the DSM definition uses terms such as "persistent" or "continued" without specifying duration of the problem. Consumption of alcohol in situations that may be hazardous or result in harmful outcomes of alcohol use is sufficient to establish a diagnosis of alcohol abuse (Table 37-1).

There is growing recognition that many people exhibit a pattern of consumption of alcoholic beverages that may be potentially hazardous without meeting criteria for alcohol abuse or alcoholism. *Hazardous drinking* is defined as consuming more than the recommended 14 drinks per week or more than 5 drinks on one occasion. Estimates of hazardous drinking in the population are as high as 20% for men and 10% for women. This definition of hazardous drinking is a subject of controversy, primarily because of the arbitrary nature of the limits for "safe consumption" and the absence of identifiable harm associated with consumption in excess of these limits. Nevertheless, the population who consumes these amounts of alcohol has been shown to have a higher risk of developing alcohol-related problems than those who consume lower amounts develop. For this reason, those who drink at levels considered hazardous are thought to represent a population that might benefit from brief interventions to reduce consumption.

SCREENING FOR ALCOHOLISM AND HAZARDOUS DRINKING

The diagnosis of alcoholism is most often based on the abnormal pattern of drinking as reflected in the definitions noted above. Frequently the affected individual may deny that he or she drinks excessively or has problems related to alcohol use. For that reason, relatives or friends may be the first to identify an abnormal pattern of drinking. Extreme

TABLE 37-1. Definitions of Alcohol Abuse (Harmful Use) and Alcoholism

Alcohol Abuse

DSM-IV A maladaptive pattern of drinking leading to clinically significant impairment as manifested by one of the following occurring within a 12 month period:
- Recurrent use of alcohol resulting in a failure to fulfill major role obligations at work, school, or home
- Recurrent alcohol use in situations in which it is physically hazardous (eg, driving or operating machinery)
- Recurrent alcohol-related legal problems
- Continued use despite persistent or recurrent social or interpersonal problems caused by alcohol
- Never met criteria for alcohol dependence

ICD-10
- Clear evidence that alcohol use contributed to physical or psychological harm, which may lead to disability/adverse consequences
- The nature of harm should be clearly identifiable
- The pattern of use has persisted for at least 1 month or has occurred repeatedly within a 12 month period
- Symptoms do not meet criteria for any other mental or behavioral disorder related to alcohol in the same time period (except acute intoxication)

Alcoholism

DSM-IV A maladaptive pattern of drinking, leading to clinically significant impairment or distress, as manifested by 3 or more of the following occurring at any time in the same 12 month period:
- Tolerance
- Withdrawal
- Impaired control
- Neglect of activities
- A great deal of time spent drinking or recovering from drinking
- Continued drinking despite problems

ICD-10 Three or more of the following occurring together for at least 1 month, or if less than 1 month, occurring together repeatedly within a 12 month period:
- Tolerance
- Withdrawal
- Impaired control
- Neglect of activities
- A great deal of time spent drinking or recovering from drinking
- Continued drinking despite problems
- A strong compulsion or desire to drink

DSM = *Diagnostic and Statistical Manual of Mental Disorders*; ICD = *International Statistical Classification of Diseases*.

---

care and diligence must be used in verifying information from these sources to avoid inappropriate labeling of an individual as alcoholic. Unfortunately, the absence of a "gold standard" test for alcoholism can make establishing the diagnosis more difficult, but certainly not impossible.

Screening Questionnaires

Screening questionnaires have been developed to detect alcoholism or hazardous consumption. These questionnaires have rates of sensitivity and specificity of approximately 50 to 80% and have been validated in a variety of clinical settings. Among the most frequently used is the *CAGE questionnaire*. This instrument uses four questions to determine the risk of alcoholism in an individual (Table 37-2). The more "yes" answers on the test, the higher the probability that an individual will meet DSM criteria for alcoholism. A second questionnaire developed by the World Health Organization, AUDIT, has been validated in six countries. Both CAGE and AUDIT are generally used to identify individuals within a general population who may not be suspected of being alcoholic before examination. They are better used as screening tests rather than as tests to confirm a diagnosis of alcoholism. The brevity of these questionnaires makes them ideal to screen for alcoholism and hazardous drinking even in busy primary care practices.

TABLE 37-2. CAGE Questionnaire

In the past year,

C Have you felt you should Cut down on your drinking?

A Have people Annoyed you by criticizing your drinking?

G Have you ever felt bad or Guilty about your drinking?

E Have you ever had a drink first thing in the morning to steady your nerves or get rid of a hangover (Eye opener)?

Other Questionnaires   The Short Michigan Alcoholism Screening Test (S-MAST) and Short Alcohol Dependence Data Questionnaire (SADD) are slightly longer questionnaires that provide useful information about the severity of physical dependence on alcohol. The length of these instruments makes them less suitable as screening tests in primary care practices.

Laboratory Tests

Although there is a need for laboratory tests to "measure" heavy drinking, most of the currently available tests are neither sensitive nor specific enough to detect heavy drinking in the general population. Both the red blood cell *mean corpuscular volume (MCV)* and γ-glutamyl transpeptidase *(GGT)* are higher in heavy drinkers than in the normal population, but there is too much overlap to make either useful as a screening test. Observing a high GGT or MCV that is otherwise unexplained in a suspected alcoholic may provide supporting evidence of heavy drinking. The *carbohydrate deficient transferrin* assay also helps to identify a population of men drinking more than 5 drinks per day for more than 1 year. However, the lack of sensitivity of this test makes its use impractical to screen for alcoholism.

Brief Interventions in Nondependent Hazardous Drinkers

Over the last decade, a large number of studies have examined the role of brief interventions to reduce alcohol consumption in those who are drinking amounts above the safe limits of consumption. Those who drink at hazardous levels are at higher risk for the future development of alcohol-related problems. The goal of brief interventions is to return alcohol consumption to more normative and safe levels and to identify situations in which individuals lose control of drinking. The National Institute of Alcoholism and Alcohol Abuse has recommended that health care providers follow these three basic steps during a brief intervention:

- State the medical concern about the level of consumption and the risk to health directly
- Advise the individual to cut down or abstain (particularly if alcohol-dependent) from consumption
- Agree on a further plan of action with the individual, such as reducing consumption to safe levels or referral for further examination as well as follow-up

Brief interventions have been demonstrated in primary and emergency care settings, as well as in college students, to reduce consumption and/or harmful consequences significantly in heavy drinkers. Despite the demonstrated effectiveness of this approach, there is still not widespread use in most practices today. It is important to recognize that there is not sufficient evidence to replace other approaches to treatment for alcohol-dependent drinkers with brief interventions. Those individuals who are known or suspected to be *alcohol-dependent* should be referred for more intensive traditional treatment of alcoholism.

Treatment of Alcoholism and Alcohol Dependence

The most important aspect of treatment of alcoholism is *recognition* of the problem and *referral for treatment*. The need to *state medical concerns* about the *level of consumption* and the *presence of any signs of physical dependence on alcohol* is a key component of the intervention. This step does not need to be carried out by a specialist in treatment of alcoholism, but can be done by any concerned health care provider. It is important that additional steps be taken to refer the individual for further treatment as soon as he or she is willing to accept the diagnosis. Patients who have developed physical complications of heavy alcohol consumption, such as *cirrhosis, pancreatitis,* or *gastritis,* are often *more amenable to beginning treatment.* The gastroenterologist has an advantage over other providers in being able to state authoritatively that a medical problem is the result of alcoholism. Using this window of opportunity often makes a difference in the likelihood of an individual beginning therapy for alcoholism. As long as appropriate steps are taken to refer the individual, it is not essential for the gastroenterologist to become personally expert in treating alcoholism.

Psychological Counseling

Psychological (counseling) approaches remain the mainstay of therapy for alcoholism. Over the years, many different approaches, including *social skills training, motivational enhancement, cognitive therapy, aversion therapy,* and *behavioral contracting,* have been used in treating alcoholism. Most approaches are more effective than no treatment, but none has been universally effective in producing long term or even short remissions. Because there are different manifestations and personality types in alcoholism, many providers within the treatment community believe that specific counseling approaches might work only within a given personality type. However, a large multicenter evaluation of matching treatment approaches to personality type in alcoholics failed to demonstrate that this approach was superior to the use of any one approach to treatment. This observation suggests *that engaging in therapy for alcoholism may be as important as the type of treatment program.*

DEPRESSION AND OTHER PSYCHOLOGICAL DISORDERS

Many alcoholics have coexistent psychiatric disorders such as depression, which require specific treatment in addition to treatment of alcoholism. *Depression* is difficult to diagnose in actively drinking alcoholics or in the early stages of abstinence. A careful history is needed to identify preexisting depression. Depression, when present, should be treated with *antidepressant medications,* such as *selective serotonin reuptake inhibitors.* Untreated depression is a potential cause of relapse or continued drinking in many alcoholics.

STRUCTURED PROGRAMS

Affiliation with Alcoholics Anonymous (AA) or similar 12 step programs is the predominant approach to treatment of alcoholism in the United States. These programs rely on development of a commitment and "therapeutic" relationship to a group of other affected individuals. Affiliation with AA does not offer success for every alcoholic, and for some this approach may be rejected because of an inability to share personal experiences openly. However, many people benefit from their affiliation with AA and all should be encouraged to attend, as AA provides a useful adjunct to other therapeutic approaches. Because AA is a volunteer administered program, there is very little cost to the individual, whereas other types of counseling may be quite expensive and therefore unavailable to many alcoholics who lack satisfactory health care insurance.

Medications for Treatment of Alcoholism

Disulfiram

Disulfiram (Antebuse) is a medication that blocks metabolism of acetaldehyde, causing an aversive reaction if alcohol is consumed while taking it. It has been used for many years, but has fallen out of favor in recent years because of problems with compliance. It may be useful in certain subsets of alcoholics or when administered under direct observation. *Drowsiness* is the most common side effect, but usually is not a problem after the first 2 weeks of therapy. There are rare reports of serious adverse reactions, including *hepatotoxicity*; therefore, monitoring liver enzymes is recommended. Stable chronic liver disease is not an absolute contraindication to treatment, but disulfiram should *not be used* during *pregnancy*, or in persons with *severe depression, severe cardiovascular disease, or dementia*. Disulfiram interferes with oxidative drug metabolism, so it should be used with caution in combination with phenytoin, warfarin, diazepam, and many other drugs that are metabolized by cytochrome P-450.

Opiate Antagonists

The opiate antagonists, *naltrexone* and *nalmefene*, were reported to reduce the euphoria associated with use of alcohol by alcoholics. This observation led to its approval by the US Food and Drug Administration (FDA) as an *adjunctive medication* in treatment of alcoholism. *Naltrexone*, (Revia) 50 mg every day, reduced the rate of relapse and extended the duration of sobriety prior to relapse compared with placebo in several clinical trials. In addition, there was a decrease in the amount of alcohol consumed and the number of days of consumption in alcoholics who relapsed while taking naltrexone. Although *naltrexone* (Revia) was approved for use more than 5 years ago, it has not been widely used in clinical practice, in part because it is relatively expensive. There is also dose-related hepatotoxicity. *Nalmefene* is not yet FDA approved. In clinical trials, it appears to be comparable in efficacy to naltrexone and does not have the dose-related hepatotoxicity reported with naltrexone.

Acamprosate

A second drug, *acamprosate* (*Campral*), affects two other neurotransmitter systems that are known to be involved in the central nervous system effects of alcohol, (1) the γ-aminobutyric acid system and (2) the glutamate system. It has been used for several years in Europe and was recently approved for use in the United States. Clinical studies there showed that approximately half of patients treated with acamprosate remained in remission after 12 weeks of medication compared with 26% on placebo. These rates are comparable to those observed with naltrexone. Currently, the NIAAA is supporting a multicenter trial *combining naltrexone with acamprosate* to determine whether there may be an additive or synergistic effect because the drugs work on different neurotransmitter systems. Although not yet approved by the FDA, *multidrug therapy* appears promising.

Management of Alcohol Withdrawal

Early Symptoms

Occurrence of *withdrawal symptoms* during abstinence from alcohol is evidence of physical dependency on alcohol and helps to confirm a diagnosis of alcoholism. Withdrawal symptoms are variable, ranging from mild tremulousness to delirium tremens (DT). Early symptoms of withdrawal, such as tremulousness and even seizures, may develop while there is still alcohol within the bloodstream. Withdrawal seizures have been noted in individuals with blood alcohol levels as high as 100 mg/dL (0.1%). In the early stages of withdrawal, alcoholics may experience nausea, vomiting, diaphoresis, mild tachycardia, hallucinations, illusions, and mild disorientation, in addition to tremor. All of these symptoms are relieved by ingestion of alcohol. Avoidance of withdrawal symptoms may be one reason why some alcoholics continue to drink despite other adverse health consequences.

Later Symptoms

The most serious consequences of alcohol withdrawal do not usually occur until 3 to 5 days of abstinence. *DT* is a potentially lethal syndrome characterized by disorientation and confusion and autonomic hyperactivity, with profuse sweating, tachycardia, and hypertension. Early withdrawal symptoms do not always precede the onset of DT. Patients with DT require *hospitalization*, treatment with *benzodiazepines* and *careful monitoring* of vital signs and *hydration* to prevent adverse cardiovascular complications. Familiarity with the syndrome and a calm, reassuring manner are essential in dealing with these patients.

Assessment of Severity

Assessment of the severity of withdrawal is an important aspect of treatment. Most units that treat alcohol withdrawal assess symptoms in a semiquantitative manner. This approach avoids under or overtreatment of patients. This author prefers the revised Clinical Institute Withdrawal Assessment for Alcohol (CIWA-r) scale. The scale employs semiquantitative estimation of 9 symptoms using a score of 1 to 7. The higher the score the greater the severity of the withdrawal. Disorientation is scored on a 1 to 4 scale (Table 37-3). Individuals with scores > 10 usually require pharmacotherapy.

BENZODIAZEPINES

Benzodiazepines have been the primary category of drugs used in treating alcohol withdrawal for many years. They are safe and effective, but require monitoring of therapy to avoid unwanted effects such as oversedation. All drugs in this category are effective in both *treating* and *preventing seizures*. In recent years, short acting drugs such as *lorazepam (Ativan)* have been used more frequently. This drug does not accumulate in those patients with chronic liver disease, such as cirrhosis or severe alcoholic hepatitis, although it can precipitate hepatic encephalopathy as easily as other drugs in this category. *Diazepam* (Valium) and *chlordiazepoxide* (Librium) have a long track record of use for treating alcohol withdrawal. Both are metabolized to active metabolites, one of which is *lorazepam*, and have a longer effective half-life than lorazepam. Some protocols for managing withdrawal take advantage of the longer half-life by using a loading dose regimen, which will "self-taper" over several days as the drugs are metabolized. *Lorazepam* (Ativan) and *oxazepam* (Serax) both require continued administration to prevent rebound withdrawal and must be tapered to prevent relapse. The CIWA-r can also be used to monitor response to treatment, allowing more than one provider to follow the patient's recovery.

TABLE 37-3. Clinical Institute Withdrawal Assessment for Alcohol—Revised

Nausea and vomiting	0 to 7
Tremor	0 to 7
Paroxysmal sweating	0 to 7
Anxiety	0 to 7
Agitation	0 to 7
Tactile disturbances	0 to 7
Auditory disturbances	0 to 7
Visual disturbances	0 to 7
Headache	0 to 7
Disorientation	0 to 4
Minimal withdrawal	0 to 9
Mild-moderate withdrawal	10 to 19
Severe withdrawal	> 20

WITHDRAWAL SEIZURES

Withdrawal seizures occur most often within the first 24 hrs of abstinence but may continue for up to 72 hrs. Seizures are a more serious manifestation of withdrawal than other early signs and symptoms. The risk of DT is increased in patients who have had seizures or previous DT. Although withdrawal seizures are usually self-limited, most experts favor drug treatment to prevent "*kindling*." Kindling increases the risk of future seizures due to past withdrawal seizures. Withdrawal seizures are best treated with *benzodiazepines*. Because of the possibility of head trauma in alcoholics, the etiology of seizures should be evaluated at least once to be certain that a structural brain injury is not the cause. Focal seizures are usually not caused solely by alcohol withdrawal; however, alcohol withdrawal can lower the threshold for focal or generalized seizures in patients with preexisting brain lesions.

Nutritional Deficiencies and Support during Alcohol Withdrawal
THIAMINE

Nutritional deficiencies are common in many alcoholics. *Thiamine deficiency* can lead to Wernicke's encephalopathy. Because of the potential for lasting brain injury, all alcoholics should be given 100 mg of thiamine daily for the first month of abstinence. Thiamine should be administered intravenously in those who are hospitalized because recent alcohol ingestion impairs the absorption of thiamine from the upper gastrointestinal tract. Pharmacologic doses of thiamine (100 mg every day) can overcome the effects of alcohol on absorption, because high concentrations are transported passively across the mucosa.

FOLATE

Folate deficiency is the most commonly observed vitamin deficiency in alcoholics. Alcohol ingestion impairs the absorption of folate and the resulting deficiency leads to loss of intestinal brush border. Damage to the intestinal villi leads to more generalized malabsorption and can result in diarrhea as well as folate deficiency in malnourished alcoholics. Mild steatorrhea, secondary to malabsorption of fat rather than pancreatic insufficiency, has been observed in malnourished alcoholics. Large doses of folate (5 mg daily) are needed initially to overcome folate deficiency, since 1 to 2 weeks is required before the intestinal lining is restored and folate absorption normalizes.

Editor's Note: I am reminded of treating the folate deficiency of tropical sprue.

Approach to the Patients Suspected of Alcoholism

When patients present with obvious medical complications of alcoholism, the gastroenterologist has an opportunity and obligation to inform the patient of the suspected cause of the problems. Use of the CAGE questions as well as an estimation of quantity and frequency of consumption of alcoholic beverages is a useful starting point in the assessment. A nonjudgmental attitude is essential in gaining the trust of the individual.

Withdrawal symptoms should be treated promptly to avoid adverse consequences. Prompt referral to AA or to other treatment programs with trained providers is helpful in initiating therapy at a time when the patient may be most amenable to treatment. At the same time as the referral is made, the gastroenterologist should advise the patient to abstain or cut down on drinking. Family members and others are often very helpful in supporting the patient in his or her decision to seek treatment. However, care should be taken to avoid discussing the patient's problems with family members in the absence of the patient's consent. Medications for alcoholism should be started only if the physician is familiar with the dosing and side effects. The outlook for successful treatment is often much better than realized, so there is never a reason to deny access to treatment on the grounds that the patient might fail or relapse.

Supplemental Reading

Beresford TP, Blow FC, Hill E, et al. Comparison of CAGE questionnaire and computer-assisted laboratory profiles in screening for covert alcoholism. Lancet 1990;336:482–5.

Buchsbaum DG, Buchanan RG, Centor RM, et al. Screening for alcohol abuse using CAGE scores and likelihood ratios. Ann Intern Med 1991;115:774–7.

Cornelius JR, Salloum IM, Ehler JG, et al. Fluoxetine in depressed alcoholics: a double-blind, placebo-controlled trial. Arch Gen Psychiatry 1997;54:700–5.

Geerlings PJ, Ansoms C, van den Brink W. Acamprosate and prevention of relapse in alcoholics: results of a randomized, placebo-controlled, double-blind study in out-patient alcoholics in the Netherlands, Belgium and Luxembourg. Eur Addict Res 1997;3:129–37.

Hasin D. Classification of alcohol use disorders. Alcohol Research and Health 2003;Vol. 27.

Marlatt GA, Baer JS, Kivlahan DR, et al. Screening and brief intervention for high-risk college student drinkers: results from an 2-year follow-up assessment. J Consult Clin Psychol 1998;66:604–15.

Mayfield DG, McLeod G, Hall P. The CAGE questionnaire: validation of a new alcoholism screening instrument. Am J Psychiatry 1974;131:1121–3.

O'Malley SS, Croop RS, Wroblewski JM. Naltrexone in the treatment of alcohol dependence: a combined analysis of two trials. Psychiatr Ann 1995;25:681–8.

O'Malley SS, Jaffe AJ, Chang G. Six-month follow-up of naltrexone and psychotherapy for alcohol dependence. Arch Gen Psychiatry 1996;53:217–24.

Project MATCH Research Group. Matching alcoholism treatments to client heterogeneity: Project MATCH three-year drinking outcomes. Alcohol Clin Exp Res 1998;22:2300–11.

Saitz R, Mayo-Smith MF, Roberts MS. Individualized treatment for alcohol withdrawal: a randomized double-blind controlled trial. JAMA 1994;272:519–23.

Sass H, Soyka M, Mann K, Zieglgansberger W. Relapse prevention by acamprosate: results from a placebo-controlled study on alcohol dependence. Arch Gen Psychiatry 1996;53:673–80.

Saunders JB, Aasland OG, Babor TF, et al. Development of the Alcohol Use Disorders Identification Test (AUDIT): WHO Collaborative Project on Early Detection of Persons with Harmful Alcohol Consumption. II. Addiction 1993;88:791–804.

Soderstrom CA, Smith GS, Kufera JA, et al. The accuracy of the CAGE, the Brief Michigan Alcoholism Screening Test, and the Alcohol Use Disorders Identification Test in screening trauma center patients for alcoholism. J Trauma 1997;43:962–9.

Anorexia Nervosa and Bulimia

Graham Redgrave, MD, and Angela Guarda, MD

Anorexia nervosa (AN) and bulimia nervosa (BN) are serious behavioral disorders associated with a wide range of gastrointestinal (GI) complications (Chami et al, 1995). Because AN and BN are characterized by frequent denial and ambivalence towards treatment, individuals with these disorders may present first (or exclusively) to gastroenterologists with secondary GI complaints (Winstead and Willard, 2001). Recognizing signs and symptoms of eating disorders, directing patients to appropriate psychiatric treatment, and assisting them in acknowledging their eating disorder is vital. For patients whose AN or BN is characterized by somatic complaints and denial of illness, a working alliance between an eating disorder specialist and a gastroenterologist is often a key factor in successful treatment.

This chapter will cover definitions of AN, BN, and other eating disorders, GI complications of eating disorders and of refeeding, management recommendations, clinical screening questions, recommendations regarding when to refer and to whom, and how to set limits on treatment of patients who refuse psychiatric intervention. Finally, we will discuss effective behavioral treatments.

Scope of the Problem

Crude mortality rates for AN are on the order of 5% per decade of follow-up, or roughly 10 times the rate for age-matched, healthy controls; causes of increased mortality include consequences of prolonged starvation and suicide (Herzog et al, 2000). The incidence of AN and BN has been increasing over the last quarter century. Among females, lifetime prevalence is 0.5% for AN and 1 to 3% for BN. Among men, prevalence rates of both disorders are roughly one-tenth those for women (American Psychiatric Association, 2000).

Definitions

AN

AN is a behavioral disorder of self-starvation motivated by an exaggerated fear of fatness in which dieting and preoccupation with thinness come to dominate life. The American Psychiatric Association (APA) defines AN as failure to maintain body weight at 85% of expected, overvalued fear of fatness, and amenorrhea for three consecutive menstrual cycles. A minimum healthy target weight should correspond to a body mass index (BMI = weight in kilograms divided by the square of height in meters) of 20 or above, age-adjusted for adolescents. Lower target weights are unlikely to result in resolution of amenorrhea (Frisch and McArthur, 1974).

All patients with AN restrict their food intake and exhibit fear of fatness; some may also excessively exercise, and engage in binge eating, self-induced vomiting, or laxative, diuretic or diet pill abuse. As many as 40% of patients with AN develop BN over time, as they become unable to restrict their intake persistently enough to maintain a very low body weight (Eckert et al, 1995).

BN

BN is characterized by frequent binge eating episodes and compensatory behaviors to avoid weight gain (eg, vomiting, laxative, diuretic or diet pill abuse, excessive exercise or fasting) and is motivated by the same fear of fatness and body dissatisfaction characteristic of AN. A binge is defined as eating more in a discrete period of time than most people would eat under similar circumstances, accompanied by a sense of loss of control. Persons who are underweight are given the diagnosis of AN, irrespective of whether they binge or purge, because AN is considered a superceding diagnosis.

Eating Disorders Not Otherwise Specified

Eating disorders occur along a spectrum. Besides AN and BN there are several variants of these disorders that may not meet full diagnostic criteria yet are associated with significant clinical impairment. Some of these may be subthreshold cases of AN or BN, whereas others may represent atypical eating disorders. All are subsumed under the diagnosis Eating Disorder Not Otherwise Specified (EDNOS). Atypical eating disorders are ones in which overvalued concern with fear of fatness is absent yet the patient develops significant eating behavior pathology. Examples include globus hystericus (phobia of swallowing or choking resulting in food refusal), rumination, or psychogenic vomiting syndromes. Binge eating disorder (BED) is also considered an EDNOS. BED is characterized by frequent binges not associated with compensatory purging behavior and is usually associated with obesity. Though treatment of EDNOS will not be covered in detail, the primary modality of treatment is behavioral and has much in common with the treatment of AN and BN.

The Nature of Behavioral Disorders

AN and BN are driven, repetitive behavioral disorders that are difficult to interrupt. They share characteristics with other pathological behavioral conditions, such as substance abuse. Excuses are made for not eating, and vomiting or hiding food is done surreptitiously. Disturbed eating and dieting behaviors gradually come to dominate the person's life, impairing physical, psychological, or social function. Persons with disorders of behavior frequently attribute their difficulties to various causes (eg, conflicts with others or circumstantial stressors) and minimize the extent to which they engage in the disturbed behavior because it is increasingly rewarding to them. Although stressors, social pressures, and individual vulnerabilities can be predisposing factors, they become irrelevant as secondary sustaining factors emerge and maintain the behavioral cycle. It is these secondary sustaining factors that account for continued engagement in the behavior in the face of mounting costs. For example, desire to drink and the physiological dependency syndrome reinforce alcoholic behavior, a fact that becomes increasingly evident as relationships and job performance are adversely affected. After years of drinking, the alcoholic drinks today because he drank yesterday. Similarly the chronic anorectic diets because she did so yesterday. In AN, desire to lose weight (or fear of gaining weight), habit, and the physiological and psychological consequences of dieting (eg, increased preoccupation with food and delayed GI transit time) sustain abnormal dieting behaviors. The characterization of AN and BN as behavioral disorders has important implications for treatment.

Gastroenterology and the Eating Disordered Patient

The GI problems of most individuals with eating disorders result from *starvation*, from *compensatory behaviors* like *vomiting, laxative* or *diuretic abuse*, or from *treatment* (eg, the *refeeding syndrome*). That *most of these problems are secondary to the behaviors* is suggested by the fact that even in nonclinical college aged women, the *severity and number of GI complaints* has been *associated with the extent of dieting* behavior (Krahn et al, 1996). *Most complaints* have been found to *reverse with normalization of eating behavior* and *do not require or respond to symptomatic treatment* with typical pharmacological agents. It is important for gastroenterologists to *be aware of common complaints in eating disordered patients* so as not to miss a diagnosis and chance for early intervention. It is also important to note that management of AN and BN may be complicated by *cardiac, metabolic,* and *endocrine sequelae*; however, the details of management of these complications are beyond the scope of this chapter.*

GI Complications

Starvation

Gastric emptying of solids, and possibly of liquids, is delayed in patients with AN (Dubois et al, 1979; Ricci and McCallum, 1988). This phenomenon presumably contributes to complaints of early satiety and fullness and may normalize *more slowly* than other markers of starvation, such as bradycardia and hypotension. *Transaminase elevations* are not uncommon in starved anorectic patients and often worsen transiently with refeeding. Compared with controls, patients are more likely to suffer from *constipation* and to demonstrate delayed whole gut and colonic transit times (Chun et al, 1997; Kamal et al, 1991). As with other eating disorder-related GI problems, slowed transit times resolve with weight restoration.

Vomiting, Laxative, and Diuretic Abuse
Oral

Anorexics and bulimics who vomit to compensate for real or perceived binges may develop *perimolysis*, a loss of the enamel and dentin on the lingual surface of the teeth caused by recurrent exposure of the teeth to gastric acids. Patients may complain of increased sensitivity to heat, cold, and acidic substances, as discussed in the chapter on oral medicine (see Chapter 7, "Oral Considerations in Patients with Gastrointestinal Disorders"). The large amounts of carbohydrates consumed by bulimic patients during binges may further exacerbate the problem, contributing to an elevated frequency of *caries*. *Parotid gland enlargement* is a common manifestation of bulimia (Cuellar and Van Thiel, 1986; Jacobs and Schneider, 1985). No treatment is required, and the parotid enlargement usually subsides over time with cessation of vomiting. Some individuals abuse syrup of *ipecac* to induce vomiting, placing themselves at risk for *cardiotoxicity* resulting from accumulation of emetine in cardiac muscle. There appears to be a dose-response curve, and ingestion of 3 to 4 bottles per day has been associated with cardiac arrest and severe cardiac arrhythmias (Sansone, 1984).

Esophageal

Patients with eating disorders suffer from a spectrum of esophageal problems, ranging from mild esophagitis and reflux to esophageal erosions, ulcers, and rupture, largely

---

*Editor's Note: Because Crohn's Disease often presents in the same age group, an occasional psychologically complex young woman with Crohn's disease will be discovered in an eating disorder clinic.

as a result of recurrent self-induced vomiting. Higher rates of dysphagia, Barrett's esophagus, and esophageal stricture are reported in bulimic patients compared with controls. As with salivary gland swelling, alcohol abuse also increases the risk of esophageal pathology (Cuellar and Van Thiel, 1986).

Gastric

Mallory-Weiss tear and even gastric rupture have occasionally been reported in patients with BN, presumably as the result of chronic vomiting (McGilley and Pryor, 1998). Data regarding gastric emptying are more mixed for BN than for AN, but at least one study revealed delayed gastric emptying in patients compared with controls. Treatment of the eating disorder improved gastric emptying time (Kamal et al, 1991).

Laxative Abuse

GI complaints associated with the abuse of laxatives, particularly the stimulant laxatives, such as bisacodyl and phenolphthalein, and the anthracene derivatives (senna, cascara, danthron), include nonspecific complaints such as constipation, diarrhea, abdominal cramping or pain, nausea and vomiting, and distention and bloating. Other sequelae of laxative abuse include steatorrhea, protein-losing enteropathy, osteomalacia and melanosis coli. Rectal prolapse secondary to severe laxative abuse can also be seen in eating disorder patients.

Amylase/Pancreatitis

Although *hyperamylasemia* is found in as many as 62% of patients with BN, it is usually *salivary* in origin. Nonetheless, Gavish and colleagues (1987) reported on 21 patients with recurrent *hyperlipidemic pancreatitis*, all of whom were subsequently diagnosed with BN, and one of whom died. It is important to reiterate the importance of assessing *alcohol use* in patients with eating disorders because of the overlap of GI pathology produced by these conditions.

Diuretic Abuse

Patients who abuse diuretics typically choose over-the-counter products, but may also use prescription medications (Roerig et al, 2003). Complications from diuretic abuse include toxicity from agents containing salicylates or acetaminophen, and hypokalemia from loop diuretics. Abrupt withdrawal from these agents may produce reflex fluid retention and edema, so diuretics should be tapered if abuse has been heavy.

Refeeding

Acute gastric dilatation has been reported both in AN and BN. This condition typically occurs anywhere from a few days to more than 3 weeks after commencement of refeeding and can usually be managed conservatively, with *intravenous (IV) fluids* and *nasogastric (NG) suction*, although there are reports of deaths and of cases requiring surgery. Pancreatitis has also been reported during refeeding in patients with AN (Cuellar and Van Thiel, 1986).

The refeeding syndrome is characterized by fluid and electrolyte shifts (especially hypokalemia, hypophosphatemia, and hypomagnesemia), hypoglycemia, low levels of thiamine, and potentially serious consequences, including severe edema, congestive heart failure, transaminitis, cardiac arrhythmias, Wernicke's encephalopathy, seizures, delirium, and death. This syndrome is encountered most frequently in patients of very low body weight (eg, < 60% of ideal body weight) who are being aggressively re-fed, and has been described in victims of famine and prisoners of war, as well as in underweight patients with eating disorders. NG and IV feeding are associated with higher risk of such complications than oral refeeding (Crook et al, 2001; Faintuch et al, 2001).

Management

Care should be coordinated to ensure consistency of recommendations between gastroenterologist, psychiatrist, therapist, and nutritionist. As a general rule, defer invasive diagnostic procedures except when absolutely necessary (eg, to rule out acute gastric distention). Reassure the patient that with weight restoration and normalization of eating patterns symptoms will subside and that if they do not do so, you will be happy to reconsider a workup for the complaints at that time. *Educate patients on the strong association between GI complaints and disordered eating behavior.*

For *reflux symptoms*, judicious use of proton pump inhibitors and H_2 blockade as needed is appropriate. We do not recommend the use of metoclopramide on a regular basis for the treatment of delayed gastric emptying because of potential side effects, including symptoms of depression and extrapyramidal symptoms; again, reassurance that feelings of fullness or discomfort will subside with refeeding is usually the best and most conservative intervention.

For treatment of *constipation*, we advocate the use of bulking agents, stool softeners, and nonstimulant laxatives. Avoid prescription of stimulant laxatives because of their abuse liability in patients with eating disorders. A *lactulose taper* can be used to wean severe laxative abusers off cathartic agents.

We do not advocate NG refeeding or the placement of percutaneous endoscopic gastrostomy (PEG) tubes, for several reasons. First, there is morbidity associated with the use of NG and PEG tubes. Second, eating disordered patients with NG tubes and PEG tubes have a tendency to "medicalize" their disorders as a means of avoiding responsibility for recovery. Third, the extinction of the drive to starve oneself is best accomplished by exposure and desensitization (ie, eating a diverse range of foods). There is no evidence that placing NG tubes improves outcomes, shortens lengths of stay, or reduces morbidity independent of refeeding itself. Enteral and parenteral feeding for weight restoration should be employed rarely and reserved for cases where treatment on a behaviorally based, dedicated eating disorder unit is not available.

Management of the *refeeding syndrome* is *prophylactic* and includes the following: (1) gradual titration of caloric intake during refeeding and low sodium intake to minimize edema, (2) continuous slow IV infusion of glucose and frequent finger sticks to manage hypoglycemia, and (3) repletion of phosphate and magnesium. Oral refeeding on a behavioral unit is the preferable setting for weight restoration; however, if despite these measures the patient develops symptomatic bradycardia or a widened QT interval, or seizures, more aggressive management, up to and including intensive care, may be required.

Screening and Referral
SCREENING

The diagnosis of AN or BN begins with a comprehensive history and physical examination. A certain amount of circumspection is helpful as some patients may be quite resistant to attempts to make an eating disorder diagnosis. The history should include careful questions about dieting and eating behavior, and screening for comorbid mood and substance abuse problems, because these often complicate the presentation of patients with eating disorders (see Table 38-1 for eating disorder-related questions we ask during an initial examination). Besides standard questions used to screen for eating disorder symptoms, we have found the following three questions to be sensitive in cases marked by denial of illness: (1) "How much would you like to weigh (desired weight)?" (2) "Exactly what (and how much) did you eat yesterday?" and (3) in the case of excessive exercisers, "If exercise did not burn calories how much time would you spend exercising?" Although emaciated anorectics will acknowledge they are too thin and express a desire to gain weight, their desired weight is usually around a BMI of 18, reflecting fear of fatness despite their insistence that they wish to weigh more. A description of the prior day's intake helps uncover avoidance of fat in the diet and narrowing of the food repertoire, and the third question helps clarify motivation for exercise in individuals who exercise excessively in order to burn calories.

On physical examination, parotid enlargement, dental erosions, lacerations on the knuckles from reflexive biting arising from self-induced vomiting (Russell's sign), starved habitus, and lanugo hair growth all help to confirm diagnosis, as can laboratory evaluations (eg, serum ketones, hypokalemia, hyperamylasemia, hypophosphatemia, elevated bicarbonate, hypochloremia, and hypomagnesemia). Once the diagnosis is made, the gastroenterologist or primary practitioner is faced with the task of engaging the patient in appropriate treatment.

WHEN AND WHERE TO REFER

If the patient is willing and the opportunity exists, it is preferable to refer the patient with AN or BN to a psychiatrist specializing in the treatment of eating disorders, as soon as possible. Data suggests earlier treatment is associated with decreased morbidity. If the patient is unwilling to see a psychiatrist, referral to a therapist (social worker or psychologist) or nutritionist with expertise in the treatment of eating disorders is appropriate.

Difficulties for the Gastroenterologist in Engaging and Maintaining Patients in Treatment

Because patients with AN and BN are strongly ambivalent about giving up dieting behavior, gastroenterologists may find themselves unwitting accomplices of *patients looking to feel better rather than to get better*. Complaints about bloating, early satiety, constipation, nausea, reflux, and abdominal pain may prompt expensive, often invasive diagnostic or therapeutic procedures, the vast majority of which are unnecessary distractions from the task of behavioral change and recovery, which usually results in the resolu-

TABLE 38-1. Important Elements of the Eating Disorder History

1. Age patient first became preoccupied with losing weight or feeling fat:
2. Age of first dieting behavior: At what weight/BMI:
3. Patient amenorrheic or oligomenorrheic > 3 months? (Note: use of oral contraceptives confounds the response to this question)
4. Patient's desired weight:
5. Maximum lifetime weight/BMI: At age:
6. Minimum lifetime weight/BMI: At age:
7. Percent of waking time spent thinking about food and weight:
8. Type of restricting (skipping meals, small meals, or narrowing food repertoire):
9. Typical day's intake:
10. Breakfast:
11. Lunch:
12. Dinner:
13. Specific eating disordered behaviors:

	Age of Onset	Frequency of Behavior in the Last 30 Days
Binging		
Vomiting		
Laxatives		
Diet Pills		
Diuretics		
Ipecac		
Exercise		

BMI = body mass index.

tion of all GI complications. Because of their *denial* and *ambivalence*, some patients may not be able or willing to accept the gastroenterologist's diagnosis and recommendations. Indeed they may seek second and third opinions and, in extreme cases, may inappropriately seek surgical intervention including colectomy or gastric bypass surgery.

These patients are clearly suffering, and the compassionate physician is faced with the difficult task of setting limits on requests for tests and procedures without being overly paternalistic and persuading patients that they would benefit most from psychiatric behavioral treatment. Because of the morbidity and mortality associated with eating disorders, we feel it is justified to exert a certain amount of pressure on patients with eating disorders to accept appropriate (ie, psychiatric) treatment.

Persuasion should consist of supportive yet repeated reminders that the cause of the patient's GI complaints is the disordered eating behavior itself, that the *recommended treatment is behavioral*, and that GI interventions are not appropriate in the absence of psychiatric treatment. Involvement of close family in this process is highly recommended, because parents and significant others may help patients accept the need for psychiatric treatment.

If the patient persists in refusing to see an eating disorder specialist, the gastroenterologist may consider terminating treatment. Termination should be framed for the patient as a consequence of his or her decision not to engage in the recommended treatment. Thus, the gastroenterologist allies him or herself with the psychiatrist, rather than allowing the illness-driven manipulation to continue.

Although patients may resist referral to an eating disorders specialist, it is our experience that when engaged in treatment many change their mind, develop increased insight, and, once they recover, are grateful for treatment (Heinberg et al, 2002). Furthermore, motivation for treatment does not appear to significantly affect rates of inpatient weight gain, which are equivalent in voluntarily admitted as compared to involuntarily admitted patients with AN (Russell, 2001).

Psychiatric Treatment of Eating Disorders

Outpatient Treatment

The mainstay of outpatient treatment for adults with AN and BN is *psychotherapy*, the goal of which is the interruption of problem behaviors and normalization of eating behavior. To recover, the patient must undergo a conversion from seeing dieting behavior as a solution to viewing it as the primary problem. *Only after behavioral change is accomplished* should treatment move on to address predisposing factors, such as family conflict, personality vulnerabilities, and a chaotic personal life. Although individuals may wish to engage in intellectual pursuit of the "causes" of their disorder rather than changing their behavior, such an approach is fruitless and similar to the alcoholic engaging in exploration of the reasons why he or she drinks while continuing to consume alcohol. Once the behaviors are extinguished, the rest of recovery can proceed.

Effective treatment depends on setting clear behavioral guidelines (eg, binging and vomiting decrement of 50% over 3 to 4 weeks, weight gain of 1 to 2 lbs/week on a prescribed diet). The patient should be weighed at the beginning of each session and be instructed to maintain a daily food log and record of abnormal behaviors, such as vomiting or use of laxatives. Triggers for eating disordered behavior and situations that sustain it are discussed and alternate thoughts and behaviors are explored. The therapeutic approach is *cognitive-behavioral* and fairly directive, with the therapist playing an active role in helping the patient problem solve, develop healthier behaviors, and challenge irrational beliefs. Although the standard course of cognitive behavioral treatment for uncomplicated BN is brief, on the order of 16 to 20 weeks, persuading patients with AN to gain weight as outpatients is difficult, and outpatient psychotherapy for AN may be more protracted.

In addition to individual therapy, *group therapy* is a powerful treatment modality for behavioral disorders of all kinds. Myths associated with eating disorders are more effectively dispelled in a group. Confrontation about maladaptive behaviors (eg, lying about caloric intake, concealing vomiting, blaming others for one's own difficulties coping with the illness) often falls on deaf ears when coming from a clinician, but is powerful when coming from a peer who has engaged in the same behaviors.

Family therapy has been demonstrated to be highly effective in the treatment of adolescent eating disorders, particularly AN (Russell et al, 1987; Eisler et al, 1997). The explicit treatment aim is to assist parents in regaining appropriate parental control over their child's eating behavior and weight gain.

Failure to achieve behavioral goals despite weekly follow-up meetings and a 1 to 2 month trial of outpatient care indicates a need for inpatient or partial hospital treatment on a dedicated eating disorders specialty unit.

Inpatient and Partial Hospital Psychiatric Treatment

Inpatient treatment for BN is uncommon and is reserved for patients who have failed outpatient interventions, are medically unstable, or have serious comorbidity (eg, suicidal symptoms, alcohol dependence, or brittle diabetes). In AN, however, a significant proportion of patients require inpatient treatment for weight restoration. Dedicated eating disorder specialty units are multidisciplinary in nature, with important contributions made by various disciplines including nursing, nutritionists, occupational therapists, psychotherapists (social workers or psychologists), medical consultants, and psychiatrists. Treatment is structured using a behavioral protocol aimed initially at blocking all eating disordered behaviors by using nursing observation and dietitian prescribed meals. Patients are gradually assisted in regaining appropriate responsibility over meal selection and preparation tasks.

For the underweight patient, hospital stays can be long. Optimum weight gain is 3 to 4 lbs/week, and some patients with AN may be 40 or 50 lbs underweight at admission. For bulimics who are not underweight, lengths of stay are typically much shorter and serve to interrupt the behavioral restrict-binge-purge cycle before transition to a less structured partial hospital setting. The focus of partial hospitalization is on supervised activities, including restaurant outings, grocery shopping, and meal preparation under staff supervision. As eating behavior and weight normalize, patients are discharged to weekly outpatient care.

Because there are few dedicated behavioral eating disorder units, patients are often treated in alternate settings including general psychiatric units, medical units, or pediatric floors. These alternate inpatient settings are less than ideal, because of the difficulty in implementing a behavioral approach, the absence of staff skilled in the treatment of these disorders, and the inability to generate the peer pressure necessary to motivate patients to change their behavior.

Although the complexity of inpatient cases and the structure of the inpatient setting make multidisciplinary treatment the standard, in the outpatient setting coordination between multiple care providers is less practical. Often simpler care is better. Although some patients benefit greatly from nutritionists, a normal weight patient, for example, should be instructed to eat a balanced and varied diet, and likely does not need specialized nutritional counseling. Furthermore, psychiatrists often do not perform psychotherapy but only manage medications, and psychotherapy is performed by a psychologist or social worker. This arrangement can work well if the psychiatrist and therapist maintain close contact and have similar views of treatment, but can be problematic if the patient is able to recruit one clinician in the service of undermining the other's recommendations. Likewise, gastroenterologists who do not coordinate care with other members of the team may be prompted by an ambivalent patient to unknowingly undermine the psychiatric treatment.

Pharmacotherapy

By far the best-studied pharmacologic agent in the treatment of AN is *fluoxetine* (Prozac and generics). The data for treatment of acutely ill, underweight patients are mixed, and there is at least some evidence that suggests if patients are treated in a sufficiently intense, multidisciplinary inpatient setting, fluoxetine does not add additional benefit (Strober et al, 1999). The APA's Practice Guidelines recommend the use of *antidepressants* as agents to aid relapse prevention, but not as the primary modality of treatment for AN.

Studies of the pharmacotherapy of BN have demonstrated efficacy for several classes of antidepressants, including *tricyclic antidepressants (TCAs)* (eg, nortriptyline [Pannelor], amitriptyline [Elavil]), monoamine oxidase inhibitors, and selective serotonin reuptake inhibitors (SSRIs) (eg, fluoxetine and related compounds). There is some evidence that treatment with *fluoxetine* (Prozac) is more effective at 60 mg daily than at 20 mg daily. There are few data on the use of other SSRIs or newer agents, such as venlafaxine (Effexor XR), and the older antidepressants, such as the TCAs, are generally felt to be relatively contraindicated because of their side effect profiles.

Outcomes: Chronicity and Relapse

Although approximately 50% of patients with AN and BN will recover in the long term, eating disorders, like substance use disorders, are best thought of as behavioral illnesses whose courses are relapsing and remitting. On the one hand, this means that clinicians treating these patients must be prepared for relapses, perhaps requiring rehospitalization; on the other hand, a certain therapeutic optimism is helpful when managing a relapse, helping the patient to "dust themselves off and get back on the wagon."

Psychiatric Comorbidity: Alcoholism, Mood, and Personality

Of particular concern to the gastroenterologist is the *high comorbidity* between eating disorders and substance abuse, especially *alcoholism*. The overall rate of all substance use disorders among eating disordered patients was 37% in one study, and rates of alcoholism among bulimics were > 40% (Braun et al, 1994). Patients abusing alcohol exhibit high rates of GI comorbidity, and women suffer adverse consequences, such as cirrhosis, from consumption of alcohol more quickly than do men. We recommend screening all eating disordered patients for alcohol abuse behaviors (Redgrave et al, 2003).

Mood disorders are highly comorbid with eating disorders; between 40 to 80% of patients with eating disorders will have an affective disorder during their lifetime (Braun et al, 1994). The presence of major depressive disorder or bipolar disorder complicates the examination and management of the patient with AN or BN. Actively depressed patients may feel hopeless and be more likely to resist treatment. In addition, because starvation is associated with a syndrome of depression, symptoms of eating disorders may mimic depression yet reverse rapidly with refeeding.

There is a strong link between *personality vulnerabilities* and eating disorders. Methods of measuring personality vary widely, so comparing studies is somewhat problematic, but it is clear that certain traits (eg, neuroticism) make recovery prolonged for patients, and that, in general, the greater the personality pathology the more complicated the management of the eating disorder (Wonderlich and Mitchell, 2001). As with eating disorders, the primary treatment of personality vulnerabilities is psychotherapy.

Conclusions

GI complaints among patients with AN and BN are the rule rather than the exception, and range from the benign (bloating and dyspepsia) to the life threatening (acute gastric distention, ipecac cardiotoxicity, and the refeeding syndrome). Gastroenterologists are frequently the first physicians to encounter these patients, and because of inherent ambivalence about weight gain that spurs patients to avoid treatment, it may fall to the gastroenterologist to educate the patient about her diagnosis and to persuade her to engage in effective behavioral treatment. Such treatment is best provided by psychiatrists and psychotherapists experienced with eating disorders. Certain aspects of care, such as requiring the keeping of food logs and weighing patients to ensure they meet behavioral expectations, are the hallmarks of effective behavioral treatment. When multiple providers (gastroenterologist, psychiatrist, therapist, and nutritionist) are working with a single patient, clear communication of expectations is vital so the patient is not afforded the opportunity to undermine one provider's treatment with the recommendation of another. Recognition and treatment of comorbid substance, mood, and personality difficulties will increase the clinician's ability to manage these challenging disorders.*

Supplemental Reading

American Psychiatric Association. Practice guideline for the treatment of patients with eating disorders (revision). American Psychiatric Association Work Group on Eating Disorders. Am J Psychiatry 2000;157:1–39.

Braun DL, Sunday SR, Halmi KA. Psychiatric comorbidity in patients with eating disorders. Psychol Med 1994;24:859–67.

Chami TN, Andersen AE, Crowell MD, et al. Gastrointestinal symptoms in bulimia nervosa: effects of treatment. Am J Gastroenterol 1995;90:88–92.

Chun AB, Sokol MS, Kaye WH, et al. Colonic and anorectal function in constipated patients with anorexia nervosa. Am J Gastroenterol 1997;92:1879–83.

Crook MA, Hally V, Panteli JV. The importance of the refeeding syndrome. Nutrition 2001;17:632–7.

Cuellar RE, Van Thiel DH. Gastrointestinal consequences of the eating disorders: anorexia nervosa and bulimia. Am J Gastroenterol 1986;81:1113–24.

Dubois A, Gross HA, Ebert MH, Castell DO. Altered gastric emptying and secretion in primary anorexia nervosa. Gastroenterol 1979;77:319–23.

Eckert ED, Halmi KA, Marchi P, et al. Ten-year follow-up of anorexia nervosa: clinical course and outcome. Psychol Med 1995;25:143–56.

Eisler I, Dare C, Russell GF, et al. Family and individual therapy in anorexia nervosa. A 5-year follow-up. Arch Gen Psychiatry 1997;54:1025–30.

Fluoxetine Bulimia Nervosa Collaborative Study Group. Fluoxetine in the treatment of bulimia nervosa. A multicenter, placebo-controlled, double-blind trial. Arch Gen Psychiatry 1992;49:139–47.

Frisch RE, McArthur JW. Menstrual cycles: fatness as a determinant of minimum weight for height necessary for their maintenance or onset. Science 1974;185:949–51.

Gavish D, Eisenberg S, Berry EM, et al. Bulimia. An underlying behavioral disorder in hyperlipidemic pancreatitis: a prospective multidisciplinary approach. Arch Intern Med 1987;147:705–8.

Heinberg LJ, Guarda AS, Marinilli AS, et al. Perceived coercion among hospitalized patients with anorexia nervosa. Paper presented at the annual meeting of the Eating Disorders Research Society; November 21–23, 2002, Charleston (SC).

Herzog DB, Greenwood DN, Dorer DJ, et al. Mortality in eating disorders: a descriptive study. Int J Eat Disord 2000;28:20–6.

Jacobs MB, Schneider JA. Medical complications of bulimia: a prospective evaluation. Q J Med 1985;54:177–82.

Kamal N, Chami T, Andersen A, et al. Delayed gastrointestinal transit times in anorexia nervosa and bulimia nervosa. Gastroenterol 1991;101:1320–4.

Krahn D, Kurth C, Nairn K, et al. Dieting severity and gastrointestinal symptoms in college women. J Am Coll Health 1996;45:67–71.

McGilley BM, Pryor TL. Assessment and treatment of bulimia nervosa. Am Fam Physician 1998;57:2743–50.

Redgrave GW, Swartz KL, Romanoski AJ. Alcohol misuse by women. Int Rev Psychiatry 2003;15:256–68.

Ricci DA, McCallum RW. Diagnosis and treatment of delayed gastric emptying. Adv Intern Med 1988;33:357–84.

Roerig JL, Mitchell JE, de Zwaan M, et al. The eating disorders medicine cabinet revisited: a clinician's guide to appetite suppressants and diuretics. Int J Eat Disord 2003;33:443–57.

Russell GF. Involuntary treatment in anorexia nervosa. Psychiatr Clin North Am 2001;24:337–49.

Russell GF, Szmukler GI, Dare C, Eisler I. An evaluation of family therapy in anorexia nervosa and bulimia nervosa. Arch Gen Psychiatry 1987;44:1047–56.

Sansone RA. Complications of hazardous weight-loss methods. Am Fam Physician 1984;30:141–6.

Strober M, Pataki C, Freeman R, DeAntonio M. No effect of adjunctive fluoxetine on eating behavior or weight phobia during the inpatient treatment of anorexia nervosa: an historical case-control study. J Child Adolesc Psychopharmacol 1999;9:195–201.

Winstead NS, Willard SG. Frequency of physician visits for GI complaints by anorexic and bulimic patients. Am J Gastroenterol 2001;96:1667–8.

Wonderlich S, Mitchell JE. The role of personality in the onset of eating disorders and treatment implications. Psychiatr Clin North Am 2001;24:249–58.

---

*Editor's Note: This is a very useful chapter that should be quite helpful to the gastroenterologist confronted with a patient with an eating disorder.

CHAPTER 39

THE IRRITABLE BOWEL SYNDROME

ROBERT S. FISHER, MD

Approach to Management

Historically, the irritable bowel syndrome (IBS) has been a disease that, once diagnosed, is difficult to treat, leaving the patient and physician less than satisfied with the outcome. With the advent of new pharmacologic therapies based on increased knowledge of the pathophysiology of IBS and the *putative role of enteric neurotransmitters* in the pathogenesis of symptoms, the therapeutic armamentarium available to the treating gastroenterologist has expanded in the last several years. New and traditional therapies for the IBS will be reviewed.

Definition

The current definition of IBS is based on the Rome II criteria, which include the following: (1) abdominal pain or discomfort for at least 12 of the preceding 52 weeks (not necessarily consecutive) and (2) at least two of the following three criteria: relief of pain/discomfort with defecation, change in the frequency of bowel movements, and change in the consistency of bowel movements (Thompson et al, 1999).

Although it is known that symptoms may change over time, recent recommendations are that patients with the IBS should be subcategorized using symptom-based criteria into the following three subgroups: (1) IBS associated with abdominal discomfort, fecal urgency, and *diarrhea*, (2) IBS associated with abdominal discomfort, bloating, and constipation, and (3) IBS *alternating* between diarrhea and constipation (Brandt et al, 2002).

Traditionally, practitioners have focused their efforts on treating the individual symptoms of IBS, including diarrhea with one medication, constipation with another medication, and pain relief with an additional medication. With the advent of serotonin receptor agonists and antagonists, multiple symptoms of IBS can be addressed with a single therapeutic agent; therefore, treatment can be approached in a more global manner (Mertz, 2003).

Pathophysiology

Rational treatment for IBS is based on our understanding of its pathophysiology (Horwitz and Fisher, 2001). *Motility dysfunction* in the colon and, perhaps, the distal small intestine have long been considered important in the genesis of IBS-associated symptoms. A second pathogenetic mechanism may be *visceral hypersensitivity* whereby nonpainful intra-abdominal stimuli become painful (*alldynia*) or painful stimuli become more painful (*hyperalgesia*). Whether visceral hypersensitivity is due to *hypervigilence* or *sensitization* of sensory pathways by an acute event has not been determined. A third potential pathophysiologic abnormality in IBS is *abnormal central processing of peripheral information* as evidenced on proton emission tomography or functional magnetic resonance imaging. Although psychiatric factors are not considered to be the major cause of IBS, there is abundant evidence that *psychological disorders* are more common in patients with IBS when compared with either the general population or with medical control patients, such as those with inflammatory bowel disease. Recently, a role for *infection* in the genesis of IBS has been suggested. Many of the treatment modalities employed in the treatment of IBS target these putative pathogenetic factors (Creed et al, 2001).

Treatment

Dietary Modification

A trial of dietary modification is a reasonable first choice in the treatment of the IBS. Patients should be encouraged to keep a diary of food intake and symptoms allowing the identification and exclusion of symptom-causing foods. Dietary modification may be useful because most IBS patients complain of symptom exacerbation after intake of certain food groups. There is a separate and highly detailed chapter on dietary-induced symptoms (Chapter 56). Some patients may benefit from avoiding or limiting intake of *caffeine, alcohol, fatty foods, gas-producing vegetables*, and/or *sorbitol-containing* products such as *sugarless gum* and *dietetic candy*. Avoiding constipating foods and the addition of *fiber* either in the diet or in the form of supplements, such as bran, polycarbophil or a psyllium derivative, equal to 20 to 30 g per day may be helpful in treating patients with constipation. In patients with diarrhea, a trial of a *lactose free diet* should be instituted in the event of a concommitent lactase deficiency in addition to the IBS.

Pain

Treatment of pain in the IBS presents a great challenge. Medications beneficial to one patient may be completely ineffectual in another. *Antispasmodics* may reduce abdominal pain via anticholinergic pathways or by direct relaxation of smooth muscles with the use of *nitrates* and *calcium channel blockers*. The latter two therapies may cause unintentional hypotension and are, therefore, rarely prescribed for IBS. Anticholinergics act by the antagonism of muscarinic receptors innervated by the parasympathetic nervous system.

In addition to the desired effect of relaxation of smooth muscle viscera, undesired effects, such as sedation, salivary hyposecretion and urinary retention, can occur; this limits the use of antispasmodics. Clinical trials of the anticholinergic medications in the United States have been of poor quality and are, therefore, difficult to evaluate. Currently the following six antispasmodic/ anticholinergic agents are available for use in the United States:

1. *Dicyclomine (Bentyl)*
2. *Hyoscyamine sulfate (Levsin, Nulev, IBS Stat)*
3. *Methscopolamine bromide (Pamine)*
4. *Glycopyrrolate (Robinul)*
5. *Clidinium bromide chlordioxipoxide (Librax)*
6. *Belladonna with phenobarbital (Donnatal)* (Table 39-1)

Psychotropic Medications

The use of psychotropic medications has become popular in the treatment of functional bowel disorders, especially the IBS. Both the *tricyclic antidepressant medications (TCAs)*, as well as the *selective serotonin reuptake inhibitors (SSRIs)*, can be used in IBS; however, the TCA medications have been more extensively evaluated for this purpose and may be more efficacious.

There is a separate chapter on the use of psychotropic drugs in patients with functional disorders (see Chapter 43, "Psychotropic Drugs and Management of Patients with Functional Gastrointestinal Disorders").

When choosing an antidepressant for therapy, the side effect profile should be used to the patient's advantage. In IBS patients with *diarrhea*, a *TCA* would be more appropriate given its side effect of constipation. Conversely, an *SSRI* should be chosen in IBS patients with *constipation*. When choosing a specific TCA, use a secondary amine with fewer overall side effects such as *nortriptyline (Pamelor)* instead of its precursor amitriptyline (Elavil) or *desipramine (Norpramin)* instead of imipramine (Tofranil). Low doses of the TCAs between 10 and 25 mg are used initially with the maximum benefit usually occurring at a dose of 50 mg/d (see Table 39-1).

Little data are currently available about the SSRI antidepressant medications. However, preliminary studies have suggested possible efficacy with the use of *paroxetine (Paxil)* (Creed et al, 2001), as well as *fluoxetine (Prozac)* (Kurken et al, 2002). Standard antidepressant doses of these SSRI medications may be necessary. Preliminary evidence suggests that the use of *naloxone*, an opioid receptor antagonist, may be useful in the treatment of pain in IBS patients with constipation, but larger scale studies are required before this recommendation can be made (Hawkes et al, 2002). As will be discussed below, the 5-HT receptor agonists and antagonists can also be used in the proper circumstances for the treatment of pain.

Diarrhea

The treatment of diarrhea can be approached in a variety of ways. Although not supported in randomized clinical trials, the use of low doses of fiber can occasionally help to reduce

TABLE 39-1. Medications for the Treatment of Pain in Irritable Bowel Syndrome

Drug		Dose
Anticholinergics/antispasmodics		
Dicyclomine	(Bentyl)	10 mg every 6 hours up to 40 mg every 6 hours, if tolerated
Hyoscyamine	(Levsin)	0.125 to 0.25 mg orally every 4 to 6 hours
	(Levsin SL,Nulev)	0.125 to 0.25 mg sublingually every 4 to 6 hours
	(Levinex,Levbid)	0.375 to 0.750 mg orally every 12 hours
	(IBS Stat)	1 to 2 sprays (1 to 2 mL) orally every 4 to 6 hours
Methscopolamine bromide		
	(Pamine)	2.5 to 5 mg every 4 to 6 hours
Glycopyrrolate	(Robinul)	1 mg orally twice daily
Clidinium bromide		
Chlordioxipoxide	(Librax)	1 cap orally 2 to 4 times daily
Belladonna with Phenobarbital		1 to 2 tabs/caps orally 2 to 4 times daily
	(Donnatal)	Extended release: 1 tab orally every 8 to 12 hours
Tricyclic compounds		
Nortriptyline	(Pamelor)	10 to 75 mg/day
Desipramine	(Norpramin)	10 to 75 mg/day

the frequency of bowel movements. Antidiarrheal medications, such as loperamide (Imodium) and diphenoxylate hydrochloride (Lomotil) may also improve stool consistency and frequency. In refractory cases of uncontrolled diarrhea, cholestyramine may bind bile acids that may be responsible for increased colonic secretion and decreased colonic absorption of water (Sciarretta et al, 1987). (Table 39-2). In some cases, a short course of antibiotics may be tried in the hope of reducing refractory diarrhea by altering the intestinal bacterial flora (Pimental et al, 2000).

Alosetron

The 5-HT$_3$ receptor antagonist alosetron (Lotronex) has been shown to be effective in the treatment of women with the IBS and diarrhea.

In addition to improving stool frequency, stool consistency and fecal urgency, alosetron has also been shown to significantly reduce abdominal pain (Camilleri et al, 2000). Unfortunately, adverse reactions, such as *severe constipation, ischemic colitis* and *bowel perforation,* caused temporary withdrawal of alosetron from use; however, in June 2002, the Food and Drug Administration approved restricted marketing of alosetron for "the treatment of women with severe, diarrhea-predominant IBS who have failed to respond to conventional IBS therapy (Brandt et al, 2002)." The starting dose is 1 mg QD for 4 weeks. The dose is then increased to 1 mg twice daily if the patient experiences only partial relief. Only physicians experienced in treating IBS patients are permitted to prescribe alosetron, and informed consent must be obtained from the patient before initiating therapy. Patients must be instructed to discontinue the medication and contact their physician if severe constipation or worsening abdominal pain occurs. Despite these restrictions, alosetron can be a very effective therapy in the properly chosen patient.

Constipation

For patients with IBS and constipation, the addition of *supplemental fiber* may help to normalize bowel movements and alleviate related symptoms, such as tenesmus, dyschezia, and abdominal pain. There are numerous fiber supplements available over the counter; the decision regarding which one to choose depends primarily on the patient's preference (ie, liquid, capsule, or wafer). It is important to instruct the patient to consume adequate amounts of water with the fiber to avoid potential side effects. If additional therapy is required, *osmotic laxatives* can be used safely and indefinitely. These include nonabsorbable carbohydrates (*lactulose* and *sorbitol*), *milk of magnesia,* magnesium citrate, or a *polyethylene glycol solution (Miralax)* (Table 39-3). There is a separate chapter on constipation.

Tegaserod

A more global approach to patients with the IBS and constipation utilizes the 5-HT$_4$ agonist tegaserod (Zelnorm). Tegaserod is approved for the treatment of women with IBS whose primary bowel symptom is constipation. In well-designed trials, tegaserod has been shown to accelerate colon and small intestine transit, increase the frequency of bowel movements, increase the softness of stools, decrease abdominal pain, reduce bloating, and improve patients overall satisfaction with bowel habits (Muller-Lissner et al, 2001). Diarrhea and headache are the most common adverse events associated with the use of tegaserod (affecting 9 and 15% of patients, respectively). Ischemic colitis and electrocardiogram changes have not been seen with the use of tegaserod. The recommended dose is 6 mg orally twice daily before breakfast and dinner. This agent is also used in smaller doses to enhance gastric emptying as discussed in the chapters on gastroparesis (Chapter 31, "Gastroparesis") and on nonulcer dysphagia (Chapter 30, The Management of Nonulcer Dypepsia").

Psychological Interventions

Patients with the IBS who actively seek care by a physician have a high incidence of psychological disorders, specifically depression and anxiety. Because of this, a variety of psychological interventions have been used to treat the symptoms of IBS. Despite methodological flaws in most studies, there are some data to support the use of relaxation exercises, *biofeedback, cognitive therapy, hypnotherapy,* and *psychotherapy* (Talley et al, 1996). The IBS-related symptoms most likely to respond to psychological intervention include abdominal

TABLE 39-2. Medications for Treatment of Diarrhea in Irritable Bowel Syndrome

Antidiarrheals	
Drug	Dose
Loperamide	4 mg/d orally up to 8 mg/d in single/divided doses
Diphenoxylate (2.5 mg) plus atropine sulfate (0.025 mg) (Lomotil)	2 tabs orally 4 times daily
Cholestyramine resin	1 packet with fluid orally 2 to 4 times daily

TABLE 39-3. Medications for the Treatment of Constipation in Irritable Bowel Sydrome

Osmotic Laxatives	
Drug	Dose
Lactulose	10 mg/15 mL of syrup; 15 to 30 mL/d orally, titrate as needed
Polyethylene glycol solution	17 g dissolved in 240 mL of water orally daily
Milk of Magnesium	15 to 30 mL/d orally as needed

pain and diarrhea. The factors influencing the choice between behavioral therapies include the availability of a skilled and interested therapist, patient preference, and cost.

Supplemental Reading

Brandt LJ, Locke GR, Olden K, et al. An evidence-based approach to the management of irritable bowel syndrome in North America. Am J Gastroenterol 2002;97:S7–26.

Camilleri M, Northcutt AR, Kong S, et al. Efficacy and safety of alosetron in women with irritable bowel syndrome: a randomized, placebo-controlled trial. Lancet 2000;355:1035–40.

Creed FH, Fernandes L, Guthne E, et al. The cost-effectiveness of psychotherapy and SSRI antidepressants for severe irritable bowel syndrome. Gastroenterol 2001;120:A619.

Hawkes ND, Rhodes J, Evans B. Naloxne treatment for irritable bowel syndrome—a pilot study. Gastroenterol 2002;122:A552.

Horwitz BJ, Fisher RS. The irritable bowel syndrome. N Engl J Med 2001;344:1846–50.

Kurken SD, Burgers P, Tytgat GN, Boeckxstaens GE. Fluoxetine (Prozac) for the treatment of irritable bowel syndrome: a randomized, controlled clinical trial. Gastroenterol 2002;122:A551.

Mertz HR. Drug therapy: irritable bowel syndrome. N Engl J Med 2003;349:2136–46.

Muller-Lissner SA, Fumigalli I, Bardhan KD, et al. Tegaserod, a 5-HT$_4$ receptor partial agonist, relieves symptoms in irritable bowel syndrome patients with abdominal pain, bloating and constipation. Aliment Pharmacol Ther 2001;15:1655–66.

Pimental M, Chow EJ, Lin HC. Eradication of small intestinal bacterial overgrowth reduces symptoms reduces symptoms of irritable bowel syndrome. Am J Gastroenterol 2000;95:3503–6.

Sciarretta G, Fagioli G, Furno A, et al. 75Se HCAT test in the detection of bile acid malabsorption in functional diarrhea and its correlation with small bowel transit. Gut 1987;28:970–5.

Talley NJ, Owen BK, Boyce P, Patterson K. Psychological treatments for irritable bowel syndrome: a critique of controlled treatment trials. Am J Gastroenterol 1996;91:277–86.

Thompson WG, Longstreth GF, Drossman DA, et al. Functional bowel disorders and functional abdominal pain. Gut 1999;45:1143–7.

CHAPTER 40

Chronic Recurrent Abdominal Pain in Childhood and Adolescence

Marvin E. Ament, MD

Chronic abdominal pain is one of the most commonly encountered symptoms in childhood and adolescence. It is believed that between 10 and 15% of school-aged children between the ages of 5 and 18 have had this condition during childhood. Most pediatricians and pediatric gastroenterologists agree that when multiple episodes or attacks of pain in the abdomen occur over a 3-month period of time, the condition is considered chronic. Patients with chronic abdominal pain typically have their normal activities affected. Occasionally, children with this condition will complain repeatedly to their parents of pain, but will not refrain from normal activities. Over 90% of children with chronic recurrent abdominal pain have a *functional gastrointestinal (GI) disorder*. The term "functional" is used if no specific structural, infectious, inflammatory or biochemical cause can be found to explain the symptoms.

Pathophysiology

The *pathophysiology* of this disorder has not been clearly identified, but it is clear that the autonomic nervous system and its connections to the cerebral cortex and mid- and hindbrain are the key parts of the nervous system involved in the condition. Many clinicians believe that functional abdominal pain represents a disturbance of GI motility that is provoked by physical and psychological stress acting through different centers in the nervous system and their connections to intestinal smooth muscle and blood vessels.

Clinical Presentations

There are three typical *clinical presentations* of chronic recurrent abdominal pain in children and adolescents, as follows: (1) *primary periumbilical paroxysmal pain*, (2) *primary mid-epigastric peptic symptoms*, and (3) *lower abdominal pain* associated with *altered bowel patterns*. The first group is by far the *most common* and is designated as being functional abdominal pain. Children with peptic symptoms complain of recurrent upper abdominal pain that may or may not be related to nausea, postprandial epigastric fullness and distension, eructations or burping, hiccups, and early satiety. This group should be considered to have "*nonulcer dyspepsia*" and is usually seen in the adolescent age group. Children who have a temporal association between lower abdominal pain and altered bowel pattern are more characteristic of *irritable bowel syndrome* (IBS) as seen in adults, and they comprise the *rarest* form of the condition. Even though patients may seem quite ill, physicians who care for them cannot find any evidence of organic disease to explain the symptoms. The symptoms are real and may be a nuisance in the lives of some, without overtly interfering with school or social activities, but in others they may be so severe as to make school attendance impossible.

Family studies have shown that there is a genetic vulnerability to the condition. Frequently, one or both parents experience symptoms similar to those of their child or experienced similar symptoms when they were children. The family dynamics may explain how a condition is experienced by the child. The best way to think about the pathogenesis of functional abdominal pain is to consider that there are heterogeneous groups of physical and psychological stressful stimuli that provoke or alter the intensity of the intestinal motor or sensory activity in susceptible children. The result of this is the development of abdominal pain. The same stimuli may elicit nausea or bloating acting through other pathways.

Role of Stress

Various physical stresses can bring about the symptoms. Sometimes a real intestinal illness provokes the onset of the condition by the family's excessive response. Examples of this would be following a viral infection of the GI tract with the development of transient lactose intolerance, or development of fecal retention following a period of diarrhea, leading to a chronic functional disorder. Psychosocial stresses that may induce the development of recurrent abdominal pain include anxiety, problems at school, and a general preoccupation with illness. Several studies have documented that functional GI disorders may be associated with both upper and lower GI manometric abnormalities and altered intestinal transit. Recurrent abdominal pain may result from dysfunction of the autonomic nervous system, which serves as an important participant in homeostasis of the intestinal tract and modulates the sensory and motor responses to various internal and external stimuli. Attempts to differentiate so-called normal individuals from those with functional abdominal pain by various measurements including pupillary dilatation and the measurement of heart rate, vasomotor tone and facial expression following a stress have been unsuccessful.

The morbidity of recurrent abdominal pain is usually not physical but may result in the child's inability to attend school regularly and to perform. Furthermore, in many children the condition interferes with peer relationships and with the youngster's participation in sports and personal and family activities.

Functional Abdominal Pain Syndrome

In children with *functional abdominal pain syndrome*, the pain episodes tend to cluster, alternating in pain-free periods of variable length. The near majority of episodes begin gradually; however they can develop suddenly. Episodes of pain last from < 1 hour in duration to at most 3 hours in most children. Continuous pain is described by 10% of patients. In over 90% of patients, the pain is periumbilical or mid-epigastric in location, or the pain is felt all over the abdomen. The child usually is only able to give a vague description of the pain, except for saying that it is constant and not crampy. Rarely, the pain is localized to a specific quadrant, which may lead to exploratory laparotomy (Table 40-1). It is unusual for the pain to radiate to the back, chest, or hips. Typically, the child does not temporally relate the pain to physical activity or the passage of bowel movements, and no consistent history of food inducing the symptoms is present. Often, the patient will be inconsistent regarding the relationship of the pain to a type of food or its temperature. Patients with recurrent abdominal pain sleep well once they fall asleep and do not awaken during the night because of pain. However, children with this condition may have difficulty going to sleep. Parents of these children usually say that during the episodes they may range from being listless to having great discomfort. During severe attacks, the child may assume the fetal position, grimace, cry, clench his/her fists, and guard when one palpates their abdomen. Headaches, skin pallor, nausea, dizziness and fatigability may be associated symptoms. Nausea and postprandial bloating can be the major symptoms, with pain being a minor component. These symptoms are found in 50 to 70% of the cases. Vomiting, regurgitation, diarrhea, or constipation, are uncommon as major parts of the symptom complex. Often the patients or parents will report a fever, but when questioned or asked to measure the temperature during these episodes, it is always < 100°F.

Organic Disorders

Weight loss, fever, arthralgia, growth failure, rectal bleeding, and sleepiness, after the episodes of course, suggest diagnoses other than functional abdominal pain. In atypical cases weight loss may develop secondary to attempts to influence the condition by diet or as a result of depression.

Careful history taking is the most important part in the examination of these patients. Information should be gathered about the family and what has recently occurred in association with this condition, such as deaths or serious illnesses in close family members and friends (Table 40-2). The physician should questions the parents about the possible financial problems and the threat they may pose to the family. Furthermore, the physician should determine whether the parents have any serious marital difficulties and if a separation is impending.

Last, it is important to ask the parents and the patient what they think is the cause of the abdominal pain and if they think

---

TABLE 40-1. Characteristics of Pain Pattern in Functional Abdominal Pain of Childhood

1. Variable in severity
   Mild: with no physical evidence of discomfort
   Severe: patient assumes fetal position, may be pale and diaphoretic.
   Physical examination of abdomen not indicative of acute abdomen.
2. Pain episodes may occur in clusters lasting weeks to months
3. Episodes of pain occur once daily to several times per day
4. Periumbilical to midepigastric in location or diffuse
5. Difficulty describing character of pain
6. No consistent relationship of pain to meals, exercise, or need to have a bowel movement
7. May occur at same time every day if specific stress factor occurs at that time
8. Typically interrupts normal activity
9. May be totally incapacitating
10. Condition in some precipitated by acute illness

TABLE 40-2. Questions To Be Asked of Parents and Children with Suspected Functional Abdominal Pain

1. Are the parents divorced?
2. Are the parents separated?
   With whom does the child live?
   What are the visiting arrangements?
3. Has a sibling left home or contemplates leaving?
4. Has a significant family member died close to the time of onset of symptoms?
5. Has a close friend of the family or patient died or been ill?
6. Has any close family member been ill or hospitalized at onset of chronic abdominal pain?
7. Do any family members have inflammatory bowel disease or peptic ulcer disease?
8. Does the patient have school problems?
   a. What are the daily after school activities of the child?
   b. What are the routine weekend activities?
   How many activities are promoted by patient/parent?
   How many hours of homework are there each day?
   Who can help the child if there is difficulty with schoolwork?
9. Does the patient have difficulty with peers?
10. Does the family have financial problems that effect the patient?
12. Has the patient or someone close to the patient moved at or close to onset of symptoms?

TABLE 40-8. Selective Tests to be Done if Indicated and/or Parents Will Not Accept Functional Diagnosis

1. Ultrasonography of upper and lower abdomen
2. Upper gastrointestinal and small bowel series
3. Barium enema
4. Liver function tests
5. Pancreatic function tests
6. C13 urea breath test for *Helicobacter pylori*
7. Fecal α-1-antitrypsin determination
8. Upper and lower gastrointestinal endoscopy

individualized. The families must be given a positive diagnosis and told the child has functional abdominal pain, with an explanation of the nature of the symptoms and their presumptive pathophysiology. Most important is to tell the family and the child that the symptoms are real and not imagined, and that they are caused by disordered intestinal function in response to a wide variety of stressful stimuli. It is appropriate to say to the child and the parents that in some individuals, certain stresses result in abnormal function that in others do not have the same effect but could result in other symptoms such as headache or skin rashes.

The test results should be presented and explained to the family and child to tell them which conditions have been excluded. Typically, I review with the family the radiographic studies and all prior tests to show that they were normal. If the family is worried about a particular condition or illness, it must be tested for or the family made aware that the symptoms do not fit the condition. Discuss with the family why the child does not have a variety of common GI disorders, including peptic ulcer disease, IBD, and cancer.

The *goals of treatment* are to *identify and clarify adverse stresses* that may provoke the pain and to *reverse environmental reinforcement* of the pain behavior. The parents and the school officials must be made aware that the child should be supported rather than the pain. The lifestyle of the child should be normal, and the child should attend school every day, regardless of the presence of pain. The physician can communicate directly with school officials to explain the nature of the problem and not to let it disrupt attendance, class activity, or performance expectations. The patients should not be sent home unless there is objective evidence of disease, such as fever or vomiting. If necessary, the child may be allowed to rest in the nurse's or school office until ready to return to class. The parent must learn not to come to school if called by their child and to work with the school to develop a plan for pain management. Giving reassurance to the patient is important. In the home, the child must learn to become independent and to develop coping skills to deal with the pain. Less attention should be directed toward the symptoms.

Medication Use

Patients with this condition are often given anticholinergics, sedatives, and even anticonvulsants. Typically, patients with this condition receive regular doses of Donnatol and Bentyl. If pain occurs regularly in response to meals and is not due to organic disease, give prophylactic treatment before each meal. Doses of antispasmodics may need to be titrated gradually to get the maximum benefit. Dicylomine, for example, may be started at 5.0 mg 15 to 30 minutes before meals and the doses gradually increased if the patient is not made comfortable by a particular dose. *Identification of stressors and teaching the entire family how to manage the problem*, however, is *more important* than using these types of medications.

Hospitalization

Hospitalization is rarely indicated, but at times, it occurs in the most disabled. Patients unquestionably get relief of their symptoms during their stay because the environment has changed and they are removed from the stressors. *Hospitalization* allows one to look at the child and family constellation in more depth and to understand more clearly what the factors are that are precipitating the episodes. Consultation with a child psychologist or psychiatrist is indicated if a conversion reaction, extreme internalized behavior or maladaptive family coping mechanisms are present, or if initial attempts at environmental modification to result in normal lifestyle fail.

Outcome

No prospective studies have been performed on the outcome of functional abdominal pain. Once diagnosed, gastroenterologists rarely identify an occult organic disorder. Many patients become asymptomatic within 2 to 6 weeks of diagnosis. Most children and parents accept the reassurance that the pain is not organic and that environmental modification is effective treatment. However, 30 to 50% of children may continue to have such problems into adult life, many of them *developing IBS*. Factors that may lead to a good prognosis for resolution of the pain include the following: (1) no family history of pain, (2) being female, (3) age of onset > 6 years of age, and (4) duration of symptoms < 6 months. Non-ulcer dyspepsia and IBS are two variants of chronic recurrent abdominal pain, usually occurring in patients > 10 years old. Some of the patients have both. Physical examination in these patients is normal. Similar to those with recurrent abdominal pain, they sleep well and are not awakened by pain. They often require full examination, including upper intestinal endoscopy, to rule out acid peptic disease in the stomach and esophagus, and even 24-hour pH monitoring to exclude reflux. Those with bowel symptoms should have stool studies and perhaps sigmoidoscopy or colonoscopy to rule out IBD, and lactose hydrogen test for lactose intolerance.

Treatment of Moderate-to-Severe Recurrent Abdominal Pain

Recognition of stressors alone may not be sufficient to alter the frequency and severity of the pain, and these patients may need psychological testing to provide additional information, such as coping and problem-solving skills, symptoms, and problems that might not have been previously determined, and other possible sources of stress. Academic testing assesses whether the child is functioning at grade level and at the expected developmental level. Learning and communication disorders might hinder academic performance and contribute to stress. The goal of this testing is to assess whether there are previously unrecognized biological, cognitive, emotional, academic, and/or social problems that might have been caused by or might contribute to a patient's stress and consequently lead to pain and disability. Although time consuming and expensive, testing is essential when a child's abdominal pain is overwhelming and disabling and fails to respond to the usual recommended measures.

Unified Plan

Ideally pharmacologic, psychological and physical interventions can be combined into a *unified plan*. Pain must be accepted as a symptom that might not be totally eradicated and the goal of treatment *focused on improvement or functioning*. As lifestyle and coping skills improve, pain may remit.

Medications

Tricyclic antidepressants such as *amitryptyline (Elavil)* are commonly used in chronic pain. This class of drugs has the added benefit of causing sedation as a side effect. However, they should be used at lowest possible doses to avoid early morning sedation and are best given before bedtime. *Selective serotonin reuptake inhibitors,* such as *fluoxetine (Prozac)*, *paroxetine* (Paxil), and *sertraline (Zoloft)*, do not show direct analgesic effects, but can be helpful when depression or anxiety contribute to the abdominal pain. *Clonidine (Catapres)*, a central α-adrenergic agent, can help wean a child from opioids when they have been used for an extended time for pain control. Clonidine comes in a topical patch-delivery system and can be quite sedating.

Occasionally patients with recurrent abdominal pain have a lowered threshold for transmission of noxious sensory information. Even non-noxious stimuli can be experienced as pain. The administration of local anesthetics through an *epidural catheter* can be useful diagnostically and therapeutically, and later, if indicated, patients can be maintained on *oral lidocaine*. If *anxiety* is a major factor in the pain, short term *benzodiazepines* can be helpful. Pharmacologic intervention has to be approached as only one part of the management plan, however, and must be integrated into a comprehensive rehabilitation program. There is a separate chapter on chronic abdominal pain (see Chapter 41, "Chronic Abdominal Pain") and on psychotropic drugs in management of patients with functional disorders (see Chapter 43, "Psychotropic Drugs and Management of Patients with Functional Gastrointestinal Disorders").

Supplemental Reading

Bayless TM, Huang SS. Recurrent abdominal pain due to milk and lactose intolerance in school-aged children. Pediatrics 1971;47:1029–32.

Burke P, Elliott M, Fleissner R. Irritable bowel syndrome and recurrent abdominal pain. A comparative review. Psychosomatics 1999;40:277–85.

Bursch B, Wlaco GA, Zeltzer L. Clinical assessment and management of chronic pain and pain associated disability syndrome. Developmental Behav Pediatr 1997;19:45–53.

Hunt S, Mantyh P. The molecular dynamics of pain control. Nat Rev Neurosci 2000;2:83–90.

Hyams JS, Burke G, Davis PM, et al. Abdominal pain and irritable bowel syndrome in adolescence: a community based study. J Pediatr 1996;129:220–6.

Hyams JS, Hyman PE. Recurrent abdominal pain and the biopsychosocial model of medical practice. J Pediatr 1998;133:473–8.

Hyams JS, Treem WR, Justinich CJ, et al. Characterization of symptoms in children with recurrent abdominal pain: resemblance to irritable bowel syndrome. J Pediatr Gastroenterol Nutr 1995;20:209–14.

Janicke DM, Finney JW. Empirically supported treatments in pediatric psychology: recurrent abdominal pain. J Pediatr Psychol 1999;24:115–27.

Price P. Psychological and neural mechanisms of the affective dimension of pain. Science 2000;288:1769–76.

Zeltzer LK, Barr R, McGrath PA, Schecter N. Pediatric pain: interacting behavior and physical factors. Pediatrics 1992;90:816–21.

CHAPTER 41

Chronic Abdominal Pain

W.A. Hoogerwerf, MD, and P. Jay Pasricha, MD

All of us have experienced acute pain, an unpleasant sensory and emotional experience that is associated with actual or potential tissue damage and which tells us that something is wrong with our body. This pain has a function because it allows for rapid identification of the site of origin of the underlying disease or injury and it allows for initiation of targeted therapy. On the contrary, *chronic* pain, one of the most common gastrointestinal (GI) conditions seen by primary care physicians and gastroenterologists, usually does not allow for rapid diagnosis of an underlying organic problem and is even less likely to lead to satisfactory therapy. Patients with chronic abdominal pain often have a track record of frequent emergency room visits and multiple physician examinations and of having been through a variety of diagnostic studies.

Pain is a subjective experience; there are no diagnostic tests that can determine the quality or intensity of an individual's pain. Regardless of whether there is an apparent so-called "organic" cause of the pain or not, the physician should bear in mind that pain often dominates the lives of patients in a negative fashion. Unfortunately, the patient with chronic abdominal pain is increasingly perceived as a clinical "liability" by the busy practitioner, with his or her symptoms either trivialized or perhaps worse, dismissed as representative of either "malingering", "psychosomatic", or "drug-seeking" behavior. These and various other, rather unscientific euphemisms of a similar nature are reflective of the physician's lack of understanding of the biological basis, as well as the psychosocial dimensions, of chronic pain and the consequent frustration of not being able to place the symptom in a conceptually familiar frame of reference (as compared with a symptom such as hematochezia). This has led to a set of physician behaviors, which are often rather irrational, towards these patients that include multiple diagnostic testing ("furor medicus"), referrals to various other specialists, and a pervasive fear of prescribing anything more than the mildest of analgesics. Ultimately, however, such behaviors do a disservice to both the medical community as well as the patients that it serves. The truth is that most patients with chronic abdominal pain are neither hypochondriacs nor drug addicts and their suffering is real and considerable. It therefore behooves the careful and compassionate gastroenterologist to remain engaged in the management of chronic abdominal pain; indeed the care of this condition can be both rewarding and relatively simple to perform, provided some basic principles are adhered to. It is the purpose of this chapter to review some of these principles and provide our own personal approach to these patients.

The Biology and Psychology of Chronic Pain

Neural Pathways

A proper understanding of the application and limitations of these approaches requires a good knowledge of the neuroanatomic pathway serving visceral pain. As with other organs, this pathway involves at least three levels of neurons. Peripheral nerve endings of the first-order neuron (the "primary nociceptor") exit from the target organ to travel along with the sympathetic nerves (but are not part of the sympathetic nervous system), passing without interruption through one of several pre-vertebral autonomic plexi associated with the corresponding visceral artery (eg, celiac, hepatic, superior mesenteric) on their way to the dorsal root ganglia where their cell bodies lie. From here, the primary nociceptors send out shorter central branches to the dorsal horn of the spinal cord where they make contact with neurons in the gray matter. Postsynaptic (ie, second-order) neurons then travel cephalad within ascending pathways to synapse in several thalamic and reticular formation nuclei of the pons and medulla, which in turn project to other parts of the brain, including the limbic system, somatosensory, and frontal cortices.

Sensitization

In the context of clinically important pain, it is also important to understand the concept of sensitization. This refers to a phenomemon in which the "gain" of the entire nociceptive system is reset upwards by neuronal changes in either the periphery or within the central nervous system (CNS). Some form of sensitization invariably accompanies any kind of chronic pain, such as that seen with persistent inflammation. The net result is that noxious stimuli now elicit a pain response that is much greater when compared with the normal state, a phenomenon termed *hyperalgesia*.

A further characteristic of the sensitized state is called *allodynia*, a phenomenon in which innocuous or physiological stimuli are perceived as painful. As an example of mechanical allodynia, patients with chronic pancreatitis may experience pain in response to physiological changes in intraductal pressure, which would be insensate in normal subjects. Similarly, subsequent minor flare-ups of inflammation in such patients could also cause the associated pain to be felt as far more severe than if being experienced for the first time (hyperalgesia).

Referred Pain: A Key Characteristic of Visceral Pain

A patient with "pure" visceral pain is seldom seen in the clinic, as this phase usually lasts only a few hours. Instead, most clinically significant forms of visceral pain are referred to somatic areas. Although the physiological basis for referred pain is incompletely understood, it is generally believed to result from the fact that nerve signals from several areas of the body may "feed" the same nerve pathway leading to the spinal cord and brain. *Visceral pain* by itself is typically felt in the midline in the epigastric, peri-umblical or hypogastric regions, reflecting the ontogenic origin of the involved organ from the fore- mid- or hind-gut respectively and is perceived as a *deep* and *dull discomfort* instead. *Referred pain*, which sets in soon after and comes to dominate the clinical picture, is perceived in overlying or remote superficial somatic structures such as skin or abdominal wall muscle, with the site varying according to the involved visceral organ. Further, referred pain is now *sharper* and assumes several of the characteristics of pain of somatic origin and indeed may dominate or even mask any underlying visceral pain.

If carefully questioned, many patients with chronic abdominal pain of visceral origin will indeed describe two types of pain, not always occurring simultaneously. However, physicians often make the mistake of lumping these together into a single pain; the result is that the disparate descriptions (eg, *one diffuse and dull*, the other *localized and sharp*) are now perceived as paradoxical and serve to reinforce the perception that the complaints are not "organic" in nature. *Referred pain* is therefore more helpful in determining the site of the underlying disorder than the original pure visceral pain, which tends to be perceived in the midline regardless of the organ involved.

Pain, Suffering, and Illness Behavior

Nociception, or the process by which the nervous system detects tissue damage, is not synonymous with pain; increased afferent signaling to the CNS by itself does not always make a patient with chronic pain seek medical attention. However, nociception can, and often does, lead to suffering, a negative response to the perceived threat to the physical and psychological integrity of the individual and made up of a combination of *cognitive* and *emotional factors* such as *anxiety, fear* and *stress*. This in turn can lead to certain patterns of *illness behavior*, which in turn determines the clinical presentation. Such behavior is a complex mixture of physiologic (eg, pain intensity/severity or associated features), psychological (mental state, stress, mood, coping style, prior memories or experiences with pain, etc), and social factors (concurrent negative life events, attitudes, and behavior of family and friends, perceived benefits such as avoidance of unpleasant duties, etc). Thus individual attitudes, beliefs, and personalities, as well as the social and cultural environment, strongly affect the pain experience. Although the biological basis of these interactions is poorly understood, it is important to understand that the clinical presentation of chronic pain represents a dysfunction of a system that is formed by the *convergence* of biological, social, and psychological factors (the so-called *biopsychosocial continuum*). These factors not only modulate each other but also together are responsible for an individual's sense of well being. In a given patient or at a given time in the same patient, the primary disturbance may disproportionately affect one component of the spectrum. An example would include intense nociceptive activity associated with an inflammatory flare-up in a patient with chronic pancreatitis; this is expected to dominate the clinical picture while the episode lasts and the physician should concentrate on suppressing pain with strong analgesics. In between such episodes, when nociceptive activity is low, the spectrum may shift towards the psychosocial end and the wise physician may focus more on counseling and behavior modification. However, in either case, the patients' suffering is equally valid.

Indeed, *most patients with chronic pain*, regardless of etiology (somatic or visceral, "organic" or " functional") frequently suffer from *depression, anxiety, sleep disturbances, withdrawal, decreased activity, fatigue, loss of libido*, and *morbid preoccupation* with their symptoms, suggesting that these features may actually be secondary to the pain and not the other way around.

Approach to the Patient with Chronic Abdominal Pain

It is not the purpose of this chapter to describe a comprehensive differential diagnosis to abdominal pain. Most experienced gastroenterologists will have no difficulty in readily identifying the underlying cause in the presence of typical clinical and laboratory features. Instead, we would like to focus on the approach to the *difficult* patient with chronic abdominal pain. These patients fall into the following three categories, as discussed in greater detail below: (1) the patient with unfamiliar or rare causes of abdominal pain, (2) the patient with a known cause of abdominal pain but one that is not easily brought under control, or (3) the patient with no apparent cause of abdominal pain.

The Patient with Unfamiliar or Rare Causes of Abdominal Pain

When a careful history and examination and routine laboratory tests fail to reveal a cause of abdominal pain, consideration must be given to rare syndromes. These include disorders that primarily affect *visceral nerves* rather than the organs themselves, such as *acute intermittent porphyria*, chronic poisoning with *lead* or *arsenic*, or *diabetic radiculopathy*. Women on *oral contraceptives* may experience mysterious attacks of abdominal pain that in some cases can be related to *mesenteric venous thrombosis*.

A clinical suspicion of "adhesions" is also often entertained by both physicians and patients with chronic abdominal pain even though the literature suggests that such a diagnosis is seldom validated. Adhesions are very common in women, even in the absence of prior surgery and are found in equal proportion in patients complaining of pelvic pain and those with other complaints. Indeed, laparoscopy for chronic pain seldom leads to a specific diagnosis and even less often to a change in management.

In contrast to the above disorders, our experience suggests it is far more fruitful to carefully examine the abdominal wall in patients with chronic pain. This is an aspect that is frequently overlooked by gastroenterologists. Pain arising primarily in the abdominal wall can result from a poorly defined group of conditions whose pathophysiology remains obscure. The diagnosis is suggested when the pain is superficial, localized to a small area that is usually significantly tender, associated with dysesthesia in the involved region, and a positive Carnett's sign (if a tender spot is identified, the patient is asked to raise his or her head, thus tensing the abdominal musculature; greater tenderness on repeat palpation is considered positive). It is postulated that such tender spots are often due to entrapment neuropathy or a neuroma; however, we speculate that they could also represent an extreme manifestation of referred pain (see above), particularly in the absence of a surgical scar or history of trauma, when they been referred to as a "*myofascial trigger points*". Regardless of etiology, it is important to make this diagnosis because such pain can often be managed in a relatively simple manner.

The Patient with a Known Cause of Abdominal Pain That Is Not Easily Brought Under Control

This type of pain is exemplified by the patient with *chronic pancreatitis*. Pain is not only the most important symptom of chronic pancreatitis but also the most difficult to treat. Pharmacologic, surgical and endoscopic approaches have been tried in this condition for many decades, with inconsistent and often less than satisfactory results. The care of these patients remains challenging and imposes a significant burden on society with the attendant problems of disability, unemployment, and ongoing alcohol or drug dependence. Pain can also be a prominent and sometimes intractable feature of other syndromes, such as gastroparesis. Although often dismissed as functional, it is quite possible that the pain in this condition can be neuropathic in origin, reflecting the underlying pathophysiology (eg, diabetes). The management of these pain syndromes is considered in greater detail below.

The Patient with No Apparent Cause of Abdominal Pain

In many patients with chronic abdominal pain, no definite abdominal pathology will be found to account for the symptoms. Indeed in the absence of obvious clinical or laboratory clues, it is relatively unusual for specialists to uncover a new pathophysiologic basis for pain in patients who have already been evaluated by their primary care physician. Although minor abnormalities in test results may be found, they may be more a reflection of statistical laws than true pathophysiology and often have questionable relevance to the pain. Eventually, many of these patients will be classified as having a "functional" pain syndrome such as noncardiac chest pain, nonulcer dyspepsia, irritable bowel syndrome (IBS), depending principally on the location of the pain and association with physiologic GI events, such as eating or defecation. In some of these patients, there is increasing evidence to support the concept of *visceral hyperalgesia*, a manifestation of *neuronal sensitization* possibly resulting from previous and remote inflammation (eg, a bout of infectious gastroenteritis). As discussed above, neuronal sensitization in these patients may not only exaggerate pain perception in response to noxious stimuli (*hyperalgesia*) but also lead to normal or physiologic events (such as gut contractions) being perceived as painful (*allodynia*). The chapter on IBS can be helpful (see Chapter 39, "Irritable Bowel Syndrome").

In a minority of patients the pain seems to be unconnected to any overt GI function such as eating or bowel movement and has been termed *functional abdominal pain syndrome (FAPS)*. This and the more well studied syndromes described in the previous paragraph have much in common including a predominance of women, heavy use of medical resources, psychological disturbances and personality disorders, and dysfunctional relationships at work, with family, and in other social settings. Conceptually, some of these patients can be perceived as occupying an extreme end of the biopsychosocial continuum of chronic pain discussed above. Thus, if patients with painful pancreatitis represent an example of a disturbance primarily (but not exclusively) affecting nociceptive signaling, then patients with FAPS can be viewed as representing a dysfunction of perception, coping, or response strategies. In either case, the net result is a patient with a hard to manage illness behavior.

Management

A readily identifiable and treatable cause of chronic abdominal pain, although uncommonly found at a tertiary care setting, is of course a straightforward problem to address. More often, however, the gastroenterologist is left dealing with a patient who falls into one of the categories discussed in the previous section. In this regard, it is important to carefully examine the patient for an abdominal wall source as this may show a gratifying response to *local neural blockade*. Our approach is to identify a trigger point by digital examination, and inject a small amount of *lidocaine* or *bupivacaine* at the site of greatest tenderness elicited by the tip of the needle. Although the response may be short-lived, it can provide valuable information as a therapeutic trial. Further, many patients get long lasting relief after one or two injections alone. In those patients in whom relief is temporary, a 1:1 mixture of *lidocaine* and steroids (eg, *triamcinolone*) can be used. More ablative chemicals (eg, *phenol*) are best left to the *anesthesiologist* to administer.

Patients with chronic pancreatitis are increasingly being approached as problems in "plumbing" with various endoscopic or surgical interventions designed to decompress what is thought to be a partially obstructive ductal system. This is discussed in greater detail elsewhere in the pancreatic and biliary sections of this book, but many of these patients remain in pain after these procedures. Other patients with chronic abdominal pain with no obvious cause are also rarely substantially pain free after 1 or more years of follow-up. In most of these cases a presumed cause of pain will have been diagnosed and treated, only to see the pain remain, or for a new type of pain to manifest itself elsewhere.

Palliation is therefore an appropriate goal, and, in most patients, it is achievable. In the following sections, we will describe the basic principles of our therapeutic approach common to both these categories of patients, realizing that some "tailoring" is appropriate depending upon the suspected underlying problem. In general, the therapeutic approach to functional forms of pain is similar to the multifactorial approach to other forms of chronic pain described below, with perhaps greater emphasis on the psychosocial dimensions. As with any chronic illness, it is essential to have a robust patient–physician relationship based on patient education, realistic goal, and clarification of mutual expectations.

Pharmacologic Therapy of Chronic Pain
Narcotics

Although narcotics are arguably the most effective of available analgesic agents, their use is commonly perceived to lead to addiction, leading to a reluctance on the part of most gastroenterologists to use these agents. We agree that such agents should be *avoided* as far as possible in patients *with the functional bowel syndromes*. However, many, if not most, other patients with chronic abdominal pain will at some point in time require their use and the compassionate physician is often faced with no other alternative to relieve suffering. The key elements that make for comfortable and judicious use of these drugs is a solid patient–physician relationship, careful patient selection, and the adherence to a fairly rigid protocol for prescription that also includes certain expectations from the patient (eg, restriction of analgesic prescribing to a single physician, return to work, etc). When *mild chronic pain* necessitates analgesic use, weak opioids such as *propoxyphene* or *codeine,* are often used, even though they are probably no more potent than simple analgesics, such as acetaminophen alone. *More severe pain* requires stronger analgesics; for short term use *meperidine* or *morphine* can be used. For patients requiring long term analgesics, sustained release preparations, such as *transdermal fentanyl* (Durgesic), are probably more useful. Agents with mixed agonist–antagonist profiles, such as *methadone* and *buprenorphine,* have been advocated by some to avoid addiction, although their use in chronic abdominal pain is not well substantiated.

Opioid analgesics have an *adverse effect* on GI motility and in addition can induce or exaggerate nausea. *Tramadol* (Ultram) is a good agent to use in patients with underlying dysmotility, such as gastroparesis, because it is reported to cause less GI disturbance. *Meperidine* (Demerol) is generally felt to be the drug of choice for patients with pancreatitis because of its lesser tendency to cause sphincter of Oddi spasm; however, this has only been shown to be true at *subanalgesic doses*. Because it is more likely to produce other side effects, however, it is seldom used for chronic pain management.

Antidepressant Agents as Analgesics

The class of agents that we prescribe most often for chronic abdominal pain is *tricyclic antidepressants (TCAs)*. The efficacy of these drugs has been best validated in patients with somatic neuropathic pain syndromes. Effective analgesic doses are significantly lower than those required to treat depression, and there is reasonable evidence to conclude that the beneficial effects of antidepressants on pain occurs independently of changes in mood. However, in this regard, diminution of anxiety and restoration of mood and sleep patterns should be considered desirable even if they represent primary neuropsychiatric effects of the drug. There are details on psychotropic medications in a separate chapter on functional GI disorders (see Chapter 43, "Psychotropic Drugs and Management of Patients with Functional Gastrointestinal Disorders").

Selective serotonin reuptake inhibitors (SSRIs), such as *paroxetine* (Paxil), *sertraline* (Zoloff), and *fluoxetine* (Prozac), which are currently the mainstay in the treatment of depression, have fewer side effects and have also been advocated for patients with chronic abdominal pain, particularly for patients with functional constipation as they can increase bowel movements and even cause diarrhea. However, they have been less well evaluated in the management of pain per se than TCAs; at the present time, the literature suggests the efficacy of these agents for chronic pain is *equivocal* at best. Newer antidepressants the *serotonin/norepinephrine reuptake inhibitors* such as *venlafaxine* (Effexor) hold more promise in this regard but have not been subjected to extensive testing in this setting. An older agent in the same class, *trazadone* (Desyrel), has been used with good effect in patients with noncardiac chest pain; although it does not have the usual side effects of the TCAs, it is more sedating and can cause priapism in males.

Before beginning antidepressants it is important to assess the psychological profile of the patient, as this may be important in determining the choice of therapy. If the patient is not depressed, it is critical to spend some time explaining the scientific rationale for the use of antidepressants, with an attempt to clearly separate the analgesic effects from the antidepressant ones. We usually begin with *nortryptiline* (Pamelor) at a dose of 10 to 25 mg/d and progress as required (and tolerated) to no more than 75 to 100 mg/d. This is given at night and will almost immediately begin helping with disturbed sleep pattern that often accompanies chronic pain. Daytime sedation may occur but tolerance develops rapidly. Tolerance to the antimuscarinic effects may take longer and it is important to advise the patients about this. In the absence of significant side effects, the dose of the antidepressant is gradually increased until adequate benefit is achieved or the upper limit of the recommended dose is reached. It is also important to tell the patient that the analgesic effect may take several days to weeks to develop and that unlike conventional analgesics, the drug is not to be taken on a as needed basis but on a fixed schedule. A trial of at least 4 to 6 weeks at a stable maximum dose is recommended before discontinuation. At that time one may consider switching to another class of antidepressants such as *nefazadone* (Serzone), *mirtazepine* (Remcron), or *venlafaxine* (Effexor). *Venflaxine* may also be substituted for a TCA if excessive sedation is observed with the latter.

If the patient is *depressed*, then it may be more appropriate to use *full antidepressant doses* of a drug that also has analgesic properties. This could be either a TCA with a low side-effect profile or perhaps one of the newer agents discussed above (not an SSRI). If the patient is already on an antidepressant, but this does not have proven analgesic activity (such as an SSRI), consideration should be given to switch to one that does or to use small doses of a TCA, if tolerated. Such decisions should be made in conjunction with the psychiatrist taking care of the patient.

OTHER DRUGS

A variety of drugs including neuroleptics (*fluphenazine* [Prolixin], *haloperidol* [Haldol]), and antiepileptics (*phenytoin* [Dilantin], *carmazepine*) have been used in chronic somatic pain with equivocal evidence of efficacy and a significant risk of adverse effects. However, we frequently use *gabapentin* (Neurontin), a drug with considerable more promise and safety that is widely used for neuropathic pain syndromes. Although admittedly anecdotal, our experience suggests that it may be useful in patients with functional bowel pain syndromes, especially in patients with *diabetic gastroparesis*. It can also be used in patients with chronic pancreatitis, in an attempt to "spare" narcotic use. Finally, mention must be made of the use of *benzodiazepines*, which are frequently used by patients with chronic pain including insomnia, anxiety, and muscle spasm. Although useful in these settings for short term use, there is a significant risk for dependence on these drugs and there is little, if any, evidence that they have any real analgesic effect.

Behavioral and Psychological Approaches

Although pharmacologic therapy has a valuable role in these patients, it is also clear that a successful outcome requires taking into consideration several, equally important, factors. As explained previously, chronic pain cannot be viewed as a purely neurophysiologic phenomenon and has many other facets, the most important of which is the psychological dimension, consisting of cognitive, emotional and behavioral processes. The combination of these factors results in *functional disability*, a third dimension of chronic pain that is often ignored. Several psychological techniques have been used with good effect in the management of a variety of chronic pain syndromes, although specific evidence for their efficacy in chronic abdominal pain syndromes is generally lacking. *Operant interventions* focus on altering maladaptive pain behaviors, such as reduced activity levels, verbal pain behaviors and excessive use of medications. *Cognitive behavioral therapy* extends beyond this to also include cognitions or thought processes, based on the premise that these closely interact with behavior, emotions, and eventually physiological sensations (ie, the biopyschosocial continuum); altering one of these components can therefore result in changes in the others. Positive cognitions include ignoring pain, using coping self-statements, and indicating acceptance of pain. Negative processes include catastrophizing (ie, viewing the pain as the worst thing in the world and believing it will never get better). *Biofeedback and relaxation* techniques teach patients to use control physiologic parameters and decrease sympathetic nervous system arousal. *Hypnosis* attempts to bring about changes in sensation, perception or cognition by structured suggestions and has recently shown promise for patients with IBS. *Group therapy* exposes patients to others with similar problems and allows them to feel less isolated. *Dynamic (interpersonal) psychotherapy* attempts to reduce the physical and psychological distress caused by difficulties in interpersonal relationships.

It is, therefore, highly desirable, and probably necessary in some cases, to involve a clinical psychologist in the care of these patients. Indeed as with somatic pain clinics, one can make a case for a broader team approach to chronic abdominal pain, involving other specialists such as anesthesiologists, occupational therapists, and pharmacists. However, in the absence of such an infrastructure, the gastroenterologist needs to assume some key responsibilities in this regard particularly in the form of ongoing patient education about the relationship of their symptoms to both underlying pathophysiology as well as to psychosocial factors. There is a chapter on exaggerated and facticious disease (see Chapter 42, "Factitious or Exaggerated Disease").

Neurolytic Blockade and Miscellaneous Approaches

The value of local blockade in abdominal wall syndromes has been described before. Theoretically, interruption of the pain pathways should provide relief of other forms of abdominal pain as well. This has led to the development of various techniques, both for diagnostic and therapeutic purposes. Neurolytic techniques are valuable for certain subsets of patients, such as those with cancer. By contrast, their use for pain relief in nonneoplastic pain, such as chronic pancreatitis, is not routinely recommended because of low efficacy ($\leq 50\%$) and the short duration of relief (around 2 months), even in those patients that initially respond. Anecdotal experience suggests a similar disappointing outcome with the use of these techniques in functional bowel pain.

Indwelling epidural and *intrathecal access systems* have been effectively used for some patients with intractable chronic pain and to deliver opiates and other drugs, such as clonidine and baclofen. A variety of *electrical stimulation techniques*, including peripheral (transcutaneous electrical nerve stimulation), spinal, and cerebral stimulations have been used for various somatic pain conditions, as well as for angina pectoris, with encouraging results. *Acupressure* is another alternative medicine technique that has been widely used for pain, with results that are mixed. However, none of these techniques have been well studied, if at all, in patients with abdominal pain.

Conclusion

The diagnosis and management of abdominal pain, particularly when chronic, is one of the most challenging clinical problems that a gastroenterologist encounters. Significant progress has been made in our understanding of the pathogenesis of somatic sensitization and it is hoped that this will lead to similar advances in visceral pain. Although there is a clear role for pharmacotherapy, the successful management of pain requires an intensely engaged physician who can interpret this symptom along with the psychosocial context of the patient.

Supplemental Reading

Cervero F, Laird JM. Visceral pain. Lancet 1999;353:2145–8.

Drossman DA. Chronic functional abdominal pain. Am J Gastroenterol 1996;91:2270–81.

Hunt S, Mantyh P. The molecular dynamics of pain control. Nature Reviews Neuroscience 2001;2:83–91.

Hyams JS, Hyman PE. Recurrent abdominal pain and the biopsychosocial model of medical practice. J Pediatrics 1998;133:473–8.

Jackson JL, O'Malley PG, Tomkins G, et al. Treatment of functional gastrointestinal disorders with antidepressant medications: a meta-analysis. Am J Med 2000;108:65–72.

Mayer EA, Gebhart GF. Basic and clinical aspects of visceral hyperalgesia. Gastroenterology 1994;107:271–93.

Pasricha PJ. Approach to the patient with abdominal pain. In: Yamada T, editor. Textbook of gastroenterology. 4th ed. Philadelphia: Lippincott Williams and Wilkins; 2003. p. 781.

Suleiman S, Johnston DE. The abdominal wall: an overlooked source of pain. Am Fam Physician 2001;64:431–8.

Wilcox G. Pharmacology of pain and analgesia. In: Committee ISP, editors. Pain 1999 — An updated review. Seattle: IASP Press; 1999. p. 573–92.

CHAPTER 42

Exaggerated and Factitious Disease

David Edwin, PhD

Gastrointestinal (GI) problems of one sort or another plague all of us throughout our lives, from our childhood bellyaches to the dyspepsia of old age. Obviously, our survival depends upon maintaining adequate nutrition, and any significant disruption of that process at any stage—from food choice and swallowing through elimination—can have serious implications. At the same time, *the act of eating* lies at the center of our lives and our relationships with others—from nursing to courting, from the family dining room to the formal banquet hall. As a result, disruptions in eating and nutrition reverberate in many other arenas of life, and disruptions in important activities and relationships may impact dramatically on eating and nutritional behavior. This is the context in which digestive symptoms develop and persist, and its interplay of biological and psychosocial influences provides opportunities for serious problems to arise.

Abnormal Illness Behavior

Pilowski (1969) coined the term "abnormal illness behavior" to encompass a variety of problems that arise out of the ways patients relate to their doctors about their health care. Physicians are the authorities who formally sanction the sick role for patients, and this certification brings with it both rewards (attention, remuneration) and relief from tiresome obligations (work, school). Indeed, some of the most vexing conflicts that arise in medical care involve disputes over the entitlement of individuals to the sick role. Some patients get caught up in abnormal "illness denying" behavior, and we are hard put to persuade them that they are really ill and need to behave accordingly. We think about these patients using concepts like denial, flight into health, and, sometimes, psychotic illness. Other patients become caught up in "illness affirming" behavior; they seem to suffer from (or even *aspire to*) illnesses they do not have or have only in mild form. A substantial, somewhat unsatisfying part of the psychiatric nomenclature is devoted to a classification of such patients; this classification describes the great diversity of problems, but its categories are neither exhaustive nor mutually exclusive and do not necessarily discriminate among cases or link them to rational interventions. It is to these persistently troubling patients that we turn our attention now.

Consider four views of patients and their symptoms that may guide responses (McHugh and Slavney, 1998; Edwin, 2001). The viewpoint of *disease* assumes that the patient's complaints are *caused by* a "broken" body part or system; this may imply either a disease of peripheral organs (inflammatory bowel disease or pancreatitis), a disease of brain (delusional depression, schizophrenia, dementing illnesses) or their interaction (metabolic encephalopathy). This is the arena in which physicians are most comfortable and effective, and in which referral or disposition becomes straightforward. The *trait* method focuses on temperamental attributes (like intelligence or dependency) that render individuals vulnerable to exaggerating, enhancing or otherwise distorting the problems and symptoms of illness. The viewpoint of *behavior* focuses attention on voluntary choices—to sustain hunger or to eat, to remain sober or to drink—and the intended and unintended consequences of these decisions. It becomes apparent that many of these problems are first and foremost behaviors, actions taken voluntarily in the service of goals that are not always obvious. The *narrative* method focuses on understanding the meanings of symptoms and illnesses, and the behaviors they engender, in the context of the patient's autobiography or subjective life story. Clinical and general life experience often provide accurate intuitions across these methods, even when the behaviors themselves seem to defy understanding.

Classic Syndromes

Primary Psychiatric Illness

First, dramatic, unlikely or even impossible physical complaints may of course be symptomatic of *primary psychiatric illness*. Somatic preoccupations are common in both schizophrenia and major depression, and may range from a chronic sense of unwellness to the fixed conviction of a dread disease (acquired immunodeficiency syndrome, cancer), to bizarre ideas of infestation, or to deliberate implantation of foreign bodies or devices. The true *anorexia* of depression, as well as the odd and rigid eating patterns seen in schizophrenia, obsessive compulsive disorder and eating disorders, may lead to weight loss and delayed transit times suggestive of primary medical illness. Indeed, some such patients may deliberately injure themselves in direct response to hallucinated commands or delusional convictions. Drawing out patients' beliefs about their illnesses may reveal these processes, but formal psychiatric consultation, including personal and family history, mental state examination, and corroborative interviews, are necessary to establish the diagnosis and institute treatment.

Somatization Disorder

Somatization Disorder (or Briquet's Syndrome) describes a chronic *pattern of behavior*—dating at least to early adulthood—of complaints about many symptoms across multiple body systems that result in medical consultation, work interruption, or self-medication, and do not lead to evidence of medical illness sufficient to justify those complaints. This behavior pattern is not uncommon; epidemiologically, it is observed in 0.1 to 2.0% of the general population, *perhaps 5% of medical outpatients, and 9% of medical inpatients*. These patients by definition do not have major psychiatric illness, and pursuit of physical causes for each of their symptoms may lead to repeated invasive procedures and the surgical removal of a great deal of healthy tissue. Recourse to physicians and pursuit of investigations indeed become habituated as a constant feature rather than a troubling interruption of normal life. There is a high proportion of *personality disorder*, including antisocial disorder, among these patients. Characteristically, they have both extraverted and obsessive traits of personality—they may be very suggestible about physical sensations and, once so impressed, they may be hard put to "let go" of their uneasy feelings even when they are reassured. Their life stories are often organized around themes of the losing struggle against encroaching illness, and family histories reveal that these dramas are often multigenerational.

Hypochondriasis

Hypochondriasis describes an attitude—a more focused preoccupation with the *conviction* or the *fear* of having a particular disease even when confronted with evidence or reassurance of its absence or mild nature. Hypochondriacal patients may be exquisitely sensitive to common normal or trivially deviant body sensations; they may enhance or distort these sensations and misinterpret them as evidence of dreaded diseases. A distinction may be drawn between individuals who have no physical disease at all and those who have a mild or manageable disease that becomes unnecessarily disabling because of the patient's preoccupation with it (eg, cardiac neurosis). Often very anxious by nature or by virtue of clinical syndromes (generalized anxiety disorder), these patients are usually *resistant to reassurance* and may in fact become angry or dismissive when offered reassurance.

Conversion Disorder

Conversion disorder (hysteria) describes symptoms or deficits, usually affecting sensation or voluntary motor performance, without underlying physiologic or anatomic abnormality. These symptoms suggest a disease that thorough investigation fails to reveal or substantiate. Often, they are inconsistent over time and may fail to map onto anatomically or physiologically coherent patterns. These symptoms are *by definition not* voluntarily produced or consciously feigned, but seem to arise in the context of a psychosocial stressor or to resolve some psychosocial dilemma confronting the patient. Suspicion is aroused when patients display personalities described as extraverted, attention-seeking, seductive, immature, and/or dependent. These stereotypical characteristics are, in fact, *not* of much diagnostic value; they produce numerous false-positive and false-negative assessments, and play into the prejudice that the concept of hysteria merely reflects "a parody of femininity." And the history of medicine is replete with reports of patients diagnosed with hysteria succumbing to undiagnosed illnesses (Shorter, 1992).*

Malingering or Factitious Behavior

The *deliberate* production of physical or psychological symptoms for an identifiable goal that makes intuitive sense (time off from work, disability compensation, or financial settlement) is referred to as *malingering,* and is regarded as criminal behavior rather than evidence of psychological disorder. On the other hand, the same behaviors, when they seem to serve no other purpose than to compel medical attention or treatment, are diagnosed as a *factitious disorder*. The most notorious factitious variant is "Munchausen syndrome" (Asher, 1951) (related terms include *pseudologica phantastica* and *hospital hobo*); these patients wander from hospital to hospital, making up elaborate histories and presenting utterly imaginary or self-inflicted symptoms, often soliciting admission and invasive investigation. They are predominantly male, socially marginal individuals many of whom have chronic psychiatric illness or profound personality disorder. Much more common are more socially integrated but personally troubled patients, more often women and frequently employed in health-related professions, who are referred to specialists by conscientious primary providers who are baffled or overwhelmed by complaints that defy diagnosis or rational treatment. This is typically a fairly chronic behavior pattern, although there are individuals who will present with problems like laxative abuse as a way of coping with situations they feel are unbearable. In retrospective reviews, as many as 40% of these patients are found on GI services (Reich and Gottfried, 1983).

---

*Editor's Note: Neurotics are not immortal.

It is important to appreciate that malingered or factitious symptoms are distinguished from conversion or hypochondriacal symptoms *only* by the patient's awareness or self-consciousness, which is ultimately a private experience that clinicians can only infer from behavior and self-report. Similarly, the only factor that discriminates malingering from factitious disorder is the presumed *goal* of the behavior, which is of course equally private and also available to others only by inference. Moreover, we are all aware that self-awareness can be a *dimension* rather that an all-or-none attribute of behavior and that intentions are very often mixed. Many patients experience genuine symptoms with exaggerated intensity in the (ultimately futile) attempt to have their lives "made whole" by litigation, and some may exacerbate such symptoms deliberately in order to compel attention to illnesses they "know" are real and threatening but unrecognized or unappreciated by physicians.

The Context and Management of Abnormal Illness Behavior

Many factors determine the intensity with which an individual experiences and responds to physical symptoms (Mechanic, 1975). Certainly, the magnitude of the stimulus is important, as is its duration. Its perceived seriousness, the degree to which it disrupts normal activity, and the knowledge, beliefs, and past experiences, of the patient are important determinants as well. Perhaps as a function of personal temperamental vulnerabilities, other contemporaneous factors in the patient's life, particularly aversive demands, current or anticipated stressors and perceived sources of available support, may more or less powerfully influence the relative weight accorded these symptoms in proportion to other life concerns. In most cases, the symptoms themselves determine the patient's presentation to the physician (and the collaboration that follows) much more than the other factors. The physician's experience and intuition often guides inquiry as the other factors come into play, but when they begin to predominate, more specialized methods are needed.

Maintaining the Therapeutic Relationship

A first principle of management is so fundamental that it merits attention *only* because these patients can render it so difficult: even as doubts grow, it is crucial to maintain the patient's confidence that you are his doctor and that you will continue to care for him. At times, these *symptom-enhancing* and *symptom-creating patients* make it *very difficult to sustain compassion and doctorly commitment*. They consume precious time and resources over "nothing" in an era of encroaching scarcity. We have undertaken to care for them, and they violate their one simple and essential obligation: to tell us the truth as they know it. *In this sense, they refuse to be patients, and yet they (and everyone else) expect us to continue to be their doctors. Indeed, this is the essence of abnormal illness behavior.*

Psychiatric consultation should be undertaken as early as possible when such a behavioral component is suspected, especially in this era when outpatient visits may be rationed and hospital stays are brief. At this point, some of these patients may become increasingly vocal about what they will and will not do. Some may become hurt or indignant at the introduction of a psychiatrist or psychologist. Some will refuse psychiatric referral, insisting that the problem is in their bodies and not in their heads. Some may respond positively to euphemisms about their being "under stress," but others will see this approach as a ruse. Some will have declined this recommendation in the past, and others may have accepted it with disappointing results for a variety of reasons. In all cases, it is crucial to provide firm assurance that you will do what is necessary to care for them and consultation is an essential part of that care.

Psychiatric Illness

When the experience of bodily symptoms or the conviction of illness seems to result from neuropsychiatric illness, patients may require a shift of focus to the treatment of that illness; they may become the primary responsibility of the psychiatrist and even need admission to a psychiatric service. Even in these cases, however, their presenting medical problems may still require investigation or management by the medical specialist, and this, too, may be facilitated by the medical specialist's reassurance of continued interest in the patient's condition. Patients with primary depressive or schizophrenic illnesses will typically become less preoccupied with their medical complaints as their affective and ideational symptoms are resolved, but these resolutions may come over a period of many weeks and may often be incomplete.

Abnormal Illness Behavior

The same principle applies to the management of illness behavior that is *not* produced by major psychiatric illness. Patients who are obsessively concerned about relatively minor problems will need *continued medical care and support* as they are helped to become reabsorbed into their work and family lives. In the absence of true psychiatric illnesses like depression, some personality traits may place patients at high risk for somatic symptoms and the conviction of illness. *Extraverted persons* tend to be vulnerable to suggestion and influence, and may report frustratingly protean symptoms. Individuals with *obsessive traits* have great difficulty accepting reassurance once a notion has taken root, and may defend the notion with endless new observations and "what ifs." Indeed, it has been observed that patients with somatization disorder often manifest both kinds of traits—extraverted dispositions that render them vulnerable to sensation and ideas about them, and obsessive traits that make it difficult to abandon these experiences. Modest intelligence and impoverished behavioral repertoires (and even very substantial resources may be taxed by some levels of challenge) may leave some individuals with few alternatives to the sick role in coping with demands the fear they cannot meet. *It is rarely helpful to try to persuade patients that their symptoms are not real.* The physician must first persuade the patient that he or she fully understands that *a psychological diagnosis provides no immunity to other medical conditions*, and that he or she has not lost interest in the patient's health and treatment. Such patients tend to do better if they are approached from a *"rehabilitation" rather than a curative perspective* and *supported* for their courage and determination in returning to their lives despite their health concerns *rather* than encouraged to relinquish those concerns altogether. It is usually much more helpful to *focus on overcoming barriers* to that re-absorption rather than on historical problems that may appear to have caused or maintained their medical preoccupations.

In some instances, conversion symptoms and even some factitious symptoms (eg, laxative abuse) may respond rapidly when the complaints are met with *studious inattention* and the patient is redirected and supported in addressing the conflicts or demands underlying their appearance. Family and other intimates may be engaged in supporting "rehabilitation" without anyone being confronted with the hypothesized "psychogenic" nature of the complaints. In most cases of somatization disorder and hypochondriasis, however, where illness has become a way of life (Ford, 1983) management becomes more a matter of long term support and "damage control" than of cure or resolution. The most effective element of treatment is the doctor–patient relationship, and it is often the doctor closest to the patient— the family or primary care physician—who carries most of the burden. It is often helpful for the primary physician to see the patient at regular intervals, even —or especially— in the absence of new complaints, so that new symptoms do not become necessary as tickets of admission to the doctor's office. The *subspecialist* then serves as a *support* and a "backup," offering occasional supplementary specialty examinations while echoing and underscoring the primary doctor's sympathetic encouragement. The importance of this support in *avoiding expensive and potentially injurious reexaminations and procedures* cannot be overestimated.†

Factitious Illness

Clinical Suspicion

The outright manufacture of symptoms by a nonpsychotic patient is a rare but serious and potentially life threatening pattern of behavior, and the most dramatic violation of the doctor–patient relationship. One of its most difficult features is that it places the physician in the role of detective as much as doctor, a very uncomfortable turn of events for most caretakers. Moreover, factitious disorder may coexist with other significant medical illnesses, and, in fact, may make them more difficult to detect and diagnose. Nonetheless, a number of features may serve as warning indicators when patients are referred for consultation (Eisendrath, 1996). A history of complaints in times of personal stress may be difficult to elicit. However, when multiple physicians have been baffled or suspicious, or when the patient has felt disappointed, abandoned or betrayed by several doctors, concern is appropriate. Symptoms that fail to respond to appropriate treatments, or that worsen when they should have improved—especially when the patient knew they would worsen— should also arouse concern. A history of "bad luck" from an early age, or of repeated treatment complications should also serve as a warning. The disproportionate representation of health care workers among factitious disorder patients is also a clue in many cases.

Psychiatric Collaboration

Based on these and other indicators, the possibility of factitious disorder should be evaluated as early as possible. Psychiatric collaboration should be engaged at the earliest point possible; euphemisms are less helpful in overcoming resistance than firm insistence along with equally firm reassurance that you are and will remain the patient's doctor. A two-track workup is crucial: the patient should be aware that the systematic evaluation of alternative *medical* diagnoses progresses along with the search for a psychological appreciation of the patient's experience. It is extremely helpful to find the "smoking gun" of contradictory or unlikely medical findings or evidence that is consistent only with factitious illness (eg, enteric organisms in the blood, contaminated syringes or phlebotomy equipment among that patient's possessions in the hospital).

Discussing Factitious Behavior

When the time comes to acknowledge explicitly the concern about self-inflicted symptoms, patients may be hurt or indignant. I have found it useful to make several points. First, factitious behavior is in fact a phenomenon that doctors encounter with some regularity. Second, certain clinical presentations (eg, recurrent fevers of unknown etiology) make it necessary and prudent to evaluate factitious behavior, and the failure to do is negligent. Third, there is no specific constellation of personal traits that is associated with factitious disorder—patients with this behavior are most often not "crazy" or bizarre in their behavior. I have found it helpful to say that I am strongly inclined to believe the patient's denials, and that I usually believe what patients tell me. However, I have learned that

---

†Editor's Note: This means not doing another endoscopic retrograde cholangiography or another colonoscopy just to "reassure" the patients.

I make mistakes in this regard, and that it would be irresponsible of me to wager patients welfare on an uncertain intuition. It may also be helpful to tell the patient, if possible, about other medical explanations that remain under investigation.

Confrontation

If you are persuaded that the patient has been producing the symptoms, and if you have ruled out all of the other reasonable possibilities, it is usually best to engage the patient in a compassionate and nonjudgmental discussion of the evidence together with the psychiatric consultant as well others who have been consistently involved in the patient's care (nurses and even family members) and who have observations to contribute. This is always a difficult and often a painful process. There is a widely circulated idea that confrontation of factitious behavior precipitates suicide; however, although patients may leave the hospital or fire their doctors when challenged or confronted with evidence, instances of suicide have not been reported.

Psychiatric Admission

Following this confrontation, our practice is to admit the patient to an inpatient psychiatric service if at all possible. I have never regretted admitting a patient to a psychiatric service but I have on several occasions sorely regretted failing to do so. Given the potentially life threatening nature of the behavior, involuntary admission is certainly a viable option if the patient cannot otherwise be persuaded. Voluntary or involuntary, psychiatric admission accomplishes several goals. It makes clear the reality and the importance of the psychiatric diagnosis in the context of the patient's ongoing medical care. It formalizes the shift of primary responsibility for the behavior to the psychiatry service while allowing the *medical subspecialist to remain an active consultant* about the medical issues, and thus to address the patient's fear of being medically abandoned. A common explanation offered by patients for this behavior is that they know they have an illness and they have been doing what was necessary to maintain their doctors' interest and involvement. Psychiatric care should not be identified with the withdrawal of that care and involvement.

Involving Family

Perhaps the most important consequence of psychiatric admission is that it becomes impossible for the patient to maintain the capsule of secrecy that has allowed the behavior to persist. Secrecy is simply incompatible with the effective management of factitious behavior. This tends to be a recurring behavior, so it is crucial for the treatment team to mobilize the patient's family and other resources to support him or her in *not* succumbing to this behavior again when stress or provocations occur, as they inevitably must. Patients are often resistant to their families being informed of their diagnosis, and it is all too easy to empathize and identify with the humiliation involved in sharing this kind information with others. It is crucial, however, that these patients continue to have the support—and sometimes the surveillance—of those who care most about them. It is awkward to negotiate such a requirement with a patient, especially in the present context of acute vigilance about confidentiality; but once a patient is safely on a psychiatric service, the staff can often help the patient and the family come to terms with the behavior and develop a plan to avoid its recurrence.

Concluding Comments

Even in the best of circumstances, it is difficult for most of us to understand the motivations of individuals who choose to organize their lives around illnesses from which they do not *need* to suffer. In this era when physicians must cope with increasing demands and diminishing resources, patients who exaggerate or even manufacture medical problems pose a frustrating challenge to our skills and our time. Nonetheless, these are patients in pain and in peril, and a careful and collaborative approach can make their care an interesting and rewarding process.

Supplemental Reading

Asher R. Munchausen's syndrome. Lancet 1951;1:339–41.

Edwin D. Psychological perspectives on patients with inflammatory bowel disease. In: Bayless T, Hanauer SB, editors. Advanced therapy of inflammatory bowel disease. Toronto: CV Mosby Co; 2001. p. 555–82.

Eisendrath SJ. When Munchausen becomes malingering: factitious disorders that penetrate the legal system. Bull Am Acad Psychiatry Law 1996;24:471–81.

Ford CV. The somatizing disorders: illness as a way of life. New York: Elsevier; 1983.

McHugh PR, Slavney PR. The perspectives of psychiatry. Baltimore (MD): Johns Hopkins University Press; 1998.

Mechanic D. The concept of illness behavior. J Chronic Dis 1975;17:189–94.

Pilowsky I. Abnormal illness behavior. Br J Med Psychol 1969;42:347–51.

Reich P, Gottfried LA. Factitious disorder in a teaching hospital. Ann Intern Med 1983;99:240–7.

Shorter E. From paralysis to fatigue: a history of psychosomatic medicine in the modern era. New York: Free Press; 1992.

Slavney PR. Perspectives on hysteria. Baltimore (MD): Johns Hopkins; 1990.

CHAPTER 43

PSYCHOTROPIC DRUGS AND MANAGEMENT OF PATIENTS WITH FUNCTIONAL GASTROINTESTINAL DISORDERS

LIN CHANG, MD, AND DOUGLAS A. DROSSMAN, MD

Functional gastrointestinal disorders (FGIDs) are defined as a "variable combination of chronic or recurrent gastrointestinal (GI) symptoms not explained by structural or biochemical abnormalities." A number of specific disorders ranging from *functional heartburn* to *functional dyspepsia* to *irritable bowel syndrome (IBS)* are considered as FGIDs. The principal underlying mechanism is felt to be a *dysregulated brain gut axis resulting* in the *alteration of gut motility, mechanoelastic properties* and *visceral perception.* Many factors (both central and peripheral) may contribute to this dysregulation, including *genetic predisposition, psychosocial factors* and *chronic stress, inflammation/infection,* and other environmental factors.

The FGIDs are best understood as a *biopsychosocial* disorder. Early life factors (eg, genetic predisposition and environmental factors) influence later psychological experiences, physiologic functioning, and the subsequent vulnerability and development of symptoms of FGIDs. The biopsychosocial model integrates *psychologic* and *physiologic* factors into the conceptual framework that helps explain the clinical symptoms, illness behavior, and treatment outcome. Thus, it is not surprising that centrally targeted medications *(psychotropics)* are frequently used to treat FGIDs because of both *central* and *visceral effects.* This chapter will include the discussion of the rationale, the evidence supporting the use of psychotropic medications, and the practical use of these agents in the treatment of FGIDs. The preceeding chapter also discusses IBS management. A recent drug therapy in IBS is reviewed by Mertz (Mertz, 2003).

Rationale for Using Psychotropics in the Treatment of FGIDs

The utility of psychotropic agents in treating the FGIDs include the following: (1) the ability to treat comorbid psychological symptoms, such as depression, anxiety, or somatization, found particularly in subjects with more severe symptoms and who are seen in tertiary referral centers, (2) their centrally mediated actions modulate visceral pain and autonomic activity of the gut, and (3) they have peripheral actions on sensory, secretory, and motor activity of the GI tract.

Comorbidity of Psychological Symptoms in FGIDs

Stress and psychological factors play a major role in the pathophysiology and clinical presentation of IBS. *Stress* may be central (eg, *psychological distress*) or peripheral (eg, *infection, surgery*) in origin. Patients with IBS report more lifetime and daily stressful events, including abuse, compared with patients with organic GI conditions or healthy individuals. A thorough history usually uncovers that stress is strongly associated with symptom onset, exacerbation, and severity in IBS.

A large proportion of patients with IBS or other functional bowel disorders have coexistent psychological disturbances, particularly those with severe symptoms or those seen in tertiary care referral centers. Psychosocial factors have been recognized to modify the illness experience and influence health care utilization and treatment outcome. These psychosocial factors include a history of emotional, sexual or physical abuse, stressful life events, chronic social stress, anxiety disorders, or maladaptive coping styles. However, the psychological profiles of individuals with IBS who have not sought health care for their GI symptoms are similar to those of healthy individuals. *Thus, although psychosocial factors are not etiologic to IBS, they appear to influence health care seeking, illness behavior, and treatment response.* Currently, the role of psychosocial factors and stress in FGIDs has been conceptualized in the following manner: adverse life experiences (past and present) influence (1) stress responsiveness, (2) physiological responses, and (3) susceptibility to developing and exacerbating FGIDs via amplification of brain-gut interactions.

The beneficial effects of psychotropic agents is most likely due to their effects on *pain modulation* (eg, *tricyclic antidepressants* [TCAs]) and, treatment of *comorbid psychological symptoms* (eg, higher doses of *TCAs and selective serotonin reuptake inhibitors* [SSRIs]).

Central Pain Modulating Effects

Ascending information from the gut to the brain is important for reflex regulation of GI function, and descending information from the brain to the gut ensures that digestive function is optimal via the modulation of motility, secretion, immune function, blood flow, and perception of incoming visceral afferent information. In IBS, neuro-imaging studies show alterations in the central registration of information within the brain-gut axis. Positron emission tomography and functional magnetic resonance imaging have demonstrated *alterations in regional brain activation* in response to *colorectal distension in IBS patients* compared with healthy individuals. Alterations in cerebral blood flow have been specifically reported in two cortical regions of the cingulate cortex, which resides just above the corpus callosum, the anterior cingulate cortex (ACC), and the midcingulate cortex (MCC). The more anterior aspects of the ACC are primarily concerned with regulation of emotion, and the dorsal subregions of the ACC, as well as the anterior MCC, are more concerned with cognitive functions, such as attentional demand and response selection. Regional cerebral blood flow to these two brain regions in IBS is significantly influenced by *psychological factors*. The perigenual subregion of the ACC showed increased *activation* in IBS patients with a history of *sexual and physical abuse*, whereas in another study it showed *deactivation* in IBS patients treated with the centrally acting TCA, *amitriptyline*. Activation of the MCC has been shown to *correlate* with subjective ratings of discomfort in response to *colorectal distension* in IBS patients. In addition, there is preliminary evidence that *resolution* of MCC activation is associated with *improvement* in psychological state and physical symptoms in IBS. These observations suggest that patients with IBS may fail to use central nervous system (CNS) downregulating mechanisms affecting emotional and cognitive processing in response to incoming or anticipated visceral pain, ultimately resulting in the amplification of pain perception. *These results support the importance of therapeutic strategies, such as TCAs, which affect CNS modulation in visceral perception and psychological distress in FGIDs.*

Peripheral Mechanisms of Altered GI Function

Peripheral abnormalities in IBS patients include alterations in *gut motility, visceral hypersensitivity, mucosal cellularity, and intestinal permeability,* which may enable changes in motor and sensory function and gut perception. Although some of these findings may be modified by centrally-mediated mechanisms, there are peripherally based abnormalities that are directly influenced by luminal factors, such as food, mechanical distension, bacteria, and toxins.

Postinfective IBS

A subset of patients associate the development of IBS symptoms with the onset of gastroenteritis. IBS-like symptoms are found in 7 to 30% of patients who have recovered from a proven bacterial gastroenteritis. Increased mucosal cellularity and intestinal permeability have been reported in these patients with *postinfective IBS (PI-IBS)*. Risk factors associated with the development of PI-IBS include *female gender, duration* of acute diarrheal illness, and the presence of *significant life stressors* occurring around the time of the infection; the latter is one of the most important predictive factors of PI-IBS. Thus, *both peripheral gut disturbances* (eg, GI infection) and *central modulating* factors (eg, psychological distress) are required for the development of persistent GI symptoms in PI-IBS.

In addition to their central effects, TCAs may in *part reduce visceral pain* by decreasing firing of *primary sensory afferent nerves,* which transmit pain signals from the gut to the spinal cord.

Lack of Effective Treatments for FGIDs

Several systematic reviews of randomized, placebo controlled treatment trials of FGIDs have been completed and attest to the limitations of treating the FGIDs by peripherally acting agents alone. Given the key pathophysiologic role of brain-gut interactions and the importance that psychosocial factors and stress play in FGIDs, it is reasonable to consider the utility of psychotropic agents in the treatment of these common GI conditions.

Psychotropic Agents

General Approach to Prescribing Antidepressants

The choice of a particular drug is based on (1) the particular symptoms that need to be treated (eg, pain, diarrhea, anxiety, or a combination of symptoms), (2) the medication's side effect profile, (3) the cost of the medications, and (4) the patient's previous medication experiences and preferences. Many patients will report a significant intolerance to medications and/or a short duration of treatment adherence. This may be avoided or minimized by *starting at low doses* of medication and *gradually increasing* to the lowest, most effective dose. Patients should understand that an initial lack of treatment response may be due to a suboptimal dose and/or that the beneficial effect of the medication usually takes at least a few weeks to occur. In addition, there are three main issues that need to be addressed when offering psychotropic medications. The first is to address any potential false beliefs or expectations that the patient may have about taking these types of medications. Many patients may have already perceived negative feedback from their health care providers and even family and friends. They commonly report being told that their symptoms "are all in their head."

Second, it is important to explain that the rationale for including psychotropic medications in the management of their GI symptoms. Third, it is valuable to *negotiate a treatment plan* that is acceptable to both the patient and physician. Involving the patient in the decision making process can empower them and allow them to feel more control over their symptoms. The unpredictability and recurrent nature of FGID symptoms can be very frustrating for patients and may cause them to feel apprehension and helplessness. Important components of instituting a successful treatment plan using psychotropic agents are shown in Table 43-1.

TCAs

Mechanism of Action

Proposed mechanisms of action for TCAs in chronic pain disorders include both *central* and *peripheral actions*. Central actions include suppression of the reuptake of amine neurotransmitters affecting ascending CNS arousal systems, as well as central analgesic and mood effects. TCAs have a peripheral inhibitory effect on primary sensory afferent nerves and therefore, these medications would relieve GI symptoms in part by reducing visceral sensorimotor afferent information from reaching higher centers of the CNS. TCAs also exert a peripheral effect because of their *noradrenergic and anticholinergic actions* that *increases* GI transit time, whereas SSRIs, because of the peripheral *serotonergic effects*, will *decrease* GI transit time. The beneficial effects of TCAs are unlikely due mainly to their effects on psychological comorbidity given their efficacy at low doses. However, the doses of these medications can be *increased* to treat *psychiatric comorbidities* if present.*

Efficacy

Approximately 30% of TCAs prescriptions are for pain conditions, including FGIDs. Low dose TCAs (eg, amitriptyline [Elavil], desipramine [Norpramine], and nortriptyline [Pamelor]) are now frequently used in the treatment of IBS and functional dyspepsia, particularly in patients with more severe or refractory symptoms, impaired daily function, and associated depression and anxiety. The temporal effects of TCAs on GI function precede those that relate to improvement in mood, which suggests that the therapeutic actions are unrelated to improvement in mental state. There was a recent systematic review of seven randomized placebo controlled trials evaluating the effect of TCAs in the treatment of IBS (Brandt et al, 2002) It was found that none of these studies were of high quality due to relatively small sample sizes (≤ 31

---

*Editor's Note: Some IBS patients already on anticholinergics for cramping will become constipated and less tolerant of the anticholingeric when placed on TCAs.

TABLE 43-1. Treatment Plan for Using Psychotropic Agents in Functional Gastrointestinal Disorders

Review Goals and Expectations

Choice depends on the type of symptoms, side effect profile, cost, and previous experience

Start with a low dose of medication and gradually increase to lowest, most effective dose

Beneficial effects may take up to 4 to 6 weeks

Most side effects diminish within 1 to 2 weeks. If persistent, best to continue same or lower dose before switching to another medication, preferably in the same class

Follow-up communication within 1st week and then 2 to 3 weeks later helps patient adherence

Treatment response depends on improvement in daily function, quality of life, and emotional state

---

patients in each arm) and poorly defined primary and secondary endpoints. However, a recently published study by Drossman and colleagues (2002), not included in the systematic review, evaluated the efficacy of the TCA (desipramine [Nonpramin]) in treating moderate to severe functional bowel disorders in a large, randomized, 12-week placebo controlled trial performed at two academic sites with known expertise in functional bowel disorders (FBD). Patients taking desipramine were started on a dose of 50 mg per day and then increased in 1 week to 100 mg per day and then to 150 mg per day from week 3 to week 12 as tolerated. Desipramine was shown to have statistically significant benefit over placebo in the per protocol analysis, which included only those patients who completed treatment (responder rate 73% vs 49%), but not in the intention-to-treat analysis. The lack of benefit in the intention to treat analysis may have related to a substantial (28%) drop out primarily due to symptom side effects, thus attesting to the value of carefully monitoring dosage and helping the patient stay on the medication long enough to achieve a treatment response. Notably, desipramine was more effective in the subgroup of patients with less severe illness (Functional Bowel Disorder Severity Index < 110) and a history of abuse (Drossman et al, 1995).

Dosage and Side Effects

Based on these data we can assume that the efficacy of TCAs as visceral analgesic agents occurs at lower doses than that used to treat major depression, and this appears related to their neuromodulatory analgesic properties. Treatment should start with *low doses* (eg, *10 to 25 mg at bedtime*) and titrate up as needed to the lowest, most effective therapeutic dose (Table 43-2). Because these agents can have sedative effects, they can be used to promote sleep with a *single nightly dose*. This is of particular value since many patients with FGIDs have sleep disturbances, and poor sleep quality correlates with increased bowel symptoms the following morning. *Desipramine* (Norpramin) and *nortriptyline* (Pamelor) are associated with *less sedation* and *constipation* than *amitriptyline* (Elavil) or *imipramine* (Tofranil), presumably because of their lower antihistaminic and anticholinergic effects. Therefore, in those patients who do not report symptoms of sleep dysfunction or feel that any sedative effect is undesirable, either of these less sedating agents can be prescribed. Whereas TCAs have proven efficacy in IBS patients, particularly those who have diarrhea-predominant symptoms, *desipramine* may be a good initial choice in patients with predominant *constipation* because of its relatively low anticholinergic effect.

SSRIs

Mechanism of Action

SSRIs inhibit the reuptake of serotonin and therefore allow greater availability of serotonin to act postsynaptically. The benefits of SSRIs in the treatment of FGIDs have not been well studied and their potential central and peripheral effects are less clear. In comparing their *indications for psychiatric conditions*, the benefits of SSRIs in FGIDs may relate to their *anxiolytic effects* and treatment of *social phobia, agoraphobia,* and *obsessive-compulsive disorders*. These conditions can occur in some patients with FGIDs.

A possible mechanism of SSRIs is through their central effects in reducing the vicious cycle of *anxiety* and *pain*. They may also have the peripheral effect of *decreasing orocecal transit time,* which is presumably the mechanism responsible for the side effect of diarrhea.

Efficacy

There is one published study comparing the efficacy of SSRIs (*paroxetine* [Paxil]) with "treatment as usual" in reducing abdominal pain, health-related quality of life and health care costs in a relatively large group of severe IBS patients at 3 months of treatment and 1 year later. Between 40 to 48% of the patients had a psychiatric disorder and 12% reported a history of sexual abuse. Paroxetine did not significantly reduce abdominal pain scores, but it did decrease days of pain compared with the treatment as usual group. Although paroxetine was significantly superior to treatment as usual in improving health-related quality of life, there was no difference between patients with and without a depressive disorder (Drossman et al, 2002). The effect of these treatment modalities on IBS symptoms, health-related quality of life and health care costs in patients with

TABLE 43-2. Antidepressant Treatment: Receptor Action Sites, Dose, and Patient Indications

Drug	Dose (mg/d)	Anticholinergic Effect	5-HT Reuptake	Antihistamine Effect	Patient Indications
TCAs					
Desipramine (Norpramin)	10 to 150	+	+++	+	Most empiric evidence for efficacy. Less sedation and constipation
Nortriptyline (Pamelor)	10 to 150	++	+	++	Least sedating
Amitriptyline (Elavil)	10 to 150	++++	+++	++++	Very sedating
Doxepin (Sinequan)	10 to 150	++	+++	++++	Very sedating
Imipramine (Tofranil)	10 to 150	–	–	–	Very sedating
SSRIs					
Citalopram (Celexa)	10 to 20	Nil	++++	Nil	Fewer side effects and drug interactions
Escitalopram (Lexapro)	10 to 20	Nil	++++	Nil	Fewer side effects and drug interactions
Fluoxetine (Prozac)	20	Nil	++++	Nil	Long half-life; less withdrawal effects
Sertraline (Zoloft)	25 to 150	Nil	++++	Nil	Requires dose ranging
Paroxetine (Paxil)	20	+	++++	Nil	Short half-life; more likely withdrawal effects. Greater anticholinergic effect; use in diarrhea-predominant patients.
Other					
Venlafaxine (Effexor)	75 to 150	Nil	++++	Nil	Similar effects to SSRIs
Mirtazepine (Remeron)	15 to 45	+	+++	++	Has 5-HT$_3$ antagonist properties and can be used to treat nausea. Use in patients with poor sleep, inability to gain weight, and diarrhea.
Buspirone (Buspar)	20 to 30	Nil	Nil	Nil	5-HT$_{1A}$ agonist. Antianxiety effects. Can augment treatment with TCAs and SSRIs. Can use for functional dyspepsia.

SSRIs = serotonin reuptake inhibitors; TCAs = tricyclic antidepressants; 5-HT = 5-hydroxytryptamine.

less severe symptoms needs further assessment.

Another smaller double blind, placebo controlled study evaluated the effect of the SSRI fluoxetine (Prozac) on symptoms and rectal sensitivity in 40 patients with varying subtypes of IBS. Patients randomized to drug treatment did not show significant differences in these outcome measures of rectal perception. Two additional preliminary studies published in abstract form evaluated the effect of the SSRI *citalopram* (Celexa) and the selective serotonin and noradrenaline reuptake inhibitor (SNRI) *venlaxafine* (Effexor) in relatively small numbers of IBS patients. In one study, oral citolapram appeared to decrease abdominal pain and bloating, but a one time dose of intravenous citalopram had no effect on rectal sensitivity. The other study found that venlafaxine appeared to reduce colonic compliance and sensation and decrease the normally increased colonic tone that occurs postprandially.

In summary, the efficacy of SSRIs and SNRIs in FGIDs has not been well studied, although there is some preliminary evidence that they may have some overall efficacy in patients with moderate to severe symptoms. It is still not clear if they are effective in patients with milder symptoms or if they exert their beneficial effect by specifically relieving GI symptoms, such as abdominal pain, versus decreasing psychological symptoms. Although it seems likely that these agents would improve overall well being in patients with FGIDs and are desirable due to their lower side effect profile compared to TCAs, the clinical impression is that a *substantial number of patients are taking these medications but reporting persistent GI symptoms.*

Dosage and Side Effects

With SSRIs, the dosage is usually similar to that used for psychological symptoms. Most patients will benefit from only *one morning dose* (10 to 20 mg *fluoxetine* [Prozac], *citalopram* [Celexa] or *escitalopram* [Lexapro], 50 mg *sertraline*, or 20 mg paroxetine) (see Table 43-2). Lower doses may be required for the elderly, or patients with liver disease, due to the prolonged half-life of the metabolites under these conditions. Treatment is continued for 6 to 12 months before tapering, and dosage adjustments can be discussed and decided mutually by the physician and patient. SSRIs are associated with fewer side effects but are more expensive than TCAs. Citalopram and escitalopram reportedly have fewer drug interactions and side effects than the other SSRIs but these have not been well studied in large trials. Side effects of SSRIs include diarrhea, nausea, diaphoresis, sexual dysfunction, and agitation. *Fluoxetine* (Prozac) has the longest half-life of the SSRIs (about 30 hours) and for that reason is not usually associated with withdrawal effects. Conversely, *paroxetine* (Paxil) has a very short half-life (about 6 hours), and when discontinuing it, the drug must be tapered slowly over several weeks.

Paroxetine (Paxil) also has more anticholinergic effects compared with other SSRIs, and so this side effect can be used as an advantage by considering it for patients with *diarrhea* as a predominant symptom.

Other Psychotropic Agents

Mirtazepine

Mirtazapine (Remeron) is a novel quadricyclic antidepressant agent that blocks pre- and postsynaptic α-2 receptors, as well as the serotonin receptors 5-HT$_2$ and 5-HT$_3$ (see Table 43-2). It also has the potentially beneficial 5-HT$_3$ receptor antagonist effect on peripheral GI symptoms and should be considered in patients who complain of *poor sleep, nausea, inability to gain weight, and diarrhea.* In contrast to TCAs, it has low affinity for α1 receptor blockade. Mirtazapine has little interaction with acetylcholine receptors, but is a potent blocker of histamine receptors.

Buspirone

Buspirone (Buspar) is a nonbenzodiazepine antianxiety agent that may take several weeks to achieve benefit. Its action as a 5-HT$_{1A}$ agonist results in *increased gastric accommodation*, and therefore, it may be beneficial in some patients with *functional dyspepsia*. In one small study comparing the effect of *venlaxafine* (Effexor), *buspirone* (Buspar) and placebo on colonic mechanoelastic properties and perception in IBS patients, buspirone was shown to have no effect on colonic sensitivity. It is relatively nonsedating and is usually well tolerated. The dosage is 20 to 30 mg in divided doses (2 to 3 times per day). This drug also has *augmentative* properties and can be combined with other antidepressants to enhance the treatment effect.

Combination Psychotropic Therapy

It is possible that *combination treatment* may enhance the effect of single drug treatment in patients with FGIDs, particularly those with more severe symptoms and/or comorbid psychological symptoms. Because of their high affinity for the cytochrome P450 system (particularly with paroxetine), the SSRIs should be used with caution if given with TCAs and benzodiazepines. Physicians can take advantage of this effect by adding a low dose SSRI when patients show an incomplete response to a TCA. A low dose TCA may more effectively treat pain-related symptoms, whereas the SSRI can be used to treat associated symptoms of anxiety. *Fibromyalgia*, a chronic somatic pain disorder that frequently coexists with FGIDs, is commonly treated with a *combined regimen* of an *SSRI* and *TCA*. Another possible therapeutic combination in patients with FGIDs is *buspirone* with an *antidepressant,* such as a TCA or SSRI. They can augment their beneficial effects so that higher doses can be avoided, thus, decreasing the side effects. *Psychotropics* can also be successfully combined with *psychotherapy* and *behavioral treatment* approaches.

Summary

Psychotropic medications are commonly used in the treatment of FGIDs. These medications include TCAs, SSRIs, SNRIs, and other psychotropics, such as *mirtazepine* (Remeron) and *buspirone* (Buspar). Psychotropics can act via central and peripheral mechanisms to decrease perception of bothersome GI symptoms. Their efficacy in FGIDs may occur via effects on pain modulatory pathways (TCAs), GI transit times (TCAs and SSRIs), and/or psychological comorbidity (TCAs and SSRIs). TCAs, such as *desipramine* (Norpramine) have the most empiric evidence for efficacy and are relatively inexpensive, but they have a significant side effect profile. The efficacy of SSRIs in FGIDs has not been as well studied but there is evidence that they may improve quality of life in these patients. SSRIs and SNRIs are useful in treating psychological symptoms such as anxiety, depression, and obsessive-compulsive behavior in patients with FGIDs. They have a lower side effect profile but are more expensive than TCAs.

Selection of the most appropriate psychotropic agent depends on the types of symptoms, the side effect profile, cost, and the patient's previous experience with these types of medications. Successful treatment of FGIDs can be achieved with psychotropics given either alone, or in combination with another psychotropic agent, or with psychological treatment via their augmentative or synergistic effects.

Supplemental Reading

Brandt LJ, Bjorkman D, Fennerty MB, et al. Systematic review on the management of irritable bowel syndrome in North America. Am J Gastroenterol 2002;97(Suppl):S7–26.

Bush G, Luu P, Posner MI. Cognitive and emotional influences in anterior cingulate cortex. Trends Cogn Sci 2000;4:215–22.

Camilleri M, Choi M-G. Review article: irritable bowel syndrome. Aliment Pharmacol Ther 1997;11:3–15.

Drossman DA, Camilleri M, Mayer EA, et al. AGA technical review on irritable bowel syndrome. Gastroenterology 2002;123:2108–31.

Drossman DA, Li Z, Toner BB, et al. Functional bowel disorders: a multicenter comparison of health status, and development of illness severity index. Dig Dis Sci 1995;40:986–95.

Drossman DA, Ringel Y, Vogt BA, et al. Alterations of brain activity associated with resolution of emotional distress and pain in a case of severe irritable bowel syndrome. Gastroenterology 2003;124:754–61.

Drossman DA, Toner BB, Whitehead WE, et .al. Cognitive-behavioral therapy vs. education and desipramine vs. placebo for moderate to severe functional bowel disorders. Gastroenterology 2003;125:19–31.

Gwee KA, Leong YI, Graham C, et al. The role of psychological and biological factors in postinfective gut dysfunction. Gut 1999;47:804–11.

Jailwala J, Imperiale TF, Kroenke K. Pharmacologic treatment of the irritable bowel syndrome: a systematic review of randomized, controlled trials. Ann Intern Med 2000;133:136–47.

Klein KB. Controlled treatment trials in the irritable bowel syndrome: a critique. Gastroenterology 1988;95:232–41.

Mertz H, Morgan V, Tanner G, et al. Regional cerebral activation in irritable bowel syndrome and control subjects with painful and nonpainful rectal distension. Gastroenterology 2000;118:842–8.

Mertz HE. Irritable bowel syndrome. N Engl J Med 2003:349:2136–46.

Naliboff BD, Derbyshire SWG, Munakata J, et al. Cerebral activation in irritable bowel syndrome patients and control subjects during rectosigmoid stimulation. Psychosom Med 2001;63:365–75.

Neal KR, Hebden J, Spiller R. Prevalence of gastrointestinal symptoms six months after bacterial gastroenteritis and risk factors for development of the irritable bowel syndrome: postal survey of patients. BMJ 1997;314:779–82.

Spiller RC, Jenkins D, Thornley JP, et al. Increased rectal mucosal enteroendocrine cells, T-lymphocytes, and increased gut permeability following acute *Campylobacter* enteritis and in post-dysenteric irritable bowel syndrome. Gut 2000;47:804–11.

Su X, Gebhart GF. Effects of tricyclic antidepressants on mechanosensitive pelvic nerve afferent fibers innervating the rat colon. Pain 1998;76:105–14.

Tack J, Piessevaux H, Caenepeel P, Janssens J. Role of impaired gastric accomodation to a meal in functional dyspepsia. Gastroenterology 1998;115:1346–52.

Talley NJ, Owen BK, Boyce P, Paterson K. Psychological treatments for irritable syndrome: a critique of controlled treatment trials. Am J Gastroenterol 1996;91:277–83.

CHAPTER 44

ROLE OF A NURSE ADVOCATE

Lisa Turnbough, RN

Inflammatory bowel disease (IBD) patients must deal with socially embarrassing, painful, and, sometimes, body image altering diseases. They experience better outcomes when they are adequately educated about their disease process and treatment and have confidence that there is a reliable contact when problems or questions arise. These patients need to feel comfortable discussing their symptoms and fears in a relaxed atmosphere of empathy, compassion, and professionalism. They deserve accurate information given in a timely manner. Unfortunately, many patients report dissatisfaction in accessing the health care system. In large institutions it is easy for the patient to feel he/she gets lost in the shuffle in the interim between regularly scheduled visits. Blaine Franklin Newman became frustrated with the inconsistent contacts and information he dealt with during his battle with Crohn's disease and vowed to help other patients avoid that distress. His generosity and foresight provided the endowment that initiated and supports the IBD nurse advocate position at the Johns Hopkins Hospital (Hunt, 2001).

Position Role

The goal of this advocacy role is to help the patient reach maximum potential in terms of achievement and maintenance of disease remission and quality of life. Through participation in clinics, urgent issue-telephone triage, and outreach activities the nurse becomes the consistent contact, provides patient education and reinforcement, and guides patients' optimum health.

This role requires professional maturity and the ability to work independently. Communication, appropriate documentation, and adherence to Practice Acts are also of paramount importance. Nursing experience in the areas of endoscopy, ostomy care, research, and patient education is advantageous in caring for the IBD patient. Patience and empathy for the chronically ill, as well as the ability to be firm and set limits as needed, are necessary with this patient population. Interpersonal skills that promote a feeling of safety and openness for patients to discuss embarrassing symptoms and honesty in compliance issues are also necessary. Of equal importance, ongoing communication between the nurse advocate and the physician is vital as the nurse promotes the adherence to the plan of care. When the patient senses a collaborative approach to their care, they are reassured and trust is developed.

The Clinic Visit

The major responsibilities of this role, as we have structured it, begin in the outpatient clinics. Through the assessment process that involves active listening, assessments, documentation and appropriate education for the individual patient, the nurse becomes an accessible link to the health care system. The clinic setting is an excellent forum for the nurse to learn, not only from the physician, but from the IBD patients as well.

The nurse sees returning clinic patients during the initial 15 minutes of the visit. Briefly the patients' IBD history is reviewed; current medical status and psychosocial issues are discussed as well as coping strategies. Reviewing the patient (health) diary can also be helpful. Medications and effectiveness, including any side effects or compliance issues, the need for prescriptions, and diagnostic or surveillance testing are also reviewed. Patients are given opportunity to ask questions.

Assessment data is presented to the physician so he or she approaches the patient better equipped to address needs in a prioritized and time efficient manner. The nurse assists with the physical examination, and the treatment plan is mutually established and documented. The nurse helps to identify the need for and facilitates referrals/appointments to other disciplines (ie, ostomy nurse, surgery, dermatology, rheumatology, endocrinology, dietetics, social work, primary care provider). Compliance with the plan is promoted further by patient education and written instructions. Patients verbalize satisfaction with the visit as they leave with their questions answered, a clear idea of the plan, and knowing that they may contact the nurse if further clarification is needed or problems arise between clinic visits. Entering visit, lab, and prescription information into a database aids patient care. Patient permission is obtained to permit use of any patient data in research.

Telephone Triage

It is in the telephone communication with patients that the IBD nurse advocate functions most in the capacity of liaison between patient and physician. The nurse must be able to quickly determine the severity of the issue prompting the call in order to prioritize the urgency. Frequent issues or requests per the phone range from new onset of symptoms, failed response to therapy, adverse events, need for refills, test results, insurance coverage problems, disability paperwork, or referral to other specialists. Often patients are asked to call the nurse for guidance in adjusting medication dosages. This is particularly important when the physician has been tapering the patient off of steroids or adjusting the dose of newly prescribed azathioprine. Documentation of the content of the calls is important for legal reasons as well as for continuity of care. Before changes in therapy or plan of care are implemented the physician approves them.

Calls that are made because of an increase in disease activity (diarrhea, cramping, urgency, etc) require an investigation that includes asking about any changes in overall health, medication compliance (nonsteroidal anti-inflammatory drug use aggravates IBD), diet, and stress level, as well as asking about the presence of other symptoms (bleeding, opening of fistulas, fevers, extra-intestinal manifestations). Even the most articulate and insightful patients can leave out important data needed to appropriately assess the situation. Conversely, patients that are known to go on and on with copious and various complaints can be under-evaluated when they have real medical needs. Good advice from Dr. Theodore Bayless: "Neurotics are not immortal." Some calls simply require an empathetic ear.

Communication with outpatients via email can be effective and timesaving in some instances. However, it does not replace the need to actually talk with patients who are experiencing a flare of disease symptoms. It is often a subtle statement made by the patient that gives a clue as to degree of disease activity or maladaptive coping.

Patient Education

Teaching that is begun at the time of diagnosis and reinforced and built upon at each clinic visit empowers the patient with judgment regarding when to call and how to manage their disease at home.

Information is given to patients keeping in mind the individual intellectual ability, age and emotional status as well as the appropriateness of the moment. Information given to a patient at the time of diagnosis or during a flare may not have been retained, as these are not optimal teachable moments. Health care providers often unintentionally talk over the heads of patients. Basic phrases used in the world of medicine sound very foreign to the layperson. It is important to recognize noncomprehension and address educational needs respectfully.

The nonemergent clinic visit is a good time to reinforce concepts related to disease process, rationale for prescribed therapies, problem solving tips, and what to do if problems do occur. A well-informed patient tends to need fewer emergent visits. Such teaching also reinforces the importance of medication compliance (Kane, 2001). Written materials and responsible Web sites can be good educational resources for the patient to further their understanding of IBD. However, newly diagnosed IBD patients can become overwhelmed and frightened with too much, too soon.

Compliance

Compliance with medical therapy is to IBD as location is to real estate. It makes all the difference! Noncompliance has been widely underestimated in treating chronically ill patients. The World Health Organization has estimated that up to 50% of patients do not take their medications as prescribed (Marcus, 2003).

The first area to explore when a patient complains of symptom recurrence is that of compliance to therapy. If nonadherence is determined further exploration can often shed light as to why the patient is not taking the prescribed medication. Some reasons for noncompliance include financial burden, side effects, and educational needs.

Loss of a job, lack of insurance coverage, other ill family members, or a change in the social/financial situation will have a huge impact on ability to pay for/obtain prescription medications (Kane, 2001). Many pharmaceutical companies offer patient assistance programs. Local, state, and federal programs may also be available. A social worker may be of benefit.

If side effects or scheduling of medications is to blame for nonadherence, alternative therapies or a change in dosing schedules can be explored. Patients who have gained remission often find it difficult to take their medication either because they forget to do so or do not see the need to continue. All too often medical noncompliance precedes disease exacerbation. The ongoing need of medications for the maintenance of remission need to be stressed with the patient.

Compliance with colonoscopy to survey for dysplasia and colon cancer in IBD patients may also be an issue (Kane, 2001). Patients need to be aware of the recommendations as well as the potential risk of noncompliance. Follow-up blood work is also necessary when the patient is on immunomodulators. Patients need to be reminded that these tests are done to detect early signs of problems, such as leukopenia. Again patient education may help the patient see the wisdom in following the recommendations.

Psychosocial Issues

Individual coping with a chronic illness varies widely. Age, maturity level, severity of disease, other medical problems, current life situation, and personal history are all factors that may either help or hinder the acceptance of an IBD diagnosis. Coexisting or newly emerging emotional issues or mental illness will affect the way in which an individual deals with IBD. If coping with the stress of IBD is overwhelming, the patient should be further examined and treated. Appropriate referrals are facilitated for psychiatry or social work. Most patients do not require such referrals. However, the health care team needs to be aware that IBD impacts upon the entire family. Support through the clergy and organizations, such as the Crohn's and Colitis Foundation (CCFA).

The nurse advocate can offer hope and some sense of control by helping the patient to realize areas where they have influence on outcomes. The nurse reinforces the need for compliance of therapy and ongoing medical care as behaviors that can impact outcomes. A letter to the employer or college housing office, to request an individual be situated so that access to a restroom is adequate, can relieve a tremendous amount of anxiety.

There are separate chapters on psychotropic drugs and management in patients with functional disorders (see Chapter 43, "Psychotropic Drugs and Management in Patients with Functional Gastrointestinal Disorders"), chronic abdominal pain (see Chapter 41, "Chronic Abdominal Pain"), abdominal pain in children and adolescents (see Chapter 40, "Chronic Recurrent Abdominal Pain in Childhood and Adolescence"), smoking cessation (see Chapter 45, "Smoking and Gastrointestinal Disease"), and factitious or exaggerated disease (see Chapter 42, "Factitious or Exaggerated Disease").

Sexual/Reproductive Issues

Even in today's postsexual revolution society there is uneasiness in talking about sexual concerns. Whereas many patients feel comfortable in bringing up the subject of sex, others do not. In the interview process the nurse can simply ask if there are sexual concerns, questions, or dysfunction. This allows the patient to express such issues if they exist. It also further assesses the overall quality of life that the patient experiences in living with the complications of IBD. Alterations in body image (from steroids, surgical scars, fistulas, or ostomies), pain, and fatigue can alter sexual functioning. Optimizing medical therapy to gain remission and steroid-sparing are the primary goals with this issue. Surgical intervention may be necessary; support groups, ostomy nurses, gynecologists, and urologists may be appropriate referrals. Often patients need an ear to talk openly to about this delicate topic in a nonthreatening environment.

Infertility, pregnancy in IBD and genetic concerns also emerge as worries. These topics are addressed in another chapter of this book (see Chapter 84, "Pregnancy and Inflammatory Bowel Disease").

Outreach

Advocacy lends itself to outreach beyond the patient population that is served by a particular physician and the nurse advocate. By increasing public awareness and deeper understanding of these diseases within the medical community and promoting research, the IBD nurse advocates for patients.

Depending on the size of the patient load, it may be unrealistic for the IBD nurse advocate to coordinate studies. At the very least though, the nurse must be aware and informed about studies involving IBD patients.

The nurse can introduce studies to patients that meet inclusion criteria and further promote research by staying in touch with investigators. At Johns Hopkins, research is being conducted on the genetics of IBD (Brant et al, 2000) and on the metabolism of azathioprine/purinethol. Information gained from studies improves patient management strategies and provides answers to patient's questions. Enzyme and metabolite levels are monitored to predict efficacy and safety of therapy. Dosages are adjusted using this information. Patients may be spared the side effects of leukopenia or liver dysfunction by monitoring the metabolite levels (Cuffari et al, 2001).

Opportunities also arise for the IBD nurse advocate to speak to groups of nurses that care for IBD patients and need more information on the unique needs of this population. Both formal and informal teaching opportunities become available for nurses on inpatient units, in the infusion room, and in endoscopy. Further opportunities to speak for the IBD patients occur with interchanges with those continuing their medical education and training (medical students, interns, residents, and fellows).

Additionally, at Johns Hopkins, the IBD nurse facilitates infliximab orders for the infusion program as well as monitoring follow-up of those patients. Long-term data is maintained to follow the progress, adverse events, and continued benefits of this therapy.

Role Impact

Patients were surveyed on their perceptions of the IBD nurse advocate role after 2 to 3 years of being in place. The completed surveys strongly supported this role.

Financial feasibility in establishing an IBD nurse advocate role is substantiated by the fact that many of the responsibilities of the role can be classified as physician-extender activities. Freeing the gastroenterologist to see more patients by reducing the amount of time spent with returning patients as well as reducing telephone time allows more patients to be seen overall. This position could also fit into a nurse practitioner's role.

Acknowledgements

I am grateful for the opportunity to work with dedicated physicians and academicians. Dr. Theodore Bayless and Dr. Mary L. Harris have patiently and diligently mentored me through the past 4 years in this position. Not only have I grown as a nurse, I have also grown as an individual from my association with these physicians.

Sincere thanks goes also to the family of Blaine Newman for providing an endowment to help support the IBD advocate position at Johns Hopkins. The Hospital, the Gastroenterology Division and the Meyerhoff IBD Center have also helped support this position. Further, the IBD patients of the Meyerhoff Digestive Disease Center at Johns Hopkins continue to teach me about the power of the human spirit.

Supplemental Reading

Barrier PA, Li J T-C, Jensen NM. Two words to improve physician-patient communication: what else? Mayo Clin Proc 2003;78:211–4.

Brant SR, Panhuysen CIM, Bailey-Wilson JE, et al. Linkage heterogeneity for the IBD1 locus in Crohn's disease. Pedigrees by disease onset and severity. Gastroenterology 2000;119:1483–90.

Cuffari C, Dassopoulos T, Turnbough L, Bayless TM. Thiropurine methyl-transferse activity influences clinical responses to azathioprine therapy in inflammatory bowel disease. Clin Gastroenterol Hepatol 2004:2.[In Press]

Cuffari C, Hunt S, Bayless T. Utilisation of erythrocyte 6-thioguanine metabolite levels to optimize azathioprine therapy in patients with inflammatory bowel disease. Gut 2001;48:642–6.

Hunt SA. Inflammatory bowel disease nurse advocate. In: Bayless TM, Hanauer SB, editors. Advanced therapy of inflammatory bowel disease. Hamilton (ON): BC Decker; 2001. p. 535–7.

Kane S. Adherence issues in management of inflammatory bowel disease. In: Bayless TM, Hanauer SB, editors. Advanced therapy of inflammatory bowel disease. Hamilton (ON): BC Decker; 2001. p. 9–11.

Marcus AD. You can write an rx, but you can't make a patient follow it. Johns Hopkins Today's News [Serial online] 2003. <http://www.jhu.edu/clips/2003_11/10/youcan.html> (accessed Nov 12, 2003).

CHAPTER 45

SMOKING AND GASTROINTESTINAL DISEASE

MICHAEL F. PICCO, MD, PHD

Cigarette smoking is the most important preventable cause of mortality in the United States. Despite the common knowledge of numerous adverse effects, it is sad that so many young people start smoking. Although smoking rates seem to be declining, in 1998 26% of adult men and 22% of adult women were current smokers. Smoking has been linked to as many as 50% of all deaths among current smokers (Burns et al, 1997). Importantly, tobacco (nicotine) is an addictive substance with a clear psychological and physical withdrawal syndrome.

Smoking Cessation

The best way to stop cigarette smoking is never to start. Of current smokers two-thirds will want to quit, three-fourths will have tried to quit and one-third will try to quit every year (Sutherland, 2003). Smoking cessation methods have limited success and the majority of patients who smoke will continue to do so even after pharmacologic and behavior therapy. Even the best methods of combined pharmacologic and intensive behavioral therapy leads to a quit rate of only 15% at 1 year. This has led some clinicians, possibly out of frustration or because of fears of straining the doctor-patient relationship, to not make smoking cessation a priority with their patients and, in some cases, to not even discuss tobacco as a threat to their patient's health. If we as clinicians do not raise this issue we miss an important opportunity. We run the risk of our patients getting the message from us that cigarettes are not an important threat to their health. We underestimate our impact on influencing and helping our patients to stop smoking especially after they have developed medical problems as a result of their smoking.

Associations With Digestive Disease

Smoking is associated with numerous digestive diseases. These associations can be divided into neoplasms, acid-peptic disorders, and chronic inflammatory disorders. In most situations the amount and duration of tobacco usage increases the risk of disease. However, paradoxically, in some disorders, such as ulcerative colitis (UC), tobacco usage can actually delay disease onset or control existing disease.

Although the illnesses discussed here are covered in other sections of this book, the purpose of this chapter is to focus on smoking and its impact on common digestive diseases.

Gastrointestinal Neoplasms

The most recognizable association of tobacco is with the development of specific gastrointestinal (GI) malignancies. Tobacco has been implicated in the development of oropharyngeal cancers and squamous carcinoma of the esophagus (Morita et al, 2002). The risk increases with amount and duration of smoking. Heavy alcohol use magnifies this risk. For esophageal adenocarcinoma (AC) the risk begins to decline only after 10 years of abstinence from tobacco. Smoking alone does not appear to be a primary risk factor for AC of the esophagus yet it may be indirectly implicated through its effect on gastroesophageal reflux disease (GERD) (Brown and Devesa, 2002). Smoking increases the risk of pancreatic cancer at least twofold and is also associated with an increased risk of anal cancer (Lowenfels and Maisonneuve, 2002; Daling et al, 1992; Konner and O'Reilley, 2002).

The associations between tobacco and cancers of the stomach and colon are not as clear. The risk for gastric cancer is higher among smokers, and smoking does increase the risk of squamous metaplasia of the gastric cardia, which is likely a premalignant condition (Brown and Devesa, 2002). Tobacco is also associated with an increased risk of colonic adenomas (Potter, 2001), which lead to colorectal cancer, but a direct link of smoking to AC of the colon has been difficult to establish.

Acid-Peptic Disorders

Smoking impacts on the development and prognosis of acid-peptic disorders. It causes hyposalivation and aerophagia and may make GERD worse by interfering with acid clearance from the esophagus and increasing the number of reflux episodes. Tobacco use is clearly associated with peptic ulcer disease, specifically duodenal ulcer (DU) (Calam and Baron, 2001). Current smokers are twice as likely to develop a DU and have impaired ulcer healing. They are also 10 times as likely to develop a perforation compared to nonsmokers and are also more prone to relapse of their ulcer disease. Long-term, male smokers have a greater likelihood of developing gastric mucinous metaplasia, which is associated with DU. In this era when we all focus on *Helicobacter pylori* and nonsteroidal inflammatory medications as causative agents, we must not overlook the contribution of smoking to DU development and complications. Tobacco does not appear to be associated with nonulcer dyspepsia.

Inflammatory Bowel Disease

Perhaps the most well established yet enigmatic relationship is between smoking and inflammatory bowel disease (IBD). IBD typically is divided into UC and Crohn's disease (CD). The onset of these disorders is influenced by both genetic and environmental factors. Surprisingly, smoking has opposite effects on CD and UC. In UC, smoking may protect against or delay onset of disease and ameliorate its course, whereas in CD smoking may lead to earlier onset and worse prognosis. These opposite effects have been the subject of intense clinical and laboratory study in hopes of better insights into the pathogenesis and treatment of these disorders.

Ulcerative Colitis

UC is typically a disease of former smokers and is rare among current smokers (Thomas et al, 1998). Never-smokers also have an increased risk compared to active smokers. Smoking may actually delay the onset of UC in susceptible individuals, with the age at diagnosis among former male smokers 17 years later than nonsmokers. Curiously, this difference does not seem to apply to females. For unclear reasons, the risk of UC is higher in former smokers than nonsmokers. Some have speculated that symptoms of UC result in patients quitting smoking whereas others suggest that smoking may keep the disease latent only for it to later emerge with tobacco cessation.

This negative association of tobacco with UC is by no means universal. Reif and colleagues (1995) found no such association among Israeli Jews. This may be because smoking is of only minor importance among this strongly ethnically predisposed group. The reasons for the development of UC and CD are multifactorial but clearly the most important risk factor is genetic predisposition.

Ex-smokers tend to develop UC soon after quitting suggesting that smoking may be protective. Many ex-smokers who return to smoking after developing UC report improvement in symptoms. Smokers with UC have been found to have lower relapse rates and lower colectomy rates as well. It is unclear as to how smoking benefits patients with UC because some have thought that nicotine may be the active ingredient. These have been trials of nicotine, usually in the form of a patch, for active UC. Some patients, in the acute setting will respond, although overall results have been inconsistent. Also two-thirds of patients, especially nonsmokers, will develop significant side effects to the nicotine. In the chapter on UC management (see Chapter 78, "Ulcerative Colitis") the use of nicotine patches is placed in perspective with other therapies. Unfortunately, once remission is established, most studies show that nicotine patches are apparently no better than placebo in maintaining remission. Among patients who do have a clinical response, the long-term effects of nicotine, especially with regard to cardiovascular side effects, are not known. As mentioned, some physicians will consider a nicotine patch in a former smoker as an adjunctive therapy. One could consider a nicotine patch (1) in a former smoker after conventional treatment had failed and (2) if there is a clear relationship of developing or worsening UC when the patient has stopped smoking.

If nicotine is the active agent in UC, smoking may provide the best delivery system and some bravely advocate smoking in UC. In his 1998 editorial "No Butts About It: Put the Fire Out By Lighting Up" Hanauer advocated smoking for ex-smokers with active UC. He took the controversial position that "low-dose" smoking (< one-half a pack of cigarettes per day) has minimal health effects and should be considered for ex-smokers before corticosteroids and immune modulation. This opinion appears to be in the minority with most physicians relying on more conventional UC therapy and avoiding the blatant health risks of smoking. Although some patients are aware of the "beneficial" effects smoking has had on their disease, most prefer to manage their disease without the risk of returning to smoking.

Sclerosing Cholangitis and Pouchitis

Smoking also appears to protect patients against developing primary sclerosing cholangitis (PSC) and pouchitis following restorative proctocolectomy. PSC is an idiopathic disease associated with inflammation and fibrosis of the bile ducts. It is associated more commonly with UC than CD. As with UC, tobacco appears to be protective against PSC probably due to the effects of nicotine (Mitchell et al, 2002).

Similarly, pouchitis, which commonly occurs after an ileo-pouch anal anastomosis, is also negatively associated with tobacco use (Sandborn, 1997). This has led some to advocate nicotine for pouchitis. To date, controlled data using nicotine prophylactically with ileal pouches is lacking.

Crohn's Disease

The association of smoking with CD is much less controversial. In contrast to UC, smoking is clearly detrimental in the patient with CD (Thomas et al, 1998). The risk of developing CD is twice as high in smokers compared to nonsmokers. CD is a heterogeneous disease that can be classified on anatomic location and clinical behavior, and location and behavior define clinical course, prognosis, and response to therapy. In addition, heavy smoking has been associated with small bowel disease, which tends to result in a worse prognosis. Heavy smoking is also associated with transmurally aggressive disease that is manifest by fistula and abscess formation, especially among patients with Jewish ethnicity. We have also found that smoking is associated with more stricturing and fistulizing complications (Picco and Bayless, 2003) as well as earlier surgery for ileal disease independent of *NOD2* status (Brant et al, 2003). Cessation of smoking is extremely important in these high risk patients especially if they have any other poor prognostic factors, such as early disease onset, Jewish ethnicity, a strong family history, and genetic abnormalities, particularly two mutations in *NOD-2/CARD15*.

Continued smoking after diagnosis of CD is associated with higher relapse rates compared to nonsmokers (Cottone et al, 1994; Cosnes et al, 1996). After resection for CD, patients who continued to smoke were at greater risk of recurrence and further surgery compared to nonsmokers. Finally, female smokers with CD were also more likely to require immunosuppressive agents compared to nonsmokers. Conversely, smokers who stop experience fewer relapses than while smoking (Cosnes et al, 2001).

Smoking Cessation

These data overwhelmingly support cessation of smoking among CD patients. I am quite surprised by the number of patients with CD who present to our center who still smoke. Some state that their physician never counseled them on the evils of smoking. Others remember that their physician mentioned smoking but did not assist them in learning to quit. Patients need our help in quitting either through our own or through the use of an integrated smoking cessation program employing physicians and mental health professionals using appropriate medical therapy. We have such an integrated plan within our institution. Although these programs may not succeed, we must convey that smoking cessation is a priority. Some patients feel that smoking makes them feel better by helping their mood. We must be aware of the psychological benefit patients get from continued smoking and educate them on the overwhelming detrimental effects tobacco has on their disease. Simply stated, I tell my patients that smoking cigarettes is the worst thing they personally can do for their CD.

Passive smoking has also been implicated in the development of IBD (Thomas et al, 1998). The relationship is strongest for CD with risk increased up to 5 times for children diagnosed before 18 years of age. For UC the risk may be slightly increased and passive smoking does not seem to protect against the development of UC. This is particularly important among my IBD patients who continue to smoke and have young children. This possible increased risk to their children is more ammunition we, as clinicians, can use to get them to stop smoking.

Osteoporosis

In addition to its harmful effect on CD, tobacco also contributes to the development of *osteoporosis* among patients with IBD. The combination of a chronic inflammatory disease, frequent use of corticosteroids, and smoking increases the risk of osteoporosis dramaticially. This is especially true for women. This is another reason for cessation of smoking in IBD. Physicians should also look for osteoporosis early because effective therapies are available and it is usually asymptomatic before serious complications occur.

Conclusions

The detrimental effects of smoking are well known and it is easy to convince patients that smoking is bad for their health. Despite this, most patients who smoke continue to do so even when faced with smoking-related illness. The reasons for this are complex and represent an interaction of physiologic (addiction) and psychosocial factors that reinforce continued smoking. We as physicians are in part to blame because we tend not make smoking cessation a priority or do not provide access to smoking cessation programs. This may be due to our own frustrations and perceived futility of these programs, lack of understanding of approaches to cessation, or fear of disturbing our relationship with the patient. We must overcome these issues and understand that we will have a significant influence on our patients stopping smoking. Although sustained quit rates are low, if we can get 15% of our smoking patients to cease and desist, that will represent a significant impact on patient welfare and public health.

Supplemental Reading

Brant SR, Picco MF, Achkar JP, et al. Defining complex contributions of NOD2/CARD15 gene mutations, age at onset, and tobacco use on Crohn's disease phenotypes. Inflamm Bowel Dis 2003;8:281–9.

Brown LM, Devesa SS. Epidemiologic trends in esophageal and gastric cancer in the United States. Surg Oncol Clin N Am 2002;11:235–56.

Burns DM, Garfinkel L, Samet JM. Changes in cigarette related disease risks and their implications for prevention and control. NCI Smoking and Tobacco Control Monographs 1997; Feb.

Calam J, Baron JH. Pathophysiology of duodenal and gastric ulcer and gastric cancer. BMJ 2001;323:980–2.

Cosnes J, Beaugerie L, Carbonnel F, et al. Smoking cessation and the course of Crohn's disease: an intervention study. Gastroenterology 2001;120:1093–9.

Cosnes J, Carbonnel F, Beaugerie L, et al. Effect of cigarette smoking on the long term course of Crohn's disease. Gastroenterology 1996;110:424–31.

Cottone M, Rosselli M, Orlando A, et al. Smoking habits and recurrence of Crohn's disease. Gastroenterology 1994; 106:643–8.

Daling JR, Sherman KJ, Hislop TG, et al. Cigarette smoking and the risk of anogenital cancer. Am J Epidemiol 1992:135:180–9.

Hanauer SB. No butts about it: put out the fire by lighting up. Inflamm Bowel Dis 1998;4:326.

Konner J, O'Reilley E. Pancreatic cancer: epidemiology genetics and approaches to screening. Oncology 2002;16:1637–8.

Lowenfels AB, Maisonneuve P. Epidemiologic and etiologic factors of pancreatic cancer. Hematol Oncol Clin North Am 2002;16:1–16.

Mitchell SA, Thyssen M, Orchard TR. Cigarette smoking, appendectomy and tonsillectomy as risk factors for the development of primary sclerosing cholangitis: a case control study. Gut 2002;51:567–73.

Morita M, Saeki H, Mori M, et al. Risk factors for esophageal cancer and the multiple occurrence of carcinoma in the aerodigestive tract. Surgery 2002;131:S1–6.

Picco MF, Bayless TM. Tobacco consumption and disease duration are associated with fistulizing and stricturing behaviors in the first 8 years of Crohn's disease. Am J Gastroenterol 2003;98:363–8.

Potter JD. Colorectal cancer: molecules and populations. J Natl Cancer Inst 2001;93:651–2.

Reif S, Klein I, Arber N, et al. Lack of association between smoking and inflammatory bowel disease among Jewish patients in Israel. Gastroenterology 1995;108:1683–7.

Sandborn WJ. Smoking benefits celiac sprue and pouchitis: implications for nicotine therapy? Gastroenterology 1997;112:1048–9.

Sutherland G. Smoking: can we really make a difference. Heart 2003;89:25–7.

Thomas GA, Rhodes J, Green JT. Inflammatory bowel disease and smoking—a review. Am J Gastroenterol 1998;93:144–9.

CHAPTER 46

Gastrointestinal and Nutritional Complications of Human Immunodeficiency Virus Infection

Donald P. Kotler, MD, and Irina Kaplounov, MD

Gastrointestinal (GI) dysfunction is common in human immunodeficiency virus (HIV)-infected patients and symptoms may arise at any time during the disease course (Kotler, 1991). GI symptoms diminish quality of life, may lead to progressive malnutrition, and be associated with increased mortality (Lubeck et al, 1993). Advances in the treatment of HIV infection with highly active antiretroviral therapy (HAART) has allowed for effective suppression of viral replication, often to undetectable levels, and immune reconstitution and spontaneous resolution of intestinal problems (Kotler et al, 1998; Palella et al, 1998). However, a substantial proportion of HIV-infected subjects are unaware of their infection status. Thus, HIV infection must now be included as part of the differential diagnosis of the causes of chronic diarrhea. In addition, some patients refuse to take HAART therapy, and antiviral drug resistance affects others. For these reasons, GI problems in HIV-infected patients continue to be seen. This chapter will discuss the diagnosis and management of GI and nutritional complications of HIV infection.

General Principles

Clinical observations have identified several characteristics typical of GI complications in HIV infection. Multiple enteric complications may coexist, reaching almost one-third of acquired immunodeficiency syndrome (AIDS) patients with chronic diarrhea in one study. A single organism, such as cytomegalovirus (CMV), may cause several different clinical syndromes, whereas many organisms can produce identical clinical syndromes, such as the malabsorption syndrome associated with intestinal protozoa. Disease complications of AIDS are notable for their chronicity, susceptibility to suppression, and resistance to cure, so that treatments must be given chronically. The specific pathogens may be typical for any one complication or related specifically to the immune deficiency.

Pathologic processes may affect the GI tract with either a focal or diffuse pattern. Focal ulcers may be found anywhere in the GI tract. They may be infectious, noninfectious, or neoplastic. Certain viral infections, such as CMV infection, and fungal infections, such as histoplasmosis, produce multifocal disease. The GI tract also can be involved diffusely. The most common diffuse lesion is candidiasis of the oral cavity and/or the esophagus. Bacteria such as *Salmonella*, *Shigella*, and *Campylobacter* may cause a diffuse colitis or enterocolitis.

Oral and Esophageal Disease

Candidiasis decreases taste sensation and affects swallowing, in addition to causing oral or substernal discomfort. Most cases are due to *Candida albicans*. Candidiasis in the esophagus and may occur in the presence or absence of thrush. Hairy leukoplakia, a hyperkeratotic lesion found along the sides of the tongue and adjacent gingiva, may be mistaken for *Candida*, but is asymptomatic. Severe gingivitis or periodontitis, infectious or idiopathic ulcers, or mass lesions, such as Kaposi's sarcoma (KS) or lymphoma, occur in the oral cavity and can cause pain or interfere with chewing and swallowing. The esophagus is affected by many of the same lesions as the oral cavity. Overall, studies have demonstrated a decline in the incidence of both oral and esophageal disease in subjects on HAART, with the possible exception of human papilloma virus (HPV)-induced lesions.

Diagnosis and Treatment

The etiologic diagnosis of disorders of food intake can be approached using a diagnostic algorithm (Figure 46-1). One should not conclude that anorexia is due to a medication until other possibilities are ruled out, or the patient responds positively to a supervised trial of medication withdrawal. In an AIDS patient with suspected esophageal candidiasis, it is advisable to treat empirically and only examine patients with persisting symptoms (Rabeneck and Laine, 1994). In contrast, all esophageal ulcerations should be investigated by direct examination and biopsy.

Oral candidiasis responds to a variety of antifungal therapies including the topical therapies, nystatin and clotrimazole, and the systemically active azole drugs. Esophageal candidiasis is best treated using systemically active compounds, because the organism is invasive. The infection may

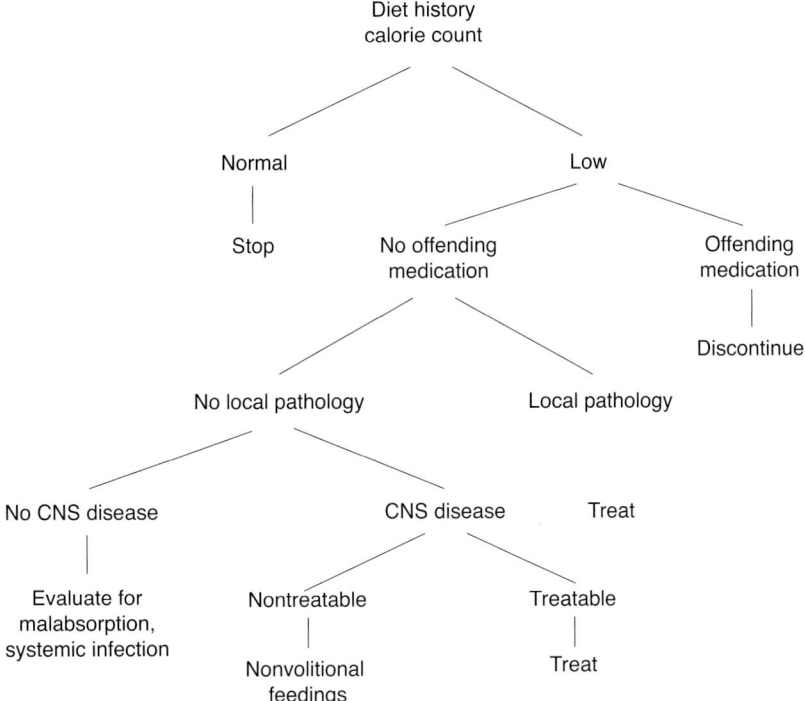

FIGURE 46-1. Diagnostic algorithm for disorders of food intake. CNS = central nervous system.

become resistant to azole therapy in some cases, or be due to other yeasts, such as *Torulopsis glabrata*, for which intravenous (IV) amphotericin B therapy is required. Therapy options for hairy leukoplakia include Acyclovir 800 mg orally 5 times per day for 2 to 3 weeks, then 1.2 to 2 g/d, or Tretinoin (Retin A) 0.025 or 0.05% solution applied 2 to 3 times per day. Herpes simplex virus (HSV) infection responds to oral treatment with acyclovir. Discontinuation of therapy after induction therapy and the use of maintenance therapy only if there are frequent relapses is recommended. Ganciclovir is an effective therapy for CMV esophageal disease (Wilcox et al, 1991). Idiopathic esophageal ulcers not due to identifiable pathogen may respond promptly to corticosteriods, though the danger of worsening immune suppression in patients with AIDS should be kept in mind. The ulcer also may recur after steroid therapy is discontinued. Studies have shown the effectiveness of thalidomide for the treatment of idiopathic esophageal ulcers. The significant neurologic and sedating side effects of thalidomide, as well as teratogenicity in women, have restricted its use to registered physicians and pharmacies.

Salivary gland enlargement frequently complicates AIDS. The concerning manifestations of this entity are cosmetic appearance, pain from distension, and xerostomia. For painful or cosmetically disfiguring cystic lesions, needle aspiration and computed tomography (CT) scan will distinguish cystic and solid lesions. For xerostomia, sugarless gum and artificial saliva may offer some relief. Pilocarpine may be necessary for refractory cases.

Nutritional Management

A major complication of oral and esophageal diseases is decreased food intake. Dietary consultation with creative diet planning and choice may be quite beneficial in milder cases. Caloric supplementation with formula diets also may be helpful. In patients with local lesions that cannot be treated successfully or in refractory cases of anorexia, some form of nonvolitional feeding is required. Nutritional repletion has been reported in response to total parenteral nutrition (TPN) and to enteral feeding regimens. Nasoenteric tubes can be used, though there are problems with cooperation in long term use and there is the possibility of precipitating or exacerbating sinus disease. Percutaneous endoscopic gastrostomy feedings are efficacious and well tolerated by AIDS patients, and can be continued indefinitely.

Diarrhea and Wasting

The ability to presumptively localize the pathologic process to the small intestine or colon is valuable in directing and streamlining a diagnostic workup. Important information often can be obtained from the clinical history. The symptoms related to small intestinal infection are typical of malabsorption. Patients complain of 3 to 10 nonbloody bowel movements per day, with urgency but no tenesmus. When severe, the diarrhea is associated with dehydration and electrolyte abnormalities. The diarrhea does not occur consistently throughout the day and is often worst at night or early in the morning. There may be no specific food intolerances, as diarrhea is worsened by any significant food intake. However, stool volumes are decreased by fasting. The infections producing malabsorption usually are not associated with fever or anorexia, though food intake may be decreased voluntarily to avoid diarrhea. A notable exception to this rule is *Mycobacterium avium* complex (MAC), a disorder in which spiking fevers may be seen. Weight loss typically is slow and progressive. In contrast, enterocolitic diseases produce numerous, small volume bowel movements that occur at regular intervals throughout the day and night. Cramping and tenesmus may occur but usually are not severe. The clinical course often is associated with fever, anorexia, rapid and progressive weight loss, and extreme debilitation.

Diagnosis

The management of acute diarrhea in HIV-infected patients is similar to that in non-HIV infected individuals, in that the presence of dehydration or other systemic toxicity is the important parameter and the focus of treatment, as opposed to the underlying infection. An algorithmic approach may be used to evaluate chronic diarrhea (Figure 46-2).

Stool examinations are an integral part of the diagnostic workup of an HIV-infected individual with diarrhea. Special diagnostic techniques are available for cryptosporidia and microsporidia, though there is relatively little clinical experience with the latter techniques (Orenstein et al, 1990). Although molecular biological techniques are available experimentally, they have not been used in clinical situations. A substantial proportion of enteric pathogens can be detected

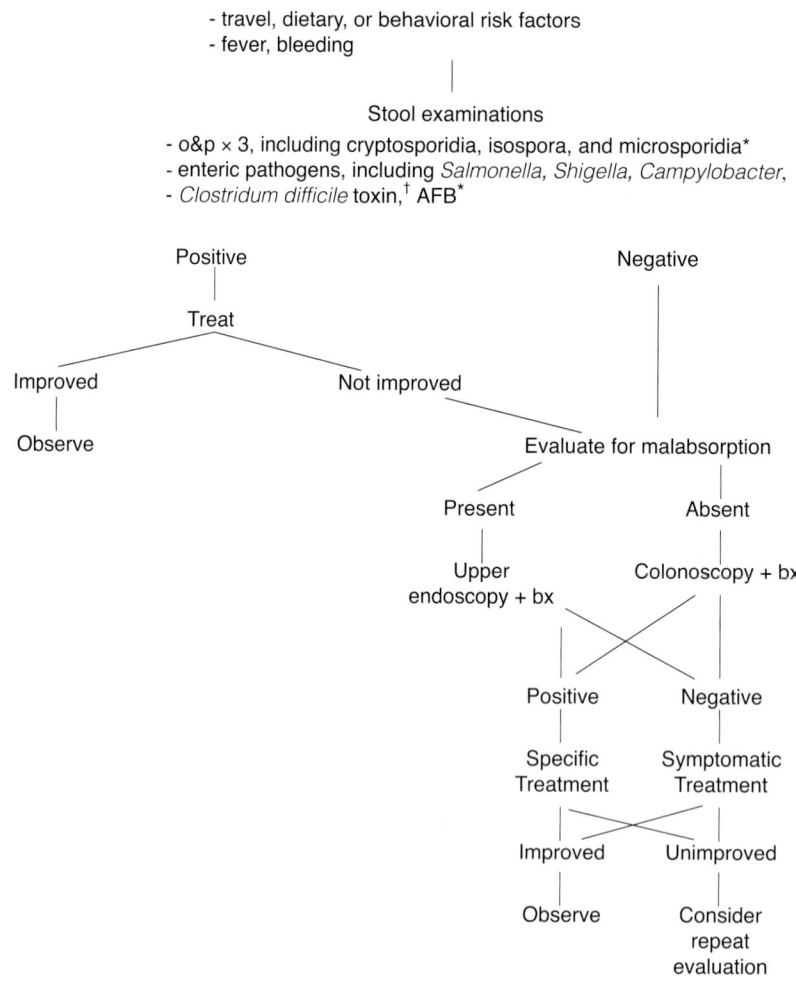

FIGURE 46-2. Evaluation of chronic diarrhea (greater than 14 days). AFB = acid fast bacilli stain; bx = biopsy; o&p = ova and parasites. *If CD4+ lymphocyte count < 100/mm³. †Concurrent or recent antibiotic use.

only by intestinal biopsy, so that negative stool examinations are incomplete as a workup.

The spectrum of endoscopic lesions in CMV colitis varies from essentially normal appearing mucosa, to scattered groups of vesicles or erosions, to broad shallow ulcerations that may coalesce (Wilcox et al, 1998). CMV usually causes a pancolitis, though the cecum and right colon may be affected earlier than elsewhere. Histopathologic examination demonstrates characteristic intracellular inclusions. Specialized immunohistochemical or in situ hybridization techniques are available and may increase the sensitivity of diagnosis.

The diagnosis of mycobacterial infection is made by culture or histology. Stool smears may demonstrate acid-fast bacilli, but the finding is not specific for tissue invasion. Mucosal thickening on barium radiographs and thickening of the intestinal wall plus enlargement of mesenteric and retroperitoneal nodes on CT scan are characteristic of MAC, though lymphoma or fungal infections have similar appearances. Histologic demonstration of acid-fast bacilli in intestinal tissue is straightforward. Diagnosis by biopsy often can be made in one day, as compared to cultures, which may take as long as six weeks to become positive.

The diagnosis of antibiotic-associated colitis is the same in AIDS and non-AIDS patients. The diagnosis of bacterial enterocolitis should be straightforward with routine examination. Blood cultures should be part of the workup of suspected infectious diarrhea with fever in an HIV-infected patient, as *Salmonella* may be cultured from blood but not from stool. An unusual feature of *Salmonella* infections in AIDS patients is the tendency for clinical and/or microbiological relapse after antibiotics are discontinued.

Diarrhea is a commonly reported complaint in subjects receiving protease inhibitors. The exact mechanisms underlying the development of drug-induced diarrhea is uncertain although fat malabsorption has been associated with HAART therapy (Poles et al, 2001).

Treatment

Therapies for the patients with diarrheal diseases can be divided into antimicrobial therapies, and therapies for the associated diarrhea, dehydration, and malnutrition. There is no known effective therapy for cryptosporidiosis. Many agents have been tried, and the results have been disappointing. Some patients improved during treatment with paromomycin (Humatin, Parke Davis, Ann Arbor, MI), whereas controlled trials showed only modest improvement and no cures. An uncontrolled trial of paromomycin plus azithromycin showed good response in terms of clinical symptoms and oocyst excretion. Clarithromycin or rifabutin prophylaxis for MAC prophylaxis may reduce risk of cryptosporidiosis. Overall, HAART with immune reconstitution is the only consistently effective treatment for cryptosporidiosis (Miao et al, 2000).

Few studies of drug treatment of *Enterocytozoon bieneusi* infection have been published. Albendazole (GlaxoSmithKline) is ineffective as treatment, but is effective therapy for *E. intestinalis* infection. Anecdotal success in the treatment of *E. intestinalis* has been reported with itraconazole, fluconazole, atovaquone, and metronidazole. Experimental drugs include Fumagillin, TNP-470, and Ovalicin. HAART with immune reconstitution is best therapy, especially for the 80 to 90% of cases involving *E. bieneusi*.

Isosporiasis may be treated with trimethoprim sulfa. Due to a high rate of recurrence, repeated courses or chronic maintenance with trimethoprim may be needed. Some have advocated treatment indefinitely unless there is immune recovery. The optimal duration of high dose therapy is not well defined. There has been one case report of refractory infection that responded to pyrimethamine plus sulfadiazine.

CMV colitis appears to occur less often in subjects taking protease inhibitors and also has a lower rate of recurrence in subjects on HAART. Survival outcomes are also significantly better in patients with CMV colitis who are on HAART. Two agents are clinically effective in the treatment of CMV colitis. The most widely used is ganciclovir. Ganciclovir therapy also has been associated with nutritional repletion and with prolonged survival. Oral ganciclovir is available for maintenance therapy. Other analogues with better bioavailability have been developed. Foscarnet has activity against CMV as well as HIV.

Several drugs have in vitro efficacy against MAC including the macrolide clarithromycin (Biaxin), ethambutal (Myambutal), rifabutin (Mycobutin), and clofazamine (Lamprene). Other drugs with in vivo or in vitro efficacy include amikacin, ciprofloxacin, cycloserine, and ethionamide. Three drugs, azythromycin, rifabutin and clarithromycin, have been shown to be effective prophylactic agents. In the setting of immune reconstitution, primary prophylaxis may be discontinued when the CD4 count increases to > $100/mm^3$ for > 3 months. It appears that secondary prophylaxis (prior disseminated MAC) may also be discontinued when the CD4 count is > 100 plus HAART for 6 to 12 months.

The treatment of enterocolitis due to *Salmonella*, *Shigella*, or *Campylopbacter* sp is modified in that IV with antibiotics is used commonly, due to the frequent occurrence of bacteremia. In addition, repeated or chronic courses of antibiotics such as trimethoprim sulfa or ciprofloxacin often are needed because of disease recurrence. Treatment of chronic bacterial enteropathy with broad spectrum antibiotics has brought clinical improvement in several patients. The difficulty in choosing antibiotics is the inability to determine which bacteria in stool are the offending organisms. In addition, the widespread use of antibiotics could lead to the development of multidrug resistance strains.

Nutritional Management

Maintenance of adequate fluid balance and nutritional status are important clinical tasks, especially in patients with malabsorption syndromes. Oral rehydration solutions may help maintain hydration status, but are hypocaloric and may promote wasting if used excessively. The goal of hydration therapy is to maximize fluid intake while minimizing diarrheal losses. A low fat, lactose-free diet may be beneficial and medium chain triglycerides are useful adjuncts in the treatment of patients with significant malabsorption. On the other hand, polymeric formula diets generally are tolerated poorly and lead to substantial diarrhea. A variety of antidiarrheal therapies may be used. Some patients with nonspecific diarrhea or ileal dysfunction respond well to the bile salt binding resin cholestyramine. The most commonly used antidiarrheal agents are loperamide and opiates, though escalating doses often are required. Octreotide has been used in the treatment of diarrhea of several etiologies, with mixed results. However, excess fluid losses from the small intestine due to malabsorption or abnormal secretion will overcome any pharmacologically produced inhibition of motility and lead to diarrhea.

Nutritional therapy of AIDS patients with diarrhea depends entirely upon the pathogenic mechanism underlying the diarrhea. Different approaches are required in patients with and without malabsorption. Nutritional maintenance may be impossible by the enteral route in patients with severe small intestinal disease, and parenteral nutrition may be required. However, the use of elemental diets, which contains simple sugars, amino acids and medium chain triglycerides, may give similar results to TPN in some cases.

Nutritional support is less effective in patients with enterocolitis associated with systemic infections. The metabolic rate is elevated, and metabolic derangements promote protein wasting irrespective of intake. Alterations in lipid metabolism often result in the development of fatty liver when nutritional support is attempted. In one study, TPN resulted in weight gain, but the increase was due entirely to an increase in body fat content. Although nutritional support might help prevent progressive protein depletion, the key to successful therapy is proper diagnosis and treatment of the specific disease complication.

Anorectal Disease

Anorectal diseases seen in AIDS patients include both infections and tumors. HSV is the most common infectious agent found. Vesicles in the anal canal may be missed as they rupture during defecation or examination. Herpes infection in AIDS patients most often presents as a painful, shallow spreading perineal ulcer. A smaller group of patients present with idiopathic ulcers, originating at the anorectal junction. Perianal and intra-anal condylomata occur in AIDS patients as well as non-AIDS patients and are related to infection with HPV. Tumors in the anorectal region include KS, lymphoma, and squamous cell carcinoma or its variants.

Hemorrhoidal disease also is seen frequently. Factors predisposing to hemorrhoids may have predated the HIV infection. Severe diarrhea or proctitis may promote local thrombosis, ulceration, and secondary infection. Fleshy skin tags, resembling those seen in Crohn's disease, are also seen. Thrombosed hemorrhoids occur frequently, but it is unclear if the incidence is higher in AIDS patients than in a comparable population.

A variety of classic venereal diseases can produce anorectal ulcerations. Diagnosis and treatment of *Neisseria gonorrhoea* proctitis is similar in AIDS and non-AIDS patients. Syphilis may have an atypical presentation in HIV-infected subjects, and serologic diagnosis is affected by the presence of immune deficiency. Chlamydia is prevalent in sexually active groups. The frequency of chancroid, caused by *Haemophilus ducreyi*, in HIV-infected patients is unknown. Rectal spirochetosis has been recognized in homosexual men with or without HIV infection (Nielsen et al, 1983). The infection usually is asymptomatic and an incidental finding on examination.

Treatment

Resolution of herpetic lesions occurs after treatment with oral or IV acyclovir. HSV resistant to acyclovir has been demonstrated in patients with refractory ulcerations. The use of foscarnet or ganciclovir may bring resolution. Anorectal ulcers containing CMV respond to antiviral therapy. Idiopathic ulcers may respond promptly to intralesional corticosteroid therapy. Areas of leukoplakia can be followed clinically, whereas large or enlarging lesions should be excised. Some caution should be placed on surgical therapy. Poor wound healing may occur, especially in severely malnourished patients, patients with serious, untreated diseases such as CMV, and patients with continued diarrhea due to nutrient malabsorption.

Epidermoid cancers, including squamous cell and cloacagenic cancer, occur in anal skin and rectal glands, respectively. Although these cancers rarely metastasize in immunocompetent persons, they may do so in patients with AIDS. For these lesions, management after diagnostic biopsy includes excision, chemotherapy, or laser photocoagulation. Laser therapy of rectal KS also is effective.

Tumors

The incidence of KS in AIDS has declined in the HAART era. KS in AIDS is indistinguishable, histopathologically, from classic KS, endemic forms of KS found in Africa, or the form that occurs during immunosuppressive therapy. Visceral involvement in AIDS patients with KS is more common than in non–HIV-infected individuals. Visceral involvement may be asymptomatic. The diagnosis is made by visual inspection and confirmed by biopsy, though endoscopic biopsy may be falsely negative if the tumor is in the submucosa. KS is responsive to chemotherapy, which can be used in symptomatic patients or in the event of rapidly progressive disease. Pegylated liposomal doxorubicin (PLD, Caelyx) in the treatment of AIDS-related KS is more effective and less toxic than bleomycin sulfate and vinblastine sulfate (BV) or Adriamycin, bleomycin sulfate, and vinblastine sulfate (ABV) combination therapy (ABV). Cost effectiveness analysis suggests that PLD is preferable over liposomal daunorubicin and other regimens, and it seems to offer a better quality of life.

A high prevalence of extranodal, high-grade non-Hodgkins B-cell lymphomas has been noted in AIDS patients. GI lymphomas in AIDS are biologically aggressive, especially the Burkitt's subtype. The lesions may respond to chemotherapy, using combination therapies. Sporadic reports of AIDS patients with carcinomas in the GI tract have been published but a heightened incidence has not been documented convincingly.

Supplemental Reading

Kotler DP. Gastrointestinal complications of the acquired immunodeficiency syndrome. In: Yamada T, editor. Textbook of gastroenterology. Philadelphia: Lippincott; 1991. p. 2086–103.

Kotler DP, Shimada T, Snow G, et al. Effect of combination antiretroviral therapy upon rectal mucosal HIV RNA burden and mononuclear cell apoptosis. AIDS 1998;12:597–604.

Lubeck DP, Bennett CL, Mazonson PD, et al. Quality of life and health service use among HIV-infected patients with chronic diarrhea. J Acquir Immune Defic Syndr 1993;6:478–84.

Miao YM, Awad-El-Kariem FM, Franzen C, et al. Eradication of cryptosporidia and microsporidia following successful antiretroviral therapy. J Acquir Immune Defic Syndr 2000;25:124–9.

Nielsen RH, Orholm M, Pedersen JO, et al. Colorectal spirochetosis: clinical significance of the infection. Gastroenterology 1983;85:62–7.

Orenstein J, Chiang J, Steinberg W, et al. Intestinal microsporidiosis as a cause of diarrhea in HIV-infected patients: a report of 20 cases. Hum Pathol 1990;21:475–81.

Palella FJ Jr, Delaney KM, Moorman AC, et al. Declining morbidity and mortality among patients with advanced human immunodeficiency virus infection. HIV outpatient study investigators. N Engl J Med 1998;338:853–60.

Poles MA, Fuerst M, McGowan I, et al. HIV-related diarrhea is multifactorial and fat malabsorption is commonly present, independent of HAART. Am J Gastroenterol 2001;96:1831–7.

Rabeneck L, Laine L. Esophageal candidiasis in patients infected with the human immunodeficiency virus. A decision analysis to assess cost-effectiveness of alternative management strategies. Arch Intern Med 1994;154:2705–10.

Wilcox CM, Chalasani N, Lazenby A, Schwartz D. Cytomegalovirus colitis in acquired immunodeficiency syndrome: a clinical and endoscopic study. Gastrointest Endosc 1998;48:39–43.

Wilcox CM, Diehl DL, Cello JP, et al. Cytomegalovirus esophagitis in patients with AIDS. A clinical, endoscopic, and pathologic correlation. Ann Intern Med 1991;113:589–93.

CHAPTER 47

Chronic Immunodeficiency Syndromes Affecting the Gastrointestinal Tract

Jimmy Ko, MD, and Lloyd Mayer, MD

The practicing gastroenterologist is frequently confronted with immune-related diseases, such as Crohn's disease (CD), ulcerative colitis (UC), celiac sprue, and pernicious anemia (PA). However, the role of the gastrointestinal (GI) tract as the body's largest lymphoid organ is often overlooked. In fact, the surface area of the GI tract could cover two tennis courts, and within that surface is a rich supply of B- and T-lymphocytes, macrophages, and dendritic cells. The number of lymphocytes in the GI tract exceeds that in the spleen, but unlike other lymphoid organs, immune-associated cells in the GI tract are constantly confronted with antigen (mainly in the form of bacteria and food). Gut-associated lymphoid tissue, generally known as mucosa-associated lymphoid tissue (MALT), regulates immune responses in the gut to maintain homeostasis. Without this tight regulation, inflammation would predominate in the GI tract. Therefore, it is not difficult to imagine how disease can result in the GI tract when immune regulation is disrupted.

Gut Immune System

The immune system in the GI tract, like in the rest of the body, can be subdivided into the following two categories: (1) cellular and (2) humoral. T-lymphocytes generally regulate cellular immune functions, such as defense against viruses, intracellular bacteria, and proteins, whereas B-lymphocytes produce immunoglobulins (Ig) to fight bacteria. Primary immunodeficiencies are the result of inherited defects in either or both the cellular or humoral branches of the immune system. In the GI tract, the major Igs are the secretory forms of IgA and IgM. These antibodies bind luminal antigens and form immune complexes, thus restricting bacterial and viral attachment to epithelium and decreasing antigen burden on the mucosal immune cells. Antibody deficiency can lead to increased antigen uptake in the GI tract, as has been demonstrated with serum levels of dietary antigens following feeding (Cunningham-Rundles et al, 1979). However, it is interesting to note in the one disease exclusively restricted to B-cells, X-linked agammaglobulinemia (XLA), there has been no significant predisposition to GI infection or disease.

Classification and Clinical Presentation of Primary Immunodeficiencies

Predominantly Antibody Deficiencies

XLA

Also known as Bruton's Disease, XLA is the prototypical antibody deficiency disease (Table 47-1). It is rare, occurring in 1 in 1 million live births. The inherited defect has been localized to a gene on the long arm of the X chromosome encoding Bruton's tyrosine kinase (Btk). Defects in Btk lead to maturation arrest of pre-B-cells, resulting in failure to generate mature B-cells and a complete lack of all classes of Igs. XLA typically presents in young males as recurrent bacterial infections, especially with encapsulated bacteria such as *Streptococcus pneumoniae* and *Haemophilus influenzae*. Standard treatment is with intravenous (IV) immunoglobulin replacement (Ammann et al, 1982).

IgA Deficiency

IgA deficiency is the most common primary immunodeficiency, found in an estimated 1 in 200 to 700 Whites and less frequently in other ethnic groups. The overwhelming majority of people with IgA deficiency are healthy and do not exhibit any illness. Serum levels of IgA are less than 5 g/L with normal or increased levels of other Igs and normal B-cell numbers. If illness occurs, the most frequent disorders associated with IgA deficiency are recurrent sinopulmonary infections. Infections are typically caused by common bacterial or viral pathogens, and it is the frequency and repetition of these infections that often lead to assessing quantitative Ig levels and a work-up. Autoimmune diseases, such as rheumatoid arthritis and lupus, and allergy have also

TABLE 47-1. Classification of Primary Immunodeficiencies

Predominantly Antibody Deficiencies	Combined or Primary T-Cell Deficiencies
X-linked agammaglobulinemia	Severe combined immunodeficiency
IgA deficiency	Ataxia telangiectasia
Common variable immunodeficiency	DiGeorge syndrome
—	Wiskott-Aldrich syndrome

been reported to be associated with IgA deficiency, and subjects with these conditions also commonly have autoantibodies (Cunningham-Rundles, 2001). IgA-deficient patients with concomitant IgG2 subclass deficiency tend to have more severe disease, and it is this subset of patients that has an increased frequency of GI manifestations, including celiac disease, inflammatory bowel disease (IBD), and giardiasis. There is a higher prevalence of IgA deficiency in patients with a family history of common variable immunodeficiency, suggesting a genetic link between the two diseases. Treatment with IV immunoglobulins (IVIG) is necessary only in patients with recurrent sinopulmonary infections and concurrent IgG2 deficiency. There is one caveat: some IgA deficient patients have anti-IgA antibodies, which may increase the risk for anaphylactic reactions to blood products (Burks et al, 1986).

COMMON VARIABLE IMMUNODEFICIENCY

Common variable immunodeficiency (CVID) is a diverse set of disorders, characterized by low levels of at least two Ig classes and recurrent infections most commonly of the upper and lower respiratory tract. With a prevalence of 1 in 50,000 (in Scandinavia), CVID is the primary immunodeficiency most often brought to clinical attention, frequently presenting in early adulthood (Spickett, 2001). Infection with encapsulated bacteria, such as *Streptococcus pneumoniae* and *Haemophilis influenzae*, reflect the defect in B-cell function. Fungal infections can be seen, in addition to other T-cell–associated infections such as *Pneumocystis carinii*. Autoimmune diseases are relatively common (found in 22% of 248 patients in one series (Cunningham-Rundles and Bodian, 1999) and an increased incidence of lymphoma and gastric carcinoma has also been reported (Kinlen et al, 1985). GI manifestations share a similar spectrum in CVID and IgA deficiency but are more common in CVID. Defects in B-cell growth and differentiation, whether primary or secondary, are often found even though B-cells numbers are generally near normal. Recurrent infections without treatment can lead to irreversible chronic lung disease with bronchiectasis and cor pulmonale. The probability of survival 20 years after diagnosis of CVID is 66% (compared with 93% for age-matched controls), which is likely a reflection of advanced progression of disease at the time of diagnosis. Although it has little effect on the GI disorders seen in CVID, the standard treatment of IVIG can help prevent recurrent sinopulmonary infections (Cunningham-Rundles et al, 1984).

Combined (B- and T-Cell) or Primary T-Cell Deficiencies

Severe Combined Immunodeficiency (SCID) is a group of congenital immune disorders in which both T-cell and B-cell development and function are disrupted. Several gene defects resulting in SCID have been isolated, including IL-2 receptor γ chain, Janus kinase 3 (*JAK3*), adenosine deaminase, and recombinase activating genes (*RAG-1* and *2*). Because SCID patients have few or no circulating B- and T-cells, they are susceptible to bacterial and opportunistic infections. SCID patients generally present in the first year of life with severe, recurrent bacterial and/or viral infections. Standard treatment is bone marrow transplant or enzyme replacement (in the case of adenosine deaminase deficiency) (IUIS Committee, 1999).

Ataxia telangiectasia (AT) is an autosomal recessive disorder usually presenting between ages 2 and 5 years with ataxia and telangiectasias of the nose, conjunctiva, ears, or shoulders. These patients have T-cell defects secondary to thymic hypoplasia, and IgA deficiency occurs in 50% of patients. A defect in the *ATM* gene, a protein kinase involved in cell cycle control and DNA repair, is the culprit in this disorder and also leads to the increased risk of malignancy (IUIS Committee, 1999). *DiGeorge Syndrome* is the result of a congenital defect in migration of the third and fourth branchial arches, leading to thymic hypoplasia and other developmental abnormalities. The severity of the T-cell defect corresponds to degree of thymic aplasia, and those patients with severe T-cell defects are susceptible to opportunistic infections. *Wiskott-Aldrich syndrome (WAS)* is an X-linked recessive disorder resulting from a defect in the WAS protein, which is involved in intracellular signaling and actin polymerization. Patients usually present with eczema, thrombocytopenia, impaired T-cell function, and recurrent infections.

GI Manifestations

GI disorders are common in primary immunodeficiencies and, at times, GI signs and symptoms, such as diarrhea or malabsorption, are the only manifestations of disease. Immune dysfunction in the GI tract can lead to infection, inflammatory disease, and malignancy, and these diseases are most prevalent in immunodeficiency states with combined B- and T-cell defects. Befitting its status as the most complex of primary immunodeficiencies, CVID has the broadest array of GI manifestations, the severity of which often leads to significant morbidity and mortality.

CVID

Both prospective and retrospective studies have shown a high rate of GI symptoms in CVID patients. Forty to 60% of patients experience chronic diarrhea, which may be accompanied by steatorrhea or other signs of malabsorption (So and Mayer, 1997). Common causes of GI symptoms are infectious, predominantly bacterial pathogens *Salmonella, Campylobacter,* and *Clostridium difficile* (from antibiotic use) or the parasite *Giardia lamblia*. However, inflammatory and malignant disorders of the GI tract also occur with increased incidence in CVID patients (Table 47-2) (Cunningham-Rundles and Bodian, 1999).

Giardia infection, though decreasing in frequency in recent years, is still an important infectious cause of diarrhea and malabsorption in CVID patients. *Giardia* is transmitted as a cyst; typically, it is consumed in water or spread by person-to-person contact. Symptoms typical of giardiasis include watery diarrhea, abdominal cramping, and bloating. Stool examination demonstrating cysts or trophozoites is indicative of infection. However, a duodenal biopsy is sometimes necessary for diagnosis. In patients with CVID, chronic or recurrent infection with *Giardia* likely related to T-cell defects, is a real concern. Therefore, prolonged treatment with *metronidazole (Flagyl)* is often required to eradicate infection and symptoms related to the infection. Empirical treatment with metronidazole is often begun following the onset of diarrhea as a therapeutic trial, given the frequent difficulty in confirming the diagnosis of *Giardia* in CVID patients. Other GI infections in CVID include *Cryptosporidium*, which was first described in a patient with CVID, and bacterial pathogens, such as *Salmonella* and *Campylobacter*, which have been found to be increased in prevalence in CVID patients (Sperber and Mayer, 1988). Additionally, infection with *C. difficile* should be considered in patients in whom antibiotics are used for recurrent infections.

Celiac-Like Conditions

Inflammatory complications in the GI tract occur with increased frequency in CVID patients. One of the most common is a celiac-like condition in which villous flattening in duodenal biopsy is found. Although the villous lesion appears similar to celiac disease, several important differences are found. Plasma cells are absent in CVID patients, whereas celiac patients have an abundance of plasma cells. Also, antigliadin and antiendomysial antibodies are not found in CVID patients. Lastly, a gluten-free diet appears to have no effect on the majority of CVID patients with sprue-like villous atrophy (Washington et al, 1996). Treatment for this condition includes steroids and immunomodulators such as azathioprine or 6-mercaptopurine (6-MP). Infectious complications are rare for patients given immunomodulators concomitantly with IVIG. Prolonged use of steroids in patients with CVID has led to reports of increased infectious complications. In one series from Mount Sinai Hospital, 4 of 248 patients receiving steroids had major complications including *Pneumocystis* pneumonia and *Nocardia* brain abscess. The authors, Cunningham-Rundles and Bodian, suggest that prolonged immunosuppression be used with caution.

Inflammatory Bowel Diseases

Inflammatory bowel disease (IBD) is also found with increased prevalence in CVID patients. In the Mount Sinai series, 16 of 248 patients with CVID (6%) had IBD. It appears that patients with CVID and IBD have more severe T-cell defects than patients with CVID alone. Both CD and UC typically respond to conventional treatment in patients with CVID. Treatment with 5-aminosalicyclic acid, azathioprine, or 6-MP can lead to long remissions. Oral steroids should be used with considerable care.*

PA

The last important inflammatory GI complication of CVID is PA. The diagnosis of PA is made at an earlier age in CVID patients (20 to 40 versus 60-years old in immunocompetent patients) (Sperber and Mayer, 1988). Plasma cells and antiparietal antibodies are absent in CVID patients with PA, suggesting a T-cell mediated mechanism. Treatment of persons with PA is the same in CVID as it is in immunocompetent patients.

Other conditions associated with CVID include *aphthous stomatitis*, which frequently responds to *sucralfate (Carafate)* suspension treatment, and *Ménétrier's disease*. Additionally, *malakoplakia*, a rare inflammatory disease characterized by granuloma formation (mostly in the bladder) and stricture formation in the bowel, can be found in CVID.

Malignancy

Malignancy is the leading cause of death in CVID, and two forms of cancer, gastric adenocarcinoma (AC) and non-Hodgkin's lymphoma (NHL), are found with increased frequency. Gastric cancer (GC) is increased by 30-fold, whereas NHL is increased by 47-fold compared with the general population (Kinlen et al, 1985). Recent studies have suggested a role for *Helicobacter pylori* in gastric carcinogenesis in CVID patients (Zullo et al, 1999). It is plausible that either impaired B- or T-cell function can lead to com-

TABLE 47-2. Gastrointestinal Complications of Common Variable Immunodeficiency

Infectious	Inflammatory
Giardia lamblia	Sprue-like disorder
Cryptosporidium	Inflammatory bowel disease
Clostridium difficile	Pernicious anemia
Atrophic gastritis	
Aphthous stomatitis	
Malakoplakia of the colon	
Ménétrier's disease	

Malignancy and Other (Benign) Lymphoproliferative
Gastric adenocarcinoma
Intestinal lymphoma
Nodular lymphoid hyperplasia

Adapted from Sperber and Mayer (1988).

---
*Editor's Note: One patient has had a long-term response while on infliximab.

promised defense against *H. pylori*. Therefore, screening for *H. pylori* in symptomatic patients and monitoring of treatment in infected individuals is advised. Atrophic gastritis with or without PA has been noted in CVID patients, and this association is also thought to play a role in the increased risk of gastric AC.

Nodular Lymphoid Hyperplasia

Benign lymphoproliferative disorders also occur with increased frequency in CVID with the main GI manifestation being nodular lymphoid hyperplasia (NLH). NLH is defined as multiple discrete nodules made up of lymphoid aggregates confined to the lamina propria and superficial submucosa. These nodules occur mostly in the small intestine and represent hyperplastic lymphoid tissue with prominent germinal centers. This hyperplastic response is thought to be a compensatory B-cell proliferative response to increase the pool of antibody producing cell precursors. NLH occurs diffusely in the gut in 10 to 20% of CVID patients. NLH was once thought to be secondary to *Giardia* infection, but antibiotic therapy does not result in resolution of nodules. Several reports suggest that NLH could be a premalignant condition leading to small intestine lymphomas (Washington et al, 1996).

IgA Deficiency

The spectrum of GI disease in IgA deficiency is similar to CVID, but is in general less severe. As in CVID, giardiasis, NLH, IBD, and celiac disease occur with increased frequency. These diseases occur almost exclusively in IgA-deficient patients with concomitant IgG2 subclass deficiency, which we and others consider a disease distinct from selective IgA deficiency and more akin to CVID. Celiac disease in IgA deficient individuals shares some features with the sprue-like illness in CVID, including no evidence of antibodies to gliadin and endomysium, and no evidence of IgA-secreting plasma cells on small bowel biopsy. Otherwise, the clinical response in IgA-deficient patients with celiac disease differs in that many IgA deficient patients with celiac disease will respond to a gluten-free diet. Giardiasis and NLH occur at a lower rate in IgA-deficient patients than in CVID patients. Management for giardiasis and IBD in IgA deficiency is subject to the same caveats noted for CVID patients. A recent study in Sweden and Denmark showed no increased risk in cancer for IgA-deficient patients, but that study noted a nonstatistically significant increase (5-fold, 95% CI = 0.7 to 19.5) in GC (2 cases of 386) (Mellemkjaer et al, 2002).

GI Manifestations in Other Primary Immunodeficiency Diseases

Other immunodeficiencies have been associated with GI disorders. Patients with XLA have intestinal biopsies that have a notable absence of lamina propria plasma cells. *Giardiasis* has been reported as a cause of chronic diarrhea, but GI complaints are rare in XLA patients. Patients with SCID often have *intractable diarrhea* resistant to medical treatment, leading to failure to thrive. Children with SCID also present with *oral candidiasis* and viral infections, including *rotavirus* and *adenovirus*. Intestinal biopsies in SCID patients show villous atrophy and are devoid of lymphocytes. Following *bone marrow transplant*, SCID patients may develop *graft-versus-host disease* in the gut leading to diarrhea and wasting (Cunningham-Rundles et al, 1984).

Patients with AT seemingly have an increased frequency of *malignancy*, as noted above, although an increased risk of GI malignancy has not been reported in the literature. GI manifestations, including *giardiasis*, occur in the subset of AT patients with IgA deficiency. Besides *oral candidiasis*, GI manifestations are not frequently seen in *DiGeorge's syndrome*. Chronic intestinal viral infections have been reported to cause diarrhea and *necrotizing enterocolitis*. The most prominent GI manifestation in WAS is *intestinal hemorrhage* due to thrombocytopenia. Of note, the mouse model of WAS has colitis, and nonspecific colitis has been reported in WAS.

Conclusion

Patients with primary immunodeficiencies often have GI manifestations. Therefore, in patients with recurrent giardiasis, celiac disease, NLH, and IBD, screening for CVID or IgA deficiency (plus IgG2 subclass deficiency) with serum Ig levels should be considered. Although treatment of inflammatory conditions with immunomodulators, such as azathioprine and 6-MP, does not lead to increased complications when given concurrently with IVIG, chronic oral steroid use in immunocompromised patients should be undertaken with extreme care. Given the increased risk of GI malignancy in CVID, periodic GI screening is warranted.

Supplemental Reading

Ammann AJ, Ashman RF, Buckley RH, et al. Use of intravenous gamma-globulin in antibody immunodeficiency: results of a multicenter controlled trial. Clin Immunol Immunopathol 1982;22:60–7.

Burks AW, Sampson HA, Buckley RH. Anaphylactic reactions after gamma globulin administration in patients with hypogammaglobulinemia. Detection of IgE antibodies to IgA. N Engl J Med 1986;314:560–4.

Cunningham-Rundles C. Physiology of IgA and IgA deficiency. J Clin Immunol 2001;21:303–9.

Cunningham-Rundles C, Bodian C. Common variable immunodeficiency: clinical and immunological features of 248 patients. Clin Immunol 1999;92:34–48.

Cunningham-Rundles C, Brandeis WE, Good RA, Day NK. Milk precipitins, circulating immune complexes and IgA deficiency. J Clin Invest 1979;64:270–2.

Cunningham-Rundles C, Siegal FP, Smithwick EM, et al. Efficacy of intravenous immunoglobulin in primary humoral immunodeficiency disease. Ann Int Med 1984;101:435–9.

DiGeorge AM. Congenital absence of the thymus and its immunologic consequences: concurrence with congenital hypoparathyroidism. Birth Defects 1968;4:1116–21.

Kinlen L, Webster ADB, Bird AG, et al. Prospective study of cancer in patients with hypogammaglobulinemia. Lancet 1985;1:263–5.

Mellemkjær L, Hammarström L, Andersen V, et al. Cancer risk among patients with IgA deficiency or common variable immunodeficiency and their relatives: a combined Danish and Swedish study. Clin Exp Immunol 2002;130:495–500.

Primary immunodeficiency diseases. Report of an IUIS scientific committee. Clin Exp Immunol 1999;118(Suppl):1–28.

So ALP, Mayer L. Gastrointestinal manifestations of primary immunodeficiency disorders. Semin Gastrointest Dis 1997;8:22–32.

Sperber KE, Mayer L. Gastrointestinal manifestations of common variable immunodeficiency. Immunol Allergy Clin North Am 1988;8:423–34.

Spickett GP. Current perspectives on common variable immunodeficiency (CVID). Clin Exp Allergy 2001;31:536–42.

Washington K, Stenzel TT, Buckley FH, Gottfried MR. Gastrointestinal pathology in patients with common variable immunodeficiency and X-linked agammaglobulinemia. Am J Surg Pathol 1996;20:1240–52.

Zullo A, Romiti A, Rinaldi V, et al. Gastric pathology in patients with common variable immunodeficiency. Gut 1999;45:77–81.

CHAPTER 48

GASTROINTESTINAL AND HEPATIC COMPLICATIONS OF STEM CELL TRANSPLANTATION

LINDA A. LEE, MD, AND GEORGIA B. VOGELSANG, MD

Stem cell transplantation (SCT) has rapidly advanced over the past 10 years, with a 5 fold increase in the frequency at which they are being performed. No longer restricted to the treatment of hematologic malignancies, aplastic anemia, and hemoglobinopathies, SCT has been used to eradicate solid tumors and autoimmune diseases. The use of nonmyeloablative SCT has expanded the age limit, so that patients 70 years and older are now transplantation candidates. SCT is generally performed at university medical centers, although recipients frequently reside in areas distant from the academic environment. Thus, with increased numbers and survival among transplantation recipients, the likelihood that a community gastroenterologist or hepatologist will confront the gastrointestinal (GI) and hepatic complications of SCT will only increase in the future.

SCT is performed with the intent of completely or partially ablating the recipient's bone marrow using high dose radiation and/or chemotherapy. Patients may receive their own stem cells (*autologous*), collected prior to the preparative regimen, or they may receive stem cells from a matched or partially matched donor (*allogeneic*). In cases where SCT is performed as consolidation therapy, the marrow may be replaced by the patient's previously removed stem cells (autologous). Although there are many preparative regimens, the most common are *total body radiation* plus high dose *cyclophosphamide* or *busulfan* plus *cyclophosphamide*. Bone marrow engraftment, as indicated by the recovery in peripheral hematologic counts, occurs by the third week after transplantation. Most SCT patients are placed on *prophylactic* antifungal, antiviral, and antibacterial agents, and allogeneic patients receive *immunosuppressive agents*, such as *tacrolimus*, *cyclosporine A*, and/or *mycophenolate mofetil* (Cellcept), to prevent graft-versus-host disease (GVHD).

Gastroenterologists and hepatologists are frequently asked to evaluate symptoms and abnormal laboratory values arising after SCT. Although transplantation physicians will commonly direct the care of the patients once the diagnosis is established, the community oncologist may increasingly rely on their GI colleagues to play an active role in management. Symptoms, such as *nausea, vomiting, diarrhea,* and *mucositis,* related to the preparative regimen may become apparent within a few days and persist for as long as 2 to 3 weeks. Thus, symptoms related to the preparative regimen can be difficult to distinguish from symptoms arising from infectious, vascular, or immune processes that often complicate SCT. When discussing diagnostic and therapeutic approaches to these symptoms, it is convenient to divide SCT into time intervals during which particular disease processes are known to be most prevalent (Figure 48-1). The challenge for gastroenterologists and hepatologists in SCT, therefore, is ascertaining the diagnosis, particularly when the use of typical diagnostic tools is limited by the critically ill conditions posed by some of these patients. For this reason, this chapter is divided into sections based on clinical presentations.

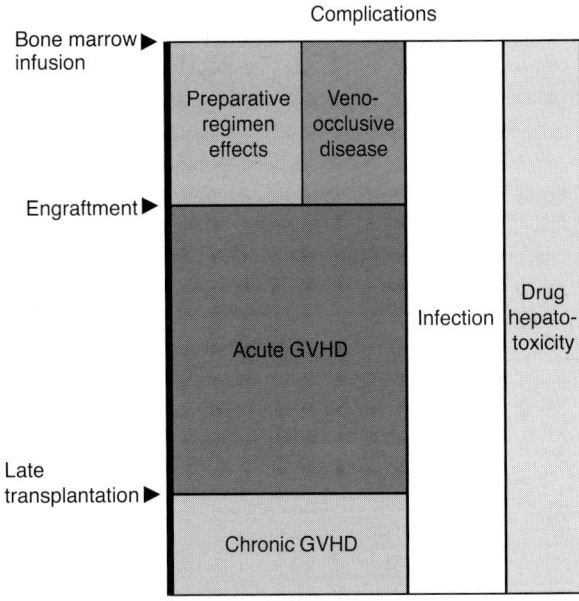

FIGURE 48-1. Timetable for gastrointestinal and hepatic complications of stem cell transplantation. Infection risk is increased in the early post-transplantation period due to neutropenia and delayed immune recovery particularly in allogeneic stem cell recipients. Later, infection risk is highest among those with graft-versus-host disease (GVHD).

Clinical Presentations

Diarrhea

PREPARATIVE PERIOD

The preparative regimen is the most common cause of diarrhea occurring within the first 2 weeks after bone marrow infusion. *Drug-induced diarrhea* occurs commonly in response to the preparative regimen that includes high dose *cyclophosphamide* and *busulfan* and may persist for 2 to 3 weeks. Sandostatin (Octreotide) (250 µg subcutaneously 3 times per day) has been reported by Morton and Durrant (1995) in a small series as being effective in loperamide-resistant preparative regimen related diarrhea. Oral glutamine supplementation has yielded mixed results when studied to determine if it could improve the nutritional status and diarrhea frequency in SCT patients (Coghlin Dickson et al, 2000). *Mycophenolate mofetil* causes diarrhea in a third of patients, inducing an enterocolitis characterized by the presence of patchy inflammation and focal crypt distortion (Maes et al, 2003). As this drug is used increasingly for GVHD prophylaxis, differentiating GVHD from the effects of the drug through use of a drug holiday is critical.

ACUTE GVHD

Diarrhea occurring after bone marrow engraftment (*about the third week after SCT*) is most likely due to *acute* GVHD, an immune mediated process triggered by activation of donor lymphocytes. Acute GVHD is a multisystemic process affecting the *skin, liver,* and *gut*. At Johns Hopkins, SCT patients with stages 2, 3, and 4 acute GVHD had median survivals of only 5.4, 3.6, and 2.5 months, respectively, despite treatment (Arai and Vogelsang, 2000). Gut involvement does *not* require the presence of skin or liver involvement, although when these organs are affected, suspicion is raised for GVHD. Acute GVHD ranges from mild, with only small increases in stool volume occurring, to severe, with the passage of several liters of watery stool per day. In its most severe form, *desquamation* of the gut mucosa occurs and the diarrhea is complicated by severe losses in *electrolytes* and *albumin*. The presence of abdominal cramping is highly variable, particularly in the less severe form of gut GVHD. However, when desquamation occurs, affected individuals may have *severe abdominal pain*, requiring the use of narcotics for relief.

The *diagnosis* of acute GVHD can only be made by endoscopic biopsy, particularly if only subtle endoscopic changes are present since there is little correlation between endoscopic appearance and degree of histologic abnormality (Cruz-Correa et al, 2002). When present in the gut, in general, the stomach, small intestine, and colon are simultaneously affected, although the extent of histologic inflammation and injury may vary from one part of the gut to another. Although acute GVHD is panintestinal, involvement may be associated with only upper or lower GI symptoms exclusively, and, therefore, endoscopic evaluation should be directed by the patient's symptoms and the *need to exclude infectious etiologies*. In the upper GI tract, the *duodenum* is often the segment that gives the most dramatic endoscopic appearance of GVHD (Figure 48-2). Excessive GI bleeding from duodenal biopsies rarely occurs if the platelet count is above 50,000/mm^3. The histologic diagnosis is based on the presence of apoptotic colonocytes, loss of crypts, and, at times, a neutrophilic or eosinophilic infiltrate. Although no definite pathognomonic endoscopic appearance of GVHD has been conclusively established, the appearance of widespread desquamation in the esophagus, duodenum or colon, is highly suspicious for the severest form of GVHD (Cruz-Correa et al, 2002).

Treatment of acute GVHD begins with *high dose steroids*, followed by the addition of other immunosuppressive agents, such as *mycophenolote mofetil* (Cellcept) or *pentostatin*. Oral *beclomethasone* should be reserved for patients that have mild to moderate GVHD isolated to the GI tract and present primarily with nausea, vomiting, or anorexia (McDonald et al, 1998). For steroid refractory GVHD, response to a *TNF-α monoclonal antibody (Infliximab)* has been encouraging (Kobbe et al, 2001). Although no randomized controlled studies exist, control of the voluminous diarrhea associated with acute GVHD has reportedly been achieved by *somatostatin* (octreotide) given at 250 to 500 µg 3 times daily subcutaneously (Ippoliti et al, 1997). Individuals with the most severe form of GVHD are at high risk of developing sepsis due to loss of the mucosal barrier and immunosuppression, so *prophylactic antibiotic use is*

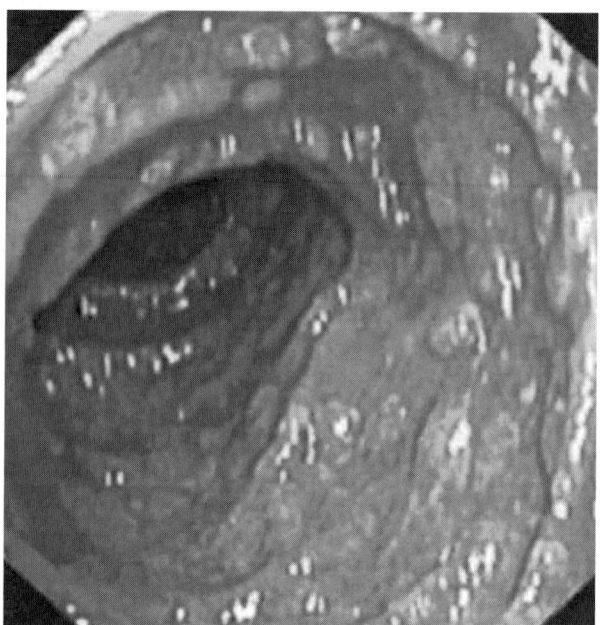

FIGURE 48-2. Endoscopic appearance of severe graft-versus-host disease in the duodenum. Histology was remarkable extensive surface erosion, inflamed granulation tissue, cryptitis, and crypt abscesses.

strongly advocated. *Total parenteral nutrition (TPN)* should also be initiated because of the tremendous protein and electrolyte losses sustained by these patients (Papadopoulou et al, 1996).

INFECTIOUS DIARRHEA

Infectious diarrhea is a less frequent complication of SCT accounting for 13% of acute diarrheal episodes in one study (Cox et al, 1994). The most common enteric viral infections were *astrovirus, adenovirus, cytomegalovirus (CMV)*, and *rotavirus*. CMV may cause colitis or gastritis, and generally occurs 4 to 5 months after transplantation in our experience, but all patients are at risk once they have engrafted. The presence of multinucleated giant cells or positive immunohistochemical stains of mucosal biopsies is diagnostic of CMV infection. On occasion the presence of CMV early antigen does not correlate with active GI involvement. Therapy for CMV is discussed in the chapter on infectious esophagitis (see Chapter 16, "Esophageal Infections"). *Clostridium difficile* is the most common cause of infectious diarrhea in the outpatient. Rare reports of *parasitic infections* occurring in the SCT patient also exist.

CHRONIC GVHD

Chronic GVHD affects 40 to 50% of SCT patients, occurring most often in those who have had acute GVHD, but can arise de novo. In contrast to acute GVHD, which is typified by mucosal injury in the gut, chronic GVHD in the gut is characterized by the presence of fibrosis and atrophy, leading to GI dysmotility syndromes such as gastroparesis or constipation. Bacterial overgrowth may complicate small bowel dysmotility. Chronic GVHD usually *does not induce* inflammatory changes in the *mucosa*, making mucosal biopsies seldom useful in making the diagnosis. However, upper endoscopy or colonoscopy is sometimes performed to evaluate for other causes of gastric outlet obstruction, diarrhea, or new onset constipation.

Most commonly, *even late diarrhea* (occurring 100 days after SCT) is due to *acute GVHD*, particularly in patients who have had GI involvement in the past, and because acute GVHD and chronic GVHD are treated differently, making the correct diagnosis very important (Akpek et al, 2002). Therapy for chronic GVHD involves *corticosteroids* usually combined with *cyclosporine A* or *tacrolimus*. Salvage therapy is *not standard* and may involve such agents as *mycophenolate mofetil, pentostatin,* and *rapamycin*.

Abdominal Pain

Abdominal pain raises a broad differential diagnosis because SCT patients, often treated with corticosteroids and having transient neutropenia, may not manifest the pain syndromes characteristic of specific GI diseases.

GRAFT VERSUS HOST DISEASE

Crampy, abdominal pain can be a prominent feature of those patients with severe gut GVHD, but usually diarrhea and or nausea and vomiting coexist. GVHD is discussed in more detail above.

CHOLECYSTITIS

SCT patients are at risk for developing both calculous and acalculous cholecystitis. Seventy percent of SCT patients develop gallbladder sludge. Patients transplanted for hematologic malignancies may develop calcium bilirubinate stones, many of which are not radiolucent. Transplantation recipients who require TPN and have no oral intake for prolonged periods of time immediately post-transplantation, also are at risk for gallbladder stasis due to the lack of food-stimulated cholecystokinin (CCK) release. Although right upper quadrant or epigastric pain are among the most common complaints, the severity and location of pain in the patient treated with corticosteroids may be atypical. If fever is present, cholecystitis should be more strongly considered in the differential diagnosis regardless of the location of the abdominal pain.

An initial examination by ultrasonography should be performed to assess for the presence of gallstones and a thickened gallbladder wall, suggestive of inflammation. If this is equivocal, biliary scintigraphy should be performed to rule out acute cholecystitis. If the gallbladder fills and CCK fails to elicit gallbladder emptying this suggests chronic cholecystitis. The sensitivity of biliary scintigraphy is preserved as long as hepatic bilirubin metabolism is intact. A total bilirubin > 10 mg/dL makes this diagnostic test less useful. Once acute or chronic cholecystitis is diagnosed, *surgical therapy* should be considered even in the SCT patient. Because thrombocytopenia frequently coexists, surgery is delayed until platelet counts can be maintained over 100 K/mm^3 with or without platelet transfusions. Such patients require *triple antibiotic therapy* until the cholecystectomy can be safely performed. Another option to consider is *endoscopic gallbladder stenting*, which has been successfully performed in high risk surgical patients with end-stage liver disease awaiting orthotopic liver transplantation (Shrestha et al, 1999).

NEUTROPENIC ENTEROCOLITIS (TYPHLITIS)

Typhlitis is an inflammatory process involving the colon that occurs in the neutropenic patient. It is associated with abdominal pain, diarrhea, and fever. Typhlitis is thought to arise by local penetration of bacteria into the colonic wall and can be treated with *antibiotic therapy* to cover gut flora. The differential diagnosis includes CMV colitis, acute GVHD, and appendicitis. Involvement is generally *limited* to the *cecum* and *right colon* and can be diagnosed by CT scan showing thickening of the colonic wall with mesenteric stranding in this area. *Pneumatosis* intestinalis may be present and complicated by *pneumoperitoneum*. Surgical intervention is often required, although case reports exist where affected individuals with isolated pneumatosis intestinalis have been treated conservatively with antibiotic therapy alone.

Viral Infection

Diffuse abdominal pain whose severity is out of proportion to the abdominal examination and negative radiologic imaging is likely to be due to disseminated varicella virus. The severity of pain requires opiates for relief in most cases. Some patients have had the misfortune of undergoing exploratory laparotomies. The abdominal pain may predate the appearance of vesicular rash by as long as 2 weeks. Serology is not useful in making this diagnosis. Empiric therapy with acyclovir may attenuate the appearance of the rash.

Pancreatitis

Chronic pancreatitis as a result of the conditioning therapy or prolonged steroid use may occur late in the posttransplantation period. Affected individuals may present with abdominal pain and/or steatorrhea. Such patients are managed similarly to standard chronic pancreatitis patients. Therapy includes pancreatic enzymes to improve malabsorption or to reduce chronic pain and endoscopic retrograde cholangiography to alleviate pancreatic duct obstruction.

Nausea and Vomiting

Nausea and vomiting in the SCT recipient is so common that it may be attributed to the preparative regimen or other immunosuppressive agents or antibiotics administered. However, *nausea* with or without vomiting may be the only manifestation of acute GVHD. Upper endoscopy with gastric and duodenal biopsies will confirm the diagnosis. Therapy for acute GVHD was discussed above. In addition, oral beclomethasone 8 mg/d allows the more rapid tapering of high dose prednisone used in the treatment of mild to moderate acute GVHD that presents primarily with nausea, vomiting, early satiety, and anorexia (McDonald et al, 1998).

Nausea and vomiting may result from *gastroparesis*, which appears to be a common complication of both autologous and allogeneic SCTs (Eagle et al, 2001). The etiology of the gastroparesis is unknown, but the preparative chemotherapy or radiation may be responsible. Rarely, coexisting *adrenal insufficiency* may contribute to GI dysmotility. Therapy should be directed at controlling gastric acid hypersecretion, a complication of gastroparesis, using *proton pump inhibitors*. Nausea may be treated with *metaclopramide* 10 to 20 mg before each meal and at bedtime, which stimulates gastric emptying in addition to centrally antagonizing nausea. *Erythromycin* 250 mg 4 times daily also has prokinetic effects but itself may provoke GI upset. *Domperidone* 10 to 20 mg before each meal also may improve gastroparesis, but is not available in the United States.

GI Bleeding

GI bleeding may complicate GVHD, and is associated with a worse prognosis overall from SCT (Nevo et al, 1999). GI bleeding may be due to severe GVHD or may result from *gastric antral vascular ectasia (GAVE)*. GAVE appears as diffuse antral telangectasias which may not be apparent due to the bright red blood adherent to the antral mucosa. Endoscopic control of bleeding in this condition is often unsuccessful, because bleeding is slow and diffuse and not readily amenable to bicap cautery or YAG laser therapy. Antrectomies have been attempted often with disastrous results. Cryotherapy, which may be effective for the control of chronic GI blood loss due to the telangectasias associated with "watermelon stomach", appears less effective in SCT patients due to prolonged thrombocytopenia. We therefore recommend supportive therapy and correction of thrombocytopenia if possible. The chapter on upper GI bleeding has a section on GAVE (see Chapter 28, "Upper Gastrointestinal Bleeding").

Esophageal Symptoms

Gastroesophageal reflux, dysphagia, and odynophagia are common complaints in the SCT patient. Severe mucositis extending down into the esophagus is common in patients receiving *methotrexate* for GVHD prophylaxis, and is usually treated with narcotics and TPN until it resolves. If given before initiation of the preparative regimen, *sulcralfate 1 g* given as an elixir 4 times a day may decrease the incidence of mucositis (Castagna et al, 2001). Dysphagia and odynophagia may result from infectious esophagitis and/or acute GVHD. Upper endoscopy should be pursued to rule out infectious esophagitis caused by herpes simplex versus, CMV, or candida. The absence of oral candidiasis should not exclude an evaluation of the esophagus for candida esophagitis. Reflux symptoms are exacerbated in those patients who develop gastroparesis, and therefore gastric acid antisecretory therapy should be instituted.

Abnormal Liver Function Tests

Abnormal liver function tests (LFTs) have been reported to occur in > 40 and 80% of patients in the first year after autologus or allogeneic SCT, respectively. Many individuals have abnormal LFTs prior to transplantation, as a result of previous chemotherapy. In addition, iron overload is commonly found among SCT patients as a result of increased red cell turnover and multiple blood transfusions. Chronic viral hepatitis B or C may also be identified prior to transplantation. Although the pattern of elevation can help distinguish between cholestatic liver disease and hepatitis, often the etiology is ambiguous without a liver biopsy. Despite the increased risk of bleeding in SCT patients, we advocate the use of *transjugular liver biopsy* whenever withdrawal of potentially hepatotoxic medications fails to improve LFT abnormalities. The transjugular liver biopsy, using a retractable Tru-Cut needle, is best performed by a skilled interventional radiologist. This approach is preferred over the percutaneous approach, which disrupts the hepatic capsule and may be complicated by subcapsular hematoma or a peritoneal bleed in these patients who have coagulopathies.

Veno-occlusive Disease

In the first 3 weeks following SCT, liver function abnormalities raise the possibility of veno-occlusive disease (VOD). VOD has been reported to occur in up to 20% of allogeneic and 10% of autologous transplantation recipients and is the most likely cause of new ascites that arises in the immediate post-transplantation period. Late-onset ascites is rare, and a diagnostic paracentesis will aid in distinguishing portal hypertension secondary to chronic liver disease, metastatic carcinoma, or myxedema ascites.

Preexisting liver disease is the major risk factor for the development of VOD. The diagnosis of VOD should be entertained if there are LFT abnormalities, ascites or a 10% increase in body weight, and hepatomegaly (Table 48-1). In the immediate post-transplantation setting, Doppler ultrasonography will demonstrate decreased or retrograde flow in the portal vein. A hepatic resistive index > 0.76 is highly suggestive of VOD, but its calculation is not particularly sensitive (Teefey et al, 1995). Although the Seattle or Baltimore VOD clinical criteria have a sensitivity and specificity > 88%, a *transjugular liver biopsy* with measurement of *hepatic vein gradient* is the best way to confirm the diagnosis. Hepatic injury occurs in zone 3 with subendothelial edema, sinusoidal congestion, hepatic venule occlusion, and hepatocyte necrosis. Severe VOD is accompanied by fibrous narrowing or terminal hepatic venules and widespread hepatocellular necrosis. VOD may result in fulminant hepatic failure, characterized by dramatic rises and falls in the serum transaminases, accompanied by prolongation of the prothrombin time and the development of hepatic encephalopathy. The prognosis is grim, but survivors may develop a nodular appearing liver, composed of regenerated liver nodules. The collapse of hepatic parenchyma may result in fibrosis and eventual portal hypertension. Transjugular intrahepatic portosystemic shunting has been attempted (Azoulay et al, 1998), as has successful orthotopic liver transplantation in patients who are free of malignancy (Rapoport et al, 1991). Therapy directed at the underlying VOD has yielded mixed results. Heparin and tissue plasminogen activator have limited efficacy and have been associated with serious bleeding complications. The experimental use of intravenous *difibrotide*, a polydeoxyribonucleotide with antithrombotic and fibrinoytic effects, shows potential promise in treating severe VOD, particularly in younger patients (Richardson et al, 2002). In one randomized, placebo-controlled study of allogeneic SCT recipients, administration of prophylactic *ursodiol* was associated with a decreased incidence of VOD (Essell et al, 1998), but no improvement in VOD incidence was observed in a more recent study by another group (Ruutu et al, 2002).

GVHD

Hepatic GVHD has two clinical presentations. Most often, cholestatic LFT abnormalities occur. This reflects the direct injury of bile duct cells by donor white blood cells. Liver biopsy is critical for making the diagnosis. Even in patients with skin and/or gut GVHD, hepatic abnormalities have many etiologies, and without a biopsy it cannot be assumed they are due to GVHD. A liver biopsy should be considered in such patients whose LFTs fail to improve in response to therapy in a manner commensurate with skin or gut improvement. Liver histology is characterized by focal or widespread bile duct epithelial injury with varying degrees of portal lymphocytic infiltration. These findings are often accompanied by interlobular bile stasis. Less commonly, usually in the setting of a donor lymphocyte infusion, an atypical lobular hepatitis occurs, with transaminases rising in some cases to > 10 times normal (Akpek et al, 2002). Treatment of GVHD is usually done at the recommendation of the transplantation center, with initial therapy usually involving high dose corticosteroids. Hepatic GVHD may progress to cirrhosis and portal hypertensive complications. In a randomized open-label study, prophylactic ursodiol administration (600 to 900 mg every day) reduced the incidence of severe GVHD and improved survival (Ruutu et al, 2002).

TPN-Associated Cholestasis

Abnormal LFTs may arise as the result of TPN (Angelico and Guardia, 2000). *Hepatic steatosis* is a common finding even 5 days after the initiation of TPN and results from an excess of calories in the form of carbohydrates. *Intrahepatic cholestasis* is typified by the presence of an

---

TABLE 48-1. Clinical Criteria for Veno-occlusive Disease

Baltimore Criteria (Jones et al, 1987)
Jaundice and any two of the following:
  Ascites
  Weight gain > 5% baseline
  Hepatomegaly
Seattle Criteria (any two prior to day 20) (McDonald et al, 1993)
  Jaundice
  Ascites ± unexplained weight gain of > 2% baseline
  Painful hepatomegaly

inflammatory periportal infiltrate and bile duct plugging. It may progress to *biliary cirrhosis*. An *excess of lipid calories* (> 50% of total calories) or *bacterial translocation* across the gut wall with resulting cytokine release are among the etiologies proposed. *Ursodiol* (Actical) 300 mg 3 times daily has been used to treat TPN-induced intrahepatic cholestasis but no randomized placebo-controlled studies have been reported. A controlled, open-label study to determine if taurine conjugated ursodeoxycholic acid (30 mg/kg/d) would protect against cholestasis in infants showed no difference in LFT abnormalities (Heubi et al, 2002).

Cholestasis of Sepsis

SCT patients are at high risk for infection due to eradication of their bone marrow and treatment with immunosuppressive drugs to control GVHD. Sepsis may be associated with profound pro-inflammatory cytokine release in response to bacterial lipopolysaccharide (Gilroy et al, 2003). Cytokines, such as tumor necrosis factor-α, interleukin 1-β, and interleukin-6, appear to interfere with sinusoidal bile transport giving rise to cholestasis. Typically there are elevations of the total bilirubin out of proportion to other LFTs. Although most commonly associated with gram-negative infections, almost any type of organism can cause the cholestasis of sepsis. The etiology is established usually by temporal correlation with other symptoms suggestive of sepsis, making liver biopsy rarely necessary. Should a liver biopsy be obtained, a fairly benign periportal inflammatory infiltrate with bile duct plugging may be observed. Fortunately, cholestasis improves with antibiotic therapy and resolution of the infection, although improvement of LFTs may lag behind clinical improvement.

Drug Hepatotoxicity

Numerous medications may cause abnormal increases in the LFTs. In patients receiving *methotrexate* for GVHD prophylaxis, an elevated bilirubin is almost universal during the first 2 weeks. A list of commonly used drugs associated with elevations in the LFTs is given in Table 48-2, along with their hepatic side effects. There is a chapter on drug-induced liver disease (see Chapter 122, "Chronic Cholestasis and its Sequelae").

Iron Overload

Hemosiderosis is a common late problem that arises from the multiple blood transfusions as well as increased red blood cell turnover as a consequence of a hematologic malignancy. Iron deposition in the liver begins in the Kupffer cells, but may eventually extend to hepatocytes. Hemosiderosis has been associated with cardiomyopathy and liver injury, such that *phlebotomy* is generally recommended for those individuals with excessive iron stores as

TABLE 48-2. Commonly Used Drugs Associated with Abnormal Liver Function Tests and Clinical Liver Disease

Drug	Cholestasis	Hepatitis	Liver Failure
Cyclosporine A			
Tacrolimus			
Trimethoprim-sulfomethoxizole	+	+	+
Piperacillin/Tobramycin	+	+	
Ciprofloxacin	+	+	+
Fluconazole			
Amphotericin B			
CotIrtimaxzole			
Ketoconazole	+	+	+
Pentostatin			
Mycophenolate mofetil			
Methotrexate	+		

determined by elevations of the serum ferritin and transferrin saturation as well by an increased hepatic iron content on liver biopsy. LFTs may improve with phlebotomy. Chapter 125, "Hereditary Hemochromatosis" is devoted to hemochromatosis.

Infections

Hepatitis B and C may result from blood transfusions particularly if they were administered prior to 1991, from an infected sexual partner, or, more rarely, from an infected donor. Importantly, previously infected SCT candidates are at higher risk for GVHD and VOD (Strasser and McDonald, 1999). Overt hepatitis may not manifest itself until after engraftment has occurred and immunosuppressive agents are tapered. Immunosuppression leads to increases in viral load, and sometimes a significant hepatitis occurs when the immunosuppressive agents are withdrawn. On occasion, a fulminant hepatitis may result. Pre-SCT treatment of hepatitis C is often not feasible because effective therapy with pegylated interferon and ribavirin usually requires 12 months of therapy. Furthermore, a complication of *interferon* therapy is *bone marrow suppression*. Strasser and McDonald (1999) suggested that therapy be attempted once patients are off immunosuppressive medications for at least 6 months. Infections with *CMV, herpes simplex virus, varicella zoster virus*, and *adenovirus* may result in a fulminant hepatitis and liver failure. Fungal infections due to *Aspergillus* or *Candida* may present as a single mass or diffuse hepatic involvement. Diagnosis is generally established by liver biopsy or recognition of the disease in another organ.

Summary

GI or hepatic complications are very common after SCT and pose significant morbidity and mortality. Diagnosis and care of these patients, who suffer from concurrent immunosuppression and coagulopathies, is a continual challenge. Additional challenges are posed by the rapid evolution of the field, with SCT protocols changing frequently with regard to preparative regimens, patient clinical characteristics, and prophylactic therapy for infectious complications, GVHD, and VOD. Fortunately, with the advent of the Internet, transplantation centers are readily accessible should further advice be necessary. Further studies are needed to better understand the pathophysiology of VOD and GVHD and to develop more effective prevention and management strategies against these conditions.

Supplemental Reading

Akpek G, Boitnott JK, Lee LA, et al. Hepatitic variant of graft-versus-host disease after donor lymphocyte infusion. Blood 2002;100:3903–7.

Akpek G, Lee SM, Anders V, et al. A high-dose pulse steroid regimen for controlling active chronic graft-versus-host disease. Biol Blood Marrow Transplant 2001;7:495–502.

Angelico M, Della Guardia P. Review article: hepatobiliary complications associated with total parenteral nutrition. Aliment Pharmacol Ther 2000;14 Suppl 2:54–7.

Arai S, Vogelsang GB. Management of graft-versus-host disease. Blood Rev 2000;14:190–204.

Azoulay D, Castaing D, Lemoine A, et al. Successful treatment of severe azathioprine-induced hepatic veno-occlusive disease in a kidney-transplanted patient with transjugular intrahepatic portosystemic shunt. Clin Nephrol 1998;50:118–22.

Castagna L, Benhamou E, Pedraza E, et al. Prevention of mucositis in bone marrow transplantation: a double blind randomised controlled trial of sucralfate. Ann Oncol 2001;12:953–5.

Coghlin Dickson TM, Wong RM, Offrin RS, et al. Effect of oral glutamine supplementation during bone marrow transplantation. J Parenter Enteral Nutr 2000;24:61–6.

Cox GJ, Matsui SM, Lo RS, et al. Etiology and outcome of diarrhea after marrow transplantation: a prospective study. Gastroenterology 1994;107:1398–407.

Cruz-Correa M, Poonawala A, Abraham SC, et al. Endoscopic findings predict the histologic diagnosis in gastrointestinal graft-versus-host disease. Endoscopy 2002;34:808–13.

Eagle DA, Gian V, Lauwers GY, et al. Gastroparesis following bone marrow transplantation. Bone Marrow Transplant 2001;28:59–62.

Essell JH, Schroeder MT, Harman GS, et al. Ursodiol prophylaxis against hepatic complications of allogeneic bone marrow transplantation. A randomized, double-blind, placebo-controlled trial. Ann Intern Med 1998;128:975–81.

Gilroy RK, Mailliard ME, Gollan JL. Cholestasis of sepsis. Best Pract Res Clin Gastroenterol 2003;17:357–67.

Heubi JE, Wiechmann DA, Creutzinger V, et al. Tauroursodeoxycholic acid (tudca) in the prevention of total parenteral nutrition-associated liver disease. J Pediatr 2002;141:237–42.

Ippoliti C, Champlin R, Bugazia N, et al. Use of octreotide in the symptomatic management of diarrhea induced by graft-versus-host disease in patients with hematologic malignancies. J Clin Oncol 1997;15:3350–4.

Jones RJ, Lee KS, Beschorner WE, et al. Venoocclusive disease of the liver following bone marrow transplantation. Transplantation 1987;44:778–83.

Kobbe G, Schneider P, Rohr U, et al. Treatment of severe steroid refractory acute graft-versus-host disease with infliximab, a chimeric human/mouse antiTNFalpha antibody. Bone Marrow Transplant 2001;28:47–9.

Maes BD, Dalle I, Geboes K, et al. Erosive enterocolitis in mycophenolate mofetil-treated renal-transplant recipients with persistent afebrile diarrhea. Transplantation 2003;75:665–72.

McDonald GB, Bouvier M, Hockenbery DM, et al. Oral beclomethasone dipropionate for treatment of intestinal graft-versus-host disease: a randomized, controlled trial. Gastroenterology 1998;115:28–35.

McDonald GB, Hinds MS, Fisher LD, et al. Veno-occlusive disease of the liver and multiorgan failure after bone marrow transplantation: a cohort study of 355 patients. Ann Intern Med 1993;118:255–67.

Morton AJ, Durrant ST. Efficacy of octreotide in controlling refractory diarrhea following bone marrow transplantation. Clin Transplant 1995;9:205–8.

Nevo S, Enger C, Swan V, et al. Acute bleeding after allogeneic bone marrow transplantation: association with graft versus host disease and effect on survival. Transplantation 1999;67:681–9.

Papadopoulou A, Lloyd DR, Williams MD, et al. Gastrointestinal and nutritional sequelae of bone marrow transplantation. Arch Dis Child 1996;75:208–13.

Rapoport AP, Doyle HR, Starzl T, et al. Orthotopic liver transplantation for life-threatening veno-occlusive disease of the liver after allogeneic bone marrow transplant. Bone Marrow Transplant 1991;8:421–4.

Richardson PG, Murakami C, Jin Z, et al. Multi-institutional use of defibrotide in 88 patients after stem cell transplantation with severe veno-occlusive disease and multisystem organ failure: response without significant toxicity in a high-risk population and factors predictive of outcome. Blood 2002;100:4337–43.

Ruutu T, Eriksson B, Remes K, et al. Ursodeoxycholic acid for the prevention of hepatic complications in allogeneic stem cell transplantation. Blood 2002;100:1977–83.

Shrestha R, Trouillot TE, and Everson GT. Endoscopic stenting of the gallbladder for symptomatic gallbladder disease in patients with end-stage liver disease awaiting orthotopic liver transplantation. Liver Transpl Surg 1999;5:275–81.

Strasser SI, McDonald GB. Hepatitis viruses and hematopoietic cell transplantation: a guide to patient and donor management. Blood 1999;93:1127–36.

Teefey SA, Brink JA, Borson RA, Middleton WD. Diagnosis of venoocclusive disease of the liver after bone marrow transplantation: value of duplex sonography. Am J Roentgenol 1995;164:1397–401.

CHAPTER 49

ACUTE INFECTIOUS DIARRHEA

BETH D. KIRKPATRICK, MD, AND W. KEMPER ALSTON, MD

Infectious diarrhea is a problem of global proportions, causing 4 to 6 million deaths each year. In North American adults, approximately 200 million cases of diarrhea occur annually, or 1.2 to 1.9 cases of diarrhea per adult. The etiologies and the spectrum of illness from acute infectious diarrhea are broad. This chapter will focus on therapies for the most common causes of infectious diarrhea in adults.

Diagnostic Approach

Acute infectious diarrhea is caused by a remarkable variety of microorganisms. The clinical presentation, however, is often nonspecific. Historical features, such as travel, ingestion of seafood, similar illnesses among close contacts, antibiotic use, and comorbidities, such as human immunodeficiency virus (HIV) infection, help guide the differential diagnosis. The physical examination permits an assessment of the degree of dehydration and malnutrition. The role of the microbiology laboratory in the diagnosis of gastroenteritis is critical. Notably, the routine "stool work-up" (bacterial cultures and examination for ova and parasites) fails to diagnose a large proportion of gastroenteritis cases. Viral infections, including rotavirus and noroviruses, *Vibrio*, *Escherichia coli*, *Clostridium perfringens*, *Staphylococcus aureus*, *Bacillus cereus*, *Clostridium difficile*, *Yersinia enterocolitica*, microsporidia, and cyclospora are among the causes of gastroenteritis that are not reliably detected by stool culture or ova and parasite examination. Because of the limitations in routine testing and the availability of selective media, rapid antigen tests, and special stains for many of these pathogens, it is important, as reviewed by Procop (2001), that the clinician communicate directly with the clinical microbiology laboratory when historical or physical findings suggest a particular diagnosis.

Therapy

Rehydration

The restoration and maintenance of adequate hydration is the most important component of the treatment of acute infectious diarrhea. Rehydration is particularly important in the elderly, pediatric, or immunocompromised patient. In otherwise healthy patients with mild to moderate diarrhea, increasing intake of most fluids is usually adequate to replace fluid losses. In moderate to severe diarrhea, however, fluids with appropriate electrolyte concentrations are needed. Water, juices, and sports drinks will not adequately replace electrolyte losses. For dehydrating diarrhea, aggressive oral rehydration with electrolyte solutions or intravenous (IV) fluids is required. The formulation of "oral rehydration solutions" (ORS), as determined by the World Health Organization (WHO), includes precise concentrations of sodium, potassium, chloride, citrate/bicarbonate, and glucose to replace fluid and electrolyte losses from diarrhea and avoid IV fluid administration (Pizarro et al, 1991). Commercial pediatric formulations are readily available (eg, Pedialyte). A home ORS recipe, based on WHO formulations, is available (Table 49-1). IV replacement of fluids and electrolytes is necessary for severe dehydration and inability to tolerate oral solutions, as well for patients with shock and metabolic acidosis.

Symptomatic Therapies

Symptomatic therapies for diarrhea include antimotility agents, antisecretory agents, adsorbants (silicates), and bulk forming agents (Powell and Szauter, 1993). Antimotility drugs, such as *loperamide* (*Imodium*), can be used safely for symptomatic relief in most cases of acute diarrhea. Antimotility agents inhibit peristalsis of the small intestinal smooth muscle and stimulate water and electrolyte absorption. The number of diarrheal stools is reduced by 80% with these agents. The recommended dose of loperamide is 4 mg initially, then 2 mg after each loose stool, to a maximum of 16 mg per day. *Diphenoxylate/atropine (Lomotil)* should be avoided because of the central opiate effect, risk of overdosage, and

TABLE 49-1. Oral Rehydration Solution Formula for Home Use

$\frac{3}{4}$ teaspoon salt
1 teaspoon baking soda
1 cup orange juice or two bananas
4 tablespoons sugar
Blend and add above to 750 cc of clean water

Adapted from Guerrant and Bobak, 1991.
Provides 90 mmol sodium, 20 mmol potassium, 80 mmol chloride, 30 mmol bicarbonate, and 111 mmol glucose.

the anticholinergic effects of the atropine, including urinary retention, mucosal and cutaneous dryness, tachycardia, and hyperthermia. Although controversial, antimotility drugs should be avoided with symptoms of inflammatory diarrhea or dysentery (ie, fever, cramps, and blood and pus in stool). However, in many cases, antimotility drugs can be used safely when used with appropriate antibiotic therapy. The antisecretory properties of salicylate in *bismuth subsalicylate (Pepto-Bismol)* can decrease diarrheal stools by 50% and is effective in decreasing symptoms of vomiting due to enteric viral infections. Salicylate overdose and bismuth encephalopathy have occurred after excessive use of bismuth subsalicylate.

Bulk forming agents add bulk and form to stool by absorbing water. Agents such as *psyllium (Metamucil), methylcellulose (Citrucel)* and *polycarbophil (FiberCon)* are safe and not systemically absorbed, but are only minimally effective. Silicate clay suspensions (adsorbents), such as activated attapulgite, also absorb water and improve stool consistency but do not decrease fecal water content.

Empiric Antibiotic Use

Use of empiric antibiotics must be weighed against potentially harmful consequences, including increases in antimicrobial resistant infections, eradication of commensal flora, cost, and side effects. As a general rule, *empiric therapy* is used in the following three patient populations: (1) *patients with acute invasive diarrhea*, (2) *patients with travelers' diarrhea*, and (3) *patients with presumed giardiasis*. These recommendations are supported by practice guidelines of the American College of Gastroenterology (Dupont, 1997) and the Infectious Disease Society of America (Dupont, 1997; Guerrant et al, 2001) For adult patients with acute invasive diarrhea, fever and signs of systemic illness are present. Stool evaluation is positive for fecal lactoferrin/white blood cells. While the diagnostic work-up for a specific pathogen is proceeding (ie, bacterial stool cultures, evaluation for ova and parasites, complete blood count, and blood cultures), treatment with a *fluoroquinolone* (eg, Ciprofloxacin 500 mg by mouth twice daily for 3 days) is appropriate. The decision to use empiric therapy in patients with bloody diarrhea and possible infection with E. coli O157:H7 should be made cautiously (especially in children), because of concerns that antibiotics may *predispose* to the *hemolytic uremic* syndrome. In *acute travelers' diarrhea*, empiric therapy with a *fluoroquinolone* is also suggested without stool culture. These infections are often due to enterotoxigenic *E. coli*, and patients have a rapid resolution of symptoms with antibiotic therapy (*Rifaxamin*). There is a separate chapter (see Chapter 50, "Traveler's Diarrhea") on traveler's diarrhea. *Metronidazole* (Table 49-2) is recommended empirically for patients with watery diarrhea lasting 10 days to > 4 weeks and with risk factors for g*iardiasis*.

Pathogen-Specific Therapy

Bacterial Pathogens

SALMONELLA

Nontyphoidal species of *Salmonella* cause *approximately 1.4 million cases* of gastroenteritis and *diarrhea annually*. Contaminated *meat, poultry,* and *eggs* are common sources of infection, although *bean sprouts, tomatoes,* and *orange juice* have also been linked to outbreaks of salmonellosis. Other than diarrhea, clinical features may include abdominal pain, fever, and chills. Grossly bloody diarrhea is uncommon. Patients may *carry Salmonella* in their stools for weeks after symptoms resolve and 0.2 to 0.6% of patients may carry *Salmonella* over 1 year (long term carriers). The majority of cases in healthy adults are self-limited and do not require antibiotics. However, *Salmonella* can invade vascular sites and cause systemic toxicity in compromised hosts. Therapy (see Table 49-2) is indicated for patients with *systemic toxicity* or *bacteremia, aged under 6 months* or *over 50 years*, and in patients with *prosthetic joints, heart valves* or *vascular grafts, severe atherosclerosis, malignancy, HIV/acquired immunodeficiency syndrome (AIDS),* or *uremia*. Typhoidal *Salmonella* is uncommon in the United States and often associated with constipation rather than diarrhea.

SHIGELLA

The four species/serogroups of *Shigella* are as follows: (1) serogroup A (*S. dysenteriae*, the agent of bacillary dysentery), (2) serogroup B (*S. flexneri*), (3) serogroup C (*S. boydii*), and (4) serogroup D (*S. sonnei*, the most common species in the United States). *Shigella* sp are extremely contagious and ingestion of < 100 bacteria may cause infection. Raw vegetables, cheeses, and eggs are common sources of infection. Shigellosis is an inflammatory colitis, often characterized by dysentery (small volume stools with abdominal cramping, fever, and tenesmus). Systemic signs of fever, toxicity, and cramping are often present, although bacteremia is rare. Unlike salmonellosis, all patients with confirmed shigellosis should be treated (see Table 49-2). Co-trimoxazole (twice daily for 3 days for normal hosts) or fluroquinolones are the agents of choice. Co-trimoxazole is preferable if the *Shigella* isolate is susceptible to this agent.

E. COLI

E. coli are aerobic gram-negative rods and normal inhabitants of the human small and large intestine. Several forms of *E. coli* cause diarrhea and distinct clinical manifestations based on the different toxins and virulence factors produced. Forms include enterotoxigenic *E. coli* (ETEC) which causes travelers' diarrhea, and enterohemorrhagic *E. coli* (EHEC), which cause a hemorrhagic colitis associated with the hemolytic uremic syndrome. The serotypes of EHEC include *E. coli* O157:H7, which has been associated with several

TABLE 49-2. Therapy of Infectious Diarrhea

Pathogen	Antimicrobial Agent	Special Circumstances
Bacterial		
nontyphoid *Salmonella*	Not recommended routinely	Ciprofloxacin 500 mg po bid for 5 days
		Treat 14 days if immunocompromised*
		Multidrug resistant *Salmonella* exists
Campylobacter species	Erythromycin 500 mg po qid	Ciprofloxacin 500 mg po bid for 5 days also effective, avoid due to resistant strains
Shigella sp	Cotrimoxazole ds po bid for 3 days (if sensitive)	Treat immunocompromised patient for 7 to 10 days
		If resistant, ciprofloxacin 500 mg bid for 3 days
Escherichia coli		
ETEC traveler's diarrhea	Ciprofloxacin 1 g po for 1 day	Ciprofloxacin 500 mg po bid for 3 days
E. coli O157:H7	Not recommended[†]	
Yersinia sp	Antibiotics not required	For serious infections: ciprofloxacin or doxycyline and AG
Clostridium difficile	Metronidazole 500 mg po tid for 10 to 14 days	In severe infections, vancomycin 125 mg po qid
		Metronidazole 500 mg IV every 8 hours[‡]
Parasitic Pathogens		
Cryptosporidium parvum	Self-limited illness in normal hosts	In immunocompromised or severe hosts, paromomycin 500 mg po tid for 14 to 28 days
Giardia lamblia	Metronidazole 250 mg po tid for 5 to 10 days	—
Cyclospora cayentensis	Cotrimoxazole 1 ds bid for 3 days	—
Isospora belli	Cotrimoxazole 2 ds po bid for 2 to 4 weeks	—
Viral Pathogens	Supportive care	—
Toxin-mediated diarrhea		
Bacillus cereus, Clostridium perfringens	Supportive care	—
Vibrio cholerae	Doxycyline 300 mg po for 1 day	Ciprofloxacin 1 mg po for one day
Vibrio parahemolyticus	Supportive care	—

Adapted, in part, from Kirkpatrick, 2003.
AG = aminoglycoside antibiotic; bid = twice daily; ds = double strength; ETEC = enterotoxigenic *Escherichia coli;* IV = intravenous; po = by mouth; qid = four times daily; tid = three times daily.
*See text for recommendations.
[†]Increased risk of hemolytic uremic syndrome.
[‡]If unable to take orally.

large-scale food and water outbreaks. Enteroaggregative *E. coli* and enteropathogenic *E. coli* are important causes of persistent and chronic diarrhea in young children, particularly in underdeveloped nations, and enteroinvasive *E. coli* causes a *Shigella*-like dysentery. As previously discussed, treatment with a *fluoroquinolone* is effective in ETEC travelers' diarrhea. *Caution* is advised when using antibiotics in EHEC infections, due to the association of antibiotic use and the development of hemolytic uremic syndrome in children.

CAMPYLOBACTER

Campylobacter jejuni is the *most commonly* identified bacterial pathogen in stool cultures and is associated with over 2 million cases of foodborne disease in the United States annually. The spectrum of illness due to *Campylobacter* ranges from mild watery diarrhea to inflammatory enteritis or colitis. Treatment is rarely needed for normal hosts, who clear the infection spontaneously. For patients with systemic symptoms, severe disease or immunosuppression, therapy is recommended with *erythromycin*. *Fluoroquinolones* are also useful to treat sensitive *Campylobacter*, however, there is a worldwide increase in fluoroquinolone *resistance* and these infections may clinically worsen when quinolones alter normal flora.

Parasitic Pathogens

The protozoans *Cryptosporidium parvum* and *Giardia lamblia* are the most common causes of diarrhea from parasites in the United States. Both occur sporadically and in outbreaks associated with contaminated food and water. Less common parasitic causes of diarrhea in North America include *Entamoeba histolytica, Cyclospora cayentensis, and Microsporidia* sp, particularly in immunocompromised patients, travelers, and patients with the AIDS. There is a separate chapter on the treatment of intestinal parasites and protozoa (Chapter 52, "Intestinal Parasites") and another on chronic immunodeficiency syndrome (Chapter 47, "Chronic Immunodeficiency Syndromes Affecting the Gastrointestinal Tract"). Giardiasis is associated with the acute onset of watery diarrhea, cramps, bloating, and flatulence. Diarrhea can persist for weeks and be associated with significant weight loss. The treatment of choice is *metronidazole* (*Flagyl*) (250 to 750 mg by mouth three times daily for 7 to 10 days), which is effective in about 80 to 90% of cases. Side effects of metronidazole, especially at higher doses, can include nausea, dizziness, and an Antabuse-like reaction when taken with alcohol. Metronidazole should be avoided in pregnancy.

C. parvum also causes a watery diarrhea that can be persistent or chronic, especially in patients with compromised immunity. There is no effective antimicrobial therapy for cryptosporidiosis. *Paromomycin* (500 mg by mouth three times daily for 7 days) has been variably reported to have clinical efficacy and has, as reported by Smith and colleagues (1998), been used with some success in combination with *azithromycin* (Zithromax) for the treatment of cryptosporidiosis in patients with AIDS. For patients with cryptosporidiosis and AIDS, improvement of immune function with highly active *antiretroviral therapy* may be successful in clearing cryptosporidial infection. There is a separate chapter on treatment of gastrointestinal in HIV-infected patients (see Chapter 46, "Gastrointestinal and Nutritional Complications of HIV Infection").

Viral Gastroenteritis

The morbidity and mortality associated with viral gastroenteritis around the world, particularly among infants and young children, cannot be overemphasized. Numerous different viruses cause a similar spectrum of illness ranging from asymptomatic infection to fatal disease from dehydration. Important viruses associated with gastroenteritis include rotavirus, noroviruses, adenovirus, and astrovirus.

Rotavirus is estimated to cause 800,000 deaths per year around the world (Parashar et al, 1998). Almost all children suffer an infection with rotavirus by the age of 5 years; many of these infections result in hospitalization or death. Disease is generally milder in adults. The incubation period is approximately 2 days, and vomiting, diarrhea, crampy abdominal pain, and fever characterize the clinical illness. A specific diagnosis can be established with rapid antigen detection on stool specimens. Treatment is supportive. A live, oral, tetravalent rotavirus *vaccine* (RRV-TV, RotaShield) was withdrawn from the market in the fall of 1999 after it was associated with intussusception (Dennehy and Bresee, 2001).

Noroviruses recently gained notoriety in association with outbreaks of gastroenteritis on cruise ships. The terminology used for these human *caliciviruses*, the prototype of which is *Norwalk virus*, has been confusing (Norwalk-like viruses, small round structured viruses, Sapporo-like viruses, etc). These highly contagious viruses are stable in the environment and are, according to Centers for Disease Control and Prevention (CDC) reports, the most common cause of gastroenteritis in the United States. After an incubation period of 1 to 2 days, patients experience nausea, vomiting, watery diarrhea, and abdominal cramps. The illness is self-limited and generally resolves within 3 days. The diagnosis can be established using reverse transcriptase polyermase chain reaction on stool specimens, and *treatment is supportive*.

Toxin-Mediated Infectious Diarrhea

BACILLUS CEREUS

B. cereus is a ubiquitous, gram-positive, spore-forming rod that causes toxin-mediated foodborne disease sporadically and in outbreaks (Mahler et al, 1997). (Please see the two CDC reports on foodborne infection in the Supplemental Reading list.) There are two clinical manifestations, a rapid onset (1 to 6 hours after incubation) emetic form resulting from the ingestion of a heat-stable, preformed toxin, and a more delayed (24 to 48 hours after incubation) diarrheal disease due to in vivo production of enterotoxins. Vomiting and cramps, typically without fever, occurring soon after ingesting a suspect meal (especially fried rice for *B. cereus*) should suggest either *B. cereus* or *S. aureus* food poisoning. Although foodborne disease is almost always self-limited (24 to 48 hours), fulminant liver failure has been reported, and *B. cereus* may cause a variety of extraintestinal infections (Mahler et al, 1997). Treatment is *supportive*.

S. AUREUS

Staphylococcal food poisoning resembles the emetic form of *B. cereus* disease, with the sudden onset of symptoms 1 to 6 hours after ingestion of contaminated food (CDC, 2001). *S. aureus* produces several enterotoxins, and outbreaks typically occur during the summer months. The disease is self-limited, often resolving within 24 hours. The diagnosis is generally a clinical one, although in the setting of an outbreak investigation the organism can be cultured from patients and food handlers, and the organism and toxin may be detected in contaminated food. Treatment is *supportive*.

C. PERFRINGENS

C. perfringens is a ubiquitous, anaerobic, gram-positive bacillus that forms heat-resistant spores. If ingested in sufficient amounts with improperly handled foods (especially inadequately stored cooked meats), it can produce an enterotoxin in vivo and cause a diarrheal illness. The disease is typically mild and self-limited, beginning after an incubation period of 6 to 24 hours with cramps and watery stools, similar to the diarrheal form of *B. cereus* (CDC, 2001). Fever and vomiting are distinctly unusual. Between 1993 and 1997 the CDC reported 57 foodborne outbreaks due to *C. perfringens* with 2,772 cases. The diagnosis is made clinically. As part of an investigation, quantitative cultures of food and stool may be performed, and the toxin can be detected. Treatment is supportive.

V. CHOLERAE

Cholera has been an acute diarrheal illness of profound public health importance since at least the 19th century.

Infections occur on an endemic basis among children and as explosive epidemics in developing countries. Approximately 120,000 deaths per year are caused by cholera. Untreated, the WHO reports that the case fatality rate may exceed 20%. *V. cholerae* is a curved gram-negative bacillus that is spread by fecal contamination of food and water. An enterotoxin produces an abrupt onset of watery diarrhea and dehydration after an incubation period of 1 to 3 days. The clinical illness may range from a mild gastroenteritis to a rapidly fatal disease with profound dehydration, acidosis, and renal failure. The illness is entirely toxin-mediated, and the organism is noninvasive. The cornerstone of treating cholera is to *replace lost fluids and electrolytes*. The *IV* route should be used for severe cases with Ringer's lactate supplemented with potassium. *Oral rehydration solutions*, such as the WHO (WHO-ORS), may reduce the fatality rate to 1%. There is a separate chapter on secretory diarrhea (Chapter 72, "Secretory Diarrhea"). *Tetracyclines, trimethoprim-sulfamethoxazole, erythromycin*, and *fluoroquinolones* have all been used successfully, guided by host factors and local resistance patterns. There is currently *no licensed cholera vaccine* in the United States.

OTHER *VIBRIO* SPECIES

Several species of *Vibrio* other than *V. cholerae* are capable of causing gastroenteritis; the most important of which is *V. parahaemolyticus*. Others include non-O1 strains of *V. cholerae, V. fluvialis, V. hollisae*, and *V. mimicus*. In addition, *V. vulnificus* is an important cause of sepsis and soft tissue infection in immunocompromised hosts, especially those with cirrhosis or advanced liver disease. Long recognized as a seafood-associated pathogen in Asia, *V. parahaemolyticus* has emerged as a significant cause of diarrhea in the United States following ingestion of raw or undercooked shellfish, such as raw oysters (Daniels et al, 2000). As with most types of foodborne gastroenteritis, the spectrum of disease ranges from quite mild to severe, bloody diarrhea. Illness due to *V. parahaemolyticus* has both a toxin-mediated and an inflammatory component. The onset of illness is generally less than 24 hours after exposure to seafood. The diagnosis can be established with stool culture, although not all laboratories routinely use selective media for *Vibrio* when processing stool specimens. The illness is generally self-limited, and severe dehydration is very uncommon. Antibiotics are not required for gastroenteritis, although some *Vibrio* (especially *V. vulnificus*) are capable of producing life threatening extraintestinal infections.

Supplemental Reading

Centers for Disease Control and Prevention. Surveillance for foodborne-disease outbreaks—United States, 1993–1997. MMWR 2000;49:1–62.

Centers for Disease Control and Prevention. Diagnosis and management of foodborne illnesses: a primer for physicians. MMWR 2001;50:1–67.

Centers for Disease Control and Prevention. Norovirus activity—United States, 2002. MMWR 2003;52:41–5.

Daniels NA, MacKinnon L, Bishop R, et al. *Vibrio parahaemolyticus* infections in the United States, 1973–1998. J Infect Dis 2000;181:1661–6.

Dennehy PH, Bresee JS. Rotavirus vaccine and intussusception: where do we go from here? Infect Dis Clin North Am 2001;15:189–207.

DuPont HL. Guidelines on acute infectious diarrhea in adults. Am J Gastroenterol 1997;92:1962–74.

Guerrant RL, Bobak DA. Bacterial and protozoal gastroenteritis. N Engl J Med 1991;325:327–40.

Guerrant RL, Van Gilder T, Steiner TS, et al. Practice guidelines for the management of infectious diarrrhea. Clin Infect Dis 2001;32:331–50.

Kirkpatrick BD. Infectious diarrhea. In: Grace CJ, editor. Medical management of infectious disease. New York: Marcel Dekker; 2003. p. 437–54.

Mahler M, Pasi A, Kramer JM, et al. Fulminant liver failure in association with the emetic toxin of *Bacillus cereus*. N Engl J Med 1997;336:1142–8.

Parashar UD, Bresee JS, Gentsch JR, Glass RI. Rotavirus. Emerg Infectious Diseases 1998;4:561–70.

Pizarro D, Posada G, Sandi L, Moran JR. Rice based oral electrolyte solutions for the management of infantile diarrhea. N Engl J Med 1991;324:517–21.

Powell DW, Szauter KE. Nonantibiotic therapy and pharmacotherapy of acute infectious diarrhea. Gastroenterol Clin North Am 1993;22:683–707.

Procop GW. Gastrointestinal infections. Infect Dis Clin North Am 2001;15:1073–108.

Smith NA, Cron S, Valdez LM, et al. Combination drug therapy for cryptosporidiosis in AIDS. J Infect Dis 1998;178:900–3.

World Health Organization. Cholera vaccines. Wkly Epidemiol Rec 2001;16:117–24.

CHAPTER 50

Traveler's Diarrhea

R. Bradley Sack, MS, MD, ScD

Travel to the developing countries is a marvelous way to experience the diversity of humankind. Visiting historic treasures, observing the wonders of nature, and experiencing the fascinations of different cultures and the taste of new cuisine are the inherent values of this type of travel. Unfortunately, along with the benefits of travel come the possibilities of unusual "tropical" illness, the most frequent of which is *travelers' diarrhea*. Although called by many colorful names (Montezuma's revenge, Delhi belly, Aztec two-step) according to location, they all represent the same illness. This type of illness was first recognized by Kean and Waters in the 1950s as a distinct entity in which large numbers of vacationers and students from the developed world began to visit the developing world, where water and sanitation were substandard (Kean and Waters, 1958). When it was first described it was attributed to changes in composition of food and water and to jet lag, and was thought generally not to be infectious or viral because bacteriological cultures were not helpful in defining an etiologic agent.

Infectious Etiology

When adequate microbiologic studies were done, beginning in the mid-1970s, it became clear that most of the episodes of travelers' diarrhea were associated with infectious agents, the primary one clearly being an *enterotoxigenic Escherichia coli* (ETEC) (Gorbach et al, 1975; Mersen et al, 1976) that was first recognized by Sack in Calcutta, India in 1968.

Immunologically Naïve

With this recognition of infectious agents being responsible for the disease, it became clear that the infectious diarrheas of travelers were basically the same as that of small children living in the areas visited. *Travelers* from developed countries were *immunologically naïve* in a way similar to *children* born into a new environment. During the first several years of life, most *children* experienced these diarrheal illnesses, thereby acquiring relative immunity if they survived. Travelers from the developed world, on the other hand, had never come into contact with these diarrheal pathogens before arriving in the developing country and, therefore, had no immunity and were unusually susceptible. It should be noted that this is not true for travelers from one developing country to another; they already have some immunity from their diarrheal exposures in their own country and, therefore, they experience travelers' diarrhea much less often.

Attack Rate

It has been estimated that during a 3-week trip in a developing country, the attack rate for travelers' diarrhea is about 30 to 40%. In fact, the diarrhea attack rates in travelers are the highest of any groups of people, with the sole exception of the effects of a single source outbreak where drinking water becomes directly contaminated with fecal material (particularly ETEC) such as happened in Crater Lake in 1977.

The Illness

Most *diarrheal illnesses* begin within a few days to a week of entering an area of poor sanitation, but may occur at any time. In fact, they may often be seen to develop on the plane while returning home, often following a large farewell party. Most episodes are acute, with watery diarrhea, nausea, occasionally vomiting, weakness, and, rarely, low grade fever. The number of bowel movements per day is usually three to eight, but may be much higher. Without specific treatment, the illness may last for an average of about 3 days, but may persist for up to 10 days. If the illness lasts greater than 14 days, it is characterized as persistent; this usually indicates that *another set* of enteric pathogens is involved.

In most cases the disease is mild, only causing the travelers to adjust their schedules so that they can be relatively close to a bathroom. It can, however, be severe enough to cause them to cancel plans for excursions in favor of staying in their hotel room. Rarely, is it severe enough to require medical attention and even hospitalization and intravenous (IV) therapy. Yet it is important for the travelers to be able to treat themselves (see later section), and thus prevent the need for hospitalization in a strange and often unsanitary hospital environment.

When the diarrhea obviously contains *blood*, it suggests an invasive pathogen, such as *Shigella* or *Campylobacter*. The patient may have fever, abdominal cramping, and tenesmus. *Antimicrobial therapy* is clearly indicated in this syndrome.

Etiologic Agents

ETEC

The known causes of travelers' diarrhea are shown in Table 50-1. Heading the list in nearly all studies is ETEC. These organisms are the *most common bacterial cause* of diarrhea in *children* living in the developing world, and they are also the most commonly seen in *travelers*. These organisms produce either one or both of two enterotoxins: a *heat labile enterotoxin* (LT), a large molecule that is very closely related to cholera toxin, and a *heat stable* enterotoxin that is a small molecular weight polypeptide. They also possess *colonization factors* (CFAs), proteins that facilitate their binding to the small intestinal mucosa. Both LT and CFAs are *antigenic*, so that infection results in some degree of *immunity*.

ENTEROAGGRATIVE *E. COLI*

A more recently discovered type of *E. coli*, called *enteroaggrative E. coli*, has also been found to be common in travelers' diarrhea. This organism was first recognized by its ability to aggregate when placed in Vero cell cultures. The mechanisms of virulence are not as well described as they are for ETEC, but they are also known to be common causes of diarrhea in children living in the developing world.

TABLE 50-1. Estimates of the Most Frequent Causes of Travelers' Diarrhea

Etiologic Agents	Frequency (%)
Enterotoxigenic *Escherichia coli*	25–40
Enteroaggregative *E. coli*	15–25
Shigella	5
Campylobacter jejuni	5*
Salmonella	< 5*
Giardia lamblia	1–2
Entameba histolytica	< 1
Cyclospora	< 1[†]
Cryptosporidium	< 1
Rotavirus	1
Norovirus	< 1[‡]
Other agents[§]	1
Unknown origin	20–30

Data from Steffen and Sack, 2003; Ericsson et al (editors), 2003; and Sack, 1990.
*These organisms are isolated much more frequently in Thailand.
[†]Found most frequently in Nepal.
[‡]Found frequently in passenger on cruise ships.
[§]These include *Vibrio* sp (including *V. cholerae, V. parahemolyticus*), *Aeromonas*, and other diarrheagenic *Escherichia coli*.

CAMPYLOBACTER

The one organism that is particularly environmentally specific is *Campylobacter jejuni*, which is found mostly as a cause of travelers' diarrhea in *Thailand*. The organism is frequently found in *meats* prepared in the markets there. Because it is also frequently antibiotic resistant, it may require some modification of antimicrobial therapy. *Campylobacter* sp are also the most frequent causes of infectious diarrhea in the United States among young adults, probably because they are widely distributed in commercially prepared (but highly contaminated) *poultry* sold in supermarkets across the United States.

SHIGELLA AND SALMONELLA

Shigella and *Salmonella* are found infrequently in travelers' diarrhea. The presence of bloody stools and/or fever should suggest the possibility of this diagnosis.

OTHER BACTERIAL PATHOGENS

Other bacterial pathogens are very infrequent. There are probably new agents yet to be found.

VIRUSES

Viruses as causes of travelers' diarrhea are *infrequent*; because most adults in the world have had rotavirus infections during their lives, they are relatively resistant to this infection, even though children living in developing countries are highly susceptible and the disease is frequent among them. Recently, however, the *Norwalk agent virus* (Norovirus) has been found to cause several outbreaks of gastrointestinal illness on *cruise ships*. The illness is characterized more by *vomiting* than diarrhea and has been called "winter vomiting disease."

PROTOZOA

With a few exceptions, protozoan parasitic infections are very rarely associated with acute travelers' diarrhea; they are more likely to be associated with persistent diarrheas. *Giardia lamblia* is probably the most frequently recognized organism in the persistent diarrhea of travelers. The organism is ubiquitous in areas where sanitation is less than optimal. *Entamoeba histolytica* is also found infrequently, but can produce severe persistent diarrhea. *Cryptosporidium* is a relatively frequent cause of acute childhood diarrhea in the developing world, but in the developed countries it is usually associated with chronic diarrhea in persons with immune deficiency disease. It may cause an acute episode of diarrhea in travelers which is short lasting. *Cyclospora* is a more recently described parasitic infection in travelers, particularly those visiting or living in Nepal. It rarely seems to be seen in other parts of the world in travelers. Usually producing a persistent diarrhea that may last months, it can be associated with considerable weight loss. *Blastocystis hominis* is frequently found in stools of returned travelers, but there is no evidence that this causes diarrhea. It should be thought of as a nondisease-associated protozoa, such as *E. coli* and *Endolimax nana*.

Epidemiology

Travelers' diarrhea occurs most frequently in areas with the most *inadequate sanitation and water supply* (Steffen and Sack, 2003). This is reflected in the *diarrhea rates of children* living in these areas; if children are frequently infected, then travelers will be also.

The *most adventurous travelers* are most likely to develop disease, particularly because they frequently like to sample exotic dishes and live in more primitive conditions.

Contaminated food and *water* are the sources of the agents that result in travelers' diarrhea. Any drinking water that has not been treated (safely bottled, heated, filtered, or chlorinated) is a potential source of diarrheal pathogens. Because freezing does not kill bacteria, *ice* made from untreated water is particularly hazardous. Foods that have been handled and perhaps rinsed in unclean water are the most dangerous. This includes *fresh vegetable salads*, such as lettuce and tomatoes. Any food that has been adequately cooked is safe. *Milk* products that have not been pasteurized are also hazardous.

The season of the year may also be important in determining when the highest incidence of diarrheal illness will occur. When the weather is warm, bacteria will grow well in food products and, therefore, the risk of ingesting them is increased.

Prevention

Dietary

Being able to eat and drink only clean food and water clearly will protect the traveler from diarrheal illness. Unfortunately this is often impossible to do, because food preparation is being done by the staff of the hotels, resorts, and cruises. A few simple suggestions may help in avoiding the riskiest foods. Avoid fresh vegetable salads, unless they have been disinfected. (This is usually not done in restaurants, but can be done easily in a home kitchen.) Avoid eating fruits that cannot be peeled, such as strawberries or grapes; fruits that can be peeled, such as bananas or oranges are safe no matter where they come from. Avoid eating poorly cooked meat or fish. Avoid eating from food vendors on the street, unless the food is piping hot. Remember that coffee and tea are always safe, because the water has been heated during preparation (Table 50-2).

Prevention with Medication

There have been several studies demonstrating that antimicrobials taken daily during a trip are highly protective (Winstrom et al, 1987). The first studies, done about 30 years ago, showed doxycycline to be highly effective; however, because many bacteria, including *E.coli*, now are resistant to doxycycline this drug is no longer used for that purpose. At present, *Ciprofloxacin* (Cipro) or other *fluoroquinolones* are the drugs of choice. They will prevent about 90% of expected episodes. If used for this purpose, they are taken once a day, beginning 1 day before travel, each day on the trip, and 1 day after leaving. In general these are not

---

TABLE 50-2. Prevention and Treatment of Travelers' Diarrhea

Prevention of Travelers' Diarrhea

    Food and Water Precautions—riskiest foods are fresh vegetable salads and untreated water
    Antimicrobials (optional, see text)—Fluroquinolones can be used od, beginning 1 day before travel, and continuing to 1 day after travel. This regimen can be used safely for at least 3 weeks. This provides about 90% protection against developing travelers' diarrhea.
    Other agents—Bismuth subsalicylate, given qid, has been found to prevent about 60% of travelers' diarrhea. It should not be taken with antibiotics.

Treatment of Travelers' Diarrhea

    Hydration
        Increase oral intake of fluids containing carbohydrates and salt to prevent/treat dehydration.
        Packets of oral rehydratrion solution are ideal for this purpose.
        IV replacement of fluids may be necessary in severe cases.
    Antibiotics*
        Ciprofloxacin (or other fluoroquinolones) bid for 1 to 2 days
        Or Azithromycin (for children or adults) daily for 1 to 2 days
        Or Rifaxamin bid or tid for 3 days
    Symptomatic treatment
        Loperamide—Imodium-like drug can be used after antibiotic started to decrease frequency of bowel movements.

Adapted from Sack, 1990; Ansdell and Ericsson, 1999.
bid = twice daily; od = once daily; qid = four times daily.
*Doxycycline and trimethoprim-sulfamethoxazol are no longer drugs of choice because of the high degree of bacterial resistance to these antimicrobials.

used for longer than 3 weeks at a time. *Pepto-Bismol* has also been used on a four times daily basis and can prevent approximately 60% of episodes. (Although the mechanism of action is not clearly understood, Pepto-Bismol has been found to have both some antibacterial and antitoxic activity.) The disadvantage of taking a medication four times daily during travel mitigates against its frequent use.

Who would benefit from prophylaxis? Only certain travelers are usually thought to be good candidates for drug prophylaxis, such as those who have scheduled appointments that cannot be missed, including musicians on concert tours or lecturers at important meetings. Other categories would include travelers with medical illnesses that could be significantly worsened by an episode of travelers' diarrhea. For most travelers, providing self-treatment is adequate (discussed below). The possible drawbacks of using this type of preventive therapy are the possibility of allergic reactions and the theoretical possibility of facilitating the emergence of antibiotic resistant enteric organisms. This latter concern, however, seems unimportant, because in most developing countries antibiotics are freely available without a prescription and are used widely by the population.

Treatment

The two goals of treatment are to *prevent dehydration* and to *eliminate* the *organisms* causing the infection (see Table 50-2).

Dehydration

Dehydration can be prevented by the intake of adequate fluids and electrolytes during the time of liquid diarrhea. In mild cases, increasing normal fluid intake (juices, soups, etc) is adequate. For more severe cases, an oral rehydration solution (ORS), which was developed to treat severe diarrhea in children, particularly in the developing world, should be taken. An ORS can be used for any type of diarrhea causing significant fluid loss. This solution contains sodium, potassium, chloride, citrate, and a carbohydrate (glucose, sucrose, or rice powder). It is available in packets (Ceralyte, Cera Products, Jessup, Maryland) that can be taken with the traveler to use as indicated. In the rare event of a cholera-like disease, where very large quantities of a watery stool are passed, IV therapy (Ringer's lactate) may be necessary. This requires a visit to a health facility, but can hopefully be avoided with the use of ORSs begun early in the course of the disease.

Antimicrobials

Antimicrobials are recommended to kill the bacterial pathogens (by far the most common cause of travelers' diarrhea) and, thus, cure the illness. The recommended drug at present for most parts of the world is *ciprofloxacin* (Cipro), 500 mg (or comparable doses of other *fluroquinolones*) given twice daily for a relatively short period of time. Initial studies were done using 5 days of therapy, which was then reduced to 3 days. Now the recommended length of treatment is basically 1 day. The drug is first taken when the traveler realizes that he/she is becoming ill, and the second dose is taken 12 hours later. The illness is usually then curtailed within less than 24 hours.

The one area of the world that deserves special mention is *Thailand* and surrounding areas. Here the most frequent organism causing travelers' diarrhea is *Campylobacter*; over the past few years antimicrobial resistance has become frequent and Cipro no longer can be relied on to be effective. In these areas, *azithromycin* (Zithromax) 500 mg per day for 1 to 2 days has been shown to be effective. In the special case of treating *small children*, because cirpofloxacin may be contraindicated, azithromycin can be used in all areas of the world.

A new *nonabsorbable antimicrobial* preparation that may be used for treatment is *Rifaxamin*. It has recently been licensed in the United States as Xifaxan (Salix Pharmaceuticals, Raleigh, North Carolina). The advantages of this drug are that it reaches high concentrations in the bowel and it is not absorbed from the gut. The concentrations achieved are 200 times more than the *minimal inhibitory concentrations (MIC's)* of any of the known bacterial diarrheal pathogens. The drug has gone through several controlled trials and seems to be equivalent to ciprofloxacin or azithromycin in treatment of travelers' diarrhea (Dupont et al, 2001). It is given 2 to 3 times per day (200 or 400 mg) for 3 days. There is the possibility that this drug could also be used for prophylaxis, although this has not yet been studied.

Antisecretory Agents

Antisecretory agents have also been studied for treatment of travelers' diarrhea and have been found to be only moderately effective. None of these preparations are on the market in the United States.

Antimotility agents, such as loperamide, may be useful, when given in addition to antimicrobials, because this combination therapy will result in a quicker resolution of the diarrhea. It is not recommended that antimotility agents be used alone because they have no antimicrobial properties and the disease may persist in spite of temporary symptomatic improvement.

Persistent Diarrhea

Treatment of persistent travelers' diarrhea depends on the identification of the etiologic agents. This, of course, requires stool evaluations for *protozoa*. The rule of thumb is still three stools collected over several days. In some instances a string capsule may be useful in identifying *Giardia* in the upper small intestine. With the exception of *Entamoeba histolytica* infection, serology is not useful in making these diagnoses. *Metronidazole* or tinidazole (Presutti Laboratories, Arlington Heights, Illinois) are the drugs of choice for both *Giardia* and *E. histolytica*. *Trimethoprim-sulfamethoxazole* is the drug for *Cyclospora*. The only drug that has been shown to be effective against *Cryptosporidium* is *nitazoxanide*, but experience with the drug has not yet been extensive.

Sequelae

In most cases, there are no significant sequelae following the diarrheal illness. However, in some cases that present as travelers' diarrhea, underlying illnesses may be unmasked. This is particularly true for irritable bowel syndrome and inflammatory bowel disease. These are usually recognized after a traveler develops a persistent diarrheal illness during travel. During the diagnostic work-up (usually done after returning from travel) these underlying diseases are identified. Tropical sprue has also occasionally been diagnosed in travelers with persistent diarrhea.

Vaccines

There is considerable work being done on the development of vaccines to prevent travelers' diarrhea. Because ETECs are most frequently involved, vaccine development has been targeted at this group of organisms. Any effective vaccine would be useful not only for travelers, but even more importantly for children of the developing world where this organism is the primary bacterial cause of their diarrheal illnesses.

The vaccines being developed are to be used *orally*, to stimulate the local immune mechanisms of the gut. Both killed and live attenuated ETEC vaccines are being studied. For their use in travelers, vaccines would need to be given some time before travel (probably 1 to 2 weeks), and they are anticipated to provide up to 1 year or more of protection. In the developing world, they would be given to children very early in life, because this is the time when the disease is most frequent. They would probably need to be repeated at intervals after that to provide continuous protection.

One travelers' vaccine (Dukoral, Chiron Corporation, Emeryville, California) is marketed in Canada and parts of Europe (not yet in the United States) for the prevention of travelers' diarrhea. The oral vaccine, originally designed for protection against cholera, contains the cholera cell-wall antigens plus the B subunit of cholera toxin (CTB), which is closely related structurally and immunologically to the LT toxin of ETEC. One such study by Peltola and colleagues (1991) in travelers has shown protection, which is thought to be due to the antibodies produced by CTB which cross-react with ETEC that produce LT, thus providing protection against these organisms.

Other vaccines against ETEC are being developed that also include the major colonization factors of ETEC.

Summary

It appears that travelers' diarrhea will be of importance to travelers to the developing world for a long time to come. Improvements in water and sanitation in the countries to be visited are the only way to decrease the frequency of this disease.

Supplemental Reading

Ansdell VE, Ericsson CD. Prevention and empiric treatment of traveler's diarrhea. Med Clin North Am 1999;83:945–73.

DuPont HL, Jiang ZE, Ericsson CD, et al. Rifaximin versus ciprofloxacin for the treatment of travelers' diarrhea: a randomized double-blind clinical trial. Clin Infect Dis 2001;33:1807–15.

Gorbach SL, Kean BH, Evans DG, et al. Travelers' diarrhea and toxigenic *Escherichia coli*. N Engl J Med 1975;292:933–6.

Kean, BH, Waters S. Diarrhea of travelers. I. Incidence in travelers returning to United States from Mexico. AMA Arch Indust Health 1958;18:148–50.

Merson MH, Morris GK, Sack DA, et al. Travelers' diarrhea in Mexico: a prospective study of physicians and family members attending a congress. N Engl J Med 1976;294:1299–305.

Peltola H, Siitonen A, Kryonseppa H, et al. Prevention of travelers' diarrhea by oral subunit/whole-cell cholera vaccine. Lancet 1991;338:1285–9.

Sack RB. Diarrhea producing factors in cultures of *Escherichia coli*. Proceedings of the 4th Joint Conference, Japan-USS Cooperative Medical Science Program 1968;23–9.

Sack RB. Travelers' diarrhea: microbiologic basis for prevention and treatment. Rev Infect Dis 1990;12 Suppl 1:S59–63.

Steffen R, Sack RB. Epidemiology, Chapter 8. In: Ericsson CD, DuPont HL, Steffen R, editors. Travelers' diarrhea. Hamilton (ON): BC Decker Inc; 2003.

Ericsson CD, DuPont HL, Steffen R, editors. Travelers' diarrhea. Hamilton (ON): BC Decker Inc; 2003.

Winstrom J, Norrby SR, Burman LG, et al. Norfloxacin versus placebo for prophylaxis against travelers' diarrhea. J Antimicrob Chemother 1987;20:563–74.

CHAPTER 51

Clostridium difficile and Antibiotic-Associated Diarrhea

John H. Kwon, MD, PhD and Ciarán P. Kelly, MD

An estimated 10 to 15% of patients experience an episode of diarrhea during or after a course of antibiotic treatment (Bartlett, 2002). Most cases of antibiotic-associated diarrhea are benign and self-limited. These require only supportive measures or, if symptoms are severe, the discontinuation of antibiotic treatment. The most serious cause of antibiotic-associated diarrhea is *Clostridium difficile* colitis.

C. difficile is an anaerobic gram-positive, spore-forming bacillus not normally part of the gastrointestinal (GI) flora in adults. Its spores are found in soil and as an environmental contaminant. *C. difficile* colitis is now the most commonly diagnosed cause of infectious diarrhea in hospitalized patients in the developed world (Warny and Kelly, 2003). It has been estimated to account for up to 15% of cases of antibiotic-associated diarrhea and to incur annual treatment costs in excess of $1.1 billion in the United States (Kyne et al, 2002).

Antibiotic administration is thought to disturb the normal colon microflora and increase susceptibility to colonization by pathogenic bacteria. Although most antibiotics have been reported to cause *C. difficile* colitis (Table 51-1), the antibiotics most commonly associated with *C. difficile* infections are amoxicillin/ampicillin, cephalosporin, and clindamycin. The subsequent colonization by *C. difficile* results from environmental exposure, with the main source being hospitals and nursing homes. The production of two exotoxins, toxin A and toxin B, results in colonic injury via the alteration of the enterocyte cytoskeleton with disruption of tight junction function and the activation of a marked inflammatory reaction. Depending on host factors, especially the immune response to *C. difficile* toxins, the outcome of colonization is either asymptomatic carriage or a spectrum of disease ranging from mild diarrhea to fulminant, life threatening pseudomembranous colitis.

Clinical Manifestations

Patients infected with *C. difficile* present with diarrhea, fever, crampy lower abdominal pain, tenesmus, nausea, vomiting, or leukocytosis. Symptoms typically occur during antibiotic treatment with the majority occurring within 14 days of antibiotic administration. However, cases have been documented to occur up to 3 months after antibiotic exposure. The diarrhea associated with *C. difficile* infection is characterized by the passage of frequent loose, foul smelling bowel movements consistent with proctocolitis. Although occult blood may be detected in the stool, visible blood is rare. Extraintestinal manifestations of *C. difficile* infection, such as bacteremia, septic arthritis, or splenic abscess, may occur but are extremely rare. An oligoarticular, asymmetric nondeforming, large joint arthropathy is more common.

Occasionally, patients may develop severe, life threatening, pseudomembranous colitis with a high fever, leukemoid reaction, lower or diffuse abdominal pain, tenderness, or distention. Diarrhea may be minimal or absent, if a toxic megacolon develops. Thus, the resolution of diarrhea with otherwise worsening symptoms or clinical signs should be a cause for major concern. An abdominal radiograph will often reveal a markedly dilated colon (> 7 cm) as well as air fluid levels consistent with an associated small bowel ileus. Complications of toxic megacolon include dehydration, hypoalbuminemia, ascites, electrolyte disturbances, bowel perforation, systemic inflammatory response syndrome, and death.

Interestingly, not all patients infected with *C. difficile* develop symptoms or signs of colitis. Asymptomatic carriage of *C. difficile* is seen in 10 to 16% of hospitalized patients. Specific antitoxin antibody production may play a role in protecting these individuals from *C. difficile* diarrhea, and patients with asymptomatic carriage of *C. difficile* should not be treated.

TABLE 51-1. Antimicrobial Agents that Predispose to *Clostridium difficile* Diarrhea

Frequently	Infrequently	Rarely or Never
Ampicillin and amoxicillin	Tetracyclines	Parenteral aminoglycosides
Cephalosporins	Sulfonamides	Metronidazole
Clindamycin	Macrolides (including erythromycin)	Bacitracin
	Chloramphenicol	Vancomycin
	Trimethoprim	
	Ciprofloxacin	
	Ureidopenicillins	

Adapted from Kelly and Lamont, 1993.

Diagnosis

C. difficile infection should be suspected in any patient presenting with diarrhea within 1 to 3 months of receiving an antibiotic, especially if this was administered in a hospital or nursing home. The diagnosis of *C. difficile* infection is confirmed by the finding of *C. difficile* toxins in the stool.

Several stool tests are available for the diagnosis of *C. difficile* infection (Kyne et al, 2001). The gold standard is the tissue culture cytotoxicity assay for toxin B, with both a high sensitivity and specificity. However, other assays have the advantages of being easier to perform, less expensive, and more rapid. The enzyme-linked immunoassay (EIA) tests for toxins A and B have a high specificity but slightly lower sensitivity. The EIA for toxins A and B is preferred over the EIA for toxin A alone because of its ability to identify toxin A negative/toxin B positive *C. difficile* strains. Polymerase chain reaction and *C. difficile* culture are also available as very sensitive diagnostic tests.

Colonoscopy is not necessary for most patients with suspected *C. difficile* diarrhea. However, gentle visualization of the colon is indicated in those situations where a rapid diagnosis is needed to distinguish pseudomembranous colitis from other causes of abdominal pain, diarrhea, or toxic megacolon. The presence of colonic pseudomembranes in a patient with a history of antibiotic therapy is virtually pathognomonic for *C. difficile* toxin-induced colitis (Figures 51-1 to 51-3). In a very few cases pseudomembranes may be present only in the proximal colon and, therefore, not evident on sigmoidoscopy. Other nonspecific colonoscopic findings include mucosal erythema, edema, and friability.

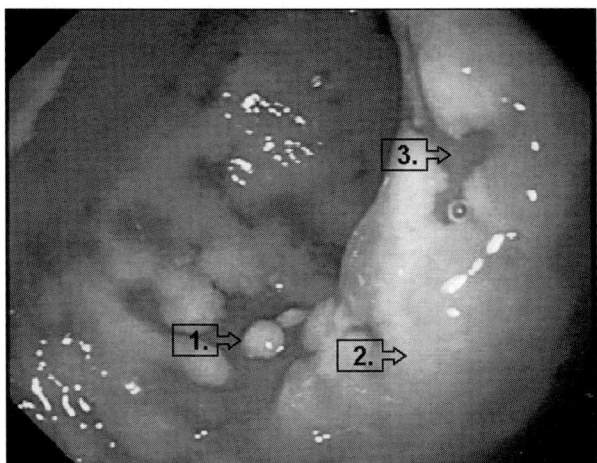

FIGURE 51-1. Colonoscopic appearance of severe pseudomembranous colitis. Raised adherent yellow pseudomembranes are visible on the colonic mucosa (*arrow 1*). In most areas, the plaques have coalesced to form a continuous pseudomembrane (*arrow 2*). There is nonspecific erythema of the colonic mucosa between the pseudomembranes (*arrow 3*).

Management of Mild to Moderately Severe *C. difficile*-Associated Diarrhea

In patients with suspected *C. difficile*-induced diarrhea, the first priority is to discontinue the inciting antibiotic, if it is safe to do so. Up to 25% of all *C. difficile* infections will resolve spontaneously upon the discontinuation of antibiotics. However, patients with more severe symptoms should be treated with specific *C. difficile*-directed antibiotics. The two most commonly used agents are metronidazole and

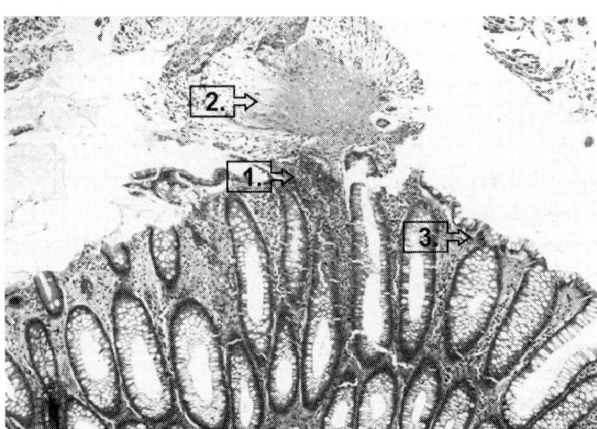

FIGURE 51-2. Specimen from an endoscopic biopsy performed on a patient with pseudomembranous colitis and a "summit" or "volcano" lesion. Focal ulceration of the colonic mucosa is evident (*arrow 1*), with exudation of a pseudomembrane made up of inflammatory cells, fibrin, and necrotic debris (*arrow 2*). The adjoining mucosa is intact (*arrow 3*). (Hematoxylin and eosin, × 55 original magnification). Reproduced with permission from Kelly CP, Pothoulakis C, Lamont JT. *Clostridium difficile* colitis. N Engl J Med 1994;330:257–62.

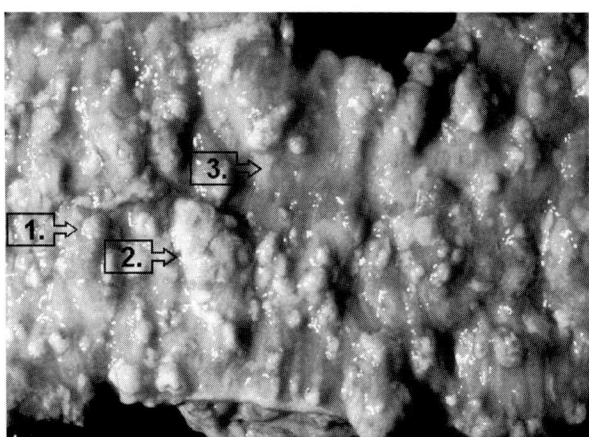

FIGURE 51-3. Colon specimen from a patient with severe, refractory *Clostridium difficile* diarrhea and colitis. Characteristic raised adherent yellow plaques that vary in size from 2 to 10 mm are visible on the colonic mucosa (*arrow 1*). In some areas, coalescing pseudomembranes are visible (*arrow 2*). There is nonspecific erythema of the colonic mucosa between the pseudomembranes (*arrow 3*). Reproduced with permission from Kelly CP, Pothoulakis C, Lamont JT. *Clostridium difficile* colitis. N Engl J Med 1994;330:257–62.

vancomycin. The advantages and disadvantages of each are described below. In addition to metronidazole and vancomycin, bacitracin, teicoplanin, fusidic acid and colestipol have been used to treat *C. difficile* infections.

Metronidazole

Metronidazole (250 to 500 mg given three to four times daily for 10 to 14 days) is now the first line agent for the treatment of *C. difficile* infection. It is less expensive and more readily available than vancomycin and is equally effective in terms of response (90%) and relapse (15 to 25%) rates.

Metronidazole can be given either orally or intravenously. Oral metronidazole is well absorbed high in the GI tract but nonetheless achieves bactericidal concentrations in the stool of patients infected by *C. difficile*. Presumably, metronidazole is secreted through an inflamed intestinal mucosa. Intravenous (IV) metronidazole (500 mg given four times daily) results in stool concentrations comparable to oral dosing and should be used in patients unable to tolerate or absorb oral medications.

Although metronidazole is relatively well tolerated, some patients experience significant side effects including nausea, vomiting, metallic taste, a disulfiram-like reaction to alcohol, and, especially with prolonged use, peripheral neuropathy. It is also contraindicated in children and is considered a class B drug for use in pregnancy and nursing.

Vancomycin

Vancomycin (125 to 500 mg given three or four times daily) is an effective treatment for *C. difficile* colitis. It is neither absorbed from nor metabolized within the GI tract and is excreted virtually unchanged. A lower dose (125 mg three times daily) is recommended for moderate to severe forms of *C. difficile* infection, whereas higher doses (up to 500 mg given four times daily) may be preferable for severe, life threatening *C. difficile* infection. In patients that are unable to tolerate oral treatment, vancomycin can be given in enema formulation (500 mg in 100 mL of normal saline administered every 6 hours) as well as via a nasogastric tube. Unlike metronidazole, vancomycin is ineffective when given intravenously because it does not reach the colonic lumen.

Although the efficacy of oral vancomycin in treating *C. difficile* colitis is excellent and side effects are rare, it should be reserved as a second line agent for two reasons. Firstly, the cost of oral vancomycin is considerably greater than metronidazole. A 10 day course of orally formulated vancomycin may cost as much as $800, whereas a 10 day course of oral metronidazole may cost as little as $20. Secondly, the risk of promoting vancomycin resistance amongst nosocomial bacteria makes metronidazole the favored first line agent. Vancomycin is reserved for patients who are intolerant to metronidazole, fail to respond to metronidazole, are pregnant, or are under the age of 10 years.

Other treatments for *C. difficile* infections that have been published include the use of bacitracin, teicoplanin, fusidic acid, and colestipol (Kyne et al, 2001). Bacitracin (25,000 U given four times a day for 7 to 10 days) is less effective than metronidazole and vancomycin. Teicoplanin, although associated with a slightly lower relapse rate (7%), is not currently available for oral administration in the United States. Fusidic acid and colestipol are associated with lower response rates as compared to metronidazole and vancomycin, and they are not recommended as primary treatments.

Management of Severe *C. difficile* Colitis

Severe, life threatening *C. difficile* colitis requiring an intensive care unit admission occurs in 1 to 3% of patients. These patients often develop high fever, leukocytosis, peritoneal signs, abdominal distention, and progressive signs of sepsis. Based on anecdotal reports of a slightly more rapid response rate, the recommended first line therapy for fulminant *C. difficile* infection is vancomycin. However, in patients unable to tolerate oral antibiotics or nasogastric delivery and in patients with an ileus, IV metronidazole may be the only available option. Additionally, in critically ill patients, combinations of antibiotics should be considered. One study demonstrated responses in 6 of 8 patients with severe *C. difficile* infection who received IV metronidazole plus vancomycin delivered via a nasogastric tube and retention enemas (Olson et al, 1994).

Based on findings of low serum and fecal concentrations of antibodies to *C. difficile* toxins in patients with severe or refractory *C. difficile* diarrhea, it was hypothesized that some patients may benefit from passive immunization with immunoglobulin products (Kyne at al, 2001). Case reports have documented clinical resolution in patients with severe and refractory pseudomembranous colitis following treatment with IV delivery of normal, pooled human immunoglobulin. Although this approach appears promising, controlled trials are required before recommending IV gamma globulin therapy for all patients with severe *C. difficile*-associated colitis.

In patients with fulminant colitis or those with progressive toxic megacolon, surgery to avert bowel perforation may be the only option to prevent death. The current most effective surgical procedure for this condition is a subtotal colectomy. Making the decision of whether and when to perform surgery is difficult due to a high mortality rate (> 40%) associated with emergent surgery for *C. difficile*-associated colitis.

Management of Recurrent *C. difficile*

Recurrence of *C. difficile* infections is seen in 15 to 25% of patients. The cause of the recurrence is thought to be due to several factors. First, the patient's colonization resistance to *C. difficile* has been reduced by treatment with antibiotics including metronidazole or vancomycin. Second, further exposure to *C. difficile* is likely to occur. This may result from the germination of antibiotic resistant spores remaining in the colon. More commonly however the patient is reinfected with *C. difficile* from their hospital or home environment. Recurrence of *C. difficile* infection is rarely caused by metronidazole or vancomycin resistance.

Several approaches to the treatment of *C. difficile* recurrence have been employed (Kyne et al, 2001). If patients experience a mild recurrence of diarrhea without concerning signs or symptoms, conservative management without antibiotics may be used. However, if symptoms are more severe or persistent, antibiotics or alternative therapies should be considered.

Patients with their first episode of *C. difficile* recurrence may receive a second course of the same antibiotic used to treat their initial infection. Most patients (92%) will respond to this treatment. However, greater than 50% of patients with at least one recurrence will have a subsequent recurrence. For patients with multiple recurrences of diarrhea and a confirmed *C. difficile* stool toxin assay, a prolonged vancomycin or metronidazole regimen has been recommended (Table 51-2).

Anion binding resins have been used as an adjunct to antibiotic treatment for recurrent *C. difficile*. Cholestyramine (4 g given 3 to 4 times a day for 1 to 2 weeks) is the most commonly used regimen. However, because of its ability to bind vancomycin, cholestyramine and vancomycin should be given 2 to 3 hours apart.

Probiotics, microbial supplements capable of colonizing the bowel with nonpathogenic strains of bacteria or yeast, are increasingly being used in the management of recurrent *C. difficile* diarrhea. *Saccharomyces boulardii* was shown in a randomized, double blind, placebo controlled trial to reduce recurrence in patients with multiple episodes of *C. difficile* diarrhea. Several other formulations have been used in uncontrolled trials, including oral administration of *Lactobacillus* gamma globulin, nontoxigenic *C. difficile*, and *Saccharomyces cerevisiae*, as well as rectal or nasogastric delivery of nonautologous feces and mixtures of colonic bacteria.

Similar to patients with severe *C. difficile* infection, patients with recurrent *C. difficile* diarrhea have low serum antibody levels against *C. difficile* toxins. Treatment with normal, pooled IV gamma globulin was associated with an increased level of serum antitoxin and reduced recurrence of *C. difficile* diarrhea in six children with relapsing *C. difficile* colitis. This approach may be promising, but controlled studies are required before recommending this as a therapeutic regimen for recurrent *C. difficile* diarrhea. A *C. difficile* vaccine, based on inactivated toxins A and B, has been produced and was well tolerated and highly immunogenic in healthy volunteers. Again, controlled trials are needed to determine whether vaccination can protect susceptible individuals against *C. difficile* infection and colitis.

Prevention

Practice guidelines for the prevention of *C. difficile* infections established by the American College of Gastroenterology (ACG) Practice Parameters Committee were published in 1997 (Fekety, 1997) (Table 51-3). Guidelines emphasized the limitation of antimicrobial usage and the use of universal precautions, including handwashing between patient contact, using gloves when handling bodily substances, using disposable thermometer covers, and using enteric isolation procedures for patients infected with *C. difficile*. The ACG also recommends disinfecting contaminated objects and surfaces with sodium hypochlorite, alkaline glutaraldehyde, or ethylene oxide. Education of physician and nursing staff regarding the disease and its epidemiology is highly recommended.

TABLE 51-2. Approach to Management of Recurrent *Clostridium difficile* Colitis

First relapse
   Confirm diagnosis
   Symptomatic treatment if symptoms are mild
   14-day course of metronidazole or vancomycin
Second relapse
   Confirm diagnosis
   Prolonged course of metronidazole or vancomycin eg, metronidazole 250 to 500 mg tid for 14 days, then 250 mg for 21 days
   or vancomycin 125 mg qid for 14 days, then 125 mg bid for 21 days
Further relapse
   Vancomycin plus cholestyramine 4 g bid
   or vancomycin 125 mg qid and rifampin 600 mg bid
   or therapy with microorganisms eg, *Saccharomyces boulardii* in combination with metronidazole or vancomycin
   or intravenous immunoglobulin

Adapted from Linevsky and Kelly, 1997.

TABLE 51-3. Practice Guidelines for *Clostridium difficile* Prevention

1. Limit the use of antimicrobial drugs
2. Wash hands between contact with all patients
3. Use enteric (stool) isolation precautions for patients with *C. difficile* diarrhea
4. Wear gloves when contacting patients with *C. difficile* diarrhea or their environment
5. Disinfect objects contaminated with *C. difficile* with sodium hypochlorite, alkaline glutaraldehyde, or ethylene oxide
6. Educate the medical, nursing, and other appropriate staff members about the disease and its epidemiology.

Reproduced with permission from Fekety, 1997.

Supplemental Reading

Bartlett JG. Clinical practice. Antibiotic-associated diarrhea. N Engl J Med 2002;346:334–9.

Fekety R. Guidelines for the diagnosis and management of *Clostridium difficile*–associated diarrhea and colitis. American College of Gastroenterology, Practice Parameters Committee. Am J Gastroenterol 1997;92:739–50.

Kelly CP, Lamont JT. Treatment of *Clostridium difficile* diarrhea and colitis. In: Wolfe MM, editor. Gastrointestinal pharmacotherapy. Philadelphia: WB Saunders; 1993. p. 199–212.

Kyne L, Farrell RJ, Kelly CP. *Clostridium difficile*. Gastroenterol Clin North Am 2001;30:753–77, ix–x.

Kyne L, Hamel MB, Polavaram R, Kelly CP. Health care costs and mortality associated with nosocomial diarrhea due to *Clostridium difficile*. Clin Infect Dis 2002;34:346–53.

Linevsky JK, Kelly CP. *Clostridium difficile* colitis. In: Lamont JT, editor. Gastrointestinal infections: diagnosis and management. New York: Marcel Dekker; 1997. p. 293–325.

Olson MM, Shanholtzer CJ, Lee JT Jr, Gerding DN. Ten years of prospective *Clostridium difficile*–associated disease surveillance and treatment at the Minneapolis VA Medical Center, 1982–1991. Infect Control Hosp Epidemiol 1994;15:371–81.

Warny M, Kelly CP. Pathogenicity of *Clostridium difficile* toxins. In: Hecht G, editor. Microbial pathogenesis and the intestinal epithelial cell. Washington: ASM Press; 2003. p. 503–23.

CHAPTER 52

INTESTINAL PARASITES

AMITA GUPTA, MD, AND ROBERT C. BOLLINGER, MD, MPH

Intestinal parasites are important causes of morbidity and mortality, particularly in resource poor settings. Disease accompanying these infections can manifest as a nutritional disturbance. Reduced food intake, impaired digestion, malabsorption, anemia and poor growth rate are among the many possible sequelae that can occur. In the United States and other developed nations, intestinal parasites are most prevalent among returning travelers, immigrant groups, and immunocompromised hosts. Domestic infection occurs in settings such as community waterborne outbreaks, persons who drink untreated stream water, children and employees of daycare centers, men who have sex with men, and persons eating raw or undercooked beef, pork, or fish.

Most intestinal parasites are treatable. Many, but not all, of the drugs discussed in this chapter are commercially available in the United States. Some are licensed for one indication, but not others. Certain drugs used to treat parasites discussed in this chapter are not commercially available in the United States, but may be obtained from the Centers for Disease Control and Prevention Drug Service at 404-639-3670 <www.cdc.gov/ncidod/dpd>.

Useful summaries of drug therapies for intestinal parasites can be found in *The Medical Letter on Drugs and Therapeutics, Sanford Guide* (Gilbert et al, 2003), *Current Medical Diagnosis and Treatment* (Goldsmith, 2003), or other references (supplemental reading).

Protozoan Infections

Balantidium coli (Balantidiasis)

Balantidium coli is a large ciliated protozoa that rarely causes disease in humans and is very rarely reported in the United States. Most infections are asymptomatic and do not need treatment. If mild to moderate diarrhea or chronic, recurrent diarrhea occurs, then the treatment of choice is *tetracycline* (500 mg 4 times daily for 10 days). Alternatively, *iodoquinol* (650 mg 3 times daily for 20 days) can be used. Occasional success has also been reported using *metronidazole* (750 mg 3 times daily for 5 days) or *paromomycin*.

Blastocystis hominis

The clinical significance of this organism is controversial. In general, symptomatic *Blastocystis hominis* infection should be a diagnosis of exclusion and not treated, until an extensive workup has been completed to rule out other pathogens. *Metronidazole* (750 mg orally 3 times daily for 10 days), *iodoquinol* (650 mg 3 times daily for 20 days), or in metronidazole-resistant cases, trimethoprim-sulfamethoxazole (*TMP-SMX*) can be used.

Cryptosporidium parvum (Cryptosporidiosis)

This organism is a spore-forming protozoan that is highly infectious and is transmitted directly from person-to-person or by contaminated water or food. An estimated 300,000 illnesses occur annually in the United States, and approximately 1 to 3% of the US population is estimated to be asymptomatic carriers. In immunocompetent persons, the illness is usually self-limited, lasting from 7 to 28 days, and ranges from mild diarrhea with flatulence to more severe nonbloody, watery diarrhea. In immunocompromised persons, particularly those with acquired immunodeficiency syndrome (AIDS), chronic diarrhea commonly occurs (accounts for 10 to 30% of AIDS patients with chronic diarrhea not on antiretroviral therapy) and a fulminant illness characterized by profuse, cholera-like watery diarrhea, electrolyte imbalance, weight loss, and malabsorption can result. Biliary tract infection (cholangitis) can also occur. Diagnosis is made by examining up to three stools for characteristic oocysts, using a modified acid-fast stain. Prior to the advent of highly active antiretroviral treatment, persons with AIDS and cryptosporidiosis had no effective treatment options. *Paromomycin* (500 mg orally 3 times daily or 1,000 mg twice daily) is of *marginal efficacy* and alternatives, such as nitazoxanide, azithromycin, octreotide, roxithromycin, and spiramycin, have been shown to be ineffective. The key to treating this illness in AIDS patients now depends on reconstituting the immune system with effective antiretroviral therapy and managing symptoms with antidiarrheals, fluids, and nutritional support. There is a separate chapter on human immunodeficiency virus (HIV) infection (see

Chapter 46, "Gastrointestinal and Nutritional Complications of HIV Infection"). Treatment for immunocompetent persons is generally targeted at symptom management, as the illness is self-limited (Chen et al, 2002).

Cyclospora cayetanensis (Cyclosporiasis)

This pathogen has a similar presentation as cryptosporidium in immunocompetent persons and is a rare cause of chronic diarrhea in immunocompromised persons. Effective treatment is with *TMP* (160 mg)-*SMZ* (800 mg) twice daily for 3 to 7 days in immunocompetent; higher doses (4 times daily) and longer maintenance treatment (3 times per week) may be needed for immunosuppressed patients.

Dientamoeba fragilis

Often asymptomatic, this organism can cause a mild-to-moderate diarrhea. It has been hypothesized that *Dientamoeba fragilis* is transmitted by the pinworm, *Enterobius vermicularis*, and therefore concomitant pinworm should be ruled out. Treatment includes *iodoquinol* (650 mg 3 times daily for 20 days) or alternatively *paromomycin, tetracycline,* or *metronidazole* (see Table 52-1 for doses).

Entamoeba histolytica and Entamoeba dispar (Amebiasis)

It is now recognized that entamoeba contains the following two morphologically identical species: (1) *Entamoeba dispar,* which colonizes the colon as an asymptomatic commensal organism and (2) *Entamoeba histolytica,* which has varying degrees of virulence ranging from asymptomatic colon colonization to invasive disease.

Entamoeba are present worldwide but are most prevalent in tropical and subtropical areas, particularly under conditions of poor sanitation, malnutrition, and crowding. An estimated 500 million persons worldwide are infected with entamoeba; 90% are *E. dispar* and 10% are *E. histolytica*. *E. dispar* does not require treatment but labs rarely differentiate between these two species. Humans are the only hosts for entamoeba. Transmission occurs through ingestion of cysts from fecally contaminated food or water; person-to-person and sexual transmission can also occur. Although entamoeba infections occur frequently among men who have sex with men, these infections are usually due to *E. dispar*. Diagnosis of intestinal amebiasis is made either by detecting the antigen or the organism in stool.

Amebiasis presents clinically as extraintestinal and intestinal disease, which is further subdivided into three clinical syndromes.

ASYMPTOMATIC INFECTION

Many entamoeba infections are asymptomatic. In asymptomatic cyst-passers, if the stool antigen and serum antibody tests are negative, it can be presumed that the patient has an *E. dispar* infection, which should not be treated. However, if asymptomatic *E. histolytica* infection is detected, treatment with one of the poorly-absorbed, luminal-acting oral drugs, such as *paramomycin* or *iodoquinol*, or alternatively *diloxanide furoate* is recommended to eliminate all cysts and prevent possible relapse (Gilbert et al, 2003).

MILD TO MODERATE COLITIS (NONDYSENTERIC)

Occasionally, *E. histolytica* infections are characterized by nonbloody diarrhea, abdominal cramps, flatulence, fatigue, and weight loss. Fever is uncommon. Treatment includes *metronidazole*, a potent, well-absorbed drug that is active both in the bowel lumen and wall, as well as in other tissues. Metronidazole, however, is often not sufficient as a luminal amebicide when used alone (up to 50% failure rate) and therefore should be followed with one of the *luminal-acting* oral drugs (*iodoquinol, paramomycin,* or *diloxinide furoate*).

SEVERE COLITIS (DYSENTERY)

Rarely, amebiasis presents with severe abdominal cramps, chills, fever, and tenesmus. Stools are liquid and contain bloody mucus. Rarely, fulminant disease can result in massive destruction of the mucosa with hemorrhage, perforation, or peritonitis. Treatment includes *metronidazole*, in addition to either *iodoquinol* or *diloxanide furoate*. If parenteral administration is required, *metronidazole* can be *administered intravenously (IV)*. But, the regimen should be switched to oral administration as soon it can be tolerated; other luminal amebicides are not available in IV formulation.

Enterocytozoan bienusi and Encephalitozoon intestinales (Microsporidiosis)

This organism's clinical presentation is similar to that of cryptosporidium and isospora. In immunocompetent patients, the diarrheal illness is usually self-limited. In immunocompromised persons, particularly AIDS patients with CD4 < 100/mm^3, it is a common cause of chronic diarrhea and can be remitting over months. Treatment depends on the species identified. For *Encephalitozoon intestinales*, the preferred regimen is *albendazole* 400 mg orally 2 times daily for at least 3 weeks; alternatively, *metronidazole* 500 mg orally three times daily has variable efficacy. Only recently, a small study among immunocomprised patients identified an effective treatment for *Enterocytozoan bieneusi*: *fumagillin* 60 mg/d for 14 days (Molina et al, 2002). Fumagillin, however, is associated with high rates of neutropenia and thrombocytopenia. For AIDS patients, again *immune reconstitution* with antiretroviral therapy is often the best therapy.

TABLE 52-1. Drug Therapy for Intestinal Protozoan Parasites

Parasite	Drug	Adult Dosage	Pediatric Dosage	Availability/Comments
Balantidium coli (Balantidiasis)				
Drug(s) of choice	Tetracycline	500 mg qid × 10 d	40 mg/kg/d (max 2 g) in 4 doses × 10 d	—
Alternative	Metronidazole	750 mg tid × 5 d	35 to 50 mg/kg/d in 3 doses × 5 d	—
Or	Iodinoquinol	650 mg tid after meals x 20 d	40 mg/kg/d (max 2 g) in 3 doses × 20 d	—
Blastocystis homini	Metronidazole	750 mg tid × 5 d	35 to 50 mg/kg/d in 3 doses × 5 d	Treatment controversial
Or	Iodoquinol	650 mg tid × 20 d	30–40 mg/kg/d (max 2 g) in 3 doses × 20 d	—
Cryptosporidium parvum (cryptosporidiosis)				
Immunocompetent	Nitazoxanide	500 mg bid × 3 d	200 mg bid (4–11 yr); 100 mg bid (1–3 yr)	Consider no treatment
HIV-infected	Paromomycin	1 g bid × 4 wks then alone	—	—
And	Azithromycin	600 mg qd × 4 wks	—	Treat with HIV antiretrovirals as most efficacious
Cyclospora cayetanensis				
Drug(s) of choice	Trimethoprim-sulfamethoxazole	160 mg TMP, 800 mg SMX bid × 7–10 d	TMP 5 mg/kg, SMX 25 mg/kg bid × 7–10 d	1 DS po bid
Dientamoeba fragilis				
Drug(s) of choice	Iodoquinol	650 mg tid × 20 d	30–40 mg/kg/d (max 2 g) in 3 doses × 20 d	
Or	Paromomycin	25–35 mg/kg/d in 3 doses × 7 d	25–35 mg/kg/d in 3 doses × 7 d	
Or	Tetracycline	500 mg qid × 10 d	40 mg/kg/d (max 2 g) in 4 doses × 10 d	
Or	Metronidazole	500–750 mg tid × 10 d	20–40 mg/kg/d in 3 doses × 10 d	
Entamoeba histolytica (Amebiasis)				
Asymptomatic				
Drug(s) of choice	Iodoquinol	650 mg tid after meals × 20 d	30–40 mg/kg/d (max 2 g) in 3 doses × 20 d	
Or	Paramomycin	25–35 mg/kg/d in 3 doses × 7 d	25–35 mg/kg/d in 3 doses × 7d	
Alternative	Diloxanide furoate	500 mg tid × 10 d	20 mg/kg/d in 3 doses × 10 d	Not commercially available but can be compounded by Medical Center Pharmacy (203-688-6816) or Panorama Compounding Pharmacy (800-292-6773)
Mild to moderate intestinal disease				
Drug(s) of choice	Metronidazole	500–750 mg tid × 7–10 d	35–50 mg/kg/d in 3 doses × 7–10 d	
Or	Tinidazole	800 mg tid × 3 d	50 mg/kg (max 2 g) qd × 3 d	Not commercially available in the US. As effective as metronidazole and better tolerated.
Plus	Iodoquinol OR Paramomycin OR Diloxanide furoate	Same as asymptomatic regimen	Same as asymptomatic regimen	
Severe intestinal disease				
Drug(s) of choice	Metronidazole	750 mg tid × 7–10 d	35–50 mg/kg/d in 3 doses × 7–10 d	
Or	Tinidazole	800 mg tid × 5 d	35-50 mg/kg/d in 3 doses × 7–10 d	
Plus	Iodoquinol OR Diloxanide furoate	Same as asymptomatic regimen	Same as asymptomatic regimen	
If parenteral therapy needed	Metronidazole IV	0.5–1g IV q12h	7.5 mg/kg q6h > 28 days old	Luminal agent helps prevent relapse/extraintestinal disease
Enterocytozoon bienusi (microsporidiosis)				
Drug(s) of choice	Fumagillin	60 mg/d po × 14 d		
Encephalitozoon [Septata] intestinalis (microsporidiosis)				
Drug(s) of choice	Albendazole	400 mg bid × 21 d		
Giardia lamblia (giardiasis)				
Drug(s) of choice	Metronidazole	250 mg tid × 5 d OR 2 g qd × 3 d	15–30 mg/kg/d in 3 doses × 5 d	
Alternatives	Albendazole	400 mg qd × 5 d	—	—
OR	Quinacrine	100 mg tid × 5 d (maximum 300 mg/d)	2 mg/kg × 5 d (max 300 mg/d)	Not available commerically in the US, but can be compounded
OR	Tinidazole	2 g once	50 mg/kg once (max 2 g)	Not available commercially in US
OR	Furazolidone	100 mg qid × 7–10 d	6 mg/kg/d in 4 doses × 7–10 d	
OR	Paramomycin	25–35 mg/kg/d in 3 doses × 3 doses × 7 d	25–35 mg/kd/d in 3 doses × 7 d	
OR	Nitazoxanide	500 mg bid × 3 d		
Isospora belli (Isosporiasis)				
Drug(s) of choice	Trimethoprim-sulfamethoxazole	160 mg TMP, 800 mg SMX bid ×10 d	TMP 5 mg/kd, SMX 25 mg/kg bid × 10 d	1 DS po bid

Adapted from *The Medical Letter on Drugs and Therapeutics*, 2002; Gilbert et al, 2003; Goldsmith, 2003.

bid = twice daily; HIV = human immunodeficiency virus; IV = intravenous; max = maximum; po = by mouth; qd = every day; qid = 4 times daily; q6h = every 6 hours; q12h = every 12 hours; SMX = sulfamethoxazole; tid = 3 times daily; TMP = trimethoprim.

Giardia lamblia (Giardiasis)

A protozoal infection of the upper small intestine, giardiasis results from ingestion of cysts that can be transmitted by fecally contaminated water or food, person-to-person contact, or oral-anal sexual contact. The parasite occurs worldwide. With an estimated 2 million infections occurring annually in the United States it is the most common intestinal protozoan pathogen in the United States. A large proportion of infected persons remain asymptomatic and the infection resolves spontaneously. Giardia can cause three clinical syndromes, including (1) acute diarrhea, which is often mild, (2) chronic diarrhea, and (3) malabsorption. The diarrhea is usually watery, nonbloody, malodorous and greasy and is often accompanied with flatulence and distension. The diagnosis can be made by *3 sequential stool examinations collected every 2 days* or more or by *stool antigen* detection using enzyme-linked immunosorbent assays (ELISA) and immunoflourescent assays (IFA). These tests have a high sensitivity (85 to 98%) and specificity (90 to 100%). But since other stool pathogens are typically being ruled out as well, stool examination is preferred.

Treatment of asymptomatic persons is controversial but can be considered if there is concern that the person may transmit the infection to others. The drug of choice in the United States is *metronidazole* (250 mg 3 times daily for 5 to 7 days) (Gardner and Hill, 2001). *Tinidazole* as a single 2 g dose is very effective as well (90 to 100% cure rates) but this drug is not available in the United States. Less commonly used regimens include *furazolidone* (100 mg 4 times daily for 7 to 10 days), which causes similar side effects to metronidazole and can cause mild hemolysis in G6PD-deficient persons. Treatment with *albendazole* (400 mg daily for 5 days) or *paramomycin* (25 to 35 mg/kg/d divided in 3 doses for 7 days) have had mixed results and are not commonly used.

Quinacrine (100 mg 3 times daily after meals for 5 to 7 days) should be used only when no other drug is available because of its rare potential for severe toxicity (toxic psychosis and exfoliative dermatitis). Other side effects include a bitter taste, gastrointestinal (GI) intolerance, headache, dizziness, and, rarely, harmless yellowing of the skin. Also this drug is not easily available in the United States and can only be obtained via two pharmacies (1-800-247-9767 or 203-688-6818). Rarely drug resistance or treatment failures occur and retreatment with an alternative drug is required.

Isospora belli (Isosporiasis)

This organism's clinical presentation is similar to that of cryptosporidium. It is an opportunistic infection that causes chronic, watery diarrhea in AIDS patients (CD4 < 100/mm^3). Unlike cryptosporidium, effective treatments for *Isospora belli* are available, including *trimethoprim* (160 mg) and *sulfamethoxazole* (800 mg) taken either as 2 double strength (DS) orally twice daily or, if immunocompromised, 1 DS 3 times daily for 10 days to 4 weeks, or *sulfadiazine* (4 g) and *pyrimethamine* (35 to 75 mg) in 4 divided doses, plus *leucovorin calcium* (10 to 25 mg daily) for 3 to 7 weeks. In immunocompromised patients, it may be necessary to use a *maintenance suppressive* therapy with preferably *TMP-SMX* either 1 to 2 DS daily or 3 times a week, or alternatively *pyrimethamine* 25 mg and *leucovorin* 5 mg/d perhaps indefinitely until immune recovery occurs.

Helminthic Infections

Trematodes (Flukes)

CLONORCHIS SINENSIS AND OPISTHORCHIS VIVERRINI (LIVER FLUKES)

Clonorchis sinensis (Chinese liver fluke) and *Opisthorchis viverrini* (Southeast Asian liver fluke) primarily infect the bile ducts. The illness usually is asymptomatic, but mild or severe illness with epigastric or right upper quadrant pain, fever, leukocytosis and eosinophilia may occur in the acute phase. A sclerosing cholangitis or choledocholithiasis can occur in the chronic phase. The diagnosis is usually made by finding eggs in the stool. The drug of choice is *praziquantel*. Alternatively, *albendazole* (10 mg/kg for 7 days) can be used for *C. sinensis*. *Fasciola hepatica* (sheep liver fluke), similarly can cause acute and chronic infections of the liver and biliary tract. The treatment of choice is *bithionol* (an investigational drug available from the Centers for Disease Control and Prevention) or *triclabendazole* (10 mg/kg once). But, this drug is only available by special request from its manufacturer, Novartis.

FASCIOLOPSIS BUSKI, HETEROPHYES HETEROPHYES, METAGONIMUS YOKOGAWAI (INTESTINAL FLUKES)

These infections are very rare in the United States. The drug of choice is 1 day of *praziquantel* (75 mg/kg/d in 3 doses). An alternative is *niclosamide* (not available in the United States) administered every other day for 3 days.

SCHISTOSOMA MANSONI AND SCHISTOSOMA JAPONICUM (SCHISTOSOMIASIS)

The most common form of intestinal schistosomiasis is due to *Schistosoma mansoni*, which is common in Africa, Arabian peninsula, South America, and the Carribean. *S. japonicum* is important in East Asia. Up to 35% of infections are asymptomatic. The disease usually causes intestinal symptoms when it is in a chronic stage, which occurs 6 months to several years after infection, presenting as diarrhea, abdominal pain, blood in stool, and hepatosplenomegaly. Treatment should be given only if live ova are identified in stool specimens. The treatment of choice for all schistosomiasis infections is one day of *praziquantel*, which has cure rates of 80 to 90%. Alternatively, *oxamniquine* can be used for *S. mansoni* infections only (see tables for exact doses).

Cestodes (Tapeworms)

Six tapeworms, three large and three small, commonly infect humans. The large tapeworms include *Taenia saginata* (beef tapeworm, up to 25 m in length), *Taenia solium* (pork tapeworm, up to 7 m), and *Diphyllobothrium latum* (fish tapeworm, up to 10 m). Infection with the large tapeworms occurs by eating raw or undercooked beef, pork, or brackish or freshwater fish, respectively. Infection with these tapeworms is generally asymptomatic or occasionally vague GI symptoms or systemic symptoms occur. The small tapeworms are *Hymenolepis nana* (dwarf tapeworm, 25 to 40 mm), *Hymenolepis dimunata* (rodent tapeworm, 20 to 60 cm), and *Dipylidium caninum* (dog tapeworm, 10 to 70 cm). A light burden of these small tapeworms is generally asymptomatic, whereas a heavy burden may cause diarrhea, abdominal pain, anorexia, weight loss, vomiting, and malaise. Diagnosis is made by stool examination for worm segments or eggs.

For treatment of all cestodes, the drug of choice is *praziquantel* and an alternative is *niclosamide* (not available in the United States). *Praziquantel* in a single dose of 10 mg/kg achieves a 99% cure for *T. saginata, T. solium* and *D. latum*, and a single dose of 25 mg/kg achieves a 95% cure for *H. nana*. Praziquantel is also effective for *H. dimunuta* and *D. caninum*, but cure rates are not known. Niclosamide, which is very well tolerated, needs to be taken on an empty stomach and chewed completely; it is taken as a single dose for *T. saginata, D. latum,* and *T. solium*, is less effective than praziquantal for *H. nana* and requires a 5 to 7 day course for treatment of *H. dimunata* and *D. caninum*.

Nematodes (Roundworms)

ANGIOSTRONGYLIASIS COSTARICENSIS (ANISAKIASIS)

Angiostrongyliasis costaricensis causes an eosinophilic ileocolitis. Infection occurs following ingestion of larva in the intermediate host (slug, snails) or from food contaminated by larvae from slug or snail mucus. Clinically, it can present as fever, right lower quadrant pain, abdominal mass, leukocytosis, and eosinophilia. Complications such as perforation, bleeding, intestinal obstruction, or infarction can occur. There is no specific treatment; mebendazole, albendazole, or *thiabendazole* can be tried and operative treatment may be necessary.

ASCARIS LUMBRICOIDES (ASCARIASIS)

With an estimated 1 billion people infected worldwide, it is among the most common intestinal helminthes. Adult worms can reach up to 20 to 40 cm. Clinically, if the worm burden is small then no symptoms are apparent. With heavy worm burden, peptic ulcer-like symptoms and vague abdominal discomfort can occur. Rarely, the worms migrate to other areas of the abdomen and the respiratory tract. Treatment of choice is *albendazole, mebendazole* or *pyrantel pamoate,* with cure rates of 85 to 100% (Bennett and Guyatt, 2000). A word of caution, treatment with antihelminthics or anasthesia can cause the worms to migrate. In pregnancy, treatment should occur after the first trimester. Stools should be rechecked at 2 weeks and patients retreated until all worms are removed.

ENTEROBIUS VERMICULARIS (PINWORM)

Children are the most commonly infected. Clinically, many infections are asymptomatic. But, when symptoms occur, perianal pruritis, especially at night, is most notable. Treatment of all symptomatic persons should occur and in some instances it is recommended to treat household contacts. Treatment is highly effective (95 to 100%), can be taken with or without food, and is easy to administer. The drugs of choice include *pyrantel pamoate*, which is available as self-medication in the United States, a single dose of *albendazole,* or a single dose of *mebendazole,* which should be chewed for best effect.

NECATOR AMERICANUS AND ANCYLOSTOMA DUODENALE (HOOKWORM)

Infections with these hookworms are very common worldwide; up to 25% of the world's population are thought to be infected with these parasites. The infection can be asymptomatic or can have skin, pulmonary or intestinal manifestations; in heavy worm burden, iron-deficient anemia is a common consequence of hookworm infection. *Mebendazole, pyrantel,* and *albendazole* are all highly efficacious treatments. All 3 drugs can be given for 1 to 3 days depending on worm burden. *Ferrous sulfate* is also recommended for 1 to 3 months if anemia is present.

STRONGYLOIDES STERCORALIS (STRONGYLOIDIASIS)

Approximately 60 million persons are infected worldwide and the disease is most common in immigrants from endemic areas. The parasite has a unique autoinfection cycle that can result in years of self-perpetuating chronic infection. Up to 30% of infections are asymptomatic. However, cutaneous, pulmonary, intestinal and hyperinfection syndromes can occur and range in severity. Diagnosis can be difficult but *ELISA* and *Western blot* have improved detection of this illness. *Ivermectin* (200 µg/kg/d for 1 to 2 days) is the drug of choice with cure rates of 82 to 95% (Gann et al, 1994). Alternatively, *thiabendazole* (50 mg/kg/d in 2 doses for 2 to 3 days, taken after meals, and repeated after 2 weeks) can be used with similar efficacy. However, it has greater potential toxicity (eg, Stephens Johnson). *Albendazole* (400 mg twice daily for 3 to 7 days and repeated in 1 week) can also be used, but it is less effective. Prolonged treatment, repeat therapy or change in therapy may be needed in those with severe infections or immunosuppression.

TRICHOSTRONGYLUS SP

The clinical symptoms of this parasite infection resemble *strongyloides* and it can cause eosinophilia. Very rare in the United States, the disease generally occurs in Iran, Korea, and Indonesia. Treatment of choice is with *pyrantel pamoate* or, alternatively, with *mebendazole* or *albendazole*.

TRICHURIS TRICHIURA (WHIPWORM)

A common parasite worldwide, whipworm is most prevalent and burdensome in children. Persons with aymptomatic, light infections do not require treatment. For heavier (30,000 or more eggs/g of feces) or symptomatic cases as manifested by abdominal cramps, tenesmus, diarrhea, nausea, and other GI symptoms, *mebendazole* or *albendazole* can be used.

Available data on safety of these drugs for use in pregnant or lactating women and young children are summarized in Table 52-3. Common side effects of important drugs are shown in Table 52-4.

TABLE 52-2. Drug Therapy for Intestinal Helminths

Parasite	Drug	Adult Dosage	Pediatric Dosage
Ancylostoma duodenale, Necator americansus (Hookworm)			
Drug(s) of choice	Albendazole	400 mg once	400 mg once
Or	Mebendazole	100 mg bid × 3 d or 500 mg once	100 mg bid × 3 d or 500 mg once
Or	Pyrantel pamoate	11 mg/kg once (max 1 g)	11 mg/kg once (max 1 g)
Ascaris lumbricoides (Ascariasis, roundworm)			
Drug(s) of choice	Albendazole	400 mg once	400 mg once
Or	Mebendazole	100 mg bid × 3 d or 500 mg once	100 mg bid × 3 d or 500 mg once
Or	Pyrantel pamoate	11 mg/kg once (max 1 g)	11 mg/kg once (max 1 g)
Clonorchis silensis (Chinese liver fluke)			
Drug(s) of choice	Praziquantel	75 mg/kg/d in 3 doses × 1 d	75 mg/kg/d in 3 doses × 1 d
Or	Albendazole	10 mg/kg × 7 d	10 mg/kg × 7 d
Enterobius vermicularis (Pinworm)			
Drug(s) of choice	Pyrantel pamoate	11 mg/kg once (max 1 g); repeat in 2 weeks	11 mg/kg once (max 1 g); repeat in 2 weeks
Or	Mebendazole	100 mg once; repeat in 2 weeks	100 mg once; repeat in 2 weeks
Or	Albendazole	400 mg once; repeat in 2 weeks	400 mg once; repeat in 2 weeks
Fasciolopsis hepatica (Sheep liver fluke)			
Drug(s) of choice	Triclabendazole	10 mg/kg once	10 mg/kg once
Alternative	Bithionol	30–50 mg/kg × 10–15 doses	30–50 mg/kg on alternate days × 10–15 doses
Fasciolopsis buski, Heterophyes heterophyes, Metagonimus yokogawi (Intestinal flukes)			
Drug(s) of choice	Praziquantel	75 mg/kg/d in 3 doses × 1 d	75 mg/kg/d in 3 doses × 1 d
Opisthorchis viverrini (Southeast Asian liver fluke)			
Drug(s) of choice	Praziquantel	75 mg/kg/d in 3 doses × 1 d	75 mg/kg/d in 3 doses × 1 d
Schistosoma japonicum, Schistosoma mansoni, Schistosoma mekongi (Schistosomiasis)			
S. japonicum, S. mekongi			
Drug(s) of choice	Praziquantel	60 mg/kg/d in 3 doses × 1 d	60 mg/kg/d in 3 doses × 1 d
S. mansoni			
Drug(s) of choice	Praziquantel	60 mg/kg/d in 3 doses × 1 d	60 mg/kg/d in 3 doses × 1 d
Alternative	Oxamniquine	15 mg/kg once	20 mg/kg/d in 2 doses × 1 d
Strongyloides stercoralis (Strongyloidiasis)			
Drug(s) of choice	Ivermectin	200 µg/kg/d × 1–2 d	200 µg/kg/d × 1–2 d
Alternative	Thiabendazole	50 mg/kg/d in 2 doses (max 3 g/d) × 2 d	50 mg/kg/d in 2 doses (max 3 g/d) × 2 d
Tapeworms			
Diphyllobothrium latum (fish), *Taenia saginata* (beef), *Taenia solium* (pork), *Dipylidium canium* (dog)			
Drug(s) of choice	Praziquantel	5–10 mg/kg once	5–10 mg/kg once
Alternative	Niclosamide	2 g once	50 mg/kg once
Hymenolepis nana (dwarf)			
Drug(s) of choice	Praziquantel	25 mg/kg once	25 mg/kg once
Trichostrongylus sp			
Drug(s) of choice	Pyrantel pamoate	11 mg/kg once (max 1 g)	11 mg/kg once (max 1 g)
Alternative	Mebendazole	100 mg once	100 mg once
Or	Albendazole	400 mg once	400 mg once
Trichuris trichiura (Trichuriasis, whipworm)			
Drug(s) of choice	Mebendazole	100 mg bid × 3 d or 500 mg once	100 mg bid × 3 d or 500 mg once
Alternative	Albendazole	400 mg × 3 d	400 mg × 3 d

Adapted from *The Medical Letter on Drugs and Therapeutics*, 2002; Gilbert et al, 2003; Goldsmith, 2003.
bid = twice daily; max = maximum.

TABLE 52-3. Use of Antiparasitic Drugs in Children and Pregnant Women

Drug	Toxicity in Pregnancy	Pregnancy FDA Category	Breastfeeding	Infants	Comments
Albendazole	Teratogenicity in lab animals when given at high doses	C	Controversial	Very little data for infants < 12 months	Recommended that pregnancy be delayed until 1 month after therapy stopped
Bithionol	Safety not established but not recommended	C	Caution	No data	—
Fumagillin	Safety not established but not recommended	?	Best not to use	No data	—
Furazolidone	Safety not established but not recommended	C	Unknown but not recommended	Contraindicated in infants < 1 month	In 132 reports of exposure, no association with malformation found. Theoretical risk of hemolytic anemia in newborn.
Iodoquinol	Safety not established but not recommended	C	Unknown but not recommended	—	—
Ivermectin	Animal data show risk of teratogenicity	C	Caution	—	In 203 reports, exposure to ivermectin (85% during 1st trimester) found no association with congenital malformations
Mebendazole	Embryotoxic and teratogenic in lab animals when given at high doses	C	Little data but considered to be "safe" due to poor absorption from the gastrointestinal tract.	Very little data for infants < 12 months	In a prospective study of 192 pregnant women using 1 to 3 days of 100 mg dose, 71% in 1st trimester, found mebendazole does not pose a risk; 2nd study of 64 first trimester exposures showed no significant teratogenic risk
Metronidazole	Carcinogen in rodents but studies demonstrate can be used in pregnancy except some caution in first trimester	B	Controversial as exposure may be high. With high doses consider expressing and discarding milk	No contraindication	The American Academy of Pediatrics has classified metronidazole as a drug "for which the effect on nursing infants is unknown but may be of concern." Discontinue breastfeeding for 12 to 24 h to allow excretion of drug.
Niclosamide	Animal data show no risk	B	No data	Children < 2 years unknown	No human data available
Oxamniquine	Mutagenic and embryotoxic effects in animal studies at 10 times human dose	C	Recommend no breastfeeding at least 4 hours postdose		No reports of abnormailites in humans
Paromomycin	Poorly absorbed, therefore thought to be safe	C	Probably safe	No contraindication	Limited information is available regarding the teratogenic potential of paromomycin. Following oral administration, minimal systemic absorption occurs, which therefore minimizes any potential teratogenic effect (Briggs et al, 1998). Paromoycin has been recommended for the treatment of infections with *Giardia lamblia* and *Entamoeba histolytica* and tapeworm infestations during pregnancy (D'Alauro et al, 1985).
Praziquantal	Animal data show no teratogenic risk	B	Probably safe	Safety in children < 2 years not well established	WHO informal consultation 2002 concludes that likely to be safe during pregencny and lactation
Pyrantel pamoate	Animal data shows no teratogenic risk	C	Controversial	Use with caution in children < 2 years	No human data available
Quinacrine	Animal data show no risk of teratogenicity	C	No data	No contraindication	no human data
Thiabendazole	Teratogenic in some animal species	C	No data	Safety in children < 15 kg not established	Case reports in humans show no fetal adverse effects.
Tinidazole	Safety not established	—	Unknown but not recommended	Unknown but not recommended	—
Trimethoprim-sulfamethoxazole	May interfere with folic acid metabolism	C	Contraindicated	Contraindicated in infants < 1 month and infants with hyperbilirubinaemia and G6PD deficiency.	—

Adapted from Savioli et al, 2003; Briggs et al (ed), 2001
FDA = Food and Drug Administration; WHO = World Health Organization.

TABLE 52-4. Common Adverse Effects of Antiparasitic Drugs

Generic Name	Trade Name	Common	Serious
Albendazole	Albenza	Headache, nausea, vomiting, abdominal pain	Rare: acute renal failure, blood dyscrasias, elevated LFTs, leukopenia, alopecia
Bithionol	Bitin	Photosensitivity, vomiting, diarrhea, abdominal pain, urticaria	—
Fumagillin	—	Thrombocytopenia, neutropenia, mild GI symptoms	—
Furazolidone	Furoxone	Common: GI symptoms, yellow to brown discoloration of urine; occasional: fever, headache, rash, disulfiram-like reaction with alcohol, mild hemolysis in G6PD-deficient persons	—
Iodoquinol	Yodoxin	Nausea, vomiting, diarrhea, cramps, acne, urticaria, pruritus, fever, headache	Rare: optic neuritis, neuropathy with long-term use
Ivermectin	Stromectol	Occasional: mild headache, pruritus, leukopenia, transient tachycardia	Rare: Mazotti reaction (hypotension, fever, pruritus, bone and joint pain)
Mebendazole	Vermox	Headache, nausea, vomiting, abdominal pain, diarrhea, constipation	Rare: hepatitis, seizures
Metronidazole	Flagyl	Nausea, vomiting, headache, metallic taste; disulfiram-like reaction in alcohol users, vaginitis, candidal overgrowth	Rare: leukopenia, thrombocytopenia, ototoxicity
Niclosamide	Yomesan; Niclocide	Occasional: nausea, vomiting, anorexia, abdominal pain, diarrhea	—
Oxamniquine	Vansil	Occassional: dizziness, drowsiness, headache, febrile reaction, urine color change, EEG and EKG changes, hallucination	Seizure
Paromomycin	Humatin	Nausea, vomiting, epigastric burning pain, abdominal cramps, diarrhea	—
Praziquantel	Biltricide	Frequent: headache, malaise, dizziness; occasional: sedation, GI intolerance, abdominal pain, fever, sweating, fatigue	—
Pyrantel pamoate	Antiminth; Reese's pinworm med	Occasional: nausea, vomiting, abdominal discomfort	—
Quinacrine	Atabrine	Frequent: bitter taste, GI symptoms, headache, dizziness. occasional: toxic psychosis, insomina, blood dyscrasias, harmless yellowing of skin, exfoliative dermatitis. Contraindicated in persons with psychosis or psoriasis.	Rare: toxic psychosis, exfoliative dermatitis
Thiabendazole	Mintezol	Dizziness, drowsiness, headache, febrile reaction, urine color change	—
Tinidazole	Fasigyn	Mild GI symptoms; headache, vertigo less common	—
Triclabendazole	Egaten	Dizziness, headache, abdominal pain; less common cough, fever	—
Trimethoprim sulfamethoxazole	Septra, Bactrim, Sulfatrim	Anorexia, nausea, vomiting, rash, urticaria	Rare: allergic reaction, fulminant hepatic necrosis, blood dyscrasias

EEG = electroencephalogram; EKG = electrocardiogram; GI = gastrointestinal.

Supplemental Reading

Bartlett JB, Gallant JE. 2003 Medical Management of HIV Infection. Johns Hopkins University (Available online <www.hopkins-aids.edu>. Treatment specific recommendations for specific intestinal parasites affecting persons with HIV are provided).

Bennett A, Guyatt H. Reducing intestinal nematode infection: efficacy of albendazole and mebendazole. Parasitol Today 2000;16:71.

Centers for Disease Control and Prevention (CDC) Division of Parasitic Diseases website. <http://www.cdc.gov/ncidod/dpd/professional/default.htm>. (Range of fact sheets, information of diagnostics and treatments available at CDC).

Chen X, Keithly JS, Paya CV, LaRusso NF. Cryptosporidiosis. N Engl J Med. 2002;346:1723–31.

Drugs for Parasitic Infections. The Medical Letter on Drugs and Therapeutics. New Rochelle: The Medical Letter, Inc; 2002. (Available online for free <www.medletter.com>. Excellent reference for particular parasites with drugs of choice and alternatives listed, with adult and pediatric dosages, adverse effects, and list of manufacturers. Updated every 2 years.)

Drugs in pregnancy and lactation. In: Briggs GG, Freeman RK, Yaffe SJ, editors. 6th ed. Lippincott Williams & Wilkins Publishers; 2001.

Gann P, Neva F, Gam A. A randomized trial of single- and two-dose ivermectin versus thiabendazole for treatment of strongyloidiasis. J Infect Dis 1994;169:1076.

Gardner TB, Hill DR. Treatment of giardiasis. Clin Microbiol Rev 2001;14:114–128.

Gilbert DN, Moellering RC, Sande MA. The Sanford guide to antimicrobial therapy. 33rd ed. Hyde Park, VT: Antimicrobial Therapy, Inc; 2003:148. (Excellent pocket reference for all infectious disease treatments. Updated annually.)

Goldsmith RS. Infectious diseases: protozoal and helminthic. In: Tierney LM, McPhee SJ, Papadakis MA, editors. Current medical diagnosis and treatment. Lange Medical Books; 2003. p. 1463–532. (Excellent comprehensive reference that is updated annually).

Haque R, Huston CD, Hughes M, et al. Amebiasis. N Engl J Med 2003;348:1565–73.

Johns Hopkins Division of Infectious Diseases Antibiotic Guide. (Available online free <http://www.hopkins-abxguide.org/> and free PDA download).

Molina J, Tourneur M, Sarfati C, et al. Fumagillin treatment of intestinal microsporidiosis. N Engl J Med 2002;346:1963–9.

Savioli L, Crompton DWT, Neira M. Use of antihelminthic drugs during pregnancy. Am J Obstet Gynecol 2003;188:5–6.

The Medical Letter on Drugs and Therapeutics, 2002.

CHAPTER 53

CURRENT MANAGEMENT OF WHIPPLE'S DISEASE

AXEL VON HERBAY, MD

With the identification of the causative bacterium, *Tropheryma whippelii*, Whipple's disease (WD) has grown out from its niche in textbooks and has colonized high ranked journals. Nevertheless, it is an uncommon multisystem disorder and not just an intestinal bacterial infection like many others. Thus, patient management is more complex. Based on lessons from history, and on new insights promoted by molecular biology in the past decade, a new concept of patient managment has emerged which is presented in this chapter.

Historical Lessons

The history of antibiotic therapy goes back to 1951, when a family physician, Dr. G. Ander in England, decided to try chloramphenicol, a new drug at the time, in a 56-year-old male with WD presenting with high fever and diarrhea. His patient's symptoms vanished and remission continued. As chroni called in Dobbins classic test, the patient was later reported (by Dr. Paulley) as an example of idiopathic steatorrhea, because the effect of chloramphenicol was considered as a control of secondary infection on the jejunal mucosa. The real implication was realized later when electron microscopy identified rod shaped bacteria in other patients' tissues. Antibiotic therapy of WD started, in fact, in 1961. During the four decades since, several drugs have been used. In retrospect, three time periods may be recognized.

In the first period, various antibiotics were applied which were available in the 1960s; penicillin, streptomycin, and tetracyline (and some additional drugs) were all given with success. A sequential combination of these 3 drugs, lasting for at least 12 months, was recommended in 1963 (ie, "Duke regimen"). To avoid possible malabsorption of antibiotics, treatment was started with parenteral administration of penicillin and streptomycin. Follow-up observations were favorable, but perhaps due to the requirement of parenteral application, this regimen was less frequently applied in the 1970s.

A second period started in 1970, when knowledge accumulated that monotherapy with tetracycline was apparently also effective. This oral regimen was widely preferred until the late 1980s, and a low rate of relapses was observed.

However, Knox and colleagues (1976) reported severe central nervous system (CNS) relapses in their patients treated with tetracycline. Indeed, in 1985 a retrospective analysis on the long term outcome (ie, after a minimum of 2 years after diagnosis) in a cohort of 88 patients by Keinath and colleagues (1985) reported that signs or symptoms attributable to WD frequently recurred; among 49 patients treated with tetracycline alone, 21 (43%) had clinically defined relapses. Seven of the 49 patients (14%) developed neurologic features suggestive of CNS relapse, and two further patients developed their second relapse in the CNS. The outcome of patients with CNS relapse was generally poor, despite new antibiotic therapies.

A third period started in the mid 1980s. To overcome the crucial problem of CNS relapse, trimethoprim-sulphamethoxazole was preferred, because this drug can penetrate the blood-brain barrier, whereas tetracyline does not. The choice of this drug was later supported by a retrospective study by Feurle and colleagues in 1976. However, with increasing usage of trimethoprim-sulphamethoxazole, several patients were observed who developed late onset CNS WD. In parallel, we observed asymptomatic CNS infection with *T. whippelii* after long term therapy with trimethoprim-sulphamethoxazole. Thus, it was felt that a more active antimicrobial regimen is necessary to prevent CNS WD.

Current Management

The management of patients with a chronic multisystem infection is more complex. Once a diagnosis of intestinal WD is reached, it is important to evaluate other commonly involved organ systems. After staging is completed, the choice and adequate duration of antibiotic treatment is critical for the patient's long term outcome. Careful monitoring is needed to ascertain its efficacy.

Staging

Diagnostic studies should evaluate tissues along the presumed route of infection, which starts with bacterial invasion in the upper small intestine (Table 53-1). Beyond endoscopy, the draining mesenteric nodes and other retroperitoneal lymph nodes should be investigated by

TABLE 53-1. Proposal for Staging of Whipple's Disease

Stage	Location of Documented Manifestation
Ia	Small intestine
Ib	Abdomincal lymph nodes
II	Extraabdominal lymph nodes
III	Extraabdominal orans (brain, heart, others)

abdominal sonography. Enlarged nodes with lipid deposits (which result in high echogenicity) are a special sign of intestinal WD. Physical examination should focus on the presence of peripheral lymphadenopathy, on evidence of cardiac involvement (pericardial effusion, valvular murmur), and also look for skin hyperpigmentation and evaluate body weight and temperature. Chest radiography should be performed, looking at heart diameter, possible pericardial calcifications, and mediastinal lymphadenopathy. Echocardiography is generally not helpful in patients without a murmur and normal chest radiography.

An essential part of staging is cerebrospinal fluid (CSF) analysis, even in the absence of neurological or psychiatric symptoms. One of the new insights gained during the 1990s was the recognition that, at the time of first diagnosis, approximately 70% of untreated patients with intestinal WD have asymptomatic ("silent") CNS infection with *T. whippelii*. These patients are considered to be at high risk of progressing from silent CNS infection to symptomatic CNS WD (or cerebral WD) unless the bacteria are eradicated. CSF analysis should be performed in parallel by means of polymerase chain reaction (PCR), which detects bacterial DNA, and by cytology of a large CSF sample which detects highly characteristic sickle-form particle containing cells. In practice, we recommend obtaining a 10 mL sample of CSF where possible; 8 mL of fresh CSF should be immediately prepared by cell concentration techniques for cytological study with PAS stain, while an aliquot of 2 mL should be fresh frozen and forwarded for PCR analysis. In our personal experience, the diagnostic yield of CSF cytology is roughly similiar with PCR analysis, but it is much less effective with samples < 5 mL (Von Herbay et al, 1997; Von Herbay, 2003). Imaging studies of the brain (computed tomography, magnetic resonance imaging) are generally not helpful in WD patients without neurological symptoms.

Additional Diagnostic Studies

Peripheral blood analysis does not contribute to staging, but it can provide other information. Most patients present with laboratory signs of inflammation (eg, elevated erythrocyte sedimentation rate, C-reactive protein), many have laboratory signs of malabsorption (eg, low iron, low betacarotene), and some may have occult intestinal bleeding (eg, low hemoglobin, low iron). Routine laboratory tests of liver function (ie, aspartate aminotransferase, alanine aminotransferase, γ-GT, AP, and albumin), renal function (ie, creatinine, sodium, potassium, and calcium), and bone marrow function (ie, blood cell counts) should be performed to recognize possible problems with drug availability.

Although an immunological deficit is likely to play a role in the pathogenesis of WD, diagnostic studies of immunological functions in individual patients are of uncertain value. A variety of cellular and humoral abnormalities may be observed. Serum electrophoresis may recognize hypogammaglobulinemia or hypergammaglobulinemia.

Antibiotic Therapy

Response of intestinal WD can be achieved with many drugs (Table 53-2), but the real challenge is to prevent late onset cerebral WD. To reach this goal, our first line recommendation is to combine an *induction therapy* with intravenous application of a *bactericidal drug*, *ceftriaxone* (2 times 1 mg/d) for 14 days, and a *maintenance* treatment with *trimethoprim-sulphamethoxazole* (2 times 160 mg, 2 times 800 mg/d by mouth) for 12 months.

Ceftriaxone, a third-generation cephalosporin, is commonly used to treat bacterial meningitis. We have 10 years of experience with its use in WD (Von Herbay et al, 1997;

TABLE 53-2. Overview of Antibiotics Used for the Treatment of Whipple's Disease

Drug(s)	Dosage	Comments
Ceftriaxone	3 mg/d IV	Induction therapy (first 14 days), good CNS penetration
Meropeneme	3 mg/d IV	Induction therapy (first 14 days), good CNS penetration, limited experience
Penicillin G plus streptomycin	6 to 24 million units/d IV plus 1 g/d IM	Induction therapy (first 7 to 14 days), moderate CNS penetration
Trimethoprim-sulfamethoxazole	320 mg/d PO, 1600 mg/d PO	Maintenance therapy, first line drug, good CNS penetration, but CNS WD may occur
Doxycycline (or tetracycline)	100 to 200 mg/d PO	Maintenance therapy; divergent reports of low and high rate of clinical relapses
Penicillin VK	500 mg 4 times daily PO	Alternative for maintenance therapy, limited experience
Cefixime	400 mg twice daily PO	Alternative for maintenance therapy, limited experience
Rifampin	600 mg 4 times daily PO	Second line drug, good CNS penetration, limited experience in CNS WD
Chloramphenicol	1000 mg 4 times daily PO	Second line drug, worrisome side effects
Erythromycin	500 mg 4 times daily PO	Second line drug, limited experience

Adapted from Maiwald et al, 2002.
CNS = central nervous system, IM = intramuscularly, IV = intravenous, PO = by mouth, WD = Whipple's disease.

Von Herbay, 2003). Alternatively, meropeneme (1 mg 3 times a day) may be given, but our experience with this drug in WD is limited to a 4-year experience. The historical "Duke regimen", previously reported to be effective, might be considered as a further alternative, although penicillin and streptomycin are considered to only moderately penetrate the normal blood-brain barrier.

Apart from common practice, our argument in favour of 1 year of maintenance treatment is derived from follow-up studies of patients with PCR analysis. Clearance of bacterial DNA from the intestinal mucosa occurs within a range of 1 to 12 months, but, in our experience, after 1 year stable intestinal remission is virtually always reached (see below). An other argument for prolonged therapy can be derived from experiments to culture *T. whippelii*, where the growth of the bacteria is very slow. The estimated duplication time of 4 days is fairly different from common enteric bacteria (eg, *Escherichia coli* has a doubling time of approximately 20 minutes). Surprisingly, there are a few reports of short term antibiotic treatment resulting in long lasting remissions (Fleming et al, 1998; Bai et al, 1991). This paradox is puzzling.

Monitoring

During antibiotic treatment, remission of symptoms and of abnormal diagnostic findings should be followed and documented at regular intervals. The initial response of patients is usually prompt. Diarrhea often resolves within several days, arthralgias within a few weeks, and significant weight gain occurs within a few months. When this clinical improvement is occuring, noninvasive laboratory examinations may be sufficient during the first 6 months.

A potential pitfall of monitoring patients is that intestinal biopsies do not equate with extraintestinal WD. It requires multiple invasive follow-up examinations in parallel. In brief, monitoring repeats staging examinations (see Table 53-1).

After 6 months, CSF analysis should be repeated, either to confirm eradication of previously detected silent CNS infection with *T. whippelii* or to ascertain its absence. Although the bactericidal effects of antibiotics will arise much earlier, there is a lag of clearance of bacterial DNA from the CSF. Up to several weeks, DNA fragments may still be detected by PCR. During this lag phase, interpretation of positive PCR results is difficult and may result in the erroneous impression of treatment failure. Similiarly, interpretation of cytologic findings is difficult during treatment and should be jointly performed with PCR results. Endoscopy with biopsies should be repeated. Although grossly visible mucosal lesions may or may not be absent, histology of biopsies should document partial remission of mucosal lesions, which indicates the common response to treatment (Von Herbay et al, 1996). At this time intestinal mucosal remission is always incomplete, but subtypes of PAS positive macrophages have significantly changed. Abdominal sonography should expect to indicate partial, but still incomplete, remission of abdominal lymphadenopathy.

After 12 months, before stopping treatment, CSF analysis should be repeated to ascertain eradication of previously detected silent CNS infection with *T. whippelii*. This is of critical importance for the patient's outcome. At this time, a DNA-negative result from PCR analysis is more important than the cytologic detection of PAS positive cells, because subtyping of PAS-positive macrophages in the CSF is not established. Endoscopy will usually be normal. When multiple biopsies are obtained, histology will document intestinal remission, although a variable number of PAS positive macrophages may still be present. Subtyping of PAS macrophages can reliably differentiate between remission and persisting infection. This can be confirmed by subsequent PCR analysis. Abdominal sonography may document complete remission of previous lesions, but, in some patients, remission is still incomplete and fibrosis may remain.

After remission is established, the physician and patients should be alert to the possible recurrance of symptoms. If this happens, it does not necessarily indicate a relapse of WD. A tissue-based diagnosis of relapse should be attempted.

Primary Nonresponders

Occasionally, diarrhea may persist (or recur) despite some weeks of treatment. We have found that this is suggestive of an associated infection with *Giardia lamblia*, rather than necessarily being refractory (or relapsing) WD. Associated *G. lamblia* may easily escape notice in PAS stained biopsies. This protozoan requires other drugs to become eradicated.

Rarely, a patient with intestinal WD does not respond to adequate primary treatment (see above) and does not reach clinical and mucosal remission after 1 year. In our personal series, there are 2 nonresponders among 162 patients (Von Herbay et al, 1996). Salvage therapy should be planed on an individual basis.

As mentioned, the real challenge of treatment is to eradicate asymptomatic CNS infection. In those patients who do not respond to initial treatment with ceftriaxone, a second course with meropeneme should follow. Further salvage therapy should be planned on an individual basis.

Cerebral WD

Some patients present initially with neurologic or psychiatric symptoms, but the majority of patients with cerebral WD develop symptoms later in the course of the disease (Knox et al, 1976). This may happen within a range of a few months to several years after the initial diagnosis of intestinal WD (Maiwald et al, 2002). At this time, a suboptimal examination may easily fail to detect residual PAS positive macrophages in intestinal mucosal biopsies. Treatment of this subset of patients is less effective and, even today, their prognosis is uncertain. One of the long term problems is differentiating persisting neurological deficits, which do not need antibiotic therapy, from persisting CNS infection.

Adjuvant Therapies

Before the historical recognition of the bacterial association, patients with WD were sometimes treated with corticosteroids, and remission was observed. Even today, some patients apparently require additive corticosteroids to control their symptoms (eg, arthralgias, pleural effusion), although antibiotic drugs alone do not achieve this effect. The background for these observations is still undefined.

Assuming an immunological basis of WD, the idea of adjuvant immunotherapy is tempting. This hypothesis was tested in one rare patient with intestinal WD who was refractory to diverse antibiotic drugs. With combined therapy of chloramphenicol and interferon-gamma, remission was eventually achieved (Schneider et al, 1998). However, in two further patients with refractory cerebral WD interferon-gamma was ineffective (unpublished). One of the latter patients later died.

Conclusions and Perspective

Treatment of WD is largely performed on a historical basis. It relies on observations from case reports, retrospective clinical series, and a meta-analysis. No evidence base is available. The recommendations and comments given in this chapter include our personal series of 162 patients studied during 1992 to 2002 at the University of Heidelberg, Germany and updated on our Web site (see below). The new concept of patient management was subjected to a prospective, randomized study, which started in September 1998 in Germany (*Studie zur Initialtherapie bei Morbus Whipple [SIMW]*). By December 31, 2002, 32 patients were enrolled. Preliminary data suggest that it works, but follow-up is still limited. Unfortunately, after some protocol violations, the study was disbanded before reaching its end point (see Web site).

Meanwhile, cultivation of *T. whippelii* is possible (but still not available clinically), and this has allowed deciphering of the complete bacterial genome. This knowledge will facilitate the establishment of new diagnostic tests, including culture systems and tests of antibiotic sensitivity in individual isolates, and will help in designing new approaches to treatment. Progress in Whipple's bacteriology has overshadowed the likely role of the immune system in the pathogenesis, which needs to be clarified. The author's Web site is Whipple's Disease online at <http://www.WhipplesDisease.net>. He can be reached at <vonHerbay@WhipplesDisease.net>.

Supplemental Reading

Bai JC, Crosetti EE, Maurino EC et al. Short-term antibiotic treatment in Whipple's Disease. J Clin Gastroenterol 1991;13:303–7.

Bentley SD, Maiwald M, Murphy LD et al. Sequencing and analysis of the genome of the Whipple's disease bacterium *Tropheryma whipplei*. Lancet 2003;361:637–44.

Dobbins WO III. Whipple's disease. Springfield (IL): Thomas; 1987.

Feurle GE, Marth T. An evaluation of antimicrobial treatment for Whipple's disease. Tetracycline versus Trimethoprim-Sulfamethoxazole. Dig Dis Sci 1994;39:1642–8.

Fleming JL, Wiesner RH, Shorter RG. Whipple's disease: clinical, biochemical, and histopathologic features and assessment of treatment in 29 patients. Mayo Clin Proc 1988;63:539–51.

Keinath RD, Merrel DE, Vlietstra R, Dobbins WO III. Antibiotic treatment and relapse in Whipple's disease. Long-term follow-up of 88 patients. Gastroenterol 1985;88:1867–73.

Knox DL, Bayless TM, Pittman FE. Neurologic disease impatients with treated Whipple's disease. Medicine 1976;55:467–76.

Maiwald M, von Herbay A, Relman DAR. Whipple disease. In: Feldman M, Friedman LS, Sleisenger MH, editors. Sleisenger & Fordtran's gastrointestinal and liver disease. 7th ed. Philadelphia: Saunders; 2002; p. 1854–63.

Schneider T, Stallmach A, von Herbay A, et al. Treatment of refractory Whipple's disease with interferon gamma. Ann Intern Med 1998;29:875–7.

Vital Durand D, Lecomte C, Cathébras P, et al. Whipple disease: clinical review of 52 cases. Medicine (Baltimore) 1997;76:170–84.

von Herbay A. Whipple's Disease Online. 2003. Available at: <http://www.WhipplesDisease.net> (accessed 2003).

von Herbay A, Ditton HJ, Maiwald M. Diagnostic application of a polymerase chain reaction assay for the Whipple's disease bacterium to intestinal biopsies. Gastroenterol 1996;110:1735–43.

von Herbay A, Ditton HJ, Schuhmacher F, Maiwald M. Whipple's disease: staging and monitoring by cytology and polymerase chain reaction analysis of cerebrospinal fluid. Gastroenterol 1997;113:434–41.

von Herbay A, Maiwald M, Ditton HJ, Otto HF. Histology of intestinal Whipple's disease revisited. A study of 48 patients. Virchows Arch 1996;429:335–43.

von Herbay A, Otto HF. Whipple's disease: a report of 22 patients. Klin Wochenschr 1988;66:533–9.

CHAPTER 54

ENTERAL AND PARENTERAL NUTRITION

Mark H. DeLegge, MD, FACG

It has long been known that the nutritional status of a patient will affect that patient's clinical outcome. Clinicians spend a considerable amount of time repairing and treating patient ills with little attention given to the more subtle signs of nutritional inadequacies or imbalances. As physicians, we have a responsibility to understand the dynamics of nutrition and the gut in both the healthy patient and in the patient under physiologic stress. In order to accomplish this task, we must be knowledgeable with regards to identifying patients at nutritional risk, determining the appropriate nutritional therapy, and capturing the right outcome measurements of our nutritional therapy.

Nutritional Assessment

Determining who is at risk for malnutrition is a complicated science. A nutritional assessment provides a mechanism by which those patients who will require nutritional support may be identified. A nutritional assessment determines not only who is at nutritional risk, but should also provide a gauge to monitor the effectiveness of the nutritional support. The most sensitive marker of malnutrition would be *percent usual body weight (UBW) loss*, or what patients have deviated from their average body weight. A > 10% UBW loss in 3 months or less is an indicator of a patient at nutritional risk. Serum albumin does not provide a good measure of a patient's nutritional status, but it does represent a measurement of their overall physiologic status (Reinhardt et al, 1980).

Nutritional Requirements

Once patients have been screened and found to be at nutritional risk, a nutritional therapy is prescribed. In order to prescribe any nutritional therapy, a patient's caloric, protein, fluid, macronutrient, micronutrient and vitamin requirements need to be considered.

Caloric Assessment

Calculation of energy requirements can be obtained through mathematical equations. The most commonly used equation for calculating energy needs is the Harris-Benedict equation. The calculation is as follows:

$$\text{Men: energy needs/24 hours} = 66 + (13.7 \times W)(5 \times L) - (6.8 \times A)$$

$$\text{Women: energy needs/24 hours} = 655 + (9.6 \times W) + (1.7 \times L) - (4.7 \times A)$$

W = weight in kg, A = age, L = height in cm

These calculations of energy needs are often multiplied by stress factors to arrive at a patient's overall calorie needs. There are alternative, simpler estimates of overall patient calorie needs dependent on whether they are in mild, moderate, or severe physiologic stress (Table 54-1).

Protein Assessment

Protein catabolism occurs at varying rates and is affected by a patient's disease status, current nutritional state, and diet. This may be calculated from a patient's daily total nitrogen losses. There are also simpler, estimated values of protein needs dependent on whether a patient is in mild, moderate, or severe physiologic stress (see Table 54-1).

Minerals

Minerals constitute an extremely important facet of metabolism although they account for only 4% of the total body weight. They serve as essential cofactors, help maintain fluid osmotic pressures and provide the proper environment for many chemical reactions (Table 54-2).

Micronutrients

The essential micronutrients are present in minute or trace amounts within the body, sometimes in quantities of less than 100 µg. Although trace elements are present in very small amounts, they often have dramatic effects. Deficiencies

TABLE 54-1. Estimated Calorie and Protein Needs

Physiologic State	Calorie Needs	Protein Needs
Mild physiologic stress	25 to 28 kcal/kg/d	0.8 to 1.0 g/kg/d
Moderate physiologic stress	28 to 32 cal/kg/d	1.0 to 1.2 g/kg/d
Severe physiologic stress	32 to 35 cal/kg/d	1.5 to 2.0 g/kg/d

TABLE 54-2. Mineral and Micronutrient Requirements

Substance	Daily Requirement	Deficiency
Calcium	1000 mg	Bone loss
Phosphorous	1000 mg	Muscle dysfunction
Magnesium	400 mg	Cardiac arrhythmias
Chromium	75 µg	Glucose intolerance
Copper	3 µg	Microcytic anemia
Iodine	150 µg	Weakness
Iron	1 mg	Microcytic anemia
Manganese	4 µg	Hair deformities
Selenium	60 µg	Muscle weakness
Zinc	10 mg	Poor wound healing

are more common than toxicity. Many of these deficiencies develop in patients who are on long term parenteral nutrition (PN) or who are severely malnourished. The assessment of trace element deficiency is extremely difficult. Serum levels may not accurately reflect body stores. Because of this, clinicians may have to depend on physical signs and symptoms to detect micronutrient deficiency (Table 54-3).

Vitamins

Vitamins are essential micronutrients involved in such basic body functions as growth, tissue maintenance and metabolism. They are broadly classified as water-soluble vitamins and fat-soluble vitamins. Absorption of fat-soluble vitamins (A, D, E, and K) requires absorption and transport of lipids. Water-soluble vitamins, except vitamin C, are part of a B-complex group.

Nutrition Interventions

After identifying a patient at nutritional risk and their daily nutritional needs, a decision must be made as to what nutritional intervention is appropriate. These decisions are based on the following tenets:
1. There is little data if any to support the efficacy of oral supplements or dietary modification in treating malnutrition.
2. There is data available demonstrating some efficacy of appetite stimulants in patients with acquired immunodeficiency syndrome (AIDS) or cancer related anorexia and a functioning gastrointestinal (GI) tract.
3. Enteral nutrition (EN), or the delivery of nutrients into the gut, requires an enteral access route, such as a nasogastric tube, percutaneous gastrostomy tube, or percurtaneous jejunostomy tube.
4. PN, or the delivery of nutrients intravenously, requires the presence of a venous access device, such as a Hickman catheter or vascular port.
5. There is a multitude of data supporting the use of EN rather than PN whenever possible because of lower cost, lower associated complications and improved gut physiologic status with the use of EN.

Oral Diet Therapy and Supplements

The general diet is designed to provide optimal nutrition to patients who do not require a therapeutic diet. It is used to promote health and contains a variety of foods low in fat and cholesterol, the use of salt in moderation and an abundance of fruits, grains and vegetables.

Oral supplements are commercially available, usually in liquid form. In general, these supplements are polypeptide in formulations of either 1 or 1.5 calories/mL. They are flavored for taste. In general, these supplements end up being a meal substitute rather than a supplement, thus minimizing their effectiveness.

Appetite stimulants have been used with some success in the AIDS and cancer populations with a functional GI tract (Kirby et al, 1995). Most of the published evidence is short term data. Long-term use of appetite stimulants as a nutritional therapy intervention has not been studied.

Enteral Nutrition

EN includes both the ingestion of food orally and the nonvolatile delivery of nutrients by a tube into the GI tract. For the purpose of further discussion, EN will refer to food entering the GI tract by means other than oral.

Contraindications to enteral feeding include patients with diffuse peritonitis, intestinal obstruction, intractable vomiting, paralytic ileus, and severe diarrhea. Other possible contraindications include enterocutaneous fistula, GI ischemia, and, in some instances, malabsorption.

After deciding to use the GI system for the delivery of nutrition, two key decisions must follow. The first is regarding the route of enteral access to the gut. The second pertains to the site of tube feeding delivery. Each route and delivery site has advantages and risks (see Table 54-3).

ENTERAL FORMULAS

Once a patient has an appropriate enteral access device in place, a decision must be made regarding the type of

TABLE 54-3. Enteral Access Decisions

Access Location	Predicted Time of Use	Tip
Nasogastric	< 30 days	Stomach
Nasojejunal	< 30 days	Jejunum
Percutaneous gastrostomy	> 30 days	Stomach
Percutaneous gastrojejunostomy	> 30 days and < 6 months	Stomach/jejunum
Direct percutaneous jejunostomy	> 30 days	Jejunum
Surgical gastrostomy	> 30 days	Stomach
Surgical jejunostomy	> 30 days	Jejunum

EN the patient should receive. This determination should be based on the patients overall caloric and protein needs. Most EN used today is in the form of pre-prepared commercial formulas. The principal categories of enteral formulas are blenderized, lactose-containing, lactose-free, elemental, modular, and specialty (Table 54-4). Each has its own potential benefits and disadvantages.

Assessment of Feeding Tolerance

Assessment of feeding tolerance is important. Stool frequency, stool consistency, abdominal distention, bowel sounds and urinary output should be monitored. Enteral formulas previously were often colored with methylene blue to monitor for gastroesophageal reflux and gastric aspiration. However, recent reports of mitochondrial injury and patient death have led to methylene blue's removal from most hospitals (Taka et al, 1996). With gastric feedings, gastric residuals should be checked every 6 hours. If residuals are > 200 mL, the tube feeding should be stopped and the residual volume replaced. The residual should be checked again in 2 hours. If it remains > 200 mL, the patient should be reassessed and considered for small bowel feedings.

Advancement of Tube Feedings

Advancement of tube feedings, once initiated, is an imperfect science. In our center, patients are initiated on continuous tube feedings at 30 mL/hr. They are advanced at a rate of 20 to 30 mL every 6 hours, until they reach their goal rate. Any sign of tube-feeding intolerance results in temporary cessation of tube feeding or a reduction in the tube-feeding rate. Once a patient has reached their goal rate, they may be maintained on continuous 24-hour tube feedings, changed to 18 or 12 hour continuous tube feedings, changed to intermittent tube feedings or changed to bolus tube feedings.

Enteral Feeding Complications

GI side effects of tube feeding are reported in 15 to 30% of patients receiving enteral feedings (Edes et al, 1990). They are listed in Table 54-5.

Parenteral Nutrition

For those patients with a non-functioning GI tract, nutrients can be delivered directly into the venous system. This is referred to as parenteral nutrition (PN). These nutrients may be delivered into a central vein, *central PN*, or peripheral vein, *peripheral PN*.

Parentral nutrition delivers a solution consisting of water, electrolytes, amino acids, carbohydrates, fats, proteins, vitamins, and trace elements. These compounds are mixed and delivered over a period of time: generally 12 to 24 hours.

The formulation of a PN solution requires the development of a solution that is six times more concentrated than blood (1800 to 2400 mOsm/L) and generally consists of approximately 30 to 50 g of protein and 1000 to 1200 kcal/L. Determination of caloric and protein needs is based on a prior nutritional assessment. Overall daily water requirements can be estimated at 25 to 30 mL/kg.

TABLE 54-4. Examples and Explanations of Enteral Formulas

Polymeric (Intact protein; 1 kcal/kg/d) (Standard tube feedings)
    Nutren 1.0
        Isocal
        Osmolite HN

Polymeric; (Intact Protein 2.0 kcal/mL) (For volume restricted patients)
        Magnal
        Two cal HN

Fiber containing (1.0 kcal/mL) (For constipation or diarrhea)
        Jevity

Free Amino Acids (Elemental; Low Fat, 1.0 kcal/mL) (For malabsorption)
        Vivonex TEN

Small Peptide Based (Moderate Fat; 1.0 kcal/mL) (For malabsorption)
        Peptamen

Specialty
    Immune Enhancing (1.0 kcal/mL, arginine, glutamine, omega-3 fatty acid fortified)
    Impact (For improving intensive care unit outcomes)

    Hepatic Formulation (Increased Branched-Chain Amino Acids)
    Nutra-Hep (For liver disease patients)

    Pulmonary (1.5 kcal/mL, Low Carbohydrate)
    Pulmocare (for lung disease patients)

    Renal (2.0 kcal/mL, Increased Essential Amino Acids)
    Amin-Aide (for renal disease patients)

    Glucose Intolerance (1.0 kcal/mL, Increased fructose component of carbohydrates)
    Glucerna (for diabetic patients)

HN = high nitrogen.

TABLE 54-5. Enteral Feeding Complications

Nausea
Vomiting
Abdominal cramping
Abdominal distention
Diarrhea
    Infectious from concurrent antibiotic use
    Sorbitol contained in other liquid medications
    Promotility agents
    Magnesium containing medications
    Hypoalbuminemia – malabsorption at the small bowel wall
    Tube feeding—least likely cause
Dehydration—Not enough free water given to the patient
Medication delivery—some medications (phenytoin) bind to the enteral formula

PN Compounding

In prescribing a total PN (TPN) formula, one must first determine the protein, carbohydrate and fat content of a formula. A representative PN formula is detailed in Table 54-6.

Vascular Access Devices

Vascular access devices have developed significantly over the past 40 years. Anatomically, the subclavian vein, internal jugular vein, and peripherally inserted central catheters provide the safest and easiest central venous access. The subclavian vein is often chosen for long term access, such as for home PN, because of a reduced incidence of complications. Multilumen catheters allow for the infusion of a number of fluids and medications at the same time.

Central Venous Catheter Complications

Central venous catheter complications occur at an incidence of 1 to 20% (Santarpia et al, 2002). Complications of subclavian vein catheterization include hemothorax, pneumothorax, brachial plexus injury, hematoma, and subcutaneous emphysema. Common long-term catheter complications include sepsis, thrombosis, and catheter occlusion.

Administration of PN

The average PN solution comprises approximately 25 to 30% solute. It should be initiated over 24 hours. Patients with glucose intolerance or those at risk for refeeding syndrome (see complications below) should have their PN infused at half their daily caloric needs for the first 24 hours. This may be increased to full caloric needs over the next 24 to 72 hours with monitoring of serum glucose, electrolytes, magnesium, phosphate, and fluid tolerance (American Gastroenterological Association, 2001). Use of the PN port or lumen for blood draws or infusion of other solutions dramatically increases the risk of catheter infection.

TABLE 54-6. Sample Central Parenteral Nutrition Order

Amino acids	55 g/L
Dextrose	555 kcal/L (163 g carbohydrates)
Lipids	400 kcal/L (40 g of lipids)
Total	1175 kcal/L
Sodium	70 meq/L
Potassium	35 meq/L
Calcium	5 meq/L
Magnesium	5 meq/L
Phosphorous	15 mmol/L
Chloride: Acetate	To balance

Volume—2000 mL (83 mL/hr over 24-hour infusion)
Multivitamins (MVI-13)
Trace elements
Drug additives/L (heparin, insulin, H_2 blockers)

Metabolic Complications

Hyperglycemia is the most common complication and is directly related to the dextrose content of the PN and the rate of infusion. Critically ill patients and patients with pre-existing glucose intolerance require the most aggressive monitoring of serum glucose. Serum glucose should be maintained below 200 mg/dL. If a patient develops hyperglycemia they should, at first, be maintained on a sliding scale of regular insulin. Two-thirds of the total amount of sliding scale insulin required over 24 hours should be added to the next day's PN formula. Further adjustments in daily insulin dosing may be required on a daily basis. It is known that failure to control blood glucose levels results in an increase of infectious complications, such as catheter sepsis.

Refeeding syndrome is a common metabolic consequence of PN. This results from the sudden provision of calories to a patient who has been previously malnourished. With PN infusion, these patients attempt to become rapidly anabolic. Insulin production is increased pushing potassium, phosphorous and magnesium into intracellular compartments with the resultant risk of hypokalemia, hypophosphatemia, and hypomagnesemia. Sodium retention and large fluid shifts may also occur and the patient may develop congestive heart failure.

Elevated liver function tests are common after initiation of TPN, and typically feature elevations in transaminases up to two times normal. These generally resolve in 10 to 15 days. A liver biopsy may ultimately be necessary to make a diagnosis. True *TPN-induced liver disease* presents as a *fatty infiltration of the liver*, especially prominent in the periportal areas. It may respond to reduction in a patient's total daily carbohydrate or total calorie infusion. Current research suggests *choline deficiency* may be playing a role in the development of liver disease associated with PN use.

Patients who develop significant complications with PN may be candidates for *small bowel transplantation*. These complications include liver failure, repeated catheter sepsis, or thrombosis of major venous systems precluding obtaining central venous access. The arrival of tacrolimus as an immunosuppressive agent has improved small bowel transplant outcomes. Current 5-year survival rates for patients receiving small bowel transplant are close to 50% (Buchman et al, 2003). There are separate chapters on short bowel syndrome (see Chapter 64, "Short Bowel Syndrome") and on small bowel transplantation (see Chapter 65, "Intestinal and Multivisceral Transplantation").

Nutrition in Specific Disease States

The impact of nutrition on various disease states remains under investigation. Although nutrition by itself may not prove curative for specific disease states, it is an important component of many therapeutic strategies. Our decisions for nutritional therapy should be outcome based.

Intestinal Failure

Is there a nutritional approach to patients with short bowel syndrome? What are the predictors to response of patient with short bowel syndrome?

Intestinal failure or short bowel syndrome results from loss and or disease of the intestine to an extent that precludes adequate digestion and absorption. There is a separate chapter on short bowel syndrome (see Chapter 64, "Short Bowel Syndrome"). Crohn's disease, intestinal trauma and intestinal infarction are the most common causes. The patient often presents with weight loss, diarrhea, and weakness. Following an extensive resection of the small intestine, intestinal rehabilitation is more likely if the colon has been preserved and the ileocecal valve is maintained (Dudrick and Latifi, 1992). The nutritional management of short bowel syndrome depends on the amount and location of small bowel removed. Initially, gastric acid suppressing agents are employed to reduce gastric hypersecretions and anticholinergic agents are used to slow transit. PN is prescribed to meet nutritional needs and to reduce gastric and intestinal secretions associated with food ingestion. Oral feedings are gradually started and the volume of PN reduced as the oral feedings are tolerated. If the patient has had an ileal resection and has fat malabsorption, a low fat diet should be utilized. Cholestyramine may be used to reduce bile-salt induced diarrhea in patients with an intact colon. However, in occasional patients with some ileum remaining, the use of cholestyramine may increase diarrhea by creating a relative bile salt deficiency. Vitamin B_{12} should be given monthly. In those patients with significant small bowel resections (80 to 100 cm left), a trial of an elemental enteral formula should be attempted. Later, a polymeric formula may be substituted. Patients with less than 80 cm of small bowel remaining are often PN-dependent for life. The use of somatostatin to reduce gut secretions and slow transit time remains controversial.

Pancreatitis

Can EN be used in pancreatitis? Do we need to use a low fat parenteral or enteral formula in the presence of pancreatitis?

In patients with pancreatitis, nutritional support is imperative. Early replacement compared to no nutrition appears to be associated with a reduction in complications and mortality associated with pancreatitis. Lipid containing PN may be used in patients without a history of hyperlipidemia or triglyceride clearance problems without worsening the pancreatic inflammation. Recently, EN has been used in patients with pancreatitis. It appears that *intrajejunal feedings are safe and well tolerated* (McClave and Dryden, 2002). The use of EN as compared with PN has been shown to result in reduced hospital length of stay, intra-abdominal abscesses, and infectious complications. The use of an elemental enteral formula is not necessary. A standard, fat containing, polymeric enteral formula may be used.

Inflammatory Bowel Disease

Is diet important in inflammatory bowel disease (IBD)? Is the use of EN as good as pharmacologic therapy? Is PN effective for the treatment of IBD?

IBD is frequently associated with malnutrition. These patients are often hypermetabolic and may have anorexia due to nausea and abdominal pain. Dietary therapy in IBD has always been considered important. However, no one specific diet can be recommended. Fat restriction may be important in patients with ileal disease or those who have undergone an ileal resection. The use of EN is an important component of IBD therapy for those patients who cannot eat. EN has not proven superior to TPN or drug therapy in inducing remissions in IBD (Lochs et al, 1990). It is, however, less costly and associated with fewer complications. The use of PN in IBD should be restricted to those who have not responded to conservative medical therapy (EN and medications) or in whom EN cannot be delivered.

Liver Disease

Are branched-chain amino acid formulas effective in patients with liver disease? Is protein restriction important in patients with hepatic encephalopathy?

Nutritional deficiencies are common in liver disease. There is an alteration in the normal serum amino acid concentrations with a rise in aromatic amino acids (tyrosine, phenylalanine, and methionine) and a fall in branched-chain amino acids (valine, leucine, and isoleucine). The aromatic amino acids are normally removed by the liver. It is postulated that the rise in aromatic amino acids precipitates hepatic encephalopathy, as these amino acids act as false neurotransmitters. In addition, branched-chain amino acids are preferentially used by patients in liver failure because they do not require the liver for metabolism. However, studies have failed to demonstrate an improved outcome in patients with liver failure who are fed a branched-chain amino acid fortified diet or enteral solution (Als-Nielsen, 2003). There is a tendency to limit protein intake in patients with cirrhosis to prevent encephalopathy. However, these patients have an increased protein demand. Further limiting their protein intake will only accelerate protein calorie malnutrition. It is preferable to feed patients according to their protein needs and treat encephalopathy with medications as it develops. The use of PN in liver failure patients should be used with caution. Liver failure is commonly associated with immune dysfunction, thus placing these PN patients at increased risk for catheter sepsis. In addition, the lack of glycogen stores can lead to episodes of hypoglycemia when patients are rapidly tapered off PN or EN.

Renal Failure

Is protein malnutrition common in this disease? Is the use of essential amino acid based nutritional formulas effective in this population? What is the indication for intradialytic PN?

Malnutrition is common in renal failure; approximately one-third of affected patients are malnourished. Severely depleted muscle mass may occur in up to 20% of these patients. Serum amino acid patterns are altered with a reduction in essential and branched-chain amino acids. Total body albumin stores are reduced due to increased catabolism and decreased protein intake. Furthermore, 6 to 9 g of protein are lost with each dialysis treatment. Glucose intolerance is common secondary to peripheral insulin resistance and increased hepatic glucose production. Vitamin D deficiency is common as is hypocalcemia, hyperkalemia, hyperphosphatemia, and hypermagnesemia, and water-soluble vitamin deficiencies are common. Nutritional therapy in these patients can be difficult. Originally, dietary protein restriction was used as a mechanism to preserve limited renal function. Although this diet does not prevent renal disease, it prolongs the time period until the patient requires dialysis. This protein restriction results in an increase in patient morbidity, a decrease in body weight, and a decrease in quality of life (Ihle et al, 1989). In general, protein restriction should not be used in patients with renal failure. The use of specialized essential amino acid diets for preserving renal function are interesting, but have little practical importance. If a patient has enteral access, commercially available enteral formulas are available that are low in potassium, magnesium, phosphorous, and free water. For those patients who cannot eat and cannot tolerate EN, PN remains an option. Concerns about fluid volume with PN can be avoided by delivering the PN during the patient's dialysis treatment (intradialytic PN [IDPN]), although outcome data with this therapy is limited. Peritoneal delivery of proteins and dextrose as a nutritional supplement has been described, although there is no convincing outcome data.

Cancer

Does nutritional therapy improve cancer treatment outcomes? What group of cancer patients would benefit from aggressive nutritional intervention?

Protein-calorie malnutrition is a common problem in cancer patients. Cancer cachexia is the consequence of multiple metabolic abnormalities induced by the tumor. The routine use of aggressive nutritional support in all patients receiving chemotherapy and radiation is controversial. Prospective, randomized studies have failed to show improved tolerance to chemotherapy with the use of nutritional support (Brennan, 1981). The use of PN in patients receiving radiation therapy has also failed to show an improvement in morbidity. PN has been shown to be beneficial in patients with small bowel obstruction from primary or metastatic tumors. EN has been shown to be of benefit in patients with head and neck or esophageal tumors with proximal GI obstruction. In summary, the use of nutritional support in the cancer patient should be restricted to those patients with a reasonable life expectancy who are likely to be unable to maintain their nutritional needs for a prolonged period of time. It is in these patients that an improved quality of life may occur.

CRITICALLY ILL PATIENTS

Does nutritional intervention improve outcomes? Is EN superior to PN in this patient population?

Providing nutritional support to seriously ill patients can alter patient outcomes in select groups, such as trauma patients, burn patients, and GI surgery patients. Unfortunately, this issue has not been extensively evaluated in other critically ill populations. EN has been shown superior to PN with regards to a reduction in infectious complications (Heyland, 2000). It is also recommended that enteral feeding be delivered via a jejunostomy tube in those patients with a history of gastric intolerance or those in whom gastric aspiration is a major concern.

Conclusion

Nutrition is an important building block that supports all other therapies in the treatment of complex disease processes. Adequately assessing a patient's nutritional status and addressing their nutritional needs is the foundation for the provision of nutritional therapy. Understanding fuel metabolism and nutrient needs is paramount for providing appropriate nutritional therapy. The delivery of EN or PN requires appropriate access. PN requires placement of a venous catheter. Either delivery system has its own advantages and disadvantages, although EN is often less costly and associated with fewer complications. Appropriate use and understanding of nutrition will result in improved patient outcomes.

Supplemental Reading

Als-Nielsen B, Koretz RL, Kjaergard LL, et al. Branched chain amino acids for encephalopathy. Cochrane Database Systemic Reviews 2003;CD001939.

American Gastroenterological Association. American Gastroenterological Association medical position statement on parenteral nutrition. Gastroenterology 2001:121:966–9.

Brennan MF. Total parenteral nutrition in cancer patient. N Engl J Med 1981;305:375–81.

Buchman AL, Scolapio J, Fryer J. AGA technical review on short bowel syndrome and intestinal transplantation. Gastroenterology 2003;124:1105–10.

Desport JC, Gory-Delbaere G, Blanc-Vincent MP, et al. Standards, options and recommendations for the use of appetite stimulants in oncology. Br J Cancer 2003;89(Suppl 1):S98–100.

Dudrick SJ, Latifi R. Total parenteral nutrition: Part II administration, monitoring and complications. Pract Gastroenterol 1992;7:29–39.

Edes TE, Walk BE, Austin JL. Diarrhea in tube-fed patients: feeding formula not necessarily the cause. Am J Med 1990;88:91–3.

Heyland DK. Parenteral nutrition in the critically-ill patient: more harm than good? Proc Nutr Soc 2000;59:457–66.

Ihle BU, Becker GJ, Whitworth JA, et al. The effect of protein restriction on the progression of renal disease. N Engl J Med 1989;321:1773–7.

Kirby DF, DeLegge MH, Fleming CR. AGA Technical Review on tube feedings and enteral nutrition. Gastroenterology 1995;108:1282–301.

Lochs H, Steinhart HJ, Lorenz-Meyer H, et al. Feasibility and effectiveness of a defined formula diet regimen in treating active Crohn's disease: ECCD study III. Scand J Gastroenterol 1990;25:235–48.

McClave SA, Dryden GW. Issues of nutrition support for the patient with acute pancreatitis. Semin Gastrointest Dis 2002;14:154–60.

Reinhardt GF, Myscofski JW, Wilkins DB, et al. Incidence and mortality of low albumin patients in hospitalized veterans. J Parenter Enteral Nutr 1980;4:357–9.

Santarpia L, Pasanisi F, Alfonsi L, et al. Prevention and treatment of implanted central venous catheter (CVC)-related sepsis: a report after six years of home parenteral nutrition (HPN). Clin Nutr 2002;21:207–11.

Taka A, Mohan V, Kashyap, et al. Pulmonary edema following intrauterine methyline blue injection. Acta Anaesth Scand 1996;40:382–4.

CHAPTER 55

METABOLIC BONE DISEASE IN GASTROINTESTINAL AND LIVER PATIENTS

MARIA T. ABREU, MD

Clinicians caring for patients with gastrointestinal (GI) or liver diseases focus primarily on the intestinal or hepatic manifestations of the disease but there are several silent extraintestinal complications that merit attention. One of these systemic consequences is bone loss. Osteopenia is defined by a WHO group as a decrease in bone mineral density (BMD) by > 1 standard deviation compared to a control population (Table 55-1), and osteoporosis is defined as a decrease in BMD by > 2.5 standard deviations compared to a control population. These cut offs were chosen to reflect an increase in fracture risk with diminished BMD, but other factors, in addition to BMD, may increase the likelihood of a fracture. Table 55-2 lists the GI or liver disorders associated with premature or excessive bone loss and the estimates of osteopenia and osteoporosis in these patients. Perhaps more important is the increased risk of vertebral or other skeletal fractures. There are morbid complications, which may contribute significantly to diminished quality of life and increased costs (Trombetti et al, 2002).

BMD is a balance between bone synthesis by osteoblasts and bone resorption by osteoclasts. Thus, low BMD may result from decreased osteoblastic activity or increased osteoclastic activity. Certain factors can increase osteoclast differentiation and survival resulting in increased bone resorption. Examples of this mechanism of osteoporosis are cytokines such as tumor necrosis factor (TNF)-α and interleukin (IL)-6. Malabsorption of calcium and vitamin D results in increased osteoclastic activity because of the body's attempt to maintain adequate serum calcium concentrations (discussed below). Certain factors can decrease osteoblastic activity. The most common cause is glucocorticoids, which can induce osteoblast apoptosis. The sections below attempt to stratify osteoporosis associated with GI and liver diseases into the distinct mechanisms that cause bone loss.

TABLE 55-1. Interpretation of Bone Test Results in Patients with Gastrointestinal-Related Metabolic Bone Disease

Test	High Value	Low Value
BMD (DXA, calcaneal U/S, quantitative CT)	—	—
T scores examine BMD compared to peak bone mass, Z scores examine BMD compared to age/gender-matched controls	N/A	Best to look at left hip and lumbar spine results, Osteopenia = −1 to −2 SD, Osteoporosis ≤ −2.5 SD, Severe osteoporosis ≤ −2.5 SD + fragility fractures
25-Hydroxyvitamin D	Increased dietary intake or supplements	Decreased absorption; decreased sun exposure or dietary intake
1,25-Dihydroxyvitamin D	Granulomatous diseases; subset Crohn's disease; secondary hyperparathyroidism (see PTH)	Decreased availability of 25-hydroxyvitamin D; renal disease
PTH	Response to low serum ionized calcium (secondary hyperparathyroidism); may also be primary hyperparathyroidism	Increased Ca; Increased 1,25(OH)$_2$D3
Ionized calcium (serum calcium may be inaccurate if albumin low)	May be elevated in granulomatous conditions such as sarcoidosis (generally accompanied by high 1,25(OH)$_2$D3)	Decreased absorption secondary to proximal small bowel disease or low 1,25(OH)$_2$D3
Urine N-telopeptide cross-linked of type 1 collagen —*marker of bone resorption*	Increased with increased bone resorption such as with inflammatory bowel disease, glucocorticoids	Decreases with bisphosphonate therapy; may be useful for monitoring therapy
Osteocalcin and Bone alkaline phosphatase —*markers of bone formation*	Increases signify increased bone formation	Decreased bone formation (osteomalacia, 1,25(OH)$_2$D3 deficiency)

Other tests are available but the ones listed are the most useful for evaluation of metabolic bone disease in the patient with gastrointestinal or liver disease.
BMD = bone mineral density; CT = computed tomography; DXA = dual-energy x-ray absorptiometry; PTH = parathyroid hormone; SD = standard deviation;

Conditions Leading to Calcium and Vitamin D Deficiency

Vitamin D is a prohormone that can be synthesized in the skin or supplied in the diet (Figure 55-1). In the United States, many foods are vitamin fortified and contain vitamin D precursors. In patients with malabsorption, vitamin D precursors (ergocalciferol) are poorly absorbed. In liver disease, hydroxylation of vitamin D3 to 25-hydroxyvitamin D may be impaired. Following 25-hydroxylation of vitamin D in the liver, 1-hydroxylation occurs in the kidney through the action of 1α-hydroxylase. 1α-Hydroxylase expression is tightly controlled by parathyroid hormone (PTH) in response to serum calcium. The hormonally active 1,25-dihydroxyvitamin D activates calcium absorption in two general ways. First it increases expression of calbindin protein required for transport of calcium through villous enterocytes. 1,25-Dihydroxyvitamin D also increases paracellular calcium uptake through tight junctions. Calcium and vitamin D precursors in foods are absorbed largely in the duodenum and jejunum although data demonstrate that calcium is also absorbed in the colon (Hylander et al, 1990).

Low serum calcium activates a variety of homeostatic mechanisms to correct extracellular calcium concentrations. These include a rise in PTH (secondary hyperparathyroidism) and increased 1 α-hydroxylase activity in the kidney resulting in increased conversion of 25-hydroxyvitamin D to 1,25-dihydroxyvitamin D. Because of the underlying malabsorption and inability to increase calcium absorption from the gut, 1,25-dihydroxyvitamin D acts on bone to stimulate osteoclast differentiation and function and mobilize skeletal calcium stores. Decreased absorption of vitamin D may result in osteomalacia (failure to mineralize new bone matrix). In conditions of malabsorption, both osteoporosis and osteomalacia may coexist. Bone biopsy is required to distinguish these entities but is generally not necessary for treatment.

Given this background, it is clear that GI diseases resulting in inflammation or pathology of the upper small bowel are particularly susceptible to osteoporosis. Examples of these include *celiac sprue, Crohn's disease (CD), pancreatic insufficiency (PI)* (Moran et al, 1997) and *postgastrectomy* (Vestergaard, 2003). CD patients are especially at risk if they have had extensive surgical resections or have diffuse intestinal disease. With improved medical and surgical therapy for CD, extensive surgical resections are thankfully the exception. Patients with *jejuno-ileal bypass* are also at risk for osteoporosis. It remains to be seen whether less drastic weight loss surgeries, such as gastric banding, will contribute to decreased BMD over time. In *chronic cholestatic liver disease*, vitamin D and calcium are malabsorbed and should be supplemented.

Because of the high risk for osteoporosis in these disorders, tests to evaluate BMD should make up part of the initial examination of the patient. Additional tests that are suggested are shown in Figure 55-1. An interpretation of bone tests is provided in Table 55-1. Improvement in the underlying malabsorption and calcium and vitamin D supplementation are required (Liedman et al, 1997). Hypocalcemia is a contraindication to the use of bisphosphonates (discussed below). Additional factors may contribute to low vitamin D and be indirectly related to GI or liver disease 7-Dehydrocholesterol

TABLE 55-2. Gastrointestinal and Hepatic Disorders Associated With Low Bone Mineral Density, Estimates of Osteopenia and Osteoporosis, and Estimates of Fracture Risk

Condition	Osteopenia	Osteoporosis	Fracture Risk
Inflammatory bowel diseases			
Crohn's disease	40 to 80%	20 to 40%	40% increase over control population; 15 to 20% (silent fractures); risk may not be directly related to BMD
Ulcerative colitis	20 to 40%	10 to 20%	No increase
Malabsorption			
Celiac sprue	35 to 38%	25 to 50%	15 to 25%
Postgastrectomy (multiple mechanisms, not all related to malabsorption)	—	40% (some studies have found little change within 5 years of surgery—long-term complication of surgery)	80% increase over control population
Pancreatic insufficiency (cystic fibrosis)	50%	20%	No data
Liver disease			
Hepatic osteodystrophy	—	10 to 20% (mostly PBC)	> 60% in postmenopausal women with chronic liver disease, 5 to 15% in younger women and men
Pre-OLT/Post-OLT	—	20 to 45%	10 to 30%

Data presented reflect population-based studies when available. In general, the data are based on Z scores of the hip. For a comprehensive detailed review please see Bernstein et al, 2003; Leslie et al, 2003.
BMD = bone mineral density; OLT = orthotopic liver transplantation; PBC = primary biliary cirrhosis.

in the skin is converted to 25-hydroxyvitamin D in response to sun exposure. Patients from northern climates with poor sun exposure or any patient that has been very ill and home or hospital bound may therefore become 25-hydroxyvitamin D deficient. Encouraging sun exposure is beneficial.

Inflammatory Cytokines

TNF receptor family members, termed osteoprotegerins (OPGs) play an integral role in bone metabolism. Receptor activator nuclear factor κB ligand (RANKL or OPG ligand) is produced by osteoblasts and binds to its receptor RANK on the surface of an osteoclast precursor. The interaction of RANKL with RANK leads to osteoclast differentiation and thereby bone resorption. Inhibition of RANKL occurs when it binds a soluble antagonist OPG. In this way, the local ratios of RANKL to OPG determine net bone synthesis. Thus cytokines or drugs affect bone remodeling through regulation of OPGs.

Several lines of evidence suggest that factors other than glucocorticoids contribute to bone loss in inflammatory conditions of the bowel. Patients with recently diagnosed inflammatory bowel disease (IBD) do not have decreased bone mass density compared with age-matched controls; however, those with symptoms of > 6 months duration have lower bone mass density than age-matched controls (Stockbrugger et al, 2002). A variety of cytokines are overproduced in IBDs and celiac disease and may have detrimental effects on BMD. The inflammatory cytokines IL-1β, IL-6 and TNF-α are elevated in the systemic circulation of patients with CD. In patients with celiac disease, there is increased IL-1β and IL-6 in the systemic circulation which correlates with osteopenia. TNF-α expression is also increased in the mucosa of celiac patients, and, recently, treatment with infliximab has been shown beneficial in a patient with gluten-insensitive, refractory disease (Gillett et al, 2002).

TNF-α has a variety of detrimental effects on bone. In vitro studies have demonstrated that TNF-α causes osteoclastic bone resorption and inhibits bone collagen synthesis. TNF-α dramatically increases the survival of osteoclasts and protects them against apoptosis. TNF-α inhibits differentiation of osteoblasts from pluripotent progenitor cells. IL-1β and IL-6 also increase bone resorption through activation of osteoclast activity. TNF-α further propagates bone resorption by stimulating IL-6 secretion by osteoblasts. Increased serum IL-6 correlates with bone loss in patients with IBD. TNF-α and IL-1β increase Fas-mediated apoptosis of osteoblasts. TNF-α inhibits the action of 1,25 (OH) vitamin D through activation of a nuclear inhibitor that antagonizes the effect of vitamin D. Inhibition of TNF-α or IL-1 in ovariectemized mice prevents bone loss, suggesting that, in animal models, blockade of high TNF-α states is beneficial to the treatment of osteopenia and osteoporosis. Thus, *treating the underlying inflammatory disorder effectively, especially suppressing TNF-α and IL-6, may have an independent effect on promoting bone synthesis and decreasing bone resorption.* Because patients with IBD have elevated levels of proinflammatory cytokines and increased bone turnover, investigators have examined genetic factors associated with increased bone loss and inflammation (Nemetz et al, 2001). Allelic variants of the IL-1 receptor antagonist (IL-1ra) and IL-6 correlate with markers of bone turnover. Carriage of the A2 allele of the IL-1ra gene and the 130-base pair allele of the IL-6 gene were independently associated with increased bone loss. The presence of both alleles led to significantly greater bone loss than either singly. Other studies have not found an association between bone loss in IBD patients and carriage of a G/C polymorphism of the IL-6 gene, which results in increased IL-6 production. Associations between bone loss and allelic variations in the IL-1β gene and the IL-1 receptor antagonist gene have also

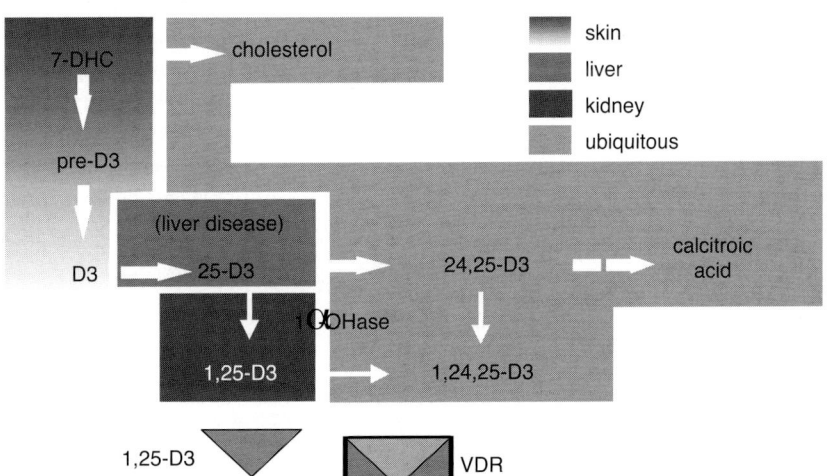

FIGURE 55-1. Vitamin D synthesis and metabolism. DHC = dihydrocalciferol; VDR = vitamin D receptor.

been studied in patients with IBD. Carriage of IL-1β-511*2 (allele *2 at the AvaI polymorphism) is associated with IL-1β hypersecretion and lower Z scores at the lumbar spine in patients with IBD. These data further substantiate the link between inflammatory mediators and osteoporosis in patients with IBD.

Hypogonadism

An under-appreciated cause of osteoporosis in patients with GI or liver disease is hypogonadism. Patients treated with glucocorticoids for any reason suppress gonadal and adrenal sex hormone production via suppression of the hypothalamic-pituitary axis. Women with CD, celiac disease or severe weight loss from any cause often do not menstruate and must be treated as if postmenopausal (Sher et al, 1994). Women that are postmenopausal and have coexistent GI diseases such as CD or celiac disease are at very high risk for osteoporosis and fractures (Clements et al, 1993). Similarly women with primary biliary cirrhosis (PBC) who are postmenopausal are at significantly higher risk than younger women for osteoporosis and fractures (Solerio et al, 2003). Estrogen replacement, especially in younger women who are not postmenopausal, should be considered. Estrogen replacement therapy has been shown to be safe and effective in patients with PBC (Monegal et al, 1997).

Men with CD, celiac disease, and liver disease may have inappropriately low levels of testosterone contributing to osteoporosis. Testosterone supplementation can be achieved through a topical gel or parenteral administration. In male liver patients in particular, hypogonadism is a principal cause of low BMD (Monegal et al, 1997). Testosterone is contraindicated, however, in patients with liver disease.

Hepatic Osteodystrophy

The mechanism of metabolic bone disease in patients with liver disease is multifactorial. The liver is a source of factors involved in bone remodeling and these factors are reduced in chronic liver disease. Patients with liver disease have impaired osteoblast proliferation and thus decreased bone formation. The liver is a source of insulin-like growth factor (IGF)-1, which is important in bone remodeling. Animal data suggest that the decrease in IGF-1 in cirrhosis results in decreased bone formation. In humans, however, the correlation between IGF-1 and osteopenia is less clear. OPG is also produced by the liver, and reductions in this may result in increased osteoclast activity. In general cholestatic liver diseases are associated with lower BMD than noncholestatic liver diseases. In particular patients with PBC appear to have decreased BMD but this may also occur because patients are generally older, postmenopausal women. There are also data to suggest that patients with PBC or autoimmune hepatitis are at an increased risk of celiac disease, both of which may contribute to low BMD. Liver transplantation, although beneficial for treatment of the underlying liver disease, appears to worsen BMD especially within the 2 years following the orthotopic liver transplantation (OLT). These data likely reflect the use of glucocorticoids and calcineurin inhibitors following OLT (discussed later in this chapter).

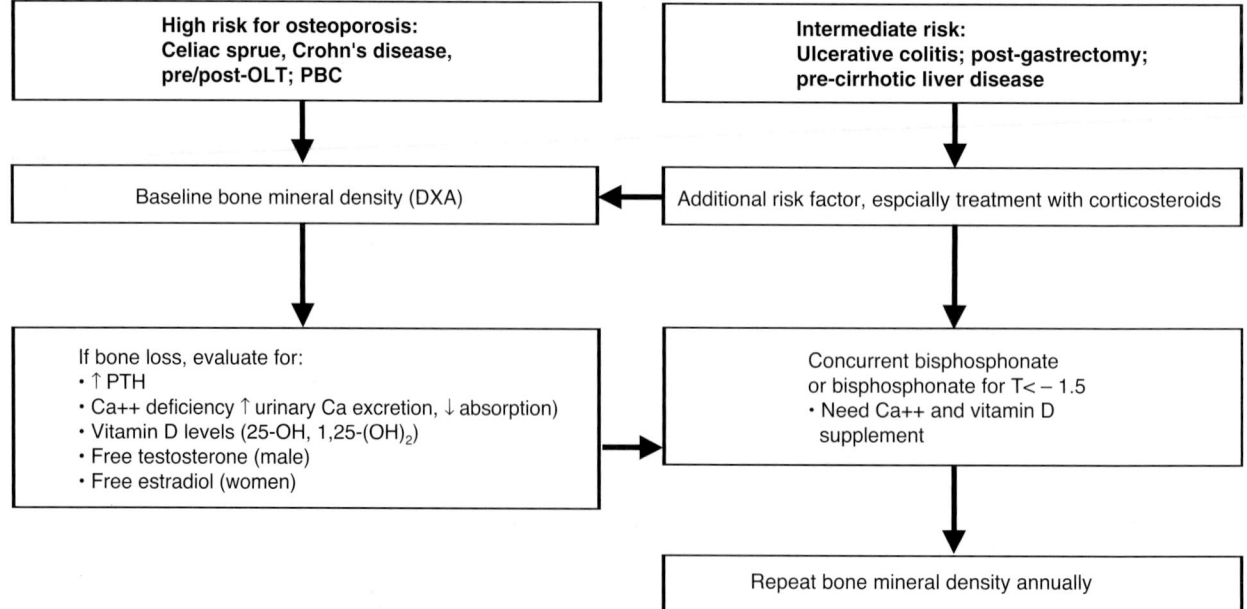

FIGURE 55-2. Diagnostic algorithm for metabolic bone disease. Ca++ = calcium; DXA = dual-energy x-ray absorptiometry; OLT = orthotopic liver transplantation; PBC = primary biliary cirrhosis; PTH = parathyroid hormone.

Drug-Induced Osteoporosis

Glucocorticoids

Glucocorticoid-induced osteoporosis occurs as a result of multiple mechanisms. Corticosteroids have multiple effects on bone including direct inhibition of bone formation, impaired calcium absorption across the intestine, and increased renal calcium excretion, all of which result in a negative calcium balance. As a result of calcium wasting, secondary hyperparathyroidism results and increases bone resorption. Corticosteroids induce a myopathy, which reduces the bone-stimulating effects of muscle activity. In animal models, corticosteroids have been shown to induce apoptosis of osteoblasts and osteocytes thereby resulting in diminished bone formation. More recently, corticosteroids have been shown to regulate bone metabolism through their effect on members of the TNF receptor family, the OPGs. Osteoclasts express the RANK receptor. Binding of RANKL to RANK activates osteoclastic activity, which can be blocked by a soluble receptor OPG (discussed above). Corticosteroids decrease OPG expression by 90% and increase RANKL expression by threefold resulting in increased osteoclastic activity. Corticosteroids also cause a threefold increase in osteoclast numbers. Finally, corticosteroids inhibit adrenal production of androgens contributing to bone loss.

The effect of corticosteroids on bone loss is most marked in the *first 6 to 12 months of therapy*; therefore, even short courses of steroids (< 6 months) will result in marked bone loss. Even within *1 week* of high dose steroid exposure, markers of bone resorption are increased. Bone loss secondary to steroids is dependent on both the *dose* and the *duration* of steroid use, with doses > 7.5 mg/d associated with 5 times the risk of fractures (Ruegsegger et al, 1983; van Staa et al, 2000). In studies of chronic exposure to steroids, average steroid doses of as little as 5.6 mg/d resulted in BMD loss of 2% per year (Buckley et al, 1996). In a large cohort of patients in the United Kingdom, the relative risk of vertebral fracture compared with a control population was 1.55 times higher with a standardized daily dose of steroids of 2.5 mg of prednisolone and increased to 5.18 for standardized doses of ≥ 7.5 mg (van Staa et al, 2000). Importantly, all fracture risks declined rapidly after cessation of steroids suggesting that therapy should be given during the time of corticosteroid use. The first decision to be made by the clinician is whether glucocorticoids are truly necessary for the management of the underlying disease. If the answer is yes, there must also be a plan in place for successfully withdrawing the glucocorticoids while maintaining remission. In the case of IBD, antimetabolites, such as 6-mercaptopurine or azathioprine and methotrexate (MTX), have been shown to be effective as steroid-sparing therapy. Infliximab is also steroid-sparing and may have independent effects on bone metabolism (Abreu et al, 2002).

Budesonide

If glucocorticoids cannot be avoided, in certain cases the clinician may choose a safer glucocorticoid alternative. *Budesonide* in a controlled ileal release (CIR) preparation (*Entocort*) is effective for mild to moderate ileal and right-sided colonic CD. This preparation is associated with fewer steroid-related side effects and less adrenocortical gland suppression. A prospective study of 98 steroid-naïve patients treated with prednisolone versus CIR-budesonide found that patients had a significantly greater drop in BMD with prednisolone treatment compared with CIR-budesonide (−1.04% versus −3.84%, $p = .0084$) (Schoon et al, 2002). Thus, whenever possible CIR-budesonide should be considered for the patient with CD. For patients with distal colonic IBD, topical rectal steroids in short courses (< 2 weeks) do not increase bone turnover in patients, but long term therapy with these agents does result in bone loss (Robinson et al, 1998). By contrast, however, oral budesonide therapy in patients with PBC or primary sclerosing cholangitis (PSC) resulted in worsening of their osteoporosis (Angulo et al, 2000). Similar to IBD, autoimmune hepatitis is treated with glucocorticoids. Patients with both PSC and underlying IBD may receive glucocorticoids and be at increased risk of osteoporosis (Angulo et al, 1998).

Cyclosporine and Tacrolimus

Cyclosporine and *tacrolimus* are calcineurin phosphatase inhibitors used in a variety of GI disorders. It is used in patients with severe ulcerative colitis (UC) to prevent colectomy. It is also commonly used post-OLT. Cyclosporine and tacrolimus both cause *osteopenia* and *osteoporosis* by increasing bone turnover, which is reflected in high levels of osteocalcin (Epstein et al, 1995; Inoue et al, 2000). Renal transplantation patients given cyclosporine alone, however, did not have sig-

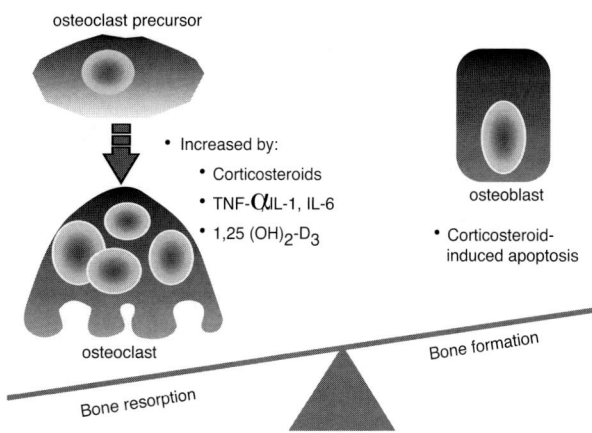

FIGURE 55-3. Determinant of bone mineral density. IL = interleukin; TNF = tumor necrosis factor.

nificant bone loss at the end of 18 months whereas those treated with corticosteroids plus cyclosporine experienced the greatest losses suggesting corticosteroids are the worst offenders in this regard (Aroldi et al, 1997). Tacrolimus is associated with less bone loss, which is probably related to a decreased requirement for concurrent steroids (Monegal et al, 2001). Although not a justification for a colectomy, UC patients post-ileal pouch anal anastomosis have an improvement in BMD, again suggesting that correction of the underlying inflammatory problem as well as avoidance of glucocorticoids and cyclosporine results in improved BMD (Abitbol et al, 1997).

MTX

Scant evidence exists that MTX contributes significantly to bone loss. In patients with rheumatoid arthritis, MTX alone is not associated with increased bone loss but the combination of MTX and prednisone > 5 mg/d led to greater bone loss than prednisone therapy alone (Buckley et al, 1997; Bianchi et al, 1999). No studies have been performed in CD patients using MTX therapy with respect to BMD.

Examination of the Gastroenterology Patient for Metabolic Bone Disease

The diseases discussed in this chapter are all associated with inappropriately low BMD resulting from a variety of distinct mechanisms. Given that the causes of bone loss are distinct, the examination of the patient with GI-related metabolic bone disease should be tailored to the particular situation. Figure 55-2 presents an algorithm that is useful in various scenarios. Diseases such as celiac disease commonly cause osteoporosis. Indeed, in studies of asymptomatic osteoporotic women, 10% demonstrate antitissue transglutaminase antibodies suggesting that celiac disease may be a contributing factor for osteoporosis in the general population (Nuti et al, 2001). Diseases such as UC and, to a lesser extent, CD result in decreased BMD because of cumulative corticosteroid use; therefore tests of BMD such as dual-energy x-ray absorptiometry (DXA) are more important following steroid exposure. In addition to DXA testing, other tests such as quantitative (usually calcaneal)

TABLE 55-3. Mechanisms of Metabolic Bone Disease in Gastrointestinal and Hepatic Diseases

Mechanism	Disorder	Bone Disease
Calcium and/or vitamin D deficiency	Intestinal malabsorption, (many causes); liver disease	Osteoporosis; osteomalacia (25-hydroxyvitamin D deficiency)
Inflammatory cytokines	Crohn's disease; celiac sprue	Osteoporosis
Drug-induced		
Glucocorticoids	IBD; Autoimmune hepatitis; post-OLT	Osteoporosis
Cyclosporine/Tacrolimus	IBD; post-OLT	Osteoporosis
Hypogonadism	IBD; celiac sprue; cirrhosis; glucocorticoid treatment	Osteoporosis
Hepatic osteodystrophy	Cholestatic liver disease; cirrhosis	Osteoporosis

IBD = inflammatory bowel disease; OLT = orthotopic liver transplantation.

Table 55-4. Choosing Bisphosphonates and Other Antiresorptive Therapies

(1) First line bisphosponates:
   Alendronate (Fosamax)—10 mg/d or 70 mg/once per week; long half-life of 10 years therefore avoid in women with child-bearing potential
   Risedronate (Actonel)—5 mg/d or 35 mg/once per week; half-life of 20 days
(2) If gastrointestinal intolerance or worsening BMD after 1 year, consider the following alternatives:
   a. Nasal calcitonin (Miacalcin)—although less effective than bisphosphonates, nasal absorption eliminates concern for poor gastrointestinal absorption.
   b. IV bisphosphonates:
      Pamidronate—although indicated for malignant hypercalcemia is also effective for glucocorticoid-induced osteoporosis (Boutsen et al, 1997, 2001) ; may use 30 mg IV given over 4 h. Half-life is 28 days. Should be repeated every 3 months.
      Zoledronic Acid (Zometa)—dose is 4 mg IV over 15 minutes; effective to increase BMD in postmenopausal women for 1 year (Reid et al, 2002)
      Teriparatide (rDNA origin) (Forteo)—black box warning regarding potential risk of osteosarcoma seen in rats; very expensive; given by daily sc injection so avoids gut absorption
(3) Special circumstances:
   Testosterone deficiency in men is suggested by low sexual drive and low BMD. Replacement can be achieved with topical gel (Androgel) or transdermal patches (many).

BMD = bone mineral density; IV = intravenous; sc = subcutaneous.

ultrasound or quantitative computed tomography may be used to assess BMD.

In addition to BMD measurements, other serum and urinary markers are available for assessment of bone turnover. Normally bone formation and bone resorption are tightly linked. N-telopeptide cross-linked of type 1 collagen is released with bone resorption and excreted in the urine. In patients with IBD, measurement of urinary N-telopeptide cross-linked of type 1 collagen was the best predictor of spinal bone loss over a 2-year follow-up period compared with other markers including bone alkaline phosphatase, osteocalcin, PTH, and vitamin D levels (Schulte et al, 2000).

For diseases in which malabsorption of vitamins and calcium may play a significant role in pathogenesis of BMD, such as celiac sprue, a baseline test of BMD is justified. Additional tests may also be necessary in order to correct the contributing metabolic deficiencies. These are shown in Figure 55-1. An interpretation of bone-related test results for common GI conditions is found in Table 55-1.

Treatment Strategies

In spite of the variety of mechanisms leading to metabolic bone disease, there are several treatment strategies that are broadly applicable. The best strategy is *prevention* (eg, avoidance of glucocorticoids to treat IBD whenever possible). Effective treatment of the underlying GI disease (eg, gluten-free diet in celiac disease) can improve BMD within a year (Mora et al, 1998; Szathmari et al, 2001; McFarlane et al, 1995). Of course, even at the time of diagnosis, bone loss may be well on its way. Low BMD is a result of decreased bone formation and/or increased bone resorption. Most therapies for osteoporosis aim to inhibit bone resorption (eg, bisphosphonates [Table 55-4]). Bisphosphonates are highly effective for both prevention (Saag et al, 1998; Cohen et al, 1999; Reid et al, 1998) and treatment of glucocorticoid and postmenopausal osteoporosis (Reid et al, 1998; Adachi et al, 1996) (see Table 55-4). As a class of drugs they are more effective than vitamin D, fluoride or calcitonin for treatment of osteoporosis (Amin et al, 1999). In addition to increasing BMD in patients receiving corticosteroids, large randomized placebo controlled trials have demonstrated a 70% reduction in the incidence of vertebral fractures in risedronate-treated (5 mg/d) patients compared with placebo-treated patients (Haderslav et al, 2000; Lindor et al, 2000). Bisphosphonates are effective for osteoporosis regardless of the cause. They have been used successfully in CD, PBC, and post-OLT (Reeves et al, 1998; Ninkovic et al, 2002). That being said, their efficacy has been most extensively studied in glucocorticoid and postmenopausal osteoporosis. Bisphosphonates as a class are themselves associated with a high degree of GI side effects, especially esophageal erosions and ulcers. Risedronate (Actonel) has been shown to have *fewer* esophageal and gastric erosions and ulcers in endoscopic studies (Lanza et al, 2000). Clinically significant GI side effects, however, are similar between risedronate (Actonel) and alendronate (Fosamax). Anecdotal data suggest that once a week preparations may have less GI toxicity because they are in contact with the esophageal mucosa for a shorter period of time. Moreover, one pill a week is desirable to improve patient adherence to the medication. Bisphosphonates are poorly absorbed drugs, generally < 1% of an oral dose is bioavailable. These drugs have not been studied in patients with malabsorption (Scott et al, 2000). Bisphosphonates should not be used in hypocalcemic patients or those with uncorrected 25-hydroxyvitamin D deficiency (Rosen and Brown, 2003). Once calcium is corrected, however, bisphosphonates may be used if osteopenia or osteoporosis is present (see Table 55-4).

Evaluation of the efficacy of bisphosphonates should be performed once a year with a repeat BMD examination. To avoid conflicting results, it is preferable if the same examination, (eg, dual-energy radiograph absorptiometry) and same machine is used in order to accurately compare results. In some cases such as very low BMD and/or the occurrence of serious fractures, it may be important prior to document that the medication is being absorbed prior to waiting a year. Because bisphosphonates are very potent antiresorptives that inhibit osteoclast function, urinary excretion of *the N-telopeptide* of type I collagen *precipitously drops* with successful uptake of the drug. This urine test may be sent 1 month after inception of bisphosphonate therapy, especially in patients suspected of upper gut malabsorption.

In patients who either do not respond to bisphosphonates or have unmanageable GI side effects from them, several options exist. The first is *nasal calcitonin*. In studies of patients with glucocorticoid-induced osteoporosis, it was effective in delaying bone loss compared to placebo (Sambrook et al, 1993; Luengo et al, 1994). The advantage is the delivery via the nasal route avoiding the need for GI absorption. It is not, however, as effective as bisphosphonates for increasing BMD. The other option that is easy to administer especially for patients who regularly require

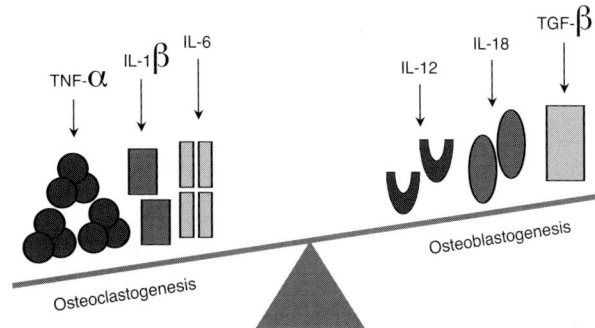

FIGURE 55-4. Chronic inflammation and bone metabolism. IL = interleukin; TGF = transforming growth factor; TNF = tumor necrosis factor.

administration of other intravenous (IV) medications (eg, infliximab) or who are hospitalized, is IV bisphosphonates. Although these are US Food and Drug Administration (FDA)-approved for malignant hypercalcemia or Paget's disease of bone, they are also highly effective for glucocorticoid-induced or postmenopausal osteoporosis. The advantages can be dramatic given that they are effective for prolonged periods of time, between *3 months (pamidronate)* (Boutsen et al, 2001) and *1 year (zoledronate)* (Reid et al, 2002). Recently, *teriparatide (Forteo)* became available for the treatment of postmenopausal osteoporosis or hypogonadal osteoporosis in men at high risk for fracture or unresponsive to other antiresorptive therapy (Body et al, 2002; Neer et al, 2001). Teriparatide is a recombinant fragment of *human PTH*. In contrast to bisphosphonates, teriparatide stimulates new bone formation through stimulation of osteoblastic activity. Studies of teriparatide have not been done in patients with GI or hepatic disease but there is no reason to believe it will be ineffective.

Calcium and vitamin D supplements should be thought of as adjunctive to the above therapies but should never be thought of as sufficiently effective to treat osteoporosis or prevent glucocorticoid-induced osteoporosis (Bernstein et al, 1996). Patients should take approximately *2 g of calcium per day*. *Calcium citrate* supplements may be better absorbed than calcium carbonate. Dairy products are an important source of calcium. Many patients with GI diseases have been told they are lactose intolerant without sufficient data to support it. Genetic testing for lactase nonpersistence and lactose breath hydrogen testing for secondary lactose intolerance may be useful to document lactose malabsorption.

Supplemental Reading

Abitbol V, Roux C, Guillemant S, et al. Bone assessment in patients with ileal pouch-anal anastomosis for inflammatory bowel disease. Br J Surg 1997;84:1551–4.

Abreu MT, Kam LY, Vasiliauskas EA, et al. Treatment with infliximab is associated with increased markers of bone synthesis in patients with Crohn's disease. Am J Gastroenterol 2002:A.

Adachi JD, Pack S, Chines AA. Intermittent etidronate and corticoisteroid-induced osteoporosis. N Engl J Med 1997; 337:1921.

Adachi JD. Corticosteroid-induced osteoporosis. Am J Med Sci 1997;313:41–9.

Adachi JD, Bensen WG, Bell MJ, et al. Salmon calcitonin nasal spray in the prevention of corticosteroid-induced osteoporosis. Br J Rheumatol 1997;36:255–9.

Adachi JD, Bensen WG, Bianchi F, et al. Vitamin D and calcium in the prevention of corticosteroid induced osteoporosis: a 3 year followup [see comments]. J Rheumatol 1996;23:995–1000.

Adachi JD, Loannidis G, Berger C, et al. The influence of osteoporotic fractures on health-related quality of life in community-dwelling men and women across Canada. Osteoporosis International 2001;12:903–8.

Adachi Y, Shiota E, Matsumata T, et al. Osteoporosis after gastrectomy: bone mineral density of lumbar spine assessed by dual-energy X-ray absorptiometry. Calcified Tissue International 2000;66:119–22.

Amin S, LaValley MP, Simms RW, Felson DT. The role of vitamin D in corticosteroid-induced osteoporosis: a meta-analytic approach. Arthritis Rheum 1999;42:1740–51.

Angulo P, Batts KP, Jorgensen RA, et al. Oral budesonide in the treatment of primary sclerosing cholangitis. Am J Gastroenterol 2000;95:2333–7.

Angulo P, Jorgensen RA, Keach JC, et al. Oral budesonide in the treatment of patients with primary biliary cirrhosis with a suboptimal response to ursodeoxycholic acid. Hepatology 2000;31:318–23.

Angulo P, Therneau TM, Jorgensen A, et al. Bone disease in patients with primary sclerosing cholangitis: prevalence, severity and prediction of progression. J Hepatol 1998;29:729–35.

Anonymous. Assessment of fracture risk and its application to screening for postmenopausal osteoporosis. Report of a WHO Study Group. World Health Organization Technical Report Series 1994;843:1–129.

Ardizzone S, Bollani S, Bettica P, et al. Altered bone metabolism in inflammatory bowel disease: there is a difference between Crohn's disease and ulcerative colitis. J Intern Med 2000;247:63–70.

Aroldi A, Tarantino A, Montagnino G, et al. Effects of three immunosuppressive regimens on vertebral bone density in renal transplant recipients: a prospective study. Transplantation 1997;63:380–6.

Bernstein CN, Blanchard JF, Leslie W, et al. The incidence of fracture among patients with inflammatory bowel disease. A population-based cohort study. Ann Intern Med 2000;133:795–9.

Bernstein CN, Leslie WD, Leboff MS. AGA technical review on osteoporosis in gastrointestinal diseases. Gastroenterology 2003;124:795–841.

Bernstein CN, Seeger LL, Anton PA, et al. A randomized, placebo-controlled trial of calcium supplementation for decreased bone density in corticosteroid-using patients with inflammatory bowel disease: a pilot study. Aliment Pharmacol Ther 1996;10:777–86.

Bernstein CN, Seeger LL, Sayre JW, et al. Decreased bone density in inflammatory bowel disease is related to corticosteroid use and not disease diagnosis. J Bone Miner Res 1995;10:250–6.

Bertolini DR, Nedwin GE, Bringman TS, et al. Stimulation of bone resorption and inhibition of bone formation in vitro by human tumour necrosis factors. Nature 1986;319:516–8.

Bianchi ML, Cimaz R, Galbiati E, et al. Bone mass change during methotrexate treatment in patients with juvenile rheumatoid arthritis. Osteoporosis International 1999;10:20–5.

Bjarnason I, Macpherson A, Mackintosh C, et al. Reduced bone density in patients with inflammatory bowel disease. Gut 1997;40:228–33.

Body JJ, Gaich GA, Scheele WH, et al. A randomized double-blind trial to compare the efficacy of teriparatide [recombinant human parathyroid hormone (1-34)] with alendronate in postmenopausal women with osteoporosis. J Clin Endocrinol Metab 2002;87:4528–35.

Boutsen Y, Jamart J, Esselinckx W, Devogelaer JP. Primary prevention of glucocorticoid-induced osteoporosis with intra-

---

Editor's Note: This is an excellent review. A complete 157-item bibliography can be obtained at <maris.abreu@cshs.org>.

venous pamidronate and calcium: a prospective controlled 1-year study comparing a single infusion, an infusion given once every 3 months, and calcium alone. J Bone Miner Res 2001;16:104–12.

Boutsen Y, Jamart J, Esselinckx W, et al. Primary prevention of glucocorticoid-induced osteoporosis with intermittent intravenous pamidronate: a randomized trial. Calcif Tissue Int 1997;61:266–71.

Buckley LM, Leib ES, Cartularo KS, et al. Effects of low dose methotrexate on the bone mineral density of patients with rheumatoid arthritis. J Rheumatol 1997;24:1489–94.

Buckley LM, Leib ES, Cartularo KS, et al. Calcium and vitamin D3 supplementation prevents bone loss in the spine secondary to low-dose corticosteroids in patients with rheumatoid arthritis. Ann Intern Med 1996;125:961–8.

Burgess TL, Qian Y, Kaufman S, et al. The ligand for osteoprotegerin (OPGL) directly activates mature osteoclasts. J Cell Biol 1999;145:527–38.

Candy S, Wright J, Gerber M, et al. controlled double blind study of azathioprine in the management of Crohn's disease. Gut 1995;37:674–8.

Cemborain A, Castilla-Cortazar I, Garcia M, et al. Effects of IGF-I treatment on osteopenia in rats with advanced liver cirrhosis. J Physiol Biochem 2000;56:91–9.

Cemborain A, Castilla-Cortazar I, Garcia M, et al. Osteopenia in rats with liver cirrhosis: beneficial effects of IGF-I treatment. J Hepatol 1998;28:122–31.

Clements D, Compston JE, Evans WD, Rhodes J. Hormone replacement therapy prevents bone loss in patients with inflammatory bowel disease. Gut 1993;34:1543–6.

Clements D, Motley RJ, Evans WD, et al. Longitudinal study of cortical bone loss in patients with inflammatory bowel disease. Scand J Gastroenterol 1992;27:1055–60.

Cohen S, Levy RM, Keller M, et al. Risedronate therapy prevents corticosteroid-induced bone loss: a twelve-month, multicenter, randomized, double-blind, placebo-controlled, parallel-group study. Arthritis Rheum 1999;42:2309–18.

Compston JE, Ayers AB, Horton LW, et al. Osteomalacia after small-intestinal resection. Lancet 1978;1:9–12.

Compston JE, Horton LW, Laker MF, et al. Bone disease after jejuno-ileal bypass for obesity. Lancet 1978;2:1–4.

Cranney A, Welch V, Tugwell P, et al. Responsiveness of endpoints in osteoporosis clinical trials—an update. J Rheumatol 1999;26:222–8.

Dickey W, McMillan SA, Callender ME. High prevalence of celiac sprue among patients with primary biliary cirrhosis. J Clin Gastroenterol 1997;25:328–9.

Dinca M, Fries W, Luisetto G, et al. Evolution of osteopenia in inflammatory bowel disease. Am J Gastroenterol 1999;94:1292–7.

Dresner-Pollak R, Karmeli F, Eliakim R, et al. Increased urinary N-telopeptide cross-linked type 1 collagen predicts bone loss in patients with inflammatory bowel disease. Am J Gastroenterol 2000;95:699–704.

Eastell R, Dickson ER, Hodgson SF, et al. Rates of vertebral bone loss before and after liver transplantation in women with primary biliary cirrhosis. Hepatology 1991;14:296–300.

Epstein S, Shane E, Bilezikian JP. Organ transplantation and osteoporosis. Curr Opin Rheumatol 1995;7:255–61.

Ezra A, Golomb G. Administration routes and delivery systems of bisphosphonates for the treatment of bone resorption. Adv Drug Deliv Rev 2000;42:175–95.

Farthing MJ, Edwards CR, Rees LH, Dawson AM. Male gonadal function in celiac disease: 1. Sexual dysfunction, infertility, and semen quality. Gut 1982;23:608–14.

Farthing MJ, Rees LH, Edwards CR, Dawson AM. Male gonadal function in celiac disease: 2. Sex hormones. Gut 1983;24:127–35.

Feagan BG, Rochon J, Fedorak RN, et al. Methotrexate for the treatment of Crohn's disease. The North American Crohn's Study Group Investigators. N Engl J Med 1995;332:292–7.

Fernandez-Martin JL, Kurian S, Farmer P, Nanes MS. Tumor necrosis factor activates a nuclear inhibitor of vitamin D and retinoid-X receptors. Mol Cell Endocrinol 1998;141:65–72.

Fornari MC, Pedreira S, Niveloni S, et al. Pre- and post-treatment serum levels of cytokines IL-1beta, IL-6, and IL-1 receptor antagonist in celiac disease. Are they related to the associated osteopenia? Am J Gastroenterol 1998;93:413–8.

Gallego-Rojo FJ, Gonzalez-Calvin JL, Munoz-Torres M, et al. Bone mineral density, serum insulin-like growth factor I, and bone turnover markers in viral cirrhosis. Hepatology 1998;28:695–9.

Gennari C. Glucocorticoids and bone. Bone Miner 1985:213.

Gilbert L, He X, Farmer P, et al. Expression of the osteoblast differentiation factor RUNX2 (Cbfa1/AML3/Pebp2alpha A) is inhibited by tumor necrosis factor-alpha. J Biol Chem 2002;277:2695–701.

Gilbert L, He X, Farmer P, et al. Inhibition of osteoblast differentiation by tumor necrosis factor-alpha. Endocrinology 2000;141:3956–64.

Gillett HR, Arnott ID, McIntyre M, et al. Successful infliximab treatment for steroid-refractory celiac disease: a case report. Gastroenterology 2002;122:800–5.

Giuliani N, Pedrazzoni M, Passeri G, Girasole G. Bisphosphonates inhibit IL-6 production by human osteoblast-like cells. Scand J Rheumatol 1998;27:38–41.

Greenberg GR, Feagan BG, Martin F, et al. Oral budesonide for active Crohn's disease. Canadian Inflammatory Bowel Disease Study Group. N Engl J Med 1994;331:836–41.

Guanabens N, Pares A, Marinoso L, et al. Factors influencing the development of metabolic bone disease in primary biliary cirrhosis. Am J Gastroenterol 1990;85:1356–62.

Guichelaar MM, Malinchoc M, Sibonga J, et al. Bone metabolism in advanced cholestatic liver disease: analysis by bone histomorphometry. Hepatology 2002;36(4 Pt 1):895–903.

Haaber AB, Rosenfalck AM, Hansen B, et al. Bone mineral metabolism, bone mineral density, and body composition in patients with chronic pancreatitis and pancreatic exocrine insufficiency. Int J Pancreatol 2000;27:21–7.

Haderslav KV, Tjellesen H, Sorensen HA, Staun M. Alendronate increases lumbar spine bone mineral density in patients with Crohn's disease. Gastroenterol 2000;119:639–46.

Hanauer SB, Feagan BG, Lichtenstein GR, et al. Maintenance infliximab for Crohn's disease: the ACCENT I randomised trial. Lancet 2002;359:1541–9.

Healy JH, Paget S, Williams-Russo P. A randomized controlled trial of salmon calcitonin to prevent bone loss in corticosteroid treated temporal arteritis and polymyalgia rheumatica. Calcif Tissue Int 1996;59:73.

Heiskanen JT, Kroger H, Paakkonen M, et al. Bone mineral metabolism after total gastrectomy. Bone 2001;28:123–7.

Hodsman AB, Toogood JH, Jennings B. Differential effect of inhaled budesonide and oral prenisolone on serum osteocalcin. J Clin Endocrinol 1991;72:530–40.

Hofbauer LC, Gori F, Riggs BL, et al. Stimulation of osteoprotegerin ligand and inhibition of osteoprotegerin production by glucocorticoids in human osteoblastic lineage cells: potential paracrine mechanisms of glucocorticoid-induced osteoporosis. Endocrinology 1999;140:4382–9.

Horowitz MC, Xi Y, Wilson K, Kacena MA. Control of osteoclastogenesis and bone resorption by members of the TNF family of receptors and ligands. Cytokine Growth Factor Rev 2001;12:9–18.

Hsu H, Lacey DL, Dunstan CR, et al. Tumor necrosis factor receptor family member RANK mediates osteoclast differentiation and activation induced by osteoprotegerin ligand. Proc Natl Acad Sci U S A 1999;96:3540–5.

Hussaini SH, Oldroyd B, Stewart SP, et al. Regional bone mineral density after orthotopic liver transplantation. Eur J Gastroenterol Hepatol 1999;11:157–63.

Hylander E, Ladefoged K, Jarnum S. Calcium absorption after intestinal resection. The importance of a preserved colon. Scand J Gastroenterol 1990;25:705–10.

Inoue T, Kawamura I, Matsuo M, et al. Lesser reduction in bone mineral density by the immunosuppressant, FK506, compared with cyclosporine in rats. Transplantation 2000;70:774–9.

Janes CH, Dickson ER, Okazaki R, et al. Role of hyperbilirubinemia in the impairment of osteoblast proliferation associated with cholestatic jaundice. J Clin Invest 1995;95:2581–6.

Jilka RL, Weinstein RS, Bellido T, et al. Increased bone formation by prevention of osteoblast apoptosis with parathyroid hormone. J Clin Invest 1999;104:439–46.

Josse R, Adachi JD, Chines AA. Prevention of corticosteroid-induced osteoporosis with etidronate: one year follow-up with calcium only. Osteoporosis International 1998;8:108.

Karbach U. Segmental heterogeneity of cellular and paracellular calcium transport across the rat duodenum and jejunum. Gastroenterol 1991;100:47.

Kemppainen T, Kroger H, Janatuinen E, et al. Osteoporosis in adult patients with celiac disease. Bone 1999;24:249–55.

Klaus J, Armbrecht G, Steinkamp M, et al. High prevalence of osteoporotic vertebral fractures in patients with Crohn's disease. Gut 2002;51:654–8.

Kong YY, Yoshida H, Sarosi I, et al. OPGL is a key regulator of osteoclastogenesis, lymphocyte development and lymph-node organogenesis. Nature 1999;397:315–23.

Kotaniemi A, Piirainen H, Paimela L, et al. Is continuous intranasal salmon calcitonin effective in treating axial bone loss in patients with active rheumatoid arthritis receiving low dose glucocorticoid therapy? J Rheumatol 1996;23:1875–9.

Kurokouchi K, Kambe F, Yasukawa K, et al. TNF-alpha increases expression of IL-6 and ICAM-1 genes through activation of NF-kappaB in osteoblast-like ROS17/2.8 cells. J Bone Miner Res 1998;13:1290–9.

Lader CS, Flanagan AM. Prostaglandin E2, interleukin 1alpha, and tumor necrosis factor-alpha increase human osteoclast formation and bone resorption in vitro. Endocrinology 1998;139:3157–64.

Lanza F, Schwartz H, Sahba B, et al. An endoscopic comparison of the effects of alendronate and risedronate on upper gastrointestinal mucosae. Am J Gastroenterol 2000;95:3112–7.

Lanza FL, Hunt RH, Thomson AB, et al. Endoscopic comparison of esophageal and gastroduodenal effects of risedronate and alendronate in postmenopausal women. Gastroenterology 2000;119:631–8.

Lee SE, Chung WJ, Kwak HB, et al. Tumor necrosis factor-alpha supports the survival of osteoclasts through the activation of Akt and ERK. J Biol Chem 2001;276:49343–9.

Leslie WD, Bernstein CN, Leboff MS. AGA technical review on osteoporosis in hepatic disorders. Gastroenterology 2003;125:941–66.

Li J, Sarosi I, Yan XQ, et al. RANK is the intrinsic hematopoietic cell surface receptor that controls osteoclastogenesis and regulation of bone mass and calcium metabolism. Proc Natl Acad Sci U S A 2000;97:1566–71.

Liedman B, Bosaeus I, Mellstrom D, Lundell L. Osteoporosis after total gastrectomy. Results of a prospective, clinical study. Scand J Gastroenterol 1997;32:1090–5.

Lindor KD, Jorgensen RA, Tiegs RD, et al. Etidronate for osteoporosis in primary biliary cirrhosis: a randomized trial. J Hepatol 2000;33:878–82.

LoCascio V, Bonucci E, Imbimbo B. Bone loss after glucocorticoid therapy. Calcif Tissue Int 1984;36:435–8.

Loftus EV Jr, Crowson CS, Sandborn WJ, et al. Long-term fracture risk in patients with Crohn's disease: a population-based study in Olmsted County, Minnesota. Gastroenterology 2002;123:468–75.

Luengo M, Picado C, Del Rio L, et al. Treatment of steroid-induced osteopenia with calcitonin in corticosteroid-dependent asthma. A one-year follow-up study. Am Rev Respir Dis 1990;142:104–7.

Luengo M, Pons F, Martinez de Osaba MJ, Picado C. Prevention of further bone mass loss by nasal calcitonin in patients on long term glucocorticoid therapy for asthma: a two year follow up study. Thorax 1994;49:1099–102.

Lukert BP, Raisz LG. Glucocorticoid-induced osteoporosis: pathogenesis and management. Ann Intern Med 1990;112:352–64.

Manolagas SC, Bellido T, Jilka RL. Sex steroids, cytokines and the bone marrow: new concepts on the pathogenesis of osteoporosis. Ciba Found Symp 1995;191:187-96; discussion 197–202.

Markowitz J, Grancher K, Kohn N, et al. A multicenter trial of 6-mercaptopurine and prednisone in children with newly diagnosed Crohn's disease. Gastroenterology 2000;119:895–902.

McFarlane XA, Bhalla AK, Reeves DE, et al. Osteoporosis in treated adult coeliac disease. Gut 1995;36:710–4.

Melton LJ III, Crowson CS, Khosla S, O'Fallon WM. Fracture risk after surgery for peptic ulcer disease: a population-based cohort study. Bone 1999;25:61–7.

Menon KV, Angulo P, Boe GM, Lindor KD. Safety and efficacy of estrogen therapy in preventing bone loss in primary biliary cirrhosis. Am J Gastroenterol 2003;98:889–92.

Menon KV, Angulo P, Weston S, et al. Bone disease in primary biliary cirrhosis: independent indicators and rate of progression. J Hepatol 2001;35:316–23.

Meyer D, Stavropolous S, Diamond B, et al. Osteoporosis in a North American adult population with celiac disease. Am J Gastroenterol 2001;96:112–9.

Michel BA, Bloch DA, Fries JF. Predictors of fractures in early rheumatoid arthritis. J Rheumatol 1991;18:804–8.

Monegal A, Navasa M, Guanabens N, et al. Bone mass and mineral metabolism in liver transplant patients treated with FK506 or cyclosporine A. Calcif Tissue Int 2001;68:83–6.

Monegal A, Navasa M, Guanabens N, et al. Osteoporosis and bone mineral metabolism disorders in cirrhotic patients referred for orthotopic liver transplantation. Calcif Tissue Int 1997;60:148–54.

Mora S, Barera G, Ricotti A, et al. Reversal of low bone density with a gluten-free diet in children and adolescents with celiac disease. Am J Clin Nutr 1998;67:477–81.

Mora S, Weber G, Barera G, et al. Effect of gluten-free diet on bone mineral content in growing patients with celiac disease. Am J Clin Nutr 1993;57:224–8.

Moran CE, Sosa EG, Martinez SM, et al. Bone mineral density in patients with pancreatic insufficiency and steatorrhea. Am J Gastroenterol 1997;92:867–71.

Motley RJ, Clements D, Evans WD, et al. A four-year longitudinal study of bone loss in patients with inflammatory bowel disease. Bone Miner 1993;23:95–104.

Neer RM, Arnaud CD, Zanchetta JR, et al. Effect of parathyroid hormone (1-34) on fractures and bone mineral density in postmenopausal women with osteoporosis. N Engl J Med. 2001;344:1434–41.

Nemetz A, Toth M, Garcia-Gonzalez MA, et al. Allelic variation at the interleukin 1beta gene is associated with decreased bone mass in patients with inflammatory bowel diseases. Gut 2001;49:644–9.

Newton J, Francis R, Prince M, et al. Osteoporosis in primary biliary cirrhosis revisited. Gut 2001;49:282–7.

Ninkovic M, Love S, Tom BD, et al. Lack of effect of intravenous pamidronate on fracture incidence and bone mineral density after orthotopic liver transplantation. J Hepatol 2002;37:93–100.

Nuti R, Martini G, Valenti R, et al. Prevalence of undiagnosed coeliac syndrome in osteoporotic women. J Intern Med 2001;250:361–6.

Ormarsdottir S, Ljunggren O, Mallmin H, et al. Circulating levels of insulin-like growth factors and their binding proteins in patients with chronic liver disease: lack of correlation with bone mineral density. Liver 2001;21:123–8.

Pollak RD, Karmeli F, Eliakim R, et al. Femoral neck osteopenia in patients with inflammatory bowel disease. Am J Gastroenterol 1998;93:1483–90.

Reeves HL, Francis RM, Manas DM, et al. Intravenous bisphosphonate prevents symptomatic osteoporotic vertebral collapse in patients after liver transplantation. Liver Transpl Surg 1998;4:404–9.

Reid D, Cohen S, Pack S, et al. Risedronate reduces the incidence of vertebral fractures in patients on chronic corticosteroid therapy. Arthritis Rheum 1998;41:S136.

Reid D, Cohen S, Pack S. Risedronate is an effective and well-tolerated therapy in both the treatment and prevention of corticosteroid-induced osteoporosis. Bone 1998;23:S402.

Reid D, Devogelaer JP, Hughes R, et al. Risedronate is effective and well tolerated in treating corticosterd-induced osteoporosis. American College of Rheumatology Annual Meeting; 1998.

Reid IR, Brown JP, Burckhardt P, et al. Intravenous zoledronic acid in postmenopausal women with low bone mineral density. N Engl J Med 2002;346:653–61.

Ringe JD, Welzel D. Salmon calcitonin in the therapy of corticoid-induced osteoporosis. Eur J Clin Pharmacol 1987;33:35.

Robinson RJ, Carr I, Iqbal SJ, et al. Screening for osteoporosis in Crohn's disease. A detailed evaluation of calcaneal ultrasound. Eur J Gastroenterol Hepatol 1998;10:137–40.

Robinson RJ, Iqbal SJ, Wolfe R, et al. The effect of rectally administered steroids on bone turnover: a comparative study. Aliment Pharmacol Ther 1998;12:213–7.

Romaldini CC, Barbieri D, Okay TS, et al. Serum soluble interleukin-2 receptor, interleukin-6, and tumor necrosis factor-alpha levels in children with celiac disease: response to treatment. J Pediatr Gastroenterol Nutr 2002;35:513–7.

Rosen CJ, Brown S. Severe hypocalcemia after intravenous bisphosphonate therapy in occult vitamin D deficiency. N Engl J Med 2003;348:1503–4.

Ruegsegger P, Medici TC, Anliker M. Corticosteroid-induced bone loss. A longitudinal study of alternate day therapy in patients with bronchial asthma using quantitative computed tomography. Eur J Clin Pharmacol 1983;25:615–20.

Saag K, Emkey R, Cividino A. Effects of alendronate for two years on BMD and fractures in patients receiving glucocorticoids. Bone 1998;23:S182.

Saag KG, Emkey R, Schnitzer TJ, et al. Alendronate for the prevention and treatment of glucocorticoid-induced osteoporosis. Glucocorticoid-Induced Osteoporosis Intervention Study Group. N Engl J Med 1998;339:292–9.

Saito JK, Davis JW, Wasnich RD, Ross PD. Users of low-dose glucocorticoids have increased bone loss rates: a longitudinal study. Calcif Tissue Int 1995;57:115–9.

Sambrook P, Birmingham J, Kelly P, et al. Prevention of corticosteroid osteoporosis. A comparison of calcium, calcitriol, and calcitonin. N Engl J Med 1993;328:1747–52.

Schoon EJ, Bollani S, Mills PR, et al. Budesonide versus prednisolone: effect on bone mineral density in patients with ileocecal Crohn's disease. Am J Gastroenterol 2002;97:A827.

Schulte C, Dignass AU, Mann K, Goebell H. Reduced bone mineral density and unbalanced bone metabolism in patients with inflammatory bowel disease. Inflammatory Bowel Diseases 1998;4:268–75.

Schulte C, Goebell H, Roher HD, Schulte KM. Genetic determinants of IL-6 expression levels do not influence bone loss in inflammatory bowel disease. Dig Dis Sci 2001;46:2521–8.

Schulte CM, Dignass AU, Goebell H, et al. Genetic factors determine extent of bone loss in inflammatory bowel disease. Gastroenterol 2000;119:909–20.

Scott EM, Gaywood I, Scott BB. Guidelines for osteoporosis in coeliac disease and inflammatory bowel disease. British Society of Gastroenterology. Gut 2000;46:1–8.

Sher KS, Jayanthi V, Probert CS, et al. Infertility, obstetric and gynaecological problems in coeliac sprue. Dig Dis 1994;12:186–90.

Solerio E, Isaia G, Innarella R, et al. Osteoporosis: still a typical complication of primary biliary cirrhosis? Dig Liver Dis 2003;35:339–46.

Stockbrugger RW, Schoon EJ, Bollani S, et al. Discordance between the degree of osteopenia and the prevalence of spontaneous vertebral fractures in Crohn's disease. Aliment Pharmacol Ther 2002;16:1519–27.

Suda T, Nakamura I, Jimi E, Takahashi N. Regulation of osteoclast function. J Bone Miner Res 1997;12:869–79.

Szathmari M, Tulassay T, Arato A, et al. Bone mineral content and density in asymptomatic children with coeliac disease on a gluten-free diet. Eur J Gastroenterol Hepatol 2001;13:419–24.

Takahashi N, Udagawa N, Suda T. A new member of tumor necrosis factor ligand family, ODF/OPGL/TRANCE/RANKL, regulates osteoclast differentiation and function. Biochem Biophys Res Commun 1999;256:449–55.

Thomason K, West J, Logan RF, et al. Fracture experience of patients with coeliac disease: a population based survey. Gut 2003;52:518–22.

Thomson BM, Mundy GR, Chambers TJ. Tumor necrosis factors alpha and beta induce osteoblastic cells to stimulate osteoclastic bone resorption. J Immunol 1987;138:775–9.

Thomson BM, Saklatvala J, Chambers TJ. Osteoblasts mediate interleukin 1 stimulation of bone resorption by rat osteoclasts. J Exp Med 1986;164:104–12.

Tidermark J, Zethraeus N, Svensson O, et al. Femoral neck fractures in the elderly: functional outcome and quality of life according to EuroQol. Qual Life Res 2002;11:473–81.

Tovey FI, Godfrey JE, Lewin MR. A gastrectomy population: 25-30 years on. Postgrad Med J 1990;66:450–6.

Trautwein C, Possienke M, Schlitt HJ, et al. Bone density and metabolism in patients with viral hepatitis and cholestatic liver diseases before and after liver transplantation. Am J Gastroenterol 2000;95:2343–51.

Trombetti A, Herrmann F, Hoffmeyer P, et al. Survival and potential years of life lost after hip fracture in men and age-matched women. Osteoporos Int 2002;13:731–7.

Tsuboi M, Kawakami A, Nakashima T, et al. Tumor necrosis factor-alpha and interleukin-1beta increase the Fas-mediated apoptosis of human osteoblasts. J Lab Clin Med 1999;134:222–31.

van Staa TP, Leufkens HGM, Abenhaim L, et al. Use of oral corticosteroids and risk of fractures. J Bone Miner Res 2000;15:993–1000.

Vasquez H, Mazure R, Gonzalez D, et al. Risk of fractures in celiac disease patients: a cross-sectional, case-control study. Am J Gastroenterol 2000;95:183–9.

Vestergaard P, Mosekilde L. Fracture risk in patients with celiac disease, Crohn's disease, and ulcerative colitis: a nationwide follow-up study of 16,416 patients in Denmark. Am J Epidemiol 2002;156:1–10.

Vestergaard P. Bone loss associated with gastrointestinal disease: prevalence and pathogenesis. Eur J Gastroenterol Hepatol 2003;15:851–6.

Vogelsang H, Klamert M, Resch H, Ferenci P. Dietary vitamin D intake in patients with Crohn's disease. Wiener Klinische Wochenschrift 1995;107:578–81.

Votta BJ, Bertolini DR. Cytokine suppressive anti-inflammatory compounds inhibit bone resorption in vitro. Bone 1994;15:533–8.

Walters J, Weiser M. Calcium transport by rat duodenal villus and crypt basolateral membranes. Am J Physiol 1987;252:G170.

Weinstein RS, Jilka RL, Parfitt AM, Manolagas SC. Inhibition of osteoblastogenesis and promotion of apoptosis of osteoblasts and osteocytes by glucocorticoids. Potential mechanisms of their deleterious effects on bone. J Clin Invest 1998;102:274–82.

West J, Logan RF, Card TR, et al. Fracture risk in people with celiac disease: a population-based cohort study. Gastroenterol 2003;125:429–36.

Westerholm-Ormio M, Garioch J, Ketola I, Savilahti E. Inflammatory cytokines in small intestinal mucosa of patients with potential coeliac disease. Clin Exp Immunol 2002;128:94–101.

Wiener H, Turnheim K. Calcium-activated potassium channels in basolateral membranes of colon epithelial cells; reconstitution and functional properties. Wien Klin Wochenschr 1990;102:622–8.

CHAPTER 56

Dietary-Induced Symptoms

Lawrence R. Schiller, MD

Most patients with gastrointestinal (GI) symptoms attribute their symptoms to "something" they ate and want advice from the doctor about what to eat to minimize their symptoms. Symptoms after food ingestion most often are due to normal food-induced physiological changes, such as the gastrocolic reflex, or to the effects of food digestion, such as the generation of gas. They rarely are due to food allergy or to immunologic reactions to food breakdown products, such as in celiac disease. Specific problems will not be discussed further in this chapter. There are separate chapters on food allergies (Chapter 57, "Gastrointestinal Food Allergy"), celiac disease (Chapter 61, "Celiac Sprue and Related Problems"), and lactose intolerance (Chapter 62, "Lactose Intolerance").

Food-related symptoms often occur when organic problems are present, but probably occur most often in patients with common functional bowel disorders, such as functional dyspepsia (FD) or irritable bowel syndrome (IBS). Patients with organic problems, such as short bowel syndrome, will have exacerbation of symptoms like diarrhea when eating, with some foods producing more problems than others. Patients with functional problems tend to be unusually sensitive to distention and other digestive events, and, therefore, may have aggravation of their basic symptoms when ingesting any foods. However some foods may be more problematic than others. It is not that these foods *cause* the fundamental functional problem, only that the offending foods aggravate the symptoms of those conditions (O'Sullivan and O'Morain, 2003).

Meal-Related Physiological Changes

Response to a Meal

Intestinal fluid and electrolyte transport and motility continue during fasting, but ingestion of a meal results in a prompt alteration of activity.

This is not different conceptually than what happens to the cardiovascular system with exercise, but it typically involves changes that are an order of magnitude greater. Thus salivary, gastric, biliary, and pancreatic secretion increase 10-fold or more over basal levels, and motility patterns abruptly change from fasting to fed patterns.

Esophagus

In the *esophagus*, the repeated swallows associated with eating and the postprandial rise in serum gastrin levels decrease lower esophageal sphincter (LES) tone. In addition, gastric distention due to ingested food and intragastric gas production as acid is neutralized by food increase the number of transient LES relaxations (the "belching reflex") and permit gastroesophageal reflux to occur. Patients with gastroesophageal reflux disease often note a distinct increase in symptoms postprandially. Fatty foods and hypertonic beverages may be particular problems (see later in chapter).

Stomach

Eating stimulates *gastric acid secretion*, increasing the volume of material in the stomach. The ability of the stomach to hold the additional fluid and the meal is due to gastric accommodation, which allows the gastric wall to relax. This vagally mediated reflex is disturbed in some patients with FD and in patients after vagotomy, who cannot accommodate large volumes in the stomach. This may aggravate gastroesophageal reflux, speed gastric emptying of liquids, and trigger sensations of bloating or early satiety. Antral motility also is stimulated by eating.

Small Bowel

In the *small bowel*, ingestion of food rapidly converts the fasting pattern of motility, which features cyclical migrating motor complexes, into the more chaotic postprandial pattern. Chyme emptied from the stomach is joined by pancreatic and biliary secretions, which distend the small bowel and stimulate peristalsis.

The bowel wall is sensitive to distention and eating activates afferent nerves that may produce painful sensations in some individuals. The entry of chyme into the duodenum also results in release of many *peptides* and other *signaling substances* that produce effects elsewhere in the gut and even outside the GI tract.

Colon

Food residues enter the *colon* hours after ingestion. Carbohydrate that is not absorbed in the small intestine (poorly absorbed carbohydrate and fiber) enters the right colon and is fermented by the colonic bacterial flora. The products of fermentation are short chain fatty acids—up to 80 g of which can be produced by the colonic flora—and voluminous amounts of gas (carbon dioxide and hydrogen gas) (Hammer et al, 1989; Hammer et al, 1990). *Every 10 g of carbohydrate can yield about 1 L of gas.* Gas can distend the colon, stimulating motility and causing *bloating, cramps and pain* in some people.

Effects of Specific Foods and Food Additives

People ingest a variety of substances that consist of mixtures of chemicals that can have specific effects on the body. These chemicals include primary macronutrients, such as carbohydrates, fats, and proteins; micronutrients, such as vitamins and minerals; and incidental chemicals that have no nutritive value, but are part of the animals and plants that we eat, such as *caffeine* in coffee or *theobromine* in chocolate. These incidental chemicals may be biologically active in the gut and elsewhere in the body and may produce symptoms.

Carbohydrates

Carbohydrates are responsible for a variety of food-induced symptoms (Table 56-1). These symptoms can be due to hypertonicity or to malabsorption of carbohydrate.

TABLE 56-1. Carbohydrate-Induced Symptoms in Specific Situations

Symptoms	Situations
Due to hypertonicity	
Dumping syndrome	Gastric surgery
Bloating	Vagotomy
Nausea	Pyloroplasty
Diarrhea	Antrectomy
Flushing	Gastrojejunostomy
Hypotension	Bariatric procedures
Dyspepsia after fruit juice	Gastroesophageal reflux disease
Due to malabsorption or ingestion of poorly absorbed carbohydrates	
Gas, bloating, diarrhea, pain	Generalized malabsorption
	Celiac disease
	Short bowel syndrome
	Specific malabsorption
	Fructose
	Sucrose
	Lactose
	Poorly absorbed substances
	Mannitol, sorbitol
	Dietary fiber

Ingestion of hypertonic carbohydrate solutions results in entry of water into the gut lumen to produce osmotic equilibration. This is mostly a problem for individuals with unregulated gastric emptying, such as those who have had gastric surgery, and can produce a dumping syndrome with bloating, nausea, diarrhea, flushing, and hypotension. Hypertonic carbohydrate solutions, such as fruit juices, also can produce dyspepsia, probably by stimulation of receptors in the esophagus and stomach.

Malabsorption of carbohydrate in the small intestine results in delivery of excess fermentable substrate to the colon. This can be due to generalized malabsorption (eg, celiac disease or short bowel syndrome) or to malabsorption of specific carbohydrate moieties. In addition, excess dietary fiber ingestion will load the colon with additional carbohydrate. When smaller amounts of carbohydrate are delivered to the colon, excess gas, bloating and cramps develop as gas is produced as a byproduct of fermentation. Diarrhea is produced when larger amounts are ingested or insufficient time is allowed for absorption due to accelerated transit. Symptoms can develop with as little as 5 to 10 g of excess carbohydrate entering the colon. Symptoms relate more to the total amount of fermentable carbohydrate entering the colon than to the specific type of carbohydrate that is malabsorbed. In some cases, "tolerance" to gradually increasing amounts of carbohydrate develops, which is probably related to changes in bacterial metabolism.

Specific carbohydrates may be incompletely absorbed by the small intestine in certain individuals. These include *fructose, sucrose, lactose,* and the sugar alcohols: *mannitol* and *sorbitol.*

MANNITOL AND SORBITOL

Absorption of *mannitol* and *sorbitol* is intrinsically limited by the absence of carriers or pores in the intestine that permit their transport. Thus, everyone malabsorbs these substances. These agents are used as non-nutritive sweeteners in a variety of dietetic foods and as sweeteners in "sugar-free" chewing gum (Carefree, Dentyne, Extra) and medicines. Sorbitol is also a natural component of some fruits and fruit juices, such as apple juice and pear juice (Rumessen and Gudmand-Hoyer, 1988; Perman, 1996).

FRUCTOSE

Fructose absorption is mediated by facilitated diffusion across the brush border, but the capacity for transport is limited. Thus, symptoms of fructose malabsorption will develop when the amount ingested is greater than a threshold amount. Fructose is found naturally in many fruits and vegetables, and high fructose corn syrup is a popular sweetener in soft drinks and processed foods (Rumessen and Gudmand-Hoyer, 1988; Perman, 1996; Ravich et al, 1983).

Sucrose is rarely malabsorbed, but some individuals have an inherited defect in sucrase-isomaltase, the brush border enzyme necessary for its absorption. Individuals with villous atrophy may have an acquired enzyme deficiency.

Lactose

There is a separate chapter on lactose intolerance (see Chapter 62, "Lactose Intolerance"). The most common carbohydrate that is malabsorbed is lactose or milk sugar (Vesa et al, 2000). Lactose is the primary carbohydrate in milk, and all mammals depend on lactase activity in the intestine to digest and absorb this substrate in infancy. Most mammals retain lactase activity until weaning and then turn off production of this enzyme, because milk is no longer a part of the diet. Most human populations retain lactase expression through adolescence and then become lactase insufficient.

In some populations (particularly the individuals in the Northern European gene pool), lactase activity is maintained into adulthood, but is typically lost gradually, producing some degree of lactose intolerance with aging.

The degree of lactose intolerance is highly variable and the development of symptoms depends not only on the amount consumed (eg, 12.5 g per glass of milk), but also on such factors as the amount of other fermentable substrates ingested with the meal, coexisting mucosal disease, and the rate of transit through the intestine. Lactose tolerance can be tested by assessing symptoms after ingestion of 1 to 2 cups of milk (240 to 480 mL) or, more formally, by breath hydrogen testing after a lactose load (typically 25 g). Use of milk that has been treated to hydrolyze the lactose can reduce symptoms. In sensitive individuals, care must also be taken with the ingestion of processed foods that have been fortified with nonfat dry milk to improve their nutritional characteristics (Paige et al, 1975).

Fats

Fats also can produce a number of symptoms (Table 56-2). Fat digestion is a complex process and the GI tract is organized to slow the movement of fats through the intestine to allow sufficient time for fat digestion to occur. Thus fatty meals slow gastric emptying and intestinal transit and, ultimately, induce satiety and stop food intake. This is mediated by duodenal receptors that recognize the presence of fat within the lumen, cause the release of cholecystokinin (CCK) into the blood, and set off neural reflexes. The consequences of reduced gastric emptying may include exacerbation of gastroesophageal reflux, bloating, and early satiety. However, as shown by Lin and colleagues (1999), fat intolerance is associated with rapid gastric emptying.

Most fat is absorbed in the jejunum and fat entering the lower ileum triggers the "ileal brake" by release of peptide YY, which inhibits gastric emptying and proximal small bowel transit. Patients who have had substantial ileal resections lack this mechanism and may flood the colon with unabsorbed nutrients after meals, producing diarrhea, gas, and cramps.

Dietary fat also has an effect on colonic motility. One of the key activators of the gastrocolic reflex is fat entering the duodenum. Because of this many patients with diarrhea have bowel movements after meals and soon learn to restrict their food intake to avoid diarrhea. This promotes development of food aversions and weight loss in patients with chronic diarrhea. An exaggerated gastrocolic reflex may also play a role in postprandial urgency in patients with IBS.*

Proteins

Proteins are less likely than other macronutrients to cause the kind of GI symptoms that we are discussing (nonimmunologically mediated symptoms) because they are ingested as large polymers that do not exert much osmotic activity, and they are efficiently digested and absorbed by the intestine. Some foods, however, contain *bioactive amines* and *peptides* that may influence gut activity. An example is *coffee*, which, in addition to *caffeine*, contains dozens of *peptides* that may influence gastric acid secretion and other GI events. Amino acids stimulate CCK secretion and may induce abdominal pain by stimulation of pancreatic exocrine secretion if the pancreatic duct is structurally or functionally obstructed.

Capsaisin, Caffeine, and Others

Other dietary components that may induce GI symptoms include capsaisin, caffeine, and various minerals. *Capsaisin* is the "active" ingredient in hot peppers and reacts with specific receptors in the mucosa that activate enteric sensory nerves. The physiological "purpose" of these receptors is not clear at the present time. *Caffeine* and other bioactive amines have pharmacological effects when ingested in milligram amounts. In addition to central nervous system effects, the co-editor of this text and his colleagues have shown that caffeine can increase intestinal chloride secretion by inhibiting phosphodiesterase, which may exaggerate diarrhea in patients with ileostomies and in those with IBS (Wald et al, 1976). Minerals such as *calcium, aluminum,* and *iron* tend

TABLE 56-2. Fat-Associated Symptoms and Situations

Symptoms	Situations
Dyspepsia	Gastroesophageal reflux disease
Bloating, early satiety	Gastric surgery
Postprandial urgency of defecation	Irritable bowel syndrome
Distension	Postprandial upper abdominal pain

---

*Editor's Note: Patients learn to eat grilled chicken breast rather than hamburger at fast food restaurants. (TMB)

to be constipating, whereas *magnesium* may cause diarrhea. Many patients ingest dietary supplements containing these elements and may not be aware of their effects on bowel function. Finally, many patients ingest "health foods" which often contain herbal products, including senna and aloe, which can have profound effects on gut function. Every patient needs to be asked about ingestion of these products. There is a separate chapter on alternative medicines (Chapter 58, "Complementary and Alternative Medicines in Gastrointestinal Disease").*

Impact of Food Intolerances in Specific Conditions

Symptoms in many GI conditions may be aggravated by food intolerance. Several disorders in which dietary factors should be explored by the physician are discussed below and summarized in Table 56-3.

Functional Syndromes

Functional syndromes, such as IBS, FD, chronic diarrhea, and chronic constipation are common disorders, affecting up to 20% of the US population. Although their pathophysiology is gradually being unraveled, management is still based on symptom control. Food intolerance may play an important role in aggravating symptoms and should be probed.

Motility Disorders

Motility disorders, such as gastroparesis and chronic intestinal pseudo-obstruction, can also be affected by diet. Although controlled clinical studies to prove efficacy have not been conducted, dietary management is key to the long term treatment of these conditions.

Post-Surgery Syndromes

Post-surgery syndromes are another fruitful area for dietary therapy. No surgical intervention on the gut is without the potential for disturbing function, and when the disturbance is severe enough to produce symptoms, careful dietary management can improve matters substantially. Conditions in which food intolerance may aggravate symptoms include postvagotomy or postgastrectomy dumping syndrome, short bowel syndrome, ileostomy diarrhea, postresection diarrhea, and ileoanal pouch dysfunction. There are separate chapters on some of those situations.

Evaluation of Symptoms That May Be Related to Food Ingestion

Many different symptoms may be due to food ingestion and its consequences. These include abdominal pain in any area, heartburn, bloating, nausea, abdominal distention,

TABLE 56-3. Potential Food Intolerance in Clinical Conditions

Condition	Potential Food Intolerance	Mechanism
Gastroesophageal reflux disease	Hypertonic, carbohydrate-rich liquids	Osmoreceptors
	Fatty foods	Delayed gastric emptying, reduced LES pressure
Gastroparesis	Hypertonic beverages	Delayed gastric emptying
	Fatty foods	Delayed gastric emptying
	Raw fruits, vegetables	Impaired trituration
Dumping syndrome	Hypertonic carbohydrate	Intestinal hormone release, osmotic fluid shifts
Functional dyspepsia	Many	Gastric distention, delayed gastric emptying, abnormal gastric motility, hypersensitivity to distention
Chronic intestinal pseudo-obstruction	Fiber	Potential substrate for bacterial overgrowth
Short bowel syndrome	Caffeine	Increased secretion, motility
	Carbohydrate	Fermentation
	Fatty foods	Accentuated gastrocolic reflex
Irritable bowel syndrome	Carbohydrate (lactose, sorbitol, fructose)	Osmotic diarrhea, fermentation
	Fatty foods	Accentuated gastrocolic reflex
Chronic diarrhea (including functional, postresection, and ileostomy diarrhea)	Fatty foods	Accentuated gastrocolic reflex
Chronic constipation	Fiber	Fermentation
Ileal pouch–anal anastomosis	Carbohydrate (lactose, sorbitol, fructose)	Osmotic diarrhea, fermentation

LES = lower esophageal sphincter.

*Editor's Note: Garlic is widely touted as a health food. However, there are numerous biologically active amines in garlic that are used as vermifuges in animals and children. Some individuals, including the aforementioned editor are, as adults, highly sensitive to an alcohol soluble fraction of garlic with a cramping laxative effect. (TMB)

gas, and diarrhea. The physician needs to establish the timing of the symptoms in relation to a meal and should try to establish a link between specific foods and the presenting symptoms. This can be done best by a diet and symptom diary in which the temporal relation between ingestion of certain foods and the onset of symptoms can be determined. However, bacterial fermentation of unabsorbed carbohydrates may occur many hours after ingestion. Reproducibility of symptom induction by specific foods should be the basis for trial of an elimination diet. Registered dietitians can be a valuable help in sorting through the patient's history and recommending alternative diets.*

---

*Editor's Note: The careful reader who employs the concepts nicely demonstrated in this chapter will help a lot of patients obtain significant relief. As stated in the first sentence of this chapter, many patients do attribute some of their symptoms to "something they ate!" (TMB)

Supplemental Reading

Burden S. Dietary treatment of irritable bowel syndrome: current evidence and guidelines for future practice. J Hum Nutr Diet 2001;14:231–41.

Hammer HF, Fine KD, Santa Ana CA, et al. Carbohydrate malabsorption. Its measurement and its contribution to diarrhea. J Clin Invest 1990;86:1936–44.

Hammer HF, Santa Ana CA, Schiller LR, Fordtrans JS. Studies of osmotic diarrhea induced in normal subjects by ingestion of polyethylene glycol and lactulose. J Clin Invest 1989;84:1056–62.

Lin HC, Van Citters GW, Zhao XT, Waxman A. Fat intolerance depends on rapid gastric emptying. Dig Dis Sci 1999;44:330–5.

O'Sullivan M, O'Morain C. Food intolerance: dietary treatments in functional bowel disorders. Curr Treat Options Gastroenterology 2003;6:339–45.

Paige DM, Bayless TM, Huang SS, Wextner R. Lactose hydrolyzed milk. Am J Clin Nutr 1975;28:898–22.

Perman JA. Digestion and absorption of fruit juice carbohydrate. J Am Coll Nutr 1996;15Suppl 5:12–17S.

Ravich WJ, Bayless TM, Thomas M. Fructose: incomplete intestinal absorption in humans. Gastroenterology 1983;84:26–9.

Rumessen JJ, Gudmand-Hoyer E. Functional bowel disease: malabsorption and abdominal distress after ingestion of fructose, sorbitol, and fructose–sorbitol mixtures. Gastroenterology 1988;95:694–700.

Vesa TH, Marteau P, Korpela R. Lactose intolerance. J Am Coll Nutr 2000;19Suppl 2:165–75S.

Wald A, Back C, Bayless TM. Effect of caffeine on the human small intestine. Gastroenterology 1976;71:738–42.

CHAPTER 57

Gastrointestinal Food Allergy

Sheila E. Crowe, MD FRCPC

Adverse reactions to food (ARF) are common, with up to 50% of some populations reporting ARF (Table 57-1). The majority of ARF are nonimmunologic in origin, but true food allergies are thought to affect up to 6 to 8% of children under the age of 10 years and 1 to 2% of the adult population (Sampson, 2003), a frequency which should result in most medical practitioners seeing cases of food allergy on a regular basis. The major difficulty in managing patients with food allergy lies in making a diagnosis of food allergy, particularly when the symptoms are primarily gastrointestinal (GI). Over 50 years ago Ingelfinger and colleagues (1949) wrote "gastrointestinal allergy is a diagnosis frequently entertained, occasionally evaluated, and rarely established" and even today this is an apt description of the problem confronting clinicians considering a diagnosis of GI food allergy. However, substantial developments have been made in our understanding of the basic biology of food allergy with implications for improved diagnostic and therapeutic strategies in the future.

Immunoglobulin E-Mediated Food Allergy Syndromes

Food allergies are often categorized for the organ systems they affect and by the immune mechanisms involved (Table 57-2) (Sicherer, 2002). Immune mediated reactions to food included immunoglobulin (Ig)E and sometimes IgG$_4$-mediated responses that degranulate mast cells and basophils, so-called type I hypersensitivity. Other forms of food allergy can involve T cells, the generation of immune-complexes, and/or the activation of eosinophils. Although the dermatologic and respiratory tract manifestations of food allergy are often better recognized, the GI tract can be affected by food allergies in various ways. IgE-mediated reactions to foods induce classic GI anaphylaxis in which food allergic reactions result in immediate hypersensitivity within the GI tract resulting in nausea, vomiting, diarrhea, cramping, and abdominal pain. Isolated GI food allergy/anaphylaxis is a relatively rare manifestation of food allergy, and, typically, the GI symptoms of food allergic reactions occur in conjunction with allergic manifestations in other target organs. GI manifestations of food allergy are reported in 30 to 70% of patients experiencing food allergy (Crowe and Perdue, 1992). The foods primarily responsible for this type of GI food allergy include cow's milk, eggs, nuts, seafood, and fish, but new allergens are emerging with the globalization of eating habits. Moreover, food allergy and allergic reactions in general are increasing worldwide, particularly in urbanized populations.

Systemic Anaphylaxis

The most important manifestation of food allergy is *systemic anaphylaxis*. It is now recognized that food allergy

TABLE 57-1. Classification of Adverse Reactions to Food or Food Additives

Food allergy (immune-mediated mechanisms)
- Immediate hypersensitivity reactions
- Allergic eosinophilic gastroenteritis
- Food protein-induced enterocolitis syndromes
- Celiac disease

Food intolerance (nonimmune mechanisms)
- Food toxicity or food poisoning
- Pharmacological reactions
- Metabolic reactions
- Idiosyncratic reactions
- Psychological reactions
- Physiological reactions

TABLE 57-2. Conditions Associated with Immunologic Reactions to Foods

Immediate gastrointestinal hypersensitivity
Oral allergy syndrome
Acute urticaria
Atopic dermatitis
Acute angioedema
Acute bronchospasm
Asthma
Celiac disease
Dermatitis herpetiformis
Cow's milk enteropathy
Food protein induced enterocolitis
Food protein induced proctocolitis or proctitis
Heiner's syndrome
Eosinophilic esophagitis
Eosinophilic gastroenteritis
Behavioral disorders

is the major cause of anaphylactic reactions in industrialized societies including the United States, Australia, and Europe. The prevalence of *peanut allergy* (0.5 to 7% of adults in the United States and the United Kingdom) and its potentially fatal consequences has had significant effect on the operational policies of groups ranging from school districts to the airline industry. Fatal anaphylaxis can result from exposure to minute amounts of antigen such as that imparted by a kiss. *Food-associated exercise-induced anaphylaxis* is a rare type of anaphylaxis in which the food only elicits an anaphylactic reaction when the subject exercises within several hours of ingesting that food. *Acetylsalicylic acid* can also augment type I allergic symptoms when combined with food and exercise in such individuals.

Pollen-Food Allergy Syndrome

The *oral allergy syndrome* or *pollen-food allergy syndrome* results from various *plant proteins* that cross-react with certain *inhalant antigens*, particularly *birch, ragweed*, and *mugwort* (Sloane and Sheffer, 2001). Exposure to the cross-reacting foods may lead to pruritus, tingling and/or swelling of the tongue, lips, palate, or oropharynx, and, occasionally, to bronchospasm or more systemic reactions. Foods that cross-react with *birch* include *raw potatoes, carrots, celery, apples, pears, hazelnuts*, and *kiwi*. Those individuals that are allergic to *ragweed* may react to fresh *melons* and to *bananas*. It is important to educate patients with inhalant allergies about potential cross-reacting foods.

Latex-Food Allergy Syndrome

Latex-food allergy syndrome, also referred to as the latex-fruit syndrome, is a specific form of food allergy in which food antigens cross-react with various latex antigens (Blanco, 2003). Natural rubber latex contains over 200 proteins, 10 of which bind IgE *Hevea brasiliensis* latex protein allergens (HEV b 1 to 10) and cross-react with a variety of food antigens including *kiwi* (HEV b 5), *potato* and *tomato* (HEV b 7), and *avocado, chestnut*, and *banana* (HEV b 6). In latex-sensitive individuals exposure to these foods can result in the same symptoms as if exposed to latex ranging from pruritus, eczema, oral-facial swelling, asthma, GI complaints, and anaphylaxis. A large number of studies from around the world indicate that the natural rubber latex allergy is increasing in prevalence and that the frequency of associated food allergy varies from 21 to 58% (Blanco, 2003). Worldwide, *banana, avocado, chestnut* and *kiwi* are the most common causes of food-induced symptoms associated with latex allergy.

Other Immune-Mediated GI Adverse Reactions to Food

Immunologic reactions to foods involving mechanisms other than immediate hypersensitivity, such as *cell-mediated immunity* (see Table 57-2), play a role in food protein-induced enterocolitis syndromes (FPIES), such as *cow's milk protein enteropathy*, and *also celiac disease*. FPIES also known as *food protein-induced enteropathies*, present in infancy or early childhood and are most commonly due to cow's milk protein followed by soy protein and less commonly, egg, fish, and other food antigens (Nowak-Wegrzyn et al, 2003). Clinical manifestations include diarrhea, vomiting, anemia, bleeding, and failure to thrive. As with many other food allergies, such cases are managed by elimination of the specific food antigen until the disease resolves with age. It is common practice to switch infants with enterocolitis from a cow's milk-based formula to a *soy-protein derived formula*, but because over half will react to soy protein, continued problems may result from the development of soy–protein-induced enterocolitis. *Hypoallergenic* or *elemental feeds* are often necessary in such cases.

Celiac Disease

Celiac disease is one of the best-recognized diseases resulting from an immunologic reaction to food. Dietary ingestion of gliadin found in wheat, hordelein in rye, and secalin on barley, induces an enteropathy in genetically susceptible individuals. Removal of the offending grains from the diet restores normal small bowel function and appearance, with improvement in symptoms that can range from diarrhea, weight loss, and failure to thrive, to the more common but less often recognized complaints of fatigue, dyspepsia, neurological dysfunction, and musculoskeletal problems. As with other immune-mediated ARF, elimination of the offending food substance (gluten) is the primary method of management in celiac disease. However, unlike most other food protein-induced enteropathies, gluten must be eliminated from the diet on a lifelong basis in celiac disease. See Chapter 61, "Celiac Sprue and Related Problems" for a more complete discussion of celiac-sprue.

Eosinophilic Gastroenteritis

Food allergy is thought to play a role in some cases of *eosinophilic gastroenteritis*, a relatively rare condition characterized by eosinophilic infiltration of the gut and, often, peripheral eosinophilia. Approximately half the patients with eosinophilic gastroenteritis have *atopic features, including food allergy*. Strategies to identify and eliminate food antigens should be followed as in other food allergic conditions, but often other measures, particularly *corticosteroids*, are necessary to manage patients with eosinophilic gastroenteritis. Even after thorough evaluation for parasites, an *empiric course* of *antihelminthic therapy* may be given before embarking on a course of corticosteroids. Allergic eosinophilic esophagitis presents in infancy through adolescence and manifests with symptoms of gastroesophageal reflux that are often refractory to typical antisecretory therapy (Hill et al, 2000). As with lower GI presentations of allergic eosinophilic conditions, this disorder is characterized by eosinophilic infiltration of the mucosa, but also the histologic hallmarks of gastroesophageal reflux disease (GERD) and abnormal 24-hour pH monitoring. Young children with this diagnosis usually have a clinical and histologic benefit from eliminating specific foods.

Nonimmune Adverse Reactions to Food

The vast majority of ARF are not immunologic in origin (see Table 57-1) and by virtue of their prevalence, are important considerations in the examination of patients complaining of ARF. Food toxicity or food poisoning results from microbial contamination of food causing primarily GI manifestations due to preformed toxins (eg, staphylococcal enterotoxin) or replication of enteric pathogens (*Campylobacter, Salmonella, Shigella, Escherichia coli*). These reactions can be distinguished from other ARF because they usually do not recur and have fairly characteristic presentations. Occasionally, a self-limited infection may result in a postinfectious irritable bowel syndrome (IBS). This is discussed in the chapter on IBS (see Chapter 39, "Irritable Bowel Syndrome") and the chapter on traveler's diarrhea (see Chapter 50, "Traveler's Diarrhea").

Anaphylactoid or Pseudoallergic

Anaphylactoid or pseudoallergic reactions to food result from foods that mimic the effects of mast cell degranulation but do not involve IgE antibodies. *Strawberries* and *shellfish* may cause this type of ARF. Certain food ingredients, including additives such as *salicylates, benzoates*, and *tartrazine*, induce pseudoallergic reactions. As with true food allergy, patients exhibiting such reactions should be instructed to avoid the offending food substance if identifiable. Pharmacological reactions to food or food additives represent a relatively common type of ARF, although most of these reactions cause symptoms outside of the GI tract. *Histamine* found in certain *cheeses* or in *scrombroid fish*, such as tuna, can cause headaches and diffuse erythema of the skin. Certain individuals develop *migraine headaches* to various foodstuffs, including those rich in *amines*. *Sulfites, tartrazine* and *monosodium glutamate (MSG)* have all been associated with asthma, and MSG can cause a characteristic syndrome consisting of a burning or warm sensation, chest tightness, headache, and gastric discomfort shortly after its ingestion.

Lactose Intolerance

Globally, lactose intolerance is the most common adverse reaction to a specific food, with most cases the result of declining levels of intestinal lactase activity in later childhood and adult life, although rare congenital deficiencies can occur. Symptoms of lactase insufficiency are usually dose related and include bloating, flatulence, and diarrhea. Secondary lactase deficiency can result from viral gastroenteritis, radiation enteritis, Crohn's disease (CD), and celiac sprue. It is important from a management standpoint to understand that individuals with constitutive lactose intolerance (1) do not suffer severe and potentially life-threatening complications of ingesting lactose and (2) are able to consume naturally lactose free diary products including most cheeses and yogurts. This contrasts with cow's milk allergic individuals who may suffer anaphylactic or asthmatic reactions to dairy products and must avoid all foods containing the culprit cow's milk protein allergen, usually casein or β-lactoglobulin. There is a chapter on carbohydrate intolerance (see Chapter 62, "Lactose Intolerance").

Psychological Reactions

In certain individuals, reactions to food may be psychological (Kelsay, 2003). This is a difficult type of ARF to diagnose because the mechanisms giving rise to such reactions are poorly understood. Individuals who are not confirmed to have ARF have higher rates of hypochondria, hysteria, somatization, and anxiety than those with ARF confirmed by food challenge. An individual who experienced a severe ARF may avoid the culprit food for fear of further reactions, and there is also some evidence that hypersensitivity reactions to food may be triggered through central neural mechanisms so that, eventually, just the thought of ingesting the food can trigger allergic symptoms in the absence of antigen. Food allergy itself may lead to psychological distress, and studies of food allergic subjects report an altered quality of life for the individual and their family, with severe manifestations such as anaphylaxis resulting in a *post-traumatic stress situation*.

Physiologic Reactions

Perhaps the most common form of ARF results from physiologic reactions to food components or additives. It is well known that starches found in legumes serve as substrate for gas production by colonic flora and many other foods are associated with "gas," including onions, cabbage, bran fiber, and other vegetables and grains. Certain foods and food additives affect the lower esophageal sphincter, whereas foods high in fat delay gastric emptying, resulting in symptoms of heartburn and dyspepsia. These physiologic reactions to foods are typically noted by patients with functional bowel disease, many of whom exhibit heightened endocrine, motor and sensory responses to normal digestive events. Because elimination of the offending food(s) may provide some benefit in select patients, it is important to determine whether specific food intolerances exist in this group of patients. The reader is referred to

Chapter 56, "Dietary-Induced Symptoms" for a further discussion of dietary-induced GI symptoms.

GI Disorders and ARF

Functional Disorders

It is human nature for patients with GI disorders to believe that something in their diet has caused their condition even in the absence of a history of food intolerance. A significant number of GI conditions are associated with ARF but food plays a causal role in only some of these disorders. For patients with GERD, nonulcer dyspepsia, IBS, and other functional conditions, nonspecific physiological reactions to food can provoke symptoms. It is generally advisable to instruct these patients to avoid foods that cause symptoms, but nondietary measures are usually also necessary to manage their complaints. However, food protein intolerance or allergy may play a role in infants with GERD symptoms. There is no generalized role for hypoallergenic diets in IBS, although a few studies report benefit from such diets (reviewed by Spanier et al, 2003) and, in some instances, instituting a rigorous diet is helpful in convincing patients that specific dietary factors are not the sole cause of their illness.

INFLAMMATORY BOWEL DISEASE

There are many studies that have examined the role of diet in inflammatory bowel disease (IBD) but there is no evidence that specific immune-mediated reactions to food play a role in the majority of patients with either CD or ulcerative colitis. Elemental enteral feeding and parenteral nutrition can assist in the management of IBD patients with benefits that appear related to improved nutrition and bowel rest (and decreased fecal flow) rather than removal of specific allergens from the diet. Patients in remission should be encouraged to eat a nutritionally balanced diet without restrictions unless they experience intolerance to specific foods. It is typical for IBD patients to be instructed to avoid dairy products but this is unnecessary in most cases. Apart from those with symptomatic lactose intolerance (in which case they should still be able to eat most cheeses and yogurts) or rare instances of cow's milk protein allergy, IBD patients should be encouraged to consume dairy products because they are excellent sources of biologically available calcium in a population at increased risk of osteoporosis.

Approach to Patients Complaining of ARF

A significant component of the difficulty in managing food allergy is determining whether the patient has food allergy or another form of ARF (Table 57-3). Guidelines for the evaluation of food allergies have recently been published as a medical position statement by the American Gastroenterological Association (Sampson et al, 2001). It is essential to obtain a careful history correlating symptoms with specific foods. Most immediate hypersensitivity reactions to food include a set of symptoms that consistently occur minutes to hours after ingesting certain foods. In some individuals, other factors, such as medications or exercise, may modulate the reaction to a specific food. Specificity of the reaction does not always imply a food allergy because patients with anaphylactoid reactions or lactose intolerance report defined reactions to specific foods. However, the nature of the reaction will help differentiate lactose intolerance (gas, bloating, diarrhea) from an allergy to cow's milk protein (often urticaria, swelling of the lips and oral mucosa, and/or asthmatic symptoms occur in addition to GI symptoms).

Dairy, Elimination, Challenge

If a specific food or group of foods cannot be identified by the initial history, the patient should keep a diet diary for several weeks in an attempt to correlate foods with GI and other symptoms. After certain foods are identified as possible culprits by history or a diet diary, these items should be eliminated from the diet for several weeks to determine the effect on symptoms. If a benefit is seen, the patient may reintroduce the putative allergen(s) in an attempt to prove the association. Such open food challenges are subject to bias and should be corroborated by another more objective method before permanent elimination from the diet, particularly if the patient is young and the food(s) in question represent a major component of the diet (eg, eggs, milk, wheat). Skin testing, in vitro testing and blinded oral challenges may be helpful in this regard and are briefly discussed below.

TABLE 57-3. Approach to Patient With Suspected Food Allergies as a Cause of Gastrointestinal Symptoms

1. Establish foods and food additives that reproducibly cause symptoms
   - Careful history
   - Diet diary
   - Elimination diet
   - Skin testing and/or RAST
   - Food antigen challenge
2. Exclude and manage other disorders that may mimic GI food allergy
   - CBC, peripheral blood eosinophil count
   - Celiac serology
   - Lactose hydrogen breath test
   - Stool studies
   - Endoscopy and biopsy
3. Initiate treatment for food allergy
   - Avoidance of specific foods
   - Medications for after accidental exposure (antihistamines, epinephrine, corticosteroids)
   - Preventive measures (Oral cromoglycate, avoid co-precipitating factors, eg, medications)
   - Education about hidden sources of antigens and cross-reacting foods

CBC = complete blood count; GI = gastrointestinal; RAST = radioallergosorbent test.

Hypoallergenic or Elimination Diet

If specific foods are not identified by the clinical history or a diet diary, a *hypoallergenic or elimination diet*, such as that shown in Table 57-4, may be tried for 2 to 3 weeks. In most cases of suspected GI adverse reactions to foods or food additives, this approach is without benefit because the majority of patients will have functional bowel disease with nonspecific reactions to foods. In cases where a benefit is seen, new foods are gradually introduced in an attempt to identify specific foods that may contribute to the illness. It should be recognized that the hypoallergenic diet can be falsely interpreted as a negative test because a minority of subjects can react to antigens contained in a typically hypoallergenic diet.

Differential Diagnosis

It is important to consider the differential diagnosis of patients who complain of food-associated GI complaints because the majority will not have food allergy. The major syndrome in which patients complain of adverse reactions to foods is *IBS*, and other functional bowel presentations.

TABLE 57-4. Elimination Diet

Food Category	Allowed	Avoid
Meat and meat alternatives	Lamb Chicken Turkey	Pork Beef Fish Eggs Milk and milk products Seafood
Grains	Rice (Barley) Tapioca Arrowroot	Wheat Oats Corn Rye
Legumes and nuts		Avoid all dried peas, beans, nuts
Vegetables	All except corn and peas	
Fruits	All except citrus fruits, strawberries, and tomatoes	
Sweeteners	Sugar (cane or beet) Maple syrup Honey	
Fats	Olive oil Safflower oil Crisco	Soy, corn, peanut oils Butter Margarine
Miscellaneous	White vinegar Water (Ginger ale) Salt (Pepper) Fruit juices	Coffee, tea Alcohol Chocolate Colas Spices Chewing gum

Note: Also known as an exclusion or hypoallergenic diet. Foods in brackets ( ) may cause adverse reactions in some individuals and these may be omitted from the trial elimination diet. If an allowed food is one that has caused a reaction in the past, it should also be omitted. While on the trial elimination diet a record of symptoms is kept, and it is also noted if there are changes from symptoms on the previous regular diet. If there are symptoms, the patient or family should note if there is any relationship to specific foods.

Lactose intolerance is the most common form of food intolerance worldwide and may coexist with other GI conditions as well as food allergy. A complete medical history is often helpful because most patients with a history of food allergy have a *family history of atopy*, and may have a personal history of *other allergic conditions*, such as asthma and dermatitis. A history of *latex allergy* should alert the practitioner to the large number of fruits that can cross-react with latex. Similarly, the *oral allergy syndrome* occurs in response to inhalant plant allergens, but cross-reactivity with fruit, nut, and certain vegetable antigens is common. Finally, it is well recognized that *exercise* and *medications* such as *aspirin* may act as *cofactors* in allergic reactions to various types of antigens.

Tests for the Diagnosis and Management of Food Allergy

Methods to detect food-specific IgE including prick skin testing and measurements in blood are helpful in clinical practice but standardized tests to detect non-IgE mediated food allergy are not as well developed. *Skin prick testing* provides a readily available and relatively inexpensive means to assess a panel of food allergens in both children and adults. The major limitation of skin testing is its *poor positive predictive value* (many asymptomatic patients exhibit reactions to food allergens) but a negative test in the absence of antihistamine drugs strongly suggests that immediate hypersensitivity is an unlikely mechanism for the patient's food-induced complaints. Skin testing is not helpful in predicting who might outgrow their food allergies, and, in fact, skin reactivity to foods can persist without clinical manifestations while the individual goes on to develop inhalant allergies. Although quite widely used by various practitioners, sublingual challenge or neuromuscular testing for food antigens are *not* considered to be scientifically acceptable methods to diagnose food allergy.

Blood Tests

A *radioallergosorbent test (RAST)* can be used as an alternative to skin testing in very young children, those with severe atopic dermatitis, those who cannot discontinue antihistamines, and those reporting anaphylactic reactions to foods or food additives. The limitations of RAST are the expense, lower sensitivity, and relatively limited number of antigens that can be tested when compared with skin testing. A modification of the traditional RAST test, the *CAP System FEIA* (Pharmacia), is reported to be more sensitive than a standard RAST. Levels of food-specific IgE above which a patient has a > 95% likelihood of experiencing an allergic reaction after the ingestion of specific food have been established (Sampson, 2002). An oral food challenge is recommended at lower levels of food-specific IgE because the clinical significance of such levels cannot be predicted.

It is important to inform patients that *unless there is clinical evidence of adverse reactions* to foods identified by skin testing or in vitro methods, these foods *do not need to be eliminated* from the diet in most instances.

Patch Testing

Diagnostic tests for non-IgE-mediated food allergies include food allergy *patch testing*, T-cell cytokine assays, and measurements of markers of eosinophil activation. Conventional patch testing is used to diagnose contact hypersensitivity reactions involving T cells and has been applied to the evaluation of food allergy in the setting of atopic dermatitis and allergic eosinophilic esophagitis, primarily to cow's milk proteins (De Boissieu et al, 2003). Other tests may be useful in specific conditions, such as 24-hour pH monitoring in eosinophilic esophagitis. Occult *parasitic infections* should be excluded in order to diagnose idiopathic or allergic eosinophilic syndromes and, occasionally, a course of empiric antihelminthic therapy may be indicated. Histological analysis is important in many presentations of food allergy including eosinophilic esophagitis, food protein-induced enterocolitis and proctocolitis, and celiac disease.

Placebo Controlled Food Challenge

Because reactions to food antigens by RAST or skin testing are neither specific nor sensitive, a double-blinded placebo-controlled food challenge (DBPCFC), in which food antigens are administered by *nasogastric tube* or *gelatin capsules,* should be performed if possible. This technique is considered the gold standard for diagnosing food allergy but is not widely available. The DBPCFC is also less reliable when assessing for delayed reactions to foods and food additives. Clinical history and the results of skin testing help guide the choice of foods to include in the oral challenge. A number of investigators have performed the GI equivalent of skin testing by *injecting* the *GI mucosa* with a panel of *antigens* and observing for a wheal-and-flare response by endoscopy but this form of testing has not been incorporated into routine clinical practice.

Treatment of Food Allergy

The cornerstone of the management of food allergy *is avoidance* of the offending allergen. This is particularly important in cases of *peanut allergy* where trace amounts of allergen can cause significant reactions. *Most fatalities due to food allergy have been due to peanut allergy.* Patients with food allergies should learn to read and understand labels for hidden food allergens and to recognize the potential for foods to cross-react with other antigens (eg, *banana and kiwi with latex,* and *birch pollen with apple, carrot, and hazel nut*).

In North America the Food Allergy and Anaphylaxis Network (1-800-929-4040, <www.foodallergy.org>) is a source of valuable information for those with various types of food allergy. Similarly, it is important for celiac patients to join local celiac disease foundations and support groups that can provide valuable information used to determine sources of gluten free foods and medications.

Infants with cow's milk protein allergy present a unique situation because avoidance of their major source of nutrition poses difficulty in this age group. Formulas with reduced antigenicity have been developed and include those in which milk proteins are partially hydrolyzed by heat or enzymes, as well as more extensively hydrolyzed preparations. It is recommended that extensively rather than partially hydrolyzed preparations are used for those who are truly allergic to cow's milk protein because only the latter are truly hypoallergenic. For the 10% of infants that still react to even the more hydrolyzed formulas, amino acid based preparations should be used. For infants with IgE-mediated cow's milk allergy there is only a small chance they will also be allergic to soy protein, whereas infants with cow's milk protein-induced enteropathy involving other immune mechanisms have a > 50% likelihood of developing soy protein-induced enterocolitis.

Anaphylactic Reactions

Because it is often difficult to prevent accidental exposure to food antigens, patients with a history of an *anaphylactic reaction* should be instructed to carry an *epinephrine-containing syringe* for emergency administration. As reactions may be biphasic in nature, patients must be instructed to go to a local emergency facility even after control of the initial symptoms. Individuals who are at increased risk of anaphylaxis include those with a past history of anaphylaxis, those with reactions with respiratory symptoms, those with episodes due the ingestion of peanuts, tree nuts, fish or seafood, and those taking β-blockers or angiotensin converting enzyme inhibitor therapy. *Antihistamines, ketotifen, oral cromolyn, leukotriene antagonists* and *corticosteroids* may modify symptoms to food allergens but apart from first generation histamine receptor antagonists, their efficacy in food allergic conditions is largely unproven. Realizing that there are limited studies available from which to make evidence-based decisions, a trial of an orally administered mast cell stabilizing drug, *sodium cromoglycate,* 100 to 200 mg up to 4 times daily, may be helpful in preventing episodes of allergy particularly for patients who have to eat outside of their own home and/or have multiple food alllergies.

Dietary Restrictions

Dietary restrictions for food allergy associated with anaphylaxis and celiac disease should be maintained on a long term basis, whereas such measures can be lessened in other types of food allergy that resolve with time, particularly those presenting in early childhood. At one time it was thought that unlike other food allergies, peanut allergy was not outgrown. However, there are recent studies that indicate that there may be as high as *a 50% chance of outgrowing* a peanut allergy. As noted above, skin testing cannot be used to predict loss of clinical reactivity because skin tests may remain positive in a child who no longer has clinical manifestations of food allergy. Instead a decline in specific IgE levels followed by a negative oral challenge provides a better index of clinical loss of reactivity to a specific food antigen.

To date, there is no definite evidence that oral desensitization, injection immunotherapy, or similar techniques used for allergies to inhalant allergens, insect venoms, and medications, are beneficial in the prevention or modulation of food allergy. One exception to this is the *oral allergy syndrome* in which *desensitization to the pollen benefits* not only the symptoms of rhinitis but also food-induced oral manifestations. *Immunomodulation* via oral, subcutaneous and sublingual desensitization remain an area of controversy and these techniques are not routinely recommended in the management of food allergy.

Prevention of Food Allergy

The optimum means to prevent the development of allergies in high risk individuals remains an area of controversy. Recommendations have been made in the United States and in Europe for infants with a strong family history of atopy at risk of developing food and other allergies and include the exclusive use of breastfeeding for at least 4 to 6 months, delayed introduction of solid foods until after 4 to 6 months of age, particularly allergenic foods such as egg, wheat, nuts, and fish, avoidance of all CMP, and if formula is needed, to use only extensively hydrolyzed or amino-acid based formulas. Partially hydrolyzed cow's milk, soy, and goat or sheep milk products are not recommended. Hypoallergenic diets have been recommended during pregnancy and with breastfeeding for atopic mothers to reduce the incidence of food allergy in their offspring.

Probiotics offer another means to prevent the development of food allergy. The rationale for using probiotics in allergic diseases is that normal enteric flora established shortly after birth provides counter regulatory signals against a sustained T-helper type 2 cell (Th2)-skewed immune response (Isolauri, 2002). A number of randomized placebo controlled studies show that *Lactobacillus GG* (also called *Lactobacillus rhamnosus* [ATCC 53103]) given to *women before and during subsequent breastfeeding reduced the occurrence of allergic eczema in their offspring.* Other studies suggest that *probiotics* such as *Lactobacillus GG* may also be beneficial in *ameliorating the severity of allergic responses in established food allergy* particularly in younger subjects.

Newer Therapies for Food Allergy

Biologic Therapy

Perhaps the most exciting developments in the field of food allergy are new therapeutic approaches that modulate immune responses to foods (Nowak-Wegrzyn, 2003). These include *tolerogenic peptides, recombinant epitopes, anti-IgE* and *DNA vaccination*, as well as administration of *Th1 type cytokines,* such as interleukin (IL)-12 and interferon-γ, or strategies to *antagonize the actions of Th2 cytokines,* such as IL-4 and Il-5. The benefit of such approaches in food allergy was recently documented in a double blind randomized, placebo controlled, dose-ranging trial, in which a humanized monoclonal IgG1 antibody against IgE that recognizes and masks an epitope in the CH3 region of IgE responsible for binding to the FcRεI on mast cells and basophils was administered subcutaneously in *peanut allergic subjects* (Leung et al, 2003). A statistically significant improvement (subjects increased their tolerance for peanuts from an average of 1.5 peanuts to 9 peanuts at one time) was seen between the highest dose and placebo. The long term benefit and practical application of this treatment is unknown but these initial results are promising for the population who are at risk of potentially fatal reactions from peanut allergy.

Modify Antigenic Structure

Methods to genetically or chemically modify the antigenic structures of foods to reduce their allergic potential are also being developed. For example, it is known that single amino acid substitutions in the IgE binding site of a peanut allergen can lead to the loss of binding to these epitopes. *Mutated protein* or *peptide immunotherapies* are promising but unproven strategies to induce desensitisation to food antigens. *Traditional Chinese medicine (herbal)* used for allergic disorders has been shown to modulate the immune response and to block anaphylaxis in a murine model of peanut allergy suggesting that such treatments may be beneficial in human food allergy. Other experimental therapies are being directed to modifying the intestinal barrier so it is less permeable to food and other types of antigens. Although all these developments hold some promise for food allergy sufferers, none are at a stage of development so as to significantly impact the current way food allergy is treated.

Summary

ARF resulting in GI symptoms are common in the general population and although only a minority of individuals will have symptoms due to food allergy, GI food allergies do exist in both children and adults. It is important to recognize potential cases of food allergy in order to correctly diagnose and manage the small subset of patients with immunologically mediated ARF. Potentially fatal reactions to food necessitate careful instruction and monitoring on the part of health care workers involved in the care of individuals at risk of anaphylaxis. This is particularly true in westernized countries where the prevalence of allergy is increasing and food allergy is now the major cause of anaphylaxis.

Supplemental Reading

American Gastroenterological Association Position Statement: Guidelines for the Evaluation of Food Allergies. Gastroenterol 2001;120:1023–5.

Blanco, C. Latex-Fruit Syndrome. Curr Allergy Asthma Rep 2003;3:47–53.

Crowe SE, Perdue MH. Gastrointestinal food hypersensitivity: Basic mechanisms of pathophysiology. Gastroenterol 1992;103:1075–v95.

De Boissieu D, Waguet JC, Dupont C. The atopy patch tests for detection of cow's milk allergy with digestive symptoms. J Pediatr 2003;142:203–5.

Hill DJ, Heine RG, Cameron DJ, et al. Role of food protein intolerance in infants with persistent distress attributed to reflux esophagitis. J Pediatr 2000;136:641–7.

Ingelfinger FJ, Lowell FC, Franklin W. Gastrointestinal allergy. N Engl J Med 1949;241:303–40.

Isolauri E, Rautava S, Kalliomaki M, et al. Role of probiotics in food hypersensitivity. Curr Opin Allergy Clin Immunol 2002;2:263–71.

Kelsay K. Psychological aspects of food allergy. Curr Allergy Asthma Rep 2003;3:41–6.

Leung DY, Sampson HA, Yunginger JW, et al. Effect of anti-IgE therapy in patients with peanut allergy. N Engl J Med 2003;348:986–93.

Nowak-Wegrzyn A. Future approaches to food allergy. Pediatrics 2003;111:1672–80.

Nowak-Wegrzyn A, Sampson HA, Wood RA, Sicherer SH. Food protein-induced enterocolitis syndrome caused by solid food proteins. Pediatrics 2003;111:829–35.

Sampson HA. Food allergy. J Allergy Clin Immunol 2003;111 (2 Suppl):S540–7.

Sampson HA. Improving in-vitro tests for the diagnosis of food hypersensitivity. Curr Opin Allergy Clin Immunol 2002;2:257–61.

Sampson HA, Sicherer SH, Birnbaum AH. AGA technical review on the evaluation of food allergy in gastrointestinal disorders. Gastroenterol 2001;120:1026–40.

Sicherer SH. Food Allergy. Lancet 2002;360:701–10.

Sloane D, Sheffer A. Oral allergy syndrome. Allergy Asthma Proc 2001;22:321–5.

Spanier JA, Howden CW, Jones MP. A systematic review of alternative therapies in the irritable bowel syndrome. Arch Intern Med 2003;163:265–74.

CHAPTER 58

COMPLEMENTARY AND ALTERNATIVE MEDICINE IN GASTROINTESTINAL DISEASE

Robert J. Hilsden, MD, PhD, FRCPC, and Marja J. Verhoef, PhD

The use of complementary and alternative medicine (CAM) by the general public is very common (Ernst, 2000). Therefore, it is not surprising that gastroenterologists frequently encounter patients who are using or want to use CAM to treat their gastrointestinal (GI) condition. Often these patients have used CAM before the development of their GI condition. Others have no prior experience with CAM but now wish to pursue it. Patients learn about CAM through friends or family, books, the media, or the Internet, or they may have seen complementary practitioners. Managing these situations can be difficult for gastroenterologists because they may not be knowledgeable about the therapy and are likely to be hesitant to support a therapy without strong scientific evidence of its efficacy and safety. We will briefly review what is currently known about the use of CAM in GI disease and provide practical guidelines for informing and counseling patients. Finally, we will recommend some useful sources of information.

CAM

The term CAM will refer to the diverse collection of health systems and diagnostic and therapeutic modalities that are not part of the conventional western medical system. Examples of CAM include alternative medical systems (eg, homeopathy, traditional Chinese medicine, and Ayurveda), products derived from nature (eg, milk thistle, aloe vera, and other herbs), probiotics, orthomolecular medicine (eg, high dose vitamin C, coenzyme Q10), pharmacological interventions (eg, antineoplastons), manipulative and physical therapies (chiropractic, massage) and various procedures and devices (eg, colonic lavage and bioresonance). Many therapies are clearly outside of conventional medicine; however, for others, the borders are blurred. Common examples of complementary therapies that are finding a role in the conventional medical care of patients with GI and liver disease include milk thistle (Silymarin), probiotics, hypnosis, and acupuncture. The ever growing number of abstracts on CAM at Digestive Disease Week is evidence of the emerging interest of biomedical scientists in CAM.

Practitioners of CAM and patients who use CAM often have a quite different view of disease and its treatment than conventional physicians. Concepts of disease and healing often emphasize holism and balance. A holistic approach is characterized by an emphasis on diagnosing and treating illness through an understanding of the whole person (ie, body, mind, and spirit) and how the individual interacts with the world around them. Health and disease are often viewed as a balance between dynamic, opposing forces. Disease may be seen as the result of a blockage or disruption of vital energy or an imbalance between two opposing forces (eg, ying and yang). Treatments are directed at restoring a healthy balance and flow in these forces and stimulating the self-healing potential of the body. These philosophies often lead to highly individualized treatments.

In many alternative medical systems, the patient plays a more active role in their treatment. The patient may be seen as the primary agent of healing helped by the guidance of the practitioner. The patient-centered focus of CAM, along with the common emphasis on health and well-being rather than on disease, may be particularly appealing to patients and may, in and of itself, have a healing effect.

Who Uses CAM and Why Do They Use It?

Several surveys have reported on the use of CAM by patients with GI diseases (Giese, 2000; Hayden et al, 2002; Hilsden et al, 2003). Each of these has reported on differences between patients who use and don't use CAM. For example, CAM users are often characterized by (1) more severe disease, (2) higher socioeconomic status, and (3) younger age. However, with the mainstreaming of CAM, it is becoming more difficult to characterize CAM users, and it may not be relevant in the clinical setting to do so. CAM use cuts across disease and sociodemographic spectrums.

It may be more important to understand the health beliefs and behaviors of those who use CAM. *CAM users often want to play a more active role in their health care.* We found that important factors leading inflammatory bowel disease (IBD) patients to use CAM included dissatisfaction with their conventional medical treatments, especially a lack of effect or side effects of medical treatments. However, other factors are also important including a patient's health beliefs, culture and knowledge and their previous experiences with CAM. Some patients' health beliefs may be more compatible with CAM, and therefore, they may use them early during the course of their disease (Astin, 1998). Others may be comfortable with conventional medicine and only seek out CAM when they believe they have seen the limitations of conventional medicine.

In general, patients do *not* abandon conventional medicine in favor of complementary therapies. Instead they tend to *use both*, often hoping that there will be a synergistic effect or that the complementary therapy will ameliorate or prevent side effects from the conventional medicine.

Patients report obtaining a number of benefits through their use of CAM. One of the most common benefits is a greater sense of being in control of their disease. They also frequently feel that by using a complementary therapy they have taken a more active role in the management of their disease. These benefits may overshadow any improvement in their symptoms resulting from their use of CAM. Therefore, a patient may not appreciate any improvement in their disease but still be satisfied and report higher quality of life with their use of CAM. Therefore, CAM use can be considered a *coping strategy* used by those with chronic diseases. It is important for the gastroenterologist to understand this because it helps explain why *rational patients* demonstrate, what is from the gastroenterologist's perspective, an irrational health behavior—the use of an unproven therapy. Understanding patients' use of CAM requires looking beyond symptoms to the impact the disease and its treatment has on every aspect of patients' lives.

We have also found that the degree of satisfaction with CAM is partly associated with the patient's *health beliefs* (Hilsden et al, 1999). Patients whose health beliefs were more congruent with CAM are more likely to report a high degree of satisfaction with the CAM they used than patients whose health beliefs were more congruent with conventional medicine.

Patients frequently *exclude their gastroenterologist* when deciding to use a CAM and then often do not inform them about using it (Hilsden and Verhoef, 1998). Patients often indicate that they withhold this information because they are afraid of their physician rejecting their use of CAM or because they do not see their physician as being knowledgeable about these therapies.

In summary, patients commonly use CAM as part of the treatment of their disease in combination with their conventional medicines, they often do so because of problems they have had with their conventional treatments, and they frequently do not include their physician in the decision making process.

Efficacy and Safety of CAM

One of the main problems facing both patients and physicians is the lack of information on the safety and efficacy of CAM. In fact, we found that GI patients rated CAM as one of their most important information needs. Gastroenterologists are well aware of the potential for severe hepatotoxicity from some herbal products. However, in general, there are no major safety concerns with the common forms of therapy (herbs and nutritional supplements) used by GI patients. Potential risks include allergic reactions, contamination or mislabeling of herbal products, nutritional deficiencies resulting from restrictive diets, and neck and spine injury resulting from spinal manipulation. However, physicians and patients should be aware that some therapies are associated with the risk of serious side effects due to the therapy's chemical constituents (eg, hepatic veno-occlusive disease from herbs such as comfrey that contain pyrrolizidine alkaloids), contamination with heavy metals (reported with some medicines prepared in Asia), and the potential risk for toxicity to the fetus.

The potential for interactions between complementary and conventional medicines exists, but is poorly documented for most therapies (Crone and Wise, 1998). Many herbs can affect the absorption or metabolism of conventional medicines. Patients on immunosuppressants or other medications with a narrow therapeutic window should be especially careful.

Many complementary therapies based on traditional healing practices have a rich folk history supporting their use, however there is little, if any, direct scientific evidence supporting the benefits of most forms of CAM. Much of the evidence that patients and physicians have access to is anecdotal. Some controlled trials of specific therapies have been conducted but these are often reported in journals unfamiliar to practicing physicians, are flawed, and examine treatments not widely used or available. Conducting randomized controlled trials of some forms of CAM are methodologically difficult due to the highly individualized nature of the therapies, lack of placebos, patient and provider preferences, and different beliefs about health and disease (Hilsden and Verhoef, 1998). There is a body of ethnopharmacology and basic science research on some herbal products that support a possible role in the treatment of IBD. Systematic reviews of some therapies used for common GI conditions are available (Spainer et al, 2003; Jacobs et al, 2002).

Approach to the Patient Using or Wishing to Use a Complementary Therapy

Counseling patients about CAM use is important and can help the patient make a more informed choice. To be effective, it must be done in a sensitive and nonjudgmental fashion. As with any attempt to modify health behavior, gastroenterologists should avoid an authoritative "advice-giving" or direct persuasion approach because this can push the patient into a more resistant and defensive position. This is not to say that physicians must agree with their patients use of CAM. In our experience, patients often recognize that they are obtaining only one side of the story from those promoting a complementary therapy. However, they want more than just a "No, don't use it" from their gastroenterologist. They value their gastroenterologist as an information source and want an open discussion of the potential value or risks associated with a therapy, even if ultimately the gastroenterologist disagrees with their use of it.

Eisenberg (1997) has written a valuable article on advising patients who seek alternative medical therapies. It is directed towards the patient who is seeking care from a complementary practitioner. Even though we find that most patients self-treat with complementary therapies rather than see a complementary practitioner, Eisenberg's guidelines are still appropriate. Below are the steps that one of us (RJH) uses when counseling a patient.

1. Document CAM use

    Determining current and past use of CAM should be part of the routine medical history for all patients. There are several reasons for doing so. First, use of a CAM may be an indication that the patient is dissatisfied with their current treatment either because they are not achieving the benefits they desire or because they are suffering side effects. Second, the use of potentially dangerous therapies can be discovered. Third, potential drug–CAM interactions can be anticipated. Finally, the effects of the CAM, either good or bad, will not be misconstrued as resulting from a conventional treatment.

    Patients, however, are reluctant to reveal their use of CAM especially if they view their gastroenterologist as being intolerant or uninformed. Therefore, this is not the correct situation to use terms such as quakery, fraudulent, or unconventional therapies. I routinely ask the patient whether they (1) use herbal or natural therapies, (2) have made any dietary changes, and (3) use any other therapies for their condition or general health.

2. Determine reasons for seeking CAM

    A patient who is using or considering using CAM should be asked about their reasons for doing so. This is important because determining specific areas of dissatisfaction with their conventional treatment could allow modifications to be made. Again careful questioning is required, as the patient may be reticent to reveal issues that they feel may be perceived as criticism by their gastroenterologist. Open-ended questions such as "What do you see as the potential benefits of using this therapy" and "Do you have any concerns about your current treatment that is leading you to consider this new therapy" allow the patient to openly discuss their perspective on their treatment. It is also valuable to obtain some sense of the patient's health beliefs. If the patient is a firm believer in the principles of complementary medicine, then it is unlikely that they will be convinced not to use one. If on the other hand the patient is more comfortable with conventional medicine but is seeking alternatives because they are experiencing problems, then they may be willing to first try a modification in their conventional medical treatment.

3. Explore the patient's knowledge and source of information about CAM

    Many sources of information available to the patient, for example books and Internet sites, provide an overly optimistic and one-sided account of the effectiveness of a therapy and are often based only on testimonials. Often information about safety is not provided. The patients understanding of how the therapy works and its potential benefits and harms should be determined. Some patients have very realistic expectations. They may understand that their chance of obtaining some benefit is low but they are willing to try it on the off chance that they do benefit. However, many patients have unrealistic expectations and expect a quick cure. In the short time available for counseling a patient, it is impossible and impractical to teach them the principles of scientific medicine and the randomized controlled trial. However, the patient should be encouraged to define realistic treatment goals and to reevaluate their use of a therapy after a set period of time.

    Many patients often believe that CAM is without risk, often because they are "natural" therapies. This belief is often promoted by advertisements for the therapy. Therefore, the patient may not have considered the possibility of side effects. Physicians should ask patients whether they know the possible side effects of a therapy and should warn patients about the possibility of interactions with alcohol or other drugs. The patient and the physician may have difficulty finding any specific information about the risks of these with a given product. Patients should be encouraged to think of any therapy in terms of a trade-off between potential benefits and potential risks. Often patients think more about the potential benefits and neglect to consider whether they are willing to incur the risks of a complementary therapy, including its cost.

4. Determine how the patient will obtain and use the therapy

    If the patient is seeing or will be seeing an alternative practitioner, the gastroenterologist can provide the patient with questions they should ask the practitioner. These would include (1) is the practitioner licensed and what was their training, (2) how experienced are they in treating patients with IBD, (3) what can the patient expect from the treatment in terms of benefits and side effects, (4) what is the basis for these expectations, and (5) what will be the cost of the treatment.

Patients should not start a number of different therapies, especially a combination of conventional and complementary therapies, at the same time. If this is done, it will be impossible to determine which therapy resulted in any benefits or side effects. Some method for monitoring for side effects should be agreed upon. This will depend upon the potential risks associated with a therapy.

Information Sources About CAM

There are a variety of valuable information sources available for physicians, although none of them are specifically focused on GI disease. Patients should not rely too heavily on the advice or recommendations provided by employees of health food stores or other stores selling herbal and nutritional supplements (Verhoef et al, 2002). Often only the owner or the manager of the store has much experience and knowledge about the therapies. Other employees may have relatively little training and may not be able to distinguish between treatments that are safe and appropriate for a given condition and those more commonly used for other GI complaints. General intestinal remedies sold at health food stores often contain laxatives.

Below are several sources of information on CAM that we find useful. We have chosen these because they critically review therapies and provide supporting evidence for any claims made. All of them are relatively inexpensive (at least compared to medical textbooks).

In conclusion, CAM is not likely to disappear in the near future. Patients will continue to incorporate it into their health care, and certain therapies such as probiotics, will be incorporated into conventional medicine if their efficacy is demonstrated. Physicians will need to address the questions and concerns of patients using CAM and will need to be able to safely manage patients using conventional and complementary therapies concomitantly.

General Sources

The American Pharmaceutical Association Practical Guide to Natural Medicines (A. Pierce). Reference book directed at potential users of natural products, includes sections on assessing safety and efficacy.

The Honest Herbal (V. E. Taylor PhD, Pharmaceutical Products Press). This comprehensive book provides a wealth of critical and referenced information on many herbs. The author describes the putative active ingredients, recommended uses and supporting evidence of efficacy for each herb, and also debunks unwarranted claims.

The Complete Book of Symptoms and Treatments (E. Ernst, Editor, Element Books Limited). This book is divided into the following three sections: (1) symptoms and disorders, (2) therapies used in complementary medicine, and (3) diagnostic techniques used in complementary medicine. Within the symptoms and disorders section, therapies used for a variety of medical conditions are discussed. There is a section on GI conditions, although neither ulcerative colitis nor Crohn's disease is specifically included. Each therapy is given a rating as to the likelihood of achieving a therapeutic benefit and potential risks are listed. The level of evidence supporting any benefits (ie, case reports, clinical trials) is given, but unfortunately no references are provided.

Professionals Handbook of Complementary and Alternative Medicines (C. W. Feltrow and J. R. Avila, Springhouse Publishers). This book describes the chemical components, actions, reported uses, and suggested doses of many herbs and alternative medicines. The authors also list potential adverse events and drug interactions. The book is less critical of claims made about the efficacy of the treatments than the above two books.

Side Effects/Drug Interventions

Herb Contraindications and Drug Interactions (F. Brinker, Eclectic Medical Publications). This book describes known and speculated side effects, contraindications, and drug interactions of herbs. The book is well referenced and indexed.

Web Sites

National Center for Complementary and Alternative Medicine <http://nccam.nih.gov/health/>. Website of National Institutes of Health that has the goals of supporting rigorous research on CAM, training researchers in CAM, and disseminating information to the public, and professionals on which CAM modalities work, which do not, and why. The Web site includes several systematic reviews of various therapies for GI conditions.

The Research Council for Complementary Medicine <www.rccm.org.uk>. Includes a centralized information service on complementary medicine with links to clinical trials and Cochrane reviews.

Quackwatch <www.quackwatch.com> Described as "Your guide to health fraud, quackery and intelligent decisions."

Supplemental Reading

Astin JA. Why patients use alternative medicine: results of a national study. JAMA 1998;279:1548–53.

Crone CC, Wise TN. Use of herbal medicines among consultation-liason populations. Psychosomatics 1998;39:313.

Eisenberg DM. Advising patients who seek alternative medical therapies. Ann Intern Med 1997;127:61–9.

Ernst E. Prevalence of use of complementary/alternative medicine: a systematic review. Bull World Health Organ 2000;78:252–7.

Giese LA. A study of alternative health care use for gastrointestinal disorders. Gastroenterol Nurs 2000;23:19–27.

Hayden CW, Bernstein CN, Hall RA, et al. Usage of supplemental alternative medicine by community-based patients with gastroesophageal reflux disease (GERD). Dig Dis Sci 2002;47:1–8.

Hilsden RJ, Scott CM, Verhoef MJ. Complementary medicine use by patients with inflammatory bowel disease. Am J Gastroenterol 1998;93:697–701.

Hilsden RJ, Meddings JB, Verhoef MJ. Complementary and alternative medicine use by patients with inflammatory bowel disease: an internet survey. Can J Gastroenterol 1999;13:327–32.

Hilsden RJ, Verhoef MJ. Complementary and alternative medicine: evaluating its effectiveness in inflammatory bowel disease. Inflamm Bowel Dis 1998;4:318–23.

Hilsden RJ, Verhoef MJ, Best A, Pocobelli G. Complementary and alternative medicine use by Canadian patients with inflammatory bowel disease: results from a national survey. Am J Gastroenterol 2003;98:1563–8.

Jacobs BP, Dennehy C, Ramirez G, et al. Milk thistle for the treatment of liver disease: a systematic review and meta-analysis. Am J Med 2002;113:506–15.

Spanier JA, Howden CW, Jones MP. A systematic review of alternative therapies in the irritable bowel syndrome [review]. Arch Intern Med 2003;163:265–74.

Verhoef MJ, Rapchuk I, Liew T, et al. Complementary practitioners' views of treatment for inflammatory bowel disease. Can J Gastroenterol 2002;16:95–100.

CHAPTER 59

Obscure Gastrointestinal Bleedings

Andrew I. Sable, MD, and Jamie S. Barkin, MD, FACP, MACG

Obscure gastrointestinal bleeding (OGIB) is defined as bleeding of unknown origin that persists or recurs after negative initial or primary endoscopy, including colonoscopy and upper endoscopy. It poses a profound diagnostic and therapeutic challenge for gastroenterologists and surgeons alike because these patients often have recurrent bleeding and use a plethora of health care resources. Bleeding may arise from virtually any location within the gastrointestinal (GI) tract and patients present with great variability, from chronic occult bleeding to acute bleeding with visible blood loss. Either of these presentations may result in iron deficiency anemia (IDA) and necessitate blood transfusion.

OGIB is categorized into the following two clinically distinct entities: (1) *obscure-occult*, which is characterized by IDA and/or recurrent positive fecal occult blood test (FOBT), and (2) *obscure-overt*, in which recurrent bleeding is clinically evident by the presence of melena, maroon stools, or hematochezia (Zuckerman et al, 2000).

There is little data regarding the frequency and natural history of OGIB. Despite timely upper endoscopy and colonoscopy, bleeding remains unexplained in approximately 5% of patients (Hayat et al, 2000). Failure to identify a bleeding source at the time of endoscopy may be the result of the following:

1. Overlooked lesions, such as nonbleeding lesions or those obscured by the presence of blood or thickened gastric folds
2. Lesions beyond the reach of traditional endoscopes (ie, third portion of duodenum)
3. Difficult to diagnose lesions (ie, Dieulafoy's malformation or gastric antral vascular ectasias (GAVE)
4. The discovery of an equivocal finding at the time of endoscopy that may or may not be the bleeding source

Colonoscopy with ileal intubation and upper endoscopy are requisite in the initial evaluation of patients with OGIB. Repeated bidirectional endoscopy may be both indicated and necessary before a diagnosis is made. A second or third endoscopic look may identify lesions that are commonly missed (ie, Cameron's erosions and arteriovenous malformations) and/or difficult to identify (ie, Dieulafoy's disease and celiac sprue). If bleeding continues and the source remains unidentified, further evaluation should be directed to the small bowel, a rare but important source of blood loss and the overwhelming location of bleeding of obscure origin (Lahoti and Fukami, 1999).

Examination of the small bowel was previously limited by the poor application of conventional studies. There is little use for radioisotope bleeding scans and angiography in OGIB of occult origin. Small bowel series and enteroclysis generally have a low diagnostic yield for lesions that commonly cause OGIB (ie, vascular ectasia and ulcerations). With the advent of wireless capsule endoscopy (WCE) direct, noninvasive examination of the entire small bowel is possible thus enabling the identification of clinically relevant lesions as well as determining their approximate location. This chapter will discuss our approach to OGIB with attention to the small bowel.

Approach to Diagnosis of Patients with OGIB

The identification of a bleeding source begins with a thorough history and physical examination. Pharmacologic agents, including aspirin and nonsteroidal antiiflammatory drugs (NSAIDs), which are cyclooxygenase-1-selective inhibitor sparing and nonselective, are toxic to the intestinal mucosa and predispose to ulceration and mucosal bleeding. The pathogenesis, although complex, is well established. In addition to the suppression of prostaglandins, there is likely local, topical mucosal injury.

These toxic effects, although well described in the stomach and duodenum, are now known to also occur in the colon (ie, NSAID-induced colitis) and small intestine (ie, erosions, ulcerations, and webs) and at a higher frequency compared with controls than previously known (58% small bowel lesions in NSAID users versus 17% in nonusers) (Graham et al, 2003). Small bowel and colonic injury may occur independently of symptoms of gastroduodenal irritation. The identification of NSAID intake is fundamental in the management of patients with bleeding of obscure origin. There is a separate chapter (Chapter 60, "Nonsteroidal Antiinflammatory Drug-Induced Small and large Intestinaal Injury") on NSAID-induced injury to the small and large intestine.

A family history may reveal hereditary disorders resulting in OGIB, including hereditary hemorrhagic telangectasias (HHT), Osler-Weber-Rendu disease (OWR) and polyposis syndromes. Patients with previous *aortic aneurysm repair* should have mandatory examination of the third portion of the duodenum to evaluate for the presence of *aortoenteric fistula*. Patients with easy bruisibility or other clinical manifestations suggesting a coagulation disorder should be examined with a coagulation profile. In addition, patients with aortic stenosis acquire defects in von Willebrand's factor.

The clinical pattern of blood loss may help localize bleeding. Hematemasis, although a rare presentation of OGIB, may help to localize bleeding proximal to the ligament of Treitz. Stool color is less helpful in predicting the site of blood loss because it is primarily a function of the transit time of the blood bolus (Hilsman, 1950). Patients with slow oozing from the distal small bowel and proximal colon can have melena, whereas those with brisk blood loss from the proximal intestine often present with hematochezia and hypotension, but without hematemasis or bloody nasogastric aspirate. The details of the history and physical examination may be helpful in providing clues to a source of bleeding as depicted in Table 59-1.

The frequency of upper intestinal lesions in patients with positive FOBT is reportedly as high as 75% (Geller et al, 1993). Furthermore, of patients with obscure-overt bleeding approximately 50% will have identifiable lesions within the reach of a standard gastroscope (Jensen, 2003).

Repeat upper endoscopy may therefore, in many cases, identify missed lesions not seen on initial evaluation. Specific lesions presenting with OGIB, occult or overt, that may be missed initially if they are not actively bleeding are in Table 59-2.

Coagulation Studies

The determination of coagulation parameters in patients with OGIB is necessary. Abnormalities in the bleeding time and partial thromboplastin time may reflect von Willebrand's disease (vWD). Whereas prolonged international normalized ratio (INR) may reflect advanced liver disease, disseminated intravascular coagulation, or surreptitious anticoagulation intake. Abnormal platelet function test (prolonged bleeding time) may indicate acetylsalicyclic acid (ASA) and/or NSAID use. Hemorrhagic tendency in vWD is variable and dependent on the type and severity of disease. Patients with Types 1 and 2 vWD may have mild, occult bleeding associated with IDA. Type 3 vWD disease is associated with telangiectasis of the small and large bowel and may present with severe obscure-overt bleeding. vWD may be acquired in individuals who were previously normal and is associated with mitral valve prolapse and aortic stenosis (Vincentelli et al, 2003; Heyde, 1958; Mant et al, 1968; Mannucci et al, 1973). Uremia in patients with acute renal failure or chronic renal insufficiency who have OGIB may indicate a need for vasopressin to correct platelet dysfunction, whereas plasma infusion and/or vitamin K supplementation may be required in patients with acute or chronic liver failure. Additionally, hospitalized patients on broad spectrum antibiotics may develop vitamin K deficiency and supplementation may be helpful in the event of bleeding.

Diagnostic Modalities

Radiologic Procedures

SMALL BOWEL SERIES/ENTEROCLYSIS

The overall yield of barium examination of the small bowel is extremely low. These techniques are employed after negative enteroscopy or when enteroscopy is not immediately

TABLE 59-1. Clues to Diagnosis

History or Physical Finding	Cause of Bleeding
GERD	Cameron's erosion/ulcers
Abdominal pain	Tumor/ischemia
Hx of pancreatic injury/pancreatitis	Hemosuccus pancreaticus
RUQ surgery/injury	Hemobilia
Arthritis/NSAIDs	SB/colon ulceration/colitis
Hx of radiation	Neovascularization
Surgery	Anastomotic
Chronic renal insufficiency	Vascular ectasia
Abdominal aortic aneurysm repair	Aorto-enteric fistula
Diarrhea	CD
Liver disease/spider angiomata	Gastro/duodenal/rectal varices
Connective tissue disorder	GAVE
Age < 40 years	Meckel's diverticulum
Aortic stenosis/MVP	Acquired von Willebrand's factor defect

CD = Crohn's disease; GAVE = gastric antral vascular ectasias; GERD = gastroesophageal reflux disease; Hx = medical history; MVP = mitral valve prolapse; NSAID = nonsteroidal anti-inflammatory drug; SB = small bowel.

TABLE 59-2. Proximal Intestinal Lesions Causing Obscure Gastrointestinal Bleeding

Esophagus	Esophagitis/ulcers
	Mallory-Weiss tear
	Cameron's erosions/ulcer
Stomach	AVM
	Dieulafoy's malformation
	GAVE
	PHG
Duodenum	Dieulafoy's malformation
	AVM
	CD
	Hemobilia
	Hemosuccus Pancreaticus
	Aorto-enteric fistula

Adapted from Mujica and Barkin, 1996.
AVM = arteriovenous malformations; CD = Crohn's disease, GAVE = gastric antral vascular ectasias; PHG = portal hypertensive gastropathy.

available. In the absence of obstructive symptoms, small bowel follow-through (SBFT) leads to a diagnosis in about 5% of patients with OGIB. The yield with enteroclysis, although better (about 10%), is still minimal, because these methods are inadequate for detecting mucosal lesions like *vascular ectasia*, which are overwhelmingly the most frequent cause for small bowel bleeding. Comparison of WCE with small bowel enteroclysis in patients with OGIB has shown the superiority of WCE for the detection of lesions (Liangpunsakul et al, 2003).

Radionucleotide Studies

Scintigraphy with technetium-labeled red blood cells may help to confirm hemorrhage that may be originating in the small bowel; however, it does not accurately locate the site of bleeding. Despite high sensitivity for detection of bleeding (positive if bleeding is less than or equal to 0.1 mL/min) (Alavi, 1982), its low specificity limits its usefulness. Its role, therefore, continues to be controversial. Delayed scans, performed at 12 to 24 hours postinjection, may be misleading by identifying luminal blood that is pooled at sites other than the bleeding source. The Meckel's scan is based on an isotope labeled compound that localizes in the ectopic gastric mucosa found in Meckel's diverticulum. As this isotope normally accumulates in the stomach and bladder, both should be empty at the time of examination to increase its diagnostic yield. Increased sensitivity is achieved by using histamine-2 receptor antagonists, which causes increased activity in the ectopic parietal cells. This test has a more specific role in the examination of patients with OGIB who are below the age of 40 years.

Angiography

Selective mesenteric angiography is expensive and invasive, yet offers both diagnostic and therapeutic modalities. Although it is not as sensitive to low rate or intermittent bleeding as bleeding scans (rate 0.5 to 1 mL/min), angiography has the potential ability to localize and treat bleeding lesions. Provocative maneuvers performed at the time of exam include the use of anticoagulants and/or vasodilators, both of which may precipitate bleeding and improve the diagnostic yield of angiography. The large arcade of mesenteric vasculature makes identification of smaller vascular ectasia difficult. The use of nuclear scans to select those actively bleeding patients who will undergo angiography is controversial but may improve diagnostic yield and lower overall cost by avoiding unnecessary exams.

Enteroscopy

In the past it was believed that asymptomatic patients with obscure-occult bleeding over 60 years of age who have undergone negative colonoscopy and upper endoscopy should only undergo small bowel examination with enteroclysis or SBFT to effectively rule out significant lesions, particularly if a response to oral iron replacement therapy was observed (Rockey and Cello, 1993.). However, in our view, this was similar to treating an automobile oil leak with oil replacement only, rather than fixing its source. In clinical practice, an occult malignancy may be missed and/or a bleeding lesion progress causing increased morbidity and mortality. Patients with OGIB and comorbid disease, and/or those who require blood transfusions, should certainly be subject to a more extensive evaluation. Our current algorithmic approach to patients with OGIB is outlined in Figure 59-1.

After they have undergone negative upper endoscopy and colonoscopy with ileoscopy (repeated if initially negative), enteroscopy, preferably performed with use of an overtube, is our standard approach (O'Loughlin and Barkin, 2004). Enteroscopes vary in length from 220 to 250 cm and with the use of fluoroscopy and an overtube, they can generally reach to a depth of 100 to 110 cm beyond the ligament of Treitz. However a physician's choice of instrument and technique (pediatric colonoscopes/use of

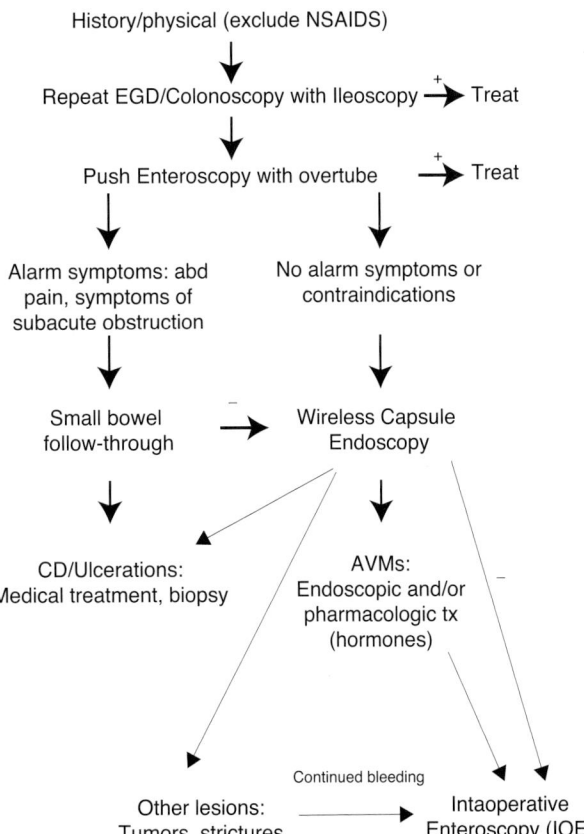

FIGURE 59-1. Schematic approach to obscure gastrointestinal bleeding. abd = abdominal; AVM = arteriovenous malformations; CD = Crohn's disease; EGD = esophagogastroduodenoscopy; NSAIDs = nonsteroidal anti-inflammatory drugs.

overtube), as well as experience, affect the depth of insertion. Regardless of technique the overall yield of diagnosis using enteroscopy in patients with OGIB is 30 to 50%. Enteroscopy has higher diagnostic yield compared with small bowel radiography and, thus, we feel that enteroscopy should be performed earlier in the evaluation of OGIB. Although this order has not been compared in randomized trials, it is generally accepted as standard of care (Zuckerman et al, 2000.)

Sonde enteroscopy permits more distal examination of the small bowel. Its insertion depth and amount of mucosa examined depends on intestinal motility. Lengthy examination, patient discomfort, and lack of therapeutic capabilities make this technique impractical and largely abandoned.

Until recently, *intraoperative enteroscopy* has been the most complete, direct diagnostic modality available for the evaluation of OGIB. It is also the most invasive and is generally reserved for patients with severe, recurrent GI bleeding in which the source remains obscure after complete, exhaustive examination. It has the considerable advantage of allowing complete small bowel examination while also directing therapy. Invariably, mucosal trauma causes artifact bleeding, which may itself obscure potential bleeding sites. Its yield varies from 77 to 87% (Bashir and Al-Kawas, 1996) and is dependent on technical expertise of the surgeon and endoscopist. To minimize artifact, the lumen should be examined in anterograde fashion as the bowel is manipulated over the scope. Potential bleeding sites identified by the endoscopist in the intestinal mucosa or on the intestinal serosa by the surgeon are marked with sutures for subsequent resection.

WCE

WCE using the M2A (Given Imaging, Yoqneam, Israel) capsule endoscope is a monumental development that allows noninvasive visualization of the entire small bowel. First approved for use in 2001, WCE has recently been recognized by the US Food and Drug Administration as a standard first line diagnostic tool for patients with suspected small bowel disorders. It is performed easily in the ambulatory setting, has few complications and/or contraindications (Table 59-3) and has opened novel diagnostic vistas in the study of small bowel disorders, including GI bleeding (see Table 59-3).

Utility of WCE in OGIB

With the introduction of capsule endoscopy, the approach to OGIB has changed. The identification and approximate location of clinically relevant lesions previously inaccessible to the "umbilicated" endoscope is possible. The capsule functions essentially as an extension of the enteroscope.

Comparison of WCE to Radiologic Techniques

Capsule endoscopy is superior to SBFT in the examination of patients with OGIB of suspected small bowel origin. The overall low diagnostic yield of SBFT and enteroclysis limit their usefulness. Costamagna and colleagues (2002) prospectively compared the yield of SBFT to WCE in patients with suspected small bowel diseases, two-thirds of whom had OGIB. They found that WCE was superior to SBFT in yielding a diagnosis (45% versus 27%). Interestingly, approximately 10% of the patients were excluded from this study secondary to suspected small bowel strictures discovered with barium SBFT radiography. This finding and the subsequent clinical investigations involving the capsule has raised awareness of the possibility of so called nonnatural excretion of the capsule (ie, hang-up of the capsule in the areas of luminal narrowing). Thus, there may be a potentially definable role for small bowel radiography prior to capsule endoscopy in certain subgroups of patients with suspected luminal narrowing. Clinically significant capsule "hang-up" (or nonnatural excretion requiring surgical intervention/retrieval) occurs in approximately 0.75% of performed studies. Barkin and Friedman (2002) reported that in each patient an intestinal structural abnormality accounted for the capsule "hang-up," including narrowing as a result of Crohn's disease, radiation, tumor, or NSAIDs.

TABLE 59-3A. Contraindication to Wireless Capsule Endoscopy

Known or suspected obstruction/stricture/fistula; extensive CD disease
Swallowing disorders
Pseudo-obstruction
Motility disorders
Cardiac pacemakers (relative)
Implanted defibrillators and electromechanical devices
Relative Contraindications
 Pregnancy
 Long-standing NSAID use
 Large and numerous diverticuli
 Zenker's diverticulum
 Gastroparesis
 Prior pelvic or abdominal surgery

CD = Crohn's disease; NSAID = nonsteroidal anti-inflammatory drug.

TABLE 59-3. Indications for Capsule Endoscopy

Absolute	Obscure gastrointestinal bleeding
Relative	Diarrhea
	Suspected Crohn's disease
Not indicated	Chronic abdominal pain

Comparison of WCE to Enteroscopy

WCE detects more distal small bowel lesions in patients with OGIB than does push enteroscopy. Lewis and Swain (2002) reported a yield of 55% (11/20) for capsule endoscopy. Ell and colleagues (2002) reported on a heterogeneous group of patients with OGIB and found a diagnostic yield of 66% for capsule endoscopy and 28% for push enteroscopy. Mylonaki and colleagues (2003) reported on 50 patients with OGIB. Using WCE, a bleeding source was discovered in the small bowel in 34 of the 50 patients (68%), whereas push enteroscopy found a source in 32% (16/50). This is not unexpected as WCE visualizes small bowel mucosa far beyond that seen with push enteroscopy. However, WCE inadequately visualizes the esophagus and stomach and lacks therapeutic capability. Therefore, these are not competitive but rather *complimentary procedures*. Ciorba and colleagues (2003) reported that push enteroscopy was recommended *after* capsule endoscopy in 16% of patients, primarily for examination and treatment. We recommend that push enteroscopy be performed before WCE, as bleeding sites in the esophagus, stomach and duodenum can be both diagnosed and treated. *WCE should not replace enteroscopy, but rather it should be viewed as its extension.*

Comparison of WCE to Intraoperative Enteroscopy

Three abstracts at *Digestive Disease Week (DDW)* 2003 reported the findings of intraoperative enteroscopy (IOE) in patients having previously undergone WCE that revealed lesions. IOE was negative in up to approximately 10% of cases (Katz et al, 2003; Hartmann et al, 2003; Wolff et al, 2003). Whether these are false positive WCE or false negative IOE remains to be determined. Obviously IOE is performed in a nonphysiologic state and lesions can be overlooked. A 10% false positive rate of WCE may be reasonable. Conversely, to our knowledge, there is no study in which patients with negative WCE and continued bleeding undergo IOE. This study may allow us to determine the false negative rate of WCE and refine its utility. Our current approach to patients with negative WCE, especially those younger than 40 years of age with severe OGIB, is early laparotomy and IOE as the frequency of small intestinal tumors and Meckel's diverticulum may be higher than those older than 40 years of age (Geller et al, 1993).

Specific Etiologies and Treatments

The small bowel is an unusual but important source of GI blood loss. In patients with negative repeat endoscopy and colonoscopy, the small bowel should become the focus of further investigation. The overwhelming majority of small bowel bleeding originates from *vascular lesions* (ie, arteriovenous malformations [AVM]) and *small bowel tumors*. Other less common sources include *drug-induced ulcerations*, *Crohn's disease (CD)*, *Dieulafoy's malformation*, and *metastatic tumors* to the small bowel. The likely bleeding source varies depending on the age of the affected individual (Table 59-4).

OGIB in patients 40 years of age and younger is more likely caused by small bowel tumors (primary and metastatic), CD, Meckel's diverticulum, and vascular malformations. Whereas patients older than 40 years of age with comorbidities, tend to have more AVMs, Dieulafoy's disease, and small bowel ulcerations secondary to NSAID use. Specific management strategies, depending on etiology, are discussed below.

INTESTINAL ANGIOECTASIAS

The etiology of AVMs is not known but there is clear association with specific clinical conditions such as valvular heart disease, chronic liver/renal disease, collagen vascular disorders, intestinal radiation, vWD, and hereditary disorders like OWR. Most AVMs remain clinically asymptomatic; therefore, their prevalence is difficult to estimate. Unless specifically identified as the cause of bleeding they should not be treated. Bleeding is typically painless, and may be chronic, subacute, or, in approximately 15% of patients, acute and massive. Treatment is directed at both the underlying condition and the AVM itself. When diagnosed as the likely cause of bleeding, endoscopic therapy seems like a reasonable approach. However, the visualized AVMs may be indicative of others located distally, which can be the source of ongoing bleeding. Endoscopic therapy with electrocoagulation may be only temporizing and repeat endoscopic sessions at regular intervals may be necessary. *Thermal contact*, which can be applied effectively with *heater probe*, *bipolar electrocoagulation* (BICAP) and *argon plasma coagulation* (APC), are generally available and easy to use. Conversely, injection sclerotherapy is

TABLE 59-4. Obscure Gastrointestinal Bleeding Etiology Depending On Age

Age 40 Years or Younger	Older Than Age 40 Years
Small bowel tumors	AVM
Crohn's disease	GAVE
Meckel's diverticulum	Cameron's ulcer
Small bowel tumors	—
Polyposis syndromes	Drug-induced small bowel injury
AVM	Dieulafoy's malformation
Dieulafoy's malformation	Amyloidosis
von Willebrand's disease	von Willebrand's disease
Drug-induced small bowel injury	Portal hypertensive intestinal "opathy"
Portal hypertensive intestinal "opathy"	Pancreatic hemosuccus
Pancreatic hemosuccus	Osler-Weber-Rendu

Adapted from Mujica and Barkin, 1996. AVM = arteriovenous malformations; GAVE = gastric antral vascular ectasias.

rather ineffective. Hemostasis can be achieved in 50 to 85% of the lesions regardless of which contact endoscopic technique is used (Van Cutsem and Piessevaux, 1996). In patients with large and multiple AVMs, such as those with OWR, coaptation in a centripetal pattern with BICAP or APC is preferred to obliterate the AVM. Control of bleeding may be difficult. Massive or recurrent, severe bleeding may warrant angiographic and/or surgical intervention with enterotomy and resection.

SMALL BOWEL TUMORS

Neoplasms of the small intestine are uncommon and often remain clinically unrecognized. Bleeding occurs in 25 to 50% of patients with small bowel tumors (Bashir and Al-Kawas, 1996) and comprises approximately 5 to 10% of cases of bleeding of obscure origin. Benign tumors are more likely to bleed than malignant lesions. When recognized, most will warrant endoscopic resection or, when not amenable to endoscopic resection, surgical evaluation and resection. Benign small bowel lesions include adenomas, leiomyomas, lipomas, hamartomas, and rarely neural tumors. Occasionally, pain or obstructive-type symptoms may lead to their diagnosis. Although a pattern of obscure-occult bleeding is more characteristic of benign small bowel tumors, lesions in the duodenum may present with frank hematemesis and those in the ileum with hematochezia. Adenomas are usually found proximal to the ligament of Treitz and account for 25% of benign lesions. All adenomas in the small bowel should be viewed as premalignant lesions and removed regardless of bleeding. Duodenoscopy with a side viewing endoscope may be necessary for diagnosis and treatment of periampullary adenomas such as those seen in familial adenomatous polyposis (FAP). Leiomyomas are the second most common tumor of the small intestine and are also the most likely small bowel tumors to bleed. They are composed primarily of smooth muscle cells and as they enlarge, tumor necrosis results in a central umbilication and ulceration that predisposes to bleeding. If they become large, small bowel series may reveal an intraluminal mass. These are very vascular tumors and 86% will demonstrate a tumor blush on angiography (Cho and Reuter, 1980). Surgical resection is mandatory for large lesions as they are grossly indistinguishable from leiomyosarcomas. Lipomas rarely bleed and, in general, require no specific treatment. When larger than 4 cm, superficial ulceration may occur that can be treated locally with injection therapy or thermal coagulation.

Small bowel malignancies are rare, accounting for < 2% of all GI cancers. Primary small bowel lesions include adenocarcinomas, carcinoid tumors, lymphoma, and leiomyosarcomas. Metastatic lesions may arise from melanoma, Kaposi's sarcoma, lung, breast, and renal cell carcinoma. They are more commonly seen in patients in their fifth to seventh decade of life. Adenocarcinomas are the most common small bowel malignant tumors to cause intestinal bleeding with an incidence approaching 60% (Bashir and Al-Kawas, 1996). In the setting of CD, adenocarcinomas tend to occur distally and are more common in the small bowel than the colon. Endoscopic treatment of small bowel malignancies is highly unsuccessful and associated with the occurrence of a high rate of complications; therefore, treatment with surgical resection, if possible, is preferred.

MISCELLANEOUS

Ulcers distal to the ligament of Treitz are rare causes of GI bleeding and are difficult to diagnose. Their multiple causes and associated conditions are reflected in Table 59-6. Recently, capsule endoscopy has shown that 58% of NSAID users develop small bowel lesions as compared to 17% of nonusers (Graham et al, 2003). Risk factors are likely similar to those for more proximal ulceration and include duration of use, age over 60 years, associated comorbidities, concurrent steroid use, and use of multiple NSAIDs, alcohol, and tobacco. Interestingly, Goldstein and colleagues confirmed that approximately *14% of healthy volunteers* also have lesions (petechiae, erosions, and mucosal breaks) on capsule endoscopy (Goldstein et al, 2003) reminding us that visualized pathology may not necessarily constitute a definitive diagnosis.

TABLE 59-5. Causes of Small Bowel Ulceration

Drugs
    NSAIDs
    Potassium
    Salicylates
Neoplasms
    Adenocarcinoma
    Lymphoma
    Melanoma
Infections
    CMV
    Tuberculosis
    Syphilis
    Yersinia
    Campylobacter
Inflammatory Diseases
    Crohn's disease
    Celiac disease
    Behçet's syndrome
    Ulcerative jejunoileitis
    Vasculitis
    Radiation enteritis

Adapted from Bashir and Al-Kawas, 1996.
CMV = cytomegalovirus; NSAID = nonsteroidal anti-inflammatory drug.

Hormonal Therapy

In addition to iron supplementation, hormonal therapy may be beneficial in patients with disseminated AVMs who have recurrent, transfusion requiring blood loss. *Combination hormone therapy (estradiol 0.035 to 0.05 mg, norethisterone 1 mg)* has been found to be highly effective in the prevention of rebleeding in patients with both suspected and verified AVMs and OGIB (Barkin and Ross, 1998). Treatment courses are recommended in six-month intervals to minimize side effects, including breast tenderness and vaginal bleeding in woman and gynecomastia and decreased libido in men.

Summary

Until recently the approach to diagnosis of OGIB has been fairly standardized, and for many physicians, often frustrating. Patients are subjected to meticulous examination that at times may seem inefficient and ineffectual. With the development of WCE, the algorithm has changed with the promise of fewer patients with obscure bleeding going undiagnosed.

Supplemental Reading

Alavi A. Radionucleotide localization of GI hemorrhage. Radiology 1982;142:801–3.

American Gastroenterological Association Medical Position Statement. Evaluation and management of occult and obscure gastrointestinal bleeding. Gastroenterology 2000;118:197–200.

Barkin JS, Friedman S. Wireless capsule endoscopy requiring surgical intervention: the world's experience. Am J Gastroenterol 2002;97:S298.

Barkin JS, Ross BS. Medical therapy for chronic gastrointestinal bleeding of obscure origin. Am J Gastroenterol 1998;93:1250–4.

Bashir RM, Al-Kawas FH. Rare causes of occult small intestinal bleeding, including aortoenteric fistula, small bowel tumors, and small bowel ulcers. Gastrointest Endosc Clin N Am 1996;6:709–38.

Cho KJ, Reuter SR. Angiography of duodenal leiomyomas and leiomyosarcomas. AJR 1980;135:31.

Ciorba M, Jonnalagadda S, Zuckerman G, et al. Capsule endoscopy: varied outcomes over short term follow-up [abstract M1876]. DDW 2003.

Coastamagna G, Shah SK, Riccioni ME et al. A prospective trial comparing small bowel radiographs and wireless capsule endoscopy for suspected small bowel disease. Gastroenterology 2002;123:999–1005.

Ell C, Remke S, May A, et al. The first prospective controlled trial comparing wireless capsule endoscopy with push enteroscopy in chronic gastrointestinal bleeding. Endoscopy 2002;34:685–9.

Geller AJ, Kolts BE, Achem SR, Wears R. The high frequency of upper intestinal pathology in patients with fecal occult blood and colon polyps. Am J Gastroenterol 1993;88:1184.

Goldstein J, Eisen G, Lewis B, et al. Abnormal small bowel findings are common in healthy subjects for a multi-center, double blind, randomized, placebo-controlled trial using capsule endoscopy [abstract 284]. DDW 2003.

Graham DY, Qureshi WA, Willingham F, et al. A controlled study of NSAID-induced small bowel injury using video capsule endoscopy [abstract 147]. DDW 2003.

Hartmann D, Schmidt H, Schilling D, et al. Proscpective controlled multicentric trial comparing wireless capsule endoscopy with intraoperative enteroscopy in patients with chronic gastrointestinal bleeding: Preliminary results [abstract M1870]. DDW 2003.

Hayat M, Axon AT, O'Mahoney S. Diagnostic yield and effect on clinical outcomes of push enteroscopy in suspected small-bowel bleeding. Endoscopy 2000;32:369–72.

Heyde EC. Gastrointestinal bleeding in aortic stenosis. N Engl J Med 1958;259:196.

Hilsman JH. The color of blood containing feces following the instillation of citrated blood at various levels of small intestine. Gastroenterol 1950;15:131–4.

Jensen, DJ. Current diagnosis and treatment of severe obscure GI hemorrhage. Gastrointest Endosc 2003;58:256–66.

Katz D, Lewis B, Katz LB. Surgical experience following capsule endoscopy [abstract M1882]. DDW 2003.

Lahoti S, Fukami N. The small bowel as a source of gastrointestinal blood loss [review]. Curr Gastroenterol Rep 1999;1:424–30.

Lewis B, Swain P. Capsule endoscopy in the evaluation of patients with suspected small intestinal bleeding: results of a pilot study. Gastrointest Endosc 2002;56:349–53.

Liangpunsakul S, Chadalawada V, Rex DK, et al. Wireless capsule endoscopy detects small bowel ulcers in patients with normal results from state of the art enteroclysis. Am J Gastroenterol 2003;98:1295–8.

Mannucci PM, Lombardi R, Bader R, et al. von Willebrand's syndrome presenting as an acquired bleeding disorder in association with a monoclonal gammopathy. Blood 1973;42:429.

Mant MH, Hirsh J, Gauldie J, et al. Acquired von Willebrand's syndrome in systemic lupus erythematosis. Blood 1968;31:806.

Mylonaki M, Fritscher-Ravens A, Swain P. Wireless capsule endoscopy: a comparison with push enteroscopy in patients with gastroscopy and colonoscopy negative gastrointestinal bleeding. Gut 2003;52:1122–6.

O'Loughlin C, Barkin JS. Wireless capsule endoscopy. Gastrointest Endosc Clin N Am.[In press]

Rockey D, Cello JP. The evaluation of the gastrointestinal tract in patients with iron deficiency anemia. N Engl J Med 1993;329:1691–5.

Van Cutsem E, Piessevaux H. Pharmacologic therapy of arteriovenous malformations. Gastrointest Clin N Am 1996;6:819–32.

Vincentelli A, Susen S, Le Tourneau T, et al. Acquired von Willebrand syndrome in aortic stenosis. N Engl J Med 2003;349:343–9.

Wolff RS, Cave D, Doherty S, et al. Surgical experience after video capsule endoscopy: the fantastic voyage to the operating room [abstract M1932]. DDW 2003.

Zuckerman GR, Prakash C, Askin MP, Lewis BS. AGA technical review on the evaluation and management of occult and obscure gastrointestinal bleeding. Gastroenterol 2000;118:201–21.

CHAPTER 60

NONSTEROIDAL ANTIINFLAMMATORY DRUG-INDUCED SMALL AND LARGE INTESTINAL INJURY

KEN TAKEUCHI, MD, SAMUEL N. ADLER, MD, AND INGVAR BJARNASON, MD, MSC, FRCPATH, FRCP DSC

"Nice to see you Mrs. Jones. I do hope that the preparation for the colonoscopy was not too taxing. As you remember, last week's endoscopy did not disclose any cause for your long standing anemia and hence your colonoscopy today."

"The colonic preparation was not as bad as the one I had 3 years ago, Doctor, when you performed these procedures on me the last time," she replied. "And it was certainly not as bad as the arthritis which has been acting up lately."

Sound familiar? Yes, chasing the cause for an iron deficiency anemia (IDA) in a rheumatic patient is common practice! At the end of the day you may be pleased because the patient did not turn out to have an underlying malignancy, but you may be slightly irritated as well because you have no apparent explanation for her iron deficiency or a treatment other than iron supplements. Well, help is at hand!

Nonsteroidal Anti-Inflammatory Drug Enteropathy

Nonsteroidal antiinflammatory drugs (NSAIDs) cause small bowel inflammation in 50 to 70% of patients on long term conventional NSAIDs. The patients with the enteropathy consequentially bleed from the small bowel (2 to 10 mL/d) and lose protein (Bjarnason et al, 1992). The bleeding is not by itself sufficiently severe to cause iron deficiency. However if there concomitant overt bleeding (heavy periods), reduced food intake, hypochlorhydria (primary or secondary to acid lowering drugs), and malabsorption of iron, then the small intestinal bleeding does become an important contributing factor to the IDA, which is very common in patients with rheumatoid arthritis. Patients with NSAID-induced enteropathy also lose protein from the inflammatory site. Similar to the blood loss, this only becomes clinically evident in a few patients, because the liver has substantial reserve capacity to produce albumin. Nevertheless about 10% of patients with rheumatoid arthritis who are sufficiently unwell as to require hospitalization have problematic hypoalbuminemia. Apart from these management problems, NSAID-induced enteropathy is associated with serious outcomes such as perforation, clinically evident bleeding, and strictures, some of which may require surgery. Although there has been some awareness of these serious outcomes for the last 20 years, it is only recently that their prevalence has been shown to be very similar to that seen in the stomach. The undue emphasis on the latter has many explanations, not least which is the difficulty of diagnosing NSAID-induced enteropathy.

Diagnosis

Faced with an arthritic patient on NSAIDs who has evidence of an IDA (or hypoalbuminemia) and a normal endoscopy and colonoscopy it is possible to make a positive diagnosis of NSAID-induced enteropathy rather than it being a diagnosis of exclusion. NSAID-induced enteropathy can now be diagnosed from analyses of a single stool sample by measurement of calprotectin (by a commercially available enzyme-linked immunosorbent assay), which is a neutrophil selective protein (Tibble et al, 1999). It is a fully validated test, correlating with the 4-day fecal excretion of ^{111}Indium white cells. Because the bleeding and protein loss correlate significantly with the severity of NSAID-induced intestinal inflammation, it can be safely assumed that those patients that have a threefold elevation or more of calprotectin have a high chance of the bleeding being contributory to their anemia.

Alternatively, it is possible to carry out an enteroscopy of the small bowel, the push enteroscopes often being unsuitable because of the distal small bowel location of the enteropathy. This technique is discussed in the preceding chapter on occult bleeding (Chapter 59, "Obscure Gastrointestinal Bleedings).

More recently it has become possible to diagnose NSAID-induced enteropathy by wireless capsule endoscopy. Here patients swallow a small camera after an overnight fast. The capsule-camera is equipped with a battery lasting 6 to 8 hours and will take approximately 50,000 pictures during its intestinal transit. These images are transmitted to an external receiver and analysed by a semiautomated computer program. NSAID-induced enteropathy has a range of appearances. First, there may be scattered petechia with or without evidence of intraluminal blood. Second, there are distinct mucosal lesions. These are probably best termed "mucosal breaks," which encompasses both erosions and ulcers. It can be difficult to distinguish between the two. Ulcers require demonstration of depth, which may not be clearly evident, unless the capsule captures the lesion at the correct angle. These mucosal breaks are often seen to bleed as the capsule irritates them mechanically. In some patients on conventional NSAIDs there is evidence of semilunar diaphragms. These appear to represent the early developmental phase of "diaphragm disease," one of the serious outcomes of NSAID-induced enteropathy, which may require surgery. Until recently NSAID-induced "diaphragm disease" was diagnosed on clinical grounds of radiology, and other conventional imaging techniques are almost invariably normal. The capsule endoscopy, with a virtual 100% detection rate, seems to be the ideal way of making a positive diagnosis of this condition. In the case that the capsule does not pass the narrowed lumen, this by itself identifies patients that are particularly likely to benefit from surgery. The preceding chapter on occult bleeding (Chapter 59) has more information on capsule endoscopy.

Treatment

The decision to treat NSAID-induced enteropathy depends on the clinical setting. The more serious the side effect the easier the decision. Hence patients with intestinal perforation require immediate surgery, those with clinically overt bleeding can usually be supported by blood transfusion over days to weeks, and those with subacute small bowel obstruction due to "diaphragm disease" can have elective surgery. If surgery is undertaken because the capsule failed to pass the diaphragm it can be milked along the small bowel tract to identify additional diaphragmatic strictures because these are almost always multiple. In the case of successful resection or stricturoplasty of the diaphragm, it is important to note that some patients have recurrent strictures if given conventional NSAIDs again. It is our practice to place all these patients on a *cyclooxygenase-2 (COX-2) selective agent* after the operation with or without a preceding course of *metronidazole* as described below.

NSAID-induced enteropathy without complications does not require treatment, because it is probably not associated with symptoms. The treatments of the more subtle complications of NSAID-induced enteropathy, namely IDA and hypoalbuminemia, require careful consideration, but are essentially similar. We have no hesitation to treat the patients with symptomatic hypoalbuminaemia (s-albumin, 20 g/L; normal 30 to 50 g/L) or those with a 3 to 4 fold elevation of fecal calprotectin with long standing or recurrent IDA. Both conditions are treated in a similar fashion. We start with *metronidazole* 400 mg (or 500 mg) twice a day for 4 to 6 weeks. The rationale for this treatment is that that the main neutrophil chemoattractant in NSAID-induced enteropathy is the commensal small bowel anaerobic bacterial flora. Metronidazole in these doses consistently decreases the inflammatory intensity and, at the same time, the bleeding and protein loss is reduced. Reversal of the low albumin levels is usually evident within 2 weeks and the effect is sustained, provided that the patients do not receive conventional NSAIDs again. In the iron deficient patient there is no immediate improvement in hemoglobin concentrations, but the efficacy of the treatment can be confirmed by repeat measure of fecal calprotectin. If placed on NSAIDs again we do *not* recommend long term metronidazole as a preventive measure because of the risk of peripheral neuropathy. Other antibiotics that have an action against anaerobes, such as the *tetracyclines* or *cipfrofloxacin*, may be effective in the long term, but this has not been studied. Rather we, in consultation with the rheumatologist in charge of the patient, may place such patients on long-term *sulphasalazine* 1 g 2 or 3 times a day. The advantage of this treatment, apart from reducing NSAID-induced intestinal inflammation and blood loss, is that it may have a disease modifying effect on the arthritis which might reduce the requirements for further NSAID treatment, although in clinical practice this is rarely the case. Side effects with sulphasalazine are predictable with 20 to 30% of patients experiencing nausea, skin rashes, and headaches; a very occasional patient may experience aplastic anemia (we have not seen a case in the last 10 years!) Failing sulphasalazine, because of side effects, it is still possible to control the enteropathy with long term coadministration of *misoprostol* with the NSAID at a dose of 200 mg 3 or 4 times a day. Again the side effects are a nuisance (ie, diarrhea) rather than serious. All of the iron deficient patients receive standard *iron supplements*.

An interesting possible treatment of the enteropathy is the use of *pro- or prebiotics*. Although not quite living up to expectations in other diseases as yet, we must emphasize that there are no reports of this treatment in patients with NSAID-enteropathy.

Since the introduction of COX-2 selective agents our practice has changed. We now as a rule (1) *stop* the conventional *NSAIDs* that the patients required, (2) treat them with *metronidazole*, as described above, and (3) place them on one of the *COX-2 selective agents* (the number of available drugs was increasing rapidly). We feel uncomfortable to make a simple switch without the metronidazole treatment because COX-2 selective agents may interfere with healing, at least in the experimental animal. The small bowel safety of COX-2 selective agents has been demonstrated in short term volunteer intestinal permeability and bleeding studies, and these drugs reduce the serious small bowel (or distal to the duodenum) outcomes by 50 to 60% as compared to conventional NSAIDs. However of note is that COX-2 selective agents *do not prevent the small bowel complications completely* and there is some intriguing data from animal studies that suggest that they may be *associated with ileocecal damage*. The ileocecal damage seen with COX-2 selective agents appears to differ from NSAID-induced enteropathy, which is mainly mid-small bowel, and it is uncertain whether it is associated with complications or if it indeed is simply a gastroenterologic curiosity.

Other Damage to the Small Bowel

Apart from causing NSAID-induced enteropathy, NSAIDs very rarely cause small bowel problems (*ie, celiac-like jejunal lesion with partial or subtotal villus atrophy*) in which case a change over to another NSAID or a COX-2 selective agent is sufficient treatment. Aggravation of preexisting disease is discussed below.

Colonic Complications of NSAIDs

Some of the side effects of NSAIDs on the large bowel are rare, such as erosions, solitary or multiple ulcers, inflammation (which may resemble classic inflammatory bowel disease [IBD]), aggravation of diverticulitis, or even appendicitis in the elderly (Bjarnason et al, 1987). Treatment is the same as for the underlying disease, with discontinuation of the particular NSAID and with COX-2 selective agents being the preferred antiinflammatory analgesic.

Relapses of IBD

One common and clinically relevant side effect of NSAIDs is to cause *relapse of classic IBD*. About 20% of patients with Crohn's disease or ulcerative colitis have a clinical relapse of their disease *within 1 week* of receiving conventional NSAIDs. This relapse is shown to be associated with escalating inflammatory activity (vastly increased fecal calprotectin). In these cases we discontinue the particular NSAID and give the patient a crash course of *prednisolone* (30 mg/d for 5 days, reducing the dose by 5 mg every 5 days). Within 4 to 5 days it is safe to give the patient the COX-2 selective agent *nimesulide* (Aulin),* because this drug is not associated with relapse of the disease (the safety of other COX-2 selective agents has not been formally tested). However, if the relapse occurs after 10 to 14 days of conventional NSAID treatment, it is most likely not due to the drug. In these cases we treat the relapse by conventional means and continue the particular NSAID. However because of the "safety" of nimesulide in patients with IBD disease we have not used conventional NSAIDs lately in these patients. Low dose aspirin for cardiovascular prophylaxis and IBD? Yes, we belief that aspirin in doses of 150 mg/d or less are perfectly safe!

Overall it is important to be aware of the side effects of conventional NSAIDs on the lower gastrointestinal (GI) tract as they are widely used, despite the availability of COX-2 selective agents. Even when patients are at serious risk of gastric bleeding, many physicians place such patients on conventional NSAIDs with a proton pump inhibitor. Whatever the rationale for this combination, remember that it does not prevent the lower GI side effects of NSAIDs.

Supplemental Reading

Bjarnason I, Zanelli G, Smith T, et al. Nonsteroidal antiinflammatory drug induced intestinal inflammation in humans. Gastroenterol 1987;93:480–9.

Bjarnason I, Zanelli G, Prouse P, et al. Blood and protein loss via small intestinal inflammation induced by nonsteroidal anti-inflammatory drugs. Lancet 1987;2:711–4.

Bjarnason I, Hayllar J, Smethurst P, et al. Metronidazole reduces inflammation and blood loss in NSAID enteropathy. Gut 1992;33:1204–8.

Bjarnason I, Hayllar J, Macpherson AJ, Russell AS. Side effects of nonsteroidal anti-inflammatory drugs on the small and large intestine. Gastroenterol 1993;104:1832–7.

Hayllar J, Price AB, Smith T, et al. Nonsteroidal antiinflammatory drug-induced small intestinal inflammation and blood loss: effect of sulphasalazine and other disease modifying drugs. Arthr Rheum 1994;37:1146–50.

Laine L, Connors LG, Reicin A, et al. Serious lower gastrointestinal clinical events with nonselective NSAID or coxib use. Gastroenterol 2003;124:288–92.

Sigthorsson G, Simpson RJ, Walley M, et al. COX-1 and 2, intestinal integrity, and pathogenesis of nonsteroidal anti-inflammatory drug enteropathy in mice. Gastroenterol 2002;122:1913–23.

Tibble J, Sigthorsson G, Foster R, et al. Faecal calprotectin: a simple method for the diagnosis of NSAID-induced enteropathy. Gut 1999;45:362–6.

---

*Editor's Note: Nimesulide (Aulin, Helsinn Healthcare, Switzerland) is not available in United State at this time.

CHAPTER 61

CELIAC SPRUE AND RELATED PROBLEMS

KAROLY HORVATH, MD, PHD, AND ALESSIO FASANO, MD

Celiac disease is characterized by the damage of the small intestinal mucosa caused by prolamins (alcohol-soluble fractions) of wheat, barley and rye in genetically susceptible subjects. It is the gliadin fraction of wheat gluten that is associated with the development of the intestinal damage. The disease is strongly associated with certain human lymphocyte antigen alleles, particularly DQA1*0501/DQB1*0201. The presence of gluten in the intestine leads to a self-perpetuating mucosal damage, whereas the elimination of gluten results in a full mucosal recovery.

The keystone treatment of celiac disease patients is a *lifelong elimination diet* in which food products containing *wheat, rye,* and *barley* are avoided. Both in vivo challenges and in vitro immunologic studies support the possibility that oat (once considered toxic for celiac disease patients) can be safely ingested. However, because of the uncontrolled harvesting and milling procedures, a cross contamination of oat with gluten is a concern.

Celiac disease has been found in approximately 0.4% of the general population worldwide. A recent study from United States reported that the overall prevalence of celiac disease in not at risk groups was 1:133 (Fasano et al, 2003).

Diagnosis

This disease often presents with vague nongastrointestinal (non-GI) symptoms. The clinical manifestations of celiac disease are protean in nature and vary markedly with the age of the patient, the duration and extent of disease, and the presence of extraintestinal pathology. In addition to the classic GI form, a variety of other clinical manifestations of the disease have been described, including atypical and asymptomatic forms. Therefore, for the *diagnosis* of celiac disease it is crucial to have a sensitive and specific algorithm that allows the identification of different manifestations of the disease. Serological tests developed in the last decade provide a noninvasive tool to screen both individuals at risk for the disease and the general population. In patients with active disease, a characteristic immunoglobulin (Ig)A antibody against endomysium is produced. The antigen recognised by IgA endomysium antibody has been identified as tissue transglutaminase (Dieterich et al, 1997). The enzyme-linked immunosorbent assay-based antihuman transglutaminase test has very high sensitivity for celiac disease. Because celiac disease treatment implies a lifelong gluten-free diet, the current gold standard for the diagnosis of celiac disease remains the histological confirmation of the intestinal evidence of disease. The need for serologic positivity is being debated.

It is known that the grains that activate celiac disease are closely related species within the grass family (Table 61-1). Significant effort has been made to understand which specific peptides of these grains are important for the development of the tissue damage in order to *engineer grains* that lack the toxic peptide sequences. However, to date, this alternative approach to the treatment of celiac disease has been *unsuccessful.*

Dietary Treatment

The lifelong abstinence of gluten ingestion remains the cornerstone treatment of the disease (Table 61-2). The diet requires an ongoing education of patients and their families by both doctors and dietitians. Regional celiac disease support groups are important sources of dietary information and provide support to new patients.

Gluten-Free versus Low Gluten

One of the major controversies of the treatment of celiac disease relates to the amount of gluten allowed in the diet of celiac disease patients. The National Food Authority has redefined the term *"gluten-free."* Previously, < 0.02% gluten was acceptable as being gluten-free, but now "gluten-free" means no gluten and < 0.02% is currently labeled as "low gluten." However, the stringency of gluten restriction (zero tolerance versus low gluten ingestion) is an issue that is far from being resolved, as the opinions differ among scientists and celiac disease support groups worldwide. These controversies are due to a lack of solid scientific evidence for a threshold of gluten consumption that does cause intestinal damage.

Editor's Note: The sensitivity and specificity of the serologic tests used for this study are the variable that influence estimates of precedence of celiac disease and the use of these tests in individual patients.

TABLE 61-1. Relationship of the Major Grains

Family	Gramineae							
Subfamily	Festucoideae					Panicoideae		
Tribe	Triticeae			Aveneae	Oryzeae	Andropogoneae		Paniceae
Common Name	Wheat	Rye	Barley	Oat	Rice	Corn	Sorghum	Millet
In Celiac Disease	Toxic					Not Toxic		

TABLE 61-2. Diet in Celiac Disease

Not Allowed		Allowed
Wheats (*Triticum* family)		Rice, wild rice
All forms including:	Einkorn wheat (*Triticum monococcum*)	Corn (maize)
- wheat flour	Emmer wheat (*Triticum dicoccon*)	Sorghum
- wheat germ	Couscous (endosperm of *Durum* wheat)	Millet
- wheat bran	Kamut (*Triticum polonicum*)	Buckwheat (kasha)
- cracked wheat, etc.	Spelt (Farro, Drinkle)	Beans, peas, and bean flours
	Semolina (*Durum* wheat)	Quinoa
Rye (*Secale cereale*)		Potato
Triticale (wheat-rye hybrid)		Soybean
Barley (*Hordeum vulgare*) and Malt		Tapioca
		Amaranth
		Teff
		Nuts
		Fruits
		Milk (Cheeses*)
		Plain meat
		Fish
		Egg
		Oat (Avena sativa)

*The coat of some cheeses may contain gluten.

Prolamins

Prolamins are found in a variety of widely used grains. Patients should be aware that products labeled "wheat free," are not necessarily gluten free. They may contain gluten as well as other grains that are not allowed. *Wheat, rye, and barley* are the predominant grains containing toxic peptides. However, *triticale* (a combination of wheat and rye), *kamut, and spelt* (sometimes called *farro*) are also toxic.

Other forms of wheat are *semolina* (durum wheat), *farina, einkorn, bulgur, couscous,* and any form that includes wheat in its name, such as *wheat germ, wheat bran, whole wheat,* and *cracked wheat, etc.*

Foods made from *rye* and *barley* are also toxic. *Malt* is toxic because it is a partial hydrolysate of barley prolamins. It may contain 100 to 200 mg of barley prolamins per 100 g of malt (Ellis et al, 1994). In general, an ingredient with *malt* in its name (eg, *barley malt, malt syrup, malt extract, and malt flavorings*) is made from *barley.*

Safe Foods

Plain meat, fish, beans, legumes, eggs, and nuts are allowed in the gluten-free diet. Other safe foods include plain vegetables, fruits, and plain peanut butter. Although dairy products and cheeses are allowed, patients should be aware that the coat of certain cheeses may contain gluten. Also acquired live lactase levels are common in active celiac disease leading to lactose intolerance.

Rice can be ingested in all its varieties including white rice, brown rice, rice bran, rice polish, sweet rice, and wild rice. Rice is the basis of many safe cereals and pastas. Different rice flours are often used in gluten-free baking and are usually combined with other gluten-free flours or baking ingredients. Also, acquired live lactase levels are common in active celiac disease leading to lactose intolerance.

Ingestion of *corn* in all of its varieties *is safe*, including corn flour, cornstarch, and corn meal. Corn is the basis of many cereals, pastas, and some tortillas. Hominy, masa, and grits are also forms of corn. *Sorghum*, a grain closely related to corn, can be used as a cereal. This grain is also available milled into flour for use in baked goods (Ellis et al, 1994). *Millet*, which is also closely related to corn, is used for cereals and other foods and the flour is used in baked goods.

Potato, in any form can be part of the celiac diet.

Buckwheat seed is used in breakfast cereals and milled into *grits* (de Francisschi et al, 1994). When roasted, the buckwheat seed is called *kasha*. Pure buckwheat flour has a very strong taste; therefore, it is only used in small quantities. Although buckwheat itself is gluten-free, *the buckwheat/wheat flour mixtures do contain gluten*. Quinoa can be used in the diet of celiac patients as a cereal, pasta, or flour.

Amaranth is a gluten-free grain-like plant used in cereals, pastas, baked goods, and other foods. *Teff* is milled into flour and used for different baked goods.

Soybean is used to make soy flour. It is a strong tasting, high protein flour best used in combination with other flours.

Several other gluten-free ingredients are used in baking, such as *tapioca, tapioca flour, tapioca starch, potato flour, potato starch*, and *arrowroot*.

Flours (and some pastas) made from *beans* are used in the American kitchen. Currently on the market are *garbanzo bean flour (chickpea flour)* alone or mixed with *fava bean flour (garfava flour)*, or *Romano bean flour*. Lentil pastas and flours are available and a few nut flours are being used for baking. Unless these flours are mixed with gluten-containing flour, they are gluten-free.

Gluten in Medications

Medications and vitamin and mineral supplements may also contain gluten as an inactive ingredient. The manufacturers can change the inactive ingredients of these products without warning, because there are no regulations on the formulation of inactive drug components. *Vegetable gum* and *modified food starch* can contain gluten. All medications should be checked for nebulous ingredients, especially if they are to be taken for a long period of time. It is imperative to know the lot number of nonprescription medications when contacting the manufacturer for clarification of the inactive ingredients. Prescription medications purchased through a pharmacy come with an ingredient list on the package insert. Different batches of medications may, however, contain different ingredients.

Information Sources

The limited expertise of health care professionals regarding celiac diet, as well as the absence of federal regulations for accurate food and drug labeling, represent significant challenges for newly diagnosed patients. Despite the efforts of celiac disease support groups there are still no laws regulating gluten-free labeling in the United States. The American Dietetic Association's National Center for Nutrition and Dietetics Consumer Nutrition Hotline at 1-800-366-1655 is a valuable source of updated information on the treatment of celiac disease. One of the functions of the Consumer Nutrition Hotline is to refer consumers and health care professionals to registered dietitians who have expertise in special diseases. The Consumer Nutrition Hotline can also provide phone numbers and addresses of companies within the food industry to help to clarify the ingredients of a given food product and how it has been processed.

Problems in the Practical Dietary Management

Possible gluten contamination of products that are presumed to be gluten free is a recurrent problem. This cross contamination can occur on farms where the grains are grown and harvested, on mills where grains are processed into flours, or on food processing lines where one line produces a food that includes gluten and the line next to it produces a gluten-free product. Contamination might also occur in stores where grains are available from open bins, in restaurants, at salad bars, or any place where a variety of different meals are produced or different ingredients come together.

Pharmalogic Treatments

Nonresponders

A minority of adult patients with celiac disease fail to respond to treatment with a gluten-free diet (Table 61-3). The most likely cause of nonresponsiveness is *continued gluten ingestion*, which can be voluntary or inadvertent. Other causes of nonresponsiveness are other *food intolerance* diseases (*eg, milk, soy*), *pancreatic insufficiency, enteropathy-associated T-cell lymphoma, refractory sprue, and ulcerative jejunitis*.

TABLE 61-3. Drug Therapies in Celiac Disease

	Medication	Dose
Lactose malabsorption	Lactase enzyme	1 to 3 tablets with dairy-containing meals
Anemia	Ferrous sulfate	3 to 5 mg (Fe^{2+})/kg/d
Pancreatic hypofunction	Pancreatic enzyme supplements	Age dependent
Lymphocytic, collagenous colitis	Antiinflammatory drugs (Pentasa, Dipentum, etc.)	30 to 70 mg/kg/d
	Prednisone (Budesonide)	2 mg/kg (maximum 60 mg/d) for 2 to 3 weeks and gradual tapering after (9 mg qid for 6 weeks, then 6 mg qid)
Refractory sprue	Prednisone (Beclemathasone)	2 mg/kg (maximum 60 mg/d) for 2 to 3 weeks and gradual tapering after equivalent dose or less
Osteoporosis	Calcium supplement Vitamin D	

qid = four times a day.

Anemia

In both children and adults, iron-deficient anemia represents the most frequent extraintestinal symptom of subclinical celiac disease. Malabsorption of iron in the duodendum, as well as occult blood loss, can contribute to iron deficiency. The majority (51 to 84%) of children have iron deficiency at the time of diagnosis. The prevalence of celiac disease in adult patients with sideropenic anemia is 5 to 6%, whereas in the group not responding to iron therapy it can reach 20%. Iron replacement therapy, in addition to diet, should be considered in most patients with celiac disease.

Lactose Malabsorption

The most frequent disaccharidase deficiency associated with untreated celiac disease is a low or missing intestinal lactase activity. It can be treated with lactase enzyme supplements or lactose-free milk. This deficit typically resolves within 2 to 3 months on a gluten-free diet, unless the patients have permanent adult-type hypolactasia. The necessity of a long term lactose-free diet should be assessed individually.

Roggero and colleagues (1989) used the breath hydrogen test to estimate the lactose absorption capacity of 42 infants and children who had flat small intestinal mucosa. All patients had positive tests when using the standard challenge dose of 2 g/kg body weight. However, most of the subjects tolerated the 0.5 to 1.5 g/kg doses. If a patient on gluten-free diet still experiences gaseousness, the possibility of lactose malabsorption should be considered.

Lymphocytic and Collagenous Colitis

Lymphocytic gastritis (LG) is associated with celiac disease and has been reported in as many as 33% of adult patients with celiac disease. Lymphocytic colitis seems to be more common (38%) in celiac disease affected by LG (Wu and Hamilton, 19990). The treatment of the colitis involves the use of antiinflammmatory agents, including mesalamine and steroids. There is a separate chapter on collagenous and lymphocytic colitis (see Chapter 87, "Microscopic Colitis: Collagenous, Lymphocytic, and Eosinophilic Colitis").

Osteoporosis

Celiac disease patients are at high risk for developing a low bone mineral density and bone turnover impairment. Persistent villous atrophy is associated with low bone mineral density. Of 86 consecutive newly diagnosed, biopsy confirmed celiac disease patients, 40% had osteopenia and 26% osteoporosis (Mora et al, 1999). There were no differences between males and females, or fertile and postmenopausal women. Bone mineral density in adult patients responsive to diet did not differ from that in healthy controls. Children maintained on a gluten-free diet for at least 5 years had normal bone mineralization and bone turnover. Even in postmenopausal women, a gluten-free diet led to a significant improvement in bone mineral density. In these cases, supplement treatment with vitamin D and calcium is indicated.

Refractory Sprue

Celiac disease patients in whom the lack of compliance to a gluten-free diet has been ruled out belong to the refractory sprue category. These patients typically undergo pharmacologic therapies, including *steroids* or immunosuppressants such as *azathioprine* and *cyclosporin*. If patients do not respond to these managements, the ultimate treatment is total parenteral nutrition. None of these therapies have been subjected to rigorous controlled studies (Horvath and Fasano, 2001).

In young children with villus atrophy who do not respond to a gluten-free diet, diseases that must be considered include the following: (1) *tufting enteropathy, (2) pancreatic insufficiency, and (3) unrecognized chronic giardiasis.*

Transient Pancreatic Insufficiency

Twenty four to 40% of patients with untreated celiac disease have temporary pancreatic hypofunction. Carroccio and colleagues (1995) performed a double-blind, placebo-controlled study on 40 patients. Half of the patients received pancreatic enzyme supplementation, while the control group was treated with placebo. After 30 days of treatment, the increase in height Z score, weight-for-height, arm circumference, and subscapular and triceps fold measurements were greater in the study group.

Emerging Therapies

Recent advances in molecular biology and genetic engineering and a better understanding of the immune mechanisms involved in celiac disease pathogenesis, represent solid bases for future alternative approaches to the treatment of the disease. It is conceivable to project innovative treatments based on either the engineering of grains that lack the toxic domains that trigger the autoimmune process or the development of vaccines that will prevent the onset of disease in genetically predisposed individuals.

Editor's Note: Oral beclamethasone in corn oil has been useful in some patients with refractory sprue.

Supplemental Reading

Baer AN, Bayless TM, Yardley JH. Intestinal ulceration and malabsorption syndromes. Gastroenterol 1980;79:754–65.

Carroccio A, Iannitto E, Cavataio F, et al. Sideropenic anemia and celiac disease: one study, two points of view. Dig Dis Sci 1998;43:673–8.

Carroccio A, Iacono G, Montalto G, et al. Pancreatic enzyme therapy in childhood celiac disease. A double-blind prospective randomized study. Dig Dis Sci 1995;40:2555–60.

de Francischi ML, Salgado JM, da Costa CP. Immunological analysis of serum for buckwheat fed celiac patients. Plant Foods Hum Nutr 1994;46:207–11.

Dieterich W, Ehnis T, Bauer M, et al. Identification of tissue transglutaminase as the autoantigen of celiac disease. Nat Med 1997;3:797–801.

Ellis HJ, Doyle AP, Day P, et al. Demonstration of the presence of coeliac-activating gliadin-like epitopes in malted barley. Int Arch Allergy Immunol 1994;104:308–10.

Ellis HJ, Doyle AP, Wieser H, et al. Measurement of gluten using a monoclonal antibody to a sequenced peptide of alpha-gliadin from the coeliac-activating domain I. J Biochem Biophys Methods 1994;28:77–82.

Fasano A, Berti I, Gerarduzzi T, et al. Prevalence of celiac disease in at-risk and not-at-risk groups in the United States: a large multicenter study. Arch Intern Med 2003;163:286–92.

Horvath K, Fasano A. Management of refractory celiac disease. Medscape Gastroenterology 2001;3:<http://www.medscape.com/Medscape/gastro/journal/2001/v2003.n2006/mgi7609.horv/mgi7609.horv-2001.html>.

Mora S, Barera G, Beccio S, et al. Bone density and bone metabolism are normal after long-term gluten-free diet in young celiac patients. Am J Gastroenterol 1999;94:398–403.

Roggero P, Ceccatelli MP, Volpe C, et al. Extent of lactose absorption in children with active celiac disease. J Pediatr Gastroenterol Nutr 1989;9:290–4.

Wu TT, Hamilton SR. Lymphocytic gastritis: association with etiology and topology. Am J Surg Pathol 1999;23:153–8.

CHAPTER 62

Lactose Intolerance

Johanna C. Escher, MD, PhD, and Hans A. Büller, MD, PhD

Lactose intolerance is a clinical diagnosis and consists of symptoms such as abdominal pain, cramps, nausea, bloating, acidic diarrhea and flatulence after the ingestion of lactose (Suarez et al, 1995). The symptoms can begin 30 minutes to 2 hours after eating or drinking foods containing lactose, primarily dairy products. The severity of symptoms varies depending on the amount of lactose each individual can tolerate. Lactose intake varies with age. Lactose is the primary carbohydrate in milk, accounting for almost 35 to 55% of the daily caloric intake in infants. As weaning foods are introduced, lactose intake falls and gradually approaches the levels ingested by adults. The carbohydrate intake of adults on a typical western diet is approximately 300 g, with a lactose content of 5% (Chitkara et al, 2003). Intolerance to lactose-containing foods is a common problem worldwide except in northern Europe. The prevalence is high in the population from eastern Asia (90% or more), among Native Americans (80 to 95%), and Blacks or African Americans (65 to 75 %) (Huang and Bayless, 1968; Bayless and Rosensweig, 1966).

Lactose malabsorption is a diagnosis that is made in patients with typical symptoms in whom the intestinal malabsorption of lactose has been confirmed by a test (such as the lactose breath hydrogen test). To be absorbed, lactose needs to be hydrolyzed by a β-galactosidase, lactase-phlorizin-hydrolase, generally called lactase. The enzyme lactase hydrolyzes lactose to glucose and galactose. Lactase is found most abundantly in the jejunum at the tip of intestinal villi.

When lactose is not absorbed in the small intestine, it arrives in the colon, where bacterial fermentation will occur. Lactose is converted to short chain fatty acids (SCFA) and hydrogen gas by the bacterial flora, producing acetate, butyrate, and propionate. This increased osmotic load will attract water, and diarrhea may develop. The production of hydrogen serves as the basis for the lactose breath hydrogen test used to diagnose lactose malabsorption. In this test, an oral dose of lactose (2 g/kg, maximum dose 25 g) is given in the fasting state, and breath hydrogen is tested before ingestion and at 30-minute intervals for 3 hours.

Lactose intolerance is not always the result of lactose malabsorption. A significant proportion of patients with suggestive symptoms have normal breath hydrogen tests. Besides a false-negative test (in subjects who are nonhydrogen producers, or after recent use of antibiotics), symptoms may be caused by psychological factors, coexistent irritable bowel syndrome, intolerance to other components in milk, or by maldigestion of other carbohydrates (Johnson et al, 1993).

Lactase deficiency exists when the enzyme lactase is absent or (more often) present in low levels in the intestine, as shown by enzymatic assay in intestinal biopsies. Symptoms of lactose intolerance may be caused by lactose malabsorption, which is usually attributed to lactase deficiency (or insufficiency). Lactase deficiency can be primary (genetically determined) or secondary (as a result of damage to the small intestinal mucosa). A genetic determinator is now available commercially.

Primary Lactase Deficiency

Congenital lactase deficiency is an extremely rare autosomal recessive disorder, described in some families in Finland. The gene for this disorder has been located on chromosome 2, in the vicinity of the lactase gene (Jarvela et al, 1998). Affected infants have diarrhea from birth, and have been reported to have hypercalcemia and nephrocalcinosis. This disorder was fatal before the development of lactose-free infant formulas. In premature infants, when born at 28 to 32 weeks gestation, lactase activity is normally low. However, most of these children (when otherwise healthy) do not have symptoms of diarrhea from lactose intolerance, because SCFAs (from bacterial fermentation of unabsorbed lactose) will be absorbed by the colonic mucosa.

The most common form of lactose malabsorption is a genetically determined reduction of enzyme activity at adult age, associated with racial or ethnic origin. Whereas infants and children (except those with congenital lactase deficiency) have normal lactase levels, the great majority of the world's population develops low levels during midchildhood. The lactase decline starts at age 2 to 5 years. In contrast, most Caucasians, especially those of northern European background, maintain intestinal lactase into adulthood.

TABLE 62-1. Underlying Causes of Secondary Lactose Malabsorption in Children

	Diagnosis
Viral gastroenteritis (eg, rotavirus)	Stool specimen for rotavirus enzyme immunoassay
	Villous atropy on duodenal biopsy
Cow's milk protein allergy	IgE + RAST, skin test, elimination and provocation
Celiac disease	Villous atrophy and increase in intraepithelial lymphocytes on duodenal biopsy
	Serologic tests (antiendomysial antibodies, antitissue transglutaminase antibodies)
Giardiasis	Stool specimen, duodenal aspirate, or duodenal biopsy
Crohn's disease (in small bowel)	Upper GI endoscopy and biopsies
Chemotherapy	Duodenal biopsy
Radiation therapy	Duodenal biopsy
Bacterial overgrowth (no mucosal injury)	Lactose or glucose hydrogen breath test

GI = gastrointestinal; Ig = immunoglobulin; RAST = radioallergosorbent test.

Secondary Lactase Deficiency

Lactase is expressed on the tip of the intestinal microvilli, and any damage to the intestinal mucosa can therefore affect the quantity of lactase enzyme. In Table 62-1, underlying causes of secondary lactase deficiency are listed. Depending on the type of mucosal injury and its treatment, lactose intolerance is temporary but may persist for months after mucosal healing has occurred. Also, bacterial overgrowth of the small intestine may lead to increased bacterial fermentation of lactose and symptoms of lactose intolerance (but not lactase deficiency).

Management of Lactose Intolerance

Infants and Young Children

In rare cases of confirmed congenital lactase deficiency, a lactose-free formula should be given. Products based on soy milk are good alternatives to lactose-containing formulas.

In most premature infants, lactase enzyme activity is temporarily low due to the immaturity of the intestine, but a normal lactose-containing formula is well tolerated by most. In infants with symptoms of lactose intolerance, the possibility of milk protein allergy should be excluded.

In children below 5 years of age, lactose malabsorption (abnormal lactose hydrogen breath test) reflects damage to the small intestinal mucosa or bacterial overgrowth, and appropriate diagnostic tests should be performed (see Table 62-1). Besides treatment of the underlying disorder, a low lactose diet should be offered for a relatively short time (6 to 8 weeks). Complete elimination of lactose is not necessary, as some lactase activity will persist in the small intestine. A low lactose diet generally eliminates only milk and milk products. However, some patients can tolerate milk in small amounts (2 oz) throughout the day or as part of a meal. Live culture yogurt contains endogenous β-galactosidase and will often be well tolerated. After healing of the mucosa, lactose can be gradually reintroduced.

Older Children and Adults

In older children (> 5 years) and adults with lactose malabsorption, this situation may be a natural condition that is permanent and genetically determined (ie, lactase deficiency is primary and not the result of underlying injury to the intestinal mucosa). Caution should be used when the patient and their family originate from a population where *lactase persistence* is prevalent (ie, Whites from northern Europe). In these patients, a diagnosis of lactose malabsorption may need further investigation.

The treatment of lactose malabsorption in the absence of underlying disease consists of the following four general principles: (1) *reduced* dietary intake of lactose, (2) *substitution* of alternative nutrients to maintain energy and protein intake, (3) *administration* of enzyme substitute, and (4) *maintenance* of calcium intake.

Complete restriction of lactose for a limited time (1 to 2 weeks) is sometimes useful to ascertain the specificity of the diagnosis. After this period, these patients can experiment to find a level of lactose they can tolerate. In some patients, dairy products like aged cheeses (cheddar, Swiss, Parmesan or Romano), ice cream, or yogurt are more easily accepted without symptoms, especially if taken with other food. Most people can build up their level of tolerance by gradually introducing the lactose-containing foods. In general, many will be able to enjoy dairy products if they take them in small amounts or eat other kinds of food at the same time in order to delay gastric emptying. People who have a very low tolerance of lactose need to know that lactose is often added to prepared foods, even to products labeled "nondairy" (Table 62-2). People with severe lactose intolerance can be even affected by lactose used as a base for more than 20% of prescription drugs (ie, birth control pills) and about 6% of over-the-counter medicines (some tablets for stomach acid and gas) (National Digestive Diseases Information Clearinghouse, 2003).

TABLE 62-2. Hidden Lactose: Food Products That Contain Small Amounts of Lactose

Bread and other baked goods
Processed breakfast cereals
Instant potatoes, soups, and breakfast drinks
Margarine
Salad dressings
Candies and other snacks
Mixes for pancakes, biscuits, and cookies
Powdered meal-replacement supplements
"Nondairy" products, such as powdered coffee creamer, whipped toppings
Prescription (> 20% lactose base or over-the-counter medications)

Calcium

A concern for both growing children and adults with lactose intolerance is getting enough *calcium* in a diet that includes little or no milk. Patients with lactose restriction are at risk for osteoporosis, osteopenia, and fracture (Infante and Tormo, 2000). Age-dependent recommendations for required daily calcium intake is shown in Table 62-3. Many nondairy foods are high in calcium, such as green vegetables and fish with soft, edible bones (Table 62-4). In patients who need a complete restriction of lactose, calcium supplementation is often recommended. Absorption of calcium from the diet is promoted by vitamin D, which is adequately supplied in a balanced diet. Sources of vitamin D include eggs and liver; sunlight helps the body to naturally absorb or synthesize vitamin D.

For patients who react to very small amounts of lactose or have trouble limiting their lactose-containing foods, bacterial or yeast β-galactosidase enzymes are available without prescription. These enzyme preparations (eg, Lactaid) can be added to milk or cream (as liquid, 14 drops/quart), which is then refrigerated overnight. Lactose will be hydrolyzed, and the milk will taste sweeter. Enzyme tablets can be taken with lactose-containing foods.

Predigested dairy products such as Lactaid milk (completely lactose-free), or Dairy Ease milk (70% lactose reduced) are commercially available. Soy milk contains no lactose.

In conclusion, for patients with lactose intolerance, a carefully chosen and often self-guided diet is the key to reducing symptoms and protecting future health.

TABLE 62-3. Calcium Intake: Recommendations*

Age group	Daily Requirement of Calcium (mg)
0 to 6 months	210
7 to 12 months	270
1 to 3 years	500
4 to 8 years	800
9 to 18 years	1300
19 to 50 years	1000
51 years and up	1200

*Reprinted with permission from the Institute of Medicine, 1999.

TABLE 62-4. Calcium and Lactose in Common Foods

Vegetables	Calcium Content	Lactose Content
Calcium-fortified orange juice, 1 cup	308 to 344 mg	0
Sardines with edible bones, 3 oz	270 mg	0
Salmon, canned, with edible bones, 3 oz	205 mg	0
Soymilk, fortified, 1 cup	200 mg	0
Broccoli, raw, 1 cup	90 mg	0
Orange, 1 medium	50 mg	0
Pinto beans, ½ cup	40 mg	0
Tuna, canned, 3 oz	10 mg	0
Lettuce greens, ½ cup	10 mg	0
Dairy Products		
Yogurt, plain, low fat, 1 cup	415 mg	5 g
Milk, reduced fat, 1 cup	295 mg	11 g
Swiss cheese, 1 oz	270 mg	1 g
Ice cream, ½ cup	85 mg	6 g
Cottage cheese, ½ cup	75 mg	2 to 3 g

Supplemental Reading

Bayless TM, Rosensweig NS. A racial difference in incidence lactase deficiency. A survey of milk tolerance and lactase deficiency in healthy adult males. JAMA 1966;197:968–72.

Chitkara DK, Montgomery RK, Grand RJ, Büller HA. Lactose intolerance. 2003. Available at: <http://www.utdol.com/application/topic.asp?file=gi_dis/13325&type=A&selectedTitle=1~15> (accessed August 29, 2003).

Huang SS, Bayless TM. Lactose intolerance in healthy orientals. Science 1968;160:8383.

Infante D, Tormo R. Risk of inadequate bone mineralization in diseases involving long-term suppression of dairy products. J Pediatr Gastroenterol Nutr 2000;30:310–3.

Institute of Medicine. Dietary reference intakes for calcium, phosphorus, magnesium, vitamin D, and fluoride. Washington: National Academy Press; 1999. p. 380.

Jarvela I, Sabri Enattah N, Kokkonen J, et al. Assignment of the locus for congenital lactase deficiency to 2q21, in the vicinity of but separate from the lactase-phlorizin hydrolase gene. Am J Hum Genet 1998;63:1078–85.

Johnson AO, Semenya JG, Buchowski MS, et al. Correlation of lactose maldigestion, lactose intolerance, and milk intolerance. Am J Clin Nutr 1993;57:399–401.

National Digestive Diseases Information Clearinghouse. Lactose intolerance. Available at: <http://digestive.niddk.nih.gov/ddiseases/pubs/lactoseintolerance/index.htm> (accessed August 26, 2003).

Suarez FL, Savaiano DA, Levitt MD. A comparison of symptoms after the consumption of milk or lactose-hydrolyzed milk by people with self-reported severe lactose intolerance. N Engl J Med 1995;333:1–4.

CHAPTER 63

CHRONIC INTESTINAL PSEUDO-OBSTRUCTION

JUSTIN ROSEMORE, DO, AND BRIAN E. LACY, PHD, MD

Chronic intestinal pseudo-obstruction (CIP) is a disorder of the gastrointestinal (GI) tract characterized by symptoms and signs (present for at least 6 months) that suggest mechanical obstruction of the intestinal tract. Although the clinical findings of CIP are usually indistinguishable from mechanical obstruction, the etiology, pathology, and treatment are quite different. The heterogeneous nature of this condition, reflected by the multiple and diverse etiologies described below, has precluded the adoption of a consensus statement on the classification and treatment of this disorder. To date, most research has focused on identifying and characterizing the underlying etiologies of CIP. The myriad of causes, including collagen vascular diseases, paraneoplastic syndromes, and primary motor and neurologic disorders, have, in general, forced clinicians to focus therapy on symptom relief, rather than treatment of the underlying disorder. We will focus on the following five aspects of CIP: (1) understanding the impact of CIP, (2) the causes and mechanisms of CIP, (3) clinical presentation (4) making the diagnosis, and (5) treatment.

The Impact of CIP

CIP was first identified by Dudley and colleagues in 1958 after a number of patients who presented with obstructive symptoms were found to have normal findings on laparotomies. The exact prevalence and incidence of CIP remains unknown, although Di Lorenzo (1999) estimates that approximately 100 infants are born each year in the United States with congenital pseudo-obstruction. This number is a gross underestimate of the total number of new cases each year, and it does not include the large number of adult patients who develop pseudo-obstruction later in life. The cost to society, including days missed from work or school, physician visits, diagnostic testing, hospital admissions and unnecessary procedures, remains to be defined.

Quality of Life

Schwankovsky and colleagues (2002) published quality of life measurements after a retrospective review of medical records of 58 patients with congenital CIP. A large number of CIP patients required central venous catheter or percutaneous gastrostomy tube placement to provide alternative routes of nutrition (parenteral or tube feeding). Furthermore, children with CIP, compared to healthy children, had lower levels of self-care and mobility, more difficulty attending school and participating in social activities, and less freedom from pain, anxiety, and depression. Parents of children with CIP had an emotional status rated as "poor" when compared with parents of healthy children. The quality of life for adults with intestinal pseudo-obstruction has not been well studied. In the one published report to date, Mann and colleagues (1997) described CIP patients as being dependent upon supplemental intravenous (IV) or enteral nutrition, requiring routine antibiotics to treat bacterial overgrowth, using multiple prokinetic agents (often without success), and often becoming dependent on narcotics due to chronic abdominal pain.

Identifying the Cause and Mechanism of Disease

Intestinal pseudo-obstruction can be divided into acute and chronic categories. CIP is generally categorized as primary (neuropathic or myopathic), secondary (collagen vascular disease, endocrine, neoplastic, neurologic, etc), or idiopathic in nature (Table 63-1). The unifying characteristic of CIP is that of disordered GI motility. In *primary* CIP this may stem from an intrinsic defect in the normal mechanisms that control GI tract motility, for example, either a muscle (*myopathy*) or nerve (*neuropathy*) injury process. To simplify an already complex classification system, we can separate the primary myopathic and primary neuropathic categories into *congenital, familial,* or *sporadic*. These subcategories may then be further divided to represent areas of intestinal involvement and potential causes. Thus, any primary CIP patient with an identifiable family history of pseudo-obstruction would be considered to have primary myopathic or neuropathic familial intestinal pseudo-obstruction, and, similarly, those patients without an identifiable family history of pseudo-obstruction would be classified as having sporadic CIP, whether it is primary or secondary in nature.

TABLE 63-1. Classification System for Intestinal Pseudo-Obstruction

ACUTE		
Ileus, Paralytic ileus, Acute colonic distension (Ogilvie's syndrome)		

CHRONIC (CIP)		
Primary	Secondary	Idiopathic
Myopathic	Collagen vascular diseases	
Congenital	Primary systemic sclerosis	
Familial	Systemic lupus erythematosus	
Sporadic	Dermatomyositis/Polymyositis	
	Periartereritis nodosa	
	Mixed connective tissue disorders	
	Rheumatoid arthritis	
	Endocrine Disorders	
	Hypothyroidism/parathyroid	
	Diabetes mellitus	
Neuropathic		
Congenital	Neurologic disorders	
Familial	Parkinson's disease	
Sporadic	Hirschsprung's disease	
	Chaga's disease	
	Intestinal hypoganglionosis	
	Viruses	
	Drug Associated	
	Opiates	
	Tricyclic antidepressants	
	Anticholinergic agents	
	Ganglionic blockers	
	Antiparkinsonian drugs	
	Phenothiazines	
	Clonidine	
	Miscellaneous*	

CIP = chronic intestinal pseudo-obstruction.
*Miscellaneous processes may include the following: celiac disease, infiltrative diseases (amyloid, lymphoma), neoplastic, familial dysautonomia, metabolic (low potassium, magnesium, phosphorous), jejunoileal bypass, short bowel syndrome, mesenteric vascular insufficiency, alcoholism, viral infections, radiation, and after organ transplant.

Familial Visceral Myopathy

Familial visceral myopathy or hollow visceral myopathy are believed to be the most common causes of primary disease (Faulk et al, 1978). Clinically affected family members may be asymptomatic or suffer from abdominal pain, dysphagia, abdominal distension, constipation, early satiety, nausea, and vomiting. Radiographic demonstration of intestinal distension via plain films or barium studies further supports the diagnosis. Involvement of the bladder and ureter commonly occurs. Gross and microscopic features, as described by Mitros and colleagues (1982), include dilatation of various segments of the intestinal tract, most commonly the duodenum (leading to megaduodenum) and microscopic changes, including fibrosis and muscle cell degeneration.

More commonly, secondary causes for CIP can be identified, such as collagen vascular disorders, endocrine disorders, neurologic disorders, or iatrogenic causes, including a variety of medications (see Table 63-1). Primary systemic sclerosis may precede the diagnosis of CIP by several years. Other common secondary causes of intestinal pseudo-obstruction include amyloidosis and small cell carcinoma of the lung. Viruses have also been implicated as a possible causative factor in CIP (Debinski et al, 1997).

Clinical Presentation

A cross-sectional analysis by Mann and colleagues (1997) demonstrated that the median age of symptom onset was 17 years with a range of 2 weeks to 59 years (11 males, 9 females). The frequency and severity of symptoms may vary remarkably depending upon the section and the extent of the GI tract involved. The most common symptoms included pain (80%), vomiting (75%), constipation (40%), and diarrhea (20%) (Stanghellini et al, 1987). When the esophagus is involved, decreased esophageal motility and lower esophageal sphincter (LES) tone may lead to complaints of dysphagia and reflux symptoms. The complete absence of bowel movements or flatus indicates complete obstruction as opposed to the more common finding of constipation. However, diarrhea may also occur in patients with CIP and is likely secondary to intestinal stasis promoting bacterial overgrowth. Some suffer from malabsorption and develop nutritional deficiencies secondary to bacterial overgrowth. Loss of appetite and weight loss can be seen as well as nausea and vomiting. Patients may complain of early satiety and epigastric fullness if the stomach is involved. Bloating and abdominal distention are frequently seen and patients may complain about "looking pregnant" or having to loosen their clothes in order to allow them to fit properly. Patients with CIP typically have complaints of abdominal pain. For some patients, the pain is episodic in nature and occurs only during an acute episode or crisis. For other patients, however, the pain is more chronic in nature. The pain can be located anywhere in the abdomen, depending on the location and the extent of the segment of bowel that is involved. Many patients characterize the pain as sharp, stabbing, or twisting, whereas others describe it as more of a pressure, ache, or discomfort. Pain typically worsens as bloating and abdominal distension progress and improves as the crisis resolves.

Extraintestinal manifestations may also be present in patients with CIP. The most common extraintestinal manifestation, as demonstrated in the Stanghellini and colleagues cross-sectional analysis, was genitourinary involvement. Genitourinary involvement may present as dilatation of the ureter, pelvis or calyces, or abnormal bladder function, and commonly leads to complaints of difficulty voiding (Sullivan et al, 1977).

Making the Diagnosis

To help distinguish the patient with CIP from the patient with mechanical obstruction, it is important to review the history (previous surgeries, the presence of adhesions, diverticula, and intestinal cancer in the family), and perform a thorough examination. Warning signs, which include weight loss, hematemesis, hematochezia, melena, obstipation, or rebound tenderness, warrant a more urgent workup and possible early surgical intervention.

Hypoactive bowel sounds may be seen in intestinal pseudo-obstruction as opposed to the high-pitched bowel sounds in mechanical obstruction. Abdominal distension and "tympany" on percussion may be seen in both disorders. Peristaltic waves are more common in mechanical obstruction.

Initially, patients should be evaluated for organic disease with laboratory tests including serum electrolytes, complete blood count, albumin, thyroid-stimulating hormone, celiac antibodies/antigens, and specialized tests to eliminate systemic diseases, including autoimmune processes, neoplastic, and endocrine disorders (Figure 63-1).

Plain Abdominal Radiograph

The initial obligatory study is a plain radiograph of the abdomen (supine, upright, and chest) to look for intestinal distension, free air, volvulus, air-fluid levels, or transition points which could identify a possible site of obstruction. CIP cannot be diagnosed if an ileus, air-fluid levels, or distended loops of bowel are not identified. In one study all 20 patients had radiological dilatation of the small intestine, usually involving the duodenal loop (Mann et al, 1997).

Imaging Studies

Computed tomography may identify bowel wall thickening, pneumoperitoneum, or pneumatosis intestinalis, which are all potential complications of intestinal pseudo-obstruction. Barium studies (enteroclysis or upper GI with small bowel follow-through) to examine the upper GI tract, followed by barium enema, is often required to rule out mechanical obstruction and provide evidence of intestinal dilatation secondary to pseudo-obstruction. Consideration must always be given to the risk of barium impaction should complete obstruction be present. Alternatives may include water-soluble contrast or small amounts of barium with air contrast. Barium studies may also demonstrate a *lack of peristalsis* (myopathic processes) or *chaotic peristalsis* (neuropathic processes). An upper GI series may demonstrate isolated megaduodenum or wide-mouthed intestinal diverticula, commonly seen with myopathic processes such as scleroderma. Loss of haustral markings, a dilated colon, or a markedly dilated and redundant colon (megacolon) may be present. Endoscopic evaluation (upper endoscopy, colonoscopy, and capsule endoscopy) for masses, strictures, or physical obstruction (or lack thereof) may aid in establishing the diagnosis of CIP.

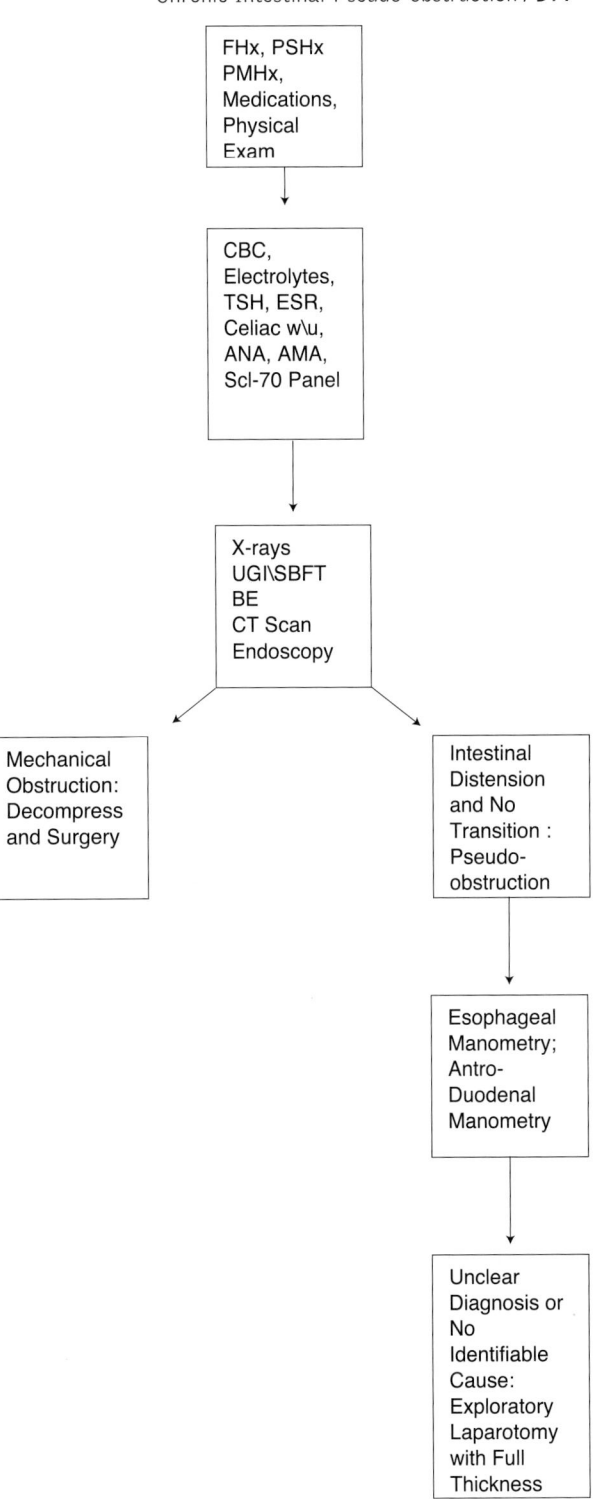

FIGURE 63-1. Algorithm: diagnosis of chronic intestinal pseudo-obstruction. CBC = complete blood cell, CT = computed tomography, UGI = upper gastrointestinal series.

Manometry

Further support for the diagnosis of CIP, and clues to the possible underlying etiology, can often be obtained from intestinal manometry. *Esophageal* manometry will reveal abnormalities in esophageal motility in approximately 80% of patients with pseudo-obstruction. Sullivan and colleagues demonstrated incomplete LES relaxation after a swallow, as well as absence of peristalsis after both a swallow and balloon distension of the upper esophagus. Studies with *antroduodenal* manometry may also reveal characteristic motility abnormalities. This may include one or more of the following:

1. Aberrant propagation and/or configuration of interdigestive migrating motor complexes
2. Bursts of nonpropagated phasic pressure activity in the fasting and fed states
3. Sustained (> 30 min) and intense phasic pressure activity occurring in a segment of intestine while normal or reduced activity is noted simultaneously at other levels of the intestine
4. Inability of the ingested meal to change fasting intestinal activity into a fed pattern (Stanghellini et al, 1987).

Laparotomy and Wall Biopsies

If after these tests are performed suspicion remains high for a mechanical obstruction, then exploratory laparotomy should be performed with full thickness biopsies of the intestinal wall. These biopsies will show smooth muscle atrophy in the primary myopathic processes, neuropathic degeneration in the primary neuropathic disorders, and various findings for the secondary causes of CIP, including fibrosis in primary systemic sclerosis or evidence of amyloid or lymphoma.*

Treatment Options

CIP remains a challenge to treat. Therapy for secondary causes of CIP should focus on the underlying disorder. This often includes correcting electrolytes, managing dehydration, treating infections, using immunosuppressants for patients with collagen vascular diseases, initiating a gluten-free diet for pseudo-obstruction associated with celiac disease, or treating the underlying cancer that has caused a paraneoplastic syndrome. *Treating idiopathic or primary CIP, however, is often quite difficult.* One important lesson to remember is the adage of *primum no nocere*. Ill-planned or repeated surgeries, radical treatments, and injudicious use of narcotics will make the patient worse. Although several large, double blind, placebo controlled studies were performed to evaluate the efficacy of medications for the treatment of CIP in the past, these agents are either no longer available (cisapride) or they lack US Food and Drug Administration approval (domperidone). Large, recent, randomized controlled trials are otherwise lacking, and the results of therapy are found only in small studies or individual case reports.

Diet

In general, treatment should attempt to correct nutritional deficiencies using either enteral or parenteral routes. As always, enteral nutrition is preferred. To maximize enteral intake patients should be encouraged to take in small, frequent meals (5 to 6 per day), with an emphasis on liquids and soft foods, while *avoiding fats and fiber*. Foods high in fat content (> 30% total calories) delay gastric emptying and cause postprandial fullness, whereas high fiber and high residue products are associated with abdominal bloating, bezoar formation, and abdominal discomfort. *Lactose* should also be avoided because of the high incidence of lactose intolerance in the general population and the potential for worsening abdominal bloating and discomfort. Numerous *nutritional supplements* are currently available and are especially useful in malnourished patients. These supplements are all high in calories and low in residue; the fat concentration varies between each supplement. A daily multivitamin should be taken, and patients should receive supplemental essential vitamins, minerals, and electrolytes as needed. *Bacterial overgrowth* and chronic diarrhea may lead to *malabsorption* of fat-soluble vitamins (A,

TABLE 63-2. Therapy for Chronic Intestinal Pseudo-Obstruction

Diet	Low residue, low fiber, low fat, low osmolality
Nutrition	Ensure adequate calories (25 kcal/kg/d)
Must have appropriate access	Ensure adequate vitamins, minerals, and electrolytes PEG, J-G tube, jejunostomy tube, central access
	Start supplemental feeding, tube feeding, or parenteral feeding based on adequacy of oral intake
Decompression	Nasogastric or nasoenteric decompression, rectal tube endoscopic decompression, "venting" enterostomy, cecostomy tube placement
Prokinetics	Erythromycin Cisapride (investigational use) Metoclopramide Domperidone (not FDA-approved) Tegaserod Octreotide
Antibiotics	Amoxicillin–Clauvanate Fluoroquinolones Cephalosporins and metronidazole Tetracycline Maintenance therapy for recurrent bacterial overgrowth Rifaximin
Surgery	Intestinal resection, intestinal transplant

FDA = US Food and Drug Administration; PEG = percutaneous gastrostomy.

---

*Editor's Note: Prolonged ileus after laparotomy can occur in these patients. Laparoscopically assisted surgery might be useful.

D, E, and K) and to B_{12} deficiency. If these dietary changes are not successful, then alternatives include *elemental feedings* with *Peptamen* and the use of supplements with *medium-chain triglycerides*. Referral to a registered dietitian can be very helpful for many patients for nutritional education and the development of a patient specific diet.

Tube Feedings and Total Parenteral Nurition

If nutritional requirements are not met by oral intake and patients continue to lose weight, enteral access with tube feedings is the next step. A retrospective study by Scolapio and colleagues (1999) demonstrated that patients with CIP can generally be successfully managed with tube feeds using a standard nonelemental formula. A trial of nasogastric or nasoenteric tube feedings should be tried before placement of percutaneous feeding tubes. If patients are able to tolerate tube feeds with low residuals, few symptoms, and regular bowel movements, then consideration should be given for placement of a percutaneous gastrostomy, G-J tube, or direct placement of a jejunostomy tube. If delayed gastric emptying is present, then direct feeding of the small intestine is preferred. Multiple methods have been described for placement of enteral access, including endoscopy, radiology, or surgery. Continuous feeding or cyclical feeding (12 hours of continuous feeding during the night) is usually better tolerated than bolus feedings (see Chapter 54 "Enteral and Parenteral Nutrition").

Ideally, parenteral nutrition should be avoided due to the risks of cellulitis, sepsis, thrombogenesis, and catheter displacement. However, a large proportion of CIP patients will eventually require parenteral nourishment at some point. Patients should receive approximately 25 kcal/kg/d and lipids should supply approximately 30% of total parenteral calories with 1.0 to 1.5 g/kg/d protein and dextrose providing the remainder of required calories (Scolapio et al, 1999).

Decompression Measures

Ideally, the best therapy for CIP would be to treat the underlying process. Unfortunately, however, for the vast majority of patients palliation of symptoms is all that can be offered at present. One such measure includes decompression of distended intestinal segments via intermittent nasogastric suction, rectal tubes, or endoscopy. A lack of clinical studies addressing this issue means there are no firm guidelines on when such intervention should be undertaken. However, most practitioners use endoscopic decompression in acute colonic distension (Ogilvie's syndrome) when there is a rapid increase in luminal distension, or when the cecum or transverse colon diameter approximates 10 cm or more. To prevent recurrence after endoscopic decompression a fluroscopically guided cecostomy tube may be placed by radiology to allow venting as needed. Other more invasive measures to provide adequate decompression of the distended intestinal segment may include a "venting" enterostomy. These are typically placed in the stomach, although some patients with feeding J-tubes also use them for venting purposes. As described by Pitt and colleagues (1985), patients with surgically placed gastrostomy tubes had a lower rate of hospital admissions (0.2 admissions per patient-year) after the procedure than before the procedure (1.2 admissions per patient-year).

Prokinetic Agents

Whether the underlying process is myopathic or neuropathic in nature, all patients with CIP have disordered GI tract motility. Multiple prokinetic agents have been used in an attempt to promote normal intestinal motility, however there are few investigational studies available to demonstrate the efficacy of any of these agents in CIP. *Erythromycin*, a macrolide antibiotic that acts as an agonist to the motilin receptor, can be given either orally or IV. Doses in the range of 50 to 200 mg orally, or 50 to 100 mg IV, approximately 30 minutes before meals, have been shown by Minami and colleagues (1996) to be effective in accelerating gastric emptying and improving the symptoms of CIP. *Cisapride*, a mixed 5-HT_4 receptor agonist/5-HT_3 receptor antagonist, is no longer routinely available for noninvestigational uses. Cisapride was found to improve symptoms of nocturnal acid reflux, and to increase gastric emptying and improve orocecal transit times. Cisapride was generally taken orally as a 10 to 20 mg dose 4 times daily. It was removed from the market in July 2000 because of drug interactions leading to prolonged QTc intervals and increased risk of ventricular tachycardia. It was available for compassionate use in selected patients. *Metoclopramide* (Reglan), a commonly used antiemetic, is a dopamine antagonist that exerts its prokinetic effects by increasing acetylcholine release. Metoclopramide is commonly given as 10 to 20 mg orally or IV 30 minutes before meals and at bedtime. Mild adverse reactions include fatigue, somnolence, anxiety, jitteriness, or depression. More severe adverse events include extrapyramidal side effects (ie, tardive dyskinesia) secondary to antidopaminergic activity. *Domperidone* is similar to metoclopramide in that it acts as an antagonist at dopamine receptors. Domperidone does *not* cross the blood-brain barrier and, therefore, does not have the potential for extrapyramidal side effects that metoclopramide does. Doses range between 10 to 20 mg orally 30 minutes before meals and at bedtime. Domperidone is

---

†Editor's Note: Some patients with intestinal failure secondary to CIP have gone on to small bowel transplantation, as discussed in Chapter 65, "Intestinal and Multivisceral Transplantation".

not FDA-approved for use in the United States. Bethanechol should be avoided as it is a poor prokinetic agent, and, in our experience, the side effects outweigh the small benefits seen only in a select group of patients. *Octreotide*, a long acting somatostatin analogue, stimulates small intestine motility when given in low doses. It is most effective in patients who have a *neuropathic* process as the underlying etiology of their CIP, because it requires the presence of smooth muscle to be effective. It is usually given in doses of 25 to 50 µg subcutaneously after both the morning and evening meals. *Tegaserod* (Zelnorm), a specific 5-HT$_4$ receptor agonist, improves gastric emptying, colonic transit, and orocecal transit time (Lacy and Yu, 2002). Although now approved for use only in women with irritable bowel syndrome and constipation (6 mg by mouth twice daily), tegaserod may improve symptoms of pseudo-obstruction by promoting small and large intestinal motility. It is important to note the major side effect of tegaserod is diarrhea and, thus, it should not be used in patients with CIP with a primary complaint of diarrhea, nor should it be used in patients with true mechanical obstruction. Tegaserod is discussed in Chapter 75, "Constipation" and in Chapter 31, "Gastroparesis."

Antibiotics

Intestinal stasis is a characteristic of intestinal pseudo-obstruction. This process may lead to bacterial overgrowth and diarrhea, with resultant malabsorption, weight loss, and the development of multiple vitamin deficiencies. Rotating antibiotics may relieve symptoms of diarrhea and bloating and improve the nutritional status in many patients with CIP. The treatment of bacterial overgrowth is discussed in Chapter 71, "Diabetic Diarrhea."

Antiemetics

Patients with CIP may suffer from recurrent bouts of nausea and vomiting during an episode of pseudo-obstruction, or they may have nausea on a near daily basis. There is no single agent particularly suited for the treatment of nausea and vomiting in CIP. Rather, each patient needs to be assessed individually to determine current medication use, previous trials of antiemetics, adverse reactions, and financial status. This area is dealt with in Chapter 31, "Gastroparesis."

Small Bowel Transplantation

This topic is discussed in Chapter 65, "Intestinal and Multivisceral Transplantation." In some series, CIP and failure of long term total parenteral nutrition has been one indication for transplantation.

Supplemental Reading

Debinski HS, Kamm MA, Talbot IC, et al. DNA viruses in the pathogenesis of sporadic chronic idiopathic intestinal pseudo-obstruction. Gut 1997;41:100–6.

Di Lorenzo C. Pseudo-obstruction: current approaches. Gastroenterology 1999;116:980–7.

Dudley HAF, Sinclair ISR, McLaren IF, et al. Intestinal pseudo-obstruction. J R Coll Surg Edin 1958;3:206–17.

Faulk DL, Anuras S, Christensen J. Clinical trends and topics: chronic intestinal pseudo-obstruction. Gastroenterology 1978;74:922–31.

Krishnamurthy S, Schuffler MD. Pathology of neuromuscular disorders of the small intestine and colon. Gastroenterology 1987;93:610–39.

Lacy BE, Yu S. Tegaserod: a new 5-HT4 agonist. J Clin Gastroenterol 2002;34:27–33.

Mann SD, Debinski HS, Kamm MA. Clinical characteristics of chronic idiopathic intestinal pseudo-obstruction in adults. Gut 1997;41:675–81.

Minami T, Nishibayashi H, Shinomura Y, Matsuzawa Y. Effects of erythromycin in chronic idiopathic intestinal pseudo-obstruction. J Gastroenterol 1996;31:855–9.

Mitros FA, Schuffler MD, Teja K, Anuras S. Pathologic features of familial visceral myopathy. Hum Path 1982;13:825–33.

Pitt HA, Mann LL, Berquist WE, et al. Chronic intestinal pseudo-obstruction: management with total parenteral nutrition and a venting enterostomy. Arch Surg 1985;120:614–8.

Schwankovsky L, Mousa H, Rowhani A, et al. Quality of life outcomes in congenital chronic intestinal pseudo-obstruction. Dig Dis Sci 2002;47:1965–8.

Scolapio JS, Camilleri M, Romano M. Audit of the treatment of malnutrition due to chronic intestinal pseudo-obstruction with enteral nutrition. Nutr Clin Prac 1999;14:29–32.

Scolapio JS, Ukleja A, Bouras EP, Romano M. Nutritional management of chronic intestinal pseudo-obstruction. J Clin Gastroenterol 1999;28:306–12.

Stanghellini V, Camilleri M, Malagelada JR. Chronic idiopathic intestinal pseudo-obstruction: clinical and intestinal manometric findings. Gut 1987;28:5–12.

Sullivan MA, Snape WJ, Matarazzo SA, et al. Gastrointestinal myoelectrical activity in idiopathic intestinal pseudo-obstruction. N Engl J Med 1977;297:233–8.

CHAPTER 64

SHORT BOWEL SYNDROME

ALAN L. BUCHMAN, MD, MSPH

The absorptive capacity of the small intestine has significant reserve capacity, and small resections are of little or no clinical consequence. However, patients that have congenital bowel atresias, or who undergo single or multiple resections that leave < 200 cm of residual and viable small intestine may develop what is known as *"short bowel syndrome."* The definition of short bowel syndrome may vary, but generally implies either malabsorption or the necessity for specific nutrient therapies. Depending upon the length and health of the remaining intestine, as well as the presence of absence of the ileocecal valve and/or colon, such patients may require various oral supplements, intravenous (IV) fluids or even total parenteral nutrition (TPN).

ADAPTATION

Bowel length may be difficult to determine because most commonly used methods, such as barium contrast studies and intraoperative measurement, are imprecise. In addition, there is significant individual variation in the adaptive response to differing lengths of residual intestine. Younger individuals, especially neonates, have a much greater capacity to adapt than adults. The adaptation phase following enterectomy may last up to 2 years in adults, during which the intestine hypertrophies by growing in diameter due to an increase in the number of villi, villus size, and crypt depth. This serves to increase the intestinal surface area and leads to enhanced nutrient absorption. In addition, colonic hypertrophy occurs, which leads to increased colonic fluid and electrolyte absorption. Several factors are important for ensuring optimal adaptation. These may be hormone-mediated responses possibly mediated by enteroglucagon, glucagon-like peptide II, secretin, cholecystokinin, and various growth factors.

ABSORPTIVE CAPACITY

Generally, virtually all digestion and nutrient absorption is completed within the first 100 to 150 cm of jejunum in a normal individual. The minimum length of residual small bowel necessary to avoid parenteral nutrition (PN) is approximately 100 cm of healthy bowel in the absence of an intact colon, and 60 cm with an intact colon. Patients who have < 100 cm of residual jejunum often exhibit a net secretory response to food. However, there is a large inter-patient variability. Equivalent proximal resections are much better tolerated than massive distal resections, because remaining ileum can take over much of the function of jejunum. In contrast, residual jejunum is incapable of either vitamin B_{12} or bile salt absorption. In addition, studies in the dog have indicated the hypermotility and, therefore, more rapid intestinal transit associated with massive bowel resections returns to normal faster with more proximal resections. Should the ileocecal valve be resected, intestinal transit time will also be decreased. It has been hypothesized that either the ileocecal valve or the colon acts as a "brake," and exhibits a negative effect on duodenal motility, perhaps mediated via peptide YY.

Medical Treatment Strategies
Treatment of Excessive Fluid Losses

Massive fluid and electrolyte losses often occur frequently during the first week or two following a massive small bowel resection, but may improve over the ensuing months. During this postoperative period, patients will usually require *parenteral fluids and nutrition*. Regardless, it is still important to institute *enteral nutrition* as soon as possible to hasten the intestinal adaptive response. Transient gastric hypersecretion also occurs for the first 6 to 12 months following a massive intestinal resection. Although the etiology for this process is unknown, it appears related to hypergastinemia. High dose H_2 antagonists and *proton pump inhibitors* are useful for decreasing jejunal fluid and potassium losses during this time. These medications are all absorbed in the proximal jejunum, but are compatible with TPN if IV delivery is necessary. Medications such as loperamide, diphenoxylate, codeine, or tincture of opium (listed in order of increasing need) may be important to slow motility and increase nutrient contact time. *Loperamide hydrochloride* or *diphenoxylate* may require doses up to 16 mg daily. If these medications are less than successful in controlling fluid losses, *codeine sulfate* (30 to 60 mg 3 times daily) or *deodorized tincture of opium* (10 drops 2 or 3 times daily) may be necessary. High doses of *calcium* (2.4 to 3.6 g/d of elemental calcium) may also be useful for decreasing diarrhea, probably because of increased binding of fatty acids. *Octreotide* (100 μg subcutaneously 3 times daily 30 min before meals) is rarely necessary, except for in some patients with high output jejunostomies. Its use should be avoided if possible because of an association with decreased pancreatic function, malabsorption, decreased intestinal adaptation, and cholelithiasis.

Malabsorption and Bacterial Overgrowth

Malabsorption develops in patients with short bowel syndrome not only because of *decreased intestinal surface area*, but also related to *bacterial colonization* of the small intestine. Normally, the ileocecal valve helps prevent the movement of bacteria from the colon into the distal ileum, but in its absence bacteria will enter the small intestine and compete for the available nutrients, such as vitamin B_{12}. *Bacterial overgrowth* may be difficult to diagnose in patients with short bowel syndrome because the rapid intestinal transit time renders breath tests difficult to interpret; *enteroscopy with jejunal aspiration* and *culture* may be necessary.

D-lactic acidosis is a rare complication of bacterial overgrowth, but may result in serious sequalae including ataxia, dysarthria, opthalmoplegia, nystagmus, stupor, and coma. It may develop when simple carbohydrates, such as glucose and lactose, are malabsorbed, leaving the anerobic flora to ferment them. Diagnosis requires the availability of a *serum d-lactic acid measurement*; the standard lactic acid laboratory test will not detect d-lactic acid.

Bacteria also deconjugate bile salts, which leads to decreased bile salt reabsorption; therefore, fewer bile salts are available for micelle formation and fat maldigestion occurs. Diarrhea may worsen in patients who have had > 100 cm of ileum resected and in whom part or all of their colon remains, in part because bile salts stimulate cyclic adenosine monophosphate and calcium-mediated chloride secretion. Unabsorbed long chain fatty acids may also stimulate colonic electrogenic anion secretion. A low fat intake (20 to 40 g) may lessen diarrhea but removes a source of calories.

Antibiotic Therapy

Treatment of bacterial overgrowth or d-lactic acidosis may be undertaken with either *metronidazole* or *tetracycline*. Unfortunately, the use of broad spectrum antibiotics may also contribute to the worsening of diarrhea because of either *Clostridium difficile* or non–*C.difficile*-associated diarrhea. Antibiotic use may also be associated with *vitamin K deficiency* because normal gastrointestinal flora synthesize at least half of the body's daily requirement.

Enhancement of Absorption

One of the most important factors for the promotion of intestinal hypertrophy and optimal adaptation of the remaining segment is the provision of *enteral feeding* as soon as possible postoperatively. The presence of growth factors, such as epidermal growth factor in the salivary glands and esophagus, makes oral feeding preferable. However, except for certain patient groups, as discussed below, there is no need for either special diets or dietary restrictions. What is important is that the patient consume as much energy and nitrogen as they can. This may mean upwards of 4,000 to 6,000 kcal and 150 g of nitrogen daily! Psychological training to induce such hyperphagia may be required. Bolus feedings should always be avoided, and the patient should be instructed to "graze" throughout the day. Although initial nonblinded studies of *glutamine* and *growth hormone* use suggested improved adaptation and absorption, two recent double-blinded, placebo-controlled studies cast doubt on whether either has any potential influence on bowel adaptation in humans. Studies with *glucagon-like peptide II* are underway, and the results are eagerly anticipated.

Diets and Specific Nutrient Requirements

All diets should be lactose-free, because the intestine will have lost a significant portion of its surface area and, therefore, its disaccharidase synthetic capacity following a massive resection. In addition, patients should avoid consumption of caffeine-containing products and osmotically active medications or sweeteners (sorbitol for example) that stimulate motility and lead to a further decrease in intestinal transit.

Oral Rehydration Solutions

Water should be avoided because additional fluid and electrolyte losses may result. Isotonic fluids such as oral rehydration solutions (ORS) should be used instead. ORSs are useful for the maintenance of normal hydrational status in short bowel syndrome as well as in acute diarrhea. Such solutions are based on the mechanism of the sodium-glucose cotransporter, whereby both solutes are actively absorbed together by the enterocyte. Water is pulled in with both sodium and glucose (solvent drag). There are several different commercially available preparations, but most importantly, for adults, these solutions should contain 90 to 120 meq/L of sodium for optimal effectiveness. *ORSs may be made up at home by dissolving sodium chloride/table salt (2.5 g), potassium chloride (1.5 g), Na_2CO_2 (2.5 g), and glucose/table sugar (20 g) in 1 L of water*. Patients should drink ORSs whenever they are thirsty because thirst is a good sign of dehydration. ORSs will not decrease fluid losses, but will enhance fluid absorption. Because ileal water absorption is unaffected by glucose, the presence of glucose in ORSs in patients without residual jejunum is not relevant. Recent data actually suggests that *hypotonic ORSs* (but not water) may be preferential because of the ability of these solutions to enhance intestinal water absorption (without sodium absorption). *Sodas and juices are quite hypertonic and should be avoided.* An attempt should be made to have the patient consume *dry solids first, followed by isotonic liquids 1 hour later.* However, this may be quite difficult in practice.

DIETS

Human studies have shown no benefit from high fat or high carbohydrate (in the absence of a colon) diets, or so-called "elemental" (small peptide or free amino acid-based enteral formulas), on stool weight, or energy, nitrogen, electrolyte, or mineral absorption. Dietary fat restriction will decrease steatorrhea, but will not increase fat absorption. *Medium-chain triacylglycerols* (MCT) are absorbed independently of bile salts and may provide a useful energy loss in patients with significant steatorrhea. There is also some colonic absorption. However, they are expensive, often unpalatable (despite modern recipes), cannot be used with cooking oil because of a low smoke temperature, may worsen diarrhea in excessive doses (> 40 g daily), and may have an adverse effect on intestinal adaptation. There have been a few case reports that suggest *replacement of bile salts with ox bile* may lead to improve in long chain triglyceride absorption (Hofmann, 2000).

FATS

Residual colon becomes an important instrument for nutrient digestion and absorption. Therefore, dietary recommendations may vary depending on whether colon is present. Unlike in the patient with a jejunostomy, dietary fat intake should be restricted in the patient with remaining colon, although not to the extent as to render the diet unpalatable. Patients should also be provided with a diet low in oxalate content.*

OXYLATES

Normally, dietary oxalate (and bile acids) is bound to calcium in the intestinal tract. This renders oxalate unavailable for absorption. However, when significant steatorrhea is present, unabsorbed fatty acids preferentially bind to calcium, the free oxalate enters the colon and is absorbed. The absorbed oxalate is then filtered by the kidneys where it becomes free to bind calcium with the potential for kidney stone formation. Foods such as chocolate, tea, cola, spinach, celery, and carrots should be avoided, as should dehydration. Although some of the vitamin C in the TPN solutions may be converted to oxalate with a resultant hyperoxaluria, patients *without* a colon do not appear at increased risk for oxalate nephrolithiasis.

*Editor's Note: Dietary fat should not be replaced with MCT because essential fat (linoleic acid) is not supplied. In order to prevent essential fatty acid deficiency, linoleic acid must constitute at least 2 to 4% of the total absorbed calories. It is presently unclear whether linolenic fatty acid is essential as well.

In the normal individual, aside from fluid and limited calcium absorption, the colon has little importance nutritionally. However, in short bowel syndrome with significant carbohydrate malabsorption, the colon plays a much greater role nutritionally. Soluble fibers (eg, pectin, but less so soy, oats, or wheat bran, but not lignin) and starch are metabolized by normal colonic flora to the short chain fatty acids (SCFAs) acetate, butyrate, and propionate. These SCFAs (most notably butyrate) are the preferred fuel for the colonocyte, stimulate sodium and water absorption (although bicarbonate secretion may increase), and may account for upwards of 1,000 kcal daily in energy absorption! Therefore, the residual colon and a diet containing, substantial amounts of soluble fiber, complex carbohydrate, and some insoluble nonstarch polysaccharides provides an opportunity for colonic energy salvage. Patients with a colonic mucus fistula should be re-anastomosed as soon as possible.

FAT-SOLUBLE VITAMINS

For the patient who can be maintained without PN, regardless of the presence or absence of a colon, various vitamin and mineral supplements are often necessary (Table 64-1). Fat-soluble vitamins (A, D, E, and K) should be routinely monitored in non-TPN dependent patients, or in those who are only partially TPN-dependent. *Vitamin A* (10,000 to 50,000 U/d), *vitamin D* (1,600 U DHT/d or 50,000 U of parent vitamin D) and/or *vitamin E* (30 U/d) supplements may be necessary. In the presence of significant steatorrhea, the *water-soluble forms* of *vitamin A and E,* as well as the $25\text{-}OH_2D_3$ form may be preferable. Patients with significant renal insufficiency may require supplementation with $1,25\text{-}OH_2D_3$ (1,25-dihydroxyvitamin D_3). Since vitamin D enhances intestinal calcium absorption, simultaneous *calcium* supplementation should also be provided. Adequate

TABLE 64-1. Vitamin and Mineral Supplements for Patients with Short Bowel Syndrome

Vitamin A	10,000 to 50,000 units daily
Vitamin B_{12}	300 µg subcutaneously monthly for those with terminal ileal resections or disease
Vitamin C	200 to 500 mg
Vitamin D	1600 units DHT daily; may require 25-OH or 1,25 $(OH_2)\text{-}D_3$
Vitamin E	30 IU daily
Vitamin K	10 mg weekly
Calcium	See text
Magnesium	See text
Iron	As needed
Selenium	60 to 100 g daily
Zinc	220 to 440 mg daily (sulfate form)
Bicarbonate	As needed

The table lists rough guidelines only. Vitamin and mineral supplementation must be routinely monitored and tailored to the individual patient because relative absorption and requirements may vary.

sun exposure may also be an inexpensive alternative to vitamin D supplementation. The serum calcium should be monitored, as well as vitamin A and D concentrations because toxicity can result from excessive intake of any of these. Vitamin E is thought to be essentially nontoxic, although the clotting activity may be further suppressed in patients taking warfarin simultaneously. Adequacy of supplementation should also be routinely monitored by *measurement* of *serum vitamin A, vitamin D (25-OH), and vitamin E* concentrations. Vitamin E concentration may vary in relation to the serum total lipid concentration. Therefore, total serum lipids should be measured simultaneously and the ratio of vitamin E to total serum lipids should actually be used as the index of vitamin E status. Because enteric bacteria synthesize much of the daily *vitamin K* requirement (approximately 1 mg/d), in addition to that contained in the diet, supplementation is not usually necessary, although the prothrombin time should be monitored.

WATER-SOLUBLE VITAMINS

Deficiencies of water-soluble vitamins are relatively rare in short bowel patients. However, they may occur and it is therefore important that patients ingest *1 or 2 B-complex vitamin supplements* and *200 to 500 mg of vitamin C daily*. *Vitamin B_{12}* should be administered at a dose of 1,000 μg intramuscularly every 3 months in patients who have had significant gastric or ileal resections, or in those who have active Crohn's disease in their remaining terminal ileum. The adequacy of vitamin B_{12} supplementation is best measured by following the serum methylmalonic acid (MMA) concentration. In the absence of sufficient B_{12}, the MMA concentration will remain elevated because it will not be metabolized to succinyl coenzyme A. Similarly, *folate* is required for the metabolism of homocysteine to methionine. The Schillings test is *not* a test to determine vitamin B_{12} status, but to determine why a particular patient *is* vitamin B_{12} deficient. Once neuropathy (B_{12}) or megaloblastic anemia (either) are present, deficiency has probably been present for some period of time. Although the B vitamins are essentially nontoxic, *excessive vitamin C ingestion* has been associated with calcium oxalate nephrolithiasis, which the patients may already have a predisposition to.

ZINC

Zinc supplements (see Table 64-1) are routinely necessary because of the significant fecal losses (17 mg/L). To put these losses in perspective, standard TPN solutions typically contain 2 mg of zinc daily. Usually one or two 220 mg zinc sulfate tablets will be sufficient. Although there is considerable debate on the appropriate test for measurement of zinc status, the serum concentration should be followed. Zinc is bound to albumin. Therefore, the serum zinc concentration may be depressed in the presence of a low serum albumin, although physiologic zinc status may be normal. Unfortunately, no conversion factor is available. *Zinc deficiency* has also been associated with *increased diarrhea*, which may be ameliorated with zinc supplementation.

ELECTROLYTES AND MINERALS

Patients with excessive fecal volume losses are also losing significant amounts of bicarbonate, magnesium, and selenium. Replacement of bicarbonate can be accomplished with *sodium bicarbonate* tablets. This may be necessary to maintain normal acid-base status, and help prevent development of osteoporosis. *Magnesium* replacement may be difficult because of the cathartic effect of all currently available oral supplements and the poor bioavailability of the enteric-coated tablets. Replacement via injection is painful. Therefore, periodic IV replacement may be required. Because the vast majority of magnesium is found intracellularly, measurement of serum concentration may not accurately reflect magnesium status. Therefore, *24-hour urine magnesium* should be routinely followed. Values above 70 mg daily suggest adequate magnesium stores.

Selenium status can be followed by measurement of the plasma selenium concentration by a laboratory experienced in the measurement of this trace metal. It can be supplemented (60 to 120 μg/d) if necessary. Deficiency has been associated with cardiomyopathy, macrocytosis, myositis, and pseudoalbinism. *Copper* deficiency is very rare, as most excretion is biliary in origin. Deficiency has been associated with anemia, cardiomyopathy, neutropenia, neuropathy, osteoporosis, retinal degeneration, and testicular atrophy.

Complications of Short Bowel Syndrome

Complications of short bowel syndrome include *dehydration* (which may result in *uric acid nephrolithiasis*), generalized *malnutrition, electrolyte disturbances*, specific *nutrient deficiencies, calcium oxalate nephrolithiasis*, and *cholelithiasis*. Those patients with significant malabsorption requiring long term TPN are at additional risk for *hepatic steatosis* and *cholestasis* with potential progression to *cirrhosis*, either *acalculous* or *calculous cholecystitis, metabolic bone disease, nephropathy*, and *central venous catheter-related problems* including infection and occlusion (thrombotic and nonthrombotic).

When TPN is Required

Patients will most likely require PN and fluids initially following massive bowel resection. This will continue for at least 7 to 10 days, and perhaps as long as 1 to 2 years during the adaptation process; it may be permanent if the bowel surface area and adaptation is insufficient. Patients should be provided with 30 to 33 kcal/kg/d (or use indirect calorimetry with an added activity factor) and 1.0 to 1.5 g/kg/d of amino acids. Energy is provided as dextrose (3.4 kcal/mL) and lipid emulsion (1.1 kcal/mL for the 10% and 2.0 kcal/mL for the 20% form). Requirements for young children and neonates are substantially greater. Electrolytes, minerals, vitamins, and trace metals are also to be provided. A further discussion of TPN requirements, management of the patient on TPN, and the management of TPN-related complications is found in Chapter 54, "Enteral and Parenteral Nutrition."

Surgical Approaches

There have been numerous reports of various bowel lengthening procedures and various other methods aimed at prolonging bowel transit time and nutrient-epithelium contact time. These have included the use of aperistaltic segments, attempts to increase surface area by "butterflying" the bowel for lack of a better description, colonic interposition, reversed intestinal segments, and recirculating small bowel loops. Although there is the isolated case report of at least temporary success, none of these procedures have been considered routinely successful. All have been associated with the potential for significant morbidity.

Intestinal transplantation (discussed in Chapter 65, "Intestinal and Multivisceral Transplantation") is an option for patients that have developed severe, chronic complications of TPN therapy.

Supplemental Reading

Buchman AL. Complications of long-term home total parenteral nutrition: their identification, prevention and treatment. Dig Dis Sci 2001;46:1–18.

Buchman AL. TPN-associated liver disease. JPEN 2002;26:S43–8.

Buchman AL, Moukarzel A. Metabolic bone disease associated with total parenteral nutrition. Clin Nutr 2000;19:217–31.

Buchman AL, Scolapio J, Fryer J. Technical review of the treatment of short bowel syndrome and intestinal transplantation. Gastroenterol 2003;124:1111–34.

Hofmann AF. Conjugated bile acid replacement therapy in short bowel syndrome. Arch Gastroenterohepatol 2000;19:2–11.

McIntyre PB, Fitchew M, Lennard-Jones JE. Patients with a high jejunostomy do not need a special diet. Gastroenterol 1986;91:25–33.

Messing B, Crenn P, Beau P, et al. Long-term survival and parenteral nutrition dependence in adult patients with short bowel syndrome. Gastroenterol 1999;117:1043–50.

Messing B, Pigot F, Rongier M, et al. Intestinal absorption of free oral hyperalimentation in the very short bowel syndrome. Gastroenterol 1991;100:1502–8.

Nordgaard I, Hansen BS, Mortensen PB. Importance of colonic support for energy absorption as small-bowel failure proceeds. Am J Clin Nutr 1996;64:222–31.

Scolapio JS, Camilleri M, Fleming CR, et al. Effect of growth hormone, glutamine, and diet on adaptation in short-bowel syndrome: a randomized, controlled trial. Gastroenterol 1997;113:1074–81.

Woolf PB, Miller C, Kurian R, Jeejeebhoy K. Diet for patients with a short bowel: high fat or high carbohydrate? Gastroenterol 1983;84:823–8.

CHAPTER 65

Intestinal and Multivisceral Transplantation

Ernesto P. Molmenti, MD, PhD, Nicholas Pyrsopoulos, MD, and Andreas G. Tzakis, MD, PhD

Intestinal allografts can be classified into the following three broad categories: (1) isolated intestine, (2) intestine and liver, and (3) multivisceral (which can include liver, stomach, pancreas, kidneys, and other organs) (Katz et al, 2002). It is estimated that two of every million live births in Western countries will develop intestinal failure (Fishbein et al, 2003).

Indications for the Procedure

Intestinal transplantation is indicated in cases of intestinal failure, defined as the irreversible inability of the intestine to adequately sustain the body's nutritional, fluid, and electrolytic balance in the absence of parenteral support. Irreversible intestinal failure can be the result of loss of surface area, functional disturbances, or the presence of unresectable tumors involving the intestine. The etiology of these in turn can be either congenital or acquired. Clinical manifestations include but are not limited to dehydration, deficiencies of nutrients and vitamins, gallstones, stomach hyperacidity, renal stones, hyperoxaluria, skin irritation, and malabsorptive diarrhea. It has been observed that < 20% of adults with < 100 cm of intestine or end jejunostomy will be able to maintain nutritional requirements in the absence of total parenteral nutrition (TPN) (Messing et al, 1999). In the pediatric population, failure to wean from TPN has been found to be associated with absence of enteral feeding tolerance early after birth, around 30 cm or less of small intestine, and absence of enterocolonic continuity (Fishbein et al, 2003; Vargas et al, 1987; Pharaon et al, 1994).

Short gut syndrome (loss of approximately 70% of the native small bowel length) is the most frequently encountered cause of irreversible intestinal failure. Causes of short gut syndrome in children include *necrotizing enterocolitis, atresia, and volvulus*. In adults, etiologies are *trauma, surgical damage, repeated resections for Crohn's disease, mesenteric vascular injuries, extensive adhesions, and desmoid tumors*. Defective motility of the gastrointestinal (GI) tract causing *pseudo-obstruction* is associated with total aganglionosis, neuropathy, and myopathy. Impaired absorptive function is found secondary to *radiation injury, autoimmune processes, extensive polyposis, and microvillus inclusion disease* (Sturm et al, 1997; Thompson, 1994; Granata and Puri, 1997; Herzog et al, 1996).

As previously mentioned, intestinal transplantation should be undertaken in those cases in which there is a life threatening complication associated with TPN treatment. Ten to 40% of patients with intestinal failure die as a result of these complications within 3 to 5 years. Such complications include cholestatic liver failure, venous thrombosis leading to loss of access, and severe line sepsis. Isolated small intestinal transplantation is also considered in cases where TPN has led to reversible liver injury (Grosfeld et al, 1986). Liver and small bowel grafts are considered in cases of irreversible liver failure. Multivisceral transplantation is undertaken in instances when individual patient characteristics have led to the loss or malfunction of the viscera being replaced (Kato et al, 2002).

Medicare-approved criteria for failure of parenteral nutrition include "impending or overt failure due to TPN-induced liver injury, thrombosis of 2 or more central veins, the development of 2 or more episodes of systemic sepsis secondary to line infection per year that require hospitalization, a single episode of line-related fungemia, septic shock, and/or acute respiratory distress, frequent episodes of severe dehydration despite intravenous fluid supplementation in addition to TPN." (Fishbein et al, 2003)

Evaluation of the Potential Candidate

When a patient presents to be examined for intestinal transplantation, it is imperative to perform a thorough evaluation of all available medical and surgical records. Evaluation of hepatic and renal function is of importance to determine the need to replace these organs. Inclusion of a kidney as part of the multivisceral transplantation is usually recommended in cases of marginal renal function because of immunosuppressive nephrotoxicity. The GI tract anatomy should be outlined in order to plan for the reconstruction at the time of transplantation. By the time of referral, most patients have undergone imaging studies, such as upper GI series and contrast enemata. On occasions, further studies are needed. Assessment of vessels patency is of great importance. Most patients have been on TPN, and as such probably have venous thrombosis to a greater or lesser degree (Kato et al, 1999).

Donor Selection

Donor selection is based on size, ABO typing, and cytomegalovirus (CMV) serology. Human leukocyte antigen typing and cytotoxic crossmatch are not universal criteria.

Although a donor somewhat smaller than the recipient is the preferred situation, the shortage of allografts makes this a limitation. Technical variations such as splitting the liver or shortening the bowel length have been adopted in order to adapt for size.

At the University of Miami, donor and recipient are chosen with identical ABO typing. Only rarely compatible but not identical combinations are undertaken (Sindhi et al, 1996).

To prevent the risk of disease in the recipient, CMV-negative donors are preferred. However, this preference does not necessarily exclude those donors with positive CMV serologies (Manez et al, 1995).

Living donation of intestinal grafts remains a controversial subject. Potential advantages include transplantation between identical twins. Other potential combinations include living donation for a liver graft and cadaver donation for an intestinal graft (Morris et al, 1996).

Transplantation

Isolated Intestinal Transplantation

The jejunum and ileum is transplanted. An ileostomy is usually created to allow for postoperative endoscopic follow up. A feeding tube is usually placed to allow for enteral feeding in cases where the patient has lost or never acquired eating habits (Nucci et al, 2002; Iyer et al, 2002). A gastrojejunostomy tube is preferred at some centers to allow for enteral feeding with simultaneous decompression of the stomach. Venous drainage of the intestinal allograft can be into the systemic (IVC) or portal (portal vein) circulation. A minimal segment of cecum may be included with the graft to preserve the ileocecal valve. This allows for better physiologic results in recipients with no functional remaining colon.

Liver–Intestine Transplantation

The liver is transplanted together with the intestine. These organs may be transplanted en bloc or as independent entities (Kato et al, 2002). The liver is usually implanted in a "piggyback" fashion. The native portal venous outflow can be directed into the allograft portal system or into the systemic circulation. Cholecystectomy is performed in all cases.

Multivisceral Transplantation

This type of transplantation involves the intestine associated with other organs, usually the stomach and pancreas. It may also include the liver and kidneys. This type of transplantation is required for patients with extensive loss of abdominal organs, for those with severe functional disorders, as well as for those in whom tumor removal compromises most of the GI tract (Giraldo et al, 2000).

Abdominal Wall Transplantation

Transplantation of a composite of abdominal wall from the donor is a novel technique developed with success at the University of Miami. It allows for the closure of the abdomen in cases in which prosthetic material would have otherwise been needed (Levi et al, 2003).

Postoperative Management

At the University of Miami, immunosuppression traditionally included tacrolimus, corticosteroids, and *mycophenolate mofetil* (Kato et al, 2002). Twelve-hour tacrolimus trough levels are aimed at 15 to 20 ng/mL. The combination of tacrolimus with *alemtuzumab* (Campath-1H) without steroids has recently been found to be effective in preventing acute rejection without an increase in opportunistic infections (Tzakis et al, 2003).

Enteral infusion of 5% dextrose in water via a feeding tube can be started immediately after surgery. This is advanced rapidly as the ostomy becomes functional. Adequate function of the graft is monitored by ostomy output volume and the presence of reducing substances. High ostomy outputs require intravenous fluid replacement. Other variables that should be taken into account include delayed gastric emptying and the lack of training for oral intake of patients on long term TPN. Caloric needs may not be met by oral intake alone sometimes for up to 12 months.

Postoperative surveillance biopsies are usually performed in the immediate postoperative period. Furthermore, changes in intestinal function manifest by increased output, bloody output, mucosal sloughing, malabsorption, changes in mucosal appearance, warrant endoscopy and biopsy. In experienced hands, the allograft can also be evaluated by the presence of magnifying, high-resolution endoscopes (Kato et al, 2002).

Some centers perform infusion of bone marrow from the donor to induce tolerance by enhancing chimerism (Ricordi et al, 1997).

Rejection

Acute rejection of the intestinal allograft is not an uncommon event. The most frequent presentation is with fever. Other presenting symptoms include abnormal liver function tests, changes in ostomy output, bloody intestinal discharge, altered intestinal motility, increased reducing substances in the stool associated with carbohydrate malabsorption, and sepsis from bacterial translocation across the bowel wall. In cases of severe rejection, it is recommended to administer an enteric decontaminant solution containing antibiotic and antifungal agents.

The classic classification of rejection is based on a histopathologic grading that encompasses mild, moderate, and severe categories. Rejection can demonstrate a geographical distribution. As such, to obtain an adequate diagnosis it is necessary to obtain multiple biopsies. Biopsy specimens at the ostomy site may show local trauma and inflammatory processes that may not reflect the status of the remaining portions of the intestine.

A more recent approach to the evaluation of rejection is by means of an endoscopic examination with visual magnification. Mucosal changes suggest the degree of damage, and, as such, the severity of rejection. It is recommended however, to perform multiple biopsies that include even normal looking mucosa to detect early changes.

Serum citrulline has also been found to be a marker of intestinal allograft rejection Treatment of rejection in with use of steroids, increases in immunosuppression levels, or administration of antibody preparations such as OKT3. According to the experience at the University of Miami, the presence of at least one episode of severe rejection is associated with diminished graft survival.

Postoperative Complications

Surgical re-intervention within the first month after transplantation is not infrequent, and may be necessary for various reasons in up to half of patients (Fishbein et al, 2003). Infections are a frequent complication after intestinal transplantation. Pathogens include bacteria, viruses, and fungi. Intra-abdominal processes are frequent, and can be associated with intestinal complications, such as anastomotic leaks, perforation, and translocation of pathogens. Infections can also arise from sites found in nontransplantation surgical patients, such as the urinary tract, respiratory system, central and peripheral lines, and wounds.

CMV remains an important pathogen in the intestinal transplantation population. It can manifest locally at the intestinal allograft as well as systemically. *Epstein-Barr virus (EBV)* infection has been reported to occur in as many as half of recipients in some series. It is considered to be associated with high levels of immunosuppression and specifically linked to the use of OKT3. EBV infection can lead to posttransplantation lymphoproliferative disease (PTLD). PTLD has been associated with delayed graft loss, as well as with a high mortality. Initial treatment of PTLD is with diminution of immunosuppression and antiviral therapy. Additional treatments available include chemo- and immunotherapies. Preemptive treatment as well as treatment with *monoclonal anti CD20* agents have shown encouraging results (Grant, 1999; Nishida et al, 2002). Adenovirus infection can be limited to the intestinal allograft or have a systemic involvement. Other infectious agents include respiratory syncitial virus and mycobacteria.

Graft-versus-host disease is encountered more frequently among recipients of intestinal allografts than among those of liver and kidney grafts. This difference in incidence has been attributed to the greater number of donor cells encountered in intestinal transplantation. At the University of Miami it has a reported incidence of 19%. Most frequently it presents with a rash and fever, and tends to respond to increased immunosuppression.

Chylous ascites after transplantation is sometimes encountered and may arise from donor or recipient lymphatic tissues. It usually becomes evident after dietary fats are introduced. Treatment is with low long-chain triglyceride diets (Nishida et al, 2002).

Recurrence of the original disease is encountered in some occasions. Reported recurrence of Crohn's disease and recurrent desmoid tumors of Gardner's disease are some examples (Kato et al, 2002).

Outcomes

According to the international intestinal transplantation registry and data from 55 centers around the world published in 1999 the overall patient and graft survival rates is 69% for isolated intestine recipients at 1 year and 66% and 63% for liver/intestine and multivisceral grafts (Grant, 1997).

The constant evolution of the surgical techniques, the better selection and preparation of the intestinal and multivisceral transplantation candidates, the discovery of new potent immunosuppressive medication, and the tendency to follow these patients closely, has resulted in a constantly improving survival rate. It was previously reported from the University of Miami that the 1-year survival rate for isolated intestinal, liver intestinal, and multivisceral transplantations prior to 1998 was 75%, 40%, and 48%, respectively. The reported 1-year patient and graft survival rates for isolated intestinal transplantations after 1998 have been 84% and 72%, respectively (Nishida et al, 2002). It seems that the introduction of *alemtuzumab* in conjunction with *tacrolimus* in the absence of corticosteroids improves the survival rate without any further compromise of the immune system or increased risk for infections. It is noteworthy that though the patient and graft survival rates remain the same a significant portion of these patients do not develop acute rejection episodes.

A recently published single-center series offers further encouraging results for isolated intestinal allograft recipients. Reported 1-year and 3-year actuarial patient survival rates were 88% for both. One-year and 3-year actuarial primary graft survival rates were approximately 78% and 71%, respectively (Fishbein et al, 2003).

Infections and rejection still remain the major lethal complications. The majority of the patients are TPN-free and have a remarkable improvement in quality of life.

Supplemental Reading

Berney T, Delis S, Kato T, et al. Successful treatment of post-transplant lymphoproliferative disease with prolonged rituximab treatment in intestinal transplant recipients. Transplantation 2002;74:1000–6.

Fishbein TM, Gondolesi GE, Kaufman SS. Intestinal transplantation for gut failure. Gastroenterol 2003;124:1615–28.

Fishbein TM, Kaufman SS, Florman SS, et al. Isolated intestinal transplantation: proof of clinical efficacy. Transplantation 2003;76:636–40.

Fontes P, Rao AS, Demetris AJ, et al. Bone marrow augmentation of donor-cell chimerism in kidney, liver, heart, and pancreas islet transplantation. Lancet 1994;344:151–5.

Giraldo M, Martin D, Colangelo J, et al. Intestinal transplantation for patients with short gut syndrome and hypercoagulable states. Transplant Proc 2000;32:1223–4.

Granata C, Puri P. Megacystis-microcolon-intestinal hypoperistalsis syndrome. J Pediatr Gastroenterol Nutr 1997;25:12–9.

Grant D. Intestinal transplantation: 1997 report of the international registry. Intestinal Transplant Registry. Transplantation 1999;67:1061–4.

Green M, Reyes J, Jabbour N, et al. Use of quantitative PCR to predict onset of Epstein-Barr viral infection and post-transplant lymphoproliferative disease after intestinal transplantation in children. Transplant Proc 1996;28:2759–60.

Grosfeld JL, Rescorla FJ, West KW. Short bowel syndrome in infancy and childhood. Analysis of survival in 60 patients. Am J Surg 1986;151:41–6.

Health Care Financing Administration (HCFA), Program Memorandum Intermediaries/Carriers. Intestinal Transplantation 2000; December.

Herzog D, Atkison P, Grant D, et al. Combined bowel-liver transplantation in an infant with microvillous inclusion disease. J Pediatr Gastroenterol Nutr 1996;22:405–8.

Iyer K, Horslen S, Iverson A, et al. Nutritional outcome and growth of children after intestinal transplantation. J Pediatr Surg 2002;37:464–6.

Kato T, Nishida S, Mittal N, et al. Intestinal transplantation at the University of Miami. Transplant Proc 2002;34:868.

Kato T, Romero R, Verzaro R, et al. Inclusion of entire pancreas in the composite liver and intestinal graft in pediatric intestinal transplantation. Pediatr Transplant 1999;3:210–4.

Kato T, Ruiz P, Thompson JF, et al. Intestinal and multivisceral transplantation. World J Surg 2002;26:226–37.

Levi DM, Tzakis AG, Kato T, et al. Transplantation of the abdominal wall. Lancet 2003;361:2173–6.

Manez R, Kusne S, Green M, et al. Incidence and risk factors associated with the development of cytomegalovirus disease after intestinal transplantation. Transplantation 1995;59:1010–4.

Messing B, Crenn P, Beau P, et al. Long-term survival and parenteral nutrition dependence in adult patients with the short bowel syndrome. Gastroenterol 1999;117:1043–50.

Morris JA, Johnson DL, Rimmer JA, et al. Identical twin small bowel transplant after resection of abdominal desmoid tumor. Transplant Proc 1996;28:2731–2.

Nery JR, Weppler D, DeFaria W, et al. Is the graft too big or too small? Technical variations to overcome size incongruity in visceral organ transplantation. Transplant Proc 1998;30:2640–1.

Nishida S, Levi D, Kato T, et al. Ninety-five cases of intestinal transplantation at the University of Miami. J Gastrointest Surg 2002;6:233–9.

Nucci AM, Barksdale EM Jr, Beserock N, et al. Long-term nutritional outcome after pediatric intestinal transplantation. J Pediatr Surg 2002;37:460–3.

Pappas PA, Saudubray JM, Tzakis AG, et al. Serum citrulline as a marker of acute cellular rejection for intestinal transplantation. Transplant Proc 2002;34:915–7.

Pharaon I, Despres C, Aigrain Y, et al. Long-term parenteral nutrition in children who are potentially candidates for small bowel transplantation. Transplant Proc 1994;26:1442.

Reyes J, Bueno J, Kocoshis S, et al. Current status of intestinal transplantation in children. J Pediatr Surg 1998;33:243–54.

Reyes J, Green M, Bueno J, et al. Epstein Barr virus associated posttransplant lymphoproliferative disease after intestinal transplantation. Transplant Proc 1996;28:2768–9.

Ricordi C, Karatzas T, Nery J, et al. High-dose donor bone marrow infusions to enhance allograft survival: the effect of timing. Transplantation 1997;63:7–11.

Sindhi R, Landmark J, Shaw BW Jr, et al. Combined liver/small bowel transplantation using a blood group compatible but nonidentical donor. Transplantation 1996;61:1782–3.

Starzl TE, Demetris AJ, Rao AS, et al. Spontaneous and iatrogenically augmented leukocyte chimerism in organ transplant recipients. Transplant Proc 1994;26:3071–6.

Sturm A, Layer P, Goebell H, Dignass AU. Short-bowel syndrome: an update on the therapeutic approach. Scand J Gastroenterol 1997;32:289–96.

Thompson JS. Management of the short bowel syndrome. Gastroenterol Clin N Am 1994;23:403–20.

Todo S, Reyes J, Furukawa H, et al. Outcome analysis of 71 clinical intestinal transplantations. Ann Surg 1995;222:270–80; discussion 280–2.

Tzakis AG, Kato T, Nishida S, et al. Alemtuzumab (Campath-1H) combined with tacrolimus in intestinal and multivisceral transplantation. Transplantation 2003;75:1512–7.

Tzakis AG, Tryphonopoulos P, Kato T, et al. Intestinal transplantation: advances in immunosuppression and surgical techniques. Transplant Proc 2003;35:1925–6.

Vargas JH, Ament ME, Berquist WE. Long-term home parenteral nutrition in pediatrics: ten years of experience in 102 patients. J Pediatr Gastroenterol Nutr 1987;6:24–32.

CHAPTER 66

Crohn's Disease of the Small Bowel

CHINYU SU, MD, AND GARY R. LICHTENSTEIN, MD

Approximately 40 to 50% of patients with Crohn's disease (CD) have disease in the terminal ileum and the colon at presentation, and another 20% of patients have disease limited to the small bowel (SB). Thus, the majority of CD patients have SB involvement. There are a number of important issues to consider in managing patients with SB CD. First, some medications are most effective for distal ileitis but not jejunitis, whereas other medications are not effective for SB disease. Thus, clinicians should have the knowledge of the site of active disease to appropriately select effective medications. Second, heterogeneity in clinical presentations is particularly important in SB CD, because both stricturing and penetrating clinical phenotypes are more common in SB than in colonic CD. In general, the clinical disease behavior for CD can be categorized into the following three patterns: (1) stricturing (fibrostenotic), (2) penetrating (perforating or fistulizing), and (3) nonstricturing, nonpenetrating (inflammatory) disease. Third, the evaluation of the active site and pattern of disease in the SB is limited by our ability to directly visualize and examine a biopsy on a large portion of the SB. Thus, correlation of the patient's symptoms with findings on endoscopy and imaging studies is crucial in determining the cause of patient's symptoms and formulating appropriate treatment plans. Fourth, patients with SB CD may develop serious metabolic complications that are not present in patients with colonic CD. These issues need to be recognized and managed appropriately.

Clinical Phenotypes

When CD is limited to the SB, it usually involves terminal ileum. The other segments of the SB are affected in approximately 20% of the cases. Given the frequent terminal ileal involvement, the classical symptoms of SB CD are right lower-quadrant abdominal pain and diarrhea. Other common symptoms include low grade fever, decreased appetite, fatigue, and weight loss. Patients with more diffuse inflammatory pattern of the SB, including fistulizing disease, have more prominent components of malabsorption, such as diarrhea and weight loss. In contrast, patients with fribrostenotic disease usually present with symptoms of partial SB obstruction, including abdominal pain, bloating, nausea, and vomiting.

NOD2

Although no single gene has been found to be responsible for the development of CD, several susceptibility gene loci have been identified. The recently discovered association of *NOD2* gene mutations with CD represents a major advancement in this regard. The Nod2 proteins encoded by *NOD2* gene bind to bacterial lipopolysaccharides (LPS) as well as activate NF-κB, a key inflammatory cytokine. Deletion of the LPS binding domain has, however, been associated with activation of NF-κB, further propagating inflammatory cascade. The prevalence of these *NOD2* variants is < 20% of the patients with CD. More importantly, mutations in *NOD2* have been associated with ileal CD, fibrostenotic disease behavior, and possibly early age at onset and, perhaps, non-perianal fistulizing disease (Brant et al, 2003; Abreu et al, 2002; Cuthbert et al, 2002). In fact, the risks of ileal disease and fibrostenotic disease are about 10-fold and 7-fold, respectively, for CD patients with 2 *NOD2* mutations compared to those without any mutation. Whether patients with SB CD may be stratified by their genotypes and managed accordingly (eg, more aggressive medical therapy and earlier surgery if mutations are identified) will need to be further examined.

Medical Therapy for SB CD

As in CD involving other parts of the gastrointestinal (GI) tract, medical therapy is the mainstay of management in patients with SB CD. Therapies can be categorized into induction and maintenance therapies, based on whether they are intended to treat active disease or to prevent recurrent disease (Hanauer and Sandborn, 2001; Stein and Lichtenstein, 2001). Choice of medication largely depends on the location, pattern, and severity of disease (Table 66-1). The general principle of a "step-up" approach whereby agents are added upon disease progression or failure to respond to existing therapy remains the prevailing strategy. The concept of earlier use during disease course of certain medications that have traditionally been reserved for more severe or refractory disease is gaining popularity; however, this has yet to be tested over long duration of time.

TABLE 66-1. Medical Options for Small Bowel Crohn's Disease

	Mild Disease	Moderate to Severe Disease	Steroid-Dependent Disease	Inactive Disease
Distal ileitis	Mesalamine Budesonide	Budesonide Conventional steroids AZA, 6-MP MTX Infliximab	AZA, 6-MP MTX Infliximab	Mesalamine AZA, 6-MP MTX Infliximab
Proximal ileitis/jejunitis	Mesalamine (Pentasa)	Budenoside Conventional steroids AZA, 6-MP MTX Infliximab	AZA, 6-MP MTX Infliximab	Mesalamine (Pentasa) AZA, 6-MP MTX Infliximab

AZA = azathioprine; 6-MP = 6-mercaptopurine; MTX = methotrexate.

Induction Therapy

Mild Disease

MESALAMINE

Mesalamine agents have traditionally been the first line therapy for patients with mildly active SB CD. Formulations that deliver 5-aminosalicylates (5-ASA) to the SB include *Asacol* and *Pentasa*. Asacol is a Eudragit-S-coated mesalamine tablet that releases the active ingredients at pH > 7 in the distal ileum and the colon. Pentasa consists of ethylcellulose-coated mesalamine microgranules that release the active ingredients in a time-dependent fashion, starting from the duodenum throughout the remainder of the bowel. High doses of mesalamines are necessary to achieve efficacy. Pentasa at 4 g/d, but not lower doses, is effective in inducing remission in patients with active CD, and may have the greatest efficacy in patients with SB CD. Asacol at 4 g/d has also been shown to have comparable efficacy as methylprednisolone at 40 mg/d for patients with Crohn's ileitis of mild to moderate severity. At doses higher than 4 g daily these agents may offer even greater benefit. This is currently being assessed in a controlled fashion.

Sulfasalazine and other 5-ASA conjugates (*olsalazine* [*Dipentum*] and *balsalazide* [*Colazal*]) have not been shown to have a role in the management of SB CD, because their delivery site of 5-ASA is the colon. The possible exception is the presence of extraintestinal manifestations, such as peripheral arthropathy, where sulfasalazine may offer benefit over the newer mesalamine preparations.†

BUDESONIDE

An alternative option to mesalamines in patients with mild distal ileitis is oral *budesonide* (Entercort), which is a glucocorticosteroid that has primarily topical actions and less toxicity than the conventional corticosteroid preparations. The use of oral budesonide is discussed in the next section.

Moderate to Severe Disease

Therapies that may be considered in patients with SB CD of moderate to severe activity or disease refractory to mesalamine therapy include *corticosteroids, azathioprine (AZA) or 6-mercaptopurine* (6-MP), *methotrexate (MTX)*, and *infliximab*.

CORTICOSTEROIDS

Conventional corticosteroids, both oral and parenteral forms, are effective for patients with moderate to severe flares. Doses equivalent to 40 to 60 mg/d (or 0.5 to 0.75 mg/kg/d) of *prednisone* are sufficient to induce remission; higher doses do not provide additional benefit and are not recommended. Parenteral corticosteroids should be initiated in patients with severe disease not responding to oral corticosteroids. Hospitalization along with a course of bowel rest is appropriate in these severely ill patients.

BUDESONIDE

Newer corticosteroid preparations such as oral *budesonide* (Entercort) have the advantage of a greater topical anti-inflammatory action and a better toxicity profile than traditional corticosteroids. In patients with mild to moderate disease activity, budesonide at 9 mg/d is superior to placebo or mesalamine, and comparable to conventional steroids at equivalent of prednisolone 40 mg/d (Greenberg et al, 1994; Thomsen et al, 1998; Rutgeerts et al, 1994). The controlled-ileal release oral budesonide (Entocort) is formulated as Eudragit-L-coated microgranules with an internal ethylcellulose component that release budesonide at pH > 5.5. The primary site of release for budesonide (Entocort) is the ileocecal region. Thus, the most appropriate candidates for this agent are patients with ileal and/or right-sided colonic CD with mild to moderate disease severity. For induction of remission, oral budesonide is administered at 9 mg/d for 8 weeks. Some individuals advocate tapering budesonide from 9 mg daily down to 6 mg/d for additional 1 to 2 weeks and then 3 mg daily for 1 to 2 further weeks and then discontinuing therapy.*

---

†Editor's Note: Some patients with ileitis did not respond to sulfasalazine.

*Editor's Note: There are some who continue budesonide, 6 mg each morning along with mesalamine because the average remission on 6 mg/d was 7 months compared with 3 months on placebo. Calcium and vitamin D should be continued and bone density monitored.

AZA 6-MP

AZA or 6-MP is also effective as primary therapy in patients with moderately to severely active CD, regardless of disease distribution. The response rate of AZA or 6-MP therapy in controlled trials is approximately 54% (Sandborn, 1996). The delayed onset of action of up to 3 to 6 months limits its use as a single therapy in patients with severely active disease. Patients with moderate disease who are willing to tolerate active symptoms for that duration of time may be managed with AZA or 6-MP as single induction therapy. The effective dosages are generally considered to be 2.0 to 2.5 mg/kg/d for AZA and 1.0 to 1.5 mg/kg/d for 6-MP. More commonly AZA is combined with corticosteroids because corticosteroids act rapidly, and as they are being tapered the onset of action of AZA occurs. It remains controversial whether clinicians should routinely phenotype thiopurine methyltransferase (TPMT) enzyme before therapy initiation, or measure levels of active metabolites, 6-thioguanine nucleotides (6-TGN), while patients are on therapy (Cuffari et al, 1996; Dubinsky et al, 2000; Cuffari et al, 2001; Cuffari et al, 2004). If pretherapy determination of TPMT phenotype or genotype is not performed, the medication frequently is started at 50 mg/d, escalating by 25 mg every 4 to 8 weeks until reaching the target dose. Complete blood counts (CBCs) need to be monitored regardless of the status of TPMT enzyme. Similarly, liver-associated laboratory chemistries should be obtained periodically as well. Measuring erythrocyte 6-TGN levels is appropriate in patients not responding to therapy and in patients suspected of noncompliance. If metabolite levels are measured, the assay should be performed at least 2 to 3 weeks following any dose change. If metabolite levels are being followed dosage should be adjusted to achieve 6-TGN levels above 235 to 250 pmoles/8×10^8 erythrocytes.[†]

MTX

MTX is another immunomodulator used for the treatment of CD of moderate to severe activity, regardless of disease location. As an induction therapy, MTX is administered *intramuscularly* at 25 mg/week for 16 weeks (Feagan et al, 2000). MTX therapy has been shown in a clinical trial to result in complete steroid withdrawal and clinical remission in 39% of patients with active CD. The response rate was over 60% in an open label study. The onset of action is approximately 8 weeks. Similar to AZA and 6-MP, liver-associated laboratory chemistries and CBCs should be monitored every 2 to 4 weeks during induction therapy.

A chest radiograph should also be obtained to assess for the presence of a relatively uncommon side effect of hypersensitivity pneumonitis in patients with a chronic cough. See later section for maintenance therapy and discussion of elevating the doses for systematic reoccurrence.

Infliximab

The newest addition to our therapy options for patients with CD is antitumor necrosis factor therapy, *infliximab* (Sandborn and Targan, 2002). In patients with moderately to severely active CD, a single infusion of 5 mg/kg of *infliximab* (*Remicade*) results in response and remission rates of 81% and 48%, respectively, at 4 weeks (Hanauer et al, 2001). The efficacy does not appear to be influenced by the disease location. The onset of action is rapid, with response within 2 weeks of therapy and lasting approximately 8 to 12 weeks. An induction regimen with 3 infusions at weeks 0, 2, and 6 is recommended because of its superior efficacy and lower immunogenicity compared with single infusions (Hanauer et al, 2002). Most patients tolerate infliximab therapy well. Common side effects include headache, myalgia, upper respiratory tract infections, fatigue, nausea, abdominal pain, and diarrhea. Acute infusion reactions occur in approximately 6 to 16% of patients, and may present with flushing, palpitation, diaphoresis, chest pain, hypotension/hypertension, or dyspnea (Cheifetz et al, 2003). These acute reactions can usually be treated with slowing or stopping infusions, acetaminophen, antihistamine, steroids, and/or epinephrine. Delayed infusion reactions ("delayed hypersensitivity-like reactions") may develop 2 to 14 days after infusion, and are characterized by polyarthralgias, myalgias, fever, rash, and malaise. They are managed with acetaminophen, antihistamines, and steroids. Although the development of antibodies against infliximab (ATF) is associated with a higher likelihood of infusion reactions, and a shorter duration response, routine determination of antibody presence is not yet recommended and many clinicians start AZA or MTX before going to infliximab. This lessens ATF formation. Cases of active tuberculosis in patients receiving infliximab have been reported. Thus, patients should be screened for latent or active tuberculosis before starting infliximab therapy. See later section on continuous versus episodic therapy.

Cyclosporine

Alternative immunomodulatory agents may be considered in patients refractory to above therapies. Intravenous (IV) cyclosporine A may be beneficial but it use is limited by the lack of sustained response following treatment cessation and potential toxicities associated with long term therapy (Sandborn, 1996). More importantly, the absorption of cyclopsorine A is dependent on the gut motility, bowel length, intact mucosa, and the presence of bile. All these factors are likely compromised in patients with SB CD.

[†]Editor's Note: There is a separate chapter on AZA use in inflammatory bowel disease (see Chapter 69) which sites a 70% response rate if TPMT actually is less than average but only a 20 to 40% response and increased toxicity if TPMT levels are above average (Cuffari et al, 2004).

Other Immunomodulators

Tacrolimus (FK 506) has similar actions as cyclosporine. It is an alternative to cyclosporine because its bioavailability is less dependent on intact bowel mucosa and bile flow. It may be considered in patients with complicated proximal SB CD. *Mycophenolate mofetil* (CellCept) has similar properties as AZA or 6-MP, and is used primarily as an alternative immunosuppressive agent for patients with perianal disease who cannot tolerate or have failed the latter. Mycophenolate may have a faster onset of action but shorter duration than AZA or 6-MP.

Maintenance Therapy

Maintenance therapy is recommended for patients with SB CD, given the recurrent nature of CD. In addition to disease location and pattern, choice of medication depends on patient compliance and the method by which remission is achieved. The efficacy of 5-ASA compounds in maintaining medically induced remission has not been *consistently* demonstrated in controlled trials. It is presumed (not yet proven in a controlled fashion) that they are alone ineffective in maintaining remission induced by immunomodulators or infliximab. For steroid-induced remission, mesalamine (Pentasa) at 4 g/d may allow steroid withdrawal and avoid steroid dependency.

Maintenance budesonide for at least 7 months is discussed in an Editor's Note earlier. In most cases of SB CD, particularly those with extensive jejunoileitis, *immunomodulatory* therapy is necessary to maintain remission. Treatment with AZA or 6-MP therapy allows maintenance of remission in approximately 67% of patients or higher. Although maintenance of remission with continued use of AZA has been demonstrated to be effective when compared with placebo for a duration of up to 5 years, many patients continue to derive benefit from this therapy beyond 5 years. Thus, AZA or 6-MP maintenance should probably be continued indefinitely unless therapy fails or patients have significant concerns regarding long term therapy.

MTX

MTX is another immunomodulatory agent that has been shown to be effective for maintaining medically induced remission (Feagan et al, 2000). The dose of MTX for maintenance therapy (15 mg/week intramuscularly) is lower than that for induction therapy. Approximately 65% of patients remain in remission at 40 weeks on such a therapy. Returning the dosage to 25 mg 1 month weekly for a number of weeks has restored remission in some patients.

Infliximab

In patients who respond to an initial infliximab infusion, repeated therapy every 8 weeks allows maintenance of remission in 28 to 38% of patients at 1 year (Hanauer et al, 2002). Although *concurrent immunosuppressive therapy* minimizes the formation of antibodies against infliximab, thereby possibly decreasing the risk of infusion reactions and prolonging the duration of response, this combination therapy theoretically may result in a greater risk of infectious complications. The optimal strategy is currently unknown (Sandborn, 2003). Owing to the issue of immunogenecity, however, maintenance therapy with infliximab administered on a regular basis instead of on demand is recommended, even if concurrent immunosuppressive therapy is employed.

In general, for patients with SB CD that require an immunosuppressant or infliximab to induce remission, therapy is continued for maintenance purpose once remission is achieved. In patients with steroid-induced remission, maintenance therapy with immunomodulatory agents or infliximab should be considered if they have had recurrent flares or if the SB disease is extensive. Traditional corticosteroids should not be used as long term therapy. Maintenance therapy with oral budesonide at 6 mg/d may increase the duration of remission, but this benefit appears to be only for short term and has not been consistently demonstrated in clinical trials. Because prolonged use of budesonide can also result in untoward toxicities as with traditional corticosteroids, budesonide maintenance therapy should be reserved for patients in whom remission cannot be maintained with other agents and surgery is not an option.[‡]

Postresection

In patients with *surgically induced remission*, mesalamine is beneficial in some patients in preventing postoperative recurrence in patients with SB CD. 6-MP at 50 mg/d may also be effective and may be superior to mesalamine (Achkar and Hanauer, 2000). Use of higher doses of 6-MP or AZA is probably appropriate but has not been adequately evaluated. Although no controlled studies have been reported for MTX and infliximab as postsurgical maintenance therapy, these agents might be considered in individuals with recurrent SB disease requiring surgery and with risk factors for early postoperative recurrence (eg, penetrating indication for initial surgery, and longer preoperative disease duration), who have failed or are intolerant of mesalamine or AZA/6-MP maintenance therapy.

Steroid-Sparing Therapy

An important aspect of managing patients with CD is minimizing steroid use. Because more than half of patients become either *steroid-resistant* or *steroid-dependent* at 1

[‡]Editor's Note: I personally use mesalamine plus budesonide plus calcium and vitamin D and follow bone density.

year after an initial course of steroid therapy, specific strategies focusing on steroid sparing need to be considered early in the management of these patients. Corticosteroid therapy should be tapered off once a good response is achieved. We typically taper steroids at a rate of 5 mg equivalent of prednisone every 1 to 2 weeks. Other standard medical therapies should be initiated before taking steroids or if disease flares up upon steroid withdrawal. *Mesalamine* (Pentasa) at 4 g/d may allow steroid-withdrawal and decrease steroid dependency following steroid-induced remission. Agents that have been shown to have steroid-sparing benefit include *AZA, 6-MP, MTX,* and *infliximab.* In pediatric population where growth retardation from corticosteroids is of particular concern, initiation of 6-MP concurrent with steroid therapy at the initial diagnosis has been recommended by some. There is a separate chapter on inflammatory bowel disease therapy in children and adolescents (see Chapter 67, "Therapeutic Strategies in Pediatric Crohn's Disease"). In general, we recommend considering steroid-sparing therapy in patients with at least 1 recurrence, particularly if the recurrence is severe and is within 1 year from the previous flare.

Jejunoileitis

Patients with *jejunoileitis* tend to be of younger age and have a more indolent course. Most patients will eventually require surgical management. Given its indolent course, steroid-sparing and preservation of bowel to minimize long term complications are critical. The use of immunomodulators or infliximab should be considered early in the disease course in these patients.

Nutritional Therapy

The role of nutritional therapy as a primary therapy for CD is controversial. There is no convincing control-trial evidence that enteral nutrition (EN) alone is effective for the treatment of active CD, and there appears to be no difference between elemental and nonelemental diets. Furthermore, both elemental and semi-elemental diets are nonpalatable and patients are unlikely to be compliant with this therapy. They may be considered in patients where other therapies, either medical or surgical, are not effective or not desired. See section below and separate chapter on enteral or parenteral therapy as an adjuvant (see Chapter 54, "Enteral and Parenteral Nutrition").

The use of growth hormone (somatotropin) in combination with nutritional therpay may be beneficial in patients with active CD, particularly in children with steroid-dependent disease. In a preliminary randomized, double blind, placebo controlled study, growth hormone was administered subcutaneously at 5 mg/d for 1 week followed by a maintenance dose of 1.5 mg/d for 4 months, while the patients increased their protein intake to > 2 g per kg of body weight per day (Slonim et al, 2000). Whether this benefit will hold up in large, randomized controlled study and the long term effect of growth hormone therapy still need to be examined.

EN, however, is an adjunct in the management of CD. This is particularly important in children or adolescents, and in patients with SB CD and compromised nutritional status. Avoidance of lactose-containing foods may be beneficial in some but not all patients. Patients with symptomatic fibrostenotic disease should be instructed to avoid high residue diets. Patients who are placed on bowel rest because of penetrating or obstructive disease should receive parenteral nutrition (PN). Routine PN supplement has no role in SB CD if patients are able to tolerate EN and maintain adequate nutrition (Ostro et al, 1985). Prolonged bowel rest and PN may be required in a small group of patients with multiple SB strictures, fistulas, and/or complications of medical therapy who are not surgical candidates. In these patients with essentially gut failure, home total parenteral nutrition (TPN) is necessary not as a primary therapy but to provide nutritional support. Whether SB transplantation may be beneficial in these patients still needs to be seen.

Surgical Therapy for SB CD

In general, surgery for CD is reserved for failure of medical therapy, intolerance to or toxicities from medical therapy, or complications of CD. Complications that may require surgical interventions include obstruction, fistulas, and abscess. Less commonly patients with SB CD may have cancerous or precancerous lesions present. When determining the need for surgery, it is important to recognize that the sequelae of chronic disease may manifest as symptoms resembling typical exacerbations of CD. On the other hand, complications such as fibrotic strictures are not amendable to medical therapy and should be managed surgically.

The overriding principle to surgery for SB CD is to minimize the length of bowel resection. Because clinical relapses occur in 20 to 40% of patients within 1 year and up to 85% at 3 years after surgery, the risk of short-gut syndrome is a serious concern in patients with SB CD. Segmental resection is performed for active SB disease. Although SB stricture can be managed with resection, stricturoplasty is an option for fibrotic strictures and has the advantage of preserving that segment of bowel (Fazio and Galandiuk, 1985). Patients with intra-abdominal fistula or abscess require surgical draining of abscess along with antibiotics, followed by resection after several weeks.

Management of Complications of SB CD

Fistulas and Abscesses

The major complications of perforating disease are fistulas and abscesses. Fistulas complicating SB CD are most commonly internal fistulas, or communications between two segments of bowel or between a segment of bowel and another organ. These fistulas in SB CD usually arise from terminal ileum. The most common enteroenteric fistulas are ileosigmoid fistulas, but ileoileal can occur. When enteroenteric fistulas are proximal or bypass a long segment of the SB, the fistula output will be greater and patients often develop malabsorption with diarrhea and weight loss. These symptomatic fistulas are typically seen with ileojejunal fistulas. In contrast, ileoileal or ileosigmoid fistulas are often asymptomatic and do not lead to malnutrition.

Fistulas arising from underlying CD rarely close spontaneously. Symptomatic fistulas can be managed medically or surgically. Mesalamine derivatives and corticosteroids are not effective for closing fistulas. Medications that can be used for managing CD fistulas, include immunomodulators such as *AZA, 6-MP, cyclosporine,* and *tacrolimus, infliximab,* and *antibiotics*. It should be noted that the data on the use of these agents for fistulizing disease are primarily for perianal fistulas, complications typically seen in patients with Crohn's colitis. The best available data for enteroenteric fistulas among these agents come from an uncontrolled report using 6-MP (Korelitz and Present, 1985). A course of bowel rest and TPN is often employed, although its benefit in closing fistula has not been consistently demonstrated. However, bowel rest temporarily decreases the output through the fistulas and improved nutritional status with PN may decrease postoperative complications. *Octeotide*, a somatostatin analogue, may be attempted in patients with high outpatient SB fistulas. In general, medical therapy alone is not sufficient, and surgery is often necessary. However, medical therapy decreases the associated inflammation and allows resection of shorter segments of bowel. Surgical resection of the fistulas and involved bowel is indicated for symptomatic fistulas refractory to conservative therapy. It should be noted that postoperative fistulas, in contrast to fistulas secondary to CD, usually respond to conservative therapy without surgery, including antibiotics, bowel rest, PN, and local wound care.

Abscesses complicating SB CD are usually intraabdominal, but retroperitoneal extension can also occur. Management of abscesses consists of antibiotics and percutaneous aspiration and drainage whenever possible. Patients should be placed on bowel rest and TPN. Oral diet may be initiated when the drainage output diminishes. Definitive surgery is usually performed after the abscess has been completely drained and the underlying CD is controlled on medications. However, early surgery may be necessary if percutaneous drainage of the abscess is not feasible or if there is evidence of peritonitis.

Obstruction

Obstruction is another common complication of SB CD. It is important, but may be difficult to differentiate, whether the stricture is due to bowel wall thickening from active inflammation or fibrosis from repeated healing process. In addition, obstruction may be secondary to adhesions, especially in CD patients who often have had prior abdominal surgery. The first line therapy should be conservative measure, with *bowel rest, nasogastric decompression,* and *IV hydration*. Medical therapy should be initiated if there is evidence of active CD. An empiric course of medical therapy is appropriate when the contribution of active inflammation to the obstruction is unclear. Patients who fail to respond to medical therapy likely have a significant fibrotic component to their stricture and require surgical therapy. Patients with mild stricturing and intermittent partial obstruction should be instructed to avoid high residue diet, and may be managed as outpatients by a brief course of clear diet or bowel rest. Recurrent obstruction despite optimal medical therapy is an indication for surgery. Surgical options for stricture include resection of the involved segment or stricturoplasty as mentioned before. There is a separate chapter on dilatation of strictures (see Chapter 85, "Intestinal and Colonic Strictures").

Nutritional Deficiency

Patients with SB CD often develop specific nutritional deficits in addition to overall malnutrition. The use of EN or PN as CD therapy or nutritional support was discussed earlier. The most common problem is anemia, which is often multifactorial in etiology. Deficiency in *iron, vitamin B_{12},* and *folate* may contribute to the development of anemia. Etiologies for these deficiencies include chronic GI blood loss, inadequate dietary iron intake or absorption, *vitamin B_{12} malabsorption* secondary to terminal ileal disease or resection, and *folate* deficiency as a result of proximal SB disease or sulfasalazine therapy. These nutritional deficiencies should be sought out and appropriately supplemented.

Calcium and Osteoporosis

Another common nutritional problem in patients with SB CD is *calcium* and *vitamin* D deficiency. Calcium deficiency is usually caused by a combination of malabsorption from the SB disease and low dietary intake. Factors contributing to the development of vitamin D deficiency include inadequate dietary intake, lack of sun exposure, fat malabsorption, and disruption of the enterohepatic circulation of vitamin D metabolites. These nutritional deficiencies may result in a number of metabolic bone complications, including *osteopenia, osteoporosis,* and *osteomalacia*. Patients with SB CD, particularly if they have metabolic bone disorders, are recommended to take supplements of calcium 1.5 g/d and vitamin D 800 U/d. There is a separate chapter on metabolic bone disease (see Chapter 55, "Metabolic Bone Disease in Gastrointestinal and Liver Patients").

Short Bowel Syndrome

Extensive bowel resections in patients with SB CD may lead to *short bowel syndrome*. Patients with < 200 cm of functioning SB are at risk for developing short bowel syndrome. Management of these patients should be focused on providing adequate nutrition, including both macro- and micronutrients, and preventing and correcting complications associated with short bowel syndrome. Common complications include the development of nephrolithiasis (calcium oxalate and uric acid stones), cholelithiasis, bacterial overgrowth, and liver disease associated with PN. Patients with oxalate stones should be placed on a low oxalate diet and increase fluid intake and take calcium supplements. There are separate chapters on "Short Bowel Syndrome (Chapter 64) and SB transplantation (see Chapter 65, "Intestinal and Multivisceral Transplantation").

Supplemental Reading

Abreu MT, Taylor KD, Lin YC, et al. Mutations in *NOD2* are associated with fibrostenosing disease in patients with Crohn's disease. Gastroenterol 2002;123:679–88.

Achkar JP, Hanauer SB. Medical therapy to reduce postoperative Crohn's disease recurrence. Am J Gastroenterol 2000;95:1139–46.

Brant SR, Picco MF, Achkar JP, et al. Defining complex contributions of *NOD2/CARD15* gene mutations, age at onset, and tobacco use on Crohn's disease phenotypes. Inflamm Bowel Dis 2003;9:281–9.

Campieri M, Ferguson A, Doe W, et al. Oral budesonide is as effective as oral prednisolone in active Crohn's disease. The Global Budesonide Study Group. Gut 1997;41:209–14.

Cheifetz A, Smedley M, Martin S, et al. The incidence and management of infusion reactions to infliximab: a large center experience. Am J Gastroenterol 2003;98:1315–24.

Cuffari C, Dassopoulos T, Turnbough L, et al. Thio methyltransferase activity affects clinical responses to azathioprine therapy in inflammatory bowel disease. Clin Gastro Hepatology, 2004:410–7.

Cuffari C, Hunt S, Bayless TM. Utilization of erythrocyte 6-thioquanine metabolite levels to optimize anathioprine therapy in patients with inflammatory bowel disease. Gut 2001;48:591–2.

Cuffari C, Theoret Y, Latour S, Seidman G. 6-mercaptopurine metabolism in Crohn's disease: correlation with efficacy and toxicity. Gut 1996;39:401–6.

Cuthbert AP, Fisher SA, Mirza MM, et al. The contribution of *NOD2* gene mutations to the risk and site of disease in inflammatory bowel disease. Gastroenterol 2002;122:867–74.

Dubinsky MC, Lamothe S, Yang HY, et al. Pharmacogenomics and metabolite measurement for 6-mercaptopurine therapy in inflammatory bowel disease. Gastroenterol 2000;118:705–13.

Fazio VW, Galandiuk S. Strictureplasty in diffuse Crohn's jejunoileitis. Dis Colon Rectum 1985;28:512–8.

Feagan BG, Fedorak RN, Irvine EJ, et al. A comparison of methotrexate with placebo for the maintenance of remission in Crohn's disease. North American Crohn's Study Group Investigators. N Engl J Med 2000;342:1627–32.

Feagan BG, Rochon J, Fedorak RN, et al. Methotrexate for the treatment of Crohn's disease. The North American Crohn's Study Group Investigators. N Engl J Med 1995;332:292–7.

Greenberg GR, Feagan BG, Martin F, et al. Oral budesonide for active Crohn's disease. Canadian Inflammatory Bowel Disease Study Group. N Engl J Med 1994;331:836–41.

Greenberg GR, Fleming CR, Jeejeebhoy KN, et al. Controlled trial of bowel rest and nutritional support in the management of Crohn's disease. Gut 1988;29:1309–15.

Hanauer SB, Feagan BG, Lichtenstein GR, et al. Maintenance infliximab for Crohn's disease: the ACCENT I randomised trial. Lancet 2002;359:1541–9.

Hanauer SB, Sandborn W. Management of Crohn's disease in adults. Am J Gastroenterol 2001;96:635–43.

Korelitz BI, Present DH. Favorable effect of 6-mercaptopurine on fistulae of Crohn's disease. Dig Dis Sci 1985;30:58–64.

Ostro MJ, Greenberg GR, Jeejeebhoy KN. Total parenteral nutrition and complete bowel rest in the management of Crohn's disease. JPEN 1985;9:280–7.

Rutgeerts P, Lofberg R, Malchow H, et al. A comparison of budesonide with prednisolone for active Crohn's disease. N Engl J Med 1994;331:842–5.

Sandborn WJ, Targan SR. Biologic therapy of inflammatory bowel disease. Gastroenterol 2002;122:1592–608.

Sandborn WJ. A review of immune modifier therapy for inflammatory bowel disease: azathioprine, 6-mercaptopurine, cyclosporine, and methotrexate. Am J Gastroenterol 1996;91:423–33.

Sandborn WJ. Preventing antibodies to infliximab in patients with Crohn's disease: optimize not immunize. Gastroenterol 2003;124:1140–5.

Slonim AE, Bulone L, Damore MB, et al. A preliminary study of growth hormone therapy for Crohn's disease. N Engl J Med 2000;342:1633–7.

Stein RB, Lichtenstein GR. Medical therapy for Crohn's disease: the state of the art. Surg Clin North Am 2001;81:71–101.

Targan SR, Hanauer SB, van Deventer SJ, et al. A short-term study of chimeric monoclonal antibody cA2 to tumor necrosis factor alpha for Crohn's disease. Crohn's Disease cA2 Study Group. N Engl J Med 1997;337:1029–35.

Thomsen OO, Cortot A, Jewell D, et al. A comparison of budesonide and mesalamine for active Crohn's disease. International Budesonide-Mesalamine Study Group. N Engl J Med 1998;339:370–4.

CHAPTER 67

THERAPEUTIC STRATEGIES IN PEDIATRIC CROHN'S DISEASE

ANTHONY P. OLIVÉ, MD, AND GEORGE D. FERRY, MD

The child with Crohn's disease (CD) poses special challenges for all involved, including parents, extended family, school personnel, and medical caretakers. The unique psychosocial and physical changes encountered during childhood and adolescence make this period of time quite vulnerable to the many complications associated with this disease. The resulting physical and emotional scars can be permanent, with lasting repercussions into one's adult life. As such, the therapeutic goals in pediatric CD can be broken down into the following three basic principles: (1) promote physical growth and development, (2) promote psychosocial growth, and (3) promote and improve quality of life. The strategies employed to achieve these goals are diverse and tailored to the individual, and include traditional medical and surgical approaches, nutritional therapies, psychological counseling, peer interaction opportunities, and aggressive involvement of the child's family and caretakers. Surgical approaches will not be included in this chapter.

Medical Therapies

Because of their state of ongoing physical and psychosocial growth, children and adolescents are quite vulnerable to side effects of the medications used to control CD, particularly corticosteroids. Our strategy is thus to minimize corticosteroid exposure by using more aggressive maintenance therapies earlier in the course of disease. Nutritional therapy with enteral formulas is an alternative method to induce remission and avoid the use of corticosteroids, but our patients are relatively resistant to this strategy because of the need to use a nasogastric (NG) tube in most cases. The rapid development of novel new therapies brings hope that alternatives to corticosteroids will soon be available as first line therapies for CD.

Corticosteroids

Corticosteroids in childhood CD are very effective in controlling the inflammatory state and inducing clinical remission. Children and adolescents, however, are adversely affected by the growth-suppressing and cosmetic side effects of corticosteroids. Avoiding repeated use of corticosteroids is thus optimal but problematic due to relatively high relapse rates. Our tendency has been to use more aggressive immunomodulator maintenance therapy earlier in the course of moderate to severe disease in the hopes of reducing long term steroid exposure. Although antibiotics are used in the initial therapy of moderate to severe disease, there is currently little data to support their use.

Tumor necrosis factor-α antibody might also be an alternative, but long-term effects are not yet known. The use of 5-aminosalicylic acid (ASA) drugs to induce and maintain remission has been successful in mild distal CD. However, many of our patients do not respond, or may relapse frequently, and will need corticosteroids.

Budesonide

The introduction of *budesonide* has created both an interest and an expectation that children with ileocecal CD might have a prompt response without, or at least with fewer, corticosteroid side effects. Due to rapid hepatic first pass metabolism of budesonide, systemic side effects are significantly reduced (but not eliminated) relative to other corticosteroids. A recent publication has looked at budesonide in pediatric CD (Table 67-1) (Levine et al, 2003). In this prospective study, budesonide 9 mg/d was compared with prednisone 40 mg/d in children with acute flares of mild to moderate ileal or ileocolonic CD. The remission rate at 12 weeks was 47% versus 50%, respectively, with medication-related side effects seen in 32% of the budesonide group versus 71% of the prednisone group. We are currently using budesonide in children with flares of ileal or ileocecal disease. We have not used it as maintenance therapy because of the potential for greater steroid side effects with long term use, including the potential for growth suppression.*

Salicylates

The efficacy of 5-ASA products, either as mesalamine encapsulated in a controlled-release form (Asacol, Pentasa), or bound via azo bond to an inert compound (balsalazide)

---

*Editor's Note: Because growth velocity is decreased in as many as 90% of prebuscent adolescents with CD, restoration of growth velocity is a key goal. Suppressing all signs of disease activity, providing adequate calories, and avoiding daily steroid use are components of successful therapy.

TABLE 67-1. Prednisone versus Budesonide in Active Crohn's Disease

	Budesonide (n = 19)	Prednisone (n = 14)
Initial dose	9 mg/d	40 mg/d
Remission at 12 weeks	9 (47%)	7 (50%)
Patient with medication side effects	6 (32%)	10 (71%)

Adapted from Levine et al, 2003.

or to a sulfapyridine group (sulfasalazine) or to itself (olsalazine), in mild to moderate CD is well documented in the adult literature. Despite paucity of data in pediatrics, these drugs have attained widespread use for these indications in our patient population. In a small prospective study, children with CD radiologically confined to the small intestine seemed to benefit from controlled-release mesalamine therapy (Griffiths et al, 1993). Our practice is to use these agents in mild disease, both acutely to induce remission as well as chronically to maintain remission. Patients that develop recurrent relapses and need for corticosteroids while on 5-ASA maintenance therapy are typically moved to immunomodulator maintenance therapy (Table 67-2).

Azathioprine and Mercaptopurine

We use these immunomodulators in corticosteroid-refractory and corticosteroid-dependent CD, and as first line therapy in combination with corticosteroids in moderate to severe disease. We have also used these successfully in perianal CD, either initially in more severe disease or when antibiotic therapy has failed in mild to moderate disease. A pediatric study by Markowitz and colleagues (2000) showed that the use of 6-mercaptopurine (6-MP) at the onset of therapy with corticosteroids in moderate to severe luminal CD resulted in relapse rates that were markedly reduced over 12 to 18 months (4% versus 28% at 12 months; 9% versus 47% at 18 months) compared with corticosteroids alone. Starting azathioprine (AZA) or 6-MP early in the course of CD is now a strategy we employ routinely, especially in children with extensive disease, growth failure, or other complications.

To monitor for toxicity, we typically follow complete blood counts (CBCs) and liver function tests every 1 to 2 weeks until stable for 1 month, then every 1 to 3 months after that. MP metabolite levels are not routinely ordered, except in individuals who are recurrently flaring, to check compliance and to see if the dose can be adjusted upward, or in individuals who display laboratory abnormalities in whom we suspect 6-MP. Besides bone marrow suppression and hepatotoxicity, we have seen pancreatitis and a rare opportunistic infection related to the use of immunomodulators.

Methotrexate

Methotrexate (MTX) is used in our pediatric population for steroid unresponsive or dependent patients despite the addition of 6-MP/AZA, or in children intolerant of 6-MP/AZA. Its effectiveness in this setting has been described in children.

There is extensive literature on the efficacy and safety of MTX in pediatric rheumatology and there is growing acceptance of its use in children with CD (Mack et al 1998; Woo et al, 2000; Giannini et al, 1992; Ravelli et al, 1998). Although uncommon, the potential risk of hepatic fibrosis with advancing accumulated dose should be monitored. Potential bone marrow toxicity and interstitial pneumonitis are also a concern. Dosing in children involves *weekly parenteral administration*, either via subcutaneous or intramuscular injection. Taking MTX orally often leads to intolerable *nausea* and absorption is variable, but no studies have been done in children comparing oral MTX with parenteral use for maintenance therapy in CD. Parenteral MTX has the added benefit of improved compliance. Because the mechanism of action of MTX is via inhibition of folate metabolism, supplementation with *folate* at a dose of 1 mg/d is a recommended. We typically dose MTX at weekly subcutaneous injections of 10 mg (for 20–29 kg of body weight), 15 mg (30–39 kg), 20 mg (40–49 kg), or 25 mg (> 50 kg) and give 50% of this dose the first week, 75% the next week, and the full dose by the third week if tolerated. Our maximum dose is 25 mg in children over 50 kg in weight. The dose can be gradually reduced after steroid withdrawal is achieved. We monitor the CBCs and alanine aminotransferase (ALT) weekly for the first 4 weeks then every 2 months, if stable. The dose is reduced by 50% for an ALT greater than 2 times baseline, white blood cells (WBC) < 4,000, absolute neutrophil count (ANC) < 1,500, or platelet count < 120,000. The dose is held for ALT > 3 times baseline, WBC < 3,000, ANC < 1,000, or platelet count < 100,000. Additionally, a chest radiograph and pulmonary function test are obtained if a child has a nonproductive cough for longer than 1 week and might be considered annually for patients on a maintenance regimen. Liver biopsy is considered when accumulated lifetime dose exceeds 1.5 g, but the data is not available to say this is necessary. Adolescent girls of childbearing age are educated about the potential *teratogenic effects* of MTX and appropriate contraceptive measures.

Infliximab

The use of infliximab in pediatric CD, both for luminal as well as perianal disease, is now widespread. For luminal disease, we have used it primarily in disease that is steroid-resistant or dependent despite the use of immunosuppressants. For perianal disease, we have used it for cases unresponsive or intolerant to antibiotics and 6-MP/AZA.

The side effect profile of infliximab has been well described through previous adult clinical trials. In children, infusion reactions may be present in as many as 10% of infusions (Crandall and Mackner, 2003). Acute infusion reactions typically involve symptoms such as flushing, headaches, tachycardia, chest tightness, and overall anxiety, and they usually resolve by stopping the infusion. Once symptoms resolve, most patients will tolerate a slower rate of infusion. Because of the frequency of this type of reaction, we routinely administer acetaminophen 15 mg/kg by mouth (650 mg maximum) and diphenhydramine 1 mg/kg by mouth (50 mg maximum) as premedication before the infusion. More severe reactions during an infusion are rare but do happen, and typically involve oxygen desaturation and hypotension. These require more aggressive resuscitative efforts, including administration of supplemental oxygen, epinephrine, and hydrocortisone. The delayed hypersensitivity reactions typically present within a few days to 2 weeks after the infusion, and may involve myalgia, arthralgia, rash, fever, headache, and fatigue. These reactions may not be as common in children as in adults (Kugathasan et al, 2002). We have not seen this complication. The optimal dosing schedule for infliximab is as yet an unresolved issue, and the diversity of approaches in clinical practice reflects this. We generally give 3 infusions at the start of therapy at 0, 2, and 6 to 8 weeks. After this, however, the strategy becomes less clear on longer term therapy, with some opting for scheduled therapy and others for episodic retreatment. Episodic retreatment greater than 20 weeks after the initial infusion appears to be associated with a higher incidence of infusion reactions in adult, but not pediatric, patients. As with adults, we maintain our patients on immunomodulators to reduce the risk of allergic reaction and increasing length of response.[†]

Antibiotics

The use of antibiotics in pediatric CD has been guided primarily by evidence from adult studies, but this evidence is not strong and there are no pediatric studies. We have used antibiotics (generally metronidazole or ciprofloxacin) primarily for mild to moderate acute Crohn's colitis or ileocolitis, as well as for perianal disease. The use of antibiotics for maintenance of remission in CD in children has not been studied, but we often use these agents for 6 to 12 months.

Future Therapies

The genetic and molecular advances being made in CD research have given hope for a brighter future regarding the therapeutic options for CD in children. For example, mutations in the *NOD2* gene on chromosome 16 have been associated with disease that is of early onset, ileal in location, and fibrostenosing and fistulizing in character (Brant et al, 2003; Cuthbert et al, 2002; Heilo et al, 2003; Lesage et al, 2003). As more gene mutations are discovered and linked to specific phenotypes, further stratification into therapeutic response categories may be possible. Ultimately, specific gene or protein replacement therapy may come to the forefront in the management of CD.

Nutritional Therapies

Existing data supports the use of primary nutritional therapy in pediatric CD and suggests equal efficacy to corticosteroids but with better growth and development and fewer side effects (Heuschkel et al, 2000). We occasionally use nutritional therapy in the form of 1 Cal/mL liquid formulas in children as the sole therapy for acute flares but more commonly in a supplemental role with other primary therapies. The volume of formula needed is often far greater than patients will take orally, thus necessitating nighttime NG feeds. Many patients cannot accept this. For maintenance of remission, given the high rate of relapse after sole primary nutritional therapy, support has been shown for the continuation of enteral nutrition as a nocturnal supplement to an otherwise normal daytime diet in children (Wilschanski et al, 1996). The further question of whether the enteral liquid formula should be elemental or polymeric is unclear, but currently there is no evidence to support that one is more efficacious than the other (Rigaud

Table 67-2. Therapy for Crohn's Disease

Mild to moderate active CD
   5-ASA drug–oral and/or rectal for active disease
   Antibiotics–for distal disease and fistulas
   Corticosteroids (budesonide) for active disease
   6-MP/AZA for corticosteroid resistance or dependence
   Methotrexate for 6-MP/AZA resistance or intolerance (less commonly used)
   Anti–TNF-α antibody in corticosteroid resistant patients, in fistulizing disease, in place of corticosteroids; after and with immunomodulators
Severe Crohn's disease
   Corticosteroids
   Anti–TNF-α antibody
   6-MP/AZA
   Elemental diet or TPN–provides nutritional support and may directly lead to decreased inflammation
Maintenance therapy
   5-ASA, 6-MP/AZA, MTX, Anti–TNF-α antibody in selected patients

5-ASA = aminosalicylic acid; AZA = azathioprine; CD = Crohn's disease; MP = mercaptopurine; MTX = methotrexate; TNF = tumor necrosis factor; TPN = total parenteral nutrition.

[†]Editor's Note: The steps to avoid the development of antibodies to infliximab include (1) induction doses at 0, 2, and 6 weeks, (2) concomitant use of immunomodulators, and (3) continuous rather than episodic dosing (TMB).

et al, 1991). In selected patients where there is an acute need for nutritional support, total parenteral nutrition (TPN) has a role and has been shown to enhance linear growth significantly (Keller and Wirth, 1992).Examples where we have used TPN include extensive small bowel disease, bowel obstruction or situations in which eliminating the fecal stream is desireable, such as fulminant colitis, fistulizing disease, or severe perianal disease.

Probiotics

Interest in probiotics has stemmed from the accumulating suggestive evidence that bacterial products play a role in the pathogenesis of inflammatory bowel disease (IBD) (Kleessen et al, 2002; Martin and Rhodes, 2000; Schultsz et al, 1999) and that certain "beneficial" bacteria may have anti-inflammatory properties (Borruel et al, 2002). A small pilot study looked at four children with mild to moderate CD treated with *Lactobacillus GG* and showed significant improvement in mucosal permeability and clinical activity over the 6-month study period (Gupta et al, 2000). Little other data is available on pediatric CD. Despite this, many of our patients are using probiotics and other complementary and alternative therapies. There is a separate chapter on alternative medicines (Chapter 58, "Complementary and Alternative Medicine in Gastrointestinal Disease"). Probiotics are discussed in chapters on ulcerative colitis (Chapter 78, "Ulcerative Colitis") and on pouchitis.

Dietary Counseling

Input from our dietitians not only serves to reinforce dietary advice we have given patients, but also gives the patients and families another source of expertise they can draw from. Generally speaking, children with active disease are placed on fiber- and residue-restricted diets. To avoid the common misperception that the patient is condemned to this diet for life, we emphasize to our patients early on that the diet can be liberalized as they improve. Lactose intolerance is another issue and is fairly common in children with CD and is included in discussions with our patients. The ethnic distribution of lactose intolerance and management in children, and adults, is discussed in a separate chapter (see Chaper 62, "Lactose Intolerance"). The main emphasis in children is to insure adequate nutrition for growth.

Psychosocial Therapies

Formal Psychological Counseling

Childhood and adolescence are unique times that make the individual quite vulnerable psychosocially. Most children with a chronic illness such as CD will periodically benefit from formal psychological assessment and counseling. A psychologist is available to see our patients at the time of the visit or, if more convenient, at a later date in the psychologist's office. Opportunities for less structured interactions exist as well.

Informal Peer Interaction Opportunities

Many opportunities exist for patients and families to interact and share experiences. Often this is the most effective approach, particularly for adolescents who may feel encumbered by the structured setting of a psychologist's office. A great deal of anxiety can be relieved as they and their families come to realize that others with IBD are leading normal and productive lives. We have "sleep over" events for adolescents, holiday parties for patients and families, a camp for patients and siblings, and a "Patient Education Day" for families that consists of formal lectures on a wide variety of IBD topics.[‡]

Family Participation Strategies

One of the most important strategies in the approach to children with CD is education of family members and any other caretakers. Children, unlike adults, often rely on others to adhere to the prescribed therapy. Although we like our patients to take this responsibility themselves, maturity and intelligence varies between patients. Educating family members and caretakers about the natural course and therapies for CD heightens their level of awareness and ultimately translates into improved compliance. This education is an ongoing and gradual process with the ultimate goal of promoting independence and a smooth transition to adulthood.[§]

Supplemental Reading

Borruel N, Carol M, Casellas F, et al. Increased mucosal tumour necrosis factor alpha production in Crohn's disease can be downregulated ex vivo by probiotic bacteria. Gut 2002;51:659–64.

Brant SR, Picco MF, Achkar JP, Bayless TM, et al. Defining complex contributions of NODz/CARD15 gene mutations, age at onset and tobacco use in Crohn's Disease phenotypes. Inflamm Bowel Dis 2003;9:281–9.

Crandall WV, Mackner LM. Infusion reactions to infliximab in children and adolescents: frequency, outcome and a predictive model. Aliment Pharmacol Ther 2003;17:75–84.

Cuthbert AP, Fisher SA, Mirza MM, et al. The contribution of NOD2 gene mutations to the risk and site of disease in inflammatory bowel disease. Gastroenterol 2002;4:867–74.

[‡]Editor's Note: The Crohn's Colitis Foundation sponsors various support groups through many of their chapters.

[§]Editor's Note: This is a nicely balanced and very useful chapter (TMB).

Giannini EH, Brewer EJ, Kuzmina N, et al. Methotrexate in resistant juvenile rheumatoid arthritis. Results of the USA-USSR double-blind, placebo-controlled trial. The Pediatric Rheumatology Collaborative Study Group and The Cooperative Children's Study Group. N Engl J Med 1992;326:1043–9.

Griffiths A, Koletzko S, Sylvester F, et al. Slow-release 5-aminosalicylic acid therapy in children with small intestinal Crohn's disease. J Pediatr Gastroenterol Nutr 1993;17:186–92.

Gupta P, Andrew H, Kirschner BS, et al. Is lactobacillus GG helpful in children with Crohn's disease? Results of a preliminary, open-label study. J Pediatr Gastroenterol Nutr 2000;31:453–7.

Heilo T, Halme L, Lappalainen M, et al. CARD15/NOD2 gene variants are associated with familially occurring and complicated forms of Crohn's disease. Gut 2003;4:558–62.

Heuschkel RB, Menache CC, Megerian JT, et al. Enteral nutrition and corticosteroids in the treatment of acute Crohn's disease in children. J Pediatr Gastroenterol Nutr 2000;31:8–15.

Kanoff ME, Lakes M, and Bayless TM. Decreased height velocity in children and adolescents before the diagnosis of Crohn's disease. Gastroenterol 1980;95:1523–7.

Keller KM, Wirth S. [Parenteral nutrition in treatment of short stature in adolescents with Crohn disease]. Klin Padiatr 1992;204:411–6.

Kleessen B, Kroesen AJ, Buhr HJ, et al. Mucosal and invading bacteria in patients with inflammatory bowel disease compared with controls. Scand J Gastroenterol 2002;37:1034–41.

Kugathasan S, Levy MB, Saeian K, et al. Infliximab retreatment in adults and children with Crohn's disease: risk factors for the development of delayed severe systemic reaction. Am J Gastroenterol 2002;97:1408–14.

Lesage S, Zouali H, Cezard JP, et al. CARD15/NOD2 mutational analysis and genotype-phenotype correlation in 612 patients with inflammatory bowel disease. Am J Hum Genet 2003;4:845–57.

Levine A, Weizman Z, Broide E, et al. A comparison of budesonide and prednisone for the treatment of active pediatric Crohn's disease. J Pediatr Gastroenterol Nutr 2003;36:248–57.

Mack DR, Young R, Kaufman SS, et al. Methotrexate in patients with Crohn's disease after 6-mercaptopurine. J Pediatr 1998;132:830–5.

Markowitz J, Grancher K, Kohn N, et al. A multicenter trial of 6-mercaptopurine and prednisone in children with newly diagnosed Crohn's disease. Gastroenterology 2000;119:895–902.

Martin HM, Rhodes JM. Bacteria and inflammatory bowel disease. Curr Opin Infect Dis 2000;13:503–9.

Ravelli A, Gerloni V, Corona F, et al. Oral versus intramuscular methotrexate in juvenile chronic arthritis. Italian Pediatric Rheumatology Study Group. Clin Exp Rheumatol 1998;16:181–3.

Rigaud D, Cosnes J, Le Quintrec Y, et al. Controlled trial comparing two types of enteral nutrition in treatment of active Crohn's disease: elemental versus polymeric diet. Gut 1991;32:1492–7.

Schultsz C, Van Den Berg FM, Ten Kate FW, et al. The intestinal mucus layer from patients with inflammatory bowel disease harbors high numbers of bacteria compared with controls. Gastroenterology 1999;117:1089–97.

Whitington PF, Bannes HV, Bayless TM. Medical management of Crohn's disease in adolescence. Gastroenterol 1977;72:1338–44.

Wilschanski M, Sherman P, Pencharz P, et al. Supplementary enteral nutrition maintains remission in paediatric Crohn's disease. Gut 1996;38:543–8.

Woo P, Southwood TR, Prieur AM, et al. Randomized, placebo-controlled, crossover trial of low-dose oral methotrexate in children with extended oligoarticular or systemic arthritis. Arthritis Rheum 2000;43:1849–57.

CHAPTER 68

SURGICAL MANAGEMENT OF CROHN'S DISEASE

MARK A. TALAMINI, MD

Crohn's disease (CD) is an inflammatory condition of the bowel that can affect the gut tube anywhere from the lips to the anus. The commonest site of pathology, however, is the small bowel (SB), and this is indeed the focus of most surgical therapy. Other sites, such as the colon and the duodenum, present unique challenges.

CD is not curable with an operation. Therefore, the goal of surgical therapy is to manage complications of the disease, or improve the patient's quality of life. Thus, decision making regarding surgery is a complex exercise, requiring data and participation from multiple physicians and often, many diagnostic studies. Because the disease has a high recurrence rate, surgeons frequently have long-term professional relationships with CD patients and often operate on the same patient multiple times.

Preoperative Examination

There is perhaps no other disease in which the teamwork between the surgeon and the gastroenterologist is so important. Thus, the first step in preoperative examination is to understand the gastroenterologist's opinion regarding the state of the patient's disease. This, of course, is most effective through direct communication.

RADIOLOGY

Preoperative radiology examination has taken on additional importance with the advent of minimally invasive surgical approaches to CD. Since the surgeon's fingers may not be feeling all aspects of the bowel, knowledge regarding the portions of bowel that are likely to be diseased is particularly important.

The mainstay of preoperative examination is the contrast gastrointestinal (GI) radiograph. Most commonly this is an upper GI and SB follow-through study. Even in patients with CD limited to the colon, the SB should be studied to avoid surprises in the operating room. Consultation with the radiologist performing the study will arm the surgeon with nuances regarding the disease and the anatomy that are not obtainable from the written radiology reports. Computed tomography (CT) scanning complements the luminal study, because it provides information regarding thickening of the bowel wall and the mesentery. This is particularly true with the current ability to synthesize three-dimensional imaging from CT scan data. CT scans also provide important information regarding the possible involvement of other organs by fistulizing CD. For instance, a CT revealing a dilated ureter on the right hand side likely means that local inflammation has created a partial ureteral obstruction. This would be an important preoperative warning that dissection in this region will be dangerous, and that placement of ureteral stents should be planned.

COLONOSCOPY

All patients undergoing abdominal surgery for CD should have the colon examined, preferably via colonoscopy in the recent past, even if no colonic involvement is suspected. In general, visual inspection of the outer colonic wall at surgery will not necessarily reflect CD within the lumen. Early mucosal CD in the colon can look quite normal from the outside. For patients anticipating surgery with known involvement of the colon, colonoscopy is particularly important to map out the diseased and nondiseased segments, and to plan the appropriate procedure.

For most patients, a SB series, CT scanning, and colonoscopy will suffice. However, additional studies to answer specific questions can be very helpful. For instance, a white blood cell tagged scan can assess the degree of active inflammation in tissues affected by CD. Magnetic resonance imaging has also been reported to be helpful in this regard, but in our experience does not add significantly to the data that good CT scanning (sometimes with water for contrast rather than normal contrast agent) provides. If the patient has symptoms referable to the upper GI tract, this should be evaluated by endoscopy. The duodenum can be afflicted with primary CD involvement, or it can suffer involvement by proximity to a diseased hepatic flexure of the colon, or even an adjacent loop of diseased SB.

Preoperative Preparation

Careful preoperative preparation can make the difference between a successful CD operation and a disaster, particularly in the setting of complex severe disease. Bowel preparation with purgatives and oral antibiotics is particularly important. We bowel prepare patients with colonic disease,

TABLE 68-1. Preoperative Preparation for Crohn's Disease Surgery

Consultation with gastroenterologist
Consider possible additional Crohn's disease sites
Appropriate imaging
Nutritional repletion
Prepare for (possible) stoma
Bowel preparation/cleansing

and those with SB disease, as many of these patients have dilated partially obstructed bowel with stagnant stool predisposed to bacterial overgrowth. Patients with high grade obstruction are prepared with an extended preoperative period of a clear liquid diet (to include tube feeding formula if the duration is long), with administration of the routine oral antibiotics. Partially obstructed patients often need to undergo their bowel preparation in the hospital with the support of intravenous fluids and antiemetics.

NUTRITIONAL SUPPORT

When preoperative studies reveal significant intra-abdominal inflammation, we will often elect to treat the patient with parenteral support and bowel rest for 4 to 8 weeks. Physical examination of the abdomen can be a guide as to whether bowel rest will be of value. If the abdomen is soft and pliable to palpation, the tissues will likely be safe to dissect. If, however, the abdomen is hard and sclerotic, either locally or throughout the abdomen, the dissection is likely to be difficult. In this case, the prolonged bowel rest might avert operative complications. Parenteral support is, of course, vital in the patient with moderate to severe malnutrition. The CD patient with high grade obstruction and severe inflammation is a case, in our judgement, where parenteral support is superior to enteral support. Nutritional support increases the number of patients who can be considered for a laparoscopically assised procedure.

INFLIXAMAB

We are beginning to have some experience with inflixamib (Remicade) in the setting of surgery for inflammatory bowel disease. It appears that patients with aggressive fistulizing CD may best be prepared for surgery by a period of treatment with Remicade to minimize inflammation and "cool off" areas of extensive fistulization. Thus far, operating upon patients recently treated with Remicade does not appear to have significant risks. The experience is early, however. A few of these patients with fistulization have been left on inflixamab postoperatively.

OSTOMY NURSE

Patients who will or might need a stoma, be it temporary or permanent, need to counsel with an enterostomal therapy nurse. The nurse provides an appropriate site for the stoma, and follows the patient through their adjustment to a stoma devise.

Surgical Approach

We attempt to perform minimally invasive surgery in all CD patients, except in patients in whom we would obviously fail. Patients with many laparotomies through multiple incisions which criss cross the abdomen are not approached laparoscopically. In many instances, use of the minimally invasive equipment may only shorten the incision needed, rather than eliminate it. This is still a worthwhile goal, particularly in this group of patients who are likely to need additional incisions and operations. In our hands, a minimally invasive approach usually consists of mobilizing the target tissue laparoscopically (with three or four port sites), creating a small incision, eviscerating the target tissue, and performing an extracorporeal resection and anastamosis. Most procedures require an incision of ≤ 2 inches for evisceration. Because the terminal ileum is the most commonly affected tissue, this usually calls for mobilization of the cecum and ascending colon. In the setting of colonic disease, mobilization of the splenic and hepatic flexures, as well as dissection of the omentum away from the transverse colon can be accomplished laparoscopically. For the experienced laparoscopic surgeon, mobilization of the splenic flexure is easier to accomplish laparoscopically than in open surgery. In some patients, safe dissection of the splenic flexure through an open laparotomy incision requires a significant extension of a midline incision well above the umbilicus. Patients done laparoscopically assisted had less blood loss than those done conventionally (14 mL vs 243 mL). There was a more rapid return of bowel function (3.7 days vs 5.1 days), shorter hospitalization (5.9 days vs 8.1 days), less use of pain medications postoperatively, and a shorter recovery period (Talamini, 2001). The key to safe minimally invasive surgery is to know when to convert, and being willing to do so (which can feel like a defeat of sorts). Patients with complicated fistulizing disease and those who required preoperative total parenteral nutrition and bowel rest were most likely to need an open laparotomy.

TABLE 68-2. Indications for Surgery in Crohn's Disease

Bowel obstruction
Reduction/elimination of medicines
Fistulization
Perforation (rare)
Bleeding (rare)
Oysplasia/cancer

Intraoperative Decision Making

The most challenging decision making in the surgical treatment of CD usually occurs in the operating room. Often faced with multiple diseased areas of varying severity, the surgeon must decide what should and should not be removed. A number of factors must be considered.

If the findings are substantially different than that anticipated based upon preoperative studies, consultation in the operating room with the gastroenterologist can be extremely helpful. The general rule regarding removal of tissue is to remove the bowel that is grossly diseased. This must, of course, be balanced against the need to maintain as much viable bowel as possible, particularly because this is a disease that tends to need multiple resections over time. Usually the outer surface of the bowel is a reliable reflection of the state of mucosal disease. So, the surgeon can assume that bowel which is soft and pliable, and without mesenteric thickening, is normal. There is no need for a "margin" of normal tissue. Similarly, there is no need for frozen section analysis of the removed bowel (Hamilton et al, 1985). It is important for the surgical team to examine the gross specimen to be sure that the removed bowel has mucosal which appears grossly normal.

Bowel Resection

Resection is the commonest procedure performed for CD. In most patients the length of diseased bowel is short, and there is more than adequate residual bowel. Our practice is to perform an anastomosis in two hand-sewn layers. We recognize that there is adequate data to support the use of stapled anastomoses. However, the degree of control when the surgeon places every stitch is comforting in the setting of CD where there is often inflamed local tissue, the presence of steroids, and nutritional issues. Stricturoplasty is an option in which the diseased bowel is not removed, but rather opened in a longitudinal fashion and closed in a transverse fashion. This has great utility when the strictured segment is short, and when there are multiple effected areas (Hurst and Michelassi, 1998). However, when the diseased segment is long, stricturoplasty becomes similar to bypass, a procedure abandoned long ago for good reason.

Fistula

A fistula can be between two portions of CD bowel, in which case both portions of diseased bowel should be removed (eg, diseased terminal ileum fistulizing to diseased sigmoid colon). More commonly the fistula is between diseased bowel and a nondiseased "innocent" organ or portion of bowel (eg, terminal ileum fistulizing into the bladder). Figure 68-1 demonstrates CD fistulization between diseased terminal ileum and appendix, and an innocent transverse colon. In this instance, the surgical objective is safe division of the fistula while avoiding damage to the innocent tissue.

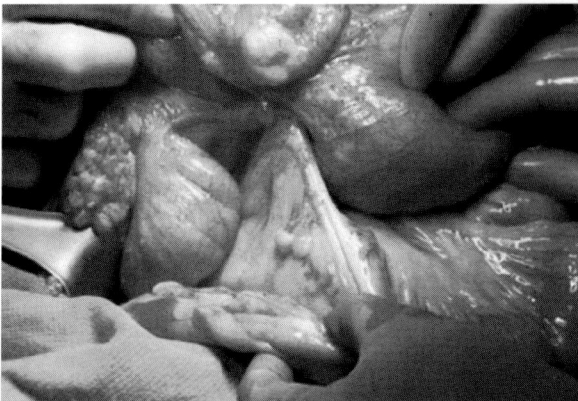

FIGURE 68-1. Crohn's disease (CD) causing fistula between the terminal ileum, appendix, and transverse colon.

This is often a point at which a laparoscopic operation may need to be converted to an open one. In all instances the innocent tissue should be carefully examined, and repaired or removed if necessary. The genitourinary system is a frequent target of fistulization, and intraoperative consultation with appropriate specialists, if available, can be enormously helpful. Figure 68-2 shows CD that has fistulized to the skin surface. Surgical correction of this severe situation takes careful planning, and great patience in the operating room.

The surgeon must also anticipate the need for additional procedures at the time of surgery. For instance, if significant portions of the bowel are to be removed, the gall bladder should probably be removed at the same time.* This is particularly true if the patient is likely to need long term parenteral support. If long term nutrition is likely to be necessary, the placement of a gastrostomy or jejunostomy might also be contemplated.

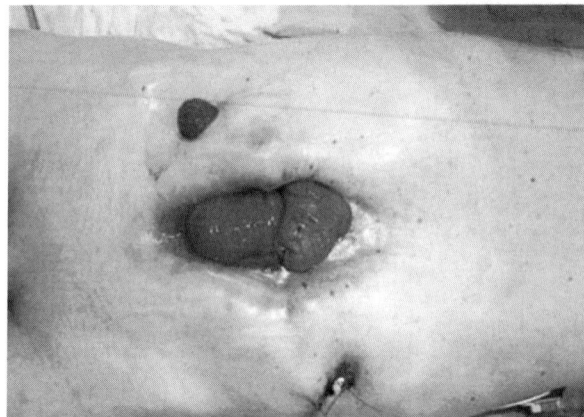

FIGURE 68-2. Enterocutaneous fistula from Crohn's disease (CD).

---

*Editor's Note: It should be recognized that bile salt-induced diarrhea will be inevitable with a cholecystectomy and a lengthy ileal resection.

Colon Resection

CD of the colon and rectum presents unique challenges. Determining the extent of disease in the colon is a challenge addressed above. In patients with skip lesions throughout the colon, the surgeon must decide whether it is worth attempting to salvage spared regions of the colon. Since the colon is not essential for nutrition, there is a tendency to be more aggressive with resection. Multiple anastomoses in the colon are worth avoiding, as they have a greater chance of anastomotic leak. However, since diarrhea is a persistent source of suffering for CD patients, salvaging colon for fluid absorption certainly has merit.

In the SB, the portion of diseased bowel can be removed and re-anastamosed. In the low rectum, this is usually not possible, leaving permanent colostomy as the only surgical option. Some centers have reported some success with restorative proctocolectomy (with ileo anal pouch anastomosis) in selected patients with CD limited to the colon. We have had patients who have undergone restorative proctocolectomy for ulcerative colitis who later were found to in fact have CD. The extremely difficult management problems with pouch function and pouch fistulas in these few patients have prevented us from offering restorative proctocolectomy to patients with even a hint of CD.

Rectal CD

Rectal CD is a particularly challenging problem. These patients suffer with pain, chronically draining fistulas, strictures, and sometimes all of the above. When Remicade fails in this group, the surgical options are few. Patients with persistent rectal structuring can be maintained for a time with intermittent dilatation under heavy sedation or anesthesia. It is extremely important in these patients to biopsy tissue in the region of any stricture any time the surgeon manipulates the tissue, as an occult adenocarcinoma can arise in these strictures. In patients with these problems, in our experience, local surgical procedures usually simply palliate the condition until the patient recognizes the need for relief in the form of a stoma. When they do so, the following two options exist: (1) proctectomy and permenant stoma or (2) stool diversion by the creation of a theoretically temporary stoma while leaving the diseased rectum in. In this latter instance, the patient is often hoping for a future breakthrough in medical therapy that will allow takedown of their stoma. When this option is chosen, the blind remaining rectum must be regularly surveyed by sigmoidoscopy and biopsy, as adenocarcinma can arise.

The duodenum, particularly the first and second portion, is another segment of gut where simple resection is not possible. In unique instances, a Whipple procedure may be appropriate as a means of removing badly diseased CD duodenum. The more common and less morbid approach is to perform a bypass in the form of a retrocolic gastrojejunostomy, usually accompanied by a vagotomy.

Summary

Surgical treatment of CD does not "cure" the disease, but the majority of patients requiring medication for CD will need surgical treatment. The appropriate treatment of these patients is challenging. It requires careful thought, careful planning, and extensive consultation between surgeon and gastroenterologist.

---

†Editor's Note: We have a rare patient whose diverting colostomy has been closed and their perianal disease has remained quirerent on Remicade and azathioprine. Follow up is < 2 years so far.

Supplemental Reading

Canin-Endres J, Salky B, Gattorno F, Edye M. Laparoscopically assisted intestinal resection in 88 patients with Crohn's disease. Surg Endosc 1999;13:595–9.

Hamilton SR, Reese J, Pennington L, et al. The role of resection margin frozen section in the surgical management of Crohn's disease. Surg Gynecol Obstet 1985;160:57–62.

Hurst RD, Michelassi F. Strictureplasty for Crohn's disease: techniques and long-term results. World J Surg 1998;22:359–63.

Ludwig KA, Milsom JW, Church JM, Fazio VW. Preliminary experience with laparoscopic intestinal surgery for Crohn's disease. Am J Surg 1996;171:52–5; discussion 55–6.

Michelassi F. Side-to-side isoperstoltic stricturoplasty for multiple Crohn's strictures. Dis Colon Rectum 1996;39:346–9.

Salky B. Severe gastroduodenal Crohn's disease: surgical treatment. Inflamm Bowel Dis 2003;9:129–30; discussion 131.

Sanfey H, Bayless TM, Cameron JL. Crohn's disease of the colon. Is there a role for limited resection? Am J Surg 1984;147:38–42.

Schmidt CM, Talamini MA, Kaufman HS, et al. Laparoscopic surgery for Crohn's disease: reasons for conversion [Erratum in Ann Surg 2001;234:following table of contents]. Ann Surg 2001;233: 733–9.

Talamini MA. Laparoscopically assisted bowel resection in advanced therapy of inflammatory bowel disease. In: Bayless TM, Hanauer SB, eds. 2nd ed. Toronto: BC Decker; 2001. p. 450–5.

Chapter 69

Monitoring of Azathioprine Metabolite Levels in Inflammatory Bowel Disease

C. Cuffari, MD

6-Mercaptopurine (6-MP) and its parent compound azathioprine (AZA) are purine analogues that have been increasingly used in the management of steroid-dependent inflammatory bowel disease (IBD). This chapter will cover the pros and cons of the routine use of metabolite testing in the monitoring of patients with IBD, as well as concepts of dosing of AZA.

The Pharmacology of 6-MP

The immunosuppressive properties of 6-MP and AZA are most likely mediated through their interference with protein synthesis and nucleic acid metabolism in the sequence that follows antigen stimulation, as well as by their cytotoxic effects on lymphoid cells (Lennard, 1992). Because 6-MP and AZA are by themselves inactive, they must be transformed intracellularly into ribonucleotides that function as purine antagonists. These antimetabolites are then incorporated into deoxyribonucleic acid (DNA) and interfere with DNA and protein interactions involved in ribonucleotide replication (Fairchild et al, 1986).

6-MP undergoes rapid and extensive catabolic oxidation to 6-thiouric acid in the intestinal mucosa and liver by the enzyme xanthine oxidase, and as a result, the bioavailability of 6-MP ranges from 5 to 37% (Zimm et al, 1983). In comparison, the intestinal absorption of AZA is somewhat better than 6-MP. Once absorbed into the circulation, AZA is rapidly converted to 6-MP and S-methyl-4-nitro-5-thioimidazole on exposure to sulfhydryl-containing compounds in the plasma and tissues. Twelve percent of AZA is excreted in the form of S-methyl-4-nitro-5-thioimidazole, and thus represents the first detoxification product known in its metabolism. This reaction has been shown to occur nonenzymatically. Beyond this metabolic step, in vivo studies in both animals and man have shown that AZA metabolism is identical to that of 6-MP. It is also important to note that AZA is 55% of 6-MP by molecular weight. All these factors may contribute to the conversion factor of 1.8 when converting a dose of 6-MP to AZA (Van Os et al, 1996).

The plasma half-life of 6-MP is very short, ranging from 1 to 2 hours on account of the rapid absorption of 6-MP into erythrocytes and organs tissues. The anabolic transformation of 6-MP into its active metabolites occurs intracellularly along the competing routes catalyzed by thiopurine methyltransferase (TPMT) and hypoxanthine phosphoribosyl transferase, giving rise to 6-methyl-mercaptopurine (6-MMP), 6-methyl-thioinosine 5′-monophosphate, and 6-thioguanine (6-TG) nucleotides, respectively (Figure 69-1) (Elion, 1977).

The 6-TG nucleotides are thought to be lymphocytoxic and beneficial in the treatment of patients with leukemia. Indeed, low erythrocyte 6-TG levels have been associated with a low 6-MP dose and with an increased risk of a disease relapse (Lennard et al, 1993). The incorporation of these antimetabolites into lymphocyte DNA and ribonucleic acid down-regulates B- and T-cell function (Stet et al, 1993). Recent in vitro studies have also shown that AZA and its metabolites induce apoptosis of peripheral blood T-lymphocytes isolated from healthy volunteers. In that study, apoptosis required costimulation with CD28 and was mediated by the specific blockade of *RAC 1* activation through the binding of 6-TG triphosphate. The inhibition of CD28 dependent *RAC 1* activation by 6-TG metabolites may also help explain the immunosuppressive effects of AZA in patients with IBD (Tiede et al, 2003).

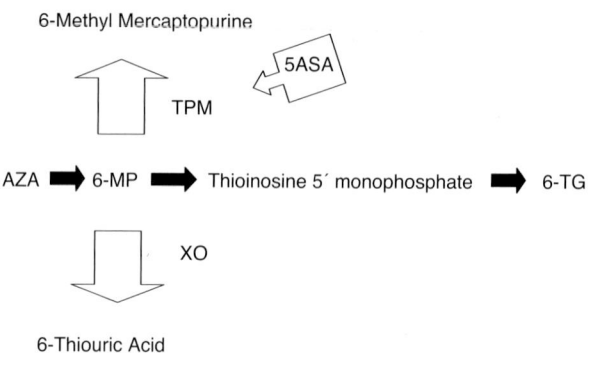

FIGURE 69-1. Azathioprine and 6-mercaptopurine metabolism. ASA = 5-acetylsalicylic acid; AZA = azathioprine; TPMT = thiopurine methyltransferase; HPRT = hypoxanthine phosphoribosyl transferase; 6-MP = 6-mercaptopurine; 6-TG = 6-thioguanine; XO = xanthine oxidase.

6-MP Metabolism in IBD

In our preliminary study in pediatric patients with IBD, there was a strong inverse correlation between erythrocyte 6-TG metabolite levels and disease activity. Although a wide range of erythrocyte 6-TG levels were associated with clinical responsiveness to therapy, patients with 6-TG levels > 235 pmol/8 × 10^8 red blood cells (RBCs) were usually asymptomatic. Moreover, the lack of clinical response and noncompliance to 6-MP therapy was associated with low erythrocyte 6-TG metabolite levels. Neither drug dose nor the level of 6-MP induced leukopenia correlated with responsiveness to therapy (Cuffari et al, 1996). Similar results have also been reported in 95 pediatric patients on long term maintenance 6-MP therapy (Table 69-1) (Dubinsky et al, 2000).

In our study of 82 adult patients with IBD on long term maintenance AZA therapy (> 3 months), an erythrocyte 6-TG level > 250 pmol/8 × 10^8 RBCs was more often associated with the maintenance of clinical remission. In that study, 18 of 22 patients who were deemed refractory to standard dosages of AZA therapy with subtherapeutic (< 250) erythrocyte 6-TG metabolite levels had their dose of AZA optimized to achieve a clinical response. 6-TG metabolite levels were used as a guide to therapy, allowing the physician to optimize the dosage of AZA without drug inducing leukopenia (Cuffari et al, 2001). Similar results were also obtained in 60 adult patients with IBD on long term 6-MP therapy. In that study, an erythrocyte 6-TG level of > 260 pmoles/8 × 10^8 RBCs was associated with the maintenance of clinical remission (Achar et al, 2000).

Adult patients with IBD on induction AZA therapy also showed a correlation between high (> 292 pmoles/8 × 10^8 RBCs) erythrocyte 6-TG metabolite levels and clinical responsiveness to therapy. An erythrocyte 6-TG > 292 pmoles/8 × 10^8 RBCs had a corresponding sensitivity and positive predictive value of clinical responsiveness to AZA therapy of 70.6% and 85.7%, respectively. In comparison, patients on maintenance AZA therapy required lower (> 234 pmoles/8 × 10^8 RBCs) 6-TG metabolite levels to maintain a clinical response (see Table 69-1) (Cuffari et al, 2004).

In comparison, several studies in both adult and pediatric patients with IBD have not shown a correlation between 6-TG and clinical responsiveness to either AZA or 6-MP therapy (Gupta et al, 2001; Belaiche et al, 2001; Lowry et al, 2001). The apparent lack of consensus over metabolite testing in clinical practice is due to patients who, despite therapeutic 6-TG levels, are still resistant to AZA therapy and require methotrexate or infliximab therapy. Moreover, it remains a common practice in most institutions, including our own to tailor the dose of either AZA or 6-MP to achieve a favorable clinical response while avoiding potential drug-induced toxicity. This treatment approach may suboptimize drug therapy and thereby lend itself to presumed subtherapeutic drug metabolite levels. Among these patients, the monitoring of 6-TG metabolite levels can be used to instill a certain level of confidence among physicians to consider escalating drug therapy, while not necessarily using leucopenia as a therapeutic endpoint. Although the measurement of erythrocyte 6-TG metabolite levels can be helpful among those patients with either active disease or steroid dependency, prospective controlled studies are needed to validate the role of metabolite testing in clinical practice.

TPMT Activity

An apparent genetic polymorphism has been observed in TPMT activity in both the white and black population. TPMT enzyme deficiency is inherited as an autosomal recessive trait, and to date, 10 mutant alleles and several silent and intronic mutations have been described (Alves et al, 2000). Negligible TPMT enzyme activity was noted in individual patients carrying 2 variant alleles (0.3%), and low levels (< 5 U/mL of blood) were noted in 11% of individuals who are heterozygotes. Individuals who are homozygous for the wild-type gene can have a wide range of TPMT phenotypic expression (> 5 U/mL of blood) (Weinshilboum and Sladek, 1980). These pharmacogenetic differences in 6-MP metabolism are known to influence clinical responsiveness to 6-MP therapy in patients with leukemia (Lennard et al, 1993). Although 6-TG ribonucleotides are thought to be lymphocytoxic, and beneficial in the treatment of patients with leukemia and lymphoma, patients with low (< 5 U/mL of blood) TPMT activity are at risk for bone marrow suppression by achieving potentially toxic erythrocyte 6-TG levels on standard doses of 6-MP (Evans et al, 1991). In these patients, therapeutic erythrocyte 6-TG metabolite levels can still be achieved without untoward cytotoxicity by lowering the dose of 6-MP 10 to 15 fold (McLeod et al, 1995). In patients with

TABLE 69-1. 6-Thioguanine Metabolite Levels: Correlation with Clinical Efficacy

Study	N	Setting	Clinical Correlation
Cuffari	25	Adolescent CD	6-TG levels
Dubinsky	95	Pediatric IBD	6-TG > 235*
Achar	60	Adult IBD	6-TG > 260*
Gupta	54	Pediatric IBD	NS
Belaiche	24	Adult IBD	NS
Lowry	170	Adult IBD	NS
Cuffari colitis/fistula	82	Adult IBD	6-TG > 250*
Cuffari (maintenance AZA therapy)	101	Adult IBD	6-TG > 234*
Cuffari (induction AZA therapy)	40	Adult IBD	6-TG > 292*

*pmoles/8 × 10^8 red blood cells.
AZA = azathioprine; CD = Crohn's disease; IBD = inflammatory bowel disease; 6-TG = 6-thioguanine.

IBD, Black and colleagues (1998) showed that patients with Crohn's disease (CD) and a "mutant" TPMT allele incurred significant drug-induced leukopenia on AZA therapy and were compelled to discontinue treatment, whereas patients with the wild-type allele achieved a good clinical response while on AZA therapy with no side effects. Conversely, in a study by Colombel and colleagues (2000), TPMT enzyme deficiency was present in just 27% of patients with AZA-induced myelosuppression. The authors concluded that TPMT genotype testing may not circumvent the need for complete blood cell count monitoring. Although a very low dosing strategy (0.25 mg/kg/d) has been reported to be acceptable in patients with IBD and the homozygous recessive TPMT genotype, it remains most authors' opinion that patients with absent TPMT enzyme activity levels should not receive antimetabolite therapy. However, a moderate dosing strategy (1 mg/kg/d) can still be applied in patients with the heterozygous TPMT genotype and low (< 5 U/mL blood) enzyme activity. This dosage has been shown to be effective in achieving therapeutic (> 250 pmoles/8 × 10^8 RBCs) 6-TG metabolite levels while achieving a favorable clinical response to therapy without drug-associated side effects (Cuffari et al, 2004).

High TMPT Activity

Patients with leukemia and high (> 12 U/mL) TPMT activity are at risk for a disease relapse despite conventional maintenance 6-MP dosing (Bostrom and Erdman, 1993). In these patients, 6-MP metabolism is believed to be shunted away from the production of 6-TG ribonucleotides and into the preferential formation of 6-MMP metabolites (McCleod et al, 1995). In patients with IBD, a recent retrospective study has shown that patients with TPMT enzyme activity levels > 14 U/mL blood were more likely to be refractory to AZA therapy (Ansari et al, 2002). A recent prospective open-labeled study showed that patients with TPMT < 15.3 U/mL of blood were 6.3 times more likely to respond to induction AZA therapy (Cuffari et al, 2004). Patients with very high (> 5700 pmoles/8 × 10^8 RBCs) erythrocyte 6-MMP levels and presumably high TPMT enzyme activity have also been shown to be at an increased risk for hepatotoxicity (Dubinsky et al, 2002).

Inhibition of TPMT Activity

The activity of TPMT is inhibited in vitro by sulfasalazine and related mesalamine compounds (see Figure 69-1) (Szumlanski et al, 1995). A recent nonrandomized 8-week drug interaction study showed that the coadministration of AZA with either mesalamine or sulfasalazine led to leukopenia, and a significant increase in erythrocyte 6-TG metabolite levels, as a result of decreased 6-MP catabolism (Lowry et al, 2001).

5-Aminosalicylic acid (5-ASA) must be metabolized by n-acetyl transferase (NAT-1) into its active n-acetyl 5-ASA metabolite. Interestingly, there are variant NAT-1 alleles present within the population that may potentially affect 5-ASA metabolism. Patients with the variant NAT-1 allele do not convert 5-ASA effectively into its active n-acetyl 5-ASA metabolite. Because 5-ASA has been shown to interfere with TPMT activity in vitro, patients with the variant NAT*1 allele may be predisposed to 6-MP induced cytotoxicity. Proujansky and colleagues (1999) have shown that inherent differences in 5-ASA metabolism may predict complications to 6-MP therapy. Patients with the NAT*1 variant allele were at a significantly increased risk for 6-MP related cytotoxicity, including pancreatitis. In contrast, patients who were identified as carriers of TPMT deficient allele responded favorably to 6-MP therapy, but were at an increased risk for developing hepatitis. Although, this study would suggest that combined TPMT genotyping and the measure of NAT*1 enzyme activity may help identify those patients susceptible to 6-MP related toxicity, further studies are required to determine whether the putative influences of the NAT*1 variant allele on 5-ASA metabolism can be correlated with alterations in erythrocyte 6-TG metabolite levels.

In a recent, prospective, noncontrolled study, AZA metabolism, drug safety and efficacy was influenced by inherent differences in TPMT activity present within the population. The response rate to induction AZA therapy was highest in patients with less than average (< 12 U/mL) TPMT activity (Figure 69-2). In that study, knowing of a low (< 5 U/mL) TPMT activity before initiating AZA therapy led to a low dosing strategy (1 mg/kg/d) with a favorable clinical response without untoward side effects (Cuffari et al, 2004). In comparison, patients with above average TPMT activity levels were less likely to respond to AZA therapy, and more likely to require higher dosages

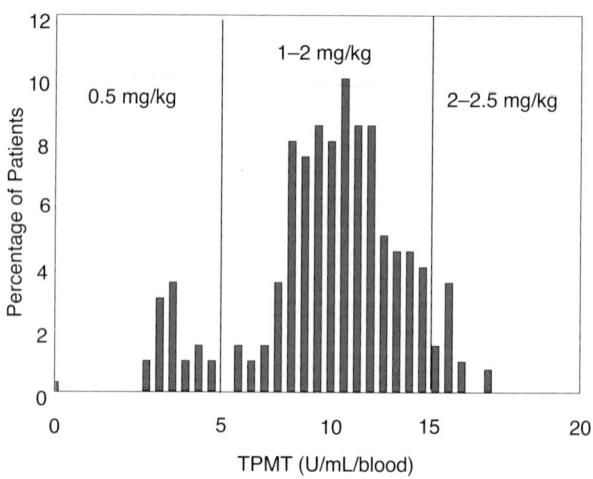

FIGURE 69-2. High thiopurine methyltransferase activity shunts azathioprine metabolism away from 6-TG production.

(2 mg/kg/d) of AZA from the outset in order to optimize erythrocyte 6-TG metabolite levels (see Figure 69-2). The careful monitoring of complete blood counts and erythrocyte 6-TG and 6-MMP metabolite levels are indicated in patients with above average (> 12 U/mL) TPMT levels to avoid the unpredictable shunting of 6-MP metabolism into the production of 6-MMP metabolites, respectively. The putative cytotoxicity of methylated metabolites in developing 6-MP induced leukopenia would suggest that leukopenia may not be an appropriate endpoint for all patients on antimetabolite therapy, especially in those patients with high TPMT activity (Dervieux et al, 2001). It remains the author's opinion that the empiric use of high AZA dosage (2 mg/kg/d) in patients with a presumed normal TPMT genotype underscores the apparent influence of TPMT polymorphisms on AZA metabolism, and may predispose patients to unnecessary AZA-related toxicity. Moreover, patients with high TPMT activity may remain refractory to therapy despite optimizing the dose of AZA.

High hepatic TPMT activity may draw most of the 6-MP from the plasma, thereby limiting the amount of substrate available for the bone marrow and peripheral leukocytes (Szumlanski et al, 1992). This concept of rapid AZA metabolism interfering with therapeutic response could explain the low (20%) remission rate in a recently published controlled trial in CD in individuals with upper normal or high levels of TPMT enzyme activity that used high dose oral (2 mg/kg/d) AZA therapy (Sandborn et al, 1999).

Clinical Parameters in IBD

Most often, physicians will measure drug efficacy, based on either an improvement in their patients' clinical symptoms and quality of life or their ability to maintain remission while weaning off of corticosteroid therapy. Colonna and Korelitz (1993) have observed that clinical responsiveness to 6-MP therapy was best in patients with leukopenia. In 51 patients with moderate to severe CD on long-term 6-MP therapy, clinical responsiveness correlated well with drug-induced leukopenia. None of their patients developed clinical signs of bone marrow suppression required hospitalization for concurrent infection or required transfusions despite total leukocyte counts < 5000. A similar strategy has also been suggested in using changes in mean corpuscular volume (MCV) to monitor clinical responsiveness to AZA therapy (Garza and Sninsky, 2001). We have seen unresponsive patients with a WBC < 6000 and MCV > 95 whose 6-TG levels are still subtherapeutic and who can tolerate and respond to additional doses of AZA (personal observation).

Concluding Remarks

The high-performance liquid chromatography measurement of erythrocyte 6-MP metabolites has now become a useful clinical tool for documenting patients' compliance to therapy as well as the adequacy of dosing. Ongoing studies have developed the notion of a therapeutic window of efficacy and toxicity based on the measure of erythrocyte 6-TG and 6-MMP levels. Moreover, prior knowledge of a patient's erythrocyte TPMT enzyme activity may allow physicians to tailor the dosage of either AZA or 6-MP to suite a patient's individual drug metabolism. Those with very low (< 5 U/mL) TPMT activity can be effectively treated (90% response) with 1 mg/kg/d while monitoring complete blood counts and erythrocyte 6-TG levels. Whereas patients with TPMT activity between 5 to 12 U/mL blood show a 70% response rate to a moderate dosing strategy, such as 1.5 mg/kg/d. In patients with above average (> 12 U/mL) TPMT activity, AZA may need to be started at 2.0 mg/kg/d in order to achieve a 40% clinical response. However, higher dosages, such as 2.5 mg/kg/d, are expected to be needed for those with very high (> 20 U/mL) TPMT enzyme activity. In these patients, the careful monitoring of 6-TG and 6-MMP levels may help to guide therapy and identify those patients that preferentially shunt AZA metabolites away from the production of 6-TG, (Cuffari et al, 2004).

Supplemental Reading

Achar JP, Stevens T, Brzezinski A, et al. 6-thioguanine levels versus white blood cell counts in guiding 6-mercaptopruine and azathioprine therapy. Am J Gastroenterol 2000;95:A272.

Alves S, Prata MJ, Ferreira F, Amorim A. Screening of thiopurine methyl s-transferase mutations by horizontal conformation-sensitive gel electrophoresis. Hum Mutat 2000;15:246–53.

Ansari A, Hassan C, Duley J, et al. Thiopruine methyltransferase activity and the use of azathioprine in inflammatory bowel disease. Aliment Pharmacol Ther 2002;16:1743–50.

Belaiche J, Desager JP, Horsmans Y, Louis E. Therapeutic drug monitoring of azathioprine and 6-mercaptopurine metabolites in Crohn's disease. Scand J Gastroenterol 2001;36:71–6.

Black AJ, McLeod HL, Capell HA. Thiopurine methyl transferase predicts therapy-limiting severe toxicity from azathioprine. Ann Intern Med 1998;129:716–8.

Bostrom B, Erdman G. Cellular pharmacology of 6-mercaptopurine in acute lymphoblastic leukemia. Am J Pediatr Hematol Oncol 1993;15:80–6.

Candy S, Wright J, Gerger M, et al. A controlled double-blind study of azathioprine in the management of Crohn's disease. Gut 1995;37:674–8.

Colombel JF, Ferrari N, DeBuysere H, et al. Genotypic analysis of thiopurine s-methyltransferase in patients with Crohn's disease and severe myelosuppression during azathioprine therapy. Gastroenterology 2000;118:1025–30.

Colonna T, Korelitz BI. The role of leucopenia in 6-mercaptopurine-induced remission of refractory Crohn's disease. Am J Gastroenterol 1993;89:362–6.

Cuffari C, Dassopoulos T, Turnbough L, et al. Thiopurine methyltransferase activity influences clinical response to azathioprine therapy in inflammatory bowel disease. Clin Gastroenterol Hepatol 2004;2:410–7.

Cuffari C, Hunt S, Bayless T. Utilisation of erythrocyte 6-thioguanine metabolite levels to optimize azathioprine therapy in patients with inflammatory bowel disease. Gut 2001;48:591–2.

Cuffari C, Theoret Y, Latour S, et al. 6-mercaptopurine metabolism in Crohn's disease: correlation with efficacy and toxicity. Gut 1996;39:401–6.

Dervieux T, Blanco JG, Krynetski EY, et al. Differing contribution of thiopurine methyltransferase to mercaptopurine versus thioguanine effects in human leukemic ells. Cancer Res 2001;61:5810–6.

Dimitriu A, Fauci AS. Activation of human B lymphocytes. Differential effects of azathioprine on B lymphocytes and lymphocyte subpopulations regulating B cell function. J Immunol 1978;121:2335–9.

Dubinsky MC, Lamothe S, Yang HY, et al. Pharmacogenomics and metabolite measurement for 6-mercaptopurine therapy in inflammatory bowel disease. Gastroenterology 2000;118;705–13.

Dubinsky MC, Yang H, Hassard PV, et al. 6-MP metabolite profiles provide a biochemical explanation for 6-MP resistance in patients with inflammatory bowel disease. Gastroenterology 2002;122:904–15.

Elion GB. The pharmacology of azathioprine. Ann N Y Acad Sci 1977;21:401–7.

Evans WE, Horner M, Chu YQ, et al. Altered mercaptopurine metabolism, toxic effects, and dosage requirements in a thiopurine methyltransferase deficient child with acute lymphoblastic leukemia. J Pediatr 1991;119:985–9.

Ewe K, Press AG, Singe CC, et al. Azathioprine combined with prednisolone or monotherapy with prednisolone in active Crohn's disease. Gastroenterology 1993;105:367–72.

Fairchild CR, Maybaum J, Kennedy KA. Concurrent unilateral chromatid damage and DNA strand breaks in response to 6-thioguanine treatment. Biochem Pharmacol 1986;35:3533–41.

Garza A, Sninsky CA. Changes in red cell mean corpuscular volume (MCV) during azathioprine or 6-mercaptopurine therapy for Crohn's disease may indicate optimal dose titration. Gastroenterology 2001;120:A3166.

Gupta P, Gokhlae R, Kirschner BS. 6-mercaptopurine metabolite levels in children with inflammatory bowel disease. J Pediatr Gastroenterol Nutr 2001;33:450–4.

Kaskas BA, Louis E, Hindorf U, et al. Safe treatment of thiopurine S-methyltransferase deficient Crohn's disease patients with azathioprine. Gut 2003;52:140–2.

Lennard L. The clinical pharmacology of 6-mercaptopurine in acute lymphoblastic leukemia. Eur J Clin Pharmacol 1992;43:329–39.

Lennard L, Rees CA, Lilleyman JS, et al. Childhood leukemia: a relationship between intracellular 6-mercaptopurine metabolites and neutropenia. Br J Clin Pharmacol 1993;16:359–63.

Lowry PW, Franklin CL, Weaver AL, et al. Leucopenia resulting from a drug interaction between azathioprine or 6-mercaptopurine and mesalamine, sulphasalazine or balsalazide. Gut 2001;49:656–64.

McLeod HL, Relling MV, Liu Q, et al. Polymorphic thiopurine methyl transferase in erythrocytes is indicative of activity in leukemic blasts from children with acute lymphoblastic leukemia. Blood 1995;85:1897–902.

Pearson DC, May GR, Fick GH, Sutherland LR. Azathioprine and 6-mercaptopurine in Crohn's disease: a meta-analysis. Ann Intern Med 1995;122:132–42.

Present DH, Korelitz BI, Wisch N. Treatment of Crohn's disease with 6-mercaptopurine. A long-term, randomized, double-blind study. N Engl J Med 1989;302:981–7.

Proujansky R, Maxwell M, Johnson J, et al. Molecular genotyping predicts complications of 6-mercaptopurine therapy in childhood IBD. Gastroenterology 1999;116:A800.

Sandborn WJ, Tremaine WJ, Wolfe DC, et al. Lack of effect of intravenous administration on time to respond to azathioprine for steroid-treated Crohn's disease. Gastroenterology 1999;117:527–35.

Stet EH, De Abreu RA, Bokkerink JPM, et al. Reversal of 6-mercaptopurine and 6-methyl mercaptopurine ribonucleoside cytotoxicity by amidoimidazole carboxamide ribonucleoside in Molt-4 human malignant T-lymphoblasts. Biochem Pharmacol 1993;46:547–50.

Szumlanski C, Honchel R, Scott MC, Weinshilboum RM. Human liver thiopurine methyl transferase pharmacogenetics: biochemical properties, liver erythrocyte correlation and presence of isozymes. Pharmacogenetics 1992;2:148.

Szumlanski C, Weinshilboum RN. Sulphasalazine inhibition of thio methyl transferase: possible mechanism of interaction with 6-mercaptopurine. Br J Clin Pharmacol 1995;39:456–9.

Tiede I, Fritz G, Strand S, et al. CD-28-dependent Rac 1 activation is the molecular target of azathioprine in primary human CD4 T lymphocytes. J Clin Invest 2003;111:1133–45.

Van Os EC, Zins BJ, Sandborn WJ, et al. Azathioprine pharmacokinetics after intravenous, oral, delayed release oral and rectal foam administration. Gut 1996;39:63–8.

Weinshilboum RN, Sladek Sl. Mercaptopurine pharmacogenetics: monogenic inheritance of erythrocyte thiopurine methyl transferase activity. Am J Hum Genet 1980;32:651–62.

Zimm S, Collins JM, Riccardi R, et al. Variable bioavailability of oral mercaptopurine. Is maintenance chemotherapy in acute lymphoblastic leukemia being optimally delivered. 1983; 308:1005–9.

CHAPTER 70

Mesenteric Vascular Ischemia

Awori J. Hayanga, MD, AFRCSI, Eugene P. Ceppa, MD, and Gregory B. Bulkley, MD, FACS

Acute intestinal vascular ischemia remains a challenging problem in modern clinical practice. The rate of missed diagnoses is high and the mortality ranges from 50 to 100%. For its most common but least lethal form, *intestinal strangulation*, the mortality rate is more than double that for unstrangulated mechanical obstruction. Successful management requires the skillful application of diagnostic and therapeutic priorities. For example, the delay of laparotomy is in some cases disastrous; in other cases it is essential to a successful outcome.

Acute mesenteric ischemia may be due either to the anatomic *occlusion* of a mesenteric vessel or to *vasospasm* of arteriolar beds that these vessels serve. Anatomic arterial occlusion is seen most commonly in the presence of atherosclerosis, where it is due either to the embolization from a proximal site or to thrombosis of or hemorrhage into an existing atherosclerotic plaque (Table 70-1). In a few patients the slow, progressive stenosis of two or three mesenteric arteries may lead to *chronic intestinal angina*, characterized by postprandial pain and weight loss. Acute vascular insufficiency may also result from the disruption of one or more mesenteric vessels due to either exogenous trauma or surgical intervention after acute surgery. Rarely, the primary vascular occlusion is due to *venous thrombosis*, precipitated by *dehydration*, a *hypercoagulable state, portal hypertension*, or *polycythemia*. In this situation, ischemic tissue injury develops more slowly, but with the same devastating effects. The most common cause of acute mesenteric vascular insufficiency is *strangulation obstruction* of the small intestine, which complicates about one-third of cases of *complete* small bowel (SB) obstruction. This may be due to a *midgut volvulus, adhesions*, or a *strangulated hernia*. Nonocclusive mesenteric ischemia (NOMI) is the result of a profound splanchnic vasospasm that can appear as an endogenous response to severe physiologic stress, such as *shock, congestive cardiac failure, sepsis, and respiratory insufficiency, or after cardiopulmonary bypass*. This condition may also be caused or exacerbated by exogenous administration of *splanchnic vasoconstrictors*, including *vasopressor agents* and *digitalis glycosides*.

General Therapeutic Principles

Early Diagnosis

Successful management of all forms of intestinal ischemia is based upon *early* diagnosis (Tables 70-2 and 70-3). This, in turn, allows prompt and definitive treatment. The high mortality associated with these diseases is not usually due to our inability to reverse the underlying vascular lesion. The surgeon is frequently able to reduce the strangulation or to anatomically revascularize. The interventional radiologist can often pharmacologically reverse the vasospasm underlying NOMI. Nevertheless, the patient often succumbs because this treatment is instituted only after irreversible intestinal tissue damage has ensued. This leaves the surgeon to choose between a massive bowel resection incompatible with a meaningful subsequent existence, or the ravages of uncontrolled ongoing sepsis. Moreover, the high overall mortality rates of these conditions, and the frequently elderly and debilitated population that they strike, have led to a depressing therapeutic nihilism on the part of many otherwise aggressive clinicians.

TABLE 70-1. Pathogenesis of Acute Mesenteric Ischemia

Condition	Primary Cause	Major Contributing Factors
Strangulation obstruction	Abdominal adhesions, hernia	Delayed laparotomy for complete small bowel obstruction
Arterial embolism	Embolus from heart (mural or valvular) or aorta	Atrial fibrillation, recent myocardial infarction, cardiac catheterization, angiography
Arterial thrombosis	Thrombosis of or hemorrhage into a preexisting atherosclerotic plaque	Dehydration, low cardiac output, hypercoagulable state
Traumatic arterial disruption	Abdominal trauma, aortic surgery	Status of collateral flow
Venous thrombosis	Venous thrombosis, trauma, (including surgery)	Dehydration, hypercoagulable state, portal hypertension, polycythemia
Nonocclusive mesenteric ischemia	Splanchnic vasospasm Endogenous: renin/angiotensin Exogenous: splanchnic vasoconstrictors	Shock, congestive heart failure, sepsis, respiratory failure

Adapted from Bulkley, 1986.

Table 70-2. Clinical Factors Predisposing to Mesenteric Ischemia

Arterial occlusion
  Embolism (15 to 40% of cases)
    Prior embolic event
    Atrial fibrillation (recent cardioversion)
    Rheumatic heart disease
    Prosthetic valve(s)
    Recent myocardial infarction
    Recent vascular instrumentation
      Cardiac catheterization
      Angiography
      Angioplasty
  Thrombosis (15 to 65%)
    Known vascular disease
      Atherosclerosis
      Aortic dissection
      Vasculitis (including systemic lupus erythematosus)
    Trauma
    Hypercoagulable states
    Dehydration
Venous thrombosis (2 to 20%)
  Hypercoagulable state
    Hormones/pregnancy
    Carcinoma and carcinomatosis
    Polycythemia
    Coagulopathies
    Protein S deficiency
    Protein C deficiency
    Factor V Leiden deficiency
    Dehydration
  Venous obstruction
    Portal hypertension
    Budd-Chiari syndrome
    Carcinoma
  Low splanchnic blood flow
    Congestive heart failure
    Shock
  Bowel obstruction
  Trauma
  Sclerotherapy
Vasospasm (5 to 25%)
  Dehydration
  Shock
  Sepsis
  Congestive failure
  Pericardial tamponade
  Cardiopulmonary bypass
  Dialysis
  Vasoconstrictive drugs
    Digitalis glycosides
    α-adrenergic agonists
    β-adrenergic antagonists
    Vasopressin
    Cocaine

Adapted from Reilly et al, 1991.

Delayed Diagnosis

Although it is undoubtedly true that mesenteric ischemia, especially NOMI, can appear as an agonal conclusion to the overall downhill course of an unsalvageable patient, in most cases a review of the hospital course reveals that timely and aggressive intervention might well have resulted in salvaging a meaningful life. The major cause of this problem is the widespread misconception that the manifestations of intestinal ischemia are so devastating and overtly explicit that they are easily recognized. This is often based on indelible impressions created by terminal patients with end-stage mesenteric vascular disease; indeed, few clinical syndromes are as dramatic as late intestinal ischemia.

Early Manifestations Versus Necrosis

What many fail to recognize is that the early, reversible, and, hence, treatable forms of mesenteric ischemia are often quite subtle in presentation and, sometimes, as in the obtunded patient, provide no symptoms, signs, nor laboratory abnormalities whatsoever as clues to the diagnosis. In fact, those signs and laboratory abnormalities that we most often associate with intestinal ischemia diseases *(fever, peritoneal signs, leukocytosis, blood in the stool, metabolic acidosis)* represent the local and systemic responses to established bowel necrosis. The early signs of decreased mesenteric blood flow are subtle and frequently masked by obtundation and coexisting and predisposing conditions. Clearly, if one waits for evidence of advanced intra-abdominal sepsis before initiating treatment, the results of therapy will remain dismal, and this therapeutic nihilism will continue to appear justified. On the other hand, an aggressive approach, based on early diagnostic studies in patients at risk and suspected of having early mesenteric ischemia, appears to improve survival.

The major clinical features of each form of acute mesenteric ischemia are summarized in Tables 70-2 and 70-3. The diagnosis can be suspected only on clinical grounds, however, usually by an astute physician with a high index of clinical suspicion, based primarily on the clinical setting (see Table 70-2). Once considered, the diagnosis must be eliminated or confirmed definitively by *computed tomography* (CT), angiography, or laparotomy. It is usually an error to depend on the passage of time to allow the diagnosis to become more obvious. The appearance of definitive physical signs and laboratory abnormalities inevitably indicates that irreversible bowel necrosis has occurred, that the opportunity for successful revascularization has been lost, and that overwhelming sepsis and cardiovascular collapse may well be imminent.

Therapy for Systemic Manifestations

The management of patients with acute mesenteric vascular disease can be considered with respect to the treatment of the underlying cause, correction of the specific anatomic lesion, and reversal or limitation of the systemic consequences. This systemic aspect can be dealt with in general terms, regardless of the particular anatomic lesion. This approach is initiated when the patient first presents and is continued through surgery and the postoperative period.

TABLE 70-3. Diagnosis of Acute Intestinal Ischemia

Condition	Clinical Setting	Symptoms	Physical Signs	Laboratory Indications	Definitive Diagnosis
Arterial thrombosis	ASCVD H/O intestinal angina Dehydration CHF Arterial fibrillation Recent MI	Severe pain sudden onset crampy, continuous nausea, vomiting abdominal distension transient diarrhea	Early: Benign abdomen Hyperactive bowel sounds Abdominal distention Stool + or – for blood Often systemically stable	Early: None Late: Leukocytosis Acidosis Hemoconcentraton Alk. Phos/CK	CT scan Angiogram Laparotomy
Arterial embolism	Recent cardioversion Arteriogram	Bloody stool	Late: Diffusely acute abdomen Ileus Sepsis Cardiovascular collapse		
Traumatic disruption	Abdominal trauma Postoperative: Abdominal aneurysm Bowel resection Colostomy/ileostomy	Usually none	Trauma: Intra-abdominal Hemorrhage Postoperative: None Ileus/distension/sepsis	Trauma: Falling Hct/Hgb Postoperative None Leukocytosis Acidosis	Laparotomy ± angiogram
Strangulation obstruction	Previous abdominal surgery Hernia H/O congenital defects	Signs of "simple obstruction" Severe pain Continuous pain Bloody stool	Early: Signs of simple obstruction Late: Acute abdomen Sepsis Cardiovascular collapse	Early: None Late: Leukocytosis Acidosis Alk. Phos/CK	Laparotomy
Nonocclusive ischemia	Shock Sepsis Respiratory failure CHF Vasoconstrictor therapy Digitalis Recent cardiopulmonary bypass	None (obtunded) Diffuse, continuous pain Abdominal distention Nausea/anorexia Ileus	Early: None Late: Acute abdomen Sepsis Cardiovascular collapse	Early: -None Late: Leukocytosis Acidosis Alk. Phos/CK	Angiogram ± Laparotomy (late)
Venous thrombosis	Dehyrdation CHF Polycythemia H/O thrombophlebitis Recent portal venous surgery Pregnancy	Subacute onset Abdominal distention Dehydration Transient diarrhea Bloody stool	Early: Abdominal distention Dehydration Ascites Late: Acute abdomen Cardiovascular collapse	Early: Hemoconcentration Late: Leukocytosis Acidosis Alk. phos/CK	CT Scan Angiogram (venous phase) ± laparotomy
Ischemic colitis	Same as nonocclusive ischemia Recent aortic surgery Recent cardiopulmonary bypass	None Distention Bloody diarrhea	Early: None Late: Acute abdomen Sepsis Cardiovascular	Early: Hemoconcentration Late: Leukocytosis Acidosis Alk. phos/CK	Sigmoidoscopy Colonoscopy

Adapted from Bulkley, 1986.
ASCVD = arteriosclerotic cardiovascular disease; CHF = congestive heart failure; CK = creatine kinase; Hct = hematocrit; Hgb = hemoglobin; H/O = history of; MI = myocardial infarction.

Dehydration and Hypovolemia

All forms of mesenteric ischemia are associated with some degree of hypovolemia, as the ischemic insult produces a marked increase in the permeability of the capillaries and the mucosa itself, with consequent losses of intravascular fluid into the bowel wall and lumen. This fluid loss can be particularly striking in cases of venous thrombosis or intestinal strangulation, in which the venous component dominates the initial occlusive process. Careful hemodynamic monitoring is thus essential, usually with at least a *central venous pressure line and a Foley catheter*, the latter to allow the hourly assessment of urinary output. Serial measurements of blood pressure and pulse, although important, are simply not adequate by themselves. In patients with significant cardiovascular disease, it is best to monitor the *pulmonary capillary wedge pressure* as well. This also facilitates the measurement of cardiac output and the calculation of peripheral resistance, parameters that must be monitored to optimize the use of cardiotonic and vasoactive agents that may be required. Vasoconstrictors,

TABLE 70-4. Organ Involvement in Multiple Organ Dysfunction Syndrome

Gastrointestinal organs
 Small intestine: nonocclusive mucosal ischemia
 Large intestine: ischemic colitis
 Stomach: stress gastritis
 Liver: ischemic hepatitis
 Gallbladder: acalculous cholecystitis
 Pancreas: ischemic pancreatitis
Nongastrointestinal organs
 Lung: adult respiratory distress syndrome
 Heart: decreased myocardial contractility
 Kidney: renal failure
 Central nervous system: obtundation
 Clotting system: disseminated intravascular coagulation
 Immune system: activation of inflammatory mediators, SIRS

SIRS = systemic inflammatory response syndrome.

such as levarterenol, and the digitalis glycosides (selective vasoconstrictors of the splanchnic bed) should be eschewed. Fluid losses, often massive, should be replaced rapidly and aggressively, using lactated Ringer's solution, continuing adequate potassium.

Sepsis

The predominant clinical feature of advanced mesenteric vascular disease is the systemic sepsis that results initially from the loss of the mucosal barrier to bacteria and endotoxin from the lumen of the intestine itself. Probably because of the size of the bacterial inoculum and the dose of endotoxin, the sepsis engendered by intestinal ischemia may be particularly fulminant, especially at later stages of the disease. It is also remarkably resistant to antibiotics, probably because the process of inoculation continues until the underlying process has been reversed. It may be particularly devastating immediately after revascularization of an ischemic bowel segment by angioplasty vascular bypass or, more often, by reduction of strangulation. All patients suspected of having ischemic bowel disease should therefore be given high intravenous (IV) doses of *broad spectrum antibiotics, including anaerobic coverage.* Nevertheless, even the most vigorous antibiotic program provides only temporary support while definitive diagnostic studies and treatment are instituted.

Metabolic Acidosis

Patients with mesenteric ischemia often manifest profound metabolic acidosis secondary to sepsis, peripheral hypoperfusion (*lactic acidosis*), and toxic products from the bowel itself. This is best managed by aggressive administration of sodium bicarbonate, with frequent monitoring of arterial blood gases. An arterial line facilitates the frequent drawing of arterial blood samples and provides for optimal monitoring of blood pressure. Because of the massive losses of isotonic saline into the bowel wall and lumen, the sodium load associated with bicarbonate administration is rarely a problem in these patients. In recent years, many intensivists have followed serum levels of lactic acid as a guide to diagnosis and the adequacy of therapy.

Multisystem Failure

Patients with ischemic bowel disease often manifest the multisystem failure syndrome (Table 70-4). Although the management of each aspect of this problem is beyond the scope of this chapter, it is worth noting here that the early forms of organ–system failure can often be reversed if the underlying lesion can be corrected and the septic source eliminated. In the interim, the massive peripheral vasodilatation of septic shock can be confirmed by measurement of peripheral resistance and treated primarily with volume support. Vasoconstrictor agents, on the other hand, can exacerbate the defect in mesenteric organ perfusion. The cardiogenic shock of late sepsis can be treated by optimizing the left atrial filling pressure and by infusing inotropic agents. Acute renal failure is managed appropriately, and in the face of oliguria or anuria this presents serious problems of fluid balance, as these patients still require large volume infusions to replace gut losses, and body weight is useless as an indicator of intravascular volume in such patients. Here again, the central venous and pulmonary capillary wedge pressures, combined with measurements of cardiac output and peripheral resistance, and hourly urine output especially, are essential as guides to fluid therapy. Respiratory failure necessitating intubation and ventilation, hepatic failure, and central nervous system dysfunction (obtundation) frequently accompany the advanced stages of this syndrome. All are managed supportively until the underlying lesion can be dealt with definitively. Overall, optimal treatment of the multisystem failure syndrome consists primarily of avoiding it by diagnosing and treating intestinal ischemia at its early stages. All too often this syndrome represents the means by which the diagnosis is first seriously entertained, and at this stage the chances for success are small.

Timing of Surgical Intervention

In most salvageable cases of intestinal ischemia, except those caused by NOMI, venous thrombosis, and ischemic colitis, early surgery offers the best means for definitive reversal of the ischemic lesion. It is therefore desirable that laparotomy proceed with a minimum of delay. Specifically, this means that a few hours, at most, should be spent setting up appropriate access for monitoring, starting IV antibiotics, improving the cardiac output, and performing angiography. It is a serious error to delay surgery in a misguided long term attempt to optimize systemic parameters, because one usually observes an initial improvement, a therapeutic plateau, and then a progressive deterioration

TABLE 70-5. Overview of Management of Acute Intestinal Ischemia

Condition	Treatment of Underlying Cause	Treatment of Specific Lesion	Treatment of Systemic Consequences
Arterial thrombosis	-	Laparotomy	Hydration
	-	Endarterectomy/thrombectomy	Antibiotics
	-	Vascular bypass	Reverse acidosis
	-	Assess viability	Support cardiac output
	-	Resect dead bowel	Ventilatory support
	-	± Anticoagulation	Avoid vasoconstrictors
Arterial embolism	Anticoagulation	Laparotomy	Hydration
	Cardioversion	Embolectomy	Antibiotics
	Proximal thrombectomy	Asess viability	Reverse acidosis
	Aneurysmectomy	Vascular bypass	Support cardiac output
	Valve replacement	Resect dead bowel	Treat other embolic sites
	-	-	Ventilatory support
	-	-	Avoid vasoconstrictors
Venous thrombosis	Hydration – often massive	Anticoagulation	Hydration – often massive
	Anticoagulation	± Laparotomy	Antibiotics
	± Portosystemic shunt	± Thrombectomy	Reverse acidosis
	-	Assess viability	Support cardiac output
	-	Resect dead bowel	Ventilatory support
	-	-	Avoid vasoconstrictors
Strangulation obstruction	Early laparotomy	Nasogastric/intestinal suction	Hydration
	Reduce incarcerated hernia	Early laparotomy	Antibiotics
	Lyse adhesions	Assess viability	Reverse acidosis
	Detort volvulus	Resect dead bowel	Support cardiac output
	-	-	Ventilatory support
	-	-	Avoid vasoconstrictors
Nonocclusive mesenteric ischemia	Hydration	Intra-arterial vasodilators	Hydration
	Support cardiac output	Delayed laparotomy	Antibiotics
	D/C splanchnic vasoconstrictors	Assess viability	Reverse acidosis
	? Ablate renin-angiotensin axis	Resect dead bowel	Support cardiac output
	-	-	Ventilatory support
	-	-	Avoid vasoconstrictors
Ischemic colitis	Same as for nonocclusive ischemia	Delayed laparotomy	Hydration – often massive
	-	Assess viability	Antibiotics
	-	Resect dead bowel	Reverse acidosis
	-	-	Support cardiac output
	-	-	Ventilatory support
	-	-	Avoid vasoconstrictors

Adapted from Bulkley, 1986.

as ongoing sepsis becomes overwhelming and the ischemic bowel lesion becomes irreversible. This plateau period can be very deceptive, lulling the less experienced clinician into a false sense of the patient's well being. In some cases it can last several days. One should try to complete diagnostic studies and initiate laparotomy during this plateau period.

An essential legitimate cause for delay is the need to obtain a preoperative arteriogram in most patients with mesenteric vascular occlusion. This is important, both as a means of definitive diagnosis and as an anatomic guide to bypass or embolectomy. In some cases it facilitates mesenteric angioplasty. In cases of suspected NOMI, initial angiography is essential for both diagnosis and treatment. Surgery in these patients is reserved for the resection of unsalvageable bowel after perfusion has been maximized by vasodilator infusion. Patients with SB obstruction do not need preoperative angiography, as the diagnosis of strangulation, so difficult to recognize preoperatively, is made easily at laparotomy.

Some cases of acute mesenteric infarction present in such a fulminant form and in such otherwise debilitated patients that consideration must be given to a nonaggressive approach that seeks only to provide comfort and ease the patient's demise. Although this decision must be an individual one, these patients have little to lose from an attempt at aggressive therapy. (In a conscious patient, the discomfort of an arteriogram or a laparotomy under general anesthesia is small in comparison with the agonizing pain of intestinal angina, peritonitis, and systemic sepsis. In an unconscious patient, the comfort question is moot.)

Intraoperative Determination of Viability

After perfusion of the intestine has been optimized by vasodilator therapy for NOMI, by reduction of a strangulation, by embolectomy, or by revascularization of an occlusion, an operative decision must be made as to whether or not to resect the injured intestine and to what extent. This decision is made by assessment of viability, determining whether or not the affected section of bowel will maintain its structural integrity and heal. Intestinal viability is assessed clinically by the observation of arterial pulsations, peristalsis, and the color and tone of the segment in question. In most cases, the result is obvious. When the surgeon feels confident of this clinic assessment of viability, he or she is usually correct. When one is unsure, the observation of the pattern of reperfusion under *ultraviolet illumination* with a standard (3,600 Å) Wood's lamp, after IV administration of 1 g of *sodium fluorescein* slowly over about 30 seconds via the IV line, is usually accurately discriminating. This technique allows rapid screening by observation of the entire area of bowel in question. Any area of nonfluorescence that is > 5 mm in diameter usually indicates impending necrosis, although occasionally an overly pessimistic assessment is made, especially cases of venous occlusion. It is important to ensure the small blood clots on the surface are not misinterpreted as areas of nonperfusion. The bowel must be laid out for observation before injection of the dye, as the transudation of the dye across the serosa may passively stain nonviable areas lying in a puddle of dye-laden peritoneal fluid. Other adjuvant methods for the assessment of viability either have proved too cumbersome for practical clinical use or, like the Doppler technique, have proved unreliable in controlled clinical trials. If doubt still exists as to intestinal viability, the abdomen should be reexplored at 24 to 48 hours to provide a *second look evaluation*.

When intestinal viability is borderline at the margin of resection, it is better to avoid anastomosis of the cut ends, and these should be exteriorized as stomas. (This measure also permits the continued assessment of the viability.) This is true whether the SB or large bowel is involved. In cases in which a high SB fistula is created, it is possible to consider early anastomosis as the patient recovers from the systemic illness. In the meantime, it is important that optimal enterostomal therapy be provided to avoid skin erosion. This is greatly facilitated by the use of gentle, continuous suction on a small sump catheter and a surrounding secure stomal appliance. Fluid losses can be easily replaced if they are accurately monitored in this manner. It is important to watch for the development of metabolic acidosis due to bicarbonate losses and to treat it appropriately.

Occasionally the extent of bowel resection required does not leave the patient with enough bowel to sustain survival by enteral alimentation. In these cases, the choice of long term or even permanent parenteral alimentation must be considered. Each decision must be made and each patient treated on an individual basis. Certainly younger patients, for example, those with a congenital midgut volvulus, deserve serious consideration for long term parenteral alimentation until SB transplantation is widely available. There is a separate chapter on short bowel syndrome (see Chapter 64, "Short Bowel Syndrome") and another on small bowel transplantation (see Chapter 65, "Intestinal and Multivisceral Transplantation").

Specific Syndromes of Mesenteric Ischemia

Acute Arterial Occlusion

When intestinal ischemia is the result of the acute occlusion of a major mesenteric artery, the diagnosis is often obvious clinically (see Table 70-3). Accordingly, many of these patients are diagnosed earlier and hence are in more stable condition at the time of diagnosis. As soon as the patient's condition has been stabilized and monitoring capabilities have been secured, he or she should be transferred to the cardiovascular diagnostic laboratory and an arteriogram obtained of the celiac, superior mesenteric artery (SMA),

TABLE 70-6. Critical Points in Management of Acute Intestinal Ischemia

Condition	Early Diagnosis	Treatment
Arterial thrombosis	CT scan	Early vascular bypass
	Angiography	Accurate assessment of viability
Arterial embolism	CT scan	Early embolectomy
	Angiography	Accurate assessment of viability
Venous thrombosis	CT scan	Anticoagulation
	Angiography	Hydration, accurate assessment of viability
Strangulation obstruction	CT scan	Early operative reduction
	Early laparotomy	Accurate assessment of viability
Nonocclusive mesenteric ischemia	Early angiography	Intra-arterial vasodilatorys
	-	Reversal of underlying systemic condition
	-	Delayed laparotomy
	-	Accurate assessment of viability
Ischemic colitis	Sigmoidoscopy	Reversal of underlying systemic condition
	-	Delayed laparotomy
	-	Accurate assessment of viability

Adapted from Bulkley, 1986.
CT = computed tomography.

and inferior mesenteric artery (IMA). Whenever a mesenteric arteriogram is obtained, it is important to obtain biplanar views. This study establishes or rules out the diagnosis and sometimes distinguishes an embolus from a thrombus. If an embolus is suspected, particularly if there is a history of a recent myocardial infarction, cardiac catheterization, angiography, endocarditis, atrial fibrillation, cardioversion, or previous embolization, anticoagulant therapy with heparin is indicated, if not immediately, then in the postoperative period.

Laparotomy should then follow directly, the leg having been prepared to provide access to a saphenous vein. The SMA is best approached by following the middle colic vessels to the root of the transverse mesocolon. Most emboli lodge just proximal to this junction. Embolectomy or thrombectomy is attempted through a transverse arteriotomy with a Number 3 Fogarty catheter. If free inflow (and backflow) are obtained, this may be sufficient. The artery is usually closed with a transverse suture line. If free inflow is not obtained, with or without the removal of an embolus, a bypass is probably required. In cases of advanced atherosclerosis of the orifice of the SMA, with or without an embolus, an endarterectomy is rarely successful, and a bypass from the aorta below the renal arteries to the distal SMA may be necessary. *Saphenous vein* is the preferred material, but expanded *polytetrafluoroethylene (GoreTex)* may also be used. In recent years, aortic thromboendarterectomy has been successfully employed from a retroperitoneal approach in elective situations. This is not the optimal approach to the patient with *acute* mesenteric ischemia, however, because it fails to afford adequate assessment of bowel viability and to provide access for resection, if necessary. Viability is assessed no less than 15 minutes after revascularization, and the appropriate resection performed if necessary. Most surgeons prefer to give heparin in the postoperative period or at least to use low molecular weight dextran. The above is the traditional paradigm for the management of acute arterial occlusion, and remains the gold standard against which other approaches are measured. Acceptable variations on this approach include immediate laparotomy (without prior angiography) in cases where the clinical setting (eg, recent cardioversion) clearly indicates an SMA embolus. Another approach to acute thrombatic (ie, hemorrhage into a preexisting plaque) occlusion is angiography with stenting. The interventional radiologist may be able to open the primarily occluded vessel, or to improve collateral flow by dilating one of the other two mesenteric vascular trunks. The long term patency of this approach remains controversial, however.

Venous Thrombosis

The less common condition of mensenteric venous thrombosis occurs in the face of a predisposing factor, such as severe, especially acute, portal hypertension, polycythemia vera, severe dehydration, and other hypercoagulable states, including, occasionally, pregnancy. In recent years, subclinical coagulopathies due to deficiencies in protein A, protein C, and factor V Leiden have been identified in many of these patients. Frequently, there is a history of (even minor) abdominal trauma. The diagnosis is suspected on the basis of the massive fluid losses and the more gradual onset of symptoms, in the presence of one of the predisposing factors. Abdominal symptoms may be subtle, but are usually progressive. After fluid resuscitation, which is often massive, the diagnosis can be confirmed by observing the venous phase of the mesenteric angiogram, but nowadays it is usually made by a CT scan with IV contrast. For the most part, treatment is by anticoagulation; surgery is reserved for the resection of dead bowel 24 to 48 hours later. There is little rationale for early laparotomy, as venous thrombectomy is rarely successful. In cases of acute portal hypertension, such as those due to the Budd-Chiari syndrome, a portasystemic shunt may be useful in combination with a successful mesenteric venous thrombectomy.

Strangulation Obstruction

Any patient with *complete* mechanical SB obstruction is at substantial risk of vascular compromise; about *one-third of patients* who *undergo laparotomy for obstruction have strangulation*. Furthermore, it is not possible to distinguish clinically those patients with early strangulation from those with simple obstruction. This fact has been repeatedly demonstrated by retrospective studies and also in a controlled, prospective study in which the clinical assessments of strangulation and no strangulation were each incorrect in about a third of the cases. *Therefore, the primary treatment of complete mechanical SB obstruction should be laparotomy, usually within 12 to 24 hours of presentation.* Delay must be justified by clinical circumstances severe enough to justify the 30% risk of delaying treatment of acute intestinal ischemia. Complete obstruction can usually be discriminated from partial obstruction clinically, and with the help of a CT scan with oral contrast. Intestinal strangulation causes both the most common and the most treatable form of mesenteric vascular disease. With prompt laparotomy, reduction of the strangulation, and judicious resection of only the nonviable bowel, recovery can usually be expected. In these cases, a primary anastomosis can usually be performed because the intestinal margins are abrupt and lie outside the area of strangulation

NOMI

NOMI represents selective vasoconstriction of the mesenteric resistance vessels in response to some form of severe physiologic stress. It is therefore essential to attempt to treat the underlying cause while addressing the disease itself. This usually includes *optimization of the cardiac output with flu-*

ids and inotropic agents, but avoidance of many vasoconstrictor agents and digitalis glycosides. Sepsis, respiratory insufficiency, metabolic acidosis, and electrolyte abnormalities must be aggressively corrected. Unfortunately, as NOMI progresses, it contributes substantially to those very factors that have caused it in the first place, and a vicious circle ensues. Therefore, management of the systemic effects of bowel ischemia must be particularly aggressive.

This disease can be diagnosed only by *angiography* in those patients in whom it is suspected by the astute clinician. The appearance of abdominal pain, distention, or ileus associated with sepsis or cardiovascular deterioration in patients in the population at risk, should immediately prompt an arteriographic study or a CT scan timed with IV contrast (see Table 70-3). Treatment consists of *selective intra-arterial infusion of a splanchnic vasodilator, usually papaverine*, via the same catheter used to establish the diagnosis. A second arteriogram is obtained 15 to 20 minutes after the start of infusion to demonstrate morphologic evidence of reversal of the previously demonstrated vasospasm. The patient is then returned to the intensive care unit (ICU), and the *infusion is continued for 24 to 48 hours*. If doubt exists as to the effectiveness of therapy, this can be reassessed at any time via the in situ catheter by repeated arteriography. The position of the infusion catheter can even be checked in the ICU by injecting a bolus of dye at the time a flat portable film of the abdomen is taken.

Surgery should be delayed initially because it adds to the level of physiologic stress and cannot reverse the primary lesion. It is an error to operate on one of these patients without first establishing and treating the diagnosis arteriographically. Because most of these patients have a substantial degree of preexisting mesenteric atherosclerosis, the situation at surgery can be quite misleading without an angiogram; in the face of severe mesenteric vasospasm, anatomic revascularization alone will not be sufficient. In such circumstances, the abdomen should be closed and the patient transported directly to the catheterization laboratory. When a patient has received optimal vasodilator therapy for a day or two and begins to show signs of increasing sepsis or of an acute abdomen, laparotomy is then appropriate to facilitate the resection of the unsalvaged, necrotic bowel. This delay also facilitates the assessment of viability because the initial laparotomy becomes, in effect, a second-look procedure.

Ischemic Colitis

Colonic ischemia may result from any of the aforementioned circumstances; the colon may even be involved in an intestinal strangulation due to *cecal or sigmoid volvulus*. Perhaps the most common cause of severe colonic ischemia is the *ligation of the IMA* during abdominal aortic surgery. It is also important to note that two common forms of infectious colitis, from *Clostridium difficile* and enteropathogenic *Escherichia coli* are manifestations of *toxin-induced tissue ischemia*. The principles of management are essentially the same as those already outlined and should be guided by the particular etiology. A substantial difference is the availability of the colonic mucosa for direct observation, and all patients suspected of having ischemic bowel disease should undergo gentle proctosigmoidoscopy with minimal air insufflation. Fiberoptic sigmoidoscopy or even colonoscopy has been found to be safe and helpful. Involvement of the colon in any diffuse ischemic process may indicate proximal SB involvement as well. The mucosa is more sensitive to ischemia than the muscularis propria, but the integrity of the muscularis determines ultimate viability; the mucosa regenerates if the muscular tube survives. One must therefore be careful not to overestimate the depth of the necrosis or to underestimate the length of bowel involved. Arteriography is rarely useful because of the high incidence of preexisting incidental occlusion of the IMA in these patients.

Unlike patients with other forms of mesenteric ischemia, many of those with ischemic colitis can be kept under observation, especially if the lesion is known to be limited to the colon. In these cases, plain abdominal films are often helpful because gas in the lumen may provide contrast for images rivaling those of a barium enema. Patients with disease limited to the mucosa sometimes recover without surgery although late strictures may form. *Serial endoscopy* is a best way to follow these patients, allowing surgery to be performed only upon those progressing to transmural ischemic necrosis. Perforation of necrotic bowel is a concern.

Some patients with a necrotic colon require a total colectomy and sometimes resection of the necrotic rectum as well. In many cases the collateral circulation of the rectum, via the inferior and middle hemorrhoidal vessels from the systemic circulation, is adequate to allow it to be left as a Hartmann's pouch. Although it is not always possible to use this segment to later restore a functioning rectum, avoidance of an abdominoperineal resection in these severely ill patients is a distinct advantage. A preoperative proctoscopic examination is essential so that the extent of the resection required can be determined.

Supplemental Reading

Abdu RA, Zakhour BJ, Dallis DJ. Mesenteric venous thrombosis—1911–1984. Surgery 1987;383–5.

Boley SJ, Sprayregen S, Siegelman SS, Veith FJ. Initial results from an aggressive approach to acute mesenteric ischemia. Surgery 1977;82:848–55.

Bulkley GB. Mesenteric vascular occlusive disease. In: Cameron JL. Current surgical therapy. 2nd ed. St Louis: Mosby-Year Book; 1986. p. 74.

Bulkley GB, Zuidema GD, Hamilton SR, et al. Intraoperative determination of small intestinal viability following ischemic injury. A prospective controlled trial of two adjacent methods (Doppler and fluorescein) compared with standard clinical judgement. Ann Surg 1981;193:628–37.

Carrico CJ, Meakins, Marshall J, et al. Multiple organ failure syndrome. Arch Surg 1986;121:196–208.

Marston A, Bulkley GB, Fiddian-Green RF, Haglund UH. Splanchnic ischemia and multiple organ failure. London: Edward Arnold; 1989.

Peters JH, Reilly PM, Merine DS, Bulkley GB. Mesenteric vascular insufficiency. In: Yamada T, editor. Textbook of gastroenterology. Philadlephia: JB Lippincott; 1991. p. 2188–217.

Reilly PM, Jones B, Bulkley GB. Noninvasive assessment of ischemic bowel syndromes. In: Ernst CB, Stanley JB, editors. Current therapy in vascular surgery. 2nd ed. Philadelphia: BC Decker; 1991. p. 718–25.

Sarr MG, Bulkley GB, Zuidema GD. Preoperative recognition of intestinal strangulation obstruction: a prospective evaluation at diagnostic capability. Am J Surg 1982;145:176–82.419

Sreenarisimhaiah J. Diagnosis and management of intestinal ischemic disorders. BMJ 2003;326;1372–6.

CHAPTER 71

Management of Diabetic Diarrhea

Michael Camilleri, MD, and Fillippo Cremonini, MD

Chronic diarrhea is a frequent manifestation in patients with diabetes mellitus, and is present in patients with type 1 or type 2 diabetes. According to some evidence, up to 15% of patients with diabetes mellitus may experience diarrhea (Bytzer et al, 2001). However, other studies have found no difference in the prevalence of diarrhea between diabetics and community control subjects (Maleki et al, 2000). Thus, in the general population there might be no increased prevalence or association between diarrhea and diabetes, and the symptoms of diarrhea might be attributable to other common conditions, such as irritable bowel syndrome (IBS), occurring in a patient with diabetes. Nonetheless, some patients with diabetes have significant diarrhea and present for examination and treatment.

Mechanisms of Chronic Diarrhea in Diabetes Mellitus

Table 71-1 provides an overview of the pathophysiological mechanisms and conditions associated with diarrhea in diabetes. The mechanisms of chronic diarrhea in diabetes are incompletely understood. However, several commonly encountered mechanisms for diarrhea in patients with diabetes should be considered. Diarrhea may result from intake of *medications* or the excessive use of dietetic foods that contain *sorbitol* as a sweetener. *Autonomic neuropathy* (Vinik et al, 2003) or diseases associated with diabetes, such as *celiac disease*, may be the underlying causes of chronic diarrhea.

Autonomic Neuropathy

Autonomic or somatic neuropathy may lead to pelvic floor dysfunction and altered small bowel and colonic motility. Alteration in bowel motor function may cause diarrhea from accelerated transit, but delayed transit may also contribute to development of *bacterial overgrowth*, resulting in deconjugation of bile salts, fat malabsorption, and diarrhea.

Some patients may have *alterations* in *intestinal transport* of water and electrolytes, resulting in diarrhea. Rarely, there is exocrine *pancreatic insufficiency*, leading to steatorrhea.

Fecal incontinence caused by pelvic floor dysfunction or anal sphincter denervation is more frequent in diabetes than in community controls and should be distinguished from "true" diarrhea.

Celiac Disease Association

The association between celiac disease and diabetes is well recognized (Walsh et al, 1978, Talal et al, 1997). Celiac disease is more prevalent in patients with diabetes than in the general population. A common underlying immunogenetic predisposition has been identified (HLA DQ_2). Conversely, the proportion of subjects with endoscopically confirmed celiac disease and concomitant diabetes mellitus is about 8%. Hence, this association with celiac disease may explain diarrhea in a small proportion of patients with diabetes.

Management of Diabetic Diarrhea

Clinical Examination and Routine Tests

An accurate clinical history should collect information on the stool form and the presence of urgency or incontinence. The chronic diarrhea of diabetes is generally watery, paroxysmal, and includes nocturnal episodes. Presence of blood per rectum, relationship of diarrhea to dietary factors including sorbitol-containing dietetic foods, and features suggestive of fecal

Table 71-1 Mechanisms, Concomitant Conditions, and Clinical Characteristics of Diarrhea in Diabetes Mellitus

Pathophysiological Mechanism	Associated Disease	Clinical Presentation
	Exocrine pancreatic insufficiency Celiac sprue SB bacterial overgrowth Bile acid malabsorption	Diarrhea, steatorrhea
SB dysmotility Colonic dysmotility Decreased α-2-adrenergic tone in enterocytes		Constipation or diarrhea
Anorectal dysfunction Sensory neuropathy IAS-sympathetic EAS-pudendal neuropathy		Diarrhea or incontinence

SB = small bowel; IAS = internal anal sphincter; EAS = external anal sphincter.

incontinence should be sought in history. Oral medications used for glycemic control, such as *metformin* (Avandemet) and *acarbose* (Precose), are often associated with bloating, diarrhea, and other gastrointestinal side effects. Other medications may cause diarrhea, including laxatives and prokinetics. The clinical examination should include a thorough neurological evaluation, with the search for signs suggesting autonomic neuropathy (such as orthostatic hypotension, lack of pupillary response to light, response of pulse and blood pressure to the Valsalva maneuver and absence of sweating), or malabsorption, such as anemia, edema, and clubbing.

The presence of an abdominal mass or tenderness suggests the presence of concomitant conditions causing diarrhea, such as inflammatory bowel disease (IBD) or a neoplasm. Since up to 20% of tertiary referral patients with diabetes may experience *fecal incontinence*, an anorectal examination should be performed (Camilleri, 1996). The anorectal examination includes inspection of the external anal area for the presence of rectal prolapse, digital assessment of the sphincter tone at rest and during squeeze, and assessment of alterations in sensation (eg, pinprick around anal verge).

Laboratory

A routine hematological and biochemical screening, serum tissue transglutaminase assay, and analysis of stool for blood, leukocytes, ova, and parasites should be performed; a flexible sigmoidoscopy or colonoscopy will exclude specific causes of chronic diarrhea, such as IBD.

Initial Management

These screening tests will indicate whether the patient needs correction of water and electrolytes imbalance in the initial management. Adequate glycemic control and nutritional support is necessary. In patients with dehydration, oral solutions containing glucose, rice powder, or glycine can be safely administered without significant fluctuation in blood glucose levels. Rarely, IV hyperalimentation or fluid replacement may be administered over a longer period to restore nutrition and hydration.

Management of Specific Causes of Diarrhea

When available, we recommend directing the therapeutic intervention to the relevant underlying mechanism of chronic diarrhea by the use of appropriate testing. We prefer this approach to sequential empiric trials with antidiarrheals and other trials (eg, with dietary alteration and antibiotics). A combined diagnostic-therapeutic algorithm is proposed in Figure 71-1.

Celiac Sprue

If the clinical examination or routine laboratory tests are suggestive of *malabsorption*, further testing should be undertaken to identify potentially relevant conditions, specifically celiac sprue, bacterial overgrowth, and pancreatic exocrine insufficiency. *Anti-endomysial* and *antitissue transglutaminase* antibodies should be sought, and, eventually, a *jejunal biopsy* will be needed to confirm any positive serological findings. In patients with concomitant diabetes and celiac disease confirmed by jejunal biopsy, the institution of a gluten-free diet leads to the regression of mucosal abnormalities and typically normalizes bowel habits. There is a separate chapter on celiac sprue (see Chapter 61, "Celiac Sprue and Related Problems").

Gut Dysmotility and Hypersecretion

The presence of *gut dysmotility* can be assessed by means of radiographic, breath or scintigraphic tests, to assess transit, or by using gastrointestinal manometry to identify abnormal contractile profiles. Compared to the more widely available, less expensive radiographic techniques, the transit techniques involving radioisotopes allow simultaneous determination of gastric emptying and small bowel and colonic transit. Figure 71-2 shows an example of markedly accelerated colonic transit. Loperamide (Imodium) (2 to 4 mg, up to 4 times a day) can prolong intestinal transit time and decrease the frequency of bowel movement.

Clonidine

Intestinal perfusion studies to detect secretory abnormalities are cumbersome and rarely available. The α-2-adrenoceptor agonist *clonidine* (Catapres) (0.05 to 0.2 mg once or twice daily) can be used on the basis of its antisecretory properties (Fedorak et al, 1985). We often administer clonidine as a patch on the skin in order to avoid its systemic side effects, such as orthostatic hypotension or bradycardia.

Octreotide

The long acting somatostatin analogue *octreotide acetate* (50 to 75 μg tid ac) is also used based on the antisecretory and motility retarding properties of somatostatin(von der Ohe et al, 1995; Mourad et al, 1992)Somatostatin can also improve gut absorptive capacity, while suppressing potentially diarrheogenic hormones. It may be administered with insulin. There is initial inhibition of pancreatic exocrine function; however, the negative effect on nutrient absorption with octreotide is short–lived (Gullo, 1996)and pancreatic secretion is enhanced over time so that iatrogenic exocrine insufficiency is not a clinical problem.

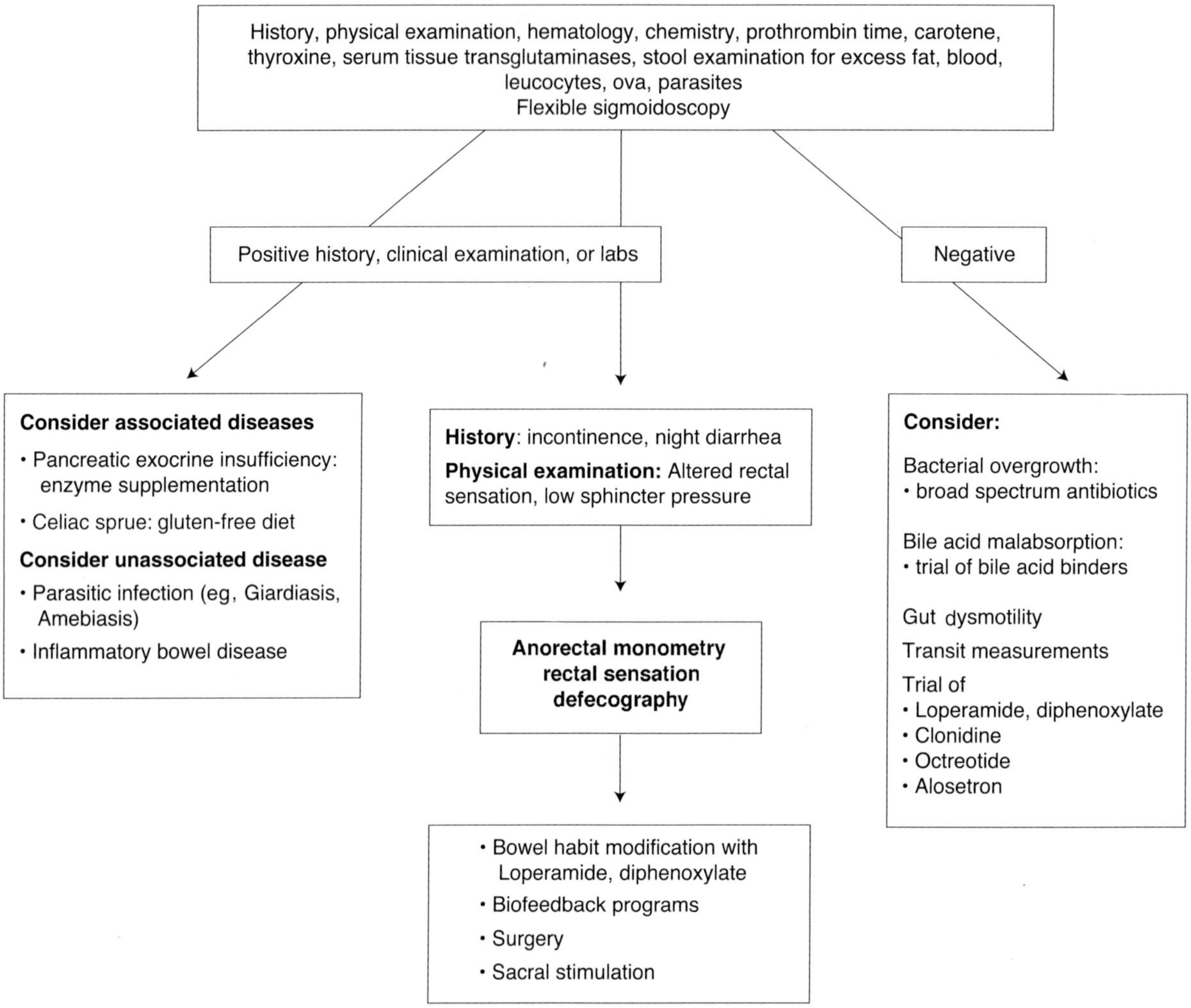

```
┌─────────────────────────────────────────────────────────┐
│ History, physical examination, hematology, chemistry,   │
│ prothrombin time, carotene, thyroxine, serum tissue     │
│ transglutaminases, stool examination for excess fat,    │
│ blood, leucocytes, ova, parasites                       │
│ Flexible sigmoidoscopy                                  │
└─────────────────────────────────────────────────────────┘
```

```
┌──────────────────────────────────────┐      ┌──────────┐
│ Positive history, clinical           │      │ Negative │
│ examination, or labs                 │      └──────────┘
└──────────────────────────────────────┘
```

Consider associated diseases
- Pancreatic exocrine insufficiency: enzyme supplementation
- Celiac sprue: gluten-free diet

Consider unassociated disease
- Parasitic infection (eg, Giardiasis, Amebiasis)
- Inflammatory bowel disease

History: incontinence, night diarrhea
Physical examination: Altered rectal sensation, low sphincter pressure

Anorectal monometry rectal sensation defecography

- Bowel habit modification with Loperamide, diphenoxylate
- Biofeedback programs
- Surgery
- Sacral stimulation

Consider:

Bacterial overgrowth:
- broad spectrum antibiotics

Bile acid malabsorption:
- trial of bile acid binders

Gut dysmotility
Transit measurements
Trial of
- Loperamide, diphenoxylate
- Clonidine
- Octreotide
- Alosetron

FIGURE 711. Diagnostic-therapeutic algorithm for the management of chronic diarrhea.

ALOSETRON

The serotonin 5HT$_3$ receptor antagonist *alosetron*, (Lotronex) at doses of 1 mg bid may retard colonic transit and reduce diarrhea, but it is approved only for severe IBS. Cases of *ischemic colitis* have been reported in the post-marketing phase of alosetron use, and this drug should be used with *extreme caution* if it is ever considered, given the great potential of microvascular complications of diabetes.

Bacterial Overgrowth

Bowel stasis may be a major contributory cause of bacterial overgrowth in diabetics. In chronic diarrhea, there are no specific clinical features suggestive of bacterial overgrowth. Bacterial overgrowth is actually quite rare in practice (Whalen et al, 1969; Valdovinos et al, 1993). The most specific technique for diagnosis of small bowel bacterial overgrowth is the quantitative culture of jejunal aspirate. An aerobic bacterial count of greater than 10^5 colony forming units/mL aspirate is regarded as the cut off for bacterial

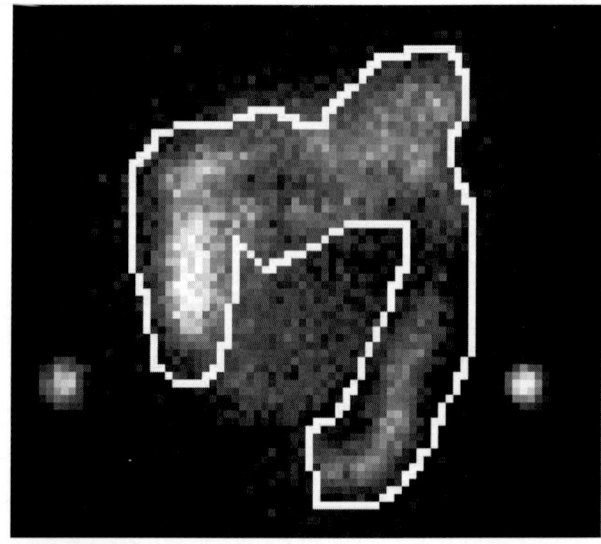

FIGURE 712. Accelerated colonic transit.

overgrowth. Noninvasive techniques, such as the 14 C-D-xylose and the H_2-lactulose breath test, have also been used. However, these techniques have poor sensitivity and may be influenced by several factors, including luminal pH, gut flora species, and alterations in motility.

ANTIBOTICS

In the presence of bacterial overgrowth, the use of broad spectrum oral antibiotics, such as *doxycycline, cephalosporins, quinolones, rifaxamin* and *nitro-imidazoles,* can resolve diarrhea and may reduce associated symptoms, such as bloating. Antibiotics are generally prescribed for 10 to 14 days, in order to avoid the development of microbial resistance. Supplementation with *probiotics*, such as *Lactobacilli* or *Saccharomyces boulardii,* can also been used in conjunction with antibiotic therapy in order to recolonize the bowel mucosa with commensal microorganisms, but the efficacy of this strategy is still unproven.

Biliary Malabsorption

Malabsorption of bile acids should be suspected when there are no elements suggestive of steatorrhea, fecal incontinence, abnormal transit, or bacterial overgrowth. The ^{75}Se-homocholic acid taurine test is the simplest method to determine bile acid absorption capacity, but it is not currently available. The abdominal retention of the radioisotope is measured after 4 and 7 days. An abdominal retention of the radioisotope of less than 10% at 7 days is considered positive for disturbance in bile acid absorption. Bile acid resin binders, such as *cholestyramine* 4 to 12 g/d, *colestipol* or *aluminium hydroxide*, may provide relief.

Pancreatic Insufficiency

A past history of heavy alcohol consumption, with recurrent abdominal pain and steatorrhea should suggest *chronic pancreatitis* as a cause for diabetes. Stool fat, pancreatic function tests (such as duodenal intubation with secretin-cholecystokinin stimulation, endoscopy-based duodenal fluid collection (Conwell et al, 2003) or less invasive techniques involving breath testing (such as 13C-mixed triglyceride breath test), confirm the diagnosis. If functional tests are suggestive of pancreatic insufficiency, *pancreatic enzymes* can be supplemented with each meal.

Fecal Incontinence

If clinical examination, routine labs, and serology fail to identify mechanisms responsible for diarrhea, the clinician should focus on possible *indicators of fecal incontinence* in the history and clinical examination. In patients with diabetes, fecal incontinence is common either alone, as a disorder of the anorectal sphincter, or in association with diarrhea. Patients most often present with nocturnal incontinence, which reflects poor rectal sensation and internal sphincter or sympathetic dysfunction. Anorectal and pelvic floor function testing techniques may be required to confirm the diagnosis and to decide on the most appropriate therapeutic strategies for fecal incontinence. Anorectal manometry and defecography are the most widely available tests. *Anorectal manometry* in patients with incontinence may demonstrate weakness of the internal anal sphincter (with reduced resting pressure), weakness of the external sphincter (reduced squeeze pressure), an increased threshold for evoking the rectosphincteric inhibitory reflex, and reduced rectal sensation. Defecography is rarely required.

PHARMACOLOGIC TREATMENT

Treatment options for fecal incontinence include pharmacological and nonpharmacological approaches (Barucha, 2003). The first step is to modify bowel habits. The peripheral opioid agonist *loperamide* (Imodium)(2 to 4 mg, ac, up to 16 mg/d) can help reduce diarrhea, and is reported to increase the anal sphincter tone, thereby reducing incontinence. The use of loperamide before social events can be encouraged to help the patients avoid episodes of incontinence and gain confidence in their ability to participate in social activities. *Diphenoxylate plasatropinal* (Lomotil®) is another opioid agonist, which can be considered as an alternative to loperamide. The topical application of *phenylephrine*, an α-1-adrenergic agonist, to the anal canal, may increase anal resting pressure(Carapeti et al, 1999) but its effect on incontinence is often unsatisfactory (Carapeti, 2000).

NONPHARMACOLOGICAL THERAPY

Nonpharmacological therapy includes biofeedback, surgical approaches, and sacral nerve stimulation. There is a separate chapter on fecal incontinence (see Chapter 88, "Fecal Incontinence: Evaluation and Treatment"). In biofeedback programs, patients are taught to contract the external anal sphincter using a rectal balloon-manometric device used for the perception of distention. Balloon volumes are progressively decreased through the training sessions to help the patient learn retention of increasingly smaller volumes of feces. An improvement in sensory discrimination after biofeedback therapy is associated with improved continence.

Surgical options should be considered a last resort for diabetic fecal incontinence, in view of the risk of surgical complications in patients with poor control of diabetes. *Sphincteroplasty* is the most frequently performed procedure and it is able to restore continence. However, 50% of patients present with recurrent incontinence at 5 years. *Sacral nerve stimulation* has received approval by the US Food and Drug Administration for patients with urinary incontinence. European multicenter studies on fecal incontinence showed encouraging results, and this technique is currently under assessment in the United States (Barucha 2003). Given the lack of data on safety and efficacy of sacral nerve stimulation, we are not able to recommend this approach at the present time.

Conclusions

The treatment of diarrhea in diabetes mellitus should be directed at the identified pathophysiology. An accurate history, clinical examination, and the use of noninvasive or minimally invasive tests can identify the mechanism of diarrhea in the majority of patients and lead to pharmacological or nonpharmacological approaches that ameliorate the patients' symptoms and quality of life.

Supplemental Reading

American Gastroenterological Association medical position statement: celiac sprue. Gastroenterology 2001;120:1522–5.

Barucha AE. Fecal incontinence. Gastroenterology 2003; 124:1672–85.

Bytzer P, Talley NJ, Leemon M, et al. Prevalence of gastrointestinal symptoms associated with diabetes mellitus: a population-based survey of 15,000 adults. Arch Intern Med 2001;161:1989–96.

Camilleri M. Gastrointestinal problems in diabetes. Endocrinol Metab Clin North Am 1996;25:361–78.

Carapeti EA, Kamm MA, Evans BK, Phillips RK. Topical phenylephrine increases anal sphincter resting pressure. Br J Surg 1999;86:267–70.

Carapeti EA, Kamm MA, Phillips RK. Randomized controlled trial of topical phenylephrine in the treatment of faecal incontinence. Br J Surg 2000;87:38–42.

Conwell DL, Zuccaro Jr G, Vargo JJ, et al. An endoscopic pancreatic function test with cholecystokinin-octapeptide for the diagnosis of chronic pancreatitis. Clin Gastroenterol Hepatol 2003;1:189–94.

Fedorak RN, Field M, Chang EB. Treatment of diabetic diarrhea with clonidine. Ann Intern Med 1985;102:197–9.

Gullo L. Somatostatin analogues and exocrine pancreatic secretion. Digestion 1996;57:93.

Maleki D, Locke GR 3rd, Camilleri M, et al. Gastrointestinal tract symptoms among persons with diabetes mellitus in the community. Arch Intern Med 2000;160:2808–16.

Mourad FH, Gorard D, Thillainayagam AV, et al. Effective treatment of diabetic diarrhoea with somatostatin analogue, octreotide. Gut 1992;33:1578–80.

Talal AH, Murray JA, Goeken JA, Sivitz WI. Celiac disease in an adult population with insulin-dependent diabetes mellitus: use of endomysial antibody testing. Am J Gastroenterol 1997;92:1280–4.

Valdovinos MA, Camilleri M, Zimmerman BR. Chronic diarrhea in diabetes mellitus: mechanisms and an approach to diagnosis and treatment. Mayo Clin Proc 1993;68:691–702.

Vinik AI, Maser RE, Mitchell BD, Freeman R. Diabetic autonomic neuropathy. Diabetes Care 2003;26:1553–79.

von der Ohe MR, Camilleri M, Thomforde GM, Klee GG. Differential regional effects of octreotide on human gastrointestinal motor function. Gut 1995;36:743–8.

Walsh CH, Cooper BT, Wright AD, et al, Diabetes mellitus and coeliac disease: a clinical study. Q J Med 1978;47:89–100.

Whalen GE, Soergel KH, Geenen JE. Diabetic diarrhea. A clinical and pathophysiological study. Gastroenterology 1969;56:1021–32.

CHAPTER 72

Secretory Diarrhea

Fathia Gibril, MD, and Robert T. Jensen, MD

Secretory diarrhea (SD) results from the active secretion of electrolytes (sodium ion [Na^+], potassium ion [K^+], chlorine ion [Cl^-], and bicarbonate ion [HCO_3^-]), the failure to absorb these electrolytes, or both processes. A secretory component can occur in diarrheal diseases owing to enteric infections, inflammatory conditions, or ectopic hormone or neurotransmitter release. The primary clinical features of SD include daily stool weights exceeding 200 g/d, watery stools, and a stool osmolarity accounted for almost entirely by twice the stool concentration of Na^+ plus K^+. This latter point is usually established by measuring stool K^+ and Na^+ concentrations and calculating the osmotic gap by subtracting twice the concentrations of stool sodium and potassium from 290 mOsm/kg, the osmolality of stool within the body. In SD, the osmotic gap is characteristically < 100 mOsm/kg and is usually < 50 mOsm/kg. In most cases, SD persists despite fasting for 1 to 2 days, although it frequently decreases in amount (Jensen, 1999).

In this chapter, treatment of SD is briefly reviewed. Not discussed are diarrheal diseases with a secretory component included in other chapters in this volume, including (1) infectious diarrheas, (2) diarrheas owing to bile salts or fatty acids, and (3) diarrhea owing to inflammatory diseases such as inflammatory bowel disease. This chapter focuses on the treatment of the remaining causes of SD, including those owing to *hormone-related diarrhea*, *surreptitious use of laxatives*, and *SD of unknown origin*. The hormone-related diarrheas include *vasoactive intestinal secreting tumors* (VIPomas), *gastrinomas* causing Zollinger-Ellison syndrome, *glucagonomas*, *somatostatinomas*, *medullary thyroid cancer*, and *systemic mastocytosis*.

General Approach to Treatment

Neuroendocrine Tumors

Many of these disorders are due to a *neuroendocrine tumor ectopically secreting* a *hormone* causing the diarrhea. Therefore, each patient has two different processes requiring treatment: *treatment of the hormone excess state* (in this article, the diarrhea) and *treatment* directed at the *tumor per se*. The latter is important because 40 to 90% of these neuroendocrine tumors are *malignant* in different series. Although complete tumor resection would accomplish both treatment aims, it is frequently not possible because of the presence of metastases at presentation resulting in unresectable disease. The clinical state owing to the ectopic release of hormone should be treated first because, in some cases (especially VIPomas, gastrinomas), it can be life threatening. Although general treatments for the diarrheal state are frequently used, definitive treatment of each of these disorders requires that the correct diagnosis is made using the appropriate laboratory methods (ie, radioimmunoassays, biochemical assays, and measurements of hormonal activity).

Diarrhea Control

The specific approach to controlling the diarrhea in each of these disorders is dictated to a large degree by its pathogenesis and the volume of the diarrhea. The approach to patients with mild to moderate diarrhea frequently differs from that of patients with more severe, large-volume diarrhea (ie, > 1/1.5 L/d). VIPomas almost invariably result in daily stool outputs > 1 L/d, and in 70% of patients, it is > 3 L/d. Although it has been proposed that a diarrhea volume < 700 mL/d excludes this diagnosis, the diarrhea can be episodic. With gastrinomas, 30 to 75% of the patients have diarrhea, but in only 10% of the patients is the stool volume > 1 L/d at present, in contrast to older studies in which 40% of patients had > 1 L/d. In carcinoid syndrome, 32 to 84% of patients have diarrhea, but in only 40% does it exceed 1 L/d. In medullary thyroid cancer, 28 to 42% of patients have diarrhea, and in 30%, it exceeds 1 L/d. In somatostatinomas and glucagonomas, 30 to 97% and 14 to 25%, respectively, have diarrhea, but it exceeds 1 L/d only in < 10% of patients. With systemic mastocytosis, 25 to 43% of patients have diarrhea, but it rarely exceeds 1 L/d. All patients with surreptitious use of laxatives or SD of unknown origin have diarrhea, which frequently exceeds 1 L/d.

Fluid and Electrolyte Replacement

Oral Rehydration Solutions

The greatest risk to life for a patient owing to SD is *dehydration* or electrolyte loss. It is, therefore, essential that these patients be adequately rehydrated and electrolyte loss corrected. In patients with *mild to moderate* SD (< 1 to 1.5 L/d), this can frequently be accomplished using *oral rehydration solutions* (*ORSs*). Some patients with severe diarrhea may have normal absorptive function retained, and oral rehydration or replacement can be effective in them. Because nutrient absorption is coupled with sodium absorption, glucose or amino acids in combination with sodium can enhance the absorption of electrolytes and water. It is important to remember that standard ORSs are primarily *designed to increase electrolyte and fluid absorption* and *may not reduce stool output*, and, in fact, *stool output may increase*. The World Health Organization's (WHO) ORS recommendation contains sodium (90 mmol/L), potassium (20 mmol/L), chloride (80 mmol/L), citrate (30 mmol/L), and glucose (111 mmol/L). This is prepared by adding 3.5 g of sodium chloride, 1.5 g of potassium chloride, 2.9 g of trisodium citrate dihydrate, and 20 g of glucose per liter of water. *Rice-based ORSs* have been shown to not only increase absorption but also to decrease stool volume. Most sport drinks, such as Gatorade, are designed to replenish electrolytes primarily lost from sweat and do not have enough sodium to fully replace diarrheal sodium loss. Commercial solutions available that approximate the WHO's ORS include Resol, Ricalyte, Ceralyte, Pedialyte, and Rehydralyte.

Intravenous Replacement

In patients with severe diarrhea, such as frequently occurs with VIPomas, with the need to adequately correct the dehydration, hypokalemia, and metabolic alkalosis, the fluid and electrolyte replacement needs to be given intravenously. This can be accomplished by using parenteral hyperalimentation or administration of saline solutions supplemented with potassium and sodium bicarbonate. Restoration of hydration and electrolytes can best be monitored by serial assessment of serum electrolytes and urine output.

Pharmacologic Control of SD

A number of different agents are used to control acute and long-term chronic diarrhea. As pointed out above, definitive treatment requires a correct diagnosis. In this section, the general use of pharmacologic agents in SD is dealt with, and in the following section, specific comments on some of the specific diseases are made. Opiates and synthetic long-acting somatostatin analogues (octreotide, lanreotide) are the most commonly used. Other agents that may be helpful are α_2-adrenergic agonists, corticosteroids, absorbent agents, prostaglandin synthetase inhibitors, calcium channel blockers, and phenothiazines. The use of each is briefly discussed below.

Opiates

Opiates are usually the first-line therapy for most mild to moderate diarrheas. Commonly used preparations include *paregoric, tincture of opium, codeine, Lomotil* (diphenoxylate with atropine), *Imodium* (loperamide), and *difenoxin with atropine*. These agents inhibit transit throughout the gastrointestinal (GI) tract; therefore, they increase the contact time between intestinal luminal contents and the mucosa, increasing absorption. Experimentally, opiates have proabsorptive and antisecretory effects, but it is unclear if these mechanisms are operative in humans. Synthetic opioids such as Lomotil (2.5 mg diphenoxylate plus 25 µg atropine per tablet) and loperamide (Imodium) (2 mg/tablet) have fewer central nervous system (CNS) side effects than morphine. The recommended doses are as follows:

1. *Loperamide*, 2 to 4 mg 4 times daily
2. Diphenyloxylate plus atropine, 1 to 2 tablets 4 times daily
3. Codeine, 30 to 60 mg 4 times daily
4. *Paregoric* (0.4 mg morphine/mL), 5 to 10 mL 4 times daily
5. *Tincture of opium* (10 mg morphine/mL), 5 to 20 drops 4 times daily

All of these drugs except loperamide are controlled substances because of their potential for misuse or addiction. At high doses, Lomotil can also cause CNS side effects, whereas loperamide, because it does not cross the blood-brain barrier as efficiently, has fewer side effects at higher doses.

The main side effects from the use of opiates are abdominal discomfort, constipation, nausea, vomiting, and CNS symptoms (drowsiness, respiratory depression, and altered mental status). Lomotil, because of the presence of atropine, can cause anticholinergic side effects. Physical dependence can occur with prolonged use, although it is reduced with Lomotil by combining the diphenoxylate with atropine.

Long-Acting Somatostatin Analogues

Octreotide and *lanreotide* are synthetic analogues of *somatostatin* that, because they are much more resistant to degradation than native somatostatin, have a much longer duration of action than native somatostatin and therefore can be used by *intermittent subcutaneous injection*. Like native somatostatin, these synthetic analogues *suppress most intestinal secretions* (gastric, pancreatic, biliary, intestinal), *inhibit release of most GI hormones and neurotransmitters*, and *can inhibit GI motility*. At present, only *octreotide* is available in the United States. *Octreotide* is the drug of choice for most large-volume, severe diarrheas. Numerous studies have demonstrated its effectiveness in *VIPomas* and *diarrhea* caused by *carcinoid syndrome*. These somatostatin analogues inhibit both the ectopic release of hormones and neurotransmitters by these tumors and secretion from the large and small intestine stimulated by a number of agents (prostaglandin E_1, serotonin, VIP); they also stimulate sodium chloride absorption in animal studies. Because of these actions, somatostatin analogues have been used to treat a number of secretory and nonsecretory diarrheal conditions, both hormonally and nonhormonally mediated. These include, in addition to *VIPomas, carcinoid syndrome, medullary thyroid carcinomas, glucagonomas, diarrhea* associated with *immune deficiency syndrome* (*AIDS*), diarrhea owing to *short bowel syndrome*, diarrhea owing to *dumping syndrome*, and diarrhea owing to *chemotherapy* or *bone marrow transplantation treatments*. The specific use of octreotide in the various secretory hormonal diarrheas is discussed in the following section on these specific diseases. Octreotide use is also discussed in the chapters on AIDS (see Chapter 46, "Gastrointestinal and Nutritional Complications of HIV Infection"), short bowel syndrome (see Chapter 64, "Short Bowel Syndrome"), and stem cell transplantation (see Chapter 48, "Gastrointestinal and Hepatic Complications of Stem Cell Transplantation").

Octreotide

Treatment with somatostatin analogues is usually limited to severe diarrheas or those refractory to other treatments because of its cost and because parenteral administration is required (Farthing, 2002). The usual starting dose of *octreotide*, which is the only synthetic analogue available in the United States, is 50 to 100 µg 2 to 4 times a day administered subcutaneously. The dose and frequency can then be titrated to control the symptoms. Doses as high as 750 µg 3 times daily have been used. The half-life of octreotide is 100 minutes compared with 2 to 3 minutes for native somatostatin, and octreotide has been shown to be 70-fold more potent than native somatostatin at inhibiting growth hormone release and 80-fold more potent at inhibiting acid secretion. There have been a small number of reports of cases in which intermittent subcutaneous administration is not effective and a continuous infusion of octreotide is more effective. With continued treatment, octreotide may become less effective and increased dosage is frequently required (Fried, 1999).

Recently, a *long-acting formulation of octreotide* (*octreotide-LAR* [long-acting release]) has become available. This formulation is administered once per month intramuscularly. Three dosage forms are available, including 10, 20, and 30 mg formulations. We usually begin with the 20 mg formulation in a patient in whom extended control of the SD will be required and who responds to the subcutaneous formulation. It is important to continue the subcutaneous formulation for at least 2 weeks after starting the octreotide-LAR because it takes that long to reach appropriate blood levels with the long-acting form. In patients with carcinoid syndrome or VIPomas, even after octreotide-LAR has been given for a number of months, it may have to be supplemented with subcutaneous octreotide periodically for acceptable symptom control (Szilagyi and Shrier, 2001).

The side effects of treatment with synthetic somatostatin analogues include cramping or nausea, which usually resolve with continued treatment, and pain at the subcutaneous injection site, which may be reduced by slow injection and warming the vial. Worsening of glucose tolerance develops in some patients, and it is advisable to obtain a serum glucose determination when beginning the medication. A small percentage of patients may develop fat malabsorption. Long term, the principal side effect is the development of *biliary sludge* or *gallstones*, thought to be due to the ability of somatostatin to inhibit gallbladder emptying. In various studies with long-term treatment, 10 to 50% of patients have developed biliary sludge or gallstones, but in only 1 to 10% is it symptomatic. With long-term treatment, an ultrasound examination of the gallbladder before the treatment and every 6 to 12 months should be considered (Redfern and Fortuner, 1995).

α_2-Adrenergic Agents

Clonidine

These agents slow GI transit as well as promote absorption. *Clonidine* is the frequently used drug in this class and has been recommended particularly for diabetic diarrhea based on a small number of reports. It also has been used to treat diarrhea associated with short bowel syndrome, usually in combination with opiates. Clonidine is usually started at 0.1 mg/d and increased slowly to 0.1 to 0.3 mg 3 times a day. A major limitation to the use of clonidine is its antihypertensive effect mediated centrally, resulting in postural hypotension. Clonidine should be reserved for patients with SDs that are refractory to opiates. When clonidine is discontinued, the dose should be tapered slowly over 3 to 5 days to avoid rebound symptoms (hypertension, nausea, vomiting, headache). This agent is discussed in the chapter on diabetic diarrhea (Chapter 71, "Management of Diabetic Diarrhea").

Glucocorticoids

Glucocorticoids stimulate absorption of water and electrolytes and have been used in refractory patients with VIPomas. The recommended dose is 60 mg of prednisone per day. If it is effective, the dosage can be decreased to the lowest level controlling the diarrhea. Glucocorticoids are now rarely needed with the availability of the somatostatin analogues, which are effective acutely and long term in most patients with VIPomas.

Prostaglandin Synthetase Inhibitors

These agents have been used in a number of SDs because prostaglandins stimulate water and electrolyte secretion. *Indomethacin* has been reported to be effective in a small number of patients with SDs.

Other Agents

Absorbent agents such as psyllium husk, kaolin, methylcellulose, and cholestyramine are frequently used in mild to moderate diarrheas. Cholestyramine and other binding resins are principally used in diarrheas for which binding bile acids may be helpful, such as after cholecystectomy or ileal resection. Some series, but not others, report that patients with *chronic diarrhea* have *idiopathic bile acid malabsorption*, and cholestyramine could reduce stool weight. It is important to remember that these agents may interfere with absorption of other drugs; therefore, the timing of their use needs to be carefully considered.

Bismuth-containing compounds such as *Pepto-Bismol* are used primarily for the prophylaxis and treatment of infectious diarrheas. They may have effects on toxin production or action as well as antibacterial effects.

Calcium channel blockers (*verapamil*) can inhibit GI motility and have an antidiarrheal effect. Hypotension may limit their usefulness.

Trifluoroperazine and *chlorpromazine* act to decrease intestinal secretion by inhibiting the calcium-calmodulin complex. They have been occasionally used in patients with VIPomas or other SDs and have been largely replaced by somatostatin analogues.

Specific Conditions

VIPomas

Almost all patients with VIPomas have large-volume diarrhea frequently resulting in hypokalemia and dehydration—hence the acronym *WDHA syndrome* (watery diarrhea, hypokalemia, achlorhydria), which is also used to name this syndrome in addition to Verner-Morrison syndrome. Diarrhea occurs in 100% of these patients and is due to the net secretion of fluid and electrolytes, primarily in the jejunum, caused by ectopic release of VIP by the tumor. In adults, 90% of these patients have a pancreatic endocrine tumor, which is usually malignant, whereas in children and a small percentage of adults, it is due to neural (ganglioneuroma) or adrenal tumors. These patients can have very large daily losses exceeding 400 mmol of potassium and 700 mmol of sodium and, therefore, require vigorous rehydration. Octreotide is the agent of choice to control the diarrhea in these patients.

In addition to controlling the diarrhea and rehydration, tumor localization studies using *computed tomography* (CT) and *somatostatin receptor scintigraphy* to define the location and extent of the tumor are indicated. In addition to medical treatment of the diarrhea, treatment directed against the tumor, including *surgical debulking*, and *chemoembolization* or *chemotherapy* for metastatic tumors are recommended.

Carcinoid Syndrome

In the 32 to 84% of patients with carcinoid syndrome with diarrhea, similar to patients with medullary thyroid cancer or thyrotoxicosis, the diarrhea is primarily caused by *increased intestinal motility and increased fluid and electrolyte secretion*. These actions are mediated in part by serotonin secretion and possibly ectopic release of *tachykinins* (*substance P, substance K, neuropeptide K*), *motilin*, and *prostaglandins*. Almost all patients with carcinoid syndrome have metastatic disease in the liver, usually from a midgut carcinoid (75 to 87%), foregut (2 to 9%), or hindgut (1 to 8%) tumor or from a carcinoid tumor of unknown location (2 to 15%). The treatment for the diarrhea is similar to that for VIPomas with *somatostatin analogues*. Octreotide controls the diarrhea in > 80% of patients by decreasing release of serotonin (5-hydroxytryptamine [HT]) and other mediators and is reported to decrease their synthesis by the tumors (O'Toole et al, 2000). Other agents that are effective are $5\text{-}HT_1$ and $5\text{-}HT_2$ *receptor antagonists*, such as *methylsergide, cyproheptadine*, and *ketanserin*. $5\text{-}HT_3$ *receptor antagonists* (*ondansetron, tropisetron, alosetron*) are now increasingly being used to control the diarrhea and also help control the nausea and occasionally the flushing. In carcinoid syndrome caused by a *foregut carcinoid* tumor of the gastric mucosa, frequently a combination of H_1 *and* H_2 *receptor antagonists* is effective. The carcinoid tumors causing carcinoid syndrome are usually unresectable because of diffuse hepatic metastases, and treatment needs to be directed against the tumor itself. The primary *antitumor* treatments are *chemoembolization*, use of *interferon* alone or in *combination with somatostatin analogues*, or somatostatin analogues alone (Jensen and Doherty, 2001).

Systemic Mastocytosis

In the 23 to 43% of patients with systemic mastocytosis, the diarrhea is mild to moderate in the majority, with > 90% having a stool volume < 1 L/d. In systemic mastocytosis, the primary cause of the most troubling diarrhea is *gastric hypersecretion* owing to hyperhistaminemia; therefore, it has a pathogenesis similar to that seen in patients with Zollinger-Ellison syndrome. However, *villous atrophy* and a *secretory component*, perhaps owing to *prostaglandins*, may be important diarrheal factors in some patients with systemic mastocytosis. The diarrhea in these patients is usually controlled by a *combination of* H_1 *and* H_2 *receptor antagonists*. The mast cell membrane-stabilizing drug *cromolyn sodium* (disodium chromoglycate) has been reported to be useful to treat diarrhea and other GI symptoms in a small number of patients with systemic mastocytosis. In patients with the malignant forms of mastocytosis, treatment with *interferon alpha-2b*, as well as *chemotherapy* and *corticosteroids*, has been used (Jensen, 2000).

Surreptitious Use of Laxatives or Diuretics

Patients with a *factitious cause* frequently have large-volume diarrhea (> 1 L/d). It should be remembered that this condition is not infrequent, occurring in 15 to 20% of patients referred to a referral center with chronic diarrhea. The primary treatment of these patients is having a high suspicion for the diagnosis because no clinical feature except for a history of psychiatric illness or macroscopic melanosis coli on sigmoidoscopy assists in the diagnosis. Some patients have a medical or veterinary background. Some laxatives increased the osmotic gap in the stool (magnesium), and its detection will help lead to the diagnosis (Phillips et al, 1995). However, with others, the osmotic gap is not increased, and only screening for laxatives in the stool or urine will establish the diagnosis. There is a chapter on managing patients with factitious or exaggerated illnesses (see Chapter 42, "Exaggerated and Factitious Disease").

Supplemental Reading

Farthing MJ. Novel targets for the control of secretory diarrhea. Gut 2002;50:III15–8.

Fried M. Octreotide in the treatment of refractory diarrhea. Digestion 1999;60:42–6.

Jensen RT. Overview of chronic diarrhea caused by functional neuroendocrine neoplasms. Semin Gastrointest Dis 1999;10:156–72.

Jensen RT. Gastrointestinal abnormalities and involvement in systemic mastocytosis. Oncol Hematol Clin North Am 2000;14:579–623.

Jensen RT, Doherty GM. Carcinoid tumors and the carcinoid syndrome. In: DeVita VT Jr, Hellman S, Rosenberg SA, editors. Cancer: principles and practice of oncology. Philadelphia: Lippincott Williams & Wilkins; 2001. p. 1813–33.

O'Toole D, Ducreux M, Bommelaer G, et al. Treatment of carcinoid syndrome: a prospective crossover evaluation of lanreotide versus octreotide in terms of efficacy, patient acceptability, and tolerance. Cancer 2000;88:770–6.

Phillips S, Donaldson L, Geisler K, et al. Stool composition in factitial diarrhea. Ann Intern Med 1995;123:97–100.

Redfern JS, Fortuner WJ II. Octreotide-associated biliary tract dysfunction and gallstone formation: pathophysiology and management. Am J Gastroenterol 1995;90:1042–52.

Szilagyi A, Shrier I. Systematic review: the use of somatostatin or octreotide in refractory diarrhoea. Aliment Pharmacol Ther 2001;15:1889–97.

CHAPTER 73

Reducing Cardiovascular Risk with Major Surgery

Michael Y. Chan, MD, and Stephen C. Achuff, MD

Background

Of the 27 million people undergoing surgery in the United States each year, approximately one-third have coronary artery disease (CAD) or significant risk factors for cardiovascular disease (Mangano and Goldman, 1995; Grayburn and Hillis, 2003). Thus it is not surprising that myocardial events are the most common serious complication of surgery. An estimated 50,000 patients per year will have perioperative myocardial infarctions (MI) with a perioperative mortality rate of approximately 20% (Fleisher and Eagle, 2001; Sprung et al, 2000; Badner et al, 1998).

Most cases occur within the first 3 days after surgery with atypical symptoms being the norm. Another 1 million patients annually will have perioperative cardiac complications with a concomitant $20 billion per year in hospital and long term care costs (Fleisher and Eagle, 2001).

The purpose of preoperative cardiovascular evaluation is more than simply "giving clearance for surgery." The goals are (1) to assess clinically the patient's current medical status and estimate a cardiac risk profile, (2) to identify patients who would benefit from further noninvasive or invasive testing, (3) to make recommendations for perioperative management that reduces risk for cardiac complications, and (4) to identify those patients who would benefit from postoperative risk stratification and modification (Cohn and Goldman, 2003).

American College of Cardiology/American Heart Association Guidelines

The American College of Cardiology (ACC)/American Heart Association (AHA) guidelines for perioperative cardiovascular evaluation for noncardiac surgery were initially published in 1996 and subsequently revised in 2002 (Eagle et al, 2002). The strategy is based on the following five factors:
1. Clinical risk predictors
2. Functional capacity of the patient
3. History of previous cardiac evaluation or treatment
4. Urgency of the surgery
5. Surgery-specific risks

Patients with no cardiac risk factors are generally at very low risk for perioperative cardiac complications and require no further evaluation or therapy (Eagle et al, 2002).

Similarly, patients who are asymptomatic with one or more coronary risk factors but who do not have established CAD also have been shown to be at very low risk. The exception is diabetic patients; those with long standing diabetes are at particularly higher risk (Eagle et al, 2002).

Clinical predictors can be classified as major, intermediate, or minor. High risk clinical predictors include the following:
1. Unstable coronary syndromes
2. Recent MI (> 7 days but < 1 month before surgery)
3. Severe angina
4. Decompensated congestive heart failure (CHF)
5. High grade atrioventricular block
6. Symptomatic ventricular arrhythmias in the presence of underlying heart disease
7. Supraventricular arrhythmias with uncontrolled ventricular rate
8. Severe valvular disease

If any of these major indicators are present, consideration should be given to delaying or canceling nonemergent surgery until medical stabilization can be achieved.

TABLE 73-1. Factors that Increase the Risk of Perioperative Cardiac Complications in Patients Undergoing Noncardiac Surgery and Indications for Use of Perioperative β-Blocker Therapy

Risk Factor	Odds Ratio (95% CI)*	Perioperative β-Blocker Indicated
Ischemic heart disease[†]	2.4 (1.3 to 4.2)	Yes
CHF	1.9 (1.1 to 3.5)	Yes
High risk surgery[‡]	2.8 (1.6 to 4.9)	Uncertain, but probably
Diabetes mellitus (especially insulin-requiring)	3.0 (1.3 to 7.1)	Yes
Renal insufficiency	3.0 (1.4 to 6.8)	Uncertain, but probably if renal insufficiency is due to diabetes or vascular disease
Poor function status[§]	1.8 (0.9 to 3.5)	Yes, if poor status is thought to be due to CAD or heart failure

From Fleisher and Eagle, 2001.
*Data from Lee et al, 1999 and Reilly et al, 1999.
CAD = coronary artery disease; CHF = congestive heart failure; CI = confidence interval.
[†]Ischemic heart disease includes angina and prior myocardial infarction.
[‡]High risk surgery includes intraperitoneal, intrathoracic, and supra-inguinal vascular procedures.
[§]Poor functional status is defined as the inability to walk four blocks or climb two flights of stairs.

The patient's functional status prior to surgery has been shown to be a strong predictor of perioperative risk. Functional status can be expressed in metabolic equivalent (MET) levels. Both perioperative and long term risks are significantly increased in those patients who are unable to achieve a 4-MET demand during most normal daily activities (Reilly et al, 1999; Older et al, 1999; Bartels et al, 1997). As a comparison, 4-METs is approximated by climbing 1 flight of stairs carrying a bag of groceries or walking on level ground at 3 to 4 mph (Cohn and Goldman, 2003).

Surgery-specific risk, grouped into high, intermediate, or minor risk procedures, is defined by the type of surgery and the associated hemodynamic stress. High risk procedures, associated with a cardiac risk of > 5%, include emergent major operations, particularly in the elderly, and prolonged operations associated with large fluid shifts and/or blood loss. Intermediate risk procedures with a cardiac complication rate of 1 to 5% include most routine intraperitoneal and intrathoracic operations. Low risk surgeries include endoscopic procedures and superficial procedures; these are associated with a cardiac risk < 1%.

Step-Wise Approach to Risk Stratification

Step 1: How urgent is the surgery? If surgery is deemed emergent, then the patient should proceed to the operating room without further assessment.

Step 2: Has the patient undergone coronary revascularization (coronary artery bypass grafting or percutaneous coronary intervention) within the past 5 years? If so, and the patient is without recurrent signs or symptoms, the patient can also proceed to the operating room directly without further cardiac testing.

Step 3: Has the patient had a coronary evaluation (cardiac stress test or coronary angiogram) in the past 2 years? If a sufficient evaluation with favorable results was performed within the past 2 years and the patient has not experienced a change or new cardiac symptoms, then no further testing is necessary.

Step 4: Does the patient have an unstable coronary syndrome or high risk features? In the setting of nonemergent surgery, any of the major clinical predictors reviewed above usually leads to cancellation or delay of surgery until correction and treatment of the problem.

Step 5: Does the patient have intermediate predictors of risk? Intermediate clinical predictors include mild angina pectoris, history of remote MI (> 1 month before surgery), compensated or prior CHF, renal insufficiency (as defined by a serum creatinine ≥ 2.0 mg/dL), and diabetes mellitus. The presence of an intermediate clinical predictor, in addition to either a high risk surgery or low patient functional capacity, would warrant noninvasive testing for further risk stratification prior to surgery.

Step 6: Patients with intermediate predictors of risk and moderate to excellent functional capacity can generally undergo intermediate-risk surgery with low likelihood of perioperative death or MI. On the other hand, further cardiac testing is often necessary in patients with low functional capacity or those undergoing high risk procedures.

Step 7: Noncardiac surgery is generally safe for patients with low risk predictors (ie, advanced age, abnormal electrocardiogram [eg, left ventricular hypertrophy (LVH), left bundle branch block (LBBB), or ST-T changes], rhythm other than sinus [eg, atrial fibrillation], history of stroke, or uncontrolled systemic hypertension) with moderate to high functional capacity (≥ 4 METs).

Step 8: The results of noninvasive testing can be used to determine the need for additional evaluation and treatment. In some patients with documented CAD, the risk of PCI or CABG may even exceed the risk of the proposed noncardiac surgery. This approach may be appropriate, however, if it increases the long term prognosis of the patient.

Noninvasive Testing

Although a careful history and physical examination are the most crucial component of any preoperative evaluation, exercise or pharmacologic stress testing can contribute significantly to a patient's risk stratification prior to surgery.

Exercise ECG Stress Testing

Exercise stress testing with or without imaging remains the test of first choice in those patients who can exercise. It provides a functional estimate of the patient's overall cardiopulmonary system and yields helpful prognostic information. The main limitation of ECG exercise testing is that only about half of the patients tested achieve peak exercise heart rates > 75% of the age-predicted maximum (Cohn and Goldman, 2003). Ischemia induced by low level exercise identifies a subset of patients at particularly high risk. However, a negative test in a patient who achieves the target blood pressure–heart rate product ratio predicts a low risk for perioperative complications.

Pharmacologic Stress Testing

Pharmacologic stress testing with imaging, primarily dobutamine stress echocardiography (DSE) and dipyridamole/exercise thallium, are excellent predictors of cardiac risk. Numerous studies have demonstrated a high negative predictive value (93 to 100%) of both thallium and DSE. The positive predictive value for thallium (4 to 67%) and DSE (7 to 23%) are much lower. The choice of the optimal test in the patient who cannot exercise depends on institutional expertise and physician comfort in interpreting results.

Specific Preoperative Cardiovascular Conditions

Hypertension

Despite earlier concerns, it is now abundantly clear that stable and reasonably well-controlled hypertension, and the drugs used to maintain this control, should not present an important risk for patients undergoing surgery. Antihypertensive medications should not be discontinued, tapered, or omitted prior to surgery because of concern over interaction with anesthetic agents. Stage 3 hypertension (systolic blood pressure ≥ to 180 mm Hg and diastolic blood pressure ≥ 100 mm Hg) should be controlled before surgery (Eagle et al, 2002). Most patients can be adequately controlled by titrating antihypertensives over days to weeks in the outpatient setting. β-Blockers are a particularly attractive choice given their perioperative protective effects (as will be discussed later). We strongly recommend preoperative antihypertensive medications be continued throughout the perioperative period to prevent a hypertensive crisis.

Valvular Heart Disease

The major complication one faces in dealing with patients with significant valvular heart disease is the potential for CHF. The indications for evaluation and treatment of valvular heart disease are identical to those in the nonpreoperative setting. Symptomatic stenotic lesions are associated with substantial risk of perioperative heart failure or shock and often require percutaneous valvulotomy or valve replacement prior to surgery (Reyes et al, 1994; Raymer and Yung, 1998; Torsher et al, 1998). In contrast, symptomatic regurgitant lesions are better tolerated perioperatively and may be stabilized with intensive medical therapy and monitoring. An exception occurs when severe regurgitation exists with reduced ventricular function in which myocardial reserve is so limited that destabilization during perioperative stresses is likely. In such cases, consideration should be given to valve repair prior to nonemergent noncardiac surgery.

Two other problems should be mentioned that are nearly unique to the patient with valvular heart disease. First is the potential risk of endocarditis, which is particularly important in patients with prosthetic heart valves. Antibiotic prophylaxis should be given prior to any surgery with even the slightest risk of bacteremia. The second area of specific concern is the management of anticoagulation therapy. This applies primarily to patients with mechanical prosthetic valves. Thomboembolic complications are an inescapable hazard of artificial heart valves, even when anticoagulation is rigorously monitored and controlled. The potential is substantially greater when normal clotting status is maintained for more than 5 to 7 days. Fortunately, the risk is relatively low if this time range is respected.

The simplest strategy for managing warfarin in the face of upcoming surgery is to discontinue the drug 2 or 3 days preoperatively, then restart it the second or third postoperative day, assuming the risk of surgical bleeding has subsided (Tinker and Tarhan, 1978). A more conservative approach from the standpoint of preventing prosthetic valve thromboembolic complications is to give heparin or low molecular weight heparin up to 6 hours preoperatively, and then again beginning 18 to 24 hours postoperatively until warfarin levels are therapeutic (Katholi et al, 1978). The latter approach may be preferable in patients with mechanical mitral valves, which are at higher risk for clotting than valves in the aortic position.

Cardiac Arrhythmias

One of the most frequent reasons for preoperative cardiology consultation is the discovery of an arrhythmia on routine ECG or the detection of some pulse irregularity on examination. This should prompt a careful search for underlying cardiopulmonary disease, drug toxicity, or metabolic abnormality (Eagle et al, 2002). In the majority of patients, these abnormalities are either intrinsically benign or are a marker of a correctable problem such as diuretic-induced hypokalemia or a relative excess of an antiarrhythmic agent (eg, digoxin). Therapy is indicated for symptomatic or hemodynamically significant arrhythmias (Eagle et al, 2002). Patients already on chronic oral antiarrhythmics should be maintained on their usual dosages that give standardized therapeutic blood levels up to the time of surgery and then have them reinstituted as promptly as possible postoperatively.

Several studies have demonstrated that frequent premature ventricular contractions or nonsustained ventricular tachycardia do not increase the risk for nonfatal MI or cardiac death in the perioperative period; therefore, aggressive monitoring or treatment is not recommended (O'Kelly et al, 1992; Mahla et al, 1998; Eagle et al, 2002). In the setting of a patient with an implantable cardiac defibrillator, the device should be programmed off immediately before surgery and reprogrammed on postoperatively (Eagle et al, 2002).

Perioperative Management

β-Blockers

Several recent trials have evaluated the benefit of medical therapy initiated in the preoperative setting in reducing cardiac events. Mangano and colleagues (1995) conducted a randomized controlled trial of atenolol versus placebo in

200 patients with or at risk for CAD undergoing noncardiac surgery and followed them for 2 years. They found that, although there was no difference in perioperative MI or death during initial hospitalization, ischemic episodes were significantly lower in the atenolol group (24% vs 39%). In addition, mortality at 2 years was 10% in the atenolol group versus 21% in controls ($p = .019$). The principal effect of atenolol was a decrease in mortality during the first 6 to 8 months. Of note, there was no difference in β-blocker use between groups over the follow-up period (approximately 15% in each treatment group).

Poldermans and colleagues (1999) randomized 173 patients undergoing major vascular surgery who had positive DSE on preoperative testing to bisoprolol versus standard care. Patients were excluded if (1) they had extensive wall motion abnormalities at rest or with dobutamine or (2) they were already on β-blocker therapy. Patients in the treatment group received bisoprolol for at least 1 week preoperatively (mean 37 days) and were continued on bisoprolol for 30 days. The primary endpoints of cardiac death and nonfatal MI occurred in only 3.4% of patients in the bisoprolol group versus 34% in the standard care group ($p < .001$). The majority of events occurred during the first 7 days after surgery. The study was subsequently extended to follow long term outcomes in 101 of 112 surviving patients remaining on bisoprolol compared with those receiving standard care (Poldermans et al, 2001). During a median follow-up period of 22 months, the bisoprolol group had a markedly decreased risk of MI and cardiac death versus standard care group (12% vs 32%).

Current recommendations suggest starting oral β-blocker therapy days to weeks before elective surgery and continuing for a week to a month postoperatively (Eagle et al, 2002). The dose should be titrated to achieve a resting heart rate of 50 to 60 bpm. There may even be benefit to starting therapy intraoperatively if it has not been initiated beforehand; evidence comes from a small study showing a decreased incidence and duration of ischemic events with intraoperative esmolol followed by postoperative metoprolol in patients undergoing total knee arthoplasty (Urban et al, 2000).

α-2 Agonist

Several trials have evaluated the use of clonidine in reducing cardiac event rates in subsets of patients with known CAD undergoing vascular surgery. Clonidine has been shown to decrease the incidence of ischemia in a study of 297 patients undergoing vascular surgery (24% vs 39%) (Stuhmeier et al, 1996). In the European Mivazerol Trial (EMIT), mivazerol, an α-2 agonist not currently available in the United States, was studied perioperatively in 2,854 patients with known CAD or significant CAD risk factors undergoing noncardiac surgery (Oliver et al, 1999). No effect was found on the rate of perioperative MI; however, a statistically significant reduced rate of cardiac death was seen in patients undergoing both general and vascular surgery.

Overall, perioperative clonidine may have a similar effect on myocardial ischemia, infarction, and cardiac death as perioperative β-blockers, but further research is needed before its role in perioperative management can be fully elucidated.

Summary

In summary, preoperative risk stratification should be undertaken with consideration of the patient's clinical markers, functional status, and surgery-specific risks. Cardiac stress tests are helpful in predicting risk but there is no clear-cut evidence they improve perioperative care. Current guidelines suggest their use in patients undergoing nonemergent surgery with two of the following three features: (1) intermediate risk profile, (2) low functional capacity, or (3) high risk surgery. The indications for coronary revascularization are the same as in the nonpreoperative setting. Lastly, perioperative β-blockers should be used in all patients with intermediate or high risk of cardiac complications in whom they are not absolutely contraindicated.

Supplemental Reading

Badner NH, Knill RL, Brown JE, et al. Myocardial infarction after noncardiac surgery. Anesthesiology 1998; 88:572–8.

Bartels C, Bechtel JF, Hossmann V, Horsch S. Cardiac risk stratification for high-risk vascular surgery. Circulation 1997;95:2473–5.

Cohn SL, Goldman L. Preoperative risk evaluation and perioperative management of patients with coronary artery disease. Med Clin North Am 2003;87:111–36.

Eagle KA, Berger PB, Calkins H, et al. ACC/AHA Guideline Update for Perioperative Cardiovascular Evaluation for Noncardiac Surgery—Executive Summary. A report of the American College of Cardiology/American Heart Association Task Force on Practice Guidelines (Committee to Update the 1996 Guidelines on Perioperative Cardiovascular Evaluation for Noncardiac Surgery). Circulation 2002;12;105:1257–67.

Fleisher LA, Eagle KA. Lowering cardiac risk in noncardiac surgery. N Engl J Med 2001;345:1677–82.

Grayburn P, Hillis LD. Cardiac events in patients undergoing noncardiac surgery: shifting the paradigm from noninvasive risk stratification to therapy. Ann Intern Med 2003 Mar 18;138:506–11.

Katholi RE, Nolan SP, McGuire LB. The management of anticoagulation during noncardiac operations in patients with prosthetic heart disease. A prosthetic study. Am Heart J 1978; 96:163–5.

Lee TH, Marcantonio ER, Mangione CM, et al. Derivation and prospective validation of a simple index for prediction of cardiac risk of major noncardiac surgery. Circulation 1999 Sep 7;100:1043–9.

Mahla E, Rotman B, Rehak P, et al. Perioperative ventricular dysrhythmias in patients with structural heart disease undergoing noncardiac surgery. Anesth Analg 1998;86:16–21.

Mangano DT, Goldman L. Preoperative assessment of patients with known or suspected coronary disease. N Engl J Med 1995; 333:1750–6.

O'Kelly B, Browner WS, Massie B, et al. Ventricular arrhythmias in patients undergoing noncardiac surgery. The Study of Perioperative Ischemia Research Group. JAMA 1992;268:217–21.

Older P, Hall A, Hader R. Cardiopulmonary exercise testing as a screening test for perioperative management of major surgery in the elderly. Chest 1999;116:355–62.

Oliver MF, Goldman L, Julian DG, Holme I. Effect of mivazerol on perioperative cardiac complications during non-cardiac surgery in patients with coronary heart disease: the European Mivazerol Trial (EMIT). Anesthesiology 1999;91:951–61.

Poldermans D, Boersma E, Bax JJ, et al. The effect of bisoprolol on perioperative mortality and myocardial infarction in high-risk patients undergoing vascular surgery. Dutch Echocardiographic Cardiac Risk Evaluation Applying Stress Echocardiography Study Group. N Engl J Med 1999;34124:1789–94.

Poldermans D, Boersma E, Bax JJ, et al. Dutch Echocardiographic Cardiac Risk Evaluation Applying Stress Echocardiography Study Group. Bisoprolol reduces cardiac death and myocardial infarction in high-risk patients as long as 2 years after successful major vascular surgery. Eur Heart J 2001;22:1353–8.

Raymer K, Yang H. Patients with aortic stenosis: cardiac complications in non-cardiac surgery. Can J Anaesth 1998;45:855–9.

Reilly DF, McNeely MJ, Doerner D, et al. Self-reported exercise tolerance and the risk of serious perioperative complications. Arch Intern Med 1999;159:2185–92.

Reyes VP, Raju BS, Wynne J, et al. Percutaneous balloon valvuloplasty compared with open surgical commissurotomy for mitral stenosis. N Engl J Med 1994;331:961–7.

Sprung J, Abdelmalak B, Gottlieb A, et al. Analysis of risk factors for myocardial infarction and cardiac mortality after major vascular surgery. Anesthesiology 2000 Jul;93(1):129–40.

Stuhmeier KD, Mainzer B, Cierpka J, et al. Small, oral dose of clonidine reduces the incidence of intraoperative myocardial ischemia in patients having vascular surgery. Anesthesiology 1996;85:706–12.

Torsher LC, Shub C, Rettke SR, Brown DL. Risk of patients with severe aortic stenosis undergoing noncardiac surgery. Am J Cardiol 1998;81:448–52.

Tinker JH, Tarhan S. Discontinuing anticoagulant therapy in surgical patients with cardiac valve prosthesis. Observation in 180 operations. JAMA 1978;239:738–9.

Urban MK, Markowitz SM, Gordon MA, et al. Postoperative prophylactic administration of beta-adrenergic blockers in patients at risk for myocardial ischemia. Anesth Analg 2000;90:1257–61.

CHAPTER 74

Acute Appendicitis

Dorry Segev, MD, and Paul Colombani, MD, FACS

Acute appendicitis continues to be one of the most common causes of abdominal pain in both the adult and pediatric populations, with a lifetime risk of about 6%. It is the most common surgical emergency in the child. The etiology of appendicitis varies from lymphoid hyperplasia in children and teenagers to appendicolith or tumor in adults, but the common pathophysiology is thought to consist of appendiceal outlet obstruction leading to inflammation, venous congestion followed by ischemia, and necrosis. The natural history includes either localized perforation, in the form of phlegmon or abscess, or free perforation with peritonitis. Diagnosis remains a clinical one and treatment remains surgical, but the roles of computed tomography (CT), percutaneous drainage, interval appendectomy, and minimally invasive surgery are evolving.

Diagnosis

Even in the era of inexpensive and easily accessible radiography, acute appendicitis is a clinical diagnosis that can often be difficult and is made with the goal of *minimizing negative appendectomies but avoiding perforation*. It is a rare patient that embodies the textbook presentation of this disease, but a combination of historical features, physical findings, laboratory values, and occasionally radiography, should reliably lead to a diagnosis and appropriate treatment.

Classic Patient

The classic patient with appendicitis complains of periumbilical pain 1 or 2 days prior to presentation that has subsequently migrated to the right lower quadrant. The patient has a low grade fever. The patient may have one or two episodes of vomiting, which are self-limiting, and is usually anorexic. Diarrhea, persistent vomiting, or a patient requesting food or drink would be unusual. A clinical course exceeding 2 or 3 days would also be unusual. A protracted course beyond 72 hours may indicate that the appendix has perforated, with the patient initially feeling better, and then worsening systemically as a phlegmon or abscess was being formed.

On physical examination, there is usually focal tenderness and localized peritoneal irritation in the right lower quadrant of the abdomen, over the appendix. Although the appendix is classically located at McBurney's point (two-thirds the distance from the umbilicus to the right anterior superior iliac spine), anatomic variations are common and include retrocecal, intrapelvic, left lower quadrant, or right upper quadrant positions.

A number of clinical signs can be used to discern localized peritonitis. Tenderness to percussion over the appendix is more sensitive, more specific, and certainly more kind to the patient being examined than rebound tenderness. The unsolicited complaint of pain in the right lower quadrant with maneuvers such as palpation of the left lower quadrant (Rovsing sign), cough (Dunphy sign), internal rotation of the flexed right thigh (obturator sign), or extension of the right hip (iliopsoas sign) all indicate an inflammatory process in the right lower quadrant.

Laboratory values can be notoriously misleading, but the classic patient has a mild leukocytosis with a left shift of neutrophils to immature forms. Urinalysis should be negative, although pyuria without bacteria can occur in the setting of appendicitis from periureteral inflammation.

Differential Diagnosis

The diagnosis can be even more difficult in a number of clinical settings. Patients who are *immunocompromised*, through diseases or medications, and patients at both *extremes of age* commonly have atypical histories and physical findings. Radiographic studies can be helpful in these patients. *Gynecological conditions* can be distracting in female patients. A pelvic examination, if not a pelvic ultrasound, is always warranted in this population. Young patients with conditions such as *otitis media, streptococcal pharyngitis, meningitis, and mesenteric lymphadenitis* may have abdominal complaints which can masquerade as appendicitis. Inflammatory bowel disease should always be considered in a patient with right lower quadrant abdominal pain. A final important consideration is the differential diagnosis of *typhlitis, or neutropenic enterocolitis,* in neutropenic patients undergoing chemotherapy for oncologic conditions.

Preoperative Management

Figure 74-1 outlines a management strategy for patients suspected to have appendicitis. Early fluid resuscitation is essential, as patients with any intra-abdominal inflammatory process will more than likely present in a dehydrated state. The mainstay of management planning is the level of clinical suspicion for appendicits, which we have divided into three categories requiring continued management.

Any patient with a 1 or 2-day textbook presentation of appendicitis as outlined above and no other distracting conditions should have an *appendectomy*. Perioperative care should depend on the presence of *peritonitis*, with *broad spectrum antibiotics* and *bowel rest* reserved for these patients. Acute appendicitis with peritonitis, even after treatment, can lead to significant morbidity and possible mortality in an elderly or debilitated patient.

The most difficult decisions arise in the patient with high suspicion for appendicitis but an atypical presentation, lack of classic physical findings, potential for gynecological etiology, or confounding medical conditions.

Common masqueraders to consider include *perforated cecal or appendiceal tumors* in the elderly, *typhlitis* in neutropenic patients, and pelvic inflammatory disease and *mittelschmerz* in females. It is for these patients that *CT scan* or *ultrasonography* should be considered, and *transvaginal pelvic ultrasound* can also be helpful in ruling out tubo-ovarian disease. The combination of a worrisome CT scan and this level of clinical suspicion would support surgical management, with other patients followed carefully by serial examinations as below.

Patients with some evidence of a right lower quadrant intra-abdominal process but little to implicate the appendix as a source should be admitted for serial observation and rehydration. There is no role for antibiotics in this scenario unless another source of infection has been documented. Most of these patients will improve in 1 to 2 days and can be discharged with precautions to return if symptoms should recur. Serious consideration should be given to operative intervention in a patient who remains undiagnosed but worsens clinically with conservative management.

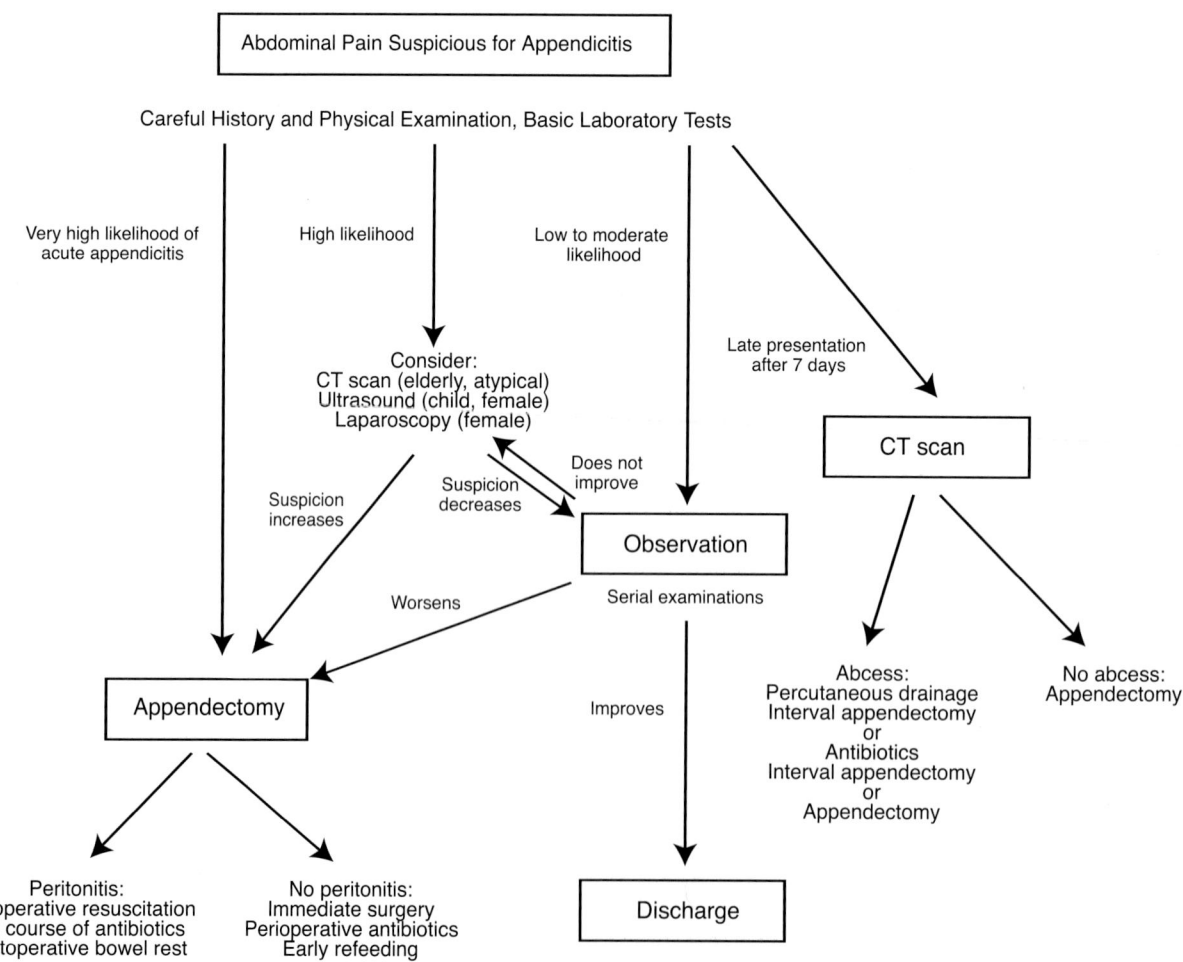

FIGURE 74-1. Management strategy for patients with suspected appendicitis. CT = computed tomography.

Special Considerations

During *pregnancy*, the gravid uterus displaces the appendix superiorly and sometimes laterally as early as the second trimester. The diagnosis can be more difficult, and the ensuing morbidity more serious if the diagnosis is missed. The fetal morbidity rate is as high as 10% for acute appendicitis and 30% when perforated, whereas morbidity to mother and fetus from negative appendectomy are minimal. As a result, there is little role for nonoperative management when the diagnosis of acute appendicits is suspected during pregnancy.

In the past, *incidental appendectomy* was a common maneuver during other surgical procedures. There is increased morbidity with an incidental appendectomy and currently *indications for such are rare* and occur mainly when appendiceal pathology is incidentally discovered.

When the *3-day window* of the acute presentation of appendicitis has passed before the patient seeks medical attention, there should be a higher index of suspicion for *peri-appendiceal phlegmon or abscess*. Patients may present with fevers and leukocytosis higher than the usual low grade nature of acute appendicitis, or be afebrile with an unimpressive examination despite a perforation and collection walled off from the peritoneum. *CT scan* plays an important role in the workup of these patients and their subsequent management. Nonoperative management of patients presenting after 7 days of symptoms may be safer with less morbidity than appendectomy.

A peri-appendiceal collection in a patient who is afebrile and nonperitonitic can be initially treated with *antibiotics and observation*. A collection in a symptomatic patient with an impressive examination warrants at least *CT guided percutaneous drainage*. Failure to resolve symptoms in a patient in these more conservative manners or clinical deterioration with the development of high fevers and peritonitis are indications for *open drainage and appendectomy*. A patient treated successfully with antibiotics or percutaneous drainage for ruptured appendicitis should undergo an *interval appendectomy* 6 weeks later.

Operative Management

The definitive therapy for appendicitis is surgical appendectomy. This can be performed either in the classic open manner using a right lower quadrant incision or laparoscopically using typically three small port incisions. The choice of surgical approach depends on a number of factors, including operator experience, need for abdominal exploration beyond the right lower quadrant, likelihood of necrosis at the base of the appendix, and size of patient and abdominal wall. On occasion a third option, exploration and appendectomy through a midline incision, should be considered in elderly patients where the diagnosis of an intra-abdominal process may be certain but involvement of the appendix is unclear.

Although the incisions for open appendectomy vary, the general principle is a small incision over McBurney's point or the area of maximal tenderness, in the direction of Langer's lines of skin tension. The incision is carried through the subcutaneous tissues and external oblique aponeurosis sharply or using electrocautery, and sequential layers of internal oblique and transverses abdominis muscles are split in the direction of the fibers. *This is known as a muscle splitting approach*, and the length of the incision depends primarily on the size of the patient and the abdominal wall. The laparoscopic approach consists of an infraumbilical camera port and at least two additional operative ports. The use of laparoscopy varies according to surgeon preferences but relative indications include obese patients who would otherwise require a large incision and female patients where exploration of the pelvis is necessary based on typical clinical presentation.

Once the abdominal cavity is entered, the appendix is identified, mobilized, and freed from the adhesions likely formed by the inflammatory process. The mesoappendix is ligated and the appendix is excised at its base. Purse string inversion of the appendiceal stump is unnecessary unless the base of the appendix is necrotic. Abdominal drains in general are not indicated.

When appendectomy is attempted and a normal appearing appendix is encountered, the abdomen is explored for the following pathologic processes, depending on patient type and presentation, including the following:

1. Terminal ileum to evaluate for *inflammatory bowel disease*
2. Distal 2 feet (60 cm) of small bowel in search of a *Meckel's diverticulum*
3. Sigmoid colon to exclude *diverticulitis*
4. Right upper quadrant to evaluate for *cholecystitis or duodenal perforation*
5. *Female adnexa* to evaluate for tubo-ovarian pathology

One of the advantages of laparoscopic appendectomy is the relative ease with which the remainder of the abdomen can be explored. If no clear cause for the patient's symptoms can be identified, an appendectomy is performed because a normal appearing appendix can later demonstrate histologic evidence of acute or chronic inflammation.

Postoperative Care

Patients with simple acute appendicitis can be treated with *one to two doses of perioperative antibiotics* and oral intake can begin on the first or second postoperative day. In the setting of peritonitis or perforation, a *5-day course* of broad spectrum antibiotics should be used, and initiation of oral intake should wait until bowel function begins to return. Ileus is not uncommon after perforated appendicitis and diet should be advanced slowly.

Complications following appendectomy include wound infection, appendiceal stump leak, and peri-appendiceal abscess or fluid collection, with a much higher incidence of these in the setting of perforation and peritonitis. Because these problems usually occur once the patient has left the hospital, it is critical to educate patients and families regarding the signs and symptoms of these complications and to return for follow up after discharge. In patients having appendectomy for perforated appendicitis and abscess, follow-up should include rectal exam to rule out recurrent abscess. Patients managed nonoperatively by antibiotics and percutaneous drainage of peri-appendiceal abscess should undergo interval appendectomy 6 weeks from the drainage procedure because of the high incidence of recurrent appendicitis.

Supplemental Reading

Emil S, Laberge JM, Mikhail P, et al. Appendicitis in children: a ten-year update of therapeutic recommendations. J Pediatr Surg 2003;38:236–42.

Jones PF. Suspected acute appendicitis: trends in management over 30 years. Br J Surg 2001;88:1570–7.

Paulson EK, Kalady MF, Pappas TN. Suspected appendicitis. N Engl J Med 2003;348:236–42.

Stephen AE, Segev DL, Ryan DP, et al. The diagnosis of acute appendicits in a pediatric population. J Pediatr Surg 2003;38:367–71.

CHAPTER 75

CONSTIPATION

ONKI CHEUNG, MD, AND ARNOLD WALD, MD

Constipation is one of the most common digestive complaints in the general population. Over 2.5 million people consult a physician and hundreds of millions of dollars are spent on laxatives each year. Although constipation is often defined as a frequency of defecation twice weekly or less, constipated patients may complain of excessive straining with defecation, passage of hard or small stools, difficulty initiating evacuation, or a feeling of incomplete evacuation. Physicians should therefore not rely only on the criteria of defecation frequency when examining patients and managing constipation.

It is important to identify treatable causes of constipation, which include many diseases and the side effects of many drugs. If these are absent, functional constipation should be considered.

The initial management of chronic constipation includes educating the patient and correcting any misconceptions as to the wide range of normal bowel habits. Broad treatment principles include increasing fluid and fiber intake, and reducing excessive or incorrect use of laxatives and cathartics. Taking advantage of normal postprandial increases in colonic motility, patients should attempt to defecate after meals, particularly in the morning when colonic motor activity is highest. Most patients will respond to these measures together with the judicious use of laxatives. A summary of available laxatives is shown in Table 75-1 followed by the approximate costs of the common laxatives summarized in Table 75-2.

TABLE 75-1. Laxatives Used in the Treatment of Constipation

Laxatives	Usual Adult Dose	Onset of Action
*Bulk-forming laxatives		
Bran	2–4 tablespoons qd	12 to 72 h
Methylcellulose	1 to 3 tbsp qd	12 to 72 h
Psyllium	1 to 3 tbsp qd	12 to 72 h
Calcium polycarbophil	2 to 4 tablets qid	24 to 48 h
*Osmotic agents		
Polyethylene glycol	17 g in 240 mL water	24 to 48 h
Sorbitol	15 to 30 mL qd	24 to 48 h
Lactulose	15 to 30 mL qd	24 to 48 h
Saline laxatives		
Magnesium sulfate	15 g qd	0.5 to 3 h
Magnesium citrate	200 mL qd	0.5 to 3 h
*Stimulant laxatives (oral)		
Senna	2 to 4 tabs qd	6 to 12 h
Cascara	1 to 2 tabs qd	6 to 12 h
Bisacodyl	30 mg qd	6 to 10 h
*Prokinetic agents		
Misoprostol	200–800 mcg qd	1 to 4 h
Tegaserod	6 mg bid	1 to 4 h
Colchicine	0.6 mg tid	1 to 4 h
Suppository		
Bisacodyl	1 every 2 to 3 days	0.25 to 1 h
Glycerine	1 every 2 to 3 days	0.25 to 1 h
Enemas		
Tap water	500 mL	0.25 h
Phosphate	45 mL	0.25 h
Mineral oil retention	100 to 250 mL	0.25 h

bid = twice daily; qd = every day; tid = 3 times daily; tbsp = tablespoon.
*In each category, laxatives are listed with the most preferred at the top and least preferred at the bottom.

TABLE 75-2. Approximate Costs of Commonly Used Laxatives

Laxatives	Monthly Costs
Osmotic agents	
Polyethylene glycol	$42 for 17 g qd
Sorbitol	$18 for 30 mL qd
Lactulose	$60 for 30 mL qd
Saline laxatives	
Magnesium citrate	$60 for 200 mL qd
Magnesium hydroxide	$27 for 30 mL qd
Stimulant laxatives	
Senna	$3 to 6 for 2 to 4 tablets every 2 to 3 days
Cascara	$2 to 4 for 1 to 2 tablets every 2 to 3 days
Bisacodyl	$3 for 30 mg every 2 to 3 days
Prokinetic agents	
Misoprostol	$45 for 200 µg qd
Tegaserod	$120 for 2 or 6 mg bid
Colchicine	$18 for 0.6 mg tid

bid = twice daily; tid = 3 times daily; qd = every day.

Agents Used in the Management of Constipation

Bulk-Forming Laxatives

Dietary fiber and *bulk laxatives* with adequate fluid intake are the most physiologic and safest of medical therapies. However, they may be *counterproductive* in patients with idiopathic slow transit constipation or with constipation associated with irritable bowel syndrome (IBS) because they often worsen bloating and abdominal distension in these populations.

DIETARY FIBER

Dietary fiber in cereals contain cell walls that resist digestion and retain water within their cellular structures, whereas those found in citrus fruits and legumes stimulate the growth of colonic flora and increase fecal mass. *Wheat bran* is the most effective fiber laxative with a clear dose response on fecal output. Patients with poor dietary habits may add 2 to 4 tablespoons of bran to each meal, followed by a glass of water or another beverage. A laxative effect may not be observed for 3 to 5 days. Patients should be cautioned that large amounts of bran can cause abdominal bloating or flatulence; therefore, they should start with small amounts and titrate slowly to the desired effect.

Psyllium (Metamucil), *calcium polycarbophil (Fiber-Con)*, and *methylcellulose (Citrucel)* are natural or synthetic polysaccharides or cellulose derivatives, which primarily exert their effects by water retention and increasing fecal mass, thus decreasing colonic transit time. They should be well diluted to ensure adequate mixing with food and may be consumed before meals or at bedtime. They are more refined and concentrated than bran but are more expensive.

Osmotic Laxatives

These agents include *magnesium salts, sorbitol, lactulose,* and *polyethylene glycol* (PEG) solutions. They may be used in patients who do not tolerate or respond poorly to fiber. The decision to use a particular laxative is often determined by individual preference, costs, and underlying medical conditions.

Sorbitol and *lactulose* are poorly absorbed sugars that are hydrolyzed to acidic metabolites by coliform bacteria, which stimulate fluid accumulation in the colon and usually produce soft, well-formed stools. As sorbitol is less expensive and as effective as lactulose, we prefer sorbitol as the low cost choice. Major side effects of these agents are *abdominal bloating* and *flatulence*.

Magnesium salts, such as *magnesium sulfate* or *citrate*, are an alternative to poorly absorbed sugars. However, they should be used with caution in patients with renal insufficiency.

PEG solutions, with or without electrolytes, have been used to treat chronic constipation. A powdered form that does not contain electrolytes (*MiraLax*) is more palatable and may be mixed with any fluid. The amount taken daily is adjusted based on clinical response. As colonic bacteria do not hydrolyze PEG, abdominal bloating or flatulence are not as problematic as with fiber or poorly absorbed sugars. This agent is costly and, as with lactulose and sorbitol, available by prescription only.

Stool Softeners

Docusates (Colace, Surfak) work by lowering the surface tension of stool and allowing water to move easily into the fecal mass. These agents have *marginal* value in treating chronic constipation.

Mineral oil also softens stool as a result of its emollient effect. It is particularly effective in enemas to soften hard impactions. However, aspiration with lipoid pneumonia is a major hazard associated with oral administration, especially in patients with impaired swallowing or severe reflux disease. Therefore we limit its use to *rectal instillation* in our practice.

Stimulant Laxatives

Stimulant laxatives, such as anthraquinone compounds, diphenylmethane derivatives and may be considered in patients who fail to respond to or are intolerant of bulk or osmotic agents. These agents alter intestinal electrolyte transport and increase intestinal motor activity. They may be used intermittently or chronically when patients fail to respond adequately to bulk or osmotic laxatives. Some physicians recommend that they be taken for no longer than several weeks. However, there is no convincing evidence that chronic use of stimulant laxatives causes damage to enteric nerves or intestinal smooth muscles nor are they associated with colorectal or other cancers. Stimulant laxatives often cause superficial damage to surface epithelial cells, but this is of no functional significance and is reversible when laxatives are discontinued. A reasonable regimen is to use stimulant laxatives when no spontaneous bowel movement occurs after 48 or 72 hours. They may be used alone or combined with bulk or osmotic laxatives. Major side effects occur only with excessive and prolonged abuse, usually by emotionally disturbed or misguided individuals.

The *anthraquinone-containing laxatives* (ie, *senna, cascara sagrada*) are widely used. *Senna* is best administered at bedtime with fluids *2 to 3 times weekly* if no defecation occurs spontaneously. *Cascara* also produces a soft or formed stool with little or no colic. Most anthraquinone-containing laxatives discolor the colonic mucosa (*melanosis coli*) if used chronically. The pale-brown to jet-black discoloration of melanosis coli occurs throughout the colon and is more prominent in the proximal colon. Withdrawal of laxatives is normally accompanied by resolution of pigmentation after many months.

Bisacodyl is the only *diphenylmethane* laxative available since the removal of phenolphthalein from the market because of a possible relationship to cancer in animal studies. The *onset* of action is between *6 to 12 hours* and the *duration* of action may be *occasionally prolonged* (3 to 4 days). It is absorbed in the upper gastrointestinal tract, undergoes an enterohepatic circulation, and is excreted largely in the stool. *Bisacodyl suppositories* may be useful in patients who prefer a rapid onset and shorter duration of bowel activity.

Prokinetic Agents

Drugs that act via *serotonin receptors (5-HT$_4$)* to stimulate acetylcholine release in the myenteric plexus and produce coordinated contraction have been studied in constipation. *Cisapride* was the best studied of these drugs, but the association with *potential lethal cardiac dysrhythmias* led to its withdrawal in the United States. *Tegaserod (Zelnorm)* is a partial 5-HT$_4$ agonist that was recently approved for treatment of constipation predominant IBS in women. In four prospective randomized placebo controlled trials, women with constipation predominant IBS reported response rates ranging from 5 to 19% in excess of placebo. Recent studies indicate that some women with functional constipation may respond as well, and is a new indication for the drug.

Another agent that is advocated for patients with chronic refractory constipation is the *prostaglandin analogue misoprostol*. Several studies have shown an acceleration of intestinal transit in healthy individuals and in those with chronic constipation. We usually start with *200 µg daily together with PEG (Miralax)* and increase the dose progressively, based on efficacy and side effects. This drug *should not be used* in young women who wish to become pregnant as stimulation of uterine contractions may result in abortion of the fetus.

Colchicine was reported to be effective in refractory chronic constipation in one small randomized double blind study in a dose of 0.6 mg by mouth 3 times daily. We have been disappointed by the failure of any of our patients to respond.

Examination and Treatment of Patients with Intractable Constipation

Testing

Patients with functional constipation who fail to respond to diet, fluids and standard laxatives should undergo testing, including *colonic transit* using *radio-opaque markers* and *anorectal manometry with balloon expulsion*, as outlined in the algorithm. Both tests must be obtained, as symptoms do not predict the underlying pathophysiology. These studies allow us to categorize such patients in what appears to us to be biologically plausible subgroups.

Slow Transit Constipation

In *slow transit constipation (STC)*, there is a failure to move luminal contents through the proximal colon. This may be associated with *dietary* factors, such as severe caloric deficiency, with *medications* that alter motility or with certain *neurologic, metabolic,* and *endocrine* disorders. Attention to such factors may lead to improvement in colonic transit. Patients with *idiopathic STC* who fail to respond to conventional laxatives may have abnormalities of the enteric nerves, such as decreased volume of interstitial cells of Cajal and reduction of myenteric neural elements. We usually start with colon cleansing using enemas with or without mineral oil. If these are unsuccessful, a water-soluble contrast enema (Gastrografin or Hypaque) administered under fluoroscopy may be very effective. After this, the colon may be further evacuated with twice daily high volume enemas or by drinking PEG solution until cleansing is complete. The patient should then be maintained on a daily osmotic agent with stimulant laxatives every 2 to 3 days if there are no spontaneous bowel movements. Other agents such as misoprostol or tegaserod may be tried if the patient responds suboptimally to osmotic and stimulant laxatives.

If a patient with disabling symptoms from STC is unresponsive to medical therapy, surgery may be considered. The most common operation recommended is subtotal colectomy with ileorectal anastomosis for which overall success rates of approximately 90% have been reported. Although our experience approximates that of the literature, we have also observed complications such as abdominal pain or bloating, adhesive obstruction and debilitating diarrhea after surgery, as have others. Because of this experience, we emphasize the importance of careful patient selection. The following four criteria should be met before surgery is undertaken: (1) chronic, severe, and disabling symptoms from constipation that are unresponsive to medical therapy, (2) slow colonic transit of the inertia pattern, (3) no evidence of intestinal pseudo-obstruction by radiologic and manometric studies, and (4) normal anorectal function. Diagnostic studies to rule out pelvic floor dysfunction are critically important, as subtotal colectomy with ileorectal anastomosis is unlikely to help if the latter is not corrected. Another reported surgical approach is antegrade colonic enema, although we use it very infrequently. For patients who have impaired continence mechanisms, an ileostomy is a viable option. We are reluctant to recommend subtotal colectomy in patients when pain is a significant component of their complaint, because it cannot be assumed that it will relieve pain.

Outlet Dysfunction Constipation

In outlet dysfunction constipation, the primary failure is an inability to adequately evacuate contents from the rectum. This may be due to failure of coordinated relaxation of the striated muscles during attempted defecation (pelvic floor dyssynergia), weak expulsion forces due to pain or neuromuscular disorders, or misdirection of expulsion forces secondary to a large rectocele. We recommend biofeedback in conjunction with conservative therapy if pelvic floor dyssynergia is demonstrated with appropriate testing (Figure 75-1). The purpose is to train patients to relax their pelvic floor muscles during straining to achieve defecation. Biofeedback sessions are held weekly or more often until abnormal defecation efforts are achieved (approximately three to eight sessions). The rate of success for biofeedback has been reported to be 60 to 90% by some, but not all, investigators, but there have been no randomized controlled studies in adults and the experience in children has been disappointing in large controlled studies. In our experience, less than 50% of patients with constipation associated with pelvic floor dyssynergia respond to biofeedback. The cost of each session is about $60 to $100. We normally refer those who are motivated and have failed conservative treatment to biofeedback.

Botulinum toxin injections into the anal sphincters for the treatment of dyssynergic defecation has been reported in small uncontrolled studies. We are not convinced that there is sufficient evidence to use botulinum toxin for this disorder nor do we recommend myotomy for the puborectalis muscle because of a high risk of incontinence.

Surgical repair of a rectocele is considered only if we can demonstrate improved rectal evacuation when pressure is placed on the posterior wall of the vagina during defecation and there is no evidence of pelvic floor dyssynergia. Most patients with megarectum can be treated conservatively with enemas or suppositories. We rarely consider proctocolectomy with an ileoanal pouch and only if anorectal continence mechanisms are intact and symptoms are intractable.

Combined Slow Colonic Transit and Outlet Dysfunction Constipation

If both outlet obstruction and slow colonic transit coexist, combined treatment with laxatives, prokinetics (see Figure 75-1), and biofeedback therapy should be offered. Failure of conservative therapy may lead to proctocolectomy with ileal pouch anal anastomosis or end ileostomy for those with untreatable anorectal dysfunction.

Normal Transit Constipation

Constipated patients with normal colon transit and normal anorectal function often misperceive bowel frequency and exhibit increased psychological distress. It is important to reassure these patients that there is no evidence of abnormal function of the colon or rectum. Patients should be educated to increase fluid and fiber intake, take advantage of gastrocolonic responses, and avoid excessive use of laxatives. We often screen these patients for underlying anxiety, depression or other psychological distress using a previously validated psychological symptom form, the SCL-90R. Pharmacotherapy to reduce underlying anxiety or depression may be helpful in some individuals.

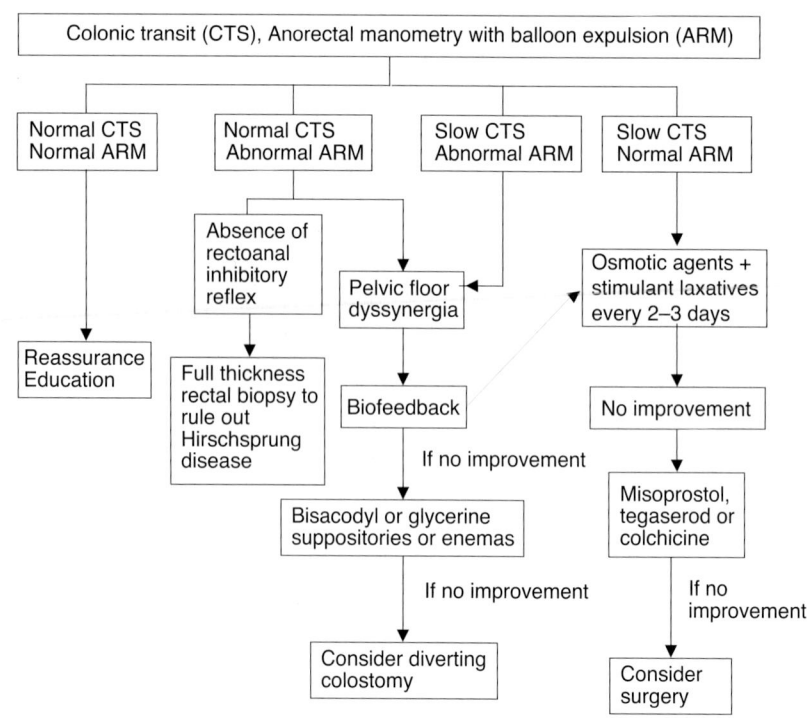

FIGURE 75-1. Diagnostic and treatment algorithm for severe constipation.

Constipation with IBS

In a patient with constipation-predominant IBS, we will attempt a high fiber diet, starting with small amounts and increasing gradually. Wheat bran, at doses of 10 to 30 g, is the best known and perhaps the most effective fiber supplement but commercial products may be more acceptable to some patients. Abdominal pain and bloating occur with fiber supplements in many IBS patients. PEG may be substituted in patients who do not tolerate fiber supplements, but we minimize the use of stimulant laxatives. Tegaserod may be useful in women with constipation-predominant IBS, although the cost of the drug far exceeds other available agents.

Constipation in Pregnancy

Dietary modifications, such as increased fluid and fiber intake, are the most physiologic and safest approachs to constipation during pregnancy. As with all patients, pregnant women should be warned that fiber can cause abdominal bloating or flatulence and that sufficient amounts of fluid should be consumed daily. Fiber supplements should be started with small amounts and gradually increased as tolerated.

In our experience, PEG is not as problematic in terms of abdominal bloating and flatulence as is sorbitol and lactulose. Although safety during pregnancy has not been established (Federal Drug Administration pregnancy Category C), PEG is inert, absorption is minuscule, and toxicity is unlikely.

Of the stimulant laxatives, senna is both safe and effective when combined with bulk-forming agents in pregnancy. Cascara is also mild and produces little or no colic. Although bisacodyl is safe for use in pregnancy, it tends to produce more colic than the anthraquinone laxatives, especially when administered orally.

Agents to be avoided during pregnancy include castor oil, which can cause premature uterine contractions, and osmotic agents such as magnesium laxatives and phosphosoda, which may produce sodium and water retention.

Chronic Megacolon

Chronic idiopathic megacolon in the adult should be viewed as chronic colon failure, which is managed by minimizing colon contents with periodic evacuations. Initial disimpaction with colon cleansing is necessary for successful long term management. We prefer to institute a low fiber diet together with daily PEG solution to minimize stool and gas buildup and to keep stools soft. Twice weekly, a glycerine suppository or a tap water enema should be administered to prompt defecation. As a rule, these patients respond poorly to stimulant laxatives and prokinetic agents.

Occasionally, surgery may be indicated for chronic megacolon when bowel distension becomes too uncomfortable. In patients with megacolon and megarectum, a diverting ileostomy or ileoanal anastomosis may be considered. For megacolon with normal anorectal function, an ileorectal anastomosis may be appropriate whereas in megarectum with normal colon, a coloanal anastomosis, diverting colostomy, or Duhamel procedure may be effective.

Supplemental Reading

Locke GR III, Pemberton JH, Phillips SF. AGA technical review on constipation. American Gastroenterological Association [review]. Gastroenterology 2000;119:1766–78.

Wald A. Slow transit constipation. Curr Treat Options Gastroenterol 2002;5:279–83.

Wald A. Constipation, diarrhea and symptomatic hemorrhoids during pregnancy. Gastroenterol Clin North Am 2003;32:301–22.

Wald A. Anorectal manometry. In: Schuster M, Crowell M, Koch K, editors. Schuster atlas of gastrointestinal motility, 2nd ed. Hamilton (ON): BC Decker Inc; 2002. p. 289–303.

Wald A, Hinds JP, Caruana BJ. Psychological and physiological characteristics of patients with severe idiopathic constipation. Gastroenterology 1989;97:932–7.

Wald A. Is chronic use of stimulant laxatives harmful to the colon. J Clin Gastroenterol 2003;36:386–9.

Wald A. Approach to the patient with constipation. In: Yamada T, editor. Textbook of gastroenterology, 4th ed. Philadephia: Lippincott, Williams and Wilkins; 2003. p. 894–910.

Wald A. Outlet dysfunction constipation. Curr Treat Options Gastroenterol 2001;4:293–7.

Management of Abdominal Wall Defects

Kurtis A. Campbell, MD, and Anthony P. Tufaro, MD, DDS

The management of the *complicated abdominal wall defect* can be quite complex. As more and more patients with an increasing number of co-morbidities undergo sophisticated abdominal operations, an increasing number of physicians will have the opportunity to participate in the management of these patients. Moreover, it is clear that a multidisciplinary approach affords the best possible outcome, particularly in those patients whose defect includes gastrointestinal (GI) complications such as enterocutaneous fistulas. The purpose of this chapter is to provide a broad discussion of the management of these problems.

Incidence

The *incidence* of incisional hernia after abdominal wall surgery is at least 10% (Mudge and Hughes, 1985). In some studies of high risk patients, the occurrence rate is as high as 20%. Repair is commonly unsuccessful, with recurrence rates ranging from 20% to greater than 50% (Flum et al, 2003; Van'T Riet et al, 2004). This obviously represents a substantial management problem for the gastroenterologist and surgeon and their associated patients. Regrettably, a large retrospective population cohort study examining over 10,000 patients demonstrated that there had been no improvement in important measures of adverse outcome in the last several decades in these patients (Flum et al, 2003).

Nomenclature

The typical definition of the complex abdominal wall defect would include one or more of the following:
1. Large sized defect (> 40 cm)
2. Absence of stable skin coverage
3. Recurrence
4. Infected or exposed prosthetic material
5. Compromised abdominal wall soft tissue secondary to co-morbidities, such as irradiation or corticosteroid dependence
6. Simultaneous visceral complication (eg, enterocutaneous fistula)
7. A systemically compromised patient (eg, posttransplant, concurrent malignancy, immunodeficiency disease) (Steinwald and Mathes, 2001).

Complex abdominal wall defects can occur both acutely and as a delayed consequence of surgery or injury. Acute defects may be the result of trauma, tumor excision, wound dehiscence and evisceration, necrotizing fasciitis, or some other intra-abdominal catastrophe. The acute complex defect may be divided into two types: (1) unstable and (2) stable. Those with unstable abdominal contents are those where urgent surgical intervention is typically required for intra-abdominal injury or the acute deterioration of intra-abdominal disease (eg, diverticular abscess). An example of an acute complex defect with stable intra-abdominal contents is necrotizing fasciitis. A detailed discussion of the management of these acute defects is more esoteric to the nonsurgeon and will not be discussed further in this chapter.

Patient Examination

A number of factors become important in the *examination of the patient* with a chronic abdominal wall defect. The location of the defect and, in particular, its relation to previous chest and abdominal scars is very important whether laparoscopic or open repair is being considered. The latter especially can involve substantial areas of tissue rearrangement and advancement. The presence of previous incisions can have a substantial impact on the blood supply to both the skin and soft tissue and the myofascial components of the abdominal wall. The extent of the fascial defect is also vitally important and is likely best determined by a combination of physical examination and radiographic imaging, particularly computed tomography or magnetic resonance imaging. In the setting of an open wound, cultures of the wound can guide antibiotic use both in the preoperative period and after surgery. In patients who have undergone previous tumor excision within the abdomen or abdominal wall, tissue biopsy within the confines of a complex wound would be important to rule out tumor recurrence.

The overall stability of the skin and soft tissue in the setting of a complex abdominal wall defect can also be classified as stable (type I) or type II, indicating absence or instability of the skin and soft tissue coverage overlying the myofascial defect (Mathes et al, 2000). As previously discussed, the perfusion of both the soft tissue and the myofascia can have a significant impact on reconstruction, and, therefore, angiography can be helpful in those patients who have undergone multiple previous procedures or in whom regional or distant tissue flaps are being considered to aid in reconstruction. Finally, an evaluation for the presence of GI pathology, including enterocutaneous fistula, inflammatory bowel disease, other inflammatory processes including diverticular disease, or recurrent tumor is vitally important before allowing the patient to enter the operating room. Optimization of these problems and their associated comorbidities, including malnutrition, abscess drainage, and assessment and control of the extent of any underlying GI pathology are of the utmost importance both in the short term postoperative outcome and in long term results of abdominal wall reconstruction.

Surgical Techniques

The appropriate *technique* for abdominal wall reconstruction has been, and continues to be, a major topic of discussion in the surgical literature. Selection for a particular patient will depend on a number of factors, including size of the fascial defect, stability or lack thereof of the skin and soft tissue, the presence or absence of complicating GI pathology, the extent of previous abdominal surgery, and surgeon experience and preference. The two most widely discussed issues are the use of *laparoscopic techniques* or *open surgery* and the performance of a *primary repair versus the use of prosthetic material*.

Laparoscopic Techniques

Laparoscopic repair of ventral and incisional hernias continues to be studied and has been demonstrated to be a safe and effective alternative to open *surgical techniques* (Franklin et al, 2004). There is, however, no consensus in the surgical literature regarding the minimum or maximum size of the fascial defect for which laparoscopic techniques should be used. Certainly this methodology would be contraindicated in those with unstable soft tissue coverage or complicating GI pathology such as enterocutaneous fistulas. Essentially all *laparoscopic techniques* employ the use of prosthetic material to achieve repair of the abdominal wall defect.

Prosthetic Material

The use of *prosthetic material* in open ventral and incisional hernia repair continues to be studied as well (Luijendijk et al, 2000). The initial report of the use of mesh in the reconstruction of large abdominal wall defects appeared in the surgical literature in 1903 and described the use of silver wire mesh (Bartlett, 1903). Use of this material was abandoned because of a significant degree of erosion into other structures. The use of modern material began in 1959 with the introduction of polypropylene (*Marlex*) mesh (Usher, 1959). This material along with polytetrafluoroethylene (*Goretex or Teflon*) or a composite material of the two represents the majority of prosthetic materials used today. The classic use of these materials is either as an inset patch or as reinforcement of a primary tissue repair of myofascia. Placement of these materials can be done extrafascial or above the fascia, extraperitoneal and subfascial, or intraperitoneal. This too continues to be a much-debated topic. Complications of the use of mesh include separation of the mesh from the fascia, contact injury (eg, adherence to other structures, erosion, and fistula formation), and infection. *Autogenous tissue* is considered by some to be the ideal material to close complex myofascial defects. The source of the tissue can be regional musculofascial flaps most commonly represented by rectus abdominis advancement, which can be achieved using one of several plastic surgery tissue advancement techniques, or the use of distant flaps, including the tensor fascia lata or rectus femoris of the thigh or latissimus dorsi.

Inguinal Hernia

Inguinal hernia, a subset or particular variety of abdominal wall defect, although usually less complicated, is a subject in the ongoing debates of prosthetic material versus primary tissue repair and laparoscopic versus open techniques. In these defects the laparoscopic repair can occur by using a transabdominal preperitoneal approach or a totally extraperitoneal technique, both of which use prosthetic mesh. The most widely accepted current open inguinal hernia technique, the *Lichtenstein repair*, as described by Amid, also uses prosthetic mesh. The appropriate methodology continues to be debated but likely involves the following two important concepts: (1) surgeon experience and (2) whether the planned procedure represents repair of a recurrence (Neumayer et al, 2004)

Summary

In conclusion durable reconstruction of a complex abdominal wall defect requires a complete evaluation of the defect and optimal preparation of the patient along with thoughtful surgical planning. Certainly a multidisciplinary approach is ideal and more times than not should likely include gastroenterology involvement, particularly in those patients who present with GI co-morbidities complicating their abdominal wall defect and its reconstruction.

Supplemental Reading

Amid PK, Shulman AG, Lichtenstein IL. Open "tension-free" repair of inguinal hernias: the Lichtenstein technique. Eur J Surg 1996;162:447–53.

Bartlett W. An improved filigree for the repair of large defects in the abdominal wall. Ann Surg 1903;38:47.

Flum DR, Horvath K, Koespell T. Have outcomes of incisional hernia repair improved with time?: a population-based analysis. Ann Surg 2003;237:129–35.

Franklin ME Jr, Gonzalez JJ Jr, Glass JL, Manjarrez A. Laparoscopic ventral and incisional hernia repair: an 11-year experience. Hernia 2004;8:23–7.

Luijendijk RW, Hop WCJ, Petrousjka van den Tol M, et al. A comparsion of suture repair with mesh repair for incisional hernia. New Engl J Med 2000;343:392–8.

Mathes SJ, Steinwald PM, Foster RD, et al. Complex abdominal wall reconstruction: a comparison of flap and mesh closure. Ann Surg 2000;232:586–96.

Mudge M, Hughes LE. Incisional hernia: a 10 year prospective study of incidence and attitudes. Br J Surg 1985;72:70-1.

Neumayer L, Giobbie-Hurder A, Jonasson O, et al. Open mesh versus laparoscopic mesh repair of inguinal hernia. New Engl J Med 2004;350:1819–27.

Steinwald PM, Mathes SJ. Management of the complex abdominal wall wound. In: Cameron JL, Evers BM, Fong Y, et al, editors. Advances in surgery. Vol 35. St. Louis: Mosby, Inc; 2001. p. 77–108.

Usher FC. A new plastic prosthesis for repairing tissue defects of the chest and abdominal wall. Am J Surg 1959;97:629–33.

Van'T Riet M, De Vos Steenwijk PJ, Bonjer HJ, et al. Incisional hernia after repair of wound dehiscence: incidence and risk factors. Am Surg 2004;70:281–6.

CHAPTER 77

LEFT-SIDED ULCERATIVE COLITIS AND ULCERATIVE PROCTITIS

PHILIP B. MINER JR, MD

Dramatic changes have occurred in the understanding and management of inflammatory bowel disease (IBD) over the past decade. The interaction of luminal contents with the gastrointestinal (GI) immune system has enhanced our understanding of mucosal inflammation and has improved the focus of general management. Biologic therapy is coming of age and dozens of new "silver bullet" compounds are being developed to treat both Crohn's disease (CD) and ulcerative colitis (UC). In the midst of the excitement about what the future holds, it is important to focus on maximizing the treatment options that are currently available. I will review the current understanding of left-sided UC and issues regarding management of mucosal inflammation and symptoms of this disease.

Pathophysiology and Diagnosis

Inflammation and Extent of Disease

Left-sided UC describes colonic inflammation that begins distal to the splenic flexure and extends in a generally uniform pattern to the anal canal margin. *Ulcerative proctitis* involves the last 15 to 20 cm of colon and always involves the junction of the anal canal and the rectum. It is often taught that left-sided UC is an extension of ulcerative proctitis. This is probably not true. The area of most severe inflammation in left-sided UC is the sigmoid colon. The rectum often is less inflamed, and may appear nearly normal. Prior to the advent of flexible endoscopy, the explanation for less active inflammation in the rectum was that the "rectal sparing" was due to topical rectal therapy. As new drugs have become available, it is clear that the rectum has less inflammation than the sigmoid colon. The other interesting observation that arose during the numerous drug studies evaluating the response to therapy in left-sided UC was that there is often a *cecal patch* of inflammation in an otherwise normal right colon. The *skip lesions* of *left-sided UC* support a unique pathophysiology that we do not fully understand. Ulcerative proctitis differs from left-sided UC because the intense inflammation does begin at the anal margin and extend for a short distance proximally. The distinction between these two disorders helps explain the different clinical courses of these two entities.

Inflammation involving only part of the colon is a curious phenomenon. The mysterious line of demarcation of disease has yet to be explained. Physiologic differences exist between the right and left sides of the colon with the dominant luminal substrate for oxidative phosphorylation being glutamine in the right colon and butyrate in the left colon. In addition, there are differences in the distribution of inflammatory cells in the right and left colon, which may provide insight into the abrupt cessation of inflammation at the line of disease demarcation. We histologically evaluated the "line of demarcation" in an attempt to understand the aggressive and protective balance occurring at the inflammatory interface. Much to our surprise, there were numerous *mast cells* on the normal side of the line of demarcation and in the terminal ileum of patients with well-defined left-sided UC. Evolving understanding of the role of the mast cells in UC suggests that the mast cells may be providing a degree of *protection* rather than active inflammation. Until recently, the homeostatic role of mast cells has been ignored because they have always been given a pathobiologic role in human physiology. The interaction between the mast cell and the eosinophil has important implications for IBD. The inflammatory response is dependent on eosinophilic chemoattractant factor released by the mast cell. The mast cell also modulates the effect of eosinophil function and engulfs major basic protein, which limits tissue injury.

From a practical perspective, the advent of videoendoscopy permits frequent assessment of the degree of mucosal inflammation and response to therapy as well as providing an opportunity to histologically evaluate a biopsy of the mucosa. Endoscopic examination is essential to the management of UC because it permits the assessment of the severity and extent of mucosal inflammation. Biopsies are easily obtainable and play an important role in distinguishing the severity and nature of the inflammation. In left-sided UC, the laboratory evaluation is often normal and the only method to assess disease severity is history, physical examination, and videoendoscopy with biopsy. During the initial evaluation, laboratory assessment is essential in order to exclude a treatable infectious cause of colitis and to assess the immunologic pressure on the patient in terms of inflammation and metabolic homeostasis. Stool studies for enteric pathogens, parasites, *Clostridium difficile*, leukocytes, eosinophils, and Charcot-

Layden crystals, provide support for idiopathic colonic inflammation as well as directing management.

IMPORTANCE OF HISTOLOGY

During the initial stage of evaluation, mucosal biopsies should be obtained to determine the chronicity of disease and to exclude other causes of colitis. The principle alternative diagnosis that needs to be considered in the first attack of UC is *acute self-limiting colitis (ASLC)*. The endoscopic appearance is indistinguishable from idiopathic UC, but the microscopic changes are more acute and the mucosal atrophy and the crypt changes of chronic colitis (crypt branching) are absent. ASLC may last for several months, but the long term prognosis is excellent with no chronic disease issues that need to be considered. For the consultant, it is often impossible to reconstruct the initial illness. Long term remission following an acute attack raises the possibility of ASLC and supports a trial period of management without maintenance therapy. *C. difficile* may masquerade as chronic colitis or may cause relapse of symptomatic disease. The characteristic "explosive volcano" seen microscopically is a useful histologic marker of this infectious colitis. All patients with distinct ulceration of the rectum require biopsies to exclude *solitary rectal ulcer syndrome (SRUS)*, which has a pathognomonic histologic picture of disrupted submucosal muscle fibers. SRUS is an ischemic lesion that does not respond to the immunosuppressive treatment offered for IBD and requires special attention to the physiology of defecation to prevent the internal prolapse of rectal mucosal into the anal canal. There is a separate chapter on this topic (Chapter 89, "Rectal Prolapse, Rectal Intussusception and Solitary Rectal Ulcer Syndrome").

EOSINOPHILS

A second issue regarding the histopathology of IBD has emerged over the past few years. In the 1950s, the *eosinophil* was recognized as a dominant cell in the microscopic picture of IBD. Because it was believed the function of the eosinophil was limited to parasitic infections and allergy, considerable research focused on identifying either of these problems as the etiology of IBD. Parasitic infections were easily dismissed, but it took over a decade to eliminate definitively the allergic etiology of IBD. The eosinophil, which had captured the interest of pathologists studying IBD, subsequently was declared to be a surrogate marker for inflammation. In the 1990s, the homeostatic role of eosinophils began to be understood. An extended pathobiologic role of eosinophil function emerged during the national epidemic of the "tryptophan-eosinophilic-myalgia syndrome" in which eosinophils caused extensive tissue injury unrelated to parasites or allergies. Tissue resident mast cells release eosinophilic chemoattractant factor to recruit eosinophils to the tissue from the circulation. Once recruited, a variety of events need to occur to activate the eosinophils, one of which is the presence of Intracellular Adhesion Molecule (ICAM-1), which not only traffics the eosinophils to the inflammatory site, but also is required for eosinophils activation. The importance of eosinophils in the activation of disease may be determined by examination of the biopsy or by stool studies. In the biopsy, the number of eosinophils gives an estimation of the intensity of the inflammatory response, but the presence of eosinophils in crypt abscesses or mucosal migration of eosinophils indicates sufficient immunologic pressure to force the eosinophils into the intestinal lumen. These histologic findings identify activated eosinophils. Eosinophils in the stool indicate migration of eosinophils. Charcot-Layden crystals, which are related to the intracellular products of the eosinophil, reflect probable eosinophil-induced tissue injury and suggest the need for aggressive treatment of the increased number of eosinophils.

Anorectal Physiology in Health and with Inflammation

The complex physiology of the anorectum is adversely influenced by inflammation with increased sensitivity to sensation and an amplification of muscular responses stimulated by stool in the rectum. Tenesmus is the sensation of incomplete evacuation of the rectum or nonproductive straining to defecate. It occurs when rectal contraction is accompanied by internal anal sphincter relaxation. In the presence of inflammation, there is sensitivity to lower than normal volumes of balloon distention and exaggerated relaxation of the internal anal sphincter (IAS). The sensations accompanying this response are perceived rectal fullness, urgency to defecate and a sense of incomplete evacuation. Occasionally, tenesmus continues when visible inflammation is no longer present. When this occurs, treatment for microscopic inflammation or pharmacologic manipulation of rectal contractility and IAS relaxation improves these symptoms. In addition to the influence of rectal inflammation on anorectal physiology, left-sided colitis changes the physiology of the normal appearing proximal colon. This was recognized as early as 1964 when Lennard-Jones described proximal constipation in patients with left-sided UC. Recent studies demonstrate inhibition of stool movement proximal to the line of demarcation of disease. The changes in motility have important implications for topical rectal therapy.

Why Patients Relapse

IBD is characterized by periods of relapse and remission. These are *not* random events although the reason an individual relapses may not be identifiable. The four most common reasons patients relapse are the following:

1. A change in medication
2. Seasonal variation
3. Infection
4. Nonsteroidal anti-inflammatory drugs (NSAIDs).

Changes in medications needs little explanation, although I emphasize to my patients that this is the only reason for a relapse in disease for which I hold responsibility because all medication changes should occur under my guidance. Seasonal variation is well recognized, however the reason this occurs remains a mystery. Seasonal variation is influenced by geographic latitude with a blunting of the seasonal variation at higher latitudes. Environmental allergens are assumed to be responsible for these relapses with nonspecific activation of the immune system through mast cells and eosinophils. When this occurs, there is an increase in intestinal permeability, which changes the relationship between the luminal contents and the mucosal immune system. The reason infection activates IBD is unclear. Enteric infections obviously activate the GI immune system with deleterious consequences for mucosal integrity. Systemic infections probably activate the immune system nonspecifically with activation of IBD related to increased immune activity. NSAIDs have numerous effects that may alter the mucosal integrity or immune activation. Of the plausible mechanisms, I favor the change in intestinal permeability because this is a common theme in activating the GI immune system with exposure to potential antigens increased in proportion to the increase in mucosal permeability. In the management of IBD patients, seeking a cause of disease relapse may guide therapy and should permit the anticipation of relapse with the potential for prophylactic intervention.

Specific Treatment of Inflammation

Aminosalicylates

The aminosalicylates are the backbone to the treatment of left-sided colitis (see Table 77-1). The special characteristics of each of the compounds, as described in the following chapter, may be used to advantage in the management of IBD, however, it is particularly important to emphasize the benefit of topical rectal therapy in proctitis and left-sided UC. The *impaired motility* of the colon proximal to the line of demarcation of active disease *decreases* the amount of medication in contact with the inflamed mucosa. During an acute relapse, rectal suppositories (500 mg) or enemas (2 to 4 g) have excellent contact with the inflamed mucosa. Oral mesalamine compounds are effective in management, but further enhances the response rate. Once in the colon, there are no differences in the medications. The therapeutic recommendation focuses on the delivery of 4 g of 5-ASA to the colon for at least 8 weeks before labeling the patient as having disease resistant to 5-ASA. 5-ASA drugs are considered very safe, although there are patients who are sensitive to the 5-ASA and develop a chemical colitis manifest by edematous and often ulcerated mucosal which appears similar to Crohn's colitis. In a careful examination of patients with indisputable mesalamine sensitivity, we were unable to identify a serologic marker or histologic findings unique to mesalamine toxicity. If mesalamine sensitivity is suspected, discontinue the mesalamine drug for 72 hours. If symptomatic improvement occurs, this withdrawal trial supports mesalamine sensitivity. The different efficacies of the various 5-ASA products are discussed in the chapter on UC (see Chapter 78, "Ulcerative Colitis).

For patients with left-sided UC, maintaining remission with mesalamine follows the guidelines that have been established for UC. Mesalamine should be continued with at least one-half of the dose required to establish a remission, or more if the initial attacks were prolonged or severe. We have successfully used 1 g mesalamine enemas and every other day 4 g enemas to maintain remission in patients with left-sided UC. The data is more ambiguous in patients with ulcerative proctitis. Primary therapy with mesalamine suppositories is favored. The direct rectal application of a 500 mg mesalamine suppository provides a concentrated dose to the distal 15 to 20 cm of the colon, which is superior to rectal mesalamine concentrations with oral medications. Because the rectum effectively moves a liquid enema out of the rectum and into the proximal sigmoid and descending colon, the concentration of mesalamine delivered to the rectum with a suppository may be higher than the dose provided by a 4 g mesalamine enema. In these patients, I treat to obtain remission and then taper the mesalamine and wait for a symptomatic relapse. Each relapse should be treated and if the interval between relapses is short, then continuous maintenance is recommended.*

TABLE 77-1. Mechanisms of Action of Aminosalicylates

Inhibition of mucosal prostaglandin production
Inhibition of leukotriene B_4 production
Decrease interleukin-1 production
Reduce the production of reactive oxygen radicals
Scavenge free oxygen radicals
Correct impaired butyrate metabolism
Modify monocyte and lymphocyte function directly as well as secondary to cytokine changes
Reduce expression of interleukin-2 receptors
Inhibit tumor necrosis factor upregulation

---

*Editor's Note: This is a realistic approach since proctitis is so variable in course and many patients do not take preventative medication until they have had several recurrences. However, occasionally that first episode proceeds into severe left-sided UC, especially in teenagers or young adults.

Glucocorticoids

The general immunosuppression caused by glucocorticoids often induces symptomatic remission in patients with left-sided UC. However, avoiding glucocorticoid therapy has become the mantra of the gastroenterologist caring for IBD patients. Many questions focus on the cost of the short term benefit of steroids in terms of changing the character of disease and the iatrogenic medical complications that arise from steroid use. Glucocorticoids follow mesalamine in the "induction of remission" treatment algorithm. Their use should be accompanied by a *strategy* to *minimize the cumulative systemic exposure to steroids*. Topical rectal therapy applies the steroid dose to the area of the inflammation with the same distribution characteristics demonstrated for mesalamine enemas. The inflamed mucosa poorly absorbs steroids and systemic glucocorticoid effects are least likely with topical rectal therapy. As the mucosa heals, glucocorticoid absorption improves and systemic effects of steroids may occur.

Role of Eosinophils in Relapses

Seasonal or infectious relapses can be linked to high numbers of eosinophils by identifying increased numbers of fecal eosinophils, Charcot-Layden crystals in the stool, or with biopsy evidence of eosinophilic mucosal migration. When eosinophils are implicated in the symptomatic relapse of disease, high dose, short-term steroids are often effective. The *diurnal variation* of *eosinophil function* often provides a useful clinical clue that eosinophil activation is related to the current flare of colitis. Eosinophils are most active *between 11 pm and 2 am*, thus a patient with dominant colitis symptoms during this time likely has active eosinophils that should be modulated. Eosinophils are usually sensitive to high plasma levels of steroids, thus an intravenous (IV) dose of steroids (eg, solumedrol 60 mg IV) or a rapidly tapering daily dose of oral steroids (eg, 60, 50, 40, 30, 20 and 10 mg of prednisone) may induce a durable remission lasting weeks, months, or until a new stimulus activates the colitis. Even without documented eosinophilic activation of a colitis flare, an excellent clinical response to the first 48 hours of steroids suggests eosinophils are pivotal in the current flare of the disease and a short course of steroid may be all that is required for inducing remission. Lessons from the tryptophan-eosinophil-myalgia syndrome include the recognition that approximately 15% of eosinophils are resistant to steroids making this subgroup of patients difficult to manage.

When chronic glucocorticoids appear necessary, I favor moving as quickly as possible to *every other day dosing* as this often controls the colonic inflammation with less acute prednisone toxicity. If continuous steroids are required to control a relapse, immunomodulation therapy should be considered because *there is no place in the treatment of IBD for maintenance steroids*.

Budenoside/Beclomethasone

Early in the development of budesonide, an enema formulation (2 mg) was determined to be beneficial, however, budesonide is only commercially available in an ileal release form for CD (Entocort EC, AstraZeneca LP, Wilmington, DE). The theoretical advantage of budesonide revolves around the efficient first pass hepatic clearance of this steroid from the portal blood. This should decrease the systemic availability of the steroid and permit local steroid suppression of the disease without systemic toxicity. It is unfortunate that further studies were not conducted with topical rectal budesonide, however, approximately 15% of the blood flow from the distal colon escapes the portal system increasing the amount of drug that may be available in the systemic circulation. *Oral beclometasone* in a delayed release formulation was successful in treating left-sided UC. The same principle of high first pass clearance resulted in few systemic side effects (Campieri et al, 2003).

Immunomodulation

Immunomodulation with *6-mercaptopurine (6-MP)* or *azathioprine (AZA)* has become the standard of practice in the management of patients with difficult CD. Initial concerns about the toxicity of these drugs has become less of an issue than the toxicity of chronic steroid use. The experience in patients with CD led to the management of pancolitis with 6-MP/AZA. Success with UC management has permitted the expansion of the patients suitable for treatment to those with relatively refractory left-sided UC. I begin with 50 mg 6-MP and increase the dose to as high as 2 mg/kg in 25 mg increments until there is control of the disease or emerging toxicity. Most of the toxicity occurs in the first few months of treatment and blood tests are followed carefully for leukopenia, hepatitis, and pancreatitis.

Methotrexate (MTX) (25 mg intramuscularly [IM] once a week) may also be used to induce remission, but many responsive patients have only a short period before a MTX-resistant relapse occurs. Once symptomatic control is achieved, the dose may be lowered to 15 mg IM a week. A return to 25 mg for a symptomatic recurrence can be helpful. The cautions advocated by the American Rheumatologic Association regarding the emergence of liver disease after a lifetime cumulative dose of 1500 mg should be applied to patients receiving MTX, although this seems to be less of an issue with once weekly IM MTX. Studies are in progress to determine if inflixamab may play a role in inducing remission in UC. The published anecdotal use of inflixamab and my experience with inflixamab in UC do not support its use for this indication at this time.

Other Treatment

Numerous new drugs are being evaluated for use in UC. Heparin was briefly advocated for management of refractory UC, but a recent properly conducted trial with low molecular weight heparin failed to demonstrate therapeutic benefit. Short chain fatty acid (SCFA) enemas are not commercially available, but have been reported to improve left-sided colitis. ICAM-1 antisense enemas were reported to induce remission as often as mesalamine enemas with the benefit of prolonged remission. Epidermal growth factor enemas have also been shown to be effective in treating left-sided UC in a small double-blind study (Sinha et al, 2003).[†]

Surgical Intervention

Occasionally, the symptoms of left-sided UC or steroid toxicity may be so severe that colectomy may be considered. The proper intervention is a total colectomy. Recently, the success of total colectomy and ileoanal pouch construction has been reported for patients with refractory left-sided UC (Hassan et al, 2003).

Modifying Symptoms

Controlling mucosal inflammation is the cornerstone of management of left-sided UC. Proper management also includes attention to the symptoms of the disease. In general, the diarrhea of left-sided UC has little to do with the accelerated passage of digested material, as the diarrhea occurs due to mucosal inflammation with blood, fluid and colonic spasm contributing to the symptoms. For this reason and the inhibition of proximal colonic motility described earlier, antidiarrheal agents are not only ineffective, but they may increase the symptoms. *Metamucil* has been used effectively in UC, although the mechanism of action is not well understood. Improved symptoms may be related to the ability of Metamucil to modulate colonic fluid, which will increase the fluid in desiccated stool proximal to the line of demarcation of disease and also absorb any excessive fluid in the lumen. Recent attention to the effect of the luminal environment offers another possible mechanism of action as Metamucil may dilute luminal contents and reduce the concentration of any proteins, chemicals or toxins that might play a role in activating the mucosal immune system. Studies in the 1960s and 1970s found disaccharidase deficiency occurred with a higher incidence in patients with IBD than in the normal population. Most believe this is a linked genetic factor, but a mucosal abnormality of the small intestine may be associated with UC. I decrease the simple sugars in the diet of patients with left-sided UC to try to reduce the symptoms of intestinal gas and some of the diarrhea.[‡]

Perineal dermatitis presents with perineal itching, pain, and occasionally bleeding. The attempt to maintain perineal hygiene in the presence of diarrhea often leads to physical trauma of the perineal cleansing. Patients should be instructed in proper perineal hygiene including gentle cleansing following a stool and with bathing. The perineum should not be scrubbed, but gently flooded with water, patted dry (not rubbed) with the use of a hair dryer to evaporate the residual moisture. Care should be taken not to burn the skin. A barrier can be gently applied to protect the skin from the acidic stool contents that remove the protective oils and injure the skin. I recommend *Balneol* (Solvay Pharmaceuticals), although recently I have been using a 3.3% concentration of *cholestyramine in white petroleum,* which is formulated locally and provides considerable symptomatic relief. In addition to the diarrheal stools, spontaneous relaxation of the IAS occurs commonly with rectal inflammation. The IAS relaxation is associated with small amounts of rectal mucus leakage, which damages the skin through the same mechanism. Because histamine is related to normal IAS relaxation, *antihistamines* are useful in decreasing the perineal soiling and injury.[§]

Tenesmus occurs with rectal contraction and IAS relaxation. In IBD patients, tenesmus is related to rectal inflammation and often improves with control of rectal inflammation. *Antihistamines* decrease rectal spasm and restore the physiologic integrity of the anal sphincter complex. Topical rectal therapy including mesalamine and/or corti-foam can be initiated to control the tenesmus or antihistamines can be used to change the anorectal dynamics and improve this troublesome symptom.

Maintaining Remission

Maintenance therapy with *mesalamine* prolongs the duration of remission and should be continued. The role of maintenance therapy in ulcerative proctitis is less clear. Many patients will have attacks of ulcerative proctitis that last for weeks or months, but they can be managed without maintenance therapy, although each episode should be aggressively treated. I recommend continued treatment with mesalamine if relapses occur within 8 weeks of discontinuing topical or oral treatment, but the data is insufficient to support this suggestion and many of my patients prefer intermittent treatment of symptomatic disease

The reasons patients relapse have been discussed. An important aspect of patient education revolves around help-

---

[†]Editor's Note: Probiotics have been shown to be effective in control trials of active UC and in preventative relapses of pouchitis in patients who were staying in remission on antibiotics.

[‡]Editor's Note: Others would point out that unabsorbed complex sugars are converted to SCFA, which may aid left colon cellular metabolism.

[§]Editor's Note: The cholestyramine paste is also helpful with bile salt-induced diarrhea.

ing each patient identify the pattern of his disease and the factors that precipitate a relapse. An example would be a patient with recurrent springtime flares. In this patient, I would recommend increasing the mesalamine dose in the weeks prior to the anticipated disease recurrence or intervene with separate therapy as close to the onset of the flare as possible.

Refractory Disease

Patients who fail to respond to treatment should be re-evaluated in order to determine whether the initial diagnosis is correct or whether there has been extension of the disease to include a larger proportion of the colon. Unrecognized problems may include infection, *SRUS* (see separate chapter), ischemic colitis, Crohn's colitis, concurrent irritable bowel syndrome, drug-induced colitis, or mesalamine sensitivity. Mesalamine sensitivity may occur at any time in the course of treatment. Our published cases were documented to be sensitive to mesalamine by withdrawing the drug and observing symptomatic improvement. This was followed by a mesalamine enema challenge and repeat assessment of symptoms and endoscopic appearance. The response to withdrawal is dramatic and usually occurs within 72 hours. Reassessment should include physical examination, laboratory tests including stool cultures with an assessment for *C. difficile*, visualizing the mucosa by flexible sigmoidoscopy, or colonoscopy with biopsy evaluation.

Supplemental Reading

Campieri M, Adamo S, Valpiani D, et al. Oral beclometasone dipropionate in the treatment of extensive and left-sided active ulcerative colitis: a multi-center randomized study. Aliment Pharmcol Ther 2003;17:1471–80.

Cohen RD, Woseth DM, Thisted RA, Hanauer SB. A meta-analysis and overview of the literature on treatment options for left-sided ulcerative colitis and ulcerative proctitis. Am J Gastroenterol 2000;95:1263–76.

Frieri G, Pimpo MT, Palumbo GC, et al. Rectal and colonic mesalzaine concentration in ulcerative colits oral vs oral plus topical treatment. Aliment Pharmcol Ther 1999;13:1413–7.

Gisbert JP, Gomollon F, Mate J, Pajares JM. Role of 5-aminosalicylic acid (5-ASA) in treatment of inflammatory bowel disease: a systematic review. Dig Dis Sci 2002;47:471–88.

Hassan I, Horgan AF, Nivatvongs S. Outcome of patients undergoing ileal pouch-anal anastamosis for left-sided chronic ulcerative colitis. J Gastrointest Surg 2003;7:567–71.

Hebden JM, Blackshaw PE, Perkins AC, et al. Limited exposure of the healthy distal colon to orally-dosed formulation is further exaggerated in active left-sided ulcerative colitis. Aliment Pharmcol Ther 2000;14:155–61.

Sandborn WJ, Hanauer SB, Katz S, et al. Efficacy and safety of ASACOL 4.8 g/day (800 mg tablet) compared to 24 g/day (400 mg tablet) in treating moderately active ulcerative colitis. Amer J gastro 2004;99:1–251.

Sinha A, Nightingale J, West KP, et al. Epidermal growth factor enemas with oral mesalamine for mild-to-moderate left-sided ulcerative colitis or proctitis. N Engl J Med 2003;349:395–7.

Sturgeon JB, Bhatia P, Hermans D, Miner PB Jr. Exacerbation of chronic ulcerative colitis with mesalamine. Gastroenterology 1995;108:1889–93.

Vecchi M, Saibeni S, Devani M, et al. Review article: diagnosis, monitoring and treatment of distal colitis. Aliment Pharmacol Ther 2003;17(Suppl 2):2–6.

CHAPTER 78

Ulcerative Colitis

Kenneth W. Schroeder, MD, PhD, and William J. Tremaine, MD

Ulcerative colitis (UC) is a chronic inflammatory disease of unknown cause, which typically affects the rectum and variable areas of the proximal colon in a continuous pattern. There is no known cure but medications are often effective in controlling the inflammation and the associated symptoms. Based on the location and extent of the inflammation, the clinician can determine which medications may be expected to provide symptomatic benefit with a minimum of adverse effects. Hence, knowledge of the disease extent and severity of activity are critical to planning a medical therapy program.

When patients present with active symptoms, the primary initial goal is to *alleviate the symptoms* and *induce remission*. The secondary goal is to plan for a treatment program to *maintain long-term remission*. These two phases of treatment may require a series of medications using different doses and routes of delivery, with a transition from induction of remission to maintenance of remission after the first few weeks.

Ideally, any medical therapy should be evidence based (see Chapter 1, "Using Evidence-Based Medicine in Patient Care"). However most therapeutic trials, including those for UC, involve a single drug given at fixed dose for a short period of time and the trials do not address the changing needs of the patient over time, through the spectrum of changes in disease activity and extent. In reality, the best therapy for an individual patient with UC is based in part on evidence-based data and in part on anecdotal clinical experience. Depending on the unique circumstances for an individual patient, treatment of UC with either a sequential or combination therapeutic approach can be effective.

Medical Therapy

Sequential versus Combination Therapy

Initial treatment with one drug at a single dose and one delivery route is the traditional and easiest way for both the clinician and patient to judge the efficacy and tolerability of a treatment. Most evidence-based data is based on this approach. Patient compliance with using a single drug is likely to be better than with multiple drugs or multiple delivery routes and the cost will probably be less. If the initial treatment is not effective or tolerable, then the dose can be adjusted, with or without starting other drugs. The main drawback to sequential therapy is that the trial and error method of adding medications may prolong the time to response compared with combining multiple drugs from the start. This sequential approach is most appropriate for mildly active disease when controlling symptoms quickly is less critical.

Combining multiple treatments at once, either with the same drug by different delivery routes, or using two or more drugs, may achieve a more prompt onset of action and better efficacy than the sequential approach. This is a common intuitive approach used by clinicians who have seen the apparent benefit of using two or more treatments at once, such as 5-aminosalicyclic (ASA, mesalamine) and prednisone. Combination therapy is most commonly used for moderate or severe disease, particularly if there is urgency to getting the symptoms controlled promptly (Table 78-1). Downsides to the combination therapy are the paucity of data from controlled trials to confirm the benefits, difficulty identifying the offending drug if adverse effects are noted, less compliance with more complicated schedules, and higher costs.

TABLE 78-1. Sequential Therapy for Ulcerative Colitis

Rectosigmoid Disease
   5-ASA suppositories/enemas
   5-ASA: enemas + oral
   5-ASA (enemas + oral) + prednisone
   5-ASA enemas + oral + prednisone + nicotine
   Stop 5-ASA and observe
   AZA/6-MP if steroid-dependent
   Surgery if poor quality of life
Extensive Disease
   5-ASA oral
   5-ASA oral + enemas
   5-ASA (oral + enemas) + prednisone
   5-ASA (oral + enemas) + prednisone + nicotine
   Stop 5-ASA and observe
   AZA/6-MP if steroid-dependent
   Intravenous steroids
   Surgery if refractory to medications
   Cyclosporine if severe disease and surgery declined

ASA = aminosalicyclic acid, AZA = azathioprine, MP = mercaptopurine.

Therapy of Distal Disease

For mildly active distal disease, 5-ASA preparations are our first choice. If the disease is limited to the distal 15 cm, a suppository preparation of 500 mg each, given 1 to 2 times daily for 2 to 4 weeks, may control the symptoms. If the disease is more extensive but limited to the colon that is distal to the splenic flexure, an enema containing 4 g of 5-ASA, given at bedtime for 3 or 4 weeks, will be effective in 80% of patients. The patient who responds with symptomatic improvement can then be switched to oral 5-ASA at a dose of 2.4 to 2.5 g/d for long-term maintenance. Flares occurring infrequently, such as once or twice yearly, can be treated with repeat suppository or enema preparations of 5-ASA for 3- to 4-week intervals when needed. If the flares recur more frequently, a higher dose of oral 5-ASA (eg, 4.8 g/d) may be necessary for maintenance treatment. This may be reduced slowly once the patient has been in remission for several months to a lower dose (2.4 to 4.8g/d) by tapering the daily dose by 1 tablet every 2 to 4 weeks. Suppositories or enemas of 5-ASA given once or twice weekly are another option for maintenance therapy of distal disease if oral 5-ASA preparations are ineffective.

When mild distal disease is not controlled with this approach, or the disease is more severe, combined rectal 5-ASA (4 g/d enema) and oral 5-ASA (2.4 to 4.8 g/d) may prove effective. Alternatively, the addition of a hydrocortisone enema or hydrocortisone foam may be given once daily in addition to the oral 5-ASA therapy for a period of 3 to 4 weeks. If remission is not accomplished with this regimen, then prednisone 40 mg/d for 2 to 4 weeks, in addition to oral 5-ASA, may be used. Once symptoms are controlled, prednisone may be reduced by decreasing the daily dose by 10 mg each week down to 20 mg/d, then reducing the daily dose by 5 mg per day each week or 2 weeks until the prednisone is stopped. Oral 5-ASA therapy (2.4 to 4.8 g/d) may be continued for long term maintenance therapy. For the patient who responds to oral prednisone but promptly worsens as the dose is reduced despite maintenance therapy with 5-ASA, then azathioprine (AZA) or 6-mercaptopurine (6-MP) can be added. We check the thiopurine methyltransferase (TPMT) red cell enzyme before starting AZA/6-MP, and if the TPMT is normal, we start with a dose of AZA 2 to 2.5 mg/kg daily or 6-MP at a dose of 1 to 1.5 mg/kg daily. A lower dose should be used in patients with a low TPMT level. There is a separate chapter on AZA use in inflammatory bowel disease (IBD) (Chapter 69, "Monitoring of Azathioprine Metabolite Levels in Inflammatory Bowel Disease"). We continue prednisone for about 2 months after starting AZA/6-MP to allow time for the drug to become effective. Occasionally, we use nicotine patches for UC, in patients who have not responded to steroids, particularly in former smokers. We start nicotine patches at an initial dose of a 7 mg/d for a week, then 14 mg/d for a week, then a 21 mg/d patch for 4 weeks as described by Sandborn and colleagues (1997). With clinical improvement, the nicotine patch dose can be reduced to the next lower dose every 2 weeks until the patches are discontinued. Once remission has been attained, prednisone can be tapered by 10 mg increments until reaching 20 mg/d and then by 5 mg/d every 1 to 2 weeks until stopped.

Unresponsive Patients

For patients who have not responded adequately to any of these measures, we recommend *proctocolectomy with ileal J pouch to anal anastomosis (IAP)* if the patient is under age 65 years and is in good health, or end *ileostomy* if the patient is obese or older. Although *cyclosporine* is an option, we consider the risks to outweigh the benefits compared with surgery and we share this opinion with the patient. We use *infliximab* for UC only within the context of an experimental trial, as it has unproved benefit for this indication.

Therapy of Extensive Disease

Mildly active extensive (extending proximal to splenic flexure) colitis is usually best treated first with oral 5-ASA. Sulfasalazine, the original 5-ASA preparation, is a prodrug that releases 5-ASA after cleavage by bacterial action on the diazo bond with sulfapyridine. However, the sulfapyridine moiety has little anti-inflammatory activity, and it causes adverse effects in up to 40% of patients. Most patients who experience adverse effects from sulfasalazine will tolerate oral 5-ASA preparations. The adverse effects from sulfapyridine can be dose related, and this prevents use of high doses of sulfasalazine, usually to a maximum of 4 g daily. Therefore, it is not possible to deliver as high a dose of 5-ASA with sulfasalazine as with other oral 5-ASA preparations. Other available oral preparations of 5-ASA include the prodrugs, olsalazine (Dipentum) and balsalazide (Colazal), as well as the targeted delivery preparation of 5-ASA (Asacol), and the continuous delivery preparation of 5-ASA (Pentasa).

One of the oral 5-ASA preparations should be used as initial therapy for *mildly active* UC. We usually start one of the newer oral 5-ASA medications such as Asacol at a dose of 2.4 g/d, balsalazide (Colazal) at 6.75 g/d (contains 2.4 g of 5-ASA), or Pentasa at a dose of 2.5 g/d. If there is no symptomatic response in 10 to 14 days, the dose may be increased to 4.8 g/d of Asacol or 4.0 g/d of Pentasa (Sutherland et al, 2000; Eaden et al, 2000). Some patients may respond well, except for persistent urgency or occasional blood streaks with mucous on stools. This usually reflects persistent distal colon inflammation, and the addition of 5-ASA suppositories (Canasa) or enemas (Rowasa) at bedtime may control these lingering symptoms.

The newer oral 5-ASA medications are several times more expensive than sulfasalazine, and when cost of the medication is a limiting factor for a patient, sulfasalazine is a reasonable choice. Sulfasalazine may be started at 1 g daily with an increase in the dose by 1 g each day up to the target dose of 3 to 4 g/d, if tolerated. The complete blood count should be checked after a week to look for toxicity, especially leukopenia. However, there are several drawbacks to using sulfasalazine instead of one of the newer 5-ASA preparations. Sulfasalazine should not be used in patients with a history of sulfa allergy. Besides allergic reactions, some patients develop headaches, nausea, anorexia, and other dose-related adverse effects. Sulfasalazine may cause reversible male infertility, which does not occur with the other oral 5-ASA medications.

For moderate symptoms, we start high dose oral 5-ASA with Asacol at 4.8 g/d (may be available as 800 mg tablets) or Pentasa at 4.0 g/d (available as 500 mg capsules); if the symptoms do not improve in a week, prednisone should be started at 40 mg/d as a single morning dose. Once symptoms come under control, the prednisone can be tapered, with reductions by 10 mg/d each week down to a dose of 20 mg/d, and with reductions of 5 mg/d each 1 to 2 weeks thereafter until prednisone is discontinued. If there is initial improvement but then symptomatic worsening while tapering prednisone or within a few weeks of stopping, the dose of prednisone can be increased again until symptoms improve and then tapered more slowly. For the patient who again flares with the second prednisone taper, the prednisone may be increased to the dose that controlled the symptoms, with AZA 2 to 2.5 mg/kg/d or 6-MP 1 to 1.5 mg/kg/d added. The prednisone may again be tapered after another 2 months. For those not responding to prednisone, nicotine patches are a consideration, gradually increased to a dose of 21 mg/d. If major symptoms persist despite these measures, consideration should be given to surgery with proctocolectomy and IAP for the patient who is less than 65 years of age, or end-ileostomy for the obese or older patient and for those with anal sphincter incompetence.*

Severe colitis symptoms can be very disabling and life threatening with risks including toxic megacolon, sepsis, and perforation. Such flares may be induced by medications, such as antibiotics and nonsteroidal anti-inflammatory drugs, or by development of an idiosyncratic reaction to sulfasalazine or 5-ASA, even in the patient who has previously tolerated these drugs for months or years. Patients with severe flares usually require hospitalization and intravenous (IV) corticosteroids. Bowel rest may be used but there is no data to support that this hastens induction of remission and patients will usually tolerate a liquid or low residue diet. With the possibility of an idiosyncratic reaction to sulfasalazine or 5-ASA, it is usually worthwhile to stop this drug for a while to make sure this is not the provoking agent. Stool cultures and assessment for *Clostridium difficile* toxin and ova and parasites should be undertaken simultaneously with initiation of the corticosteroids. Daily monitoring of the patient should include examination of the abdomen and plain films of the abdomen daily or on alternate days. If symptoms do not improve with 5 days of IV steroids, such as Solu-Medrol at doses of 60 mg over 24 hours up to 40 to 60 mg each 8 hours, then proctocolectomy or IV cyclosporine should be considered. Although surgery may be the best alternative, some patients are unwilling to proceed with surgery, and IV cyclosporine (2 to 4 mg/d) is a reasonable alternative for 7 to 10 days. Initial combined therapy with steroid and cyclosporine does not appear to be more advantageous than starting with steroids and later adding the cyclosporine, if needed. After the patient improves from the severe flare, AZA (2 to 2.5 mg/kg) or 6-MP (1 to 1.5 mg/kg)[†] should be overlapped with oral cyclosporine (5 mg/kg/d) with intended blood levels of cyclosporine of 150 to 300 ng/mL for 3 to 6 months. While the patient is on cyclosporine, antibiotic prophylaxis for *Pneumocystis carinii* with trimethoprim 160 mg/sulfamethoxazole 800 mg (one double strength tablet) once daily should be given. For the patient who responds to this program, AZA or 6-MP should be continued for years. For some patients intolerant of AZA, 6-MP may be better tolerated (Boulton-Jones et al, 2000). Concomitant 5-ASA seemingly adds little to the immunomodulatory drug regimen. Initial use of IV cyclosporine without corticosteroids may be reasonable therapy for severe UC in the patient with a history of steroid-induced psychosis, avascular necrosis, or other severe side effects from corticosteroids.

Medical Therapy during Pregnancy and Nursing

5-ASA and corticosteroids are safe to use during pregnancy and during nursing. There is reassuring retrospective data that AZA/6-MP and cyclosporine are safe and do not need to be stopped if pregnancy occurs while on such therapy. Nicotine should not be used during pregnancy and nursing. There is a separate chapter (Chapter 84, "Pregnancy and Inflammatory Bowel Disease") on pregnancy and IBD.

Long-Term Maintenance Therapy

Inducing a remission can be a challenge and long-term remission is an important goal for all patients. Both sulfasalazine and the newer generation of 5-ASA preparations are comparably effective for maintenance of remission. Effective 5-ASA maintenance doses are usually in the range of 2 to 4 g/d of sulfasalazine (Azulfidine), 2 to 4 g/d of Pentasa (available as 500 mg capsules), 2.4 to 4.8 g/d of

---

*Editor's Note: I am also concerned about IAP anastomosis in patients with severe co-existent irritable bowel syndrome.

[†]Editors Note: AZA/6-MP dosage variation based on TPMT and later 6-TG/6-MMP levels can also be used. There is a separate chapter on this approach.

Asacol (available as 800 mg tablets), 1 g/d of olsalazine (Dipentum), or 6.75 g/d of balsalazide (Colazal). Another benefit is that recent studies have demonstrated an association between maintenance treatment with an oral 5-ASA drug (over 1.2 g) and a reduction in the risk of colorectal cancer in patients with UC (Eaden et al, 2000). For patients who eventually require immunomodulatory therapy with AZA/6-MP, these drugs should be continued indefinitely. It is usually unnecessary to continue 5-ASA along with AZA or 6-MP. For most patients, a lifelong maintenance treatment program will prove beneficial and should reduce the frequency of flares considerably (Kamm, 2002). Frequent flares despite adequate doses of maintenance medications are an indication for colectomy

Supplemental Reading

Boulton-Jones JR, Pritchard K, Mahmoud AA. The use of 6-mercaptopurine in patients with inflammatory bowel disease after failure of azathioprine therapy. Aliment Pharmacol Ther 2000;14:1561–5.

Campbell S, Ghosh S. Effective maintenance of inflammatory bowel disease remission by azathioprine does not require concurrent 5-aminosalicyate therapy. Eur J Gastroenterol Hepatol 2001;13:1297–301.

Cohen RD, Stein R, Hanauer S. Intravenous cyclosporine in ulcerative colitis: a five-year experience. Am J Gastroenterol 1999;94:1587–92.

Cohen RD, Woseth DM, Thisted RA, Hanauer SB. A meta-analysis and overview of the literature on treatment options for left-sided ulcerative colitis and ulcerative proctitis. Am J Gastroenterol 2000;95:1263–76.

Connell WR. Safety of drug therapy for inflammatory bowel disease in pregnant and nursing women. Inflamm Bowel Dis 1996;2:33–47.

Eaden J, Abrams K, Ekbom A, et al. Colorectal cancer prevention in ulcerative colitis: a case-control study. Aliment Pharmacol Ther 2000;14:145–53.

Kamm MA. Review article: maintenance of remission in ulcerative colitis. Aliment Pharmacol Ther 2002:16 Suppl 4:21–4.

Sandborn WJ, Hanauer SB, Katz S, et al. Efficacy and safety of ASACOL 4.8 g/day (800 mg tablet) compared to 24 g/day (400 mg tablet) in treating moderately active ulcerative colitis. Amer J gastro 2004;99:1–251.

Sandborn WJ, Tremaine WJ, Offord KP, et al. Transdermal nicotine for mildly to moderately active ulcerative colitis (UC): a randomized, double-blind, placebo-controlled trial. Ann Intern Med 1997;126:364–71.

Sutherland L, Roth D, Beck P, et al. Oral 5-aminosalicylic acid for inducing remission in ulcerative colitis (Cochran Review). The Cochrane Library. Issue 4. Oxford: Update Software; 2000.

Vecchi M, Meucci G, Gionchetti P, et al. Oral versus combination mesalazine therapy in active ulcerative colitis: a double-blind, double-dummy, randomized multicentre study. Aliment Pharmacol Ther 2001;15:251–6.

CHAPTER 79

Ileoanal Pouch Anastomosis

FEZA H. REMZI, MD, AND VICTOR W. FAZIO, MB, MS

Restorative proctocolectomy (RP) with ileal pouch anal anastomosis (IPAA) has become the gold standard of surgical treatment for ulcerative colitis (UC) (Parks and Nicholls, 1978). In many series, > 90% of procedures for UC involve RP/IPAA. This may be performed as (1) a primary procedure, of total proctocolectomy (TPC) and IPAA, with temporary loop ileostomy or (2) a multistaged with subtotal colectomy oversew of rectal stump and end ileostomy, followed by completion proctectomy IPAA and loop ileostomy, with final (third) procedure being closure of loop ileostomy. Figure 79-1 outlines indications for surgery.

In a few cases (up to 10% of RP cases) the procedure is done in one stage, TPC and IPAA without loop ileostomy (Fazio et al, 1995). This is an alternative we will use in well-motivated and informed patients who are:

1. Aware of the 5 to 10% leak rate from the pouch anal anastomosis and the possibility that an urgent ileostomy may be required in the early postoperative period (Tjandra et al, 1993; Remzi et al, in press).
2. Aware that recovery—both hospital stay and recovery time (return of stamina) to return to work and social activities—may be double that of the usual 6 to 7 day

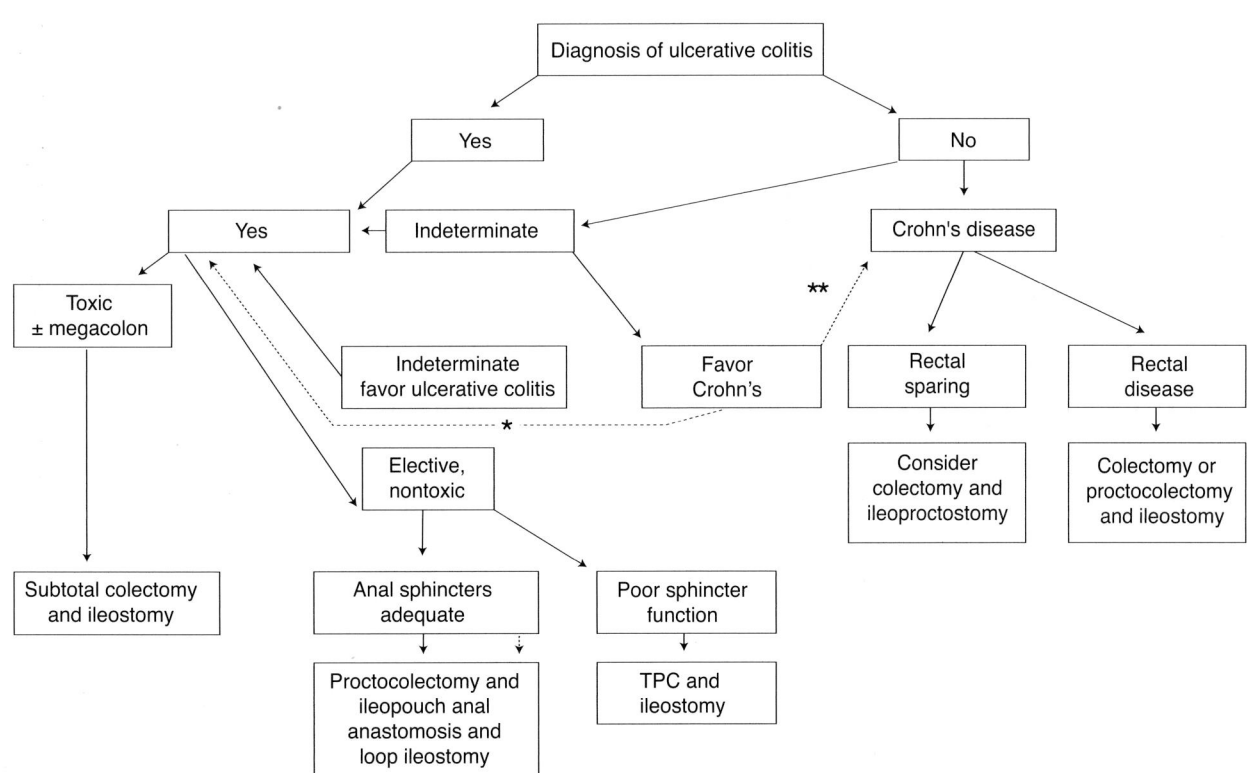

FIGURE 79-1. Legend: Indications for surgery. IPAA= ileal pouch-anal anastomosis; TPC= total proctocolectomy.
*Absence of perianal or small bowel disease.
**Presence of adverse/clinical/radiologic indicators.

hospital stay and the 2-month normal recovery time. This is due to the combination of recovery from a major abdominal procedure as well as from the obligatory early excessive stool frequency accompanying a one-stage operation due to undesirable consequences of early postoperative sphincter function.

Thus, we will consider the one-staged operation

3. Where there is no toxicity or features adverse to tissue healing (prednisone dose < 20 mg/d, diabetes, immunosuppressive therapy)
4. Where the operation has proceeded effortlessly with minimal blood loss (no transfusion requirement) and hemostasis is considered excellent
5. Where there has been no difficulty in getting the pouch to reach the anus without excessive tension
6. Where intact tissue rings (doughnuts) have been obtained using the double stapled technique
7. Where on table pouch/anastomotic testing with air has shown no anastomotic or pouch leak.

Paradoxically, this may be the procedure of choice in obese patients who cannot lose weight preoperatively. In those individuals, addition of a temporary ileostomy may produce such tension on the superior mesenteric artery (the determining factor for the ease of reach of the pouch to the anus) that we believe the completed IPAA may be excessively vulnerable to leak or disruption.

In our recent review, patients who had one-stage pouch procedure were younger, more often female, smaller in body surface area, on lesser doses of steroids, and required less blood transfusions at the time of their surgery than those who had required ileostomy at the time of the IPAA (Remzi et al, in press). We believe avoidance of diverting ileostomy with these stringent criteria is pivotal to prevent postoperative septic complications and potentially pouch loss in the long term.*

OTHER PROCEDURES FOR UC PATIENTS

1. Subtotal or total colectomy and ileostomy. This is preferred in patients:
   - Where there is a diagnostic dilemma (features that are ambiguous for Crohn's disease [CD] versus UC, eg, patchy colonic disease, backwash ileitis)
   - Patients on very large doses (eg, 50 to 60 mg/d) of prednisone
   - Patients with toxic colitis or megacolon
   - Gross obesity, where ability to lose weight is precluded by high dose steroid
   - Malnutrition, especially hypoalbuminemia

We prefer suturing the stapled-across rectosigmoid stump to the distal aspect of the incision. This places the suture line extraperitoneally, and if breakdown at the staple line occurs, drainage from the rectal stump can be controlled via a lower incisional fistula without the patient becoming septic. Following subtotal colectomy (STC) and ileostomy, and favorable histology review, patients may undergo completion proctectomy and IPAA some 5 to 6 months later.

2. Total colectomy and ileorectal anastomosis: This may be the procedure of choice in two situations, both requiring absence of florid or significant rectal disease.
   - Patients with distant metastases (liver, lung) where colon cancer complicates UC
   - The young(er) woman who is anxious to maximize her chances of child bearing.

There is evidence that RP/IPAA with its necessary pelvic adhesions postoperatively will diminish fertility due to peritubal and peri-ovarian adhesions (Ording et al, 2002). Additionally, we usually do oophoropexy and apply hyaluronidase/methyl cellulose film (Seprafilm, Genzyme, Cambridge, MA) to the gonadal structures to limit such adhesions. Patients may undergo rectal resection and conversion to a pelvic pouch in 30 to 50% of cases—should disabling proctitis occur or rectal cancer risk become significant with future pregnancies. Following RP and IPAA, we recommend cesarean section due to the risk of sphincter injury with episiotomy or prolonged or difficult labor. Although data from several sources attest to the early good pouch function with vaginal delivery, the studies are flawed by the lack of adequate follow up of pouch function in the middle-aged woman, many years "out" from IPAA (Juhasz et al, 1995).

3. TPC and ileostomy: This has been the standard surgical treatment of UC and is appropriate when:
   - The patient is not unduly concerned about having a permanent ileostomy.
   - Anal sphincter function is poor. We note however, that preoperative anal incontinence may be due to very active rectal disease reflecting urgency, rather than true sphincter deficiency. Such patients merit anal physiology testing, with particular emphasis on resting pressure. Values above 35 to 40 mm of mercury do not contraindicate RP when the concern is preoperative sphincter function (Halverson et al, 2002).
   - Cancer of the lower third of the rectum is present.
   - There is a history of radiation to the abdomen and concern for radiation enteritis at the time of the laparotomy.
   - The patient is elderly. Our studies show that when patients over the age of 70 years undergo RP/IPAA, although they perceive quality of life to be good/satisfactory, pad usage and continence is considerably greater than in their younger counterparts. Careful discussion must be had with these older patients before offering them RP (Delaney et al, 2002).

---

*Editor's Note: Patients and referring doctors should, as stated, realize that the period of adjustment postoperatively can last 4 months. However, they have avoided an ileostomy.

The Current Operation of RP and IPAA

Indications

It follows that RP/IPAA is a suitable and preferred operation for patients where subtotal colectomy or TPC and Brooke ileostomy are not indicated. In general, these are patients who:
- are in good condition mentally and physically
- have had no previous small bowel (SB) resections
- have good anal sphincter function
- are without evidence of CD, such as perianal fistula (past or present)
- may be diagnosed of indeterminate colitis
- have no history of radiation to the abdomen
- may undergo RP with curative intent if colorectal cancer is present
- are particularly eligible if portal hypertension is present in association with UC (Kartheuser et al, 1996).

Issues and Controversies

POUCH CONSTRUCTION

A variety of pouch techniques and configurations have been described including the J, S, W, and lateral isoperistaltic (H) types. The functional results of these various pouch designs appear to be comparable, where the *J pouch* is easiest to construct and has functional outcomes identical to those of more complex designs (Johnston et al, 1996). We prefer the J pouch, as it is simple to make using a linear stapler cutting technique, can be done rapidly in ≤ 5 minutes, and has no obstructive defecation sequelae. The S pouch is occasionally used when excessive anastomotic tension is predictable in a given patient. It usually reaches 2 to 4 cm farther than does the J pouch and is useful in patients with a short fat mesentery, and long, narrow pelvis when the reach of the ileal pouch to the anal canal can be a problem. In our practice, this is especially true in patients who are obese or where mucosectomy and hand-sewn anastomosis is indicated due to neoplasia. Care is exercised to limit the exit conduit to ≤ 2 cm as obstructive defecation—necessitating pouch emptying by periodic catheter intubation—may ensue.

ANASTOMOTIC ISSUES

The two main ways in which the pouch can be joined to the anal canal are by stapling and by hand sutured techniques. For a stapled anastomosis, it is necessary to leave a 1 to 2 cm strip of anal transitional mucosa to allow transanal insertion of the staple head. This zone is usually referred to as the *anal transitional zone* (ATZ). This creates a controversy, which centers on the potential advantages and disadvantages of leaving a mucosal cuff of rectal mucosa. The potential advantages include better functional results, lower rate of septic complications, and ease of construction, whereas disadvantages include possible malignant or premalignant transformation of the columnar epithelial cells in the retained mucosal cuff, cuffitis, and a longer, more difficult surgery. The prospective randomized trials have not shown a difference in functional outcome and septic complications between the two methods (Sonoda and Fazio, 2000). However these studies warrant careful analysis, because of relatively short term follow up and because the small number of cases studied make them vulnerable to type II error. Our initial studies comparing the two types of techniques showed less septic complications and better functional outcome favoring stapled anastomosis (Ziv et al, 1996). The most recent study of over 2,000 patients from our institution continued to show superior functional results in patients with stapled anastomosis, where the septic complications showed some increased trend in mucosectomy group but did not reach the statistical difference of the prior study from our institution (Remzi et al, 2002).

We believe that the major complication of pouch surgery is sepsis secondary to anastomotic dehiscence and this, in turn, is due to excessive anastomotic tension. We believe, the least septic complication rates occur when the ileal pouch is stapled to the top of the anal columns 1 to 2 cm above the dentate line.

This ATZ is vulnerable to neoplastic and/or acute symptomatic inflammatory change. Our studies show that in the absence of synchronous colonic carcinoma at the time of index TPC and IPAA for UC, the risk of dysplasia is negligible and cancer in the ATZ has yet to be reported. From an oncogenic standpoint, stapled IPAA is therefore safe (Remzi et al, 2003). We do, however, recommend ATZ surveillance and biopsy. Our current recommendation for the management of risk of ATZ dysplasia and selection of type of anastomosis to be used in creation of IPAA is summarized in Figure 79-2. Further data is needed before this examination frequency can be relaxed, in our view. For patients with synchronous colorectal cancer, dysplasia in lower two-thirds of rectum or primary sclerosing cholangitis, postoperative ATZ dysplasia is a substantial risk and complete anal mucosectomy is recommended at time of RP (Kartheuser et al, 1996; Remzi et al, 2003; Marchesa et al, 1997).

If a patient has undergone stapled IPAA for cancer complicating UC (usually first diagnosed in the colectomy specimen), then close follow up (eg, annual or 6-month biopsies) is recommended. We were successful in preserving the pelvic pouch in two patients who underwent late transanal mucosectomy and pouch advancement for late development of ATZ dysplasia (Fazio and Tjandra, 1994). So, why not do mucosectomy in every case? We believe that anal sphincter stretch is considerable and protracted when hand-sewn techniques with mucosectomy are used. This produces significant and prolonged reduction in resting sphincter tone and is associated with higher rates (compared to stapled IPAA) of nocturnal incontinence, seepage, and pad usage, by

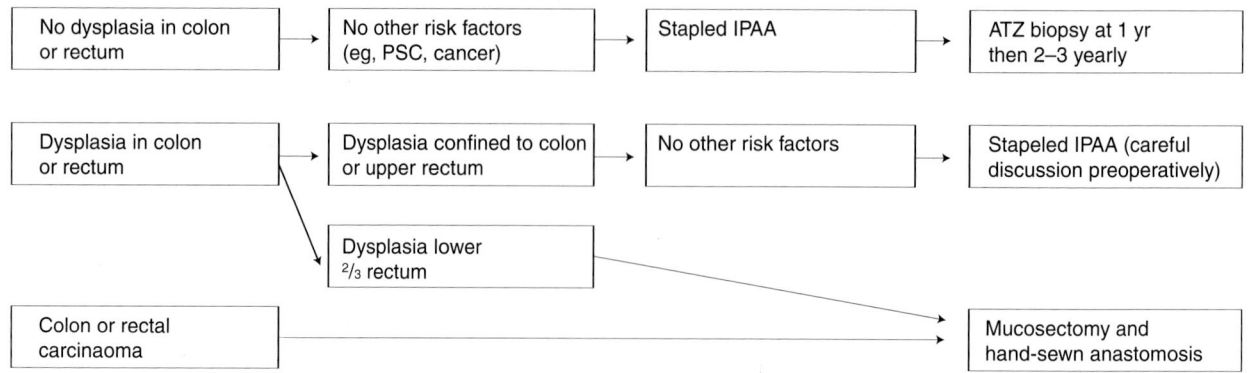

FIGURE 79-2. Management of risk of anal transitional zone (ATZ) dysplasia. IPAA = ileal pouch-anal anastomosis; PSC = primary sclerosing cholangitis.

patients during daytime and nighttime (Remzi et al, 2002; Tuckson et al, 1991). In the patients without risk factors for ATZ dysplasia (absence of synchronous cancer or dysplasia in the rectum), the continence factor is a compelling one in our advocating stapled IPAA. When the risk factors for ATZ dysplasia are present, the balance of risk/benefit comes down in favor of complete mucosectomy in our view.

A final point on this issue: if we see a patient whose body habitus suggests that anastomotic tension will be excessive with a hand-sewn anastomosis, we will lay out the pros and cons of a stapled alternative even if adverse oncologic indicators are present. We believe the patient should be given full data on this issue to allow a measured decision to be made along with the caveats (viz surveillance) attendant with a decision to pursue restorative proctocolectomy.

Perioperative and Postoperative Issues

Sepsis Pelvic sepsis is the most serious early complication of ileal pouch operations and is one of the main causes of pouch failure. The rate of sepsis after ileoanal pouch construction ranges from 5 to 24% (Fazio et al, 1995). It may be due to suture line leaks, or bacterial contamination of the surgical space during the operation. Etiologic risk factors predisposing to pelvic sepsis are local and general inflammatory changes, such as malnutrition, prolonged steroid usage, hypoalbuminemia, anemia, and hypoxemia. Fever, perineal pain, purulent discharge, and leukocytosis are the most common presenting symptoms of sepsis.

Leaks may develop from the pouch-anal anastomosis, from the pouch itself or from tip of the J pouch. Anastomotic tension and bowel ischemia are the two main factors associated with high leakage rates after IPAA.

Anastomotic leaks may be asymptomatic "sinuses" that originate from the anastomosis, and they are most often diagnosed at the time of pouchography when the patient returns for the takedown of the ileostomy. Such radiologically detected leaks represent incomplete healing of the anastomosis or the ileal pouch. The leaks will usually heal spontaneously by deferring the closure of the ileostomy for a few months. A repeat Gastrografin enema should be performed 3 to 6 months later for evaluation. If no abscess cavities are present and the sinus track leading from the anastomosis is narrowed or obliterated, then ileostomy closure can be performed.

In a symptomatic patient who is stable, not septic, and has no peritonitis, initial treatment for a leak should include intravenous (IV) antibiotic therapy, drainage, and bowel rest. Antibiotic coverage should include both aerobic gram-negative and anaerobic organisms. In the presence of a sizeable pelvic abscess, percutaneous drainage under computed tomography guidance may prevent the need for re-laparotomy.

In some instances, a minor leak results in a small presacral collection. Examination under anesthesia allows evaluation of the abscess collection and passage of a transanal catheter into the cavity for daily irrigation. The catheter may be safely removed when there is clinical and radiologic evidence of resolution of the abscess cavity.

Emergent surgical intervention may be required for patients who are treated with nonoperative therapy whose signs and symptoms worsen and those with generalized peritonitis or high output pouch-cutaneous fistulas, although this is uncommon, especially in the presence of a diverting ileostomy. The surgical intervention should be preceded by immediate fluid resuscitation and administration of IV broad spectrum antibiotics.

Sinuses, fistulas, or leaks that persist after treatment, may require repeat IPAA or permanent ileostomy (Baixauli et al, 2004). They may also suggest the presence of underlying CD. Sepsis, sinuses, or fistulas (eg, pouch anastomotic vaginal fistulas), which appear late (over 6 months) from

IPAA, are often indicative of CD, although not always (Shah et al, 2003). The management ranges from intermittent antibiotic therapy (ciprofloxacin and metronidazole with or without local seton drainage) pouch advancement flap-through to repeat IPAA with fistula exclusion. The latter is used if the former is unsuccessful.

Bowel Obstruction

Patients undergoing RP are at particularly high risk for SB obstruction because of the combined abdominal and pelvic dissection, the need for multiple operations, and the possibility of septic complications. SB obstruction is the commonest reason for unplanned major re-operation on RP patients, occurring in 10 to 20% of cases, half of which require surgery to release the adhesion(s) causing the obstruction (Fazio et al, 1995). So far, the only factor associated with lessening this risk is ileostomy avoidance at the time of pouch construction, but at the price of possible sepsis, symptomatic anastomotic leak, and prolonged patient adjustment with ileostomy avoidance.

Evacuation Disorders

Strictures are usually secondary to fibrosis followed by partial dehiscence of the IPAA or ischemia. If severe, the stricture may obstruct the outlet of the pouch and result in evacuation problems, pouch dilatation, and bacterial overgrowth. The anal canal typically narrows by some degree after IPAA. Short strictures at the anastomosis generally respond to careful dilatation. Many strictures are webs and can be either dilated by fingers or dilators. For this reason, either at the initial 6-week postoperative visit or at the time of the ileostomy closure, it has been our practice to perform a routine digital and proctoscopic assessment and dilatation. We believe that this practice prevents fibrous webs from progressing to subsequent stricture development. Transanal stricture lysis is occasionally necessary for recurrent short strictures. Long strictures (> 1 to 2 cm) require stricture excision and neopouch anal anastomosis either transanally or by abdomino anal approach. Ischemia and sepsis are the two commonest causes.*

Long exit conduit of S or H pouches. These obstructions are managed by intermittent catheter intubation about 4 times a day. If this is deemed disabling by the patient or perforative complication occurs, repeat IPAA or ileostomy is usually needed (Baixauli et al, 2004).

Paradoxical Puborectalis Contraction

This is an infrequent cause of evacuation disorder, often associated with pouchitis. Diagnosis is readily made with electromyelogram or pouchography. Biofeedback is usually successful but requires 4 to 6 sessions (Hull et al, 1995).

*Editor's Note: Regular anal examinations and dilatation, if needed, has been used by some surgeons after mucosal stripping to lessen stricture occurrence (Sitzmann et al, 1999).

"Cuffitis" or Inflammation of ATZ

The preservation of ATZ after stapled anastomosis is meant to optimize anal canal sensation, to minimize sphincter injury and septic complications, and to maximize the preservation of normal postoperative resting and squeeze pressures. This zone is susceptible to inflammation (cuffitis). This rarely reaches significant proportions, and can be managed by topical agents such as corticosteroids or 5-aminosalicylic acid (5-ASA) preparations. Patients with symptomatic cuffitis have similar symptoms to those with pouchitis. However, bloody bowel movements are more commonly seen in patients with cuffitis. This problem rarely required the need for further mucosectomy in our experience. Also, in our recent experience with usage of topical mesalamine suppositories (500 mg twice daily) in 14 consecutive patients with symptomatic cuffitis was safe and effective (Shen et al, 2003).

Pouchitis

This term covers a spectrum of symptomatic inflammatory conditions of the ileal pouch mucosa. We understand this to be a syndrome combining histopathologic evidence of ileal pouch mucosal inflammation with clinical features characterized by one or more of the following:
1. Significant increase in stool frequency above the patient's usual base level
2. Low grade fever and malaise
3. Bleeding
4. Dull pelvic pressure/pain

Most cases respond to metronidazole with or without ciprofloxacin given over a 5 to 10 day period. A chronic variety of pouchitis is much less common. We usually will treat such patients with initial long term (6 months plus) antibiotic therapy. Probiotics have been used to replace long term antibiotics in some patients. If there is little or no response, we will use, 5-ASA orally and/or by enema. The next chapter (Chapter 80, "Crohn's Colitis") details treatment of pouchitis, including a discussion of CD in IPAA. Occasionally ileostomy with pouch excision is necessary.

Irritable Pouch Syndrome

Diarrhea, abdominal pain, urgency, and pelvic discomfort are common after surgery. Pouchitis with those symptoms is the most common long term complication. However, these most frequently reported symptoms in patients with IPAA are not specific for pouchitis. Shen and colleagues (2001) showed that symptom assessment alone is not sufficient for the diagnosis of pouchitis, and that pouch endoscopy and biopsy may be required for diagnosis. Based on symptom, endoscopy and histology assessment using the Pouchitis Disease Activity Index criteria (the most commonly used and validated diagnostic instrument for pouchitis), we examined 61 consecutive symptomatic patients with UC and IPAA, and found that 43% of patients with symptoms suggestive of pouchitis had no endoscopic or histologic evidence of pouchitis or cuffitis. These patients have a condition resembling irritable bowel syndrome (IBS), which we termed it irritable pouch syndrome (IPS) (Shen et al, 2002).

IPS is common in patients with IPAA, and this new disease category has become increasingly recognized. Patients with IPS comprise a substantial portion of outpatient clinic visits in tertiary care centers. Clinical features of pouchitis, cuffitis, and IPS overlap, with the most common symptoms being increased stool frequency, abdominal cramps, and pelvic discomfort. The only way to differentiate the three disease entities is by pouch endoscopy. Patients with IPS also share clinical features of IBS, such as abdominal pain, bloating, urgency, and pelvic discomfort, which are largely relived with defecation. Similar to IBS, weight loss, bloody bowel movement, and fever are not features of IPS.

In a recent study, we found patients with IPS, similar to those with pouchitis or cuffitis, had significantly poorer quality of life scores than patients with normal pouches. Appropriate diagnosis and treatment are important for improving a patient's quality of life. Currently, the diagnosis of IPS is based on the exclusion of structural and inflammatory conditions (such as pouchitis, cuffitis, anastomotic stricture or CD) using pouch endoscopy. We prefer the test-first strategy with diagnostic pouchoscopy rather than the treat first strategy (empiric antibiotics for 5 to 7 days) in the management of patients who present pouchitis-like symptoms. We have recently shown that test-first strategy with pouch endoscopy without biopsy is cost effective and it avoids both diagnostic delay and adverse effects associated with unnecessary antibiotics (Shen et al, 2003). If a patient has symptoms of abdominal or perianal pain, diarrhea, or pelvic discomfort while having a normal pouch endoscopy, he or she is diagnosed as having IPS.

There are no published controlled drug trials for the treatment of patients with IPS. In our institution, we have adopted some safe and effective drug regimens in patients with IBS to treat patients with IPS. The first line therapy includes low dose antidepressants and antispasmodic agents. We believe that safer and more effective agents will become available once we learn more about the cause and mechanism of this new disease.*

---

*Editor's Note: Sometimes a "predict-first" strategy is helpful because some of the IBS patients give a very clear history of irritable bowel type symptoms for many years before they developed recognized UC. Because the small bowel is also "irritable", an IPAA may not be the best option for such patients (Bayless), one can expect more than 10 evacuations per day in some because the irritable or "spastic" pouch can only hold 90 to 100 cc in contrast to the "normal" pouch capacity of 300 to 400 cc. In addition, the patient with irritable pouch can only expel half of the diminished pouch contents, thus this patient may have more than 10 movements per day (Schmidt et al, 1996). The next chapter (Chapter 80, "Crohn's Colitis") has more details in high output IPAAs.

Postoperative Management

After RP and IPAA with loop ileostomy, patients invariably have high ileostomy outputs of from 1,000 to ≥ 2,000 cc per 24 hours. Effectively the "high" ileostomy bypasses ≥ 20% or more of the distal SB and this sets the stage for dehydration. The following advice is given our patients:

- Be aware of added risk factors for dehydration (hot weather, exercise, air conditioning)
- Be aware of symptoms of dehydration (ie, lassitude, fatigue, headache, nausea)
- Maintain intake of adequate oral liquids, especially salty soups, electrolytes supplements. Minimize caffeine intake.
- Avoid high solid fiber/indigestible foods for 6 weeks (as with all new ileostomates)
- Use bulking agents (eg, Konsyl, Citrucel, Metamucil)
- Use liquid loperamide or atropine diphenoxylate dosed on a weight basis to thicken enteric output
- Be aware of the fact that external ileostomy pouches may stay on for only 2 days or so (compared with 5 to 7 days for end ileostomies). Loop ileostomies tend to be flush with the skin
- Follow the steroid-tapering schedule prescribed on discharge
- Recognize symptoms of post discharge bowel obstruction
- After the ileostomy is closed, a similar program is instituted.

Long-Term Follow-Up

In patients with ATZ preservation, recommendations for follow up surveillance are outlined in Figure 79-2. It should be noted that not all patients reported to have total mucosectomy in fact have had this done. Theoretically, if the patient has undergone mucosectomy as part of the RP and remains well, no follow-up is necessary after bowel function has stabilized (usually within 6 to 12 months). Although stapled anastomosis with ATZ preservation has been the focus of risk of neoplasia, the majority of the described cases of adenocarcinoma in UC patients arising at the pouch anal anastomosis have been in those who had undergone mucosectomy (Ooi et al, 2003). The answer may relate to the longevity of the follow-up and the number of patients in each group. It is likely that diseased epithelium was left behind by incomplete mucosectomy. Thus mucosectomy with a hand-sewn anastomosis may give a false sense of security as compared to stapled anastomosis where good visualization and biopsy of the ATZ can be performed. Thus these patients may be vulnerable to ATZ neoplasia development as monitoring is rarely done, least of all with biopsy surveillance. As a separate issue, patients with a chronic type of pouch inflammation, characterized by severe villous atrophy and crypt hyperplasia, may be vulnerable to the complications of pouch "colon-ization", including dysplasia. This type C pouch inflammation has been reported to develop such dysplasia (Gullberg et al, 1997). Also, the recent reports of the malignant potential of the pouch mucosa itself do not eliminate the necessity of pouch surveillance (Ooi et al, 2003). Thus we recommend that all of our patients have pouch surveillance and biopsy at regular intervals. There is no good data as to how frequently this should be done, but every 2 to 3 years seems reasonable unless risk factors for dysplasia in the preserved ATZ are significant, in which case prudence dictates a closer surveillance schedule.

Conclusion

Our long-term follow-up of pouch function and quality of life indicates a very high degree of acceptance and happiness level of the patients undergoing restorative proctocolectomy. This is on a par with age and sex matched US citizens using SF36 assessment tool (Fazio et al, 1999). Bowel movement frequency ranges from 3 to 9 per 24 hours, averaging 6 times per day. This however is not a good indication of success as many patients will evacuate their pouches when it is convenient to do so, rather than defer defecation. Urgency, defined as inability to defer defecation for 15 minutes, is a major concern for many patients preoperatively, yet invariably this is negated by the pouch procedure (the exception is when patients develop pouchitis).

Pad use, either due to need or for sense of security, increases with age, episodes of pouchitis, and the proportions of patients with mucosal stripping of the anal canal as well as decreasing sphincter function. Operative mortality remains < 0.5%, and we have reported impotence rates of < 1% (Fazio et al, 1995). Although dyspareunia may occur post–pouch construction (Bambrick et al, 1996), overall, there is an improvement in female sexual function post-pouch compared to pre-pouch. There are some reports of infertility post-TPC.

Perhaps the most singled out problem of the pelvic pouch procedure is that of pouchitis; by eliminating one disease, the patient is set up for another! Yet this has to be viewed with the perspective that 90% of pouchitis cases are transient and easily treated and that < 10% of patients are subject to repeated episodes. Also, patients, in their quest for preservation of their anal function, understand and generally believe they get a good deal with the trade off of RP.

In conclusion, IPAA provides a very satisfactory quality of life and functional outcome in patients who require proctocolectomy for their disease. Patients < 45 years of age at the time of surgery experience the best functional result. Careful discussion of the procedure and outcome with individual patients allows prudent case selection, yielding a high percentage of patients of all ages who are happy with their postoperative outcome and are happy to recommend it to other patients with the same diagnosis (Delaney et al, 2003).

Supplemental Reading

Baixauli J, Delaney CP, Wu JS, et al. Functional outcome and quality of life after repeat ileal pouch-anal anastomosis for complications of ileoanal surgery. Dis Colon Rectum 2004;47:2–11.

Bambrick M, Fazio VW, Hull TL, et al. Sexual function following restorative proctocolectomy in women. Dis Colon Rectum 1996;39:610–4.

Bayless TM. Coexistant irritable bowel syndrome and inflammatory bowel disease. In: Bayless TM, Hanauer SB, editors. Advanced therapy of inflammatory bowel disease. Hamilton (ON): BC Decker; 2001.

Delaney CP, Dadvand B, Remzi FH, et al. Functional outcome, quality of life, and complications after ileal pouch-anal anastomosis in selected septuagenarians. Dis Colon Rectum 2002;45:890–4.

Delaney CP, Fazio VW, Remzi FH, et al. Prospective, age-related analysis of surgical results, functional outcome, and quality of life after ileal pouch-anal anastomosis. Ann Surg 2003;238:221–8.

Fazio VW, O'Riordain MG, Lavery IC, et al. Long term functional outcome and quality of life after stapled restorative proctocolectomy. Ann Surg 1999;230:578–86.

Fazio VW, Tjandra JJ. Transanal mucosectomy; ileal pouch advancement for anorectal dysplasia or inflammation after restorative proctocolectomy. Dis Colon Rectum 1994;37:1008–11.

Fazio VW, Ziv Y, Church JM, et al. Ileal pouch anal anastomosis: complications and function in 1005 patients. Ann Surg 1995;222:120–7.

Gullberg K, Stahlberg D, Liljeqvist L, et al. Neoplastic transformation of the pelvic pouch mucosa in patients with ulcerative colitis. Gastroenterology 1997;112:1487–92.

Halverson AH, Hull TL, Remzi FH, et al. Perioperative resting pressure predicts long-term postoperative function after ileal pouch-anal anastomosis. J Gastrointest Surg 2002;6:316–20.

Hull TL, Fazio VW, Schroeder T. Paradoxical puborectalis contraction in patients after pelvic pouch construction. Dis Colon Rectum 1995;38:1144–6.

Johnston D, Williamson MER, Lewis WG, et al. Prospective controlled trial of duplicated (j) versus quadruplicated (W) pelvic ileal reservoirs in restorative proctocolectomy for ulcerative colitis. Gut 1996;39:242–7.

Juhasz ES, Fozard B, Dozois RR, et al. Ileal pouch anal anastomosis function following childbirth: an extended evaluation. Dis Colon Rectum 1995;38:159–65.

Kartheuser AH, Dozois RR, LaRusso NF, et al. Comparison of surgical treatment of ulcerative colitis associated with primary sclerosing cholangitis: ileal pouch-anal anastomosis versus Brooke ileostomy. Mayo Clin Proc 1996;71:748–56.

Marchesa P, Lashner BA, Lavery IC, et al. The risk of cancer and dysplasia among ulcerative colitis patients with primary sclerosing cholangitis. Am J Gastroenterol 1997;92:1285–8.

Ooi BS, Remzi FH, Gramlich T, et al. Anal transitional zone cancer following restorative proctocolectomy and ileoanal anastomosis in familial adenomatous polyposis. Dis Colon Rectum 2003;46:1418–23.

Ording OK, Juul S, Berndtsson I, et al. Ulcerative colitis: female fecundity before diagnosis, during disease, and after surgery compared with a population sample. Gastroenterology 2002;122:15–9.

Parks AG, Nicholls RJ. Proctocolectomy without ileostomy for ulcerative colitis. BMJ 1978;2:85–8.

Remzi FH, Fazio VW, Ooi B, et al. Prospective evaluation of functional outcome and quality of life in patients undergoing mucosectomy hand-sewn (MHS) versus stapled pouch-anal anastomosis (IPAA). Presented at the Tripartite Colorectal Meeting; 2002 Oct 27–30; Melbourne, Australia.

Remzi FH, Fazio VW, Delaney CP, et al. Dysplasia of the anal transitional zone after ileal pouch-anal anastomosis. Dis Colon Rectum 2003;46:6–13.

Remzi FH, Fazio VW, Madbouly K, et al. Omission of temporary diversion (TD) after restorative proctocolectomy (RP) and ileal pouch anal anastomosis (IPAA): surgical complications, functional outcome and quality of life analysis. Dis Colon Rectum. [In press]

Schmidt CM, Horton KM, Sitzmann JV, et al. Simple radiography evaluation of iela-anal pouch volume. Dis Colon Rectum 1996;39:66–75.

Shah NS, Remzi FH, Massmann A, et al. Management and treatment outcome of pouch-vaginal fistulas following restorative proctocolectomy. Dis Colon Rectum 2003;46:911–7.

Shen B, Achkar JP, Lashner, et al. Irritable pouch syndrome: a new category of diagnosis for symptomatic patients with ileal pouch-anal anastomosis. Am J Gastroenterol 2002;97:972–7.

Shen B, Achkar JP, Ormsby AH, et al. Endoscopic and histologic evaluation together with symptom assessment are required for diagnosis of pouchitis. Gastroenterology 2001;121:261–7.

Shen B, Lashner BA, Bennett A, et al. Treatment of rectal cuff inflammation (cuffitis) in patients with ulcerative colitis following total proctocolectomy and ileal pouch-anal anastomosis. Presented at the 67th Annual Meeting of American College of Gastroenterology; 2003 Oct 12; Baltimore (MD).

Shen B, Shermock KM, Fazio VW et al. A cost-effectiveness analysis of diagnostic strategies for symptomatic patients with ileal pouch-anal anastomosis. Am J Gastroenterol 2003;98:2460–7.

Sitzmann JV, Buano RC, Bayless TM. Rectal squamous-mucosectomy and ilo-anal pull through procedures. Single Surgeon Experience in 105 patients. In: Becker J, editor. Med problems in general surgery. Philadelphia: Lippincott. 1999:115–23.

Sonoda T, Fazio VW. Controveries in the construction of the ileal pouch anal anastomosis. Sem Gastrointest Dis 2000;11:33–40.

Tjandra JJ, Fazio VW, Milsom JW, et al. Omission of temporary diversion in restorative proctocolectomy—is it safe? Dis Colon Rectum 1993;36:1007–14.

Tuckson WB, Lavery IC, Oakley J et al. Manometric and functional comparison of ileal pouch anal anastomosis with and without anal manipulation. Am J Surg 1991;161:90–6.

Ziv Y, Fazio VW, Church JM, et al. Stapled ileal pouch anal anastomoses are safer than handsewn anastomoses in patients with ulcerative colitis. Am J Surg 1996;171:320–3.

CHAPTER 80

Crohn's Colitis

MILES SPARROW, MD, AND STEPHEN B. HANAUER, MD

Crohn's disease (CD) is a chronic, often granulomatous, inflammatory disease with the potential to affect any part of the gastrointestinal (GI) tract, from mouth to anus. It was not until the 1960s that CD, isolated to the colon, was described and distinguished from ulcerative colitis (UC). In a series by Farmer and colleagues (1975), of 615 CD cases from the Cleveland Clinic the anatomical location of disease was described and found to involve the small intestine in 29% of cases, the ileum and colon in 41% of cases, and the large intestine alone in 27% of cases. These figures have been replicated in subsequent series, such that roughly one-fourth of patients have disease isolated to the colon. Subtle but important differences exist in the presentation and management of CD of the small and large bowel.

Features Unique to Colonic Crohn's Disease

Crohn's colitis has several features, both in diagnosis and management, which differentiate it from CD elsewhere in the GI tract.

Clinical Features

The symptoms of large bowel CD are similar to those of UC, usually presenting with diarrhea and rectal bleeding. In contrast, however, because of the transmural nature of CD, there is a greater likelihood that the symptoms will be associated with abdominal pain, fever, and weight loss. The distinction between UC and Crohn's colitis, although not possible in up to 10 to 15% of cases, is important with regard to potential medical interventions (eg, antitumor necrosis factor [TNF] therapy) and surgical management (the potential for creation of an ileal pouch anal anastomoses is less with CD due to disease recurrence in the ileal pouch). Perianal disease, present in 30 to 40% of patients with Crohn's colitis, is another differentiating feature from UC and is present in up to 80% of cases of Crohn's proctitis. Crohn's colitis is also more common in older patients (> 80% of Crohn's patients older than 40 years have colonic involvement) and in this population it must be differentiated from ischemic colitis and diverticulitis. Crohn's colitis can also present with, or evolve to, toxic megacolon.

The extra-intestinal manifestations of inflammatory bowel disease (IBD) including inflammatory symptoms of the joints, eyes, skin and liver are more common in patients with colonic disease than in patients with disease limited to the small bowel. There are also environmental factors contributing to CD of the colon; cigarette smoking protects against UC such that patients with indeterminate colitis who are smokers are much more likely to "evolve" to CD. In contrast, the *NOD2* genotype is not seen to the same degree in patients with Crohn's colitis compared to CD disease patients with ileal disease (Brant et al,). Similarly, serologic markers to distinguish UC from CD are not as reliable in Crohn's colitis due to the lack of specificity of myeloperoxidase (pANCA) antigen to distinguish UC from Crohn's colitis and the lack of sensitivity for anti-saccharomyces cerevisiae antibodies (ASCA) in colonic CD. Crohn's colitis patients positive for pANCA tend to have left-sided UC-like colitis, whilst those who are ASCA positive tend to have complicated small bowel disease.

MANAGEMENT IMPLICATIONS

The anatomical site of disease has implications related to both medical and surgical therapies. Medically, aminosalicylate therapies must deliver 5-aminosalicylic acid to the colon, and sulfasalazine has been more effective for patients with CD involving the colon than for patients with isolated small bowel disease. Response to antibiotic therapy also is improved with Crohn's colitis versus small bowel disease.

In contrast to small bowel CD, surgery for Crohn's colitis is more often for fulminant or refractory inflammatory colitis rather than for fistulas, abscesses, or obstruction. Postoperative recurrence is less common after colonic resections than after ileocolonic anastomoses and may also occur less often after proctocolectomy and ileostomy for Crohn's colitis than after resections and anastomoses. The latter is also the reason why Crohn's colitis is a relative contraindication for colectomy and ileal pouch anal anastomosis because of the likelihood of pouch complications related to recurrent CD.

Management of Colonic CD

The management goals for treating Crohn's colitis are the same as for CD elsewhere in the gastrointestinal tract; in general, they are to *induce* and *maintain remission (now including mucosal healing)*, to improve quality of life, and to optimise timing of surgery if and when an operation proves necessary to achieve the aforementioned. General treatment measures include correction of anemia and nutritional deficiencies, antidiarrheal medications if required, and cessation of smoking if at all possible. Infectious complications, in particular *Clostridium difficile*, should be excluded. Specific medications used depend on disease features such as site, extent, severity, presence of extra-intestinal manifestations or complications, disease behaviour (inflammatory, fibrostenosing or fistulizing), and previous response to different classes of drugs. The aim is to deliver the maximum dose of the drug to the site of maximal mucosal inflammation.

Medical Management

Figure 80-1 shows a treatment algorithm for induction and maintenance medical therapy for Crohn's colitis, which for simplicity and practicality divides severity into either mild/moderate or severe disease.

Mild/Moderate Acute Crohn's Colitis

AMINOSALICYLATES

Although debate continues regarding the role of aminosalicylates for the treatment of mild-moderate CD, there is good evidence that *sulfasalazine* is efficacious for the treatment of colonic CD. There is less substantial evidence for alternative mesalamine agents. Nevertheless, the aminosalicylates are advocated as a first line therapy for mild-moderately active CD. The use of sulfasalazine in divided doses of 3 to 6 g/d, supported by the National Cooperative Crohn's Disease Study (NCCDS), is compromised, in up to 25% of patients, by side effects attributable to the sulfapyridine carrier molecule, such as headache, nausea, GI upset, and, in males, a transient reduction in number and motility of sperm. Rare but more serious hypersensitivity reactions include hemolytic anemia, neutropenia, rash, and hepatitis. In contrast to UC, where alternative azo bond delivery systems such as olsalazine and balsalazide are effective alternatives, in Crohn's colitis these agents have not been shown to be effective. There is more evidence, however, that alternative *mesalamine* formulations are comparable to sulfasalazine or antibiotics in Crohn's colitis, but less efficacious than corticosteroids. *Mesalamine* in doses up to 4.8 g/d has a similar side effect profile as placebo in clinical trials. Also, despite general use, there is scant available data regarding the utility of *rectal mesalamine suppositories* (1 to 1.5 g/d) for Crohn's proctitis or *mesalamine enemas* (1 to 4 g/d) for left-sided colitis.

ANTIBIOTICS

Metronidazole (0.75 to 2 g/d) and *ciprofloxacin* (1 g/d), alone or in combination, are also commonly used as an alternative or in addition to aminosalicylates for mild-moderate colonic CD, particularly for patients with accompanying perianal disease or for individuals who have failed to respond to aminosalicylates and are not "sick enough" to warrant corticosteroid therapy. Colonic disease responds better to antibiotics than small bowel disease, and *metronidazole* is effective in treating perianal CD. The Cooperative Crohn's Disease Study in Sweden (CCDSS) showed 800 mg daily of *metronidazole* to be successful in Crohn's colitis that had failed to respond to sulfasalazine. Approximately 55% or patients randomized to *ciprofloxacin*, 1 g/d, or mesalamine, 4 g/d, will respond with clinical remissions. The *combination* of *sulfasalazine* and *corticosteroids* in the European Cooperative Crohn's Disease Study and a combination of *antibiotics* with *budesonide* are more effective that either agents alone for patients with CD of the colon.

CORTICOSTEROIDS

Corticosteroids are effective inductive therapies for patients with moderate-severe Crohn's colitis or for patients with mild-moderate disease that has not responded to aminosalicylates and/or antibiotics. Controlled release *budesonide* formulations are also efficacious for mild-moderate CD involving the right colon, but are not effective for more distal colonic disease. Doses of 40 to 60 mg daily of *prednisone* (or up to 1 mg/kg/d) are initiated until a clinical response has been established. Subsequent tapering is "individualized" according to the rate of response. Generally, the dosage is gradually reduced by 5 mg/week until the drug can be ceased or symptoms flare. In the NCCDS, 78% of patients responded to steroids given in this way. The response to budesonide is somewhat less and neither systemic nor nonsystemic steroids are efficacious at preventing relapse. Indeed, after a course of corticosteroids, approximately 75% of patients will either have a flare of disease activity or become *steroid-dependent* within a year. The use of corticosteroids is further limited by their significant acute and chronic side effect profiles, including short term side effects of emotional lability, insomnia, hypertension, glucose intolerance, and acne; and long term complications that include cataracts, accelerated osteoporosis, avascular necrosis, and growth impairment in children. Glucocorticoid side effects are significantly reduced with *budesonide* formulations, but there is still a risk for systemic side effects, particularly if the 9 mg dosage is used as maintenance therapy. There is substantial empiric use, but no clinical trial data regarding the efficacy of *topical (rectal) steroid applications* for Crohn's colitis.

NUTRITIONAL THERAPIES

Nutritional therapy with elemental or polymeric oral or enteral feeding has been shown to be beneficial to small bowel CD, but the benefits for Crohn's colitis have yet to be established. Their utility has, primarily, been limited to pediatric use where elemental or polymeric diets may be initiated as an alternative to steroids for children and adolescents. Total parenteral nutrition is only indicated for severely malnourished patients or those unable to tolerate enteral feeding.

Moderate-Severe Acute Crohn's Colitis

Moderate-severe Crohn's colitis includes a spectrum of patients that have not responded to treatment for mild-moderate disease or individuals who are acutely ill with fever, dehydration, malnutrition, anemia, diarrhea, abdominal tenderness, or an inflammatory mass. Patients

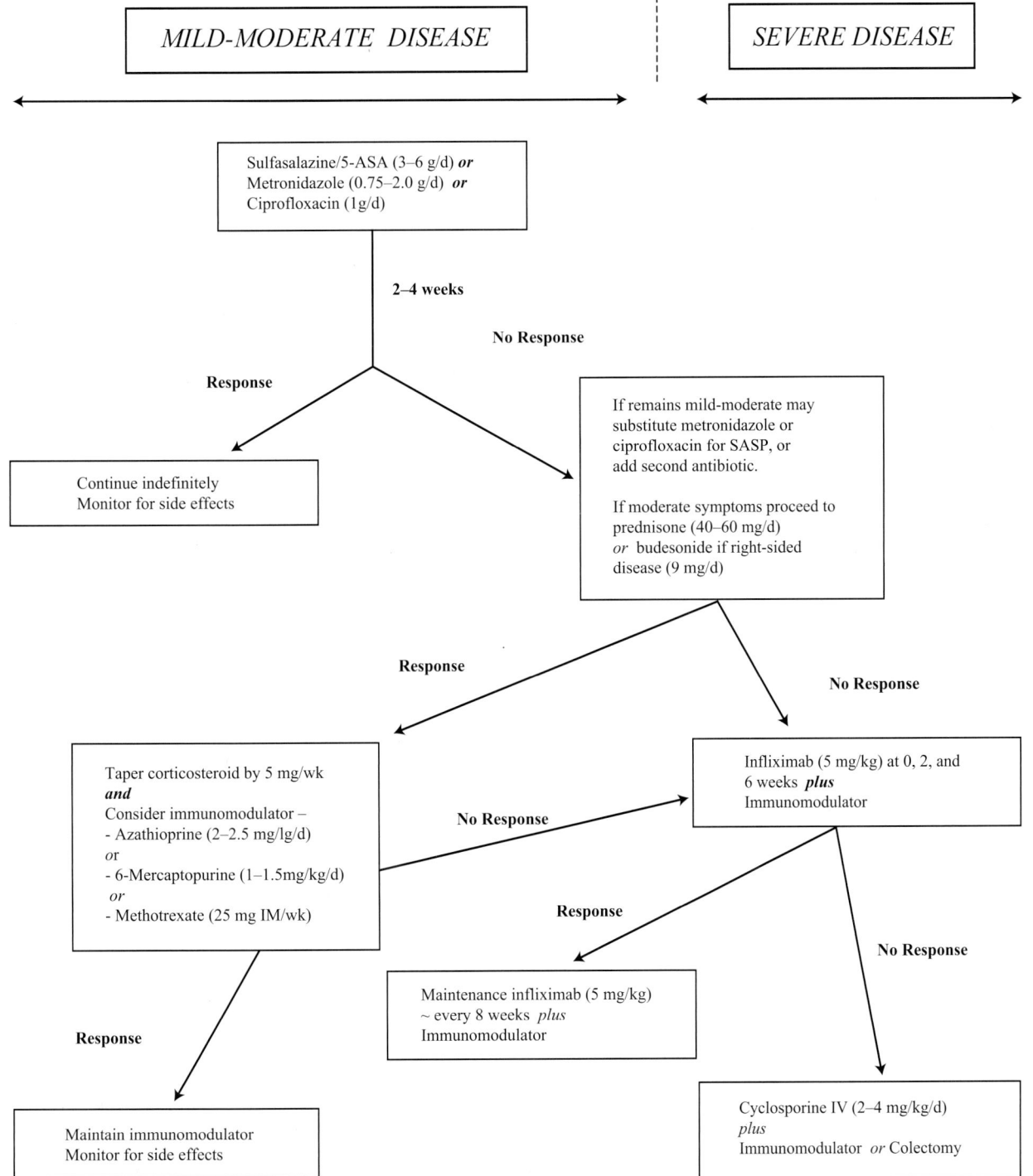

FIGURE 80-1. Treatment algorithm for induction and maintenance medical therapy for Crohn's colitis. ASA = aminosalicylic acid; IV = intravenous; 6-MP = 6-mercaptopurine.

with an incomplete response to corticosteroids are candidates for infliximab therapy, usually given as an outpatient, whereas those presenting with severe-fulminant symptoms or evidence of an abscess or peritoneal signs require hospitalization.

Infliximab

Anti-TNF therapy with the chimeric monoclonal antibody, infliximab, has been embraced as an inductive and maintenance therapy for patients with active luminal CD not responding to the above therapies (steroid-refractory or dependent) or for patients with fistulizing disease. Enthusiasm for its' efficacy must be tempered by knowledge of the potentially serious side effects, limitations in availability due to its high cost, and need for long-term therapy. The clinical response is rapid and usually noted within the first days or weeks after infusion. Up to 80% of patients with active CD will respond and over 50% of patients with fistula have complete cessation of drainage after a series of infusions at 0, 2, and 6 weeks with 5 mg/kg doses.

Infliximab should be administered initially, at a dose of 5 mg/kg with the 3-dose induction regimen to reduce immunogenicity, and the majority of patients who respond will require continued maintenance therapy at an average interval of every 8 weeks. There is growing recognition and acceptance that *concurrent administration* with an *immunomodulator and/or corticosteroids* improves the long term outcome of therapy by reducing antibody-to-infliximab formation. Potential side effects include immunogenicity to infliximab, development of autoantibodies, and the risk of opportunistic infections.*

Up to 3% of patients develop an acute, anaphylactoid, infusion reaction that can usually be managed conservatively by temporarily stopping the infusion, treatment with *diphenhydramine*, and restarting the infusion at a slower rate. The acute infusion reactions have been associated with anti-infliximab antibodies and are also associated with decreased duration of response to infliximab. The acute infusion reactions are in contrast to *delayed hypersensitivity reactions* that occur in up to 19% of patients, many of whom who have had a significant *delay* of many months to years between infusions. This serum sickness-like reaction is thought to be due to the development of high-titer, anti-infliximab antibodies. The incidence of antibodies to infliximab is reduced by concomitant corticosteroids, azathioprine (AZA) or 6-mercaptopurine (6-MP) administration, and continuous rather than episodic administration.

Infliximab and other anti-TNF agents have also been associated with increasing titers of antinuclear and anti-double stranded DNA (dsDNA) antibodies that, rarely, can be associated with a drug-induced lupus syndrome that resolves with discontinuation of anti-TNF therapy. Immunosuppression and opportunistic infection can occur, particularly intracellular infections such as *Mycobacterium tuberculosis*, histoplasmosis, cryptococcidiosis, and listeriosis, related to anti-TNF therapy such that skin testing and chest radiographs are recommended prior to initiating therapy with infliximab or other anti-TNF agents.

Cyclosporine

Cyclosporine, used successfully in severe UC, can also be used in colonic CD. Continous intravenous infusion at doses of 2 to 4 mg/kg/d may avoid colectomy, although oral dosing has not proved effective for either induction or maintenance of remission. Immunosuppression and nephrotoxicity are the primary side effects. Renal function and serum drug levels must be monitored regularly. Other significant side effects are hypertension, seizures (especially in hypocholesterolemic patients) (< 120 mg/dL), and opportunistic infection.

Refractory Disease and Steroid-Dependent Disease

In patients whose disease becomes either steroid-resistant or steroid-dependent, additional immunomodulatory drugs have been shown to be effective in inducing remission, reducing corticosteroid doses, or avoiding surgery. The purine antimetabolites AZA and 6-MP, are the first line choices in this regard, but alternatives exist if patients are unresponsive or intolerant to these drugs.

AZA and 6-MP

The purine antagonists *AZA* (2.0 to 2.5 mg/kg daily) and *6-MP* (1.0 to 1.5 mg/kg daily) have become accepted therapies for steroid-dependent CD and to maintain remission after steroid-withdrawal. Because of the high risk of relapse or steroid-dependence they should be introduced with the first evidence of steroid-dependence (relapsing symptoms during or shortly after steroid-tapering). Cochrane analyses have confirmed their utility for inductive therapy when coadministered with steroids and for maintenance of remission after steroid tapering. Historical concerns regarding potential side effects have been abrogated by the expanding experience with these agents over the past decade. Still, debate continues regarding optimization of dosing according to a mg/kg schedule, monitoring of the white blood cell count or measurement of the thioguanine metabolites. All methods have been successful and none has been evaluated prospectively, as yet, with pre-defined outcomes. These agents are generally well tolerated, although up to 20% of patients discontinue therapy due to some form of intolerance, usually nausea or abdominal pain. Pancreatitis occurs in 3 to 15% of patients after several weeks of therapy, resolves spontaneously on their cessation, but recurs again with reintroduction of either agent. Bone marrow suppression, particularly neutropenia, is dose

---

*Editors Note: Some physicians utilize azathioprine or methotrexate therapy before starting infliximab.

related and requires monitoring with full blood counts weekly for the first month and then subsequently at least four times annually. *Thioguanine* has been used successfully for patients with allergies to AZA or mercaptopurine, or for patients with high functional thiopurine methyltransferase activity; however, the risk of hepatic complications such as veno-occlusive disease or nodular regenerative hyperplasia has limited the utility of this end product of mercaptopurine metabolism. AZA and 6-MP are also beneficial in perianal disease, including fistulas, and should be continued if tolerated as first line maintenance therapy. There is a separate chapter on AZA use in IBD (see Chapter 69, "Monitoring of Azathioprine Metabolite Levels in Inflammatory Bowel Disease").

METHOTREXATE

Parenteral methotrexate (MTX), a dihydrofolate reductase inhibitor, at a dose of 25 mg/week administered either intramuscularly or subcutaneously for 16 weeks has been shown to be superior to placebo and to have steroid-sparing effects in refractory CD. The benefits noted were with regard to disease activity, quality of life, and reduced steroid requirements. Oral administration is less efficacious, and with either route folic acid supplementation is recommended to reduce bone marrow toxicity. Other significant side effects include hepatotoxicity (including hepatic fibrosis) and an allergic pneumonitis. MTX at a dose of 15 mg, administered parenterally, weekly has been shown to be successful in maintaining remissions for patients who initially responded to acute therapy. Dosage can be increased back to 25 mg weekly for symptomatic recurrences.

Maintenance of Remission

The role of the aminosalicylates in maintenance of remission for Crohn's colitis is controversial, although they are frequently used for this means given their relatively good safety profile. They are usually continued at the same dose after inductive therapy for as long as they are effective. None of the aminosalicylates have been found to be effective for patients who have required steroids to induce remission.

The primary drugs with evidence supporting maintenance benefits are *AZA* and *6-MP*. As previously stated, the trend has been to introduce the purine antagonists earlier in the course of disease, usually at initiation of steroids, or after the first relapse during steroid tapering. *MTX* has also been effective for at least 1 year for patients responding to introduction by successfully weaning of steroids.

Most recently, *infliximab* has also been demonstrated to have maintenance benefits for patients responding to initial dosing. The average dose is 5 mg/kg every 8 weeks, although many patients will benefit from shorter intervals between infusions or increased dosing to 10 mg/kg (30% in ACCENT I) to prolong the benefits, which have also included mucosal healing, reduced hospitalisations, and reduced surgeries.

Surgical Management of Crohn's Colitis

Surgery for colonic CD is indicated when medical treatment fails or complications of the disease develop. Rarely, toxic megacolon or fulminant colitis requires a colectomy. The most common indications for surgery include refractory steroid-dependent disease, obstructing strictures, hemorrhage, internal fistulas, or abscesses. Compared to small bowel disease, operations for abscesses and fistulas are less common for colonic disease. Similar to UC, dysplasia and cancer of the colon are related to disease extent, duration and the presence of primary sclerosing cholangitis. Thus, patients with long-standing Crohn's colitis should be entered into a surveillance colonoscopy program even though stricturing disease may preclude complete examination of the colon in all patients. Whether segmental resection is adequate for colonic dysplasia, or whether colectomy is required, remains controversial.

The choice of operation and preoperative patient examination is of paramount importance with Crohn's colitis. All patients require small bowel follow through and colonoscopy prior to surgery, and during colonoscopy the distal limit of disease and condition of the rectum must be noted as rectal involvement may necessitate a permanent stoma. The choice of operation depends on the location and extent of disease, previous resections, rectal compliance, and adequacy of fecal continence.

A few scenarios specific to colonic CD deserve special mention. Pancolitis with rectal sparing occurs in 20% of cases of colonic CD, and in the presence of patent anal sphincters and the absence of perianal disease, subtotal colectomy and ileorectal anastomosis can be performed if over 15 to 20 cm of rectum is available. Patients are thus able to avoid a permanent stoma and yet retain adequate bowel function. Rectal disease recurrence is possible and hence further medical or surgical therapy, including ileostomy, may be required.

Crohn's proctocolitis requiring surgery necessitates a total proctocolectomy and permanent ileostomy. In up to 80% of patients without evidence of small bowel involvement, this procedure provides a long term "cure." Restorative surgery such as the ileal pouch-anal anastomosis (IPAA) is relatively contraindicated in CD due to the risk of ileal disease recurrence in the pouch and the difficulty of treating this without pouch excision. This illustrates the importance of making a correct diagnosis prior to surgery, as IPAA for "indeterminate colitis," although almost as successful as for UC, can bring about pouch problems including perianal disease, chronic pouch dysfunction, or recurrence proximal to the pouch should the diagnosis in fact be CD. Fortunately, infliximab therapy has been effective for many patients who have developed CD in an ileoanal pouch. More detailed discussions of perianal disease management of CD and of dysplasia surveillance are discussed in other chapters (see Chapter 81, "Perianal Complications in Crohn's Disease," Chapter 82, "Perianal Disease in Inflammatory Bowel Disease" and Chapter 83, "Dysplasia Surveillance Programs").

Supplemental Reading

Connell WR, Kamm MA, Dickson M, et al. Long-term neoplasia risk after azathioprine treatment in inflammatory bowel disease. Lancet 1994;343:1249–52.

Connell WR, Kamm MA, Ritchie JK, Lennard-Jones JE. Bone marrow toxicity caused by azathioprine in inflammatory bowel disease: 27 years of experience. Gut 1993;34:1081–5.

Cottone M, Brignola C, Rosselli M, et al. Relationship between site of disease and familial occurrence in Crohn's disease. Dig Dis Sci 1997;42:129–32.

Farmer RG, Hawk WA, Turnbull RB. Clinical patterns in Crohn's disease: a statistical study of 615 cases. Gastroenterol 1975;68: 627–35.

Feagan BG, Fedorak RN, Irvine EJ, et al. A comparison of methotrexate with placebo for the maintenance of remission in Crohn's disease. North American Crohn's Study Group Investigators. N Engl J Med 2000;342:1627–32.

Feagan BG, Rochon J, Fedorak RN, et al. Methotrexate for the treatment of Crohn's disease. The North American Crohn's Study Group Investigators. N Engl J Med 1995;332:292–7.

Hanauer SB, Feagan BG, Lichtenstein GR, et al. Maintenance infliximab for Crohn's disease: the ACCENT I randomised trial. Lancet 2002;359:1541–9.

Hanauer SB, Sandborn W. Management of Crohn's disease in adults. Am J Gastroenterol 2001;96:635–43.

Pearson DC, May GR, Fick G, Sutherland LR. Azathioprine for maintaining remission of Crohn's disease. Cochrane Database Syst Rev 2000:CD000067.

Prantera C, Zannoni F, Scribano ML, et al. An antibiotic regimen for the treatment of active Crohn's disease: a randomized, controlled clinical trial of metronidazole plus ciprofloxacin. Am J Gastroenterol 1996;91:328–32.

Sandborn WJ, Hanauer SB. Infliximab in the treatment of Crohn's disease: a user's guide for clinicians. Am J Gastroenterol 2002;97:2962–72.

Sandborn W, Sutherland L, Pearson D, et al. Azathioprine or 6-mercaptopurine for inducing remission of Crohn's disease. Cochrane Database Syst Rev 2000;2.

Simms L, Steinhart AH. Budesonide for maintenance of remission in Crohn's disease (Cochrane Review). Cochrane Database Syst Rev 2001;1.

Steinhart AH, Ewe K, Griffiths AM, et al. Corticosteroids for maintaining remission of Crohn's disease. Cochrane Database Syst Rev 2001:CD000301.

Ursing B, Alm T, Barany F, et al. A comparative study of metronidazole and sulfasalazine for active Crohn's disease: the cooperative Crohn's disease study in Sweden. II. Result. Gastroenterol 1982;83:550–62.

…

Perianal Complications in Crohn's Disease Patient Management

Daniel H. Present, MD

Since the classic paper published by Crohn and colleagues in 1932 describing the chronic inflammatory process of the bowel there have been multiple articles published on the complications of this illness. The description of perianal fistula was followed 6 years later with the incorrect concept that the inflammatory process extended from the bowel down to the perianal area. There are multiple problems that can affect the perianal area, including simple skin tags, fissures, hemorrhoids, high and low fistulas, strictures, rectovaginal fistulas, and, finally, neoplasia. Severe perianal skin excoriation can result in significant discomfort and impaired quality of life. The main purpose of this article is to review the perianal complications with a focus on management of fistulas.

Incidence and Pathogenesis

There has been great variation in the reported incidence of fistula in patients with Crohn's disease (CD) ranging from a low of 17% up to almost 50% (Allan and Keighley, 1988). There have been several population-based studies reporting that the overall incidence of fistulas was 35% in patients with CD with perianal fistulas occurring in 20% (Schwartz et al, 2002). A cumulative incidence of fistulizing CD appeared in 33% of patients after 10 years and 50% of patients after 20 years (Hellers et al, 1980). Perianal fistulas were much more common in patients with colonic disease (41%) versus those with ileal disease (12%). The highest incidence occurred in those patients with CD involving the colon and rectum. It is interesting to note in this population-based study that recurrent fistulas occurred less frequently in patients who were placed on maintenance therapy with an immunosuppressive agent.

Often confusing to the practicing physician is the development of a perianal fistula in a patient who demonstrates no involvement of their bowel with CD. In 10% of patients the fistula may precede the onset by several years. Another confusing diagnostic problem is the female patient who develops an abscess in the labial area and a diagnosis of a Bartholin cyst is incorrectly made. Gynecologists should be fully aware that patients with CD may develop fistulas in this area.

Regarding pathogenesis, it is now quite clear that fistulas occurring in the perianal area do not arise from the small intestine or the sigmoid colon but rather develop locally, starting either as a deep penetrating ulcer in the anus or rectum or secondary to an anal gland abscess. There are various classification schemes for describing perianal fistulas, with some surgeons classifying them as either low or high, depending upon whether they are above or below the dentate line. What has been accepted recently as more precise is the Parks classification, which uses the external sphincter as the point of reference (Parks et al, 1976). This classification describes five types of fistula, which include the following:

1. superficial (low),
2. intersphincteric (low or high),
3. transphincteric (low or high),
4. suprasphincteric (high),
5. extrasphincteric (high).

Following this classification, fistulas can be more specifically identified as simple or complex. Surgical management will depend on the site and classification of the perianal fistula.

Diagnostic Modalities

The first, and most important, diagnostic modalities are clinical history and physical examination by the practicing gastroenterologist. The development of large anal tags (often referred to as "elephant ears") is associated with CD in the perianal area. Fistulas may hide between these large folds, but the patient should either have had a rectal abscess or have pain and stricturing on physical examination. As noted earlier the diagnosis of a Bartholin abscess that has failed to heal in a patient with CD suggests a perivaginal fistula. The intermittent passing of air through the vagina indicates a rectovaginal fistula. This question should be asked of female patients because it is often not volunteered. Rectovaginal fistulas are usually small and derive from the distal portion of the rectovaginal septum with induration palpable on physical examination. Any patient with a suspected fistula should have a complete bowel evaluation, including colonoscopy and small bowel series.

A more precise diagnosis can be made after a colorectal surgeon has performed an examination under anesthesia (EUA). This procedure has been the gold standard for assessing fistulas, but more recently rectal endoscopic ultrasonography (EUS) and pelvic magnetic resonance imaging (MRI) have been able to more definitively identify a fistula. A small study of 34 patients found that the accuracy of EUS, pelvic MRI, and surgical EUA all exceeded 85% (Schwartz et al, 2001). However, when any 2 of the diagnostic modalities were combined, the accuracy increased to 100%. All of the above modalities are very helpful in planning whether medical therapy or surgical therapy is most appropriate. The diagnosis of simple fistula by physical examination and endoscopy may be adequate when medical therapy is the initial strategy. However, it is often necessary to perform the above studies to decide whether surgical intervention is required (complex fistulas).

There have been several instruments that have been used to quantify disease activity of fistulas and to assess clinical response. These include the perianal disease activity index, as well as a more recent index used in the infliximab study, which looks at drainage and tenderness (Present et al, 1999). Much has been made of the fact that the patient's closed fistula can still be detected on MRI. I think this is important academically but of little importance clinically because the patient cares only about whether he or she is having pain and/or drainage.

Surgical therapy will be covered in another chapter (see Chapter 68 "Surgical Management of Crohn's Disease") and the reader can refer to a recent American Gastroenterological Association technical review of the subject (American Gastroenterological Association, 2003). I would, however, point out that a frequent error in surgical management is the performance of diverting ostomy in the hope that the perianal fistula will heal. In my experience, this will provide only short term relief and the majority of patients will subsequently require a proctectomy. Likewise many anal strictures do not require any therapy. Physicians are often surprised to find that they cannot perform a digital rectal exam and yet the patient is having relatively normal bowel movements. Retrograde passage of a finger or a scope does not always correlate with antegrade progression of stool. The same concept can be applied when colonoscopy is ineffective in entering the terminal ileum. This does not mean obstruction.

Medical Management

General

As noted, an adequate history and physical examination is essential. If the patient has an abscess, it should be adequately drained before proceeding with medications. Not all patients require a colorectal surgeon, that is if the abscess has either drained spontaneously or been drained by incision. On the other hand, if there is persistent rectal pain and/or tenderness, or there are multiple draining sites, then a colorectal surgeon should be consulted to be certain that all pus has been adequately drained. In this situation, an EUA and/or MRI is indicated.

Although there have been multiple trials conducted throughout the world using sulfasalazine or mesalamine in the treatment of CD, there have never been any studies designed to study or reports indicating that these agents are efficacious in the treatment of perianal fistula (Present, 2003). In the vast majority of cases, mesalamine or sulfasalazine will be maintained as part of the management of the active bowel disease, but again there is no reason to institute these agents if the major problem is perianal fistula.

In looking at the control trials using corticosteroids in the treatment of CD, neither the National Cooperative Crohn's Disease Study, nor the European Cooperative Crohn's Disease Study randomized patients for fistula, and there is, therefore, no data available for this subgroup of patients. In these two steroid placebo controlled trials the only deaths occurred in patients who were receiving steroids and who had internal fistula with the subsequent development of an abscess and overwhelming sepsis. Multiple controlled trials have been performed evaluating a newer steroid, budesonide, in the treatment of CD. Efficacy has been demonstrated. However, all patients with a fistula were excluded from these placebo controlled trials. There is, therefore, no control data suggesting that steroids should be instituted in patients who developed perianal complications and fistula. I have experienced multiple patients with longstanding disease going on to develop fistulas and abscesses for the first time after steroids are introduced. I have also seen a significant lack of healing when patients are taking steroids and attempts are made for closure with immunomodulatory agents (Present, 2002). It is my personal opinion that steroids are "contraindicated" when trying to manage perianal fistulas, and if the bowel symptoms allow, I quickly withdraw them from the therapeutic regimen.

Effective Therapeutic Agents

ANTIBIOTICS

The first step in the management of perianal CD is usually the institution of antibiotics. Although there have been several control trials looking at the efficacy of metronidazole in the treatment of active CD, none of them have randomized for fistula response. Because there are no controlled trials showing efficacy we must rely on open-label studies and personal experience. For example, in an uncontrolled study reported by Bernstein and colleagues (1987), 21 patients with fistula were evaluated, with clinical response being observed in 20 of the 21. Complete healing was seen in 10 of 18. High dose metronidazole was used in these studies, which can produce significant side effects in a large percentage of patients. Improvement was seen in about 6 to 8 weeks; however, my personal experience is that response is observed more quickly, usually within 2 to 3 weeks. A follow-up report of 17 of these patients with 9 additional patients showed that relapse frequently occurred but patients often responded to restarting the metronidazole. Unfortunately, only about one-third of patients could successfully stop the metronidazole without experiencing a relapse. As noted, with the high dose administered, neuropathy may be encountered which may persist for years. Nausea, vomiting, and fatigue are also common side effects with metronidazole.

Although ciprofloxacin is now widely used for the treatment of CD fistulas, there are only anecdotal reports of response and closure. In these small studies, approximately 70% of patients responded to 1 to 1.5 g of cipro when used for up to 1 year (Turunen et al, 1989). As with metronidazole, exacerbations were seen after the ciprofloxacin was withdrawn. The combination of ciprofloxacin and metronidazole was reported in an uncontrolled study to show approximately 85% response rate, with healing seen in slightly over 20% of the patients (Solomon, 1993).

In summary, although lacking controlled data, current clinical experience, including my own, indicates that antibiotics are effective in the treatment of perianal CD and can be used for long periods of time. The dose of metronidazole should be maintained at < 1 g daily to prevent neuropathy. For patients who do not respond to either ciprofloxacin or metronidazole, the combination is indicated. Antibiotics are not likely to close a fistula but can be used to control this complication while awaiting more potent immunomodulatory therapy.

6-Mercaptopurine/Azathioprine

The first control trial designed to evaluate for fistula response in patients with CD was a randomized double blind placebo controlled trial studying 6-mercaptopurine (6-MP) versus placebo (Present et al, 1980). This was a 2-year study in which patients were crossed over after 1 year. In addition to demonstrating clinical response and steroid sparing, 9 of 29 patients (31%) who received 6-MP closed their fistula. Only 1 of the 17 (6%) placebo patients showed closure. Additional healing was observed in 34% with 6-MP as compared with 18% with placebo. Although showing a strong trend to healing, the numbers of the study were not large enough to show statistical significance. Subsequent data looking at this problem in an uncontrolled manner showed complete closure in 39% of patients with a response in another 26% (Korelitz and Present, 1985). Of major importance was the slow response to this medication, which took 2 to 4 months to be effective. Of the 13 patients in this open-label study whose fistula closed completely, the fistula continued to be closed in 6 of the 13. This is contrasted with seven patients who stopped the drug and only two whose fistula remained closed and five whose fistula reopened. A subsequent meta-analysis showed that 54% (22 of 41) patients treated with 6-MP responded compared with only 6 of 29 (21%) treated with placebo (Pearson et al, 1995). The pooled odds ratio favoring fistula healing was 4.44. In the gastrointestinal (GI) community the dosing and administration of 6-MP or azathioprine (AZA) has significant variation. Control trials used AZA in doses of 2 to 3 mg/kg daily, whereas 6-MP was used at a dose of 1.5 mg daily. My experience has suggested that < 1.5 mg/kg of 6-MP is required for a therapeutic response, and the mean dose that is needed is 75 mg daily. There is some synergistic effect when using 5-aminosalicylates with 6-MP, and this should be taken into account in looking at the dose of the immunosuppressive.

There is no question but that 6-MP/AZA is an effective agent both in closing and maintaining closure of fistulas. These agents are quite safe long term with no definite evidence of the development of neoplasia or superinfections. Toxicity is mainly limited to allergic reactions, including rash, fever, pancreatitis, and to those patients who are thiopurine methyl transferase deficient. In this group lower doses must be used to prevent the development of leukopenia.

In summary, 6-MP/AZA should be instituted if fistulas do not close spontaneously or do not close with antibiotics. The presence of multiple fistulas is also an urgent indication for the institution of 6-MP/AZA. It is difficult to predict which patients are going to go on to a chronic course and my clinical experience suggests that 6-MP/AZA can alter the natural history of these fistulas. I have seen maintenance of closure for 20 plus years in many patients who continue to take these agents.

Methotrexate

Although there have been several controlled and uncontrolled studies evaluating the efficacy of methotrexate (MTX) in the management of CD, none of them were designed to look at the response of fistula. In a small recently published study of 37 courses of MTX in CD patients, 4 of 16 (25%) had complete closure of fistula, whereas 5 of the 16 (31%) had partial response (Mahadevan et al, 2003). The overall rate of fistula response was, therefore, 56%. Several of these patients had not responded to prior treatment with cyclosporin and/or 6-MP. With the limited available data it would appear that 6-MP/AZA would be the first choice in the management of perianal fistulas. However, if patients are allergic or fail to respond then MTX in a dose of 25 mg administered intramuscularly on a weekly basis should be instituted. The toxicity of MTX is well known, including GI upset, interstitial pneumonitis, and possible hepatic fibrosis. This medication is also contraindicated in those patients attempting to conceive.

Cyclosporin

There are currently no control trials demonstrating that cyclosporin is an effective therapy for CD perianal fistula. Multiple uncontrolled studies showed an overall clinical response rate of around 80%. When cyclosporin has been administered in low doses (≤ 5 mg/kg daily), it is ineffective. However, administration of the drug intravenously in a dose of 4 mg/kg has shown efficacy both in clinical response and in the management of fistula. This intravenous (IV) dose is comparable to an oral dose of 8 mg/kg. In a personal series of 16 patients, 14 (88%) responded to this regimen (Present and Lichtiger, 1994). Complete closure of fistula was observed in 44% and moderate improvement in about 44%. The mean time to respond was slightly over 7 days. A recent study looking at IV cyclosporin in ulcerative colitis showed that a dose of 2 mg/kg was equally effective to 4 mg/kg, but this has not been studied in CD patients. We have usually tried to obtain monoclonal levels of cyclosporin between 300 to 500 ng/mL during the 7 to 10 day hospitalization with a trough level of approximately 300 ng/mL after discharge. We have seen relapse in 36% after discharge, but 64% maintain their response and allowed us to discontinue steroids, which may facilitate healing of fistulas. In order to avoid cyclosporin toxicity, experience is essential in dosing regimens. Access to a laboratory that can give same day results is quite important, and we usually recommend referral to a tertiary center if experience is lacking in the gastroenterologist's clinical practice. The main adverse effects of cyclosporin are abnormal renal function, hypertension, headache, and gingival hyperplasia. When used in combination with steroids *Pneumocystis carinii* pneumonia has been observed and prophylaxis should be instituted with Septra. After the steroid dose is lowered or discontinued, the Septra can also be stopped. We advise an EUA prior to instituting cyclosporin therapy to ensure all abscesses have been drained.

Tacrolimus (FK506)

Several uncontrolled case series have been published suggesting that tacrolimus may be beneficial in the treatment of perianal fistulas. A small placebo controlled trial evaluated 43 patients with perianal fistula and compared tacrolimas with placebo (Sandborn et al, 2003). The dose of the oral tacrolimus was 0.20 mg/kg/d. Closure of at least 50% of fistulas at 2 visits 4 weeks apart occurred in 8% of placebo patients compared with 43% of patients treated with tacrolimus. On the other hand, closure of all fistulas occurred in only 10% of tacrolimus-treated patients compared with 8% with placebo. Adverse events occurred, the most important being an increased serum creatinine level. This was the major toxicity but others were observed, including paresthesias, tremors, and leg cramps. Nephrotoxicity was observed in 38% of patients compared with 0% with placebo. At the current time tacrolimus cannot be recommended for the management of perianal fistulas.

Infliximab

Infliximab, a chimeric monoclonal antibody, has shown efficacy not only in the treatment of active CD but also in the management of perianal fistula. An initial randomized double-blind placebo controlled trial was carried out on 94 patients who received infusions at weeks 0, 2, and 6 (Present et al, 1999). The primary endpoint was the reduction in the number of draining fistulas of ≥ 50% on 2 visits 4 weeks apart. Fistulas were considered to be closed if drainage had stopped and could not be observed with gentle finger compression. At a 5 mg/kg dose the primary endpoint was achieved in 62% of patients, with complete closure of fistula in 46% of patients compared with 13% receiving placebo. The 5 mg/kg dose was the most effective and closed 55% of all fistula. The vast majority of fistulas closed after the second infusion. The main complication was the occasional development of a perianal abscess, which may have been related to the very rapid closure of the cutaneous end of the fistula tract before the rest of the fistula had healed. It is my habit to use concurrent antibiotics when trying to close perianal fistula with infliximab, as well as trying to discontinue steroids.

There has been an abstract report of a second control trial studying 306 patients who were initially treated with 3 doses of 5 mg/kg at 0, 2, and 6 weeks (Sands et al, 2002). Patients who responded were then randomized into maintenance infliximab every 8 weeks compared with placebo. The primary endpoint was the "time to loss of response" through week 54. The median time to lose response in infliximab patients was > 40 weeks, whereas with placebo it was 14 weeks. At week 54, 39% of patients who were receiving maintenance had complete closure of all draining fistula compared with only 19% of those receiving placebo. Despite this response rate, some patients treated with infliximab for fistulas may still ultimately require surgical intervention.

Our personal experience is to have a patient undergo an EUA prior to instituting infliximab to ensure that all abscesses are being drained. The placement of setons may help in maintaining drainage while waiting for the infliximab to be effective (Dawnelle et al, 2003). The development of human antichimeric antibodies in high percentages of patients receiving infliximab indicates that a concurrent immunomodulatory agent (such as 6-MP) be given so that the degree and duration of response may be enhanced. Infliximab has shown to increase the overall rate of infections, and serious complications, such as tuberculosis, histoplasmosis, coccidiomycosis, and others, have been observed following administration of this agent.

Miscellaneous Medical Therapies

Through the years there have been several reviews evaluating the benefit of various therapies in CD patients with fistulization (Lichtenstein, 2000; Schwartz et al, 2001). A commonly used agent is total parenteral nutrition with bowel rest. In my experience this is never effective if there is active CD in the bowel, whereas it may be effective in postoperative fistula management. Other agents used have been elemental diet, thalidomide, and hyperbaric oxygenation. Control trials are required before any of these agents are considered effective therapy and we should use those agents that have shown efficacy.

Summary

In the management of perianal CD, when a fistula develops appropriate diagnosis should be made by history, physical, colonoscopy, and small bowel series. If the fistula is simple, it should be drained and treated with antibiotics. If there is healing, it is my opinion that one or two antibiotics should be maintained for at least 6 to 12 months. I would use low doses of metronidazole 250 mg 3 times daily or ciprofloxacin 250 to 500 mg twice daily. If there is recurrence of the fistula and it drains freely, I would then add 6-MP/AZA to the regimen. If pain persists or the fistula occurs in a new site, I prefer to obtain an examination by a colorectal surgeon with an EUA. If the surgeon is not certain of the status, then an MRI should be added to the regimen. Setons should be placed to allow time for the 6-MP/AZA to promote healing. If the fistula heals with 6-MP/AZA, I would maintain this agent for 5 years or longer. If healing is not induced or maintained with 6-MP/AZA, a 3-course infusion of infliximab is indicated. I do not continue infliximab every 8 weeks, but rather maximize all therapy by giving adequate doses of antibiotics and 6-MP, then treat only after recurrence. It is my experience that not all patients will relapse and require infliximab every 8 weeks. If infliximab fails, a 7- to 10-day course of IV cyclosporin in a dose of 4 mg/kg is indicated.

Failure to respond to all of the above medical therapies would dictate proctectomy and a total colectomy if the CD is active in the remaining colon.

Supplemental Reading

Allan A, Keighley RB. Management of perianal disease. World J Surg 1988;12:198–202.
American Gastroenterological Association Medical Position Statement: Perianal Crohn's disease. Gastroenterology 2003;125:1503–7.
Bernstein LH, Frank MS, Brandt LJ, et al. Healing of perineal Crohn's disease with metronidazole. Gastroenterology 1987;79:357–65.
Dawnelle R, Tapstad MD, Panaccione R, et al. Combined Seton placement, Infliximab infusion and maintenance of immunosuppressives improve healing rate in fistulizing anorectal Crohn's disease. Dis Colon Rectum 2003;46:577–83.
Hellers G, Bergstrand O, Ewerth S, et al. Occurrence in outcome after primary treatment of anal fistulae in Crohn's disease. Gut 1980;21:525–7.
Korelitz BI, Present DH. The favorable effects of 6-mercaptopurine on the fistulae of Crohn's disease. Dig Dis Sci 1985;30:58–64.
Lichtenstein GR. Treatment of fistulizing Crohn's disease. Gastroenterology 2000;119:1132–47.

TABLE 81-1. Perianal Fistulas—Crohn's Disease

Effective for closure
  6-MP/Azathioprine
  Methotrexate
  Cyclosporin
  Infliximab
Effective for clinical response
  Ciprofloxacin
  Metronidazole
Not effective
  Mesalamine
  Steroids

6-MP = 6-mercaptopurine.

Mahadevan V, Marion JF, Present DH. Fistula response to methotrexate in Crohn's disease: a case series. Aliment Pharmacol Ther 2003;18:1003–8.
Parks AG, Gordon PH, Hardcastle JD. A classification of fistula-in-ano. Br J Surg 1976;63:1–12.
Pearson DC, May GR, Fick GH, et al. Azathioprine and 6-mercaptopurine in Crohn's disease—a meta-analysis. Ann Intern Med 1995;123:132–42.
Present DH. Crohn's fistula: current concepts in management. Gastroenterology 2003;124:1629–35.
Present DH. Urinary tract fistulas in Crohn's disease: surgery versus medical therapy. Am J Gastroenterol 2002;97:2165–7.
Present DH, Korelitz BI, Wisch N, et al. Treatment of Crohn's disease with 6-mercaptopurine. A long term randomized double-blind study. N Engl J Med 1980;302:981–7.
Present DH, Lichtiger S. Efficacy of cyclosporine in the treatment of fistula of Crohn's disease. Dig Dis Sci 1994;39:374–80.
Present DH, Rutgeerts P, Targan S, et al. Infliximab for the treatment of fistulas in patients with Crohn's disease. N Engl J Med 1999;340:1398–405.
Sandborn WJ, Present DH, Isaacs KL, et al. Tacrolimus for the treatment of fistulas in patients with Crohn's disease. A randomized placebo controlled trial. Gastroenterology 2003;125:380–8.
Sands B, Vandeventer S, Bernstein C, et al. Long term treatment of fistulizing Crohn's disease: response to infliximab in the Accent II trial through 54 weeks. Gastroenterology 2002;122:A81.
Schwartz DA, Loftus Jr EV, Tremaine WJ, et al. The natural history of fistulizing Crohn's disease in Olmstead County, Minnesota. Gastroenterology 2002;122:875–80.
Schwartz DA, Permberton JH, Sandborn WJ. Diagnosis and treatment of perianal fistulas in Crohn's disease. Ann Intern Med 2001;135:906–18.
Schwartz DA, Wiersema MJ, Dudiak KM, et al. A comparison of endoscopic ultrasound, magnetic resonance imaging, and exam under anesthesia for evaluation of Crohn's perianal fistulas. Gastroenterology 2001;121:1064–72.
Solomon MJ. Combination of ciprofloxacin and metronidazole in severe perianal Crohn's disease. Can J Gastroenterol 1993;7:571–3.
Turunen V, Farkkila M, Seppala K. Long term treatment of perianal or fistulous Crohn's disease with ciprofloxacin. Scand J Gastroenterol Suppl 1989;24:11.

Perianal Disease in Inflammatory Bowel Disease

David W. Larson, MD, and John H. Pemberton, MD

The proper surgical management of perianal Crohn's disease (CD) is controversial. Ever since fistulas were first recognized as a manifestation of CD by Penner and Crohn, the specter of incontinence from aggressive perianal surgery has haunted its operative management. Given the often extensive presentation of CD, the decision of when to operate must be a collaborative effort among the patient, gastroenterologist, and surgeon.

CD typically presents in the following three ways: (1) ulceration, (2) fistula, and (3) stricture. There are reviews by Frizelle and colleagues (1996) and by Hughes (1978). The criteria for such a diagnosis include typical perianal lesions with histologic evidence of granulomata. Michelassi and colleagues (2000) observed that 23% of patients with CD manifested perineal fistulas, 18% stenosis, 16% abscess, 9% rectovaginal fistula, 5% incontinence, and 29% from a combination of problems. The cumulative incidence of perianal fistulas in CD has been estimated by two population-based studies. Hellers and colleagues (1980) reported a cumulative incidence of perianal fistulas of 23%. In a Mayo series, Schwartz and colleagues (2002), showed that the cumulative incidence of fistulizing CD in Olmsted County, Minnesota, between 1970 and 1993, was 38%. The lifetime risk for developing a fistula is 20 to 40%.

The presence of perianal disease may also be affected by the location of proximal disease. Patients with disease confined to the colon have a higher incidence of perianal fistulas, with a rate approaching 100% in those with rectal involvement. Although rare, up to 5% of patients with perianal CD will have no evidence of proximal disease. Once treated the risk of recurrence remains high. It is estimated that the rate of recurrence of CD is 70% by 20 years (Agrez et al, 1982).

Substantial morbidity, including scarring, continual seepage, and fecal incontinence, complicate perianal CD. Therapy is not standardized and debate continues on the role of operative intervention. The aim of this review is to discuss the perianal complications of inflammatory bowel disease (IBD) and provide appropriate surgical solutions.

Anatomy

The anal canal consists of two separate and distinct muscles (Figure 82-1). The internal anal sphincter is a continuation of the circular smooth muscle of the rectum. The outer external sphincter is a continuation of the puborectalis muscle. Overlying the internal sphincter is the mucosa and the submucosa of the anal canal. The dentate or pectinate line separates the transitional and columnar epithelium of the

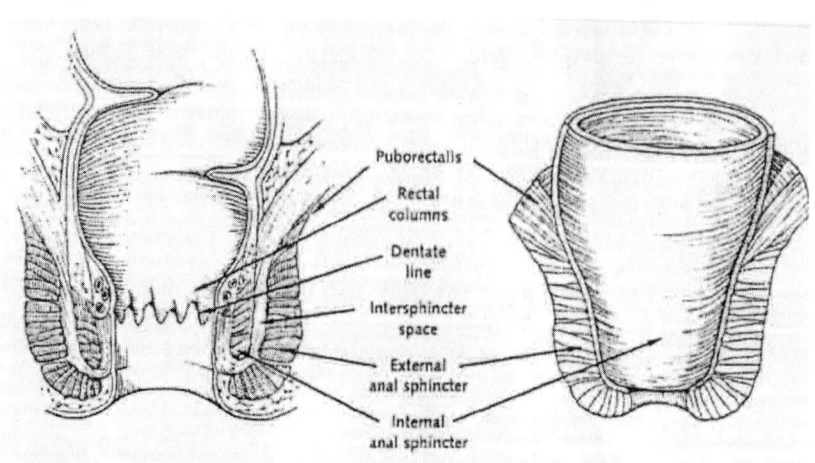

FIGURE 82-1. Anal anatomy. Anatomic relationships in the perianal region.

rectum. It is at this level that the anal crypts and glands may become infected, leading to perianal fistulas.

The appearance of active CD is classic. In active perianal disease, the lesions are swollen and take on a translucent pink or bluish hue. As inflammation resolves, the tissues become opaque and the ulcers heal with a fragile layer of epithelium. Chronically, the tissues become thickened, fibrotic, and scarred. When CD is in an active state, wound healing is significantly prolonged, but may be relatively normal when the disease is quiescent.

Classification

Hughes developed the first pathologic classification of fistula in ano based on morphology. This classification was based on structural abnormalities such as (1) ulceration, (2) fistula/abscess, and (3) stricture. More recently, several classification systems have been proposed. The most well known is, of course, Parks classic description of 1976. Park and colleagues developed the most anatomic and clinically relevant classification. Their use of the anatomy of the sphincter muscles as a reference point has made it the most surgically useful description to date (Figure 82-2). It is important to remember that fistulas associated with CD rarely follow classically described pathways; indeed, it is the rare CD fistula that has a primary opening at the dentate line. Most fistulas associated with CD have a primary opening in the rectum proper and a secondary opening quite far removed (> 4 cm) from the anal verge.

MEASUREMENT OF FISTULA DISEASE ACTIVITY

The Perianal Disease Activity Index (Irvine, 1995) provides the most comprehensive measure of the morbidity caused by perianal CD. This index evaluates fistula disease in the following five categories:
1. Discharge
2. Pain
3. Restriction of sexual activity
4. Type of perianal disease
5. Degree of induration (Table 82-1).

Diagnostic Methods

Adequate evaluation of perianal disease in the setting of IBD usually requires an examination under anesthesia (EUA). As is typical with perianal disease, an examination

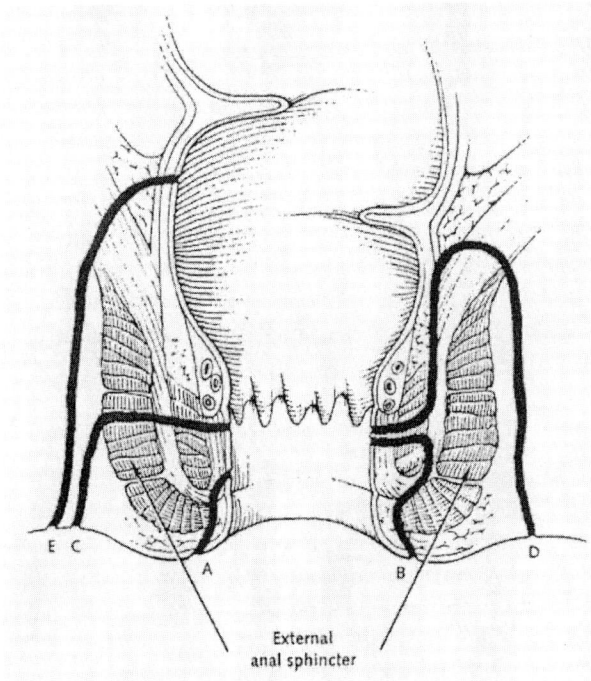

FIGURE 82-2. Classification of Parks and colleagues. A, A superficial fistula tracks below both the internal anal sphincter and external anal sphincter complexes. B, An intersphincteric fistula tracks between the internal anal sphincter and the external anal sphincter in the intersphincteric space. C, A transsphincteric fistula tracks from the intersphincteric space through the external anal sphincter. D, A suprasphincteric fistula leaves the intersphincteric space over the top of the puborectalis and penetrates the levator muscle before tracking down to the skin. E, An extrasphincteric fistula tracks outside of the external anal sphincter and penetrates the levator muscle into the rectum.

TABLE 82-1. Perianal Crohn Disease Activity Index

Categories Affected by Fistulas	Score
Discharge	
None	0
Minimal mucous discharge	1
Moderate mucous or purulent discharge	2
Substantial discharge	3
Gross fecal soiling	4
Pain and restriction of activities	
No activity restriction	0
Mild discomfort, no restriction	1
Moderate discomfort, some limitation of activities	2
Marked discomfort, marked limitation of activities	3
Severe pain, severe limitation of activities	4
Restriction of sexual activity	
No restriction	0
Slight restriction	1
Moderate limitation	2
Marked limitation	3
Unable to engage in sexual activity	4
Type of perianal disease	
None or skin tags	0
Anal fissure or mucosal tear	1
< 3 perianal fistulas	2
≥ 3 perianal fistulas	3
Anal sphincter ulceration or fistulas with substantial undermining skin	4
Degree of induration	
None	0
Minimal	1
Moderate	2
Substantial	3
Gross fluctuance or abscess	4

in the office setting is not only painful, but yields little. EUA facilitates the examining of the anal canal and distal rectum digitally; proctoscopical examination remains the current gold standard for assessment of perianal disease. EUA not only lends itself to the diagnosis of perianal pathology, but also provides an opportunity to treat any pathology encountered.

Other nonsurgical methods of assessing perianal disease include fistulography, computed tomography (CT), magnetic resonance imaging (MRI), and endoscopic ultrasound (EUS). Fistulography has an accuracy ranging from 16 to 50%. Like fistulography, CT is an imprecise test, providing accurate diagnoses in only 24 to 60% of patients (Yousem et al, 1988). However, MRI and EUS accurately delineate fistulas in 76 to 100% of patients (Schratter-Sehn et al, 1993; Haggett et al, 1995; Orsoni et al, 1999).

The Mayo series reported by Schwartz and colleagues (2001) is the most helpful study regarding accurate diagnostics. In this series, the accuracy of EUA, MRI and EUS were all equal ranging from 87 to 91%. The differences between modalities were found to be insignificant. The interesting finding was that using any 2 of these 3 modalities increased the accuracy to 100%. MRI or EUS combined with EUA provides the highest diagnostic accuracy for perianal fistulous disease with the added benefit of enabling concomitant surgery if needed. As stated above, CT scan was only accurate in about half the patients with perianal abscesses.

Surgical Treatment

Because CD cannot be cured by surgery, the guiding surgical principle is to do as little as possible while relieving symptoms as completely as possible. Risks of iatrogenic injury combined with disappointing surgical results prompt a conservative approach in nearly all patients. We agree completely with Alexander-Williams' observation that "fecal incontinence is the result of aggressive surgeons and not progressive disease."

Although some perianal lesions heal spontaneously without specific treatment, surgery has an important role. Anorectal surgery in IBD is primarily a management tool for complications. The goal of operative intervention is preservation of sphincter function along with elimination of perianal symptoms.

Which patient deserves operative intervention? First, perianal pathology must be *symptomatic*. Many CD patients will have what has been coined as a "dry fistula." These asymptomatic patients have no current complaints, and therefore, no treatment is warranted or prudent. Second, all *perianal sepsis* must be *drained* or *controlled*. Third, *rectal disease must be absent* or in a state of *quiescence*. Fourth, the diagnosis must be *secured*. As previously discussed, the use of MRI or EUS and EUA increases the accuracy of our diagnostic skills. Once the diagnosis has been made, the proper surgical intervention can be undertaken. There is also a separate chapter on anorectal disease with and without IBD (see Chapter 91, "Anorectal Diseases").

Hemorrhoids

Is it prudent to perform a hemorrhoidectomy in a CD patient? In the past, complications such as fistula, stricture, abscesses, and need for proctectomy (Jeffery et al, 1977) precluded hemorrhoidectomy in patients with CD. In contrast, Wolkomir reported successful outcomes in healing in 15 of 17 patients undergoing hemorrhoidectomy. Nonetheless, hemorrhoids generally are not removed in patients with CD, because of potential imperfect wound healing and stricture formation. There is a separate chapter on hemorrhoids (see Chapter 92, "Hemorrhoids").

Fissures

Fissures in CD typically appear in positions *other* than anterior and posterior. But, like non-IBD fissures, most heal spontaneously and require no surgical therapy (Allan and Keighley, 1988). Some fissures in perianal CD are asymptomatic whereas others cause significant discomfort. In general, fissures in CD are managed conservatively. For those who fail conservative management, surgical intervention is indicated. Wolkomir and Luchtefeld (1993) treated 25 patients with symptomatic fissures surgically and complete healing occurred in 22. Fleshner and colleagues (1995) compared medical with internal sphincterotomy for fissures in CD patients. They found healing in only 49% of those treated medically, but 88% of fissures healed in those undergoing surgery.

Anal Stenosis

Anorectal strictures are commonly found on digital rectal examination in patients with perianal CD. Most patients with mild stenosis are asymptomatic. When the degree of stenosis becomes severe enough to cause difficulty with evacuation, most patients respond to simple finger dilatation. In 1986, Bernard and colleagues reported on seven patients with anal stenosis. Patients eventually responded to anal dilation. The historical four-finger dilatation should, of course, be avoided in patients because risk of incontinence is prohibitive.

Although short, mild strictures respond to gentle dilatation, long strictures in general do not. Patients with these more problematic strictures have a very high likelihood of coming to proctectomy. Keighley and Allen in 1986 and Linares and colleagues in 1988 documented that up to 86% of their patients with severe stenosis had to be diverted.

Perianal Abscess

When a patient with IBD presents with perianal pain, perianal sepsis is the most common cause. In turn, the two most common causes of perianal abscess are *cryptoglandular infection* or an *obstructed fistula tract*. The treatment of perianal abscess includes prompt and adequate surgical drainage. The location of the abscess will determine the surgical approach. For superficial abscesses, simple incision and drainage is effective in the majority of cases. Abscesses which are deep to the sphincter mechanism (supralevator or ischiorectal) should be drained using a mushroom catheter (Figure 82-3) and/or a noncutting Seton to provide adequate and continued drainage with as little tissue disruption as possible (Makowiec et al, 1997).

Fistulas

Low Fistulas

The surgical treatment of perianal fistulas in CD is based on the fistula type (low or high) and, more importantly, the presence of active proctitis. For those with low fistula in ano, fistulotomy still has a role. The data to date support the conclusion that, for low fistulas with no active disease, surgery for CD patients is as effective as in non-IBD patients (Figure 82-4). Interestingly, a University of Minnesota series of 41 fistulas in 33 patients without active proctocolitis showed a 93% healing rate at 6 months with standard fistulotomy (Williams et al, 1981). As expected, Nordgren and colleagues (1992) found a healing rate of only 27% in those treated with fistulotomy who had active proctocolitis and 83% in those without active disease. More recently, Scott and Northover (1996) documented in patients with CD that in simple fistula, low fistulas without active disease, fistulotomy is acceptable treatment. For those with active disease, the fistula should be treated with a noncutting Seton (Radcliffe et al, 1988) and concomitant medical therapy.

High or Complex Fistula

Those fistulas which involve a significant portion of the anal sphincter, such as high transsphincteric, suprasphincteric, or extrasphincteric, including rectovaginal and anal vaginal fistula, as well as those with primary openings in the rectum, require a more thoughtful approach. The type of surgical treatment is again dependent on the type of fistula and the presence and severity of rectal disease. Patients with complex fistulas often required proctectomy because of the failure of both medical and surgical therapy. More recently, techniques such as Seton placement, fibrin glue, advancement flaps, and, of course, anti-tumour necrosis factor-α infusion therapies, have all been used successfully.

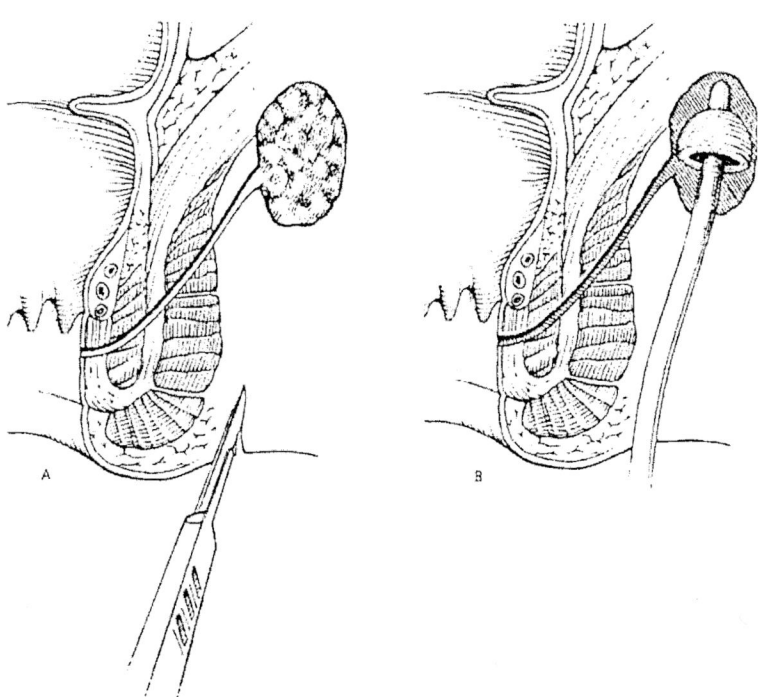

FIGURE 82-3. Surgical approach to perianal abscess drainage. *A*, Simple incision and drainage procedure for an abscess. *B*, Incision and drainage followed by placement of a mushroom drainage catheter for an abscess.

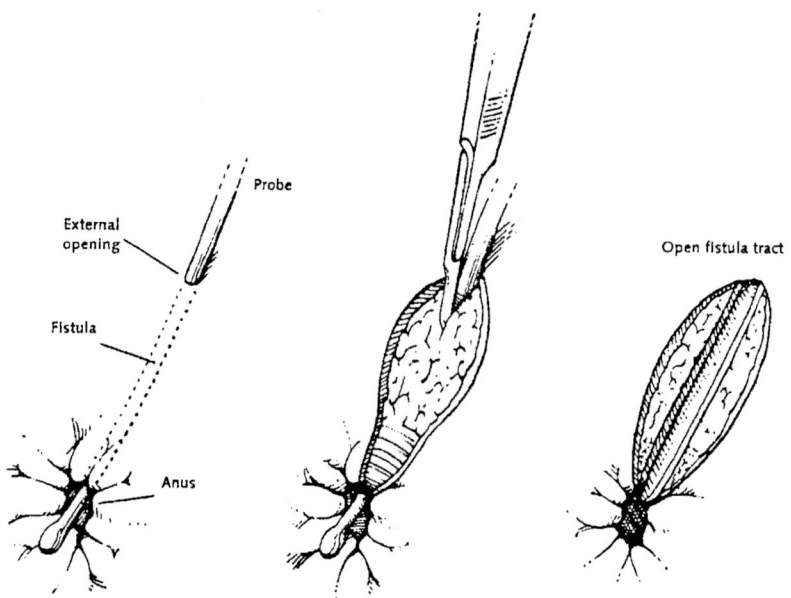

FIGURE 82-4. Fistulotomy. In the absence of active proctocolitis, simple low transsphincteric, intersphincteric, and superficial fistulas can be treated with a fistulotomy.

Setons

The use of a *noncutting Seton* is the most common and effective treatment modality in use for CD patients with complex fistula in ano (Scott and Northover, 1996; Takesue et al, 2002; Koganei et al, 1995). A Seton is a nonabsorbable suture (or vessel loop) that is placed through the fistula tract (Figure 82-5). Passing it through the cutaneous opening of the fistula and out of the associated anal canal opening allows the two ends to be tied loosely together. Although sometimes these draining setons are uncomfortable for the patient, the risk of recurrent abscess is minimized while aggressive medical therapy is being instituted.

In a case series of 27 patients with fistulizing CD, Scott and Northover reported that 85% of patients treated with noncutting Setons experienced fistula closure. Others (White et al, 1990; Pearl et al, 1993) have looked at long-term Seton placement and have reported excellent initial results. However, rates of fistula recurrence may be as high as 39% after Seton removal, highlighting the need for concomitant medical therapy with antibiotics, azathioprine, or 6-mercaptopurine and infliximab (Schwartz et al, 2001; Pearl et al, 1993). More recently the approach of combining medicine and surgery has offered greater success. Our own experience with infiximab and surgery has lead to the resolution of perianal fistulas in 68% of patients (Ricart et al, 2001). We also found that the adding Seton placement to infiximab therapy decreased the rate of recurrent abscesses. Others have found similar results; Topstad and colleagues (2003) found 67% of the 29 patients studied had a complete response to combination therapy and 19% had a partial response. In a comparative study by Regueiro and Mardini (2003), perianal fistulas were treated with infliximab alone versus combination therapy with Seton placement. The findings showed that initial response was improved with Seton placement (100% versus 82.6%), lower recurrence rates (44% versus 79%), and longer time to recurrence (13.5 months versus 3.6 months). The preceding chapter (see Chapter 81, "Perianal Complications in Crohn's Disease Patient Management") is on medical aspects of perianal disease treatment.

In our practice, after Seton placement, medical therapy is instituted to decrease the inflammatory process. Once the inflammation subsides, the Seton is down sized as the fistula fibroses and narrows in caliber, or it is removed.

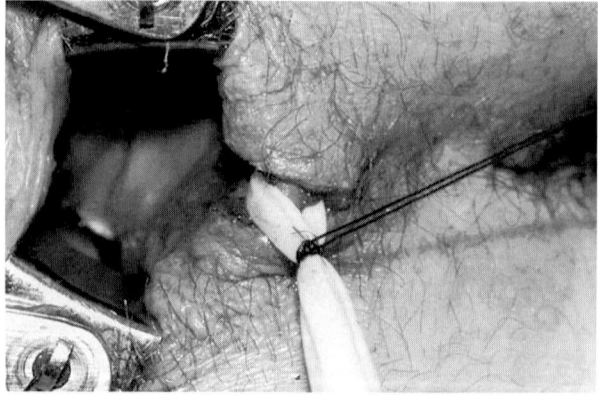

FIGURE 82-5. A transsphincteric perianal fistula with a draining Seton placed through the fistula tract.

Fibrin Glue

A recent addition to our armamentaria is fibrin glue. Our technique is to place a noncutting Seton into the tract leaving it in place for 6 to 8 weeks. The Setons are removed and fibrin glue injected into the fistula tract. The internal opening is suture closed whereas the cutaneous one is left open.

Lindsey and colleagues (2002) performed a randomized trial of fibrin glue versus conventional fistula treatment in patients with and without CD. One hundred percent of simple fistulas healed with standard treatment and only 33% healed with fibrin glue injection. Of the complex fistulas, the cumulative healing rate after 1 to 2 treatments with fibrin glue was 69%. Sentovich (2003) reported on 48 patients with fistulas, among whom 10% were CD patients. The closure rate was 85%. Interestingly, the failure rate in their CD patients was only 20%. Over all, the healing rates of fistulas vary between 40% for CD patients and 80% for cryptoglandular fistulas. Fibrin glue along with Seton placement may have a role to play in the treatment of complex perianal fistula with long tracts in patients with CD.

Rectovaginal Fistula

About 2% of women with CD will develop a rectovaginal fistula (RVF). Surgical as well as medical treatment may be unnecessary as many of these fistulas are very low and have no associated symptoms. Surgical treatment is reserved for those patients with an unacceptable quality of life in whom medical treatment has failed. Unfortunately, the development of a RVF is a poor prognostic sign and may require proximal diversion to decrease local sepsis and/or eventual proctectomy. In patients undergoing RVF repair, the disease should be quiescent and the rectum distensible. In general, for low RVF (< 15% of the sphincter involved) and normal sphincter function, simple fistulotomy is a viable option. However, some surgeons advocate use of an endorectal advancement flap as an alternative to fistulotomy or noncutting Setons in patients with a simple fistula who do not have active rectal inflammation (Joo et al, 1998; Makowiec et al, 1995). An advancement flap involves creating a flap of tissue around the internal opening of a fistula (Hobbiss and Schofield, 1982) (Figure 82-6). Reports of its efficacy vary widely; in our experience, this approach yields unpredictable results.

Joo and colleagues (1998) reported sustained closure in 74% of 26 patients with fistulizing CD treated with endorectal advancement flap. Hull and Fazio (1997) reported that, among 35 patients with an advancement flap for low anovaginal fistulas, the initial healing rate was 54%, and an ultimate healing rate after > 1 procedure was 68%, but few others have such outcomes. Even more aggressive options can be considered in a few selective patients (Radcliffe et al, 1988; Halverson et al, 2001). Procedures such as an *advancement sleeve flap* can be used for larger perianal fistula dis-

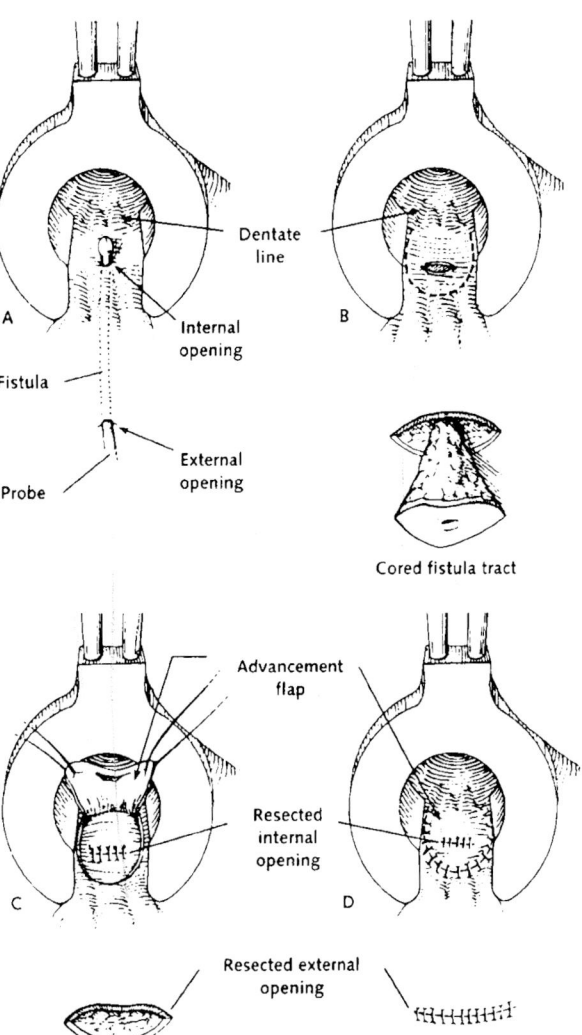

FIGURE 82-6. Endorectal advancement flap. *A,* The fistula tract is probed to identify the internal opening of the fistula. *B,* The internal opening of the fistula tract is incised. *C,* A flap of tissue (including mucosa, submucosa, and circular muscle) around the site of the resected internal opening of the fistula is incised. *D,* The flap is pulled down to cover the site of the resected internal opening of the fistula.

ease, as long as the rectum is spared. A report from Hull and Fazio (1997) looked at five patients with CD vaginal fistulas where four of the five have had resolution of their fistulas. Another 13 with complex fistulas have been treated in this manner, with 61% having resolution of symptoms. Although these results seem reasonable, we are unable to achieve anything near these outcomes and *do not* perform flap advancement for patients with RVF caused by CD.*

---

*Editor's Note: The role of aggressive medical therapy and of fecal diversion will have to be considered in the future, as mentioned below.

Influence of Proximal Disease

Does removal of proximal disease improve perianal disease in patients with CD? It has been shown that removal of all proximal disease does in fact promote healing in the perineum. Moreover, if proximal disease recurs, then the chance of recurrence in the perineum is also increased. Wolff and colleagues (1985) supported this conclusion with a report of 86 patients. In those patients with complete resection of proximal disease, only 29% developed recurrence. In those who had incomplete resections, 63% developed recurrent anorectal disease. However, in our opinion, proximal disease should be removed only when symptomatic as the influence of proximal resection or perineal disease is uncertain.

Fecal Diversion

The effect of fecal diversion or activity of perineal CD is controversial. Yamamoto and colleagues (2000) found no improvement in perianal disease with proximal diversion. Over the years, this practice had been frowned upon because of the historically low rates of restoration of continuity. This negative experience, however, *predates combination therapy* using antibiotics, azathioprine or 6-mercaptopurine, infliximab, cyclosporine, or tacrolimus. Given the current ease of laparoscopic loop ileostomy and the use of these newer medications, fecal diversion may again have a place in our overall treatment of perianal CD.

Proctectomy

Proctectomy is uncommonly performed in patients with perineal CD; between 5 to 25% of patients will ultimately require proctectomy. In our own long term series of patients with anorectal CD, two groups have emerged. The first had suffered severe rectal involvement and proceeded to proctectomy very early in the disease process. The second group had more limited rectal disease and has been managed well with conservative treatment. Within this series, the cumulative probability of avoiding proctectomy was 92% at 10 years and 83% at 20 years (Wolff et al, 1985). Despite good results with intensive medical and surgical therapy, a small percentage of patients will ultimately require proctectomy. As perineal wound complications are a major source of morbidity, an intersphincteric dissection to decrease morbidity is performed routinely (Lubbers, 1982). In patients with severe perianal sepsis, a diverting laparoscopic ileostomy followed by proctocolectomy in 6 to 12 weeks results in fewer wound complications. For patients who have persistent perianal pain, discharge, or incontinence despite maximal medical therapy, proctectomy offers a substantially improved quality of life.

Oncologic Risk of Perianal Disease in IBD

The risk of cancer developing in longstanding (decades) perianal disease is low indeed. There have been a few case reports of CD fistulas developing adenocarcinoma. Malignant degeneration should be considered in the differential diagnosis of all chronic nonhealing fistulas. If cancer is suspected, patients should undergo EUA with curettage of the fistulous tract for diagnosis. There is a separate chapter by Brentrall on surveillance for dysplasia in CD, as well as in ulcerative colitis (see Chapter 83, "Dysplasia Surveillance Programs").

Comments

Most patients with rectal CD have concomitant perianal involvement. Conservative medical management works well in most patients and there is little risk of progression to proctectomy. In more complex disease, sepsis continues to cause discomfort and morbidity. Management of perianal disease continues to evolve. Aggressive surgical treatment alone has invariably lead to the serious complications of healing, incontinence, and need for permanent fecal diversion. Combining surgical drainage with aggressive anti-inflammatory and/or immunomodulators has become a powerful tool in the management of perianal CD. Surgery is indicated for the treatment of complications of perianal CD, and only when such combination therapy fails is proctectomy indicated.

Editor's Note: There are separate chapters on anorectal disease (see Chapter 91, "Anorectal Diseases") and medical treatment of perianal disease (see Chapter 81, "Perianal Complications in Crohn's Disease Patient Management"). A complete 80-item reference bibliography for this detailed chapter can be obtained at Pemberton, John@mayo.edu.

Supplemental Reading

Agrez MV, Valente RM, Pierce W, et al. Surgical history of CD in a well-defined population. Mayo Clin Proc 1982;57:747–52.

Alexander-Williams J. Fistula-in-ano: management of Chrohn's fistula. Dis Colon Rectum 1976;19:518–9.

Allan A, Keighley MR. Management of perianal CD. World J Surg 1988;12:198–202.

Bayer I, Gordon PH. Selected operative management of fistula-in-ano in CD. Dis Colon Rectum 1994;37:760–5.

Berliner L, Redmond P, Purow E, et al. Computed tomography in CD. Am J Gastroenterol 1982;77:548–53.

Bernard D, Morgan S, Tasse D. Selective surgical management of CD of the anus. Can J Surg 1986;29:318–21.

Buchmann P, Keighley MR, Allan RN, et al. Natural history of perianal CD. Ten year follow-up: a plea for conservatism. Am J Surg 1980;140:642–4.

Farmer RG, Hawk WA, Turnbull RB Jr. Clinical patterns in CD: a statistical study of 615 cases. Gastroenterol 1975;68:627–35.

Fazio VW, Wilk P, Turnbull RB Jr, Jagelman DG. The dilemma of CD: ileosigmoidal fistula complicating CD. Dis Colon Rectum 1977;20:381–6.

Fielding JH. CD in London in the latter half of the nineteenth century. Ir J Med Sci 1984;153:214–20.

Fishman EK, Wolf EJ, Jones B, et al. CT evaluation of CD: effect on patient management. AJR Am J Roentgenol 1987;148:537–40.

Fleshner PR, Schoetz DJ Jr, Roberts PL, et al. Anal fissure in CD: a plea for aggressive management. Dis Colon Rectum 1995;38:1137–43.

Frizelle FA, Santoro GA, Pemberton JH. The management of perianal CD. Int J Colorectal Dis 1996;11:227–37.

Fry RD, Shemesh EI, Kodner IJ, Timmcke A. Techniques and results in the management of anal and perianal CD. Surg Gynecol Obstet 1989;168:42–8.

Fuhrman GM, Larach SW. Experience with perirectal fistulae in patients with CD. Dis Colon Rectum 1989;32:847–8.

Glass RE, Ritchie JK, Lennard-Jones JE, et al. Internal fistulae in CD. Dis Colon Rectum 1985;28:557–61.

Goldberg HI, Gore RM, Margulis AR, et al. Computed tomography in the evaluation of Crohn disease. AJR Am J Roentgenol 1983;140:277–82.

Haggett PJ, Moore NR, Shearman JD, et al. Pelvic and perineal complications of CD: assessment using magnetic resonance imaging. Gut 1995;36:407–10.

Halme L, Sainio AP. Factors related to frequency, type, and outcome of anal fistulae in CD. Dis Colon Rectum 1995;38:55–9.

Halverson AL, Hull TL, Fazio VW, et al. Repair of recurrent rectovaginal fistulae. Surgery 2001;130:753–7.

Harper PH, Kettlewell MG, Lee EC. The effect of split ileostomy on perianal CD. Br J Surg 1982;69:608–10.

Hellers G, Bergstrand O, Ewerth S, Holmstrom B. Occurrence and outcome after primary treatment of anal fistulae in CD. Gut 1980;21:525–7.

Hobbiss JH, Schofield PF. Management of perianal CD. J R Soc Med 1982; 75:414–7.

Hughes LE. Clinical classification of perianal CD. Dis Colon Rectum 1992; 35:928–32.

Hughes LE. Surgical pathology and management of anorectal CD. J R Soc Med 1978;71:644–51.

Hull TL, Fazio VW. Surgical approaches to low anovaginal fistula in CD. Am J Surg 1997;173:95–8.

Irvine EJ. Usual therapy improves perianal CD as measured by a new disease activity index. McMaster IBD Study Group. J Clin Gastroenterol 1995;20:27–32.

Jeffery PJ, Parks AG, Ritchie JK. Treatment of haemorrhoids in patients with inflammatory bowel disease. Lancet 1977;1:1084–5.

Joo JS, Weiss EG, Nogueras JJ, Wexner SD. Endorectal advancement flap in perianal CD. Am Surg 1998;64:147–50.

Kangas E. Anal lesions complicating CD. Ann Chir Gynaecol 1991;80:336–9.

Keighley MR, Allan RN. Current status and influence of operation on perianal CD. Int J Colorectal Dis 1986;1:104–7.

Kerber GW, Greenberg M, Rubin JM. Computed tomography evaluation of local and extraintestinal complications of CD. Gastrointest Radiol 1984;9:143–8.

Koelbel G, Schmiedl U, Majer MC, et al. Diagnosis of fistulae and sinus tracts in patients with Crohn disease: value of MR imaging. AJR Am J Roentgenol 1989;52:999–1003.

Koganei K, Sugita A, Harada H, et al. Seton treatment for perianal Crohn's fistulae. Surg Today 1995;25:32–6.

Kuijpers HC, Schulpen T. Fistulography for fistula-in-ano. Is it useful? Dis Colon Rectum 1985;28:103–4.

Levien DH, Surrell J, Mazier WP. Surgical treatment of anorectal fistula in patients with CD. Surg Gynecol Obstet 1989;169:133–6.

Linares L, Moreira LF, Andrews H, et al. Natural history and treatment of anorectal strictures complicating CD. Br J Surg 1988;75:653–5.

Lindsey I, Smilgin-Humphreys MM, Cunningham C, et al. A randomized, controlled trial of fibrin glue vs. conventional treatment for anal fistula. Dis Colon Rectum 2002;45:1608–15.

Lubbers EJ. Healing of the perineal wound after proctectomy for nonmalignant conditions. Dis Colon Rectum 1982;25:351–7.

Makowiec F, Jehle EC, Becker HD, Starlinger M. Clinical course after transanal advancement flap repair of perianal fistula in patients with CD. Br J Surg 1995;82:603–6.

Makowiec F, Jehle EC, Becker HD, Starlinger M. Perianal abscess in CD. Dis Colon Rectum 1997;40:443–50.

Marchesa P, Hull TL, Fazio VW. Advancement sleeve flaps for treatment of severe perianal CD. Br J Surg 1998;85:1695–8.

Marks CG, Ritchie JK, Lockhart-Mummery HE. Anal fistulae in CD. Br J Surg 1981;68:525–7.

McLeod RS. Management of fistula-in-ano: 1990 Roussel Lecture. Can J Surg 1991;34:581–5.

Michelassi F, Melis M, Rubin M, Hurst RD. Surgical treatment of anorectal complications in CD. Surgery 2000;128:597–603.

Nordgren S, Fasth S, Hulten L. Anal fistulae in CD: incidence and outcome of surgical treatment. Int J Colorectal Dis 1992;7:214–8.

Orsoni P, Barthet M, Portier F, et al. Prospective comparison of endosonography, magnetic resonance imaging and surgical findings in anorectal fistula and abscess complicating CD. Br J Surg 1999;86:360–4.

Parks AG, Motson RW. Peranal repair of rectoprostatic fistula. Br J Surg 1983;70:725–6.

Pearl RK, Andrews JR, Orsay CP, et al. Role of the seton in the management of anorectal fistulae. Dis Colon Rectum 1993;36:573–7.

Penner A CB. Perianal fistulae as a complication of regional ileitis. Ann Surg 2003;108:867–73.

Pomerri F, Pittarello F, Dodi G, et al. [Radiologic diagnosis of anal fistulae with radio-opaque markers]. Radiol Med (Torino) 1988;75:632–7.

Radcliffe AG, Ritchie JK, Hawley PR, et al. Anovaginal and rectovaginal fistulae in CD. Dis Colon Rectum 1988;31:94–9.

Rankin GB, Watts HD, Melnyk CS, Kelley ML Jr. National Cooperative CD Study: extraintestinal manifestations and perianal complications. Gastroenterol 1979;77:914–20.

Regueiro M, Mardini H. Treatment of perianal fistulizing CD with infliximab alone or as an adjunct to exam under anesthesia with seton placement. Inflamm Bowel Dis 2003;9:98–103.

Ricart E, Panaccione R, Loftus EV, et al. Infliximab for CD in clinical practice at the Mayo Clinic: the first 100 patients. Am J Gastroenterol 2001; 96:722–9.

Schratter-Sehn AU, Lochs H, Vogelsang H, et al. Endoscopic ultrasonography versus computed tomography in the differential diagnosis of perianorectal complications in CD. Endoscopy 1993;25:582–6.

Schwartz DA, Loftus EV Jr, Tremaine WJ, et al. The natural history of fistulizing CD in Olmsted County, Minnesota. Gastroenterol 2002;122:875–80.

Schwartz DA, Pemberton JH, Sandborn WJ. Diagnosis and treatment of perianal fistulae in Crohn disease. Ann Intern Med 2001;135:906–18.

Schwartz DA, Wiersema MJ, Dudiak KM, et al. A comparison of endoscopic ultrasound, magnetic resonance imaging, and exam under anesthesia for evaluation of Crohn's perianal fistulae. Gastroenterol 2001;121:1064–72.

Scott HJ, Northover JM. Evaluation of surgery for perianal Crohn's fistulae. Dis Colon Rectum 1996;39:1039–43.

Sentovich SM. Fibrin glue for anal fistulae: long-term results. Dis Colon Rectum 2003;46:498–502.

Skalej M, Makowiec F, Weinlich M, et al. [Magnetic resonance imaging in perianal CD]. Dtsch Med Wochenschr 1993;118:1791–6.

Sohn N, Korelitz BI, Weinstein MA. Anorectal CD: definitive surgery for fistulae and recurrent abscesses. Am J Surg 1980;139:394–7.

Sugita A, Koganei K, Harada H, et al. Surgery for Crohn's anal fistulae. J Gastroenterol 1995;30 Suppl 8:143–6.

Takesue Y, Ohge H, Yokoyama T, et al. Long-term results of seton drainage on complex anal fistulae in patients with CD. J Gastroenterol 2002;37:912–5.

Tio TL, Mulder CJ, Wijers OB, et al. Endosonography of peri-anal and peri-colorectal fistula and/or abscess in CD. Gastrointest Endosc 1990;36:331–6.

Topstad DR, Panaccione R, Heine JA, et al. Combined seton placement, infliximab infusion, and maintenance immunosuppressives improve healing rate in fistulizing anorectal CD: a single center experience. Dis Colon Rectum 2003;46:577–83.

White RA, Eisenstat TE, Rubin RJ, Salvati EP. Seton management of complex anorectal fistulae in patients with CD. Dis Colon Rectum 1990;33:587–9.

Williams DR, Coller JA, Corman ML, et al. Anal complications in CD. Dis Colon Rectum 1981;24:22–4.

Williams JG, Rothenberger DA, Nemer FD, Goldberg SM. Fistula-in-ano in CD. Results of aggressive surgical treatment. Dis Colon Rectum 1991;34:378–84.

Winter AM, Banks PA, Petros JG. Healing of transsphincteric perianal fistulae in CD using a new technique. Am J Gastroenterol 1993;88:2022–5.

Weisman RI, Orsay CP, Pearl RK, Abcarian H. The role of fistulography in fistula-in-ano. Report of five cases. Dis Colon Rectum 1991;34:181–4.

Van Outryve MJ, Pelckmans PA, Michielsen PP, Van Maercke YM. Value of transrectal ultrasonography in CD. Gastroenterol 1991;101:1171–7.

Wolff BG. CD: the role of surgical treatment. Mayo Clin Proc 1986;61:292–5.

Wolff BG, Culp CE, Beart RW Jr, et al. Anorectal CD. A long-term perspective. Dis Colon Rectum 1985;28:709–11.

Wolkomir AF, Luchtefeld MA. Surgery for symptomatic hemorrhoids and anal fissures in CD. Dis Colon Rectum 1993;36:545–7.

Yamamoto T, Allan RN, Keighley MR. Effect of fecal diversion alone on perianal CD. World J Surg 2000;24:1258–62.

Yousem DM, Fishman EK, Jones B. Crohn disease: perirectal and perianal findings at CT. Radiology 1988;167:331–4.

Zelas P, Jagelman DG. Loop illeostomy in the management of Crohn's colitis in the debilitated patient. Ann Surg 1980;191:164–8.

Dysplasia Surveillance Programs

Teresa A. Brentnall, MD

Does Surveillance Save Lives?

Several studies now show the benefits of endoscopic surveillance for neoplasia in ulcerative colitis (UC). The cancers that develop in patients under surveillance are detected at an earlier stage than those in patients who are not under surveillance (Choi et al, 1993; Nugent et al, 1991). This earlier detection of cancer translates into improved 5-year survival rates—77% for those in surveillance versus 36% for those who are not. Do the benefits of surveillance outweigh the costs? Two decision analyses by Provenzale and colleagues (1995, 1998) suggest that *not only does surveillance increase life expectancy, it ultimately costs less than no surveillance* (Provenzale et al, 1995; Provenzale et al, 1998).

The Dilemmas

The current standard of practice in all patients with extensive UC of 8 or more years of duration is to perform lifelong colonoscopic biopsy surveillance. Yet, the optimal protocol for this surveillance has not been established. The lack of consensus on *which* patients warrant frequent colonoscopy is compounded by the divergent opinions regarding *what* constitutes adequate colonoscopic surveillance. A major problem in surveillance is the large surface area of the colon, which ranges from 0.5 to 1.0 m^2. Dysplasia may arise anywhere within this large area and frequently produces no endoscopically visible lesion.

Surveillance Protocol

As indicated above, the current standard of practice is to perform lifelong annual or biannual colonoscopic biopsy surveillance in patients with extensive colitis of 8 or more years of duration (Figure 83-1). Many physicians perform colonoscopy annually, taking an average of 3 to 8 biopsy samples. The current guidelines from the World Health Organization (WHO) recommend annual to biannual colonoscopy with unspecified numbers of biopsies, taken from normal appearing mucosa at 10 to 12 cm intervals throughout the colon and extra biopsies taken from areas of mucosal irregularity (Winawer et al, 1995). The American Gastroenterologic Association (AGA) has suggested a similar guideline, however, neither of these recommendations is based on a scientific data analysis (Winawer et al, 1997). Our prospective studies have shown that to detect focal dysplasia in UC with 90% confidence, *33 colonoscopic biopsies must be examined histologically* (Rubin et al, 1999). The acquisition of this many biopsies is both time and cost intensive, *however once the patient's histologic diagnosis is established with confidence, it may be possible to extend the surveillance intervals*.

Our current protocol is to obtain biopsies at 4 quadrants every 10 cm from the cecum through the descending

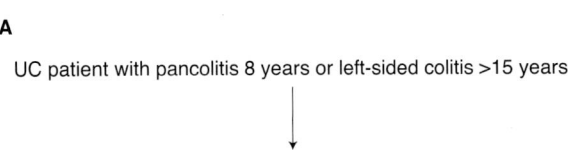

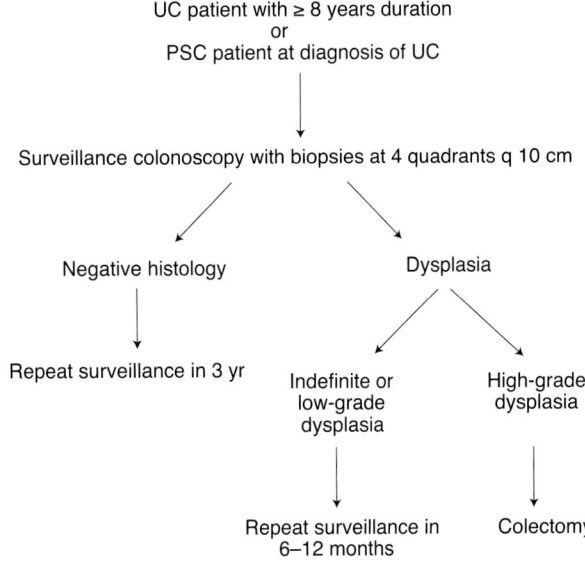

FIGURE 83-1. Surveillance strategies for inflammatory bowel disease. Strategy A requires annual to biannual colonoscopy for the lifetime of the patient; Strategy B stratifies patients according to neoplastic risk. PSC = primary sclerossing cholangitis; UC = ulcerative colitis.

colon and at 5 cm intervals from the rectosigmoid, where cancer is most common. This provides an average of 44 biopsies per procedure. The biopsies are taken with jumbo biopsy forceps, to provide a sample that is large enough to orient correctly and to minimize crush artifact. The biopsies are orientated (straightened out from the forceps cup) and mounted flat on monofilament mesh prior to fixation. Four biopsy samples from each level are placed in a single fixative bottle (Hollande's gives the best nuclear detail) and labeled as to their location in the colon. After fixation, the four biopsy samples from each level are placed in a single paraffin block, serially sectioned, and interpreted by an experienced gastrointestinal (GI) pathologist.

Patients who have mucosal irregularities, bumps or polyps, have the lesion sampled, and when possible, removed in its entirety for histologic evaluation. Samples from visible lesions are taken in addition to the usual number of surveillance biopsies and are placed in a separately labeled bottle of fixative. The location of the lesion is noted and described in the colonoscopy report.

The Importance of Interpretation by an Experienced Pathologist

The diagnosis of dysplasia in inflammatory bowel disease (IBD) is a subjective interpretation and requires an experienced pathologist for optimum accuracy. Because major clinical decisions rest on the histologic diagnosis, it is imperative that the colonic biopsies be evaluated by a pathologist who has expertise in the diagnosis of IBD and the associated neoplastic transformation. This caution is especially true when the diagnosis of dysplasia is made. For example, we recommend colectomy for high grade dysplasia (HGD), but usually not for low grade dysplasia (LGD). Thus, unless the pathologist is experienced in the interpretation of dysplasia, get a second opinion on biopsies that will change clinical management.

Surveillance Intervals

According to WHO guidelines, if biopsies are classified as negative or indefinite for dysplasia then surveillance colonoscopy should be repeated every 1 to 2 years. The current AGA guidelines suggest annual colonoscopy for IBD patients. *If the physician is only taking 8 to 10 biopsies per procedure, I think this is sage advice.* If, however, you perform a more thorough sampling of the colon, with more than 33 biopsies taken per procedure, the clinician and the patient can have confidence that dysplasia is less likely to have been missed. Our current recommendations are outlined in Table 83-1 and are based on the histologic findings at colonoscopy, with the intervals longer for patients who are negative for dysplasia. This approach has several advantages; it costs less and it focuses the physicians time and effort on those patients who are most likely to progress to cancer (Provenzale et al, 1998).

High Risk Patients

Patients with UC *and Crohn's colitis* have an increased risk of colorectal cancer. The following two chief factors determine which patients are at increased risk: (1) disease *duration* of more than 8 years and (2) disease *extent* proximal to the sigmoid colon. Primary sclerosing cholangitis (PSC) has been identified as a third factor; the risk of neoplasia approaches 50% after 25 years duration of UC in these patients (Brentnall et al, 1996; Broomé et al, 1992; D'Haens et al, 1993; Gurbuz et al, 1995). Patients with PSC have an 80 to 90% probability of having UC, but *are often asymptomatic,* and the duration of UC may be difficult to determine. Therefore, PSC patients who have not been diagnosed with UC should have periodic flexible sigmoidoscopy with 5 to 10 biopsies performed to determine whether UC has developed. PSC patients found to have UC should then undergo surveillance colonoscopy as soon as they are diagnosed, rather than waiting for the usual 8-year duration before initiating surveillance. The reasons for this are because (1) the duration of UC cannot be accurately determined in patients who may be asymptomatic and (2) these patients have the highest risk of developing neoplasia. The concept of chemoprevention is discussed later.

Management of LGD

The optimal management of UC patients with LGD is controversial. Some experts recommend colectomy, because a high probability of finding an occult cancer in the colectomy specimen from these patients has been reported. However, the retrospective studies upon which these recommendations are based used a variable number of biop-

---

TABLE 83-1. Time Intervals between Surveillance Colonoscopies Assuming Adequate Sampling Has Been Achieved

Histology	Interval between Colonoscopies
Negative for dysplasia	3 years
Indefinite for dysplasia	1 year
LGD	6 to 12 months
HGD	Colectomy; for those who refuse colectomy then colonoscopy every 3 to 6 months

HGD = high grade dysplasia; LGD = low grade dyplasia.

---

*Editor's Note: Oh, that all colonoscopists and pathologists were as compulsive and experienced as the Seattle groups. Incomplete preps, rushed endoscopy schedules, variable patient compliance, and increasing risk with time would seen to justify more frequent surveillance after 20 years of colitis, especially with childhood onset or with advanced chronologic age. It is also difficult to set the date of onset for patients with Crohn's colitis diagnosed after age 40 or, as below, patients with coexistent primary sclerosing cholangitis.

sies (average 13 to 30 biopsies per 100 cm colon) obtained at inconsistent colonoscopic intervals varying from 1 month to 5 years. Thus the finding of occult cancers in these studies is not surprising because insufficient numbers of biopsies were taken to make the correct histologic diagnosis.

Although colectomy may be the least costly method for managing patients with LGD, many patients are reluctant to undergo this surgery. Patients who have had UC for 20 years, which is the average duration of disease prior to the development of dysplasia, often have minimal or no symptoms, and it can be difficult to convince them that a colectomy will benefit them. An informed discussion of the risks and benefits of colectomy for LGD requires an understanding of its natural history. Important questions about the biology of LGD include the following:

1. Do all patients with LGD develop cancer?
2. If so, over what time frame?
3. Does LGD ever regress?
4. Is HGD always an intermediate step between LGD and cancer?
5. Can it be detected with confidence?
6. Are there patient characteristics that predict who will progress to cancer?

We performed a prospective evaluation of the natural history of LGD in 18 UC patients. The preliminary results suggest that only one-third of these LGD patients will progress in the short term, and those who do progress usually do so within 18 months of the diagnosis of LGD. With our protocol of 4 quadrant biopsies every 10 cm and follow-up intervals occurring at least annually, none of the 18 LGD patients developed cancer while under surveillance. Six patients who progressed in the study developed HGD and underwent colectomy; none had an unsuspected carcinoma in their colectomy specimen. Characteristics of those who were more likely to progress to HGD included (1) patients with three or more biopsies with LGD per colonoscopy and (2) *younger* patients. Two-thirds of LGD patients did not progress, but rather continue to have LGD or downgraded to indefinite or negative for dysplasia during an average follow-up of 3 years. Because of these data, we do not routinely recommend colectomy for UC patients with LGD, but rather follow them endoscopically every 6 to 12 months, taking an adequate number of biopsies so that HGD or cancer will be detected if it is present.

The surveillance protocol described above is time intensive, expensive, and requires collaborative commitment from the physician, the patient, and the pathologist; moreover, one cannot absolutely guarantee that the patient will not develop cancer. If the gastroenterologist takes fewer biopsies, does not have access to a good GI pathologist, or if the patient is unwilling to adhere to a strict surveillance protocol, then colectomy is probably the safest plan of action in the setting of LGD found in flat mucosa. For dysplasia found in a polyp, see guidelines below.

Management of Polyps

Part of the controversy regarding the management of polypoid lesions found in UC patients is embedded in the nomenclature associated with IBD neoplasia. Until recently, the finding of a dysplasia-associated lesion or mass (DALM) in the colon has been considered an indication for colectomy; however, the dilemma arises when trying to differentiate a sporadic adenoma (removed by polypectomy) from a DALM (requires colectomy). Many UC patients undergoing surveillance are in the age range to have a 30% probability of sporadic adenoma. There are many approaches to the problem of polypoid lesions in the IBD patient. One approach is to perform a *polypectomy* on lesions that arise in a field of normal colon (IBD-free) and a *colectomy* for dysplastic lesions that arise in a field of colitis. This approach is based on the concern that occult cancer is present, either in the lesion itself or elsewhere in the colon. The problem of this approach is that colectomies will be performed on many patients who would otherwise have a benign course. The reason for this problem is, again, one of sampling error; if the endoscopist fails to remove the entire lesion for full histologic examination and/or fails to take sufficient biopsies to find dysplasia in the remaining colon, then a missed diagnosis of HGD or cancer can occur.

An alternative approach is the performance of a complete *colonoscopic* resection of sessile and pedunculated polyps, regardless of whether they occur in IBD-affected colon or not, while at the same time taking sufficient numbers of biopsies to evaluate the remaining colon (Figure 83-2). If the biopsies of the lesion reveal invasive adenocarcinoma (AC) *or* if biopsies of the *flat* mucosa reveal dysplasia, then a colectomy is warranted. If histologic examination of the polyp reveals a completely resected dysplastic lesion, and if the remaining colon is dysplasia-free, then the patient should have a repeat surveillance colonoscopy in 1 year. Two recent studies have

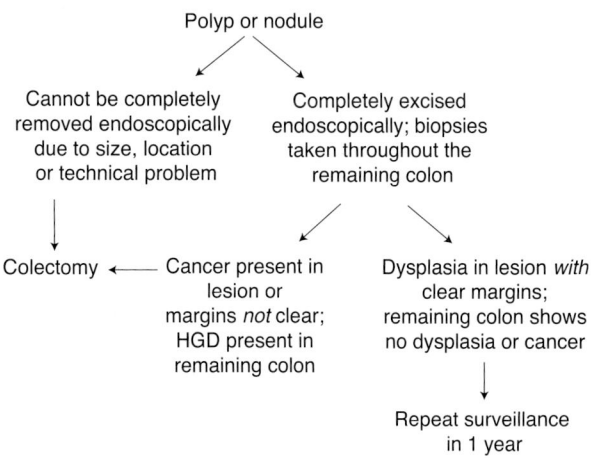

FIGURE 83-2. Management of polypoid lesions. HGD = high grade dysplasia.

used this paradigm. The studies involved 24 and 73 polypoid lesions, respectively, from colitic sites (Engelsgjerd et al, 1999; Rubin et al, 1992). A large number of the polypoid lesions were sessile. Approximately half of the patients had recurrent polyps on follow-up colonoscopy, often in the same location, which required repeated polypectomy. However, the patients had a benign course; *no patients developed cancer and few patients developed flat dysplasia outside the polypoid lesion.*

We use this strategy for management of polypoid lesions and have found it to be successful (ie, patients have not developed cancer and have avoided colectomy), provided that the entire lesion is excised with clean margins and the patient continues in annual surveillance. If patients have dysplasia both in a polyp and in flat mucosa, colectomy should be considered. Please refer to Chapter 6 "Endoscopic Mucosal Resection" which is relevant to this discussion.

Surveillance of Pouches

AC of the ileal reservoir of pouches has been reported. These reports are relatively uncommon, but the risk is present. Risk factors for the development of dysplasia and cancer may include the age of the pouch, chronic pouchitis, and the codiagnosis of PSC. Studies performed in Sweden suggest that the primary risk factor of neoplastic progression in the pouch is associated with chronic pouchitis resulting in permanent subtotal or total villous atrophy (Veress et al, 1995). Such atrophic changes set the stage for metaplasia (change in epithelial type in the pouch) and neoplastic transformation; therefore, patients with chronic pouchitis and villous atrophy are likely the subset best suited for pouch surveillance. The second major risk factor involves patients who have PSC and UC and have undergone an ileoanal anastomosis with pouch construction of 8 or more years duration. These UC/PSC patients develop moderate or severe atrophy in the pouch significantly more often ($p < .01$) than UC patients without PSC who have similar characteristics (Stahlberg et al, 2003). Otherwise, the yield for dysplasia/cancer during pouch surveillance is likely to be very low (Herlin et al, 2003; Thompson-Fawcett et al, 2001; Hulten et al, 2002).

Chemoprevention

Multiple molecular and epigenetic steps underlie the process of tumorigenesis in IBD, thus chemoprevention is a realistic proposition. Biochemical targets of chemopreventive agents include drugs that alter bile acid metabolism, arachidonic acid metabolism, and drugs that effect proliferation and cell death (apoptosis) of precancerous cells. Aspirin, cyclooxygenase-2 (COX-2) inhibitors, and calcium are examples of drugs that have undergone clinical testing in sporadic colorectal cancer and may have a chemopreventive role in IBD-associated colon cancers.

IBD patients have multiple reasons for folate depletion, including inadequate diet, malabsorption, and rapid epithelial cell turnover. Although there are no prospective studies using folate as a chemopreventive agent in UC, there are retrospective studies demonstrating a trend toward a lower prevalence of colonic dysplasia in UC patients who use folate supplements, with the risk of neoplasia inversely related to the dose (Lashner et al, 1997).

Ursodiol has been traditionally used for its very positive effects on the hepatobiliary system. It has multiple mechanisms of action, including: (1) acting as a chemopreventive agent, in animal models, (2) acting as an antioxidant, and (3) inhibiting cellular proliferation and being cytoprotective. Two studies have demonstrated the chemoprotective effect of ursodiol in UC/PSC patients, a subgroup of UC patients that has a 50% risk of colonic neoplasia after 25 years of UC. A retrospective study demonstrated that patients with PSC/UC had a significant reduction in dysplasia (*odds ratio, 0.18* [95% CI, 0.05 to 0.61]; $p = .005$) (Tung et al, 2001). A second prospective study also demonstrated a similar risk reduction of neoplasia in UC/PSC patients who were taking ursodiol (Pardi et al, 2003). Whether ursodiol can prevent dysplasia in UC patients who do not have PSC, or prevent *progression* of dysplasia that is already present in UC/PSC patients, remains to be determined.

COX-2 overexpression occurs early in UC-associated neoplasia, and the increase cannot be explained by inflammatory activity alone. The laboratory data suggests that COX-2-specific inhibitors celecoxib (Celebrex) and rofecoxib (Vioxx) may have a chemopreventive role in UC, but the possibility that they could exacerbate UC inflammatory activity needs to be tested. In the same vein, anti-inflammatory agents, such as 5-acetylsalicylic acid (ASA), have been reported in retrospective studies to reduce the incidence of dysplasia. Two case control studies suggest that regular 5-ASA therapy (including sulfasalazine) reduces cancer risk by 60 to 75% (Eaden et al, 2000; Pinczowski et al, 1994).

Odds and Ends

A few important caveats are worth mentioning. Patients should have their colitis in remission prior to surveillance colonoscopy. It is difficult for the pathologist to interpret the subtleties of dysplasia when moderate to severe inflammation is present in the biopsy specimen. Therefore, every effort should be made to bring inflammation under control *prior to* surveillance colonoscopy. If the patient has active disease clearly evident at a scheduled surveillance colonoscopy, I postpone the procedure until I can bring it under control. If inflamma-

---

[†]Editor's Note: I am a worrier. I worry about patients who had a cuff of colonic mucosa left at time of a stapled anastomosis rather than a mucosal stripping. If there was dysplasia or cancer in the resected colon, I worry even more.

tion cannot be suppressed, the patient may be a candidate for a colectomy on the basis of intractable disease and an inability to monitor the mucosa histologically for dysplasia.

When in doubt about management or pathology, get a second opinion. Biopsies with dysplasia should be assessed by a pathologist with expertise in IBD. Barium enema should *not* be substituted for colonoscopy in IBD patients because dysplasia may not cause a visible defect. Patients with ulcerative proctitis do not require surveillance because there appears to be no increased risk of colorectal cancer (Ekbom et al, 1990; Farmer and Brown, 1966). Patients with Crohn's colitis have the same elevated neoplastic risk as those with UC and, thus, should be under similar surveillance protocols (Ekbom et al, 1990).

Acknowledgment

I would like to thank the late Dr. Rodger Haggitt‡ for his sage advice and thoughtful comments regarding the information in this manuscript.

---

‡Editor's Note: We are all in debt to Dr Haggitt.

Supplemental Reading

Bernstein CN, Shanahan F, Weinstein WM. Are we telling patients the truth about surveillance colonoscopy in UC? Lancet 1994;343:71–4.

Brentnall TA, Haggitt RC, Rabinovitch PS, et al. Risk and natural history of colonic neoplasia in patients with primary sclerosing cholangitis and UC. Gastroenterology 1996;110:331–8.

Broomé U, Lindberg G, Lofberg R. Primary sclerosing cholangitis in UC: a risk factor for the development of dysplasia and DNA aneuploidy? Gastroenterology 1992;102:1877–80.

Choi PM, Nugent FW, Schoetz DJ, et al. Colonoscopic surveillance reduces mortality from colorectal cancer in UC. Gastroenterology 1993;105:418–24.

Dawson IM, Pryse-Davies J. The development of carcinoma of the large intestine in ulcerative colitis. Br J Surg 1959;47:113–28.

D'Haens GR, Lashner BA, Hanauer SB. Pericholangitis and sclerosing cholangitis are risk factors for dysplasia and cancer in UC. Am J Gastroenterol 1993;88:1174–8.

Eaden J, Abrams K, Ekbom A, et al. Colorectal cancer prevention in UC: a case-control study. Aliment Pharmacol Ther 2000;14:145–53.

Ekbom A, Helmick C, Zack M, Adami H-O. Increased risk of large-bowel cancer in Crohn's disease with colonic involvement. Lancet 1990;336:357–9.

Ekbom A, Helmick C, Zack M, Adami HO. UC and colorectal cancer. A population-based study. N Engl J Med 1990;323:1228–33.

Engelsgjerd M, Torres C, Farraye F, Odze D. Adenoma-like polypoid dysplasia in chronic UC: a follow up study of 23 cases. Gastroenterology 1999;116:A2100.

Farmer RG, Brown CH. Ulcerative proctitis: course and prognosis. Gastroenterology 1966;51:219–23.

Goldgraber MB, Kirsner JB. Carcinoma of the colon in UC. Cancer 1964;15:657–65.

Gurbuz AK, Giardiello FM, Bayless TM. Colorectal neoplasia in patients with ulcerative colitis and primary sclerosing cholangitis. Dis Colon Rectum 1995;38:37–41.

Herlin AJ, Meisinger LL, Rusin LC, et al. Is routine pouch surveillance for dysplasia indicated for ileoanal pouches? Dis Colon Rectum 2003;46:156–9.

Hulten L, Willen R, Nilsson O, et al. Mucosal assessment for dysplasia and cancer in the ileal pouch mucosa in patients operated on for UC–30-year follow-up study. Dis Colon Rectum 2002;45:448–52.

Lashner BA, Provencher KS, Seidner DL, et al. The effect of folic acid supplementation on the risk for cancer or dysplasia in UC. Gastroenterology 1997;112:29–32.

Lennard-Jones JE. Cancer risk in UC: surveillance or surgery. Br J Surg 1985;72(Suppl):84–6.

Nugent FW, Haggitt RC, Gilpin PA. Cancer surveillance in UC. Gastroenterology 1991;100:1241–8.

Pardi DS, Loftus EV Jr, Kremers WK, et al. Ursodeoxycholic acid as a chemopreventive agent in patients with UC and primary sclerosing cholangitis. Gastroenterology 2003;124:889–93.

Pinczowski D, Ekbom A, Baron J, et al. Risk factors for colorectal cancer in patients with UC: a case-control study. Gastroenterology 1994;107:117–20.

Provenzale D, Kowdley KV, Arora S, Wong JB. Prophylactic colectomy or surveillance for chronic UC? A decision analysis. Gastroenterology 1995;109:1188–96.

Provenzale D, Wong J, Onken J, Lipscomb J. Performing a cost-effectiveness analysis: surveillance of patients with UC. Am J Gastroenterol 1998;93:872–80.

Ransohoff DF. Colon cancer in UC. Gastroenterology 1988; 94:1089–91.

Rubin PH, Friedman S, Harpaz N, et al. Colonoscopic polypectomy in chronic colitis: are we removing adenomas or "DALMS"? Gastroenterology 1999;116:A807.

Rubin CE, Haggitt RC, Burmer GC, et al. DNA aneuploidy in colonic biopsies predicts future development of dysplasia in UC. Gastroenterology 1992;103:1611–20.

Stahlberg D, Veress B, Tribukait B, Broome U. Atrophy and neoplastic transformation of the ileal pouch mucosa in patients with UC and primary sclerosing cholangitis: a case control study. Dis Colon Rectum 2003;46:770–8.

Thompson–Fawcett MW, Marcus V, Redston M, et al. Risk of dysplasia in long-term ileal pouches and pouches with chronic pouchitis. Gastroenterology 2001;121:275–81.

Tung BY, Emond MJ, Haggitt RC, et al. Ursodiol protects against neoplastic progression in ulcerative colitis patients with primary sclerosing cholangitis. Ann Int Med 2001;134:89–95.

Veress B, Reinholt FP, Lindquist K, et al. Long-term histomorphological surveillance of the pelvic ileal pouch: dysplasia develops in a subgroup of patients. Gastroenterology 1995;109:1090–7.

Winawer SJ, Fletcher RH, Miller L, et al. Colorectal cancer screening: clinical guidelines and rationale. Gastroenterology 1997;112:594–642.

Winawer SJ, St. John DJ, Bond JH, et al. Prevention of colorectal cancer: guidelines based on new data. Bull WHO 1995;73:7–10.

Woolrich AJ, DaSilva MD, Korelitz BI. Surveillance in the routine management of UC: the predictive value of low-grade dysplasia. Gastroenterology 1992;103:431–8.

CHAPTER 84

Pregnancy and Inflammatory Bowel Disease

Mary Lawrence Harris, MD

Ulcerative colitis (UC) and Crohn's disease (CD), collectively referred to as inflammatory bowel disease (IBD), are diagnosed most commonly in patients in their childbearing years. The incidence of CD in young adults is increasing, whereas the incidence of UC affecting patients in their reproductive years has remained stable. The etiology of IBDs is unknown, but clearly genetic factors and tobacco use have been implicated. Women routinely express concern about sexual intimacy, self-esteem, marriage, fertility, offspring inheritance of IBD, role of disease activity during pregnancy, safety of medications, and, finally, outcome or general health of the fetus. The most important issues for the patient are education and optimal timing of the pregnancy.

Fertility and Disease Activity

Most studies support normal fertility rates in females with UC. However, Swedish physicians (Olsen et al, 2002) report a markedly reduced potential of reproductive capacity of women after restorative proctocolectomy. It has been noted that women with IBD have fewer children than unaffected individuals. This may reflect decreased libido, dyspareunia, abdominal pain, diarrhea, or a conscious decision not to procreate.

Active CD does impair fertility (Khosla et al, 1984). Ileal inflammation can involve the ovaries and fallopian tubes resulting in scarring and obstruction. In addition, rectovaginal and perianal fistulizing disease may contribute to fear of intimacy, and dyspareunia, and vaginal candidiasis may follow medical therapy. In general, patients with UC and CD should have a quiescent disease interval of at least 3 months prior to conception. The course of IBD during pregnancy usually correlates with disease activity at time of conception. Patients with active disease may continue with symptoms one-third of the time and may actually have worsening of disease. Women with disease quiescence typically remain in remission during the pregnancy. Additionally, the gastroenterologist should be vigilant for possible disease recurrence in the puerperium.

Studies suggest that smoking supports active CD, affecting fertility and reducing fetal growth. Most patients are aware of tobacco's ill effects and consider cessation prior to conception. Alternatively, the UC patient risks disease flare with smoking cessation. The physician should prescribe adequate medical maintenance therapy to avoid reactivation of symptoms and disease during tobacco withdrawal, pregnancy, and postpartum.

In male patients with IBD, impotence from proctocolectomy may be an unspoken issue regarding fertility. Compassionate inquiry may be helpful; some patients respond to Viagra therapy. It is known that sulfasalazine may cause reversible oligospermia and impair sperm morphology and motility (Narendranathan et al, 1989).

Inheritance

Because of the well-described concept of genetic predisposition to CD, and less commonly UC, patients inquire about disease transmission to their offspring. The risk of inheriting CD is four times greater in Ashkanazae Jewish families. A positive family history, greater risk when a first degree relative, coupled with location, extent and behavior of CD influence risks. These phenotypes may provide future basis for molecular classification of IBD.

Recent data suggests that when the affected non-Jewish parent has CD the child has a 5% lifetime risk. The offspring has a 1.6% risk when the affected parent has UC (Orholm et al, 1999). Another study reports that with Jewish parents, lifetime risk to child for CD is 7.8%; if both parents have IBD, the risk to offspring may exceed 35%. The risk to the child for UC is lower in all scenarios (Yang et al, 1993).

Medications During Pregnancy

Most women do not want to ingest any medications or products such as alcohol or tobacco when conceiving. With quiescent IBD, many patients consider discontinuation of maintenance treatments. However meta-analysis data clearly supports maintenance medications such as *sulfasalazine* or *mesalamine* products. Relapsing IBD symptoms during pregnancy should be aggressively managed with *corticosteroids* and perhaps antibiotics. As discussed earlier, most physicians feel that it is not advisable to initiate *azathioprine* (AZA) or 6-mercaptapurine (6-MP) during a pregnancy but maintenance use of AZA to continue remission during pregnancy is reasonable (Table 84-1). Sachar (1998) has stated that "disease activity is more threatening to the pregnancy than most medical treatments".

Sulfasalazine and Mesalamine

Sulfasalazine has been prescribed for decades in pregnant IBD patients with no evidence of teratogenicity (Diav-Citrin et al, 1998). Oral and topical *mesalamine* agents are not associated with congenital anomalies. However, as sulfasalazine interferes with folate metabolism, *folic acid* must be prescribed prior to conception to avoid neural tube defects. Again, education and planning are essential. *High dose aminosalicylates* should be avoided during pregnancy because of reported fetal nephrotoxicity.

Antibiotics

Metronidazole and ciprofloxacin after the first trimester, are considered to be safe in pregnancy. Metronidazole, though it crosses the placenta, has been used to treat vaginal trichomonas during the first trimester without evidence of congenital anomalies. Quinolones have been associated with fetal animal musculoskeletal problems but have not been associated with birth defects in humans. Penicillin's and cephalosporins are pregnancy category B and maybe useful in perianal disease.

Corticosteroids

Prednisone has been used extensively in pregnancy without teratogenesis or fetal adrenocortical insufficiency. Corticosteroids cross the placental barrier and animal studies report an increase of cleft palate and stillbirth. These agents are used for moderate to severe disease in the pregnant patient (Mogadam et al, 1981).

AZA and Metabolites

Experience with immunomodulators in pregnant patients with renal transplants and systemic lupus erythematosis yields no teratogenecity or other adverse events. Physicians and patients should discuss the use of AZA and 6-MP for maintenance of remission during pregnancy especially if the disease activity was severe prior to beginning the medication. Controversy exists in the literature regarding the safety of AZA and 6-MP for childbearing female and male patients. In a recent publication, Francella, Present and colleagues reviewed the records of 155 IBD patients who had conceived at least one pregnancy after developing IBD. There were 325 pregnancies and 18 elective abortions. Seventy-nine of the patients were female and they had 171 pregnancies (median 2). There were 154 pregnancies from the 76 male patients. One involved 65 pregnancies with parents who had not been on 6-MP. There was no statistical difference in spontaneous abortions, abortions sec-

TABLE 84-1. Safety of Inflammatory Bowel Disease Medications during Pregnancy

Safe	Limited Data	Contraindicated
Oral mesalamine	Azathioprine	Methotrexate
Topical mesalamine	6-Mercaptopurine	Thalidomide
Sulfasalazine	Cyclosporine	Diphenoxylate
Ciprofloxacin, metronidazole (after first trimester)	Infliximab	–
Corticosteroids	–	–

ondary to a birth defect, major congenital malformations, neoplasia, or increased infections among female or male patients taking 6-MP compared with controls. The authors concluded that 6-MP use before (40 pregnancies), at conception (24 pregnancies) or during pregnancy (15 pregnancies) appears to be safe. They felt that discontinuation of 6-MP before and during pregnancy was not indicated. Personally, I believe disease activity to be far more detrimental than AZA/6-MP and I usually advise patients to continue this medication both before and during pregnancy if they need an immunomodulator to remain in remission.*

Cyclosporine

Cyclosporine has been used again extensively during pregnancy in renal transplant patients and patients with systemic lupus erythematosus (SLE) (Bermas and Hill, 1995). The medical literature reports cyclosporine use to avoid colectomy in a few pregnant patients without fetal loss. However, nephrotoxicity, hypertension, and hepatoxicity are commonly reported in the pregnant patient and these are potential side effects of cyclosporine. One must therefore weigh the risk of medication toxicity versus urgent colectomy in the pregnant patient with severe colitis.

Methotrexate

Methotrexate (MTX) a folic acid antagonist is contraindicated before conception or during pregnancy. The drug is mutagenic and teratogenic with a high incidence of neural tube defects (Donnenfield et al, 1994). In male patients, MTX can produce oligospermia and chromosomal damage. If a patient has received MTX prior to attemting conception, folic acid should be prescribed (Narendranathan et al, 1989).

---

*Editor's Note: As mentioned, this issue is still controversial and most women want to stop the use of AZA/6-MP before conceiving. I share the author's view of staying on AZA, if needed, to maintain remission. To repeat, disease activity seemingly poses greater risks than immunomodular toxicity in most cases.

Infliximab

The Food and Drug Administration has classified infliximab as pregnancy category B; however, animal reproduction studies have not been conducted as infliximab does not cross react with tumor necrosis factor (TNF)-α in species other than humans and chimpanzees. Toxicity studies have been conducted in mice using an analogous antibody with no evidence of maternal toxicity or teratogenicity. A safety database is maintained by Centocor (Malvern, PA). Outcomes data in direct exposure to infliximab report similar live births, miscarriage rates and therapeutic termination to the general population. Pharmacokinetics of this chimeric antibody to TNF-α suggests a 3 to 6 month washout period to ensure infliximab is no longer present in circulation.

Disease Activity Assessment

Pregnant women by nature may have intermittent abdominal discomfort from the enlarging gravid uterus, pre-existing fibroids, changing bowel habits particularly constipation, bladder compression and gastroesophageal reflux. Other more serious causes of accelerating abdominal pain include cholelithiasis or choledocholithiasis, sphincter of oddi dysfunction, intra-abdominal or retroperitoneal abscess, and toxemia of pregnancy.

Because anemia and erythrocyte sedimentation rate (ESR) elevations occur in pregnancy, basic laboratory parameters (complete blood count, ESR, and albumin) are usually of little value unless there is a dramatic fall of hemoglobin or albumin or a rise of two to three fold of the erythrocyte sedimentation rate.

Diagnostic imaging by either transabdominal ultrasound or magnetic resonance are considered safe in the pregnant patient. If concern for an acute complication such as perforation exists, the suprapubic area can be shielded with a lead apron, and an obstruction series to rule out pneumoperitoneum can be performed. Risk to the fetus from the radiograph is considered minimal when clinical necessity is paramount.

Upper endoscopy may be indicated in the patient with intractable nausea and vomiting in the setting of hematemesis. Note that intravenous *propofol (diprovan)* for sedation is pregnancy category B, *demerol (meperidine)* category C, and versed (*midazolam*) category D. Flexible sigmoidoscopy may be safely performed in the patient with UC. Colonoscopy is rarely necessary in pregnancy though some clinicians feel that it can be performed safely.

Perforation, hemodynamically significant or transfusion dependent gastrointestinal bleeding and severe medication refractory disease are absolute indications for surgery. If invasive intervention is necessary, the "safest" opportunity, according to surgeons and obstetricians, is the *second trimester* though fetal demise can approach 50%.

Women with ileo-anal anastomotic pouches and conventional Brooke ileostomies are often concerned about abnormal bowel function during pregnancy. Several of my patients have developed parastomal hernias requiring revision of the ileostomy at cesarean delivery. One patient developed distal small bowel obstruction postpartum as the boggy uterus compressed the ileal pouch. This resolved in time with nasogastric suction and pharmacologic assistance to the uterus.

Outcome of Pregnancy

In quiescent IBD epidemiologic and case controlled studies suggest that birth weight, prematurity, spontaneous abortion and congenital anomalies are no different from the general population. Importantly, active CD prior to conception and/or during the pregnancy may account for adverse events of pre-term delivery or fetal loss. Thus, both delaying pregnancy when the IBD is active and using maintenance therapy during pregnancy are good pieces of advice. However, a Swedish prospective population-based study reports increases in pre-term birth and small gestational size of babies with IBD mothers. Steroid use could be one factor in decreased birth weights.

Mode of Delivery

Population-based cohort studies reveal an increased rate of cesarean section for both patients with UC and CD versus the general population, 26% versus 13% respectively. Cesarean section is not necessary if there is no perineal disease or if the perianal disease is inactive. Mediolateral episiotomy is recommended to avoid rectal sphincter damage. However, Brandt and others report vaginal delivery and episiotomy may lead to perineal involvement in women with no prior perianal disease.

Summary

Pregnancy and IBD requires education and planning with the patient and physician. Folic acid supplementation prior to conception is essential. Disease activity should be managed expediently. I personally see my pregnant patients in each trimester and 6 to 8 weeks postpartum.

Supplemental Reading

Ahmad T, Armuzzi A, Bunce M, et al. The molecular classificaction of the clinical manifestations of Crohn's disease. Gastroenterology 2002;122:854–66.

Bermas BL, Hill JA. Effects of immunosuppressive drugs during pregnancy. Arthritis Rheum 1995;38:1722–32.

Brandt LJ, Estabrook SG, Reinus JF. Results of a survey to evaluate whether vaginal delivery and episiotomy lead to perineal involvement in women with Crohn's disease. Am J Gastroenterol 1995;90:1918–22.

Brant SR, Picco MF, Achkar JP, et al. Defining complex contributions of NOD2/CARD gene mutations, age at onset and tobacco cases on Crohn's disease phenotypes. Inflamm Bowel Dis 2003;9:381–8.

Diav-Citrin O, Park YH, Veerasuntharam G. The safety of mesalamine in human pregnancy: a prospective controlled cohort study. Gastroenterology 1998;114:23–8.

Donnenfield AE, Pastuszak A, Nash JS, et al. Methotrexate exposure prior to and during pregnancy. Teratology 1994;49:79–81.

Francella A, Dylan A, Bodian C, et al. The safety of 6-mercaptopurine for childbearing patients with inflammatory bowel disease: a retrospective cohort study. Gastroenterology 2003;124:9–17.

Khosla R, Willoughby CP, Jewell DP. Crohn's disease and pregnancy. Gut 1984;25:52–6.

Mogadam M, Dobbins WO, Korelitz BI. Pregnancy and inflammatory bowel disease: effect of sulfasalazine and corticosteroids on fetal outcome. Gastroenterology 1981;80:72–6.

Narendranathan M, Sandler RS, Suchindran M. Male infertility in inflammatory bowel disease. J Clin Gastroenterol 1989;11:403–6.

Ogura Y, Bonen DK, Inohara N, et al. A frameshift mutation in NoD2 associated with susceptibility to Crohn's disease. Nature 2001;411:603–6.

Olsen KO, Juul S, Berndisson, et al. Ulcerative colitis: female fecundity before diagnosis, during disease, and after surgery compared with a population sample. Gastroenterology 2002;122:15–9.

Orholm M, Fonager K, Sorensen HT. Risk of ulcerative colitis and Crohn's disease among offspring of patients with chronic inflammatory bowel disease. Am J Gastroenterol 1999;94:3236–8.

Sachar D. Exposure to mesalamine during pregnancy increase preterm deliveries (but not birth defects) and decrease birth weight. Gut 1998;43:316.

Yang, H, McElree C, Roth MP, et al. Familial empirical risks for inflammatory bowel disease: differences between Jews and non-Jews. Gut 1993;34:517–24.

CHAPTER 85

INTESTINAL AND COLONIC STRICTURES

RICHARD KOZAREK, MD

Fixed strictures of the small or large intestine need to be distinguished from extrinsic compression or acute gut angulation as a consequence of adhesions. They must also be distinguished from dynamic processes to include mural spasm, intussusception, and volvulus. Colonic strictures are most common, particularly following anastomoses in which there is a postoperative leak, pelvic abscess, or previous pelvic irradiation (Kozarek, 2001; Kozarek, 2003). Table 85-1 outlines additional causes of benign and malignant colonic strictures. Intestinal strictures, in turn, are mostly inflammatory and are the consequence of acid-peptic disease and nonsteroidal anti-inflammatory drug (NSAID) use in the proximal gut and inflammatory bowel disease (IBD) and anastomotic cicatrization in the mid and distal small bowel. Other etiologies are listed in Table 85-2.

As important as defining the presence of a gut stenosis by endoscopy, barium contrast studies, or abdominal computed tomography (CT) is the delineation of its etiology and clinical significance. Is it simply a radiographic phenomenon with marginal clinical importance? Or are there true obstructive symptoms, which might include pain, nausea and vomiting plus early satiety in intestinal stenoses, and obstipation, tenesmus and passage of small or ribbon-like stools in more distal bowel obstruction? Evidence of concomitant weight loss and bleeding may be particularly important signs that push the clinician into an aggressive workup that requires full examination of the stricture in question. Whether the latter occurs endoscopically using small caliber instruments, contrast injection through a catheter placed within a stricture, or even a capsular endoscope for mid to distal strictures (recognizing impaction and obstruction as a potential problem) or occurs with radiologic imaging in conjunction with tumor markers (eg, CEA, CA19-9, CA-125), it is most important to rule out a malignant etiology of the stricture. The latter may be relatively evident such as the invariable young and female patient who develops gastric outlet obstruction in the setting of chronic NSAID use for headaches or the individual who develops an anastomotic leak or pelvic abscess following bowel resection for diverticulitis. Alternatively, a stricture in an area of diverticulosis, as well as in the setting of chronic ulcerative colitis, is considered malignant until proven otherwise. Diagnosis depends, therefore, on endoscopically assessing the entire stricture with histologic confirmation of benignity. Even then, sometimes ambiguous strictures remain which may require open or laparoscopic examination for definitive diagnosis.

Management

The correct management of gut stenoses presupposes that a correct diagnosis has been made. Asymptomatic strictures in which benignity has been defined with certainty usually need no treatment.

Upper Gastrointestinal Strictures

The most common benign causes of proximal gut obstruction are iatrogenic and best treated by prevention (Table 85-3). These include absolute NSAID interdiction in the patient with recurrent peptic ulcer disease and pyloric channel or postbulbar stenoses (Kozarek et al, 1990; Solt et al, 2003). They also include ulcer (and subsequent stricture) prophylaxis in patients who undergo a pylorus-preserving Whipple procedure or total pancreatectomy. Both of the latter procedures predispose to ulceration because decreased bicarbonate secretion by the pancreas and ulcer risk with or without concomitant stricture, approximate 20% and 50%, respectively, in my medical center.

TABLE 85-1. Common Causes of Colonic Strictures

Cancer
    Colon
    Ovarian
    Drop metastases (gastric)
Inflammatory bowel disease
    Crohn's
    Ulcerative colitis
Ischemic colitis
    Occlusive/nonocclusive
    Abdominal aortic aneurysm repair
Postoperative/anastomotic
Diverticulitis
Irradiation
Miscellaneous
    Infections
    Caustic enemas
    Circumferential endotherapy

TABLE 85-2. Common Causes of Intestinal Strictures

Proximal gut
   Acid peptic
   NSAIDs
   Anastomotic
   Miscellaneous, eg, annular pancreas, duodenal web
   Malignancy
      Primary duodenal/jejunal adenocarcinoma
         Metastatic infiltration; eg, pancreatic, gallbladder, bile duct
Mid-distal gut
   Crohn's disease
   NSAIDs
   Anastomotic strictures
   Malignancy
      Jejunal adenocarcinoma
      Ileal lymphoma/carcinoid
   Miscellaneous
      Infectious
      Ischemic

NSAIDs = nonsteroidal anti-inflammatory drugs

Proximal intestinal stenoses, including anastomotic strictures initially only amenable to surgical therapy, have primarily been treated with dilatating balloons (Figure 85-1). The latter technology has evolved from single diameter balloons placed over an endoscopically or fluoroscopically placed guide wire to single diameter through-the-scope (TTS) balloons to dilatating balloons that have a variable diameter contingent upon balloon insufflation pressure (eg, continuous radial expansion [CRE] balloons, Microvasive Inc., Natick, MA). Whatever dilatation technique or technology is adopted, however, the goals are the following: (1) luminal enlargement safely and (2) prevention of restenosis.

Benign Strictures

As dilatation has been available for almost two decades, most of the series attesting to its efficacy in 80 to 90% of patients are older (Kozarek et al, 1990). Nevertheless, several issues deserve mention. On the one hand, it is important to recognize that extrinsic lesions, including annular pancreas as well as malignancies, cause proximal C loop obstruction, and other abdominal imaging procedures (eg, CT scan) should be considered before treatment in all but the most obvious cases of proximal gastric outlet obstruction. On the other hand, there are certain situations in which dilatation is much less likely to be successful. The latter include long, acutely angulated stenoses and situations in which ongoing intestinal insult occurs. Occasionally the consequence of ongoing acid secretion surreptitious NSAID use is actually a considerably more common cause. Finally, from a technical standpoint, taking a 2 mm stricture to 15 to 20 mm in a single dilatating session seems risky and is likely to increase the 1 to 5% perforation rate quoted by most authors. As such, multiple dilatating sessions over a period of weeks or even months, perhaps accompanied by four quadrant steroid injections, seems preferable to perforation (Miyashita et al, 1997). By way of example, a recent publication by Solt and colleagues (2003) reported 177 dilatation procedures in 72 patients with benign disease. At a mean follow-up of 98 months, symptomatic relief was noted in 80%, and 70% maintained that relief at 3 months. There were two perforations and one case of procedure-related bleeding, and approximately one-quarter of patients developed recurrent stenosis requiring repeat dilatation.

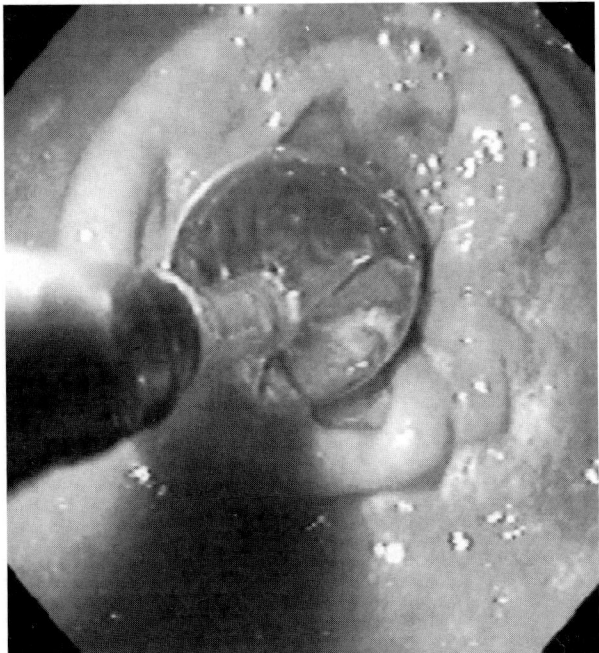

FIGURE 85-1. Balloon dilatation of benign gastric outlet obstruction in a patient with chronic aspirin ingestion.

TABLE 85-3. Endoscopic Therapies Available for Benign Intestinal and Colonic Strictures

Upper intestinal tract
   Prevention
        NSAID interdiction, chronic ulcer disease
        Acid suppression, pylorus-preserving Whipple
   Dilatation
        Balloon; eg, TTS/CRE
        Corticosteroid injection into stricture
   Surgery
Mid-distal small bowel/colon
   Dilatation
      Savary versus balloon type
      ± Corticosteroid injection
   Radial incisions
   SEMS
   Surgery

CRE = continuous radial expansion; NSAID = nonsteroidal anti-inflammatory drug; SB = small bowel; SEMS = self-expandable metallic stent; TTS = through-the-scope.

Malignant Strictures

Proximal and unresectable malignant strictures, in turn, have usually been treated with surgical bypass or, occasionally, palliative resection (Table 85-4). The latter has been associated with morbidity of 20 to 40% and mortality rates ranging from 0 to 20% (Nassif et al, 2003). As a consequence, self-expandable metal stents (SEMS) have been used with increased frequency, particularly in patients with late stage gastric outlet obstruction in the setting of pancreaticobiliary malignancy (Wong et al, 2002; Adler and Baron, 2002; Nassif et al, 2003; Mosler et al, 2004). Although many esophageal prostheses have been used (Z stent, Wilson-Cook, Inc., Winston-Salem, NC; Ultraflex, Microvasive, Inc., Natick, MA; and EsophaCoil, Medtronics, Inc., Eden Prairie, MN), most US series have used the only TTS prosthesis currently released by the Food and Drug Administration, the Enteral Wallstent (Microvasive, Inc., Natick, MA) (Figure 85-2). The latter prosthesis, ranging between 6 to 9 cm in length and 18 to 22 mm in diameter, is released after stricture delineation by contrast injection through the stenosis or submucosal injection of contrast proximally and distally at the margins of the tumor (Figure 85-3).

Technical success rates for stent placement approximate 90 to 95%, although a second stent is needed in up to one-third of placements (Mosler et al, 2004). Functional success rates allowing intake of soft foods or full liquids, in turn, have been reported to be 80 to 90% (Nassif et al, 2003) and complications include both short term (bleeding, perforation, and malplacement) as well as long term (erosion/perforation, migration, bleeding, and obstruction). Most series

TABLE 85-4. Treatment Modalities for Malignant Intestinal and Colonic Stenoses

Upper intestinal tract
    Surgery
        Resection
        Bypass
    Endoscopic Rx
        Dilatation/enteric stent placement
        ± Diverting PEG/feeding PEJ
Mid-distal SB/Colon
    Surgery
    Endoscopic Rx
        Dilatation – balloon versus Savary-type
        SEMS
            Palliative Rx
            Preoperatively

PEG = percutaneous endoscopic gastrostomy; PEJ = percutaneous endoscopic jejunostomy; SB = small bowel; SEMS = self-expandable metal stent.

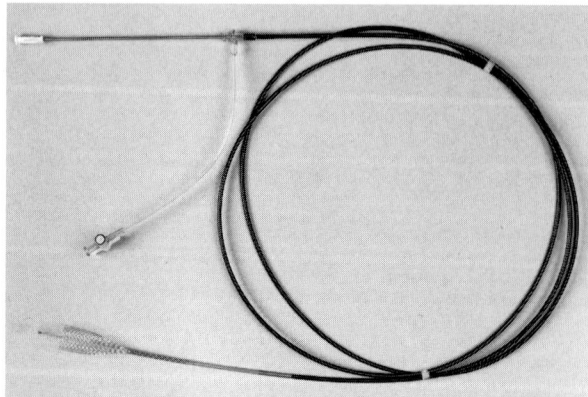

FIGURE 85-2. Enteral Wallstent delivery system.

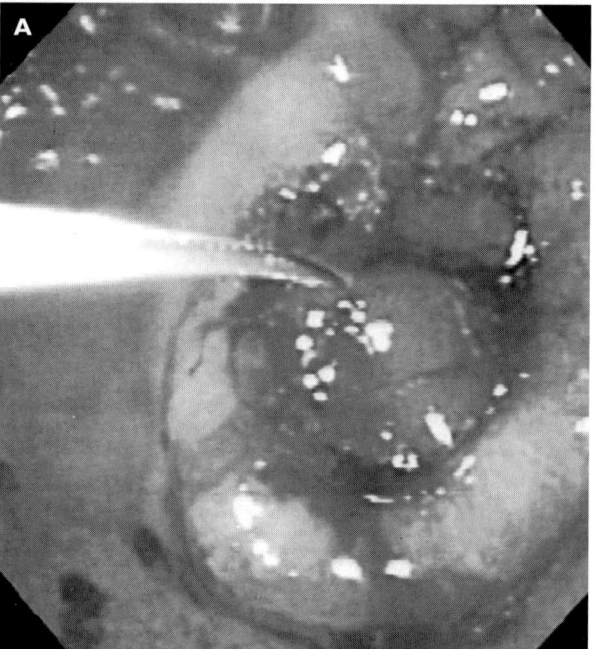

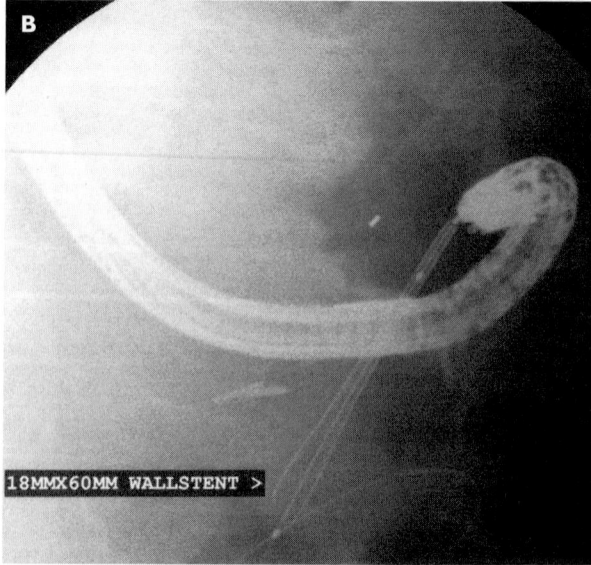

FIGURE 85-3. C-loop Wallstents in patient with primary pancreatic malignancy (A to F). Note incomplete distal prosthesis expansion (B) treated with second prosthesis (D,E, and F). *Continued on next page.*

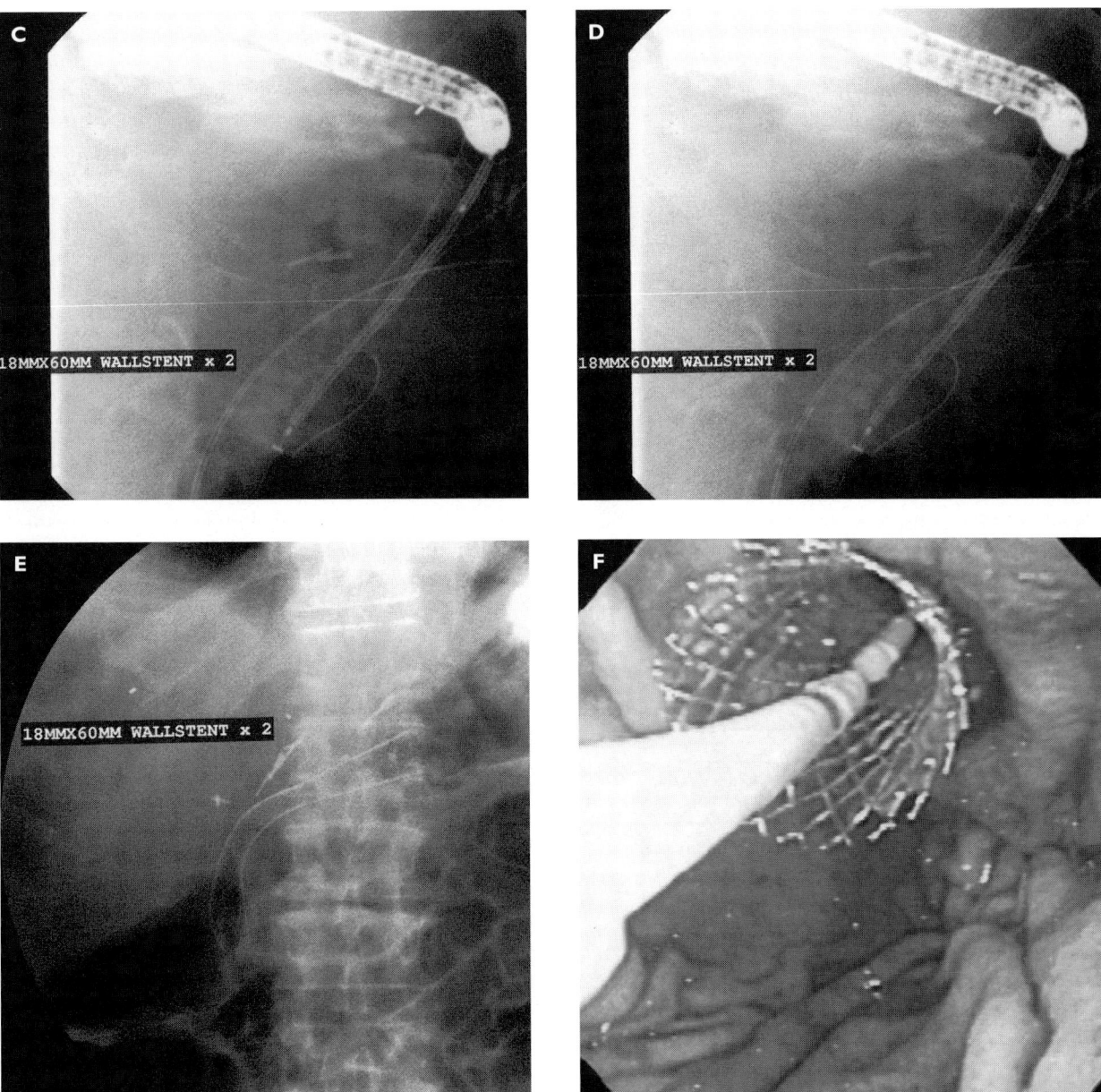

FIGURE 85-3 Continued. C-loop Wallstents in patient with primary pancreatic malignancy (A to F). Note incomplete distal prosthesis expansion (B) treated with second prosthesis (D,E, and F).

cited earlier report a survival approximating only 2 to 4 months after SEMS insertion for upper gastrointestinal (GI) malignancies, and, at the time of this writing, there have been no randomized studies comparing upper GI tract stenting to palliative surgery. There have, however, been large single center series, and a recent multicenter trial by Nassif and colleagues (2003) reported 63 patients in whom stent placement was attempted. Successful in 60 (95%), there was no procedure-related mortality, but 30% of the patients developed complications including 13 stent obstructions, 4 migrations, and 2 duodenal perforations. Median survival was 7 weeks.

Colonic Strictures

As in the upper GI tract, symptomatic strictures of the colon were traditionally treated surgically (Cappell and Friedel, 2002). Not only did surgery allow definitive diagnosis of malignancy or benignity, particularly in the setting of IBD, it could also theoretically be "curative" in contrast to dilatation. Several problems were noted, however. There was significant procedural morbidity, particularly when operating on an acutely obstructed patient necessitating performance of a two-stage operation in an attempt to minimize anastomotic leak. Nor was palliative resection a "cure" for patients with malignant ascites or liver metastasis or even in patients with Crohn's stenosis in whom recurrence, usually proximal to the anastomosis, is invariable (Kozarek, 2001). Finally, surgery has been associated with further stenosis with anastomotic leak, pelvic abscess, and local anastomotic ischemia (Porcellini et al, 1996). All of the above have helped push endoscopic therapy to the forefront in many cases of colonic stricture.

Benign Disease

Comparable to upper GI tract stenoses, the evolution of balloon technology has allowed dilatation of previously inaccessible colon strictures, although distal lesions had previously been amenable to Savary-type dilators placed over a guide wire (Morini et al, 2001). Although stricture delineation can be done using an initial water-soluble or barium contrast study, it can also be done endoscopically. Techniques include use of a pediatric colonoscope or small caliber upper endoscope to fully visualize and biopsy the stenosis or injection of contrast through the scope using a combination of fluoroscopic and endoscopic control. Currently, I prefer endoscopically placed CRE-type balloons over a guide wire and rely on fluoroscopic control to assure obliteration of the balloon waist as a measure of efficacy (Figure 85-4). Whether the balloon needs to be fully inflated for 15, 30, 60, or 300 seconds for improved efficacy has not been studied and it is my personal opinion that waist effacement of the balloon resulting in stricture fracture (as opposed to simple stretch) is the therapeutic goal.

Most anastomotic strictures, short (< 5 cm) Crohn's strictures, and some ischemic strictures, particularly those that are the consequence of abdominal aneurysm resection, have proven amenable to balloon endotherapy, whereas long, ischemic and diverticular strictures of the intraperitoneal colon are best left to surgical or conservative management.

Comparable to treatment of benign upper GI strictures, most endoscopists use balloon dilatation as primary therapy, ultimately trying to achieve luminal enlargement to a

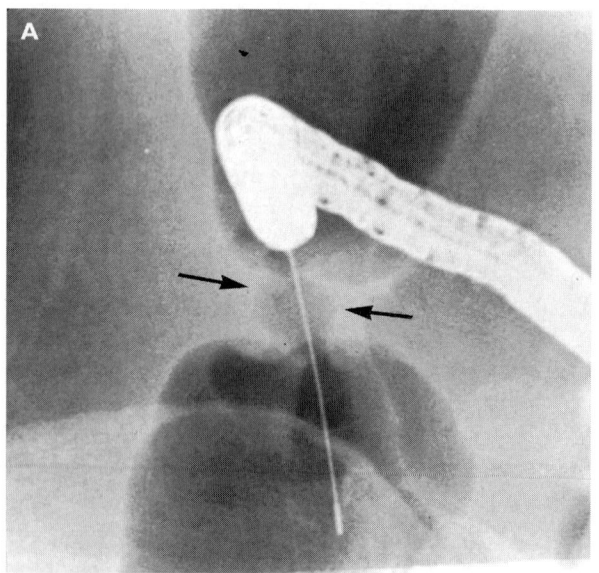 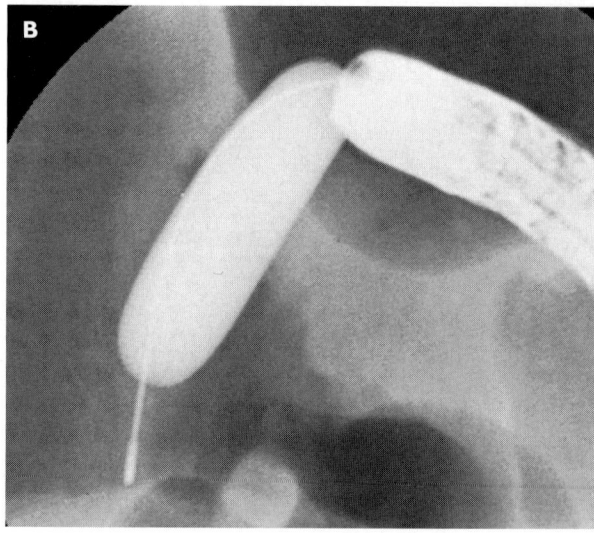

FIGURE 85-4. Arrows delineate short, annular stricture in a patient with obstructive Crohn's (A), treated with 12 to 15 mm CRE balloon (B). CRE = continuous radial expansion.

TABLE 85-5. Use of Balloon Dilatation for Anastomotic and Ileocolonic Stenoses

Author	Number of Patients	Successful Dilatation (%)	Successful Treatment (%)	Complications (%)	Follow-Up (months)
Couckayt et al	55	90	62	11	12
Ramboer et al*	13	85	85	0	7
Rolny et al	27	100	66	15	7 to 38
Unereset al	33	100	51	NS	NS

NS = not specified.
*Includes radial cautery incisions.

*Editor's Note: The results with anastomotic strictures in Crohn's disease have been best if it was over 7 years since surgery (TMB).

TABLE 85-6. Self-Expandable Metallic Stents Marketed/Used for Colonic Stenoses

SEMS	Stent Diameters (mm)	Length Delivery Catheter (cm)	Delivery Catheter Size (F)	Material
Z	25	40	31	Stainless steel
Memotherm	25, 30	120	14.5	Nitinol
Enteral Wallstent	18, 20, 22	135, 255	10	Elgiloy
CoRectCoil	18,20	80	32	Nitinol
Choostent	22	75, 120	12	Nitinol
Niti-S	20, 22, 24	100	24	Nitinol

final diameter of 15 to 20 mm, although use of achalasia dilatators up to 30 to 40 mm have been reported in stenoses below the peritoneal reflection (Virgilio et al, 1995). Table 85-5 outlines some of the series reporting results of balloon dilatation.* Benign colonic and anastomotic strictures have also been dilated with Savary-type dilatators, particular with distal lesions, injected with long acting corticosteroids after initial stricture split, and even treated with SEMS (Luck et al, 2001; Kozarek, 2001). There have been no controlled trials using steroid injections but there are parallels to such treatment to include corticosteroid injection into keloids or refractory and acid-peptic strictures. In contrast, SEMS placement is clearly investigational and, from a personal perspective, should not be used in otherwise good-risk surgical patients or those patients with a prolonged survival prognosis.

Malignant Disease

Malignant colon strictures can also be dilatated with the above-mentioned technologies but results are transient and usually done in conjunction with other treatment modalities. Historically, unresectable or poor surgical risk patients presenting with bleeding or obstruction were invariably treated with Nd:YAG laser ablative therapy (Figure 85-5). More recently, however, SEMS insertion has evolved both to treat unresectable malignancies in patients who would have historically undergone palliative decompressive colostomy and as a preoperative procedure in obstructed, resectable patients conventionally treated with two-stage operations (Kozarek, 2001; Martinez-Santos et al, 2002; Khot et al, 2002; Dauphine et al, 2002; Kozarek, 2000; Kozarek, 2002). A recent meta-analysis of the latter approach suggests a 20 to 60% morbidity and a 5 to 20% mortality in patients with obstructing colorectal cancer treated surgically (Keymling, 2003).

Colorectal Prostheses

A number of prostheses have been used worldwide for obstructing colorectal neoplasms (Table 85-6). Technically, strictures are usually delineated using a small caliber endoscope or a combination of endoscopy and contrast injected fluoroscopically. Prostheses should be 4 to 5 cm longer than the stricture to be stented, and technically stents can be inserted through the scope (eg, Enteral Wallstent), alongside it over a previously placed guide wire using a combination of endoscopy and fluoroscopy, or using fluoroscopy alone (Figure 85-7).

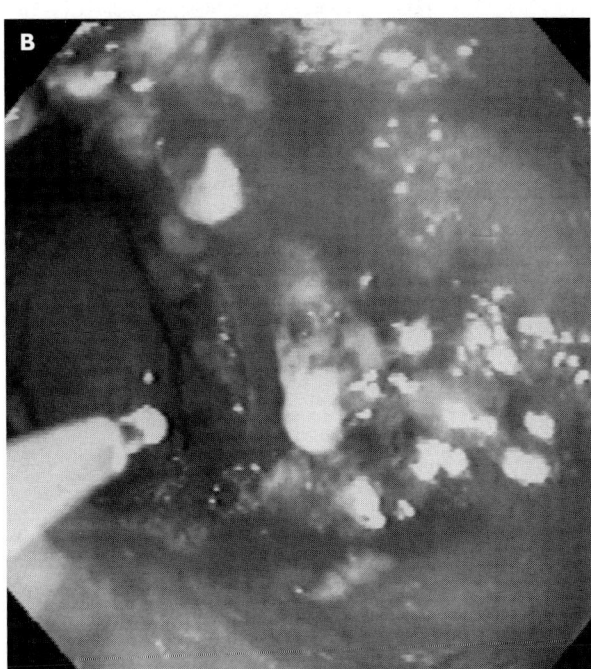

FIGURE 85-5. Bulky intraluminal tumor undergoing photoablation with Nd:YAG laser fiber (A, B).

In a recent analysis of multiple series using prostheses for obstructing colorectal neoplasms, there was a 93% technical success rate in 234 patients in whom stenting was attempted (Khot et al, 2002). There was a 90% success rate clinically and a 9% total complication rate (bleeding, perforation, malplacement, migration). Fifty-eight percent of patients were stented under fluoroscopic control alone, 11% under endoscopic control, and 31% underwent insertion using both modalities.

Despite the encouraging data noted above, it should be stressed that there have been no controlled trials randomizing stent insertion versus surgery in patients with unresectable, malignant colon obstructions (intrinsic or extrinsic). Nor have controlled trials been done randomizing stent insertion preoperatively in resectable but obstructed individuals versus two-stage surgery. Nevertheless, as the technology continues to improve and techniques become standardized, SEMS insertion for malignant colorectal obstruction is only likely to increase. There is a separate chapter on palliation for colorectal cancer (see Chapter 99, "Palliative Therapy for Rectal Cancer").

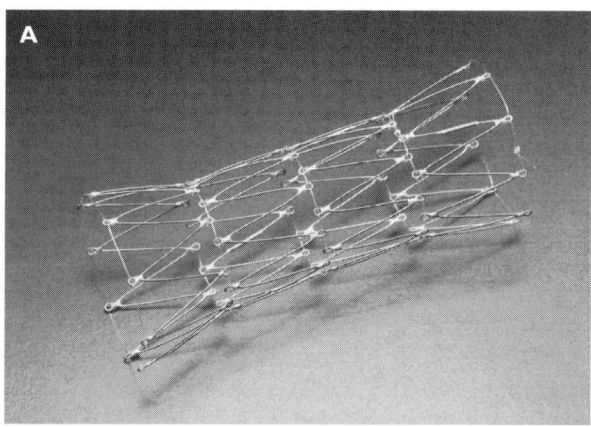

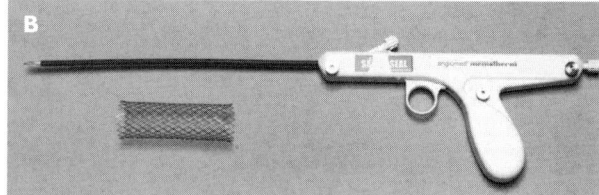

FIGURE 85-6. Colonic Z (A) and Memotherm (B) SEMS. The latter is released using a "pistol-type" delivery system. SEMS = self-expandable metal stent.

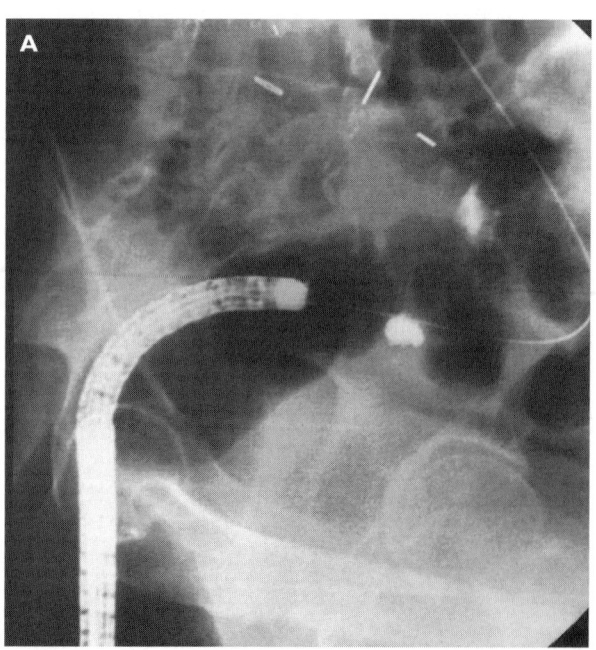

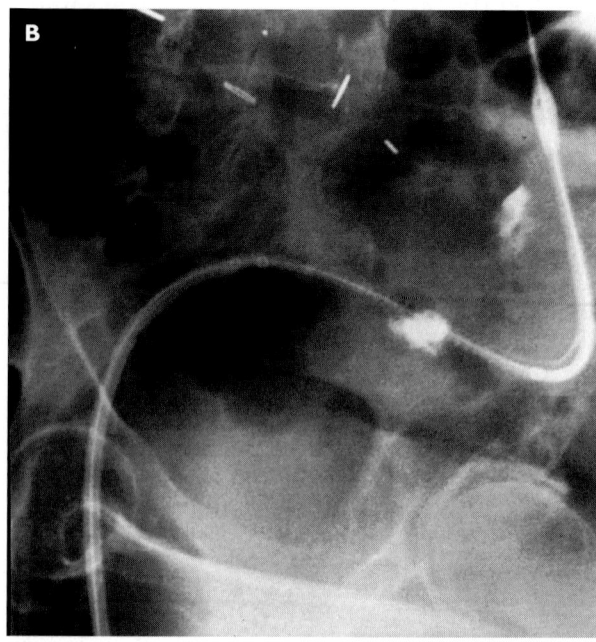

FIGURE 85-7. Malignant sigmoid stricture is delineated using a small caliber upper endoscope, the tumor margins marked with contrast injection (A), followed by fluoroscopic release of Ultraflex stent placed over an endoscopically placed guidewire (B, C, and D). Arrows outline expanded stent. *Continued on next page.*

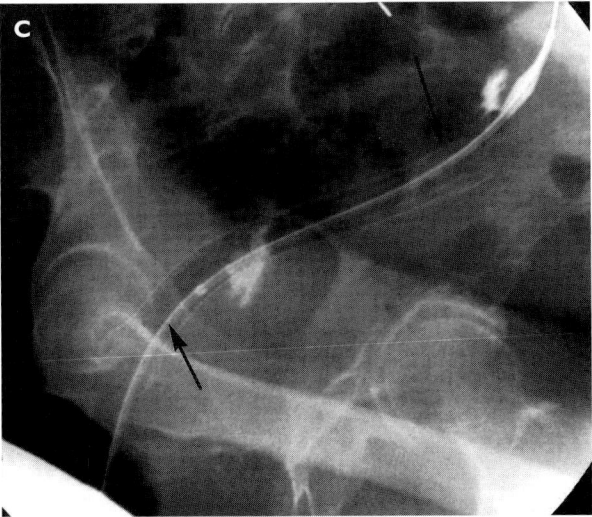
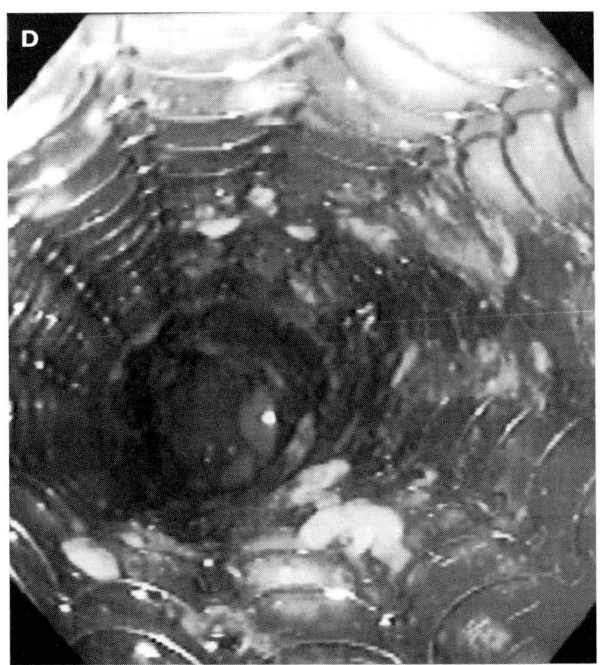

FIGURE 85-7 Continued. Fluoroscopic release of Ultraflex stent placed over an endoscopically placed guidewire (C, and D). Arrows outline expanded stent.

Conclusions

Intestinal and colonic strictures require thorough evaluation using endoscopic and other imaging modalities to define benign versus malignant disease. Good surgical risk patients with potentially resectable malignancy should undergo resective surgery, although preoperative decompression with nasogastric suction, stricture dilatation, a colon decompression tube, or preoperative SEMS insertion may decrease postoperative complications or need for a two-stage operation. In unresectable patients with malignant strictures, SEMS offer an alternative to current surgical bypass, decompressive gastrostomy, or comfort care measures. With technologic refinements to include smaller delivery devices and increased use of TTS technology as well as refinements in the prostheses and the accuracy in their delivery, I predict that SEMS will be used with increased frequency, despite the lack of controlled clinical trials.

Supplemental Reading

Adler DG, Baron TH. Endoscopic palliation of malignant gastric outlet obstruction using self-expandable metal stents: experience in 36 patients. Am J Gastroenterol 2002;97:72–8.

Cappell MS, Friedel D. The role of sigmoidoscopy and colonoscopy in the diagnosis and management of lower gastrointestinal disorders: endoscopic findings, therapy, and complications. Med Clin North Am 2002;86:1253–88.

Dauphine CE, Tan P, Beart RW Jr. Placement of self-expanding metal stents for acute malignant large bowel obstruction: a collective review. Ann Surg Oncol 2002;9:574–9.

Keymling M. Colorectal stenting. Endoscopy 2003;35:234–8.

Khot UP, Lang AW, Murali K, Parker MC. Systematic review of the efficacy and safety of colorectal stents. Br J Surg 2002;89:1096–102.

Kozarek RA. Bridging intestinal narrowings with prostheses. In: Tytgat GNJ, Classen M, Waye J, Nakazawa H, editors. Therapeutic endoscopy. 2nd ed. Philadelphia: WB Saunders; 2000. p. 39–58.

Kozarek RA. Endoscopic management of small bowel, anastomotic, and colonic strictures in Crohn's disease. In: Bayless TM, Hanauer SB, editors. Advanced therapy of inflammatory bowel disease. 2nd ed. Hamilton (ON): BC Decker, Inc.; 2001. p. 509–13.

Kozarek RA. Gastrointestinal dilation and stent placement. In: Yamada T, Alpers DH, Kaplowitz N, et al, editors. Textbook of gastroenterology. 4th ed. Philadelphia: Lippincott Williams & Wilkins; 2003. p. 2988–99.

Kozarek RA. Intestinal tract stenting. In: Classen M, Tytgat GNJ, Lightdale C, editors. Gastroenterological endoscopy. New York: Georg Thieme Verlag; 2002. p. 372–86.

Kozarek RA. Treatment of malignant colonic stenosis with self-expandable metallic stents. In: Galmiche JP, Tytgat GNJ, editors. Management of gastrointestinal lesions with malignant potential. Paris: John Libbey Eurotext; 2001. p. 93–9.

Kozarek RA, Botoman VA, Patterson DJ. Long-term follow-up in patients who have undergone balloon dilation for gastric outlet obstruction. Gastrointest Endosc 1990;36:558–9.

Luck A, Chapins P, Sinclair G, Hood J. Endoscopic laser stricturotomy and balloon dilation for benign colorectal strictures. A NZ J Surg 2001;71:594–7.

Martinez-Santos C, Lobato RF, Fradyas JM, et al. Self-expandable stent before elective surgery vs emergency surgery for the treatment of malignant colorectal obstructions: comparison of primary anastomosis and morbidity rates. Dis Colon Rectum 2002;45:401–6.

Miyashita M, Onda M, Okawa K, et al. Endoscopic dexamethasone injection following balloon dilation of an anastomotic stricture after esophagogastrostomy. Am J Surg 1997;174:442–4.

Morini S, Hassan C, Cerro P, Lorenzetti R. Management of an ileocolonic anastomotic stricture using polyvinyl over-the-guidewire dilators in Crohn's disease. Gastrointest Endosc 2001;53:384–6.

Mosler P, Mergener KD, Brandabur J, et al. Palliation of gastric outlet obstruction and proximal small bowel obstruction with self-expandable metal stents – a single center series. J Clin Gastroenterol 2004. [In press]

Nassif T, Prat B, Meduri J, et al. Endoscopic palliation of malignant gastric outlet obstruction using self-expandable stents: results of a multicenter study. Endoscopy 2003;36:483–9.

Porcellini M, Rend A, Selvetalla L, et al. Intestinal ischemia after aortic surgery. Int Surg 1996;81:195–9.

Solt V, Bayer J, Szabo ÖM, Horvath G. Long-term results of balloon catheter dilation for benign gastric outlet stenosis. Endoscopy 2003;35:490–5.

Virgilio C, Cosentino S, Favara C, et al. Endoscopic treatment of postoperative colonic strictures using an achalasia dilator: short-term and long-term results. Endoscopy 1995;27:219–22.

Wong YT, Brams DM, Munson L, et al. Gastric outlet obstruction secondary to pancreatic cancer: surgical vs endoscopic palliation. Surg Endosc 2002;16:310–2.

CHAPTER 86

ACUTE COLONIC PSEUDO-OBSTRUCTION

Parviz Nikoomanesh, MD, and Salim A. Jaffer, MD

Acute pseudo-obstruction of the colon is the massive dilatation of the colon without evidence of mechanical obstruction. When acute pseudo-obstruction occurs without evidence of colonic disease, it is known as Ogilvie's syndrome, and occurs as a complication of an underlying clinical condition. If perforation, usually of the cecum, occurs, the mortality rate can be as high as 50%.

Patients with acute colonic pseudo-obstruction are usually postoperative or critically ill. The numerous conditions associated with pseudo-obstruction include recent surgery, trauma, metabolic disturbances, electrolyte imbalance, sepsis, infections, narcotics and other medications, hypothyroidism, diabetes, renal failure, myocardial infarction, inflammatory processes, and prolonged bed rest. It is more predominant in males and is most commonly reported in the sixth decade of life. It is almost always temporary and reversible. Acute pseudo-obstruction is believed to result from an imbalance between neurotransmitters of the sympathetic and the parasympathetic neurons.

Patients with acute pseudo-obstruction have a soft, but distended, and tympanic abdomen. Bowel sounds are high pitched to absent. Patients usually do not have peritoneal signs or colicky pain, but may precipitate vague abdominal pain as the cecum distends. Nausea and vomiting may be present. Patients may pass flatus and liquid stools or they may be obstipated. White blood cell (WBC) count is usually normal.

Radiographs

Plain abdominal roentgenographs are the most useful tests in the diagnosis and the management of acute pseudo-obstruction. The dilatated colon is gas filled with small amounts of fluid. The haustral and the mucosal pattern are maintained. The cecum is dilatated. Importantly, the abdominal radiograph provides information on the degree of dilatation. It also allows the clinician to follow the day-to-day progression or regression of the colonic dilatation. The cecum has the largest diameter and is most susceptible to *perforation*. The risk increases as the cecum dilatates to > 12 cm. Application of the law of Laplace predicts that the tension on the colonic wall is directly proportional to the diameter of the cecum as well as the pressure within it and is inversely proportional to the thickness of the cecal wall. As the diameter and the pressure of the cecum increases, the tension of the cecal wall increases. The risk of *spontaneous perforation* is about 3% and carries a *mortality* of 50%. Hence, early diagnosis and effective management is critical.

Conservative Management

Initial conservative management of acute pseudo-obstruction is appropriate in the absence of significant abdominal pain and peritoneal signs, and with cecal diameter < 12 cm. This approach is successful in 86 to 96% of the cases within 3 days of management. There are no controlled data available comparing the efficacy of initial conservative treatment with interventional management. Initial management aims at correcting and managing underlying clinical complications and withdrawing offending agents. A meticulous chart review and a careful history and physical examination are performed to elucidate the etiologies of pseudo-obstruction. The principles of conservative management of pseudo-obstruction are based on the knowledge of these risk factors. The following must be accomplished promptly:

1. Oral feedings discontinued, the patient admitted to the intensive care unit (ICU), and an intravenous (IV) line placed for hydration.
2. Nasogastric tube placed for gastric decompression and a rectal tube placed to decompress the rectum and the colon.
3. Rectal enemas used to liquefy the stools. This will also aid in colonic decompression and increase the visibility during endoscopy if required in the future.
4. All *narcotic analgesics* and *opioids discontinued* immediately.
5. All *anxiolytics, anticholinergics, calcium channel antagonists,* and *antidepressant agents* also are discontinued.
6. Any medication that effects the colonic motility discontinued. Common miscellaneous drugs including chemotherapeutic agents, phenothiazines and *antidiarrheal* medications (eg, loperamide, diphenoxylate plus atropine) have also been implicated in the precipitation of acute pseudo-obstruction. Only essential medications are continued in the ICU.
7. All electrolyte imbalances, especially hypokalemia, cor-

rected promptly. Also abnormalities of calcium, magnesium, phosphate, bicarbonate, sodium and other electrolytes are potentially important in the precipitation of pseudo-obstruction.

8. All sources of infections sought and treated with appropriate IV antibiotics. If the WBC count is elevated, this should raise an index of suspicion for an underlying infection as an etiology for pseudo-obstruction. A chest radiograph may aid in making a diagnosis of pneumonia in a hospitalized patient. A urine analysis will detect an underlying urinary tract infection. A diagnostic paracentesis is required in a patient with ascites and elevated WBC, fever, or peritoneal signs.
9. Analysis of cerebrospinal fluid in a patient with neurological signs and symptoms of meningitis is necessary. A two-dimensional echocardiogram of the heart in a patient with new onset murmur is justified.
10. Prolonged bed rest avoided. Frequent turning of the patient and early ambulation is desirable and encouraged.

Abdominal radiographs, metabolic panel, and a complete blood count with differential are obtained on a daily basis in the ICU. Daily abdominal radiography allows the clinician to follow the course of colonic dilatation. If the patient has no peritoneal signs and the cecum is < 12 cm, the patient is followed and observed conservatively for 48 to 72 hours in the ICU. If the caliber of colonic distension is regressing, conservative management with daily problem focused physical examination is continued. Abdominal sounds are auscultated daily to assure peristalsis and functioning bowel. The patient should be passing gas and fecal material, and improving clinically. IV fluid is continued, as are all conservative measures.

Pharmacologic Management

The success of pharmacologic treatment of acute pseudo-obstruction of the colon has been reported in a number of studies. Most experience comes from the use of the parasympathomimetic drug neostigmine as an early alternative to colonoscopic decompression or surgery (Ponec et al, 1999). The aim is to increase the peristaltic activity of the colon and promote decompression. Neostigmine competes with acetylcholine for binding at acetylcholinesterase receptor sites. This increases acetylcholine and the excitatory parasympathetic effects on the colon. If the patient is not improving following 48 to 72 hours of conservative management and the cecal diameter is < 12 cm, pharmacologic treatment with neostigmine should be considered before interventional or surgical decompression. The clinical condition of each patient should be given specialized attention and the treatment tailored individually. The indications for pharmacologic management are as follows: (1) colonic distension progressively increasing beyond 10 cm up to 12 cm and (2) conservative management failing after 48 hours of treatment.

There should be no peritoneal signs, blood pressures must be > 90/60 mm Hg, and pulse > 60 beats/min. Contraindications to neostigmine use include recent use of β-blockers, bradycardia, hypotension, acidosis, recent myocardial infarction, renal failure, acute bronchospasm, and signs of bowel perforation. Mechanical obstruction must first be excluded by a Gastrografin study. Atropine must be available. Neostigmine is given intravenously at a dose of 2.5 mg in 100 mL saline infused over 5 minutes with electrocardiographic monitoring in the ICU. Neostigmine is effective and rapid decompression can be expected after a single dose. Median time to clinical response varies from 4 to 30 minutes as measured by time to pass flatus or stool. An abdominal film is obtained in 60 minutes to assess radiographic response. A second dose may be required and should be given 3 hours following the first dose. Side effects include postural hypotension, symptomatic bradycardia requiring atropine, abdominal pain, excessive salivation, and vomiting. Bradycardia can be avoided by prophylactically administering an antimuscarinic anticholinergic drug such as atropine (1 mg IV × 1) or glycopyrrolate (500 × μg IV × 1) prior to neostigmine use. Patients must remain supine for 1 hour after neostigmine use and vital signs checked every 10 minutes. Sustained response is seen more frequently in the elderly females, and those not on narcotics and not postsurgery.

Anecdotal success of *erythromycin* and *cisapride* use has been reported. Cisapride, no longer available in the United States, releases acetylcholine from the myenteric plexus and stimulates gastrointestinal motility. Erythromycin is a motilin agonist. However, there are no large controlled studies of either cisapride or erythromycin for treating acute colonic pseudo-obstruction.

Interventional Management

The colon and the cecum should be quantified with a measuring ruler and compared with previous abdominal radiographs each morning in the ICU. Each patient is given individualized care, and treatment is based not only on cecal diameters, but also on clinical history and condition. If the caliber of the cecum has surpassed 12 cm, or if cecal diameter is geometrically progressing beyond 10 cm, interventional measures are needed. The risk of cecal perforation does not have a linear relationship to its diameter. It is the rate of progression of cecal dilatation, the length of time the cecum has dilatated, and the clinical condition of the patient taken together which allows the clinician to assess the emergence of an impending rupture.

Colonoscopic Decompression

Colonoscopy is the initial invasive therapeutic modality when conservative management is no longer appropriate or has failed. However, controlled studies are lacking to define the colonoscopic standard of care in patients with pseudo-obstruction. The purpose of colonoscopy is to promptly decompress the colon and avoid colonic ischemia and cecal perforation. It has an initial success rate of 76 to 95% in achieving decompression. Colonoscopy also excludes a mechanical etiology of obstruction. The criteria used at our institution for performing colonoscopic suction decompression with or without endoscopic rectal tube placement include the following:

1. The caliber of cecal distension shows a geometric progression beyond 12 cm based on daily abdominal radiography at any point during hospitalization.
2. Patient continues to deteriorate clinically despite conservative and pharmacologic management, irrespective of the caliber of the cecum.
3. Colon shows persistent dilatation beyond 72 hours despite conservative and pharmacologic managements.

Colonoscopy in these patients may need to be done without bowel preparation, but is technically difficult; hence, it should be performed by an experienced endoscopist. One critical risk of colonoscopy is perforation, which carries a morbidity of 2.9% and mortality of 1%. Benefits achieved must be assessed against the risk of perforation and mortality. Common contraindications to endoscopy include perforated colon or suspicion of perforation, peritonitis with peritoneal signs, myocardial infarct, and patient noncompliance. As each and subsequent section of the colon is entered, air is suctioned to near collapse and the scope is advanced gently. Gas and liquid stool is suctioned until the colonic wall nearly collapses. It is optimal, but not necessary to reach the cecum. The colonoscope can be positioned at the hepatic flexure with no or minimal air insufflation. Colonoscopic suction decompression is very effective. Recurrences range from 0 to 65%, with a mean of 25%. Hence, repeat decompressions are often necessary. This recurrence can be minimized by the placement of the rectal tube endoscopically. A catheter is endoscopically placed deep within the colon for continuous drainage and decompression. Technically exhausting, rectal tubes are usually placed in one of three methods. Tubes may be carried into the colon along with the colonoscope during insertion, by direct placement through the channel of the scope, or over the endoscopically inserted guide wire following withdrawal of the colonoscope. Disposable colonic decompression tubes with 480-cm catheters (Wilson–Cook) uses a 0.035 inch guide wire and comes in 7.0, 8.5, 10.0, and 14.0 F sizes. Tubes passed through the channel of the endoscope are only about 2 mm in diameter and frequently get obstructed with fecal material. The tube is left in place until it is expelled by the peristaltic activity of the colon.

Surgery

Surgical intervention is necessary when colonoscopic decompression has failed on three attempts, there is a danger of impending cecal perforation, or when the patient has signs and symptoms or peritonitis and cecal perforation. Surgical intervention is associated with mortality of 20 to 40%. Right hemicolectomy, ileostomy and mucus fistula is performed for complicated pseudo-obstruction with perforation. In patients with ischemic bowel without perforation, a surgical consultation should be obtained. In patients without ischemia or perforation, percutaneous or laparoscopic cecostomy has been used to decompress the colon.

Supplemental Reading

ASGE Standard of Practice Committee statement: acute colonic pseudo-obstruction. Gastroendoscopy 2002;56:789–92.

Bode WE, Beart RW Jr, Spencer RJ, et al. Colonoscopic decompression for acute pseudo-obstruction of the colon (Ogilvie's syndrome). Am J Surg 1984;147:243.

Hutchinson R, Griffiths C. Acute colonic pseudo-obstruction: a pharmacological approach. Ann R Coll Surg Engl 1992;74:364–7.

Ponec RJ, Saunders MD, Kimmey MB. Neostigmine for the treatment of acute colonic pseudo-obstruction. N Engl J Med 1999;341:137–41.

Rex DK. Colonoscopy and acute colonic pseudo-obstruction. Gastrointest Endosc Clin N Am 1997;7:499–508.

Sloyer AF, Panella VS, Demas BE, et al. Ogilvie's syndrome. Successful management without colonoscopy. Dig Dis Sci 1988;2:1391–6.

Stephenson BM, Morgan AR, Salaman JR, Wheeler MH. Ogilvie's syndrome: a new approach to an old problem. Dis Colon Rectum, 1995;38:424–7.

Stephenson KR, Rodriguez-Bigas MA. Decompression of the large intestine in Ogilvie's syndrome by a colonoscopically placed long intestinal tube. Surg Endosc 1994;8:116.

CHAPTER 87

MICROSCOPIC COLITIS: COLLAGENOUS, LYMPHOCYTIC, AND EOSINOPHILIC COLITIS

MARCIA CRUZ-CORREA, MD, PHD, AND FRANCIS M. GIARDIELLO, MD

Definition

Microscopic colitis is a term encompassing collagenous and lymphocytic colitis. It denotes the absence of endoscopic (macroscopic) abnormalities in the presence of microscopic histopathology.

Collagenous and lymphocytic colitis are clinicopathologic syndromes that represent distinct, possibly autoimmune, forms of idiopathic inflammatory colonic bowel disease. Both disorders present as chronic, watery, noninfectious diarrhea in middle-aged patients with negative radiographic and endoscopic studies. Collagenous colitis predominantly occurs in women; lymphocytic colitis is found equally in both genders. Often there is intermittent, diffuse abdominal pain, and, not surprisingly, some patients have a previous diagnosis of irritable bowel syndrome (IBS). Routine blood studies generally show normal results, but elevations in the Westergren sedimentation rate and eosinophil count are not uncommon. Abnormalities in complement levels, serum immunoglobulins (Igs), and pANCA (antineutrophil cytoplasmic antibodies) may be found. Although stool studies are negative for pathogens and blood, up to 55% of patients have white blood cells in stool samples. Other medical conditions reported to occur concomitantly with collagenous and lymphocytic colitis include thyroid disease, inflammatory arthropathies, pernicious anemia, urethral fibrosis, vitiligo, and small bowel villous atrophy. This association is discussed in the chapter on celiac disease (Chapter 61, "Celiac Sprue and Related Problems").

Gastrointestinal (GI), radiographic, and endoscopic examinations are not diagnostic with collagenous colitis. By endoscopic examination, the colorectal mucosa is usually normal, although some nonspecific findings, such as erythema, paleness, and edema, have been reported in up to one-third of cases.

Mucosal Lacerations

Mucosal lacerations occurring during colonoscopic examination were recently described in three patients with collagenous colitis (Cruz-Correa et al, 2002).

The diagnosis of microscopic colitis is based on histologic examination of colorectal biopsies. A diffuse colitis is present with *lymphocytic infiltration* of the surface epithelium and lamina propria. The characteristic histopathologic finding in collagenous colitis is a distinctive *band of collagen* beneath the surface epithelium in colonic mucosa. The banding is most consistently noted in the right and transverse colon. Also, occasional damage to, flattening of, and/or detachment of the surface epithelium can be found. Rectal biopsies may show the lymphocytic colitis but little or no collagen banding, in contrast to samples taken in the more proximal colon.

Lymphocytic Colitis

In lymphocytic colitis, the colitis component is similar to collagenous colitis except that collagenous thickening does not occur. Because of the clinical and histopathologic similarity in these disorders, we currently consider them a single category of inflammatory bowel diseases (IBDs), "collagenous-lymphocytic colitis," for the purposes of treatment.

Diarrhea Pathogenesis

The pathogenesis of chronic diarrhea in collagenous lymphocytic colitis is multifactorial. Primarily, diarrhea appears to result from *net colonic fluid secretion*. This occurs from decreased luminal absorption secondary to damaged surface epithelium and collagen deposition, combined with a continued normal rate of secretion from intact crypts. In some patients, small bowel dysfunction has been noted, including *bile salt wasting*, *fatty acid malabsorption*, *small bowel net secretion*, and, rarely, *villous atrophy*. These additional abnormalities may exacerbate the diarrhea.

Underlying IBS and thyroid disease must also be considered as possible elements in the diarrheal diathesis. Because fecal diversion with an ileostomy leads to improvement in the diarrhea and histology, a role for the luminal contents and gut bacteria must be considered.

Medical Management

General Concepts

Limited experience exists in the treatment of collagenous lymphocytic colitis. There are single case reports and several small series but few randomized studies from which to draw firm conclusions. However, the following concepts to guide therapy can be gleaned from examination of the literature and the personal experience of the authors. First, collagenous lymphocytic colitis is an IBD that clinicopathologically responds to anti-inflammatory medications as used in idiopathic IBD (Crohn's disease and ulcerative colitis). Prompt improvement in diarrhea is noted in most patients, and histopathologic resolution of collagen banding is noted in some. Second, literature reports note a dramatic clinicopathologic response with remission to antibacterial agents such as bismuth subsalicylate (Pepto-Bismol) in some patients. For these reasons, it may be prudent to attempt an initial trial of antibacterial treatment before using anti-inflammatory treatment. There are no studies of probiotics. Third, unless the patient has only mild diarrhea easily controlled by dietary restrictions, cholestyramine, and bulk or antimotility agents, a course of anti-inflammatory therapy with large doses of 5-acetylsalicylic acid (ASA) compounds, prednisone, or budesonide seems justified. Fourth, in mildly symptomatic patients, physicians may feel that the side effects of prolonged therapy with anti-inflammatory agents and adrenocorticoids outweigh the benefits of relieving mild diarrhea. Finally, redirection of the small bowel effluent by diversion ileostomy results in clinicopathologic resolution. Our approach to treatment is outlined in Table 87-1.

Because experience is limited and largely anecdotal, the answers to several questions remain unknown. The danger of leaving this disorder untreated by antibacterial or anti-inflammatory medication has not been determined. Our study did not demonstrate an increased risk of colon cancer (Chan et al, 1999). Because, on the one hand, spontaneous clinicopathologic remissions have been documented in some patients and, conversely, exacerbation after removal of anti-inflammatory medication in others, the appropriate duration of anti-inflammatory therapy is difficult to define. In the future, double-blind randomized trials using both clinical and histopathologic criteria should allow the determination of reasonable courses of therapy.

Symptomatic Therapy

In patients with symptomatic collagenous lymphocytic colitis, several factors should be considered. Because small bowel secretion has been noted in some patients, dietary secretagogues such as *caffeine-* or *lactose-containing foods* should be eliminated from the diet. Because of a possible association between collagenous colitis and *nonsteroidal anti-inflammatory drugs*, these agents should be discontinued. If *steatorrhea* is documented, *a low-fat diet* may be helpful. In the presence of bile salt malabsoption, binding resins such as *cholestyramine* have been useful. Some patients are helped by *bulking agents* and by *antidiarrheal medications* such as loperamide hydrochloride (Imodium), diphenoxylate hydrochloride and atropine (Lomotil), deodorized tincture of opium, or codeine.

Antibacterial Agents

Investigators have treated collagenous colitis patients with antibacterial agents with remarkable results.

In an open-label trial, Fine and Lee (1998) reported a trial of bismuth subsalicylate (8 chewable 262 mg tablets per day for 8 weeks) in 12 patients, which included those with collagenous and lymphocytic colitis. Eleven patients had resolution of diarrhea and histopathologic changes, with no recurrence 7 to 28 months after treatment. In this study, no side effects were reported. However, there are two case reports of bismuth nitrate (used for treatment of gastritis) causing dementia, both of which resolved after the discontinuation of the drug. In collagenous lymphocytic colitis, response rates of 60% have been seen with metronidazole (250 mg 3 or 4 times daily) and erythromycin antibiotics. There are no treatments with probiotics.

Sulfasalazine and Other 5-ASAs

Sulfasalazine has been used as the initial anti-inflammatory agent because of documented effectiveness in colonic idiopathic IBD, low cost, and a comparative lack of side effects. The usual dose of sulfasalazine is 2 to 4 g/d administered by mouth in divided doses with meals and at bedtime. The full dosage should be achieved slowly, starting with 1 tablet (0.5 g) daily and adding 1 tablet per day until the desired dosage is achieved. This may help avoid nausea and, perhaps, headaches. Conventional folic acid administration, 1 mg/d, seems reasonable. Abatement of diarrhea in 1 to 2 weeks with sulfasalazine as a single agent has been noted in approximately 50% of patients so treated. Patients have been continued on this agent or other 5-ASA drugs for 3 months and then tapered to a maintenance dose of 1 g twice a day. Some patients require higher doses of 5-ASA.

In persons with a history of sulfa allergy and those who

TABLE 87-1. Treatment Approach in Collagenous Lymphocytic Colitis

1. Eliminate secretagogues (lactose, caffeine, fat) and stop NSAIDs. Rule out thyroid dysfunction.
2. Trial of bismuth subsalicylate 262 mg 3 tablets in am, 2 tablets at noon, 3 tablets pm qd for 8 weeks

If no resolution,

3. 5-ASA drugs ± antimotility agents × 1 to 2 months (mesalamine [Asacol] 800 to 1,200 mg tid, sulfasalazine [Azulfidine] 2 g bid)

If no resolution,

4. Add/substitute adrenocorticoid ± antimotility agents (prednisone 20 to 40 mg qd; budesonide 3 mg tid)

If no resolution,

5. Rule out small bowel disease, steatorrhea

If no resolution,

6. Immunosuppressive therapy (methotrexate) or surgery (diverting ileostomy versus colectomy)

ASA = acetylsalicylic acid; bid = twice daily; NSAID = nonsteroidal anti-inflammatory drug; qd = every day; tid = 3 times daily.

have had adverse reactions to sulfasalazine (not infrequent circumstances) or are unresponsive, other 5-ASA mesalamine compounds may be used. Two oral mesalamine preparations are available (Asacol and Pentasa).

The usual dose of Asacol is 800 to 1,200 mg 3 times a day; the usual dose of Pentasa is 500 to 1,000 mg 2 to 3 times a day. Because the initial site of action of Pentasa is the small intestine, it may be less effective than other 5-ASA–continuing compounds. Patients who respond usually improve within 2 to 3 weeks. Maximum doses may be needed in some patients. Once symptomatic control is achieved, the dose may be gradually tapered, but most require the dose used for remission medicine. Because Dipentum (olsalazine) can cause net small bowel secretion, it is best avoided with microscopic colitis. Because collagenous lymphocytic colitis usually involves the proximal colon, 5-ASA enemas and suppositories are unlikely to be effective.

As a guide to therapy, repeat colonic biopsies can be taken after 2 to 3 months of treatment to assess resolution of collagen banding and the inflammatory infiltrate in the surface epithelium and lamina propria. If clinical and histologic benefits are evident, 6 to 12 months of empiric treatment has been given in an attempt to maximize histologic improvement. Subsequently, we have maintained the sulfasalazine or 5-ASA with continued attention to dietary factors and the use of antidiarrheal agents. Unfortunately, in some patients, diarrhea has recurred after lowering the dose or cessation of these agents.

Adverse Events

Major side effects attributable to sulfasalazine include allergic skin reactions, hemolysis, neutropenia, and mild allergic reactions with rash and fever. During sulfasalazine therapy, the patient's hematologic status should be monitored. Sulfasalazine may interfere with dietary folate absorption, and routine oral folate replacement with 1 mg/d is suggested unless red blood cell folate levels are monitored. Fortunately, serious idiosyncratic reactions (eg, hepatitis, pancreatitis, alveolitis, and serum sickness) are very uncommon.

Side effects occur with the oral 5-ASA drugs in less than 5% of patients. These include diarrhea, nausea, vomiting, abdominal pain, dyspepsia, and rash.

Adrenocorticoids

If no clinical improvement is noted after 2 to 4 weeks of sulfasalazine and/or 5-ASA therapy, adrenocorticoid medication is added or substituted. Most of our patients with collagenous lymphocytic colitis have received prednisone. Dramatic resolution of diarrhea in 80 to 90% of individuals has been noted within 5 days of the start of treatment. Additionally, in patients with lymphocytic colitis, histologic improvement has been seen. Disappearance of the collagen banding and repair of the surface epithelial damage have also been documented in those with collagenous colitis.

Most individuals have been treated as outpatients with prednisone in a morning oral dosage of 20 to 40 mg. An occasional patient with more than 2 L of stool a day has been hospitalized and treated with intravenous prednisolone, 60 mg/d, or hydrocortisone. Once control of diarrhea is achieved, patients have been maintained on 20 to 30 mg of prednisone for 3 months, and repeat colonic biopsies are obtained. After 3 months, we have attempted to change to an alternate-day dose or to discontinue prednisone. However, recurrence of diarrhea has been noted in most patients. In these cases, small doses of 10 to 15 mg of prednisone daily or alternate-day steroids have been administered with success. In addition, other antidiarrheal agents described above have been added to the regimen to minimize prednisone dosage and adverse side effects.

Recently, budesonide (Entocort), an oral medication with topical corticoid released in the small intestine and ascending colon, has been incorporated in the treatment of collagenous lymphocytic colitis. Budesonide has a topical effect and a low bioavailability of about 10%.

This drug is therapeutically similar to prednisone, but with fewer side effects. In a randomized, double-blind, placebo-controlled trial, 20 patients with collagenous colitis were randomized to either placebo or budesonide (Entocort) 9 mg/d for 8 weeks. Clinical improvement was achieved in 10 (100%) patients receiving budesonide compared with 2 (20%) patients in the placebo group ($p < .001$). The histologic inflammation grade in the sigmoid mucosa and the thickness of the collagen layer were significantly reduced ($p < .02$) in those receiving budesonide. Symptoms relapsed in 8 of 10 patients within 8 weeks after discontinuation of budesonide, suggesting that most may need sustained treatment to remain asymptomatic. Further studies and long-term follow-up are warranted.*

In our experience with the above therapeutic approach, symptomatic improvement has occurred in most patients, and histologic improvement has occurred in some. However, in only a few patients has total histologic reversal occurred, even in those who are asymptomatic for many months. Therefore, questions still remain as to the duration of therapy and the utility of histologic appearances as a guide to treatment.

Other Agents

Several case reports have suggested improvement with *octreotide*. Also, *methotrexate* has been used with dramatic reduction of symptoms in a patient refractory to antidiarrheal, 5-ASA, and corticosteroid agents. Case reports doc-

---

*Editor's Note: Anecdotally, 6 mg of budesonide (Entocort) plus 3,200 to 4,800 mg of mesalamine (Asacol) have been associated with 3-year clinical remissions. All patients are on calcium plus vitamin D and are followed with bone density measurements.

umenting improvement of collagenous colitis have been noted with *chlorpheniramine* (an H_1-histamine antagonist), *quinacrine, mepacrine,* and *ketotifen* (a mast cell stabilizer).

Surgery

Colectomy has been performed in a handful of patients. In one patient, diarrheal symptoms were eliminated, and in another, diarrhea and extraintestinal manifestations of collagenous colitis were abated. However, one patient continued with diarrhea after colectomy for unclear reasons. Diverting ileostomy has regressed the clinicopathologic findings in this disorder. Jarnerot and colleagues (1995) reported nine women with collagenous colitis unresponsive to medical therapy (sulfasalazine, mepacrine, corticosteroids, mesalamines, metronidazole [Flagyl]). An ileostomy was performed in eight patients and a sigmoidostomy in one patient. Postoperatively, diarrhea ceased in all patients, with histologic resolution of the collagen layer. The ileostomy was reversed in three patients after a diversion period of 4 to 15 months, and clinical symptoms and the abnormal collagen layer recurred in all.

Other Considerations

Villous atrophy of the small bowel has been documented in some cases of lymphocytic and collagenous colitis. This probably represents another entity rather than concomitant celiac disease because several of these patients with collagenous colitis have been given gluten-free diets without improvement. Consequently, the possibility of small bowel disease should be investigated in a medically unresponsive patient with collagenous lymphocytic colitis. Conversely, collagenous lymphocytic colitis should be considered in a patient with refractory malabsorption and/or diarrhea and small bowel villous atrophy. This is discussed in the chapter on celiac disease (Chapter 61, "Celiac Sprue and Related Problems").

Because thyroid disease has been associated with this syndrome, attention should be paid to the thyroid hormone status, and any abnormalities should be treated.

Long-term experience is limited, but retrospective analysis of patients with collagenous lymphocytic colitis reveals a benign and chronic course. A few case reports of rectal or colonic cancer in elderly patients with coexistent collagenous colitis are likely coincidental. In a study by Chan and colleagues (1999), 117 patients diagnosed with collagenous colitis were reviewed. No cases of colorectal cancer were diagnosed during a mean follow-up period of 7 years after the diagnosis of colitis, and the relative risk of colon cancer in collagenous colitis patients was similar to that of the general population. There was no regular surveillance schedule.

Eosinophilic Colitis

Infiltration of the GI tract with eosinophils may involve the entire GI tract but usually entails the stomach and small intestine. Isolated colonic involvement (eosinophilic colitis) is limited to sporadic case reports. Eosinophilic colitis can occur as a component of the inflammatory response in Crohn's disease, ulcerative colitis, parasitic diseases, milk protein–induced colitis, and eosinophilic gastroenteritis. Eosinophilic GI disease is estimated to have an incidence of 1:100,000, whereas isolated colonic involvement appears to be very sporadic.

There is no clear definition of eosinophilic gastroenteritis, but most authorities agree that the diagnosis of this syndrome should include the following: (1) the presence of GI symptoms (diarrhea, abdominal pain), (2) biopsies showing eosinophilic infiltration of one or more areas of the GI tract from the esophagus to the colon, and (3) peripheral eosinophilia and no evidence of parasitic or extraintestinal disease. The diagnosis of eosinophilic colitis rests on peripheral blood eosinophilia and eosinophilic tissue infiltration with the exclusion of other diseases that may mimic eosinophilic gastroenteropathy.

Eosinophilic colitis may be patchy; hence, colonic mucosal biopsies may miss the diagnosis. Additionally, elevated serum IgE levels may be present in some patients. However, the peripheral eosinophilic count seems to be *normal* in 20 to 40% of patients considered to have eosinophilic colitis.

The etiology of eosinophilic colitis is unknown, and the disorder is considered to be idiopathic. Approximately 30 to 50% of patients with eosinophilic gastroenteritis have a history of allergies to medications, food proteins, or worms. Similarly, the pathogenesis of eosinophilic colitis is unclear. Eosinophilic gastroenteritis is a treatable disease; patients generally respond to steroid therapy, although relapse is common. The use of nonenteric-coated budesonide may be an alternative to steroid treatment, but very limited data are available. Elimination of the precipitating agent, including dietary modifications and amino acid–based diets, may lead to resolution of this disorder. Use of antiallergic medications such as ketotifen, with or without steroids, has been recommended. Promising new drugs for eosinophilic gastroenteritis include montelukast, a selective leukotriene receptor antagonist, and suplaplast tosilate, a selective T helper 2 cytokine inhibitor with inhibitory effects on allergy-induced eosinophilic infiltration and IgE production.

Acknowledgment

Supported by National Institutes of Health grants K07 CA092445 (to M.C.C.) and P50 CA–62924-10, The John G. Rangos, Sr. Charitable Foundation (to F.M.G.), and The Clayton Fund.

Supplemental Reading

Bohr J, Tysk C, Eriksson S, Jarnerot G. Collagenous colitis in Orebro, Sweden, an epidemiological study 1984–1993. Gut 1995;37:394–7.

Bonderup OK, Hansen JB, Birket-Smith L, et al. Budesonide treatment of collagenous colitis: a randomized, double blind, placebo controlled trial with morphometric analysis. Gut 2003;52:248–51.

Chan JL, Tersmette AC, Offerhaus GJA, et al. Cancer risk in collagenous colitis. Inflamm Bowel Dis 1999;5:40–3.

Cruz-Correa M, Giardiello FM. Lymphocytic and collagenous colitis. Curr Treat Options Gastroenterol 2000;3:243–8.

Cruz-Correa M, Milligan F, Giardiello FM, et al. Collagenous colitis with mucosal tears on endoscopic insufflation: a unique presentation. Gut 2002;51:600.

Daneshjoo R, Talley JN. Eosinophilic gastroenteritis. Curr Gastroenterol Rep 2002;4:366–72.

Fine KD, Lee EL. Efficacy of open-label bismuth subsalicylate for treatment of microscopic colitis. Gastroenterology 1998;114:29–36.

Giardiello FM, Bayless TM, Jessurun J, et al. Collagenous colitis: physiologic and histopathologic studies in seven patients. Ann Intern Med 1987;106:46–9.

Jarnerot G, Tysk C, Bohr J, Eriksson S. Collagenous colitis and fecal stream diversion. Gastroenterology 1995;109:449–55.

Miehlke S, Heymer P, Bethke B, et al. Budesonide treatment for collagenous colitis: a randomized, double-blind, placebo-controlled, multicenter trial. Gastroenterology 2002;123:978–84.

CHAPTER 88

Fecal Incontinence: Evaluation and Treatment

Arden M. Morris, MD, MPH, and Robert D. Madoff, MD

Fecal incontinence is the inability to control discharge of anal contents, which may be gas, liquid, or solid. Episodes of incontinence vary in frequency and often have a profoundly negative impact on both physical and psychological well-being. Patients with fecal incontinence may limit their social interaction, change or reduce activities of daily living, and experience grave health side effects. Given the associated social stigma, patients are often reluctant to discuss symptoms of fecal incontinence, and health care providers often fail to appreciate its impact (Madoff et al, 1992). Population-based surveys indicate a prevalence rate of 2 to 7% in the general population and a roughly 10-fold higher rate among nursing home residents. Clinicians accordingly must be sensitive to the issue of incontinence and pay particular attention to code words and euphemisms (eg, "diarrhea") that indicate its presence. Fortunately, for most patients who do seek treatment, a host of therapeutic options, including several promising newer interventions, are available.

Evaluation

A methodical evaluation is crucial to developing a successful treatment plan. At the University of Minnesota, our initial goals are to establish the etiology of fecal incontinence and to assess its severity and impact on the patient's lifestyle.

Etiology

Myriad underlying disorders, singly or combined, may lead to fecal incontinence (Table 88-1). Our evaluation begins with a clinical history, physical examination, and appropriate objective testing. For many nursing home patients, the workup can stop as soon as a history of constipation is elicited and a stool ball in the rectal vault is found, indicating *overflow incontinence*. Such patients may be treated by digital disimpaction, under anesthesia if necessary, and then by a bowel management regimen, including a fiber supplement, stool softeners, and possibly a cathartic. For young patients with no history of trauma or underlying disease who experience incontinence due to severe diarrhea, evaluation should focus on determining the *cause of the diarrhea* rather than investigating possible pelvic floor dysfunction.

Endoanal Ultrasound

The most important information needed to treat incontinence is the anatomic status of the anal sphincter. Sphincter anatomy is best visualized using *endoanal ultrasonography*. Ultrasonography is particularly informative (1) if a large sphincter defect is identified, clearly indicating sphincteroplasty as the appropriate therapy, (2) as a "road map" for sphincteroplasty, for example, in the case of previous sphincterotomy, and (3) as a contraindication to sphincteroplasty if the suspected defect is not identified.

TABLE 88-1. Causes of Fecal Incontinence

Normal pelvic floor
Diarrhea
Infection
IBD
Laxative abuse
Radiation enteritis
Short-gut syndrome
Dietary intolerance or malabsorption
Overflow or decreased rectal compliance
Constipation or impaction
Encopresis
Rectal mass
Rectal scarring due to IBD or radiation injury
Previous rectal resection with sphincter sparing
Collagen vascular or autoimmune diseases
Systemic or neurologic disease
Congenital anomalies
Central nervous system disease or injury
Collagen vascular or autoimmune diseases
Neuropathy (eg, diabetes)
Abnormal pelvic floor
Congenital malformation
Sphincter trauma
Obstetrical injury
Previous anorectal surgery
Other anorectal trauma
Pudendal nerve injury
Vaginal delivery
Chronic straining during defecation
Rectal prolapse
Other (aging, idiopathic causes)

Adapted from Madoff et al, 1992. IBD = inflammatory bowel disease.

Anorectal Hystolgic Function

We next assess anorectal physiologic function using a series of objective tests. Anal manometry can help determine resting tone and voluntary contraction pressure, indicative of internal and external sphincter function, respectively. *Rectal sensitivity* is determined by use of an *inflatable rectal balloon*. The *rectoanal inhibitory reflex (RAIR)* causes the anal canal to relax when the rectum is distended. The RAIR is absent in patients with *Hirschprung's disease* and is often lost following *low anterior resection* of the rectum. Absence of a normal RAIR indicates loss of the normal sampling reflex, which is associated with diminished postoperative continence. *Electromyography* can help document pelvic floor reinnervation, a marker of a previous denervating injury. Denervation is due to traction injury of the pudendal nerve, most commonly caused by stretching of the nerve during vaginal delivery or chronic straining during defecation. Most laboratories now use *pudendal nerve terminal motor latency testing* as a measure of pudendal nerve function, but the sensitivity and predictive capabilities of this test are controversial.

Cinedefecography is a dynamic radiologic test that demonstrates the anatomic relationships of the pelvic floor organs during rectal evacuation. We use a barium oatmeal paste administered by rectal enema; in female patients, a radiopaque vaginal contrast should also be used to clarify anatomic relationships. Defecography is unnecessary if anorectal physiology tests and ultrasonography have delineated an unequivocal diagnosis and treatment plan. However, defecography can be an invaluable aid to planning when incontinence is associated with other hard-to-define disorders, such as internal prolapse.

SEVERITY AND IMPACT

The evaluation of fecal incontinence is incomplete without measuring its severity and subjective impact on the patient. Such clinical issues inform patients' motivation to seek treatment and clinicians' motivation to provide it. Experienced practitioners informally measure severity while obtaining every patient's history, in order to formulate the most appropriate treatment plan. Using a reliable, validated measurement tool confers the advantages of a formalized method, comparison with other patients, assessment of treatment effectiveness, ability to follow results over time, and individual provider feedback. Furthermore, evidence suggests that clinical assessment, in contrast to physiologic testing, is the only truly meaningful way to predict treatment success (Buie et al, 2001). Numerous measurement tools of varying simplicity, reliability, validity, and sensitivity have been devised; unfortunately, no consensus regarding a criterion standard has been reached. A more complete discussion of fecal incontinence measurement tools is in the excellent review by Baxter and colleagues (2003).

The clinical evaluation of fecal incontinence should include measures of both severity and impact on quality of life. Although these factors are closely intertwined, they may show surprising divergence in many cases. For example, one patient may refuse to leave her home due to fear of incontinence to flatus, whereas another may be little impacted by occasional episodes of complete incontinence. Accordingly, severity and quality of life should be measured separately (Shelton and Madoff, 1997) Even in the absence of a commonly accepted standard measure of incontinence severity, the key features (frequency and nature of incontinent episodes) are largely agreed upon. We measure the impact of incontinence on quality of life using the validated Fecal Incontinence Quality of Life Scale (FIQL) (Rockwood et al, 2000).

Taken together, anorectal physiology testing and incontinence measurement tools provide essential guidance for treatment planning and are the key to meaningful review and comparison of treatment effectiveness.

Treatment

Our fundamental treatment goal for patients with fecal incontinence is to control their symptoms. For a significant proportion of patients, an underlying medical problem, such as gastrointestinal infection, first led to diarrhea and then to fecal incontinence; their symptoms generally resolve with medical correction of the underlying problem and control of diarrhea. However, for most of our referred patients, treatment of underlying medical disorders has already failed, so interventional therapy must be considered. Treatment options range from noninvasive frontline therapy to interventional salvage procedures, alone, combined, or repeated.

Medical Management

Even patients with anatomic or physiologic abnormalities may benefit from maximizing medical therapy. Dietary counseling regarding diarrhea-producing foods, food intolerance, and fiber intake is virtually risk-free and may ameliorate symptoms during the workup process. We counsel most patients to maximize dietary fiber intake, including use of a bulking agent. The goal is eventual intake of 25 to 30 g of fiber daily; most patients start at levels substantially lower than this, and they should be counseled to increase their intake gradually to avoid excessive gassiness.

Selection of an antidiarrheal agent depends on the severity of incontinence. Adsorbing or coating agents are generally used for infrequent episodes. Medications that increase colonic transit time and adsorption are effective for moderate to severe symptoms. We prefer Imodium because of its combined effects on adsorption, transit time, and sphincter agonist activity. Diphenoxylate is a useful second line agent with a similar profile but more atropine-neutral side effects.

Topical sphincter agonists such as phenylephrine gel have been disappointing in randomized trials. However, novel medical therapies such as the L-erythro *methoxamine isomer* are in development and may prove more effective (Parker et al, 2003).

For *alternating diarrhea and constipation conditions*, such as irritable bowel syndrome or overflow incontinence due to obstipation or spinal cord injury, we recommend a bowel management regimen. We start with rectal disimpaction and a whole bowel cathartic, such as polyethylene glycol, followed by regular laxatives combined with suppositories or enemas if necessary.

Biofeedback

Biofeedback therapy confers the distinct advantage of a noninvasive intervention that is safe, that allows (requires) active patient participation, and that may enhance the effects of other treatments (Jensen and Lowry, 1997). Patients perform *anal sphincter contraction exercises* and receive computerized visual or auditory responses; thus, they learn muscle control by means of sensory feedback. Anorectal biofeedback therapy specifically aims (1) to augment external anal sphincter function, resulting in successful voluntary delay of defecation, (2) to improve rectal sensation, thereby alerting patients to the presence of stool in the vault and the need for voluntary sphincter contraction, and (3) to coordinate sensation and contraction, thereby overcoming reflexive relaxation in the presence of rectal contents (Loening-Baucke, 1990).

We use a two-channel electromyography electrode with one sensor placed in the anal canal and the other surface electrode placed on the gluteus muscles for strength and endurance training. Patients practice maximum squeeze and muscle isolation in the upright position, which facilitates coordination training and enhances feedback. When patients demonstrate adequate understanding and ability to perform exercises, they are assigned to continue strength training at home, using gradually increasing daily exercises. We have found that patients relearn sensitivity to smaller filling volumes and sensation improves without formalized training.

A trained, dedicated, and sensitive therapist is essential in biofeedback therapy. To qualify for biofeedback therapy, patients must be capable of the required cognitive function and have some degree of rectal sensation and of external anal sphincter function. Despite a lack of a standardized biofeedback method, outcomes have been highly encouraging. Pager and colleagues (2002) recently reported long term results for 83 incontinent patients who completed a 4-month biofeedback training program. At a median of 42 months, patients demonstrated ongoing significant improvements in all outcome measures; many improved further after completing the program. However, a recent randomized controlled trial of biofeedback versus standard conservative therapy failed to show a difference between these approaches (Norton et al, 2002). This finding calls into question the exact role of biofeedback itself and emphasizes the importance of ancillary therapy (such as dietary counseling and drug therapy) in the conservative management of incontinent patients. We have seen substantial clinical improvement in our biofeedback patients (Jensen and Lowry, 1997), but a decline in function may occur over time. We have found that performance may be bolstered by intermittent supplementary training sessions.

Surgical Intervention

Traditionally, surgical intervention has been based on the following two simple underlying concepts: (1) introducing mechanical obstruction, via encirclement with native or prosthetic materials, or (2) decommissioning the anorectum, via creation of a diverting stoma. Sphincteroplasty, historical and novel encirclement methods, and interesting new techniques still under investigation are discussed below.

Sphincteroplasty For incontinent patients with a sphincter defect, our initial intervention is usually *overlapping sphincteroplasty*. With the patient in prone jackknife position, we sharply dissect the internal and external sphincters, mobilizing for an overlapping plication. An anterior levatoroplasty can be performed to lengthen the anal canal at the discretion of the surgeon; some advise against levatoroplasty because it may contribute to postoperative dyspareunia. Significant improvement in continence with minimal morbidity is achieved in approximately 70% of patients who undergo sphincteroplasty. Recent data, however, suggest that the results of sphincteroplasty *deteriorate with time*. We reviewed our long term (median 10 years) results of overlapping sphincteroplasty in 191 consecutive patients and found that only *40% of patients maintained long-term continence* (Baxter et al, 2003). Older patients were more likely to develop recurrent incontinence to solid stool. Surprisingly, despite the deterioration of continence with time, *74% of patients still stated that they were satisfied with their treatment* at 10 years postoperation.

Encirclement Procedures The concept of circumferential anal sphincter support began in 1891 with the *Thiersch wire*, a silver wire tunneled subcutaneously around the external anal sphincter. Because of a high rate of local complications, this technique is now of historical interest only. Both *dynamic graciloplasty* and the *artificial bowel sphincter* work on the same principle as the Thiersch wire; in contrast, however, these newer techniques each work dynamically to permit both closure and relaxation of the anal canal.

Dynamic Graciloplasty. Encirclement using native muscle has been a trial-and-error process. Both *gracilis* and *gluteus maximus wraps* have been used. From the technical perspective, the gracilis is well suited for transposition because of its proximal neurovascular bundle, superficial location, and lack of important function in humans. The muscle is mobilized, tunneled subcutaneously in the upper thigh, and wrapped around the external sphincter. The muscle works largely as a passive barrier, though some contraction is possible by adduction of the leg. In an effort to improve the functional results of gracioloplasty, electrical stimulation is applied to convert from fast-twitch, fatigue-prone fibers to slow-twitch, fatigue-resistant fibers over an 8-week period. After 8 weeks, the neosphincter muscle is maintained in tonic contraction, except when the implanted pulse generator is magnetically deactivated.

Outcomes of *dynamic gracioloplasty* are mixed. Although approximately two thirds of patients who undergo the procedure achieve successful results (Madoff et al, 1999), complication rates have been prohibitively high. Accordingly, the technique remains available in a small number of highly specialized centers worldwide, but is not approved by the Food and Drug Administration for use in the United States.

ARTIFICIAL ANAL SPHINCTER. The *artificial anal sphincter* (Acticon Neosphincter, American Medical Systems, Minnetonka, MN) consists of a silicone elastomer cuff tunneled around the external anal sphincter. The cuff is connected to a pump in the labia or scrotum, with a reservoir balloon placed in the preperitoneal space (Figure 88-1).

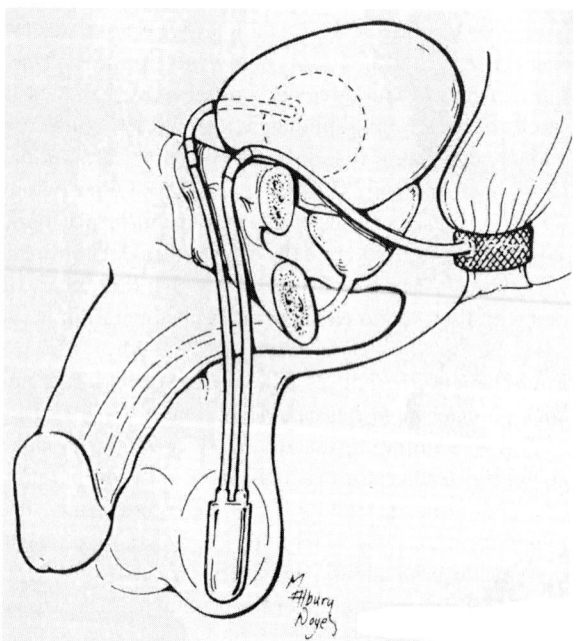

FIGURE 88-1 Acticon artificial bowel sphincter. Reproduced with permission from: Wong WD, Rothenberger DA. Surgical approaches to anal incontinence. In: Bock C, editor. Neurobiology of incontinence (Ciba Foundation Symposium 151). Chichester, England: John Wiley and Sons; 1990. p. 246–66.

Repetitive compression of the pump causes fluid efflux from the cuff to the balloon, allowing rectal evacuation, followed by slow return of fluid from the balloon to the cuff.

A multicenter trial of the artificial anal sphincter ended recently, with results somewhat similar to those for dynamic gracioloplasty (Wong et al, 2002). Success was defined as a decrease of at least 24 points on the Fecal Incontinence Scoring System designed for that trial (range 0 to 120 points). In all, 46% of patients required reoperation, primarily because of infection; 37% required device explantation, 20% of whom were reimplanted with a new device. In patients with a functioning device, 85% achieved continence; the success rate was only 53%, however, if all treated patients were included in the calculation. The artificial anal sphincter has now been approved by the Food and Drug Administration in the United States.

Although neosphincter outcomes may appear less than encouraging at first glance, one must remain mindful that these are patients with substantial incontinence who have failed or are not candidates for standard therapy such as sphincteroplasty or biofeedback. For either neosphincter procedure (ie, dynamic gracioloplasty or the artificial anal sphincter), patient selection should be based on the presence of severe incontinence refractory to other therapy, otherwise good performance status, adequate cognitive ability, and psychological stability. Trained practitioners who reserve these treatments for appropriate patients under rigorously controlled conditions can have an extremely positive impact on their patients' quality of life (Madoff et al, 2000). Furthermore, among our patients at the University of Minnesota with established artificial sphincters, full functioning has been ongoing for several years postimplantation (Parker et al, 2003).

Neuromodulation Sacral nerve stimulation (SNS), initially developed for urinary incontinence, represents a departure from previous models of fecal incontinence therapy. Instead of correcting or replacing defective morphology, this treatment aims to augment physiologic function by recruiting and stimulating S2, S3, or S4 nerves as they exit the sacral foramina. The three-part procedure begins with placement of a subcutaneous electrode in the sacral foramina to identify the site of maximal pelvic floor and minimal lower extremity stimulation. Next, the lead is connected to an external pulse generator for a 3-week test period. After 3 weeks, if functional improvement is adequate, we implant a permanent pulse generator (Figure 88-2).

Initially, the consistent reduction in incontinent episodes was attributed to electrical recruitment of striated muscle fibers in the pelvic floor and external sphincter (Matzel et al, 1995). More recent data suggest other possible mechanisms of action, including improved rectal sensation, enhanced resting anal tone, alteration in local reflexes, and dampening of rectal activity. Kenefick and colleagues (2002)

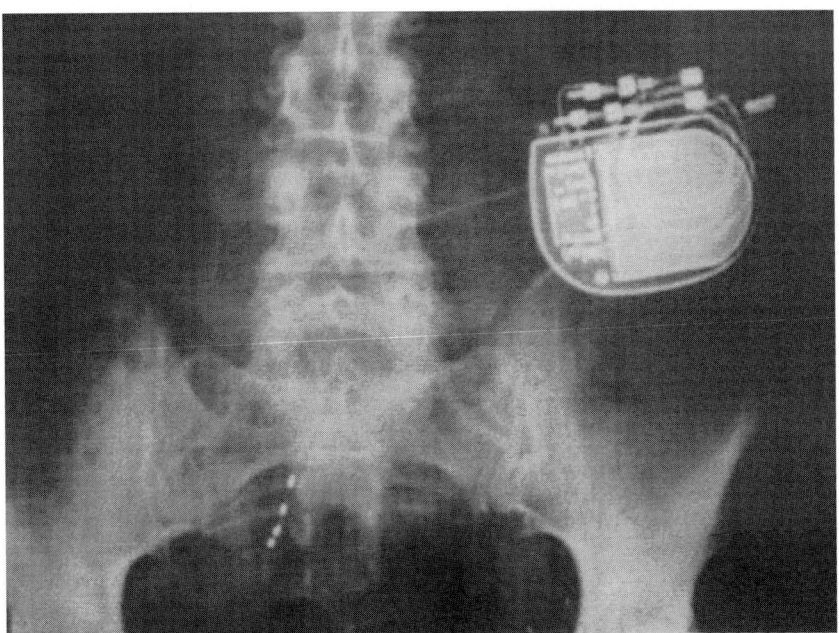

FIGURE 88-2 Radiograph of an implanted sacral nerve stimulator device. Courtesy of Robert D. Madoff, MD.

recently reported excellent results; at a median of 2 years, 73% of previously incapacitated patients achieved full continence; symptoms markedly improved for the others. Unlike the neosphincter procedures, SNS has been associated with minimal morbidity. This fact suggests that indications for the procedure might reasonably be broadened, at least on an investigational basis, in the future.

Radiofrequency Energy Delivery Submucosal radiofrequency energy delivery to the anal canal (also known as the Secca procedure) is a thermal technique currently under investigation in a multicenter trial. The procedure consists of anal insertion of a heat-controlled probe. The probe then deploys electrodes that pierce the mucosa and heat the muscularis, resulting in collagen contraction. However, the exact mechanism of action using this technique is unknown. Early results have shown modest improvement in incontinence severity.

Anal Canal Bulking and Obstructing Agents In contrast to stool bulking agents, anal canal bulking agents are made of implanted natural or synthetic materials, such as collagen, silicone, or carbon coated beads, that are injected into the intersphincteric space to bolster function of the internal anal sphincter. We do not perform this procedure, although good outcomes in very small series have been reported. Obstructing agents, such as pliable rubber balloons, are placed in the anus; they can be removed by the patient for controlled defecation (Norton and Kamm, 2001; Mortensen and Humphreys, 1991). Such an intervention might be useful for patients who are at very poor risk for surgery.

Stoma For patients with refractory incontinence, a properly placed and well-constructed stoma offers restoration of bowel control (if not true continence) with minimal associated morbidity. Although the presence of a stoma admittedly distorts an individual's body image, this disadvantage is usually outweighed by the patient's enhanced ability to function normally (or nearly so) in social, work, and sexual situations without fear of loss of bowel control.

Summary

Fecal incontinence is a prevalent and frustrating problem that has a profound impact on physical and psychological well-being. Appropriate care relies on systematic evaluation and application of a tailored treatment plan. Figure 88-3 presents a systematic algorithm for care of patients with persistent fecal incontinence. Although we champion the methodical approach, we frequently encourage a combined treatment plan, such as medical optimization, biofeedback, and sphincteroplasty, depending on the needs and abilities of individual patients. Broad adaptation of a standardized pre- and postintervention evaluation system will enhance the individual patient's experience and our understanding of treatment effectiveness.

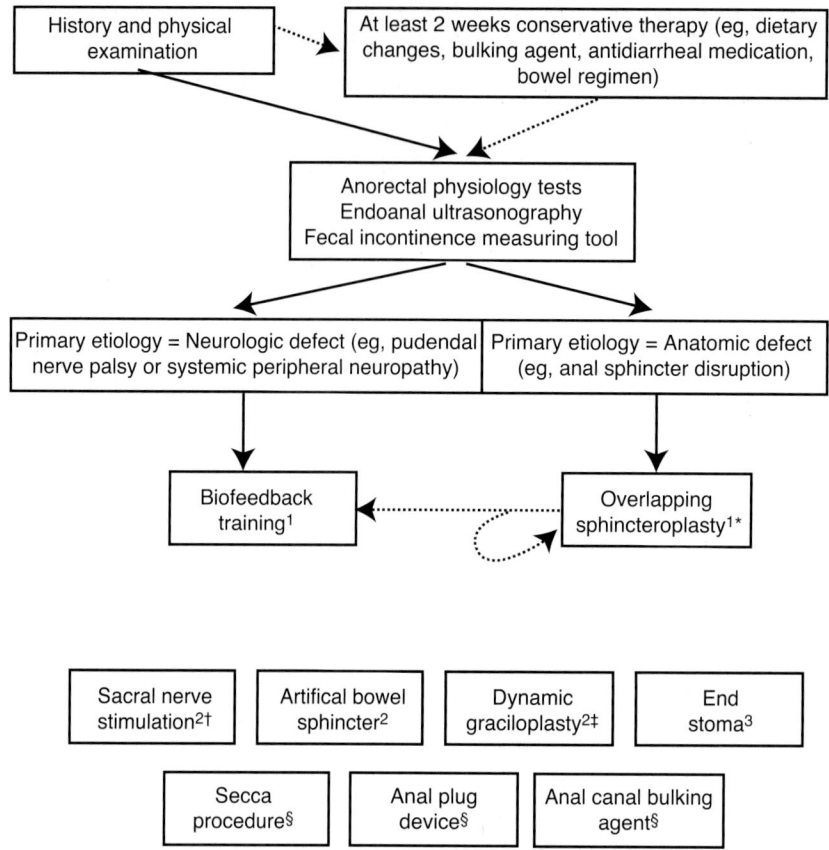

FIGURE 88-3 An evaluation and treatment algorithm for fecal incontinence. [1]Indicates first line therapy, with conservative management as above. *Failed sphincteroplasty should be re-evaluated. Good results may still be achieved with a re-wrap or with biofeedback therapy. [2]Second line therapy. ‡Available on protocol only. †Not available in the United States. [3]Permanent stoma represents a definitive therapy option for many patients, especially those with reduced medical access, limited mobility, or impaired cognitive or psychological function. §Available off protocol but limited efficacy data available at this time.

Supplemental Reading

Baxter NN, Bravo Guittierez A, Lowry A, et al. Long-term results of sphincteroplasty for acquired fecal incontinence. American Society of Colon and Rectal Surgeons Annual Meeting; 2003 June 24; New Orleans, LA.

Baxter NN, Rothenberger DA, Lowry AC. Measuring fecal incontinence. Dis Colon Rectum 2003;46:1591–605.

Buie WD, Lowry AC, Rothenberger DA, Madoff RD. Clinical rather than laboratory assessment predicts continence after anterior sphincteroplasty. Dis Colon Rectum 2001;44:1255–60.

Jensen LL, Lowry AC. Biofeedback improves functional outcome after sphincteroplasty. Dis Colon Rectum 1997;40:197–200.

Kenefick NJ, Vaizey CJ, Cohen RC, et al. Medium-term results of permanent sacral nerve stimulation for faecal incontinence. Br J Surg 2002;89:896–901.

Loening-Baucke V. Biofeedback therapy for fecal incontinence. Dig Dis 1990;7:112–24.

Madoff RD, Baeten CG, Christiansen J, et al. Standards for anal sphincter replacement. Dis Colon Rectum 2000;43:135–41.

Madoff RD, Rosen HR, Baeten CG, et al. Safety and efficacy of dynamic muscle plasty for anal incontinence: lessons from a prospective, multicenter trial. Gastroenterology 1999;116:549–56.

Madoff RD, Williams JG, Caushaj PF. Fecal incontinence. Current concepts. N Engl J Med 1992;326:1002–7.

Matzel KE, Stadelmaier U, Hohenfellner M, Gall FP. Electrical stimulation of sacral spinal nerves for treatment of faecal incontinence. Lancet 1995;346:1124–7.

Mortensen N, Humphreys MS. The anal continence plug: a disposable device for patients with anorectal incontinence. Lancet 1991;338:295–7.

Norton C, Chelvanayagam S, Kamm M. Randomised controlled trial of biofeedback for fecal incontinence [abstract]. J Neurosurg 2002;122:A–70.

Norton C, Kamm MA. Anal plug for faecal incontinence. Colorectal Dis 2001;3:323–7.

Pager CK, Solomon MJ, Rex J, Roberts RA. Long-term outcomes of pelvic floor exercise and biofeedback treatment for patients with fecal incontinence. Dis Colon Rectum 2002;45:997–1003.

Parker SC, Morris AM, Thorson AJ. New developments in anal surgery: incontinence. Seminars in Colon & Rectal Surgery 2003;14:82–92.

Parker SC, Spencer MP, Madoff RD, et al. Artificial bowel sphincter: long-term experience at a single institution. Dis Colon Rectum 2003;46:722–9.

Rockwood TH, Church JM, Fleshman JW, et al. Fecal Incontinence Quality of Life Scale: quality of life instrument for patients with fecal incontinence. Dis Colon Rectum 2000;43:9–16; discussion 16–7.

Shelton AA, Madoff RD. Defining anal incontinence: establishing a uniform continence scale. Seminars in Colon & Rectal Surgery 1997;8:54–60.

Whitehead WE, Norton NJ, Wald A. Introduction. Advancing the treatment of fecal and urinary incontinence through research. Gastroenterology. 2004;126(1 Suppl 1):S1–2.

Wong WD, Congilosi SM, Spencer MP, et al. The safety and efficacy of the artificial bowel sphincter for fecal incontinence: results from a multicenter cohort study. Dis Colon Rectum 2002;45:1139–53.

CHAPTER 89

Rectal Prolapse, Rectal Intussusception, and Solitary Rectal Ulcer Syndrome

ANDERS MELLGREN, MD, PHD, JOHAN POLLACK, MD, AND INKERI SCHULTZ, MD, PHD

Rectal Prolapse

The word prolapse comes from the Latin term "prolapsus" and means "falling down." Rectal prolapse was described in 1500 BC in the Ebers papyrus, and Mr. Frederick Salmon, the founder of the famous St. Marks Hospital in London, wrote his classic article "Practical observations on prolapsus of the rectum" in 1831.

Rectal prolapse is a benign disorder that is frequently associated with disturbed bowel function. Rectal prolapse can be treated surgically by many different techniques and results regarding recurrence rate and mortality are generally good. Unfortunately, anal incontinence and/or constipation sometimes continue to bother the patients after otherwise successful correction of the prolapse.

Epidemiology

Rectal prolapse is most commonly found in elderly and the peak incidence is found after the fifth decade. Being female is one of the highest risk factors for development of rectal prolapse and women represent approximately 90% of the patient population. Rectal prolapse in elderly women is frequently accompanied with poor sphincter function and fecal incontinence. In the rather few younger women with rectal prolapse, continence function is frequently preserved. A background history of lifelong straining is common in these patients. Rectal prolapse is sometimes associated with underlying psychiatric illness.

Etiology

There are two theories regarding development of rectal prolapse. Moschowitz proposed in 1912 that rectal prolapse is a sliding hernia that protrudes through a defect in the pelvic floor. He found that patients with rectal prolapse have a deep cul-de-sac, which he believed resulted from herniation of the small intestine into the anterior wall of the rectum. He suggested that the herniation pushed the rectum down, resulting in rectal prolapse. This idea is supported by the finding of a deep cul-de-sac in many prolapse patients.

Brodén and Snellman (1968) used defecography and could demonstrate that rectal prolapse starts as an internal rectal intussusception. They demonstrated that rectal prolapse starts as anorectal intussusception 6 to 8 cm up in the rectum and as the patient strains, the intussusception progresses and extends down through the rectum and out through the anus.

The underlying mechanism for the rectum to prolapse remains unclear. A mobile rectum, a weak pelvic floor, and excessive straining at stool, all predispose for development of rectal prolapse. Lack of rectal support is of etiological importance, but rectal prolapse also develops in young men and in nulliparous women with normal pelvic floor and anal sphincter function.

Symptoms

Rectal prolapse is a full-thickness, circumferential intussusception of the entire rectal wall through the anal canal and anus. The prolapsing bowel itself, mucosanguineous discharge, bleeding, constipation and/or incontinence, and a feeling of incomplete evacuation, are the most frequent complaints. The incidence of preoperative incontinence and constipation has only been reported prospectively in a few studies and definitions vary. Allen-Mersh and colleagues (1990) studied 57 patients with rectal prolapse prospectively and found fecal incontinence symptoms in 49% and constipation symptoms in 30% of the patients. Madden and colleagues (1992) reported some degree of anal incontinence in 17 of 23 patients (74%) and constipation in 11 (48%) of their patients. In another prospective study, Huber and colleagues (1995) included 42 patients, 5 of whom had internal rectal intussusception. They found fecal incontinence in 54% and some degree of constipation in 44% of the patients.

The underlying mechanism for incontinence symptoms in approximately 50% of patients with rectal prolapse is not fully understood. Porter used needle electromyography and noted excessive reflex inhibition in prolapse patients. Recently, it has been demonstrated that patients with rectal prolapse have a thickened internal anal sphincter at endo-anal ultrasound (Marshall et al, 2002). Several mechanisms have been proposed to explain prolapse-associated incontinence. These include direct sphincter trauma caused by repeated stretching by the intussuscepting rectum or that the intussuscepting rectum leads to chronic stimulation of the rectoanal inhibitory reflex. Constipation, defined either as abnormally few stools per week or increased straining at stool may be explained by the presence of the intussuscepting bowel in the rectum, colonic dysmotility or inappropriate puborectalis contraction.

Preoperative Evaluation

Verification of the *rectal prolapse* and differentiating it from hemorrhoids and/or mucosal prolapse is usually the first step in the examination of patients with a history suggestive of rectal prolapse. Rectal prolapse is identified as a circular, full-thickness prolapse extending outside the anal verge when the patient strains. Occasionally the patient is unable to reproduce their prolapse at clinical examination in the left lateral position. Examination in the sitting position on a commode or diagnosis using defecography may then be quite helpful (Mellgren et al, 1994).

The patient history should include preoperative constipation and incontinence symptoms, bowel frequency, obstetric history, and other associated pelvic floor disorders, such as co-existing urinary incontinence or genital prolapse. Patients with rectal prolapse are at an increased risk for other concomitant pelvic floor abnormalities.

The clinical examination includes inspection of the perineum. Digital examination will assess the resting and squeeze tones of the anal sphincters. Proctoscopy or endoscopy will frequently reveal an area of mild erythema within the lower rectum. Sometimes a *solitary rectal ulcer* will be found in the mid-rectum. This may sometimes be difficult to distinguish from a polyp or tumor, and biopsies may therefore be needed. Evaluation of the remaining colon is encouraged, to exclude any coexisting colorectal pathology, particularly cancer. *Solitary rectal ulcer syndrome (SRUS)* is discussed later in this chapter.

Colon transit studies, anorectal manometry, pudendal latencies and endo-anal ultrasound may also be used in the examination of prolapse patients, but they are usually not essential for the preoperative assessment.

Surgical Therapy

Rectal prolapse in children is generally treated conservatively, whereas surgical repair is suggested for adults. In 1912, Moschcowitz presented his theory that rectal prolapse is a sliding hernia and he suggested obliteration of the deep cul-de-sac of Douglas as treatment, but this method had a high recurrence rate.

Today both abdominal and perineal approaches are used. Abdominal approaches include different types of rectal suspension and fixation and they usually have low recurrence rates (Table 89-1). Perineal approaches have higher recurrence rates and they are usually reserved for elderly patients or patients with concomitant health problems.

Abdominal Rectal Prolapse Repair

Most authors advocate complete posterior mobilization of the rectum to the coccyx, and some recommend partial anterior mobilization as well. The extent of lateral mobilization has been debated and there is little data reported in the literature. It has been found in patients undergoing posterior mesh rectopexy for prolapse that division of lateral ligaments may contribute to the development of onset constipation. A marked increase of constipation has been found in patients who had undergone Wells rectopexy with division of lateral ligaments, when they were compared

TABLE 89-1. Recurrence Rates After Treatment of Rectal Prolapse

	Number of Patients	Mean Follow-Up (years)	Recurrence (%)
Abdominal Procedures			
Ripstein			
Holmström 1986	82	6.9	5
Roberts 1988	130	3.4	10
Tjandra 1993	129	4.2	8
Winde 1993	35	4.2	0
Posterior rectopexy with mesh			
Mann 1988	51	4.8	0
Yoshioka 1989	135	3	2
McCue 1991	53	3.1	2
Suture rectopexy			
Ejerblad 1988	—	6.8	4
Blatchford 1989	51	2.3	2
Graf 1996	135	5.3	9
Resection rectopexy			
Madoff 1992		5.4	6
Huber 1997	51	4.5	0
Anterior resection			
Schlinkert 1985	53	7	9
Perineal Procedures			
Perineal recto-sigmoidectomy	51	—	—
Altemeier 1971	135	?	3
Williams 1992	53	1	10
Delorme			
Uhlig 1979	51	—	7
Monson 1986	135	—	7
Senapati 1994	53	2	22
Oliver 1994	—	3.9	13
Tsunoda 2003	31	3.3	13
Watkins 2003	52	5	6

with patients who had undergone Ripstein's operation with the lateral ligaments preserved. Preservation of the lateral ligaments may therefore be recommended.

Ripstein Rectopexy

After mobilization, the rectum is usually suspended to the sacrum, but the optimal technique for this suspension is still debated. Ripstein (1965) described a repair based on the theory that prolapse is caused by rectal attachment to the sacrum. This repair has been used extensively in the United States.

The rectopexy is performed by suturing an approximately 5 cm wide piece of mesh to the sacrum. The mesh is wrapped around and sutured to the anterior wall of the rectum. The wrap should be loose enough to avoid stricturing of the rectum.

The Ripstein rectopexy has sometimes been accused of causing obstructed defecation, but early reports of postoperative constipation following this procedure were not controlled for preoperative symptoms. However, the technique includes a risk for infection and fistula formation because of the circular mesh and the recurrence rate, and functional outcome does not differ from other techniques. Its popularity has therefore decreased.

Wells' Rectopexy

The Ivalon sponge procedure is similar to the Ripstein procedure, but the mesh is placed partially around the bowel instead of circumferentially. This technique was popularized because of concerns over sling obstruction with a circumferential mesh.

The technique was described by Wells in 1959. Wells based his procedure on the use of a polyvinyl alcohol sponge (Ivalon) with its tendency to create a reactive fibrotic response. It is, however, unclear whether this reactive response is needed, as techniques such as suture rectopexy seem to offer the same low recurrence rates as the Wells' procedure.

Suture Rectopexy

Direct *suture rectopexy* was first advocated by Cutait in 1959. The suture rectopexy is used as a temporary suspension of the rectum while adhesions form between the rectum and the presacral fascia. This technique has gained renewed interest after the introduction of laparoscopic surgery (see below). After mobilization, the rectum is suspended to the sacrum with 2 to 4 sutures that are anchored in the mesorectum and the presacral fascia.

Suture rectopexy seems to offer similar recurrence and complication rates as techniques involving mesh. Suture rectopexy is therefore an attractive alternative and it may also be used together with simultaneous sigmoid resection (see below) because no foreign material is used.

Resection Rectopexy

Another topic of debate is whether the redundant sigmoid colon should or should not be resected at suture rectopexy. When Frykman and Goldberg (1969) described resection rectopexy, the original rationale of the resection was to suspend the left colon from the splenic flexure to prevent recurrence.

It is apparent today that this is not needed when the low recurrence rates in most series evaluating abdominal prolapse repair. On the other hand, the use of resection may decrease the risk for postoperative constipation symptoms. A higher rate of new or persisting constipation has been reported in three additional trials in patients treated with sling rectopexy alone versus those treated with suture rectopexy and sigmoid resection.

Sometimes patients are not relieved of preexisting constipation despite a sigmoid resection at the time of rectopexy and on occasion subtotal colectomy with rectopexy may be the appropriate surgical method for carefully selected patients with severe slow transit constipation (Madoff et al, 1992). The risk for postoperative fecal incontinence may however be substantial, as many of these patients will have loose stools postoperatively.

Anterior Resection

Schlinkert and colleagues (1985) have reported the Mayo Clinic experience with anterior resection as therapy for rectal prolapse and found an acceptable recurrence rate (9%). They found that a low anastomosis increased morbidity without significantly decreasing recurrence when compared with high anterior resection. The effects of repair on patient continence were unpredictable.

Laparoscopic Prolapse Repair

Laparoscopic abdominal repair represents a new development in rectal prolapse surgery. Laparoscopy offers improved patient comfort, better cosmetic result, and decreased lengths of hospital stay and disability (Solomon and Eyers, 1996; Kellokumpu et al, 2000) and most of the procedures described above may be performed with this technique. In two recent studies (Heah et al, 2000; Zittel et al, 2000), it was reported that functional outcome after laparoscopic rectopexy was comparable with open surgery.

Perineal Rectal Prolapse Repair

Perineal prolapse repair is usually reserved for elderly patients or patients with concomitant health problems, because the recurrence rate is substantially higher. The recurrence rates in different series range from 5 to more than 50% (Williams et al, 1992; Senapati et al, 1994; Tsunoda et al, 2003; Watkins et al, 2003; Frykman and Goldberg, 1969) and there is a tendency that series with longer follow-up time have higher recurrence rates. In a recent study from our institution (Kim et al, 1999), perineal rectosigmoidectomy had a recurrence rate of 16% compared with 5% after rectopexy. Functional outcomes were similar following either operation. The results suggest that perineal rectosigmoidectomy may not be the ideal operation for healthy patients due to its relatively high recurrence rate.

Most authors currently favor either perineal rectosigmoidectomy or Delorme's operation and the choice between these two types of procedures usually depends upon individual surgeon training and preference. Series comparing different perineal operations are rare.

Perineal procedures are well tolerated by most patients. The postoperative course is usually benign and most patients tolerate the procedure quite well and the postoperative stay is usually short.

Perineal Rectosigmoidectomy

Perineal rectosigmoidectomy was first described by Mikulicz in 1889. Renewed interest in this procedure, particularly in the United States, can be attributed to W.A. Altemeier, whose 1971 report claimed only 3 recurrences in a series of 106 patients. A few series have recurrence rates comparable to those seen after abdominal repairs, but several reports have considerably higher recurrence rates. The variability in results reported by different centers stands in contrast to the marked uniformity and predictability of success seen after abdominal repairs.

Perineal rectosigmoidectomy can be done under regional or regional anesthesia in the lithotomy or prone position. The rectum is externalized as far as possible, and an incision is made approximately 1 to 2 cm from the dentate line. The incision is made full thickness through the outer bowel wall, entering the space between the external and internal bowel tubes of the prolapsed rectum. The rectal and sigmoid mesenteric vessels are divided with ligatures or using a harmonic scalpel and the prolapsed segment of rectum is folded down as far as possible. Resection of 20 to 40 cm of rectum and sigmoid colon is not uncommon. After mobilizing the maximum length of bowel, the prolapsed segment is resected and an anastomosis is sutured.

Addition of a levatoroplasty to the procedure might influence recurrence rates by tightening the levator hiatus and providing a new anorectal angle that contrasts with the "straight" rectal contour typically seen in prolapse patients (Williams et al, 1992; Agachan et al, 1997).

Delorme's Operation

Delorme described an alternative perineal repair and the method was popularized after the report of Uhlig and Sullivan (1979). This procedure can also be done under regional or regional anesthesia in the lithotomy or prone position. The submucosa above the dentate line is injected with an epinephrine solution where after the rectal mucosa on the external side of the prolapse is dissected free from the underlying muscle. The rectal muscle is then vertically plicated in all four quadrants, usually by using eight plicating sutures. As these sutures are tied, the muscle is plicated, and the excess mucosa is then excised and the mucosa is closed with a mucosa-to-mucosa closure.

Functional Outcome After Rectal Prolapse Surgery

Several attempts have been made to predict postoperative outcome with physiologic testing. Preoperative manometry results have generally not been predictive of the functional outcome regarding continence, though patients with very severe physiologic abnormalities may have a worse prognosis (Williams et al, 1992; Yoshioka et al, 1989).

A majority of studies report that approximately 50% of incontinent patients improve after surgery. Restoration of internal anal sphincter function plays probably an important role in this process, as improved continence after surgery is often accompanied by increased resting pressures (Schultz et al, 1996). The removal of the prolapsing may also be an important reason, as the prolapse disturbs the sphincter function by repetitive sphincter dilatation. Other important factors may be postoperative improvements in anal sphincter electomyogram and improved sensation (Duthie, 1992).

The frequency of postoperative constipation varies greatly between studies. Some studies report increased incidence (Graf et al, 1996; Aitola et al, 1999), whereas others report an unchanged (Tjandra et al, 1993), or decreased (Roberts et al, 1988; Winde et al, 1993) incidence. Possible reasons for postoperative constipation include colonic denervation, rectal denervation by division of the lateral ligaments, or a redundant sigmoid that may contribute to rectosigmoid kinking.

Rectal Intussusception

Internal rectal intussusception is sometimes labeled "occult rectal prolapse" as the conditions are quite similar at defecography, with the only difference that rectal intussusception does not extend beyond the anal verge.

Internal intussusception is associated with several different functional complaints. Johansson and colleagues (1985) examined 190 patients with rectal intussusception and found that 57% of patients experienced a sensation of obstruction, 44% had fecal incontinence, 43% had painful defecations, and 27% had anal bleeding. Mucous discharge and diarrhea have also been reported.

The most common symptom associated with internal intussusception is, thus, obstructed defecation. This can be explained by several mechanisms. The intussusception, sometimes together with a concomitant enterocele and/or rectocele, may restrict emptying or produce a sensation of rectal fullness. The intussuscepting bowel, present in the rectum, may be experienced by the patient as fecal material that cannot be expelled. Continued straining will then increase the size of the intussusception and further worsen symptoms.

The association between the internal rectal intussusception and the above-mentioned symptoms remains unclear. Surgical correction of the anatomical intussusception does not always alleviate symptoms and rectal intussusception is a frequent finding in patients with defecation disorders. In an evaluation of 2,816 defecography investigations, we found that 31% of the patients had a circumferential rectal intussusception (Mellgren et al, 1994). Rectal intussusception has also been reported to be a frequent finding in defecography studies of healthy volunteers (Shorvon et al, 1989; Goei, 1990).

Diagnosis

Rectal intussusception is usually diagnosed at defecography as a circumferential infolding of the rectal wall that does not pass beyond the anal verge. However, at rectal examination the intussusception may be palpated or inspected with a proctoscope. A distal proctitis or a solitary ulcer may also be seen.

Treatment

Patients with internal rectal intussusception have often a long history of anorectal problems and they have consulted several physicians. After establishing the diagnosis, management is usually conservative. Patients are informed about the condition and they are advised to avoid straining at stool, as this may increase symptoms. Bulking agents may be beneficial and, sometimes, small enemas may facilitate rectal emptying.

Indications for surgical treatment vary in different studies, as do the surgical results. Unfortunately most published studies are retrospective and they include relatively small numbers of patients. Fecal incontinence in patients with rectal intussusception is an indication for surgical treatment and most studies (Table 89-2) report improved postoperative anal continence. Outlet obstruction is often unchanged or may even deteriorate after surgery (see Table 89-2), and patients should be counseled regarding this before surgical treatment. However the effect on outlet obstruction is unpredictable and some patients improve after rectopexy (Schultz et al, 1998).

As mentioned, rectal intussusception and rectal prolapse are quite similar at defecography, with the only difference being that rectal intussusception does not extend beyond the anal verge. Sometimes the risk for developing rectal prolapse is used as a surgical indication in patients with rectal intussusception. This risk seemed however to be quite limited, when we followed rectal intussusception patients over time (Mellgren et al, 1997).

SRUS

SRUS is a proctologic disease characterized by erythema and/or one or several ulcerations of the rectal wall. It is a benign condition with a characteristic histologic picture, and patients usually have associated disordered defecation. The ulcer is usually located anteriorly in the rectum, and instead of an ulcer, the lesion may also be polypoid.

The histologic characteristics of the lesion were first described by Madigan and Morson in 1969 and they include a thickened muscularis mucosa, a lamina propria expanded by fibroblasts, and smooth muscle cells arranged to point towards the lumen. Colitis cystica profunda is a form of the SRUS, with dilated displaced glands filled with mucus and lined with normal colonic epithelium in the submucosa. Frequently the lesion at SRUS can be difficult to distinguish from adenomateus polyps or tumors, and biopsies are therefore essential to verify the diagnosis.

The etiology of SRUS remains obscure and patients frequently have concomitant pelvic floor disorders. There is an association between SRUS, rectal prolapse, internal rectal intussusception, paradoxical sphincter reaction (PSR), and outlet obstruction. The symptoms are similar and the conditions sometimes coexist, but the relationship between these disorders is not fully understood, as all can exist alone.

TABLE 89-2. Treatment Results of Rectal Intussusception

	Technique	Number of Patients	Mean Follow Up (years)	Incontinence	Constipation
Ihre 1975	Ripstein	36	2 to 13	Improved	Worse
Johansson 1985	Ripstein	63	—	Improved	Worse
Lazorthes 1986	Post. Recopexy	14	> 0.5	Improved	Improved
Berman 1990	Delorme	21	> 3	—	Improved
McCue 1990	Wells	12	2.2	Improved	Worse
Christiansen 1992	Wells + Orr	9 + 15	1 to 8	Improved	45% Improved
van Tets 1995	Post. Rectopexy	21	6	—	Improved
Briel 1997	Suture rectopexy	13	5.6	38% improved	—

Excessive straining causing trauma and ischemia of the prolapsed mucosa is probably one of the pathogenetic factors and self-digitation has also been discussed as a possible causative factor (Rutter and Riddell, 1975).

Symptoms

SRUS affects both men and women, usually with onset before the age of 50 years. Typical symptoms include evacuation difficulties with prolonged straining at bowel movements, passage of blood and mucous per rectum, tenesmus, and, sometimes, anorectal pain. Digitation for evacuation of feces is considered to be common. SRUS may, however, also be found in asymptomatic patients.

Treatment

Nonsurgical options are usually preferred as initial treatment (Vaizey et al, 1997). Retraining of bowel habits, decrease of straining efforts, and a high fiber diet, is generally recommended. Biofeedback-training might be helpful, especially if the patient has PSR (Binnie et al, 1992). Abdominal rectopexy offers long term symptom improvement in approximately 50% of patients (Vaizey et al, 1998). Rectal ulceration may persist after any treatment, even if symptoms improve.

Surgery is frequently recommended when SRUS is accompanied by rectal intussusception or rectal prolapse. Reports on surgical outcome are, however, usually based on small series with limited follow-up time. Successful outcome has been reported after Ripstein rectopexy in 9 of 10 patients with concomitant rectal prolapse (Schweiger and Alexander-Williams, 1977), after posterior rectopexy with Marlex mesh in 5 of 6 patients with rectal prolapse (Keighley and Shouler, 1984), and after Wells' posterior rectopexy in 17 of 17 patients with concomitant internal rectal intussusception. Other reports have not found the same excellent results. Marchal and colleagues (2001) reviewed 13 patients operated on for SRUS with a mean FU of 57 months. The authors operated with various techniques and they found a high failure rate after surgery. They therefore recommend surgical therapy only in patients with total rectal prolapse or intractable symptoms.

Editor's Note: A complete 110-item bibliography is available at <mellgren@umn.edu>.

Supplemental Reading

Agachan F, Reissman P, Pfeifer J, et al. Comparison of three perineal procedures for the treatment of rectal prolapse. South Med J 1997;90:925–32.

Aitola PT, Hiltunen KM, Matikainen MJ. Functional results of operative treatment of rectal prolapse over an 11-year period: emphasis on transabdominal approach. Dis Colon Rectum 1999;42:655–60.

Allen-Mersh TG, Turner MJ, Mann CV. Effect of abdominal Ivalon rectopexy on bowel habit and rectal wall. Dis Colon Rectum 1990;33:550–3.

Binnie NR, Papachrysostomou M, Clare N, Smith AN. Solitary rectal ulcer: the place of biofeedback and surgery in the treatment of the syndrome. World J Surg 1992;16:836–40.

Brodén B, Snellman B. Procidentia of the rectum studied with cineradiography: a contribution to the discussion of causative mechanism. Dis Colon Rectum 1968;11:330–47.

Cutait D. Sacro-promontory fixation of the rectum for complete rectal prolapse. Proc R Soc Med 1959;52:105.

Delorme E. On the treatment of total prolapse of the rectum by excision of the rectal mucus membranes or recto-colic. Dis Colon Rectum 1985;28:544–53.

Frykman HM, Goldberg SM. The surgical treatment of rectal procidentia. Surg Gynecol Obstet 1969;129:1225–30.

Goei R. Anorectal function in patients with defecation disorders and asymptomatic subjects: evaluation with defecography. Radiology 1990;174:121–3.

Heah SM, Hartley JE, Hurley J, et al. Laparoscopic suture rectopexy without resection is effective treatment for full-thickness rectal prolapse. Dis Colon Rectum 2000;43:638–43.

Huber FT, Stein H, Siewert JR. Functional results after treatment of rectal prolapse with rectopexy and sigmoid resection. W J Surg 1995;19:138–43.

Johansson C, Ihre T, Ahlbäck SO. Disturbances in the defecation mechanism with special reference to intussusception of the rectum (internal procidentia). Dis Colon Rectum 1985;28:920–4.

Keighley MRB, Shouler PJ. Clinical and manometric features of the solitary rectal ulcer syndrome. Dis Colon Rectum 1984;27:507–12.

Kellokumpu IH, Vironen J, Scheinin T. Laparoscopic repair of rectal prolapse: a prospective study evaluating surgical outcome and changes in symptoms and bowel function. Surg Endosc 2000;14:634–40.

Kim DS, Tsang CB, Wong WD, et al. Complete rectal prolapse: evolution of management and results. Dis Colon Rectum 1999;42:460–6; discussion 466–9.

Madden MV, Kamm MA, Nicholls RJ, et al. Abdominal rectopexy for complete prolapse: prospective study evaluating changes in symptoms and anorectal function. Dis Colon Rectum 1992;35:48–55.

Madigan MR, Morson BC. Solitary ulcer of the rectum. Gut 1969;10:871–81.

Madoff RD, Williams JG, Wong WD, et al. Long-term functional results of colon resection and rectopexy for overt rectal prolapse. Am J Gastroenterol 1992;87:101–4.

Marchal F, Bresler L, Brunaud L, et al. Solitary rectal ulcer syndrome: a series of 13 patients operated with a mean follow-up of 4.5 years. Int J Colorectal Dis 2001;16:228–33.

Marshall M, Halligan S, Fotheringham T, et al. Predictive value of internal anal sphincter thickness for diagnosis of rectal intussusception in patients with solitary rectal ulcer syndrome. Br J Surg 2002;89:1281–5.

Mellgren A, Bremmer S, Johansson C, et al. Defecography, results of investigations in 2,816 patients. Dis Colon Rectum 1994;37:1133–41.

Mellgren A, Schultz I, Johansson C, Dolk A. Internal rectal intussusception seldom develops into rectal prolapse. Dis Colon Rectum 1997.[In press].

Plusa SM, Charig JA, Balaji V, Watts A. Physiological changes after Delorme's procedure for full-thickness rectal prolapse. Br J Surg 1995;82:1475–8.

Porter NH. A physiological study of the pelvic floor in rectal prolapse. Ann R Coll Surg Engl 1962;31:379–404.

Ripstein CB. Surgical care of massive rectal prolapse. Dis Colon Rectum 1965;8:34–8.

Roberts PL, Schoetz DJ, Coller JA, Veidenheimer MC. Ripstein procedure. Lahey Clinic experience: 1963–1985. Arch Surg 1988;123:554–7.

Rutter KRP, Riddell RH. The solitary ulcer syndrome of the rectum. Clin Gastroenterol 1975;4:505–30.

Schlinkert RT, Beart RW, Wolf BG, Pemberton JH. Anterior resection for complete rectal prolapse. Dis Colon Rectum 1985;28:409–12.

Schultz I, Mellgren A, Johansson C, et al. Continence is improved after the Ripstein rectopexy. Different mechanisms in patients with rectal prolapse and rectal intussusception? Dis Colon Rectum 1996;39:300–5.

Schultz I, Mellgren A, Nilsson BY, et al. Preoperative electrophysiologic assessment cannot predict continence after rectopexy. Dis Colon Rectum 1998;41:1392–8.

Schweiger M, Alexander-Williams J. Solitary ulcer of the rectum. Its association with occult rectal prolapse. Lancet 1977;1:170–1.

Senapati A, Nicholls RJ, Thomson JPS, Phillips RKS. Results of Delorme's procedure for rectal prolapse. Dis Colon Rectum 1994;37:456–60.

Shorvon PJ, McHugh S, Diamant NE, et al. Defecography in normal volunteers: results and implications. Gut 1989;30:1737–49.

Solomon MJ, Eyers AA. Laparoscopic rectopexy using mesh fixation with a spiked chromium staple. Dis Colon Rectum 1996;39:279–84.

Tjandra JJ, Fazio VW, Church JM, et al. Ripstein procedure is an effective treatment for rectal prolapse without constipation. Dis Colon Rectum 1993;36:501–7.

Tsunoda A, Yasuda N, Yokoyama N, et al. Delorme's procedure for rectal prolapse: clinical and physiological analysis. Dis Colon Rectum 2003;46:1260–5.

Uhlig BE, Sullivan ES. The modified Delorme operation: its place in surgical treatment for massive rectal prolapse. Dis Colon Rectum 1979;22:513–21.

Vaizey CJ, Roy AJ, Kamm MA. Prospective evaluation of the treatment of solitary rectal ulcer syndrome with biofeedback. Gut 1997;41:817–20.

Vaizey CJ, van den Bogaerde JB, Emmanuel AV, et al. Solitary rectal ulcer syndrome. Br J Surg 1998;85:1617–23.

Watkins BP, Landercasper J, Belzer GE, et al. Long-term follow-up of the modified Delorme procedure for rectal prolapse. Arch Surg 2003;138:498–502; discussion 502–3.

Wells C. New operation for rectal prolapse. Proc R Soc Med 1959;52:602–3.

Williams JG, Rothenberger DA, Madoff RD, Goldberg SM. Treatment of rectal prolapse in the elderly by perineal rectosigmoidectomy. Dis Colon Rectum 1992;35:830–4.

Winde G, Reers B, Nottberg H, et al. Clinical and functional results of abdominal rectopexy with absorbable mesh-graft for treatment of complete rectal prolapse. Eur J Surg 1993;159:301–5.

Zittel TT, Manncke K, Haug S, et al. Functional results after laparoscopic rectopexy for rectal prolapse. J Gastrointest Surg 2000;4:632–41.

Chapter 90

Ileoanal Pouch: Frequent Evacuation

L.J. Egan, MD, and S.F. Phillips, MD

Proctocolectomy with ileal pouch-anal anastomosis (IPAA) is the most popular surgical option when colonic resection is necessary for the treatment of ulcerative colitis (UC) and familial adenomatous polyposis. However, after IPAA, patients will always defecate more frequently than do healthy people. Thus, after proctocolectomy, whether surgical continuity is restored with a terminal ileostomy or with a pouch, daily fecal volumes will be 500 to 700 mL (Metcalf and Phillips, 1986). In health, fecal volumes do not often exceed 200 mL. Moreover, the reservoir of an ileoanal pouch is smaller than that of a normal rectum. IPAA patients complaining of frequent bowel movements must recognize their symptoms in this context; they will never have only one or two solid stools daily! Although patients who complain of frequent defecation after IPAA may have no identifiable pathology, they can, nevertheless, be helped to accept a new lifestyle by being taught to understand the postoperative physiology (Dean and Dozois, 1997; Levitt and Kuan, 1998). Moreover, simple antidiarrheal therapy may significantly improve their lifestyle.

The majority of patients with normally functioning IPAAs should evacuate between four and eight times per day, and once or twice at night. After the initial postoperative phase, IPAA patients should not have extreme fecal urgency and should be able to distinguish between the urges of flatus and feces. Approximately 10 to 20% of IPAA patients experience minor leakage of stool, especially at night, when they may need to wear a pad (Meagher et al, 1998). However, they should be continent during the day. Passage of stools should be painless, should not be accompanied by the need to strain, and should feel complete. In taking the history, the features of "diarrhea" need to be defined precisely; increased fecal frequency needs to be distinguished from urgency, fecal leakage, or gross incontinence.

Importance of an Adequate History

The key to helping IPAA patients who complain of excessive bowel movements is to make an accurate diagnosis. Disorders of the pouch outlet (the anal sphincter segment), the pouch itself, or of the ileum proximal to the pouch may be the cause of an increased stool frequency. In many patients, a careful history will provide the astute clinician with a short list of diagnostic possibilities. The most important element of the history is to determine precisely what it is about pouch function that is unsatisfactory to the patient. A typical complaint might be of having to "go all the time." The physician must then determine exactly what the patient means. Is the patient having true watery diarrhea, or is the main complaint urgency or leakage? Is an inability to completely empty the pouch with consequent leakage of retained stool the real problem? Careful evaluation of the patient's complaints, in conjunction with knowledge of the likely causes of symptoms, should point to the correct diagnosis. In practice, it is advantageous to divide the clinical picture into those patients who are distressed soon after surgery from those who present later.

Excessive or Uncontrolled Bowel Movements with Newly Formed Pouches

General Approach

Problems occurring soon after the operation (0 to 6 months) present more often to surgeons, but gastroenterologists need also to be aware of these issues (Table 90-1). It is helpful to

TABLE 90-1. Approach to Patients After Ileal Pouch-Anal Anastomosis With Excessive Bowel Movements in the First 6 Months of Pouch Reanastomosis

Cause	Diagnostic Approaches	Treatment
Unrealistic expectations	Exclude pathology by physical examination; ± Endoscopy, ± Pouchogram	Education and reassurance Fiber supplements, antidiarrheals
Anastomotic leak	Endoscopy Pouchogram	Intestinal diversion, abscess drainage Pouch revision (late decisions)
Defective sphincter function and anal incontinence	Physical examination Anal manometry	Antidiarrheals, fiber supplements Biofeedback
Anastomotic stricture	Physical examination Endoscopy	Dilatation
Pouchitis	Pouchoscopy and biopsy	Antibiotics
Cuffitis	Pouchoscopy and biopsy	Mesalamine, steroids

consider the time of onset of increased bowel frequency in relation to the age of the pouch. The first few weeks after closure of the temporary ileostomy and restoration of the fecal stream to the pouch are often marked by frequent loose stools, to which the pouch and the patient must be helped to adapt. The sensation of a full ileal pouch may be qualitatively different from that of a full rectum, and patients must learn to recognize those sensations that indicate that they need to empty the pouch.

Thus, some patients, if they have not received adequate preoperative counseling, have unrealistic expectations about the functional outcomes after "curative" IPAA surgery. They need to be educated; they will always have a high fecal volume, and their stools will never be fully formed. Moreover, it is important to reassure patients that a healthy pouch and anal sphincter will *gradually adapt postoperatively* and, consequently, bowel function should be expected to improve. In addition to reassurance and education, simple measures can significantly help patients with a new IPAA to learn to compensate. For example, *fiber supplements,* such as methylcellulose or psyllium, of 1 g in a large glass of water once or twice per day, will increase the consistency of stools. *Loperamide* 2 to 4 mg taken 30 minutes before meals will reduce postprandial urgency. Although many IPAA patients find that certain foodstuffs increase stool, it is not particularly helpful to counsel individual patients on the consumption of specific items of food. One patient's experience is likely to differ so much from another's. Rather, patients should experiment, be moderate, and be guided by their own experience in choosing a lifestyle that minimizes any negative impacts of the pouch. It is important not to promote compulsivity in dietary or other habits.

Although many patients complaining of excessive bowel frequency, diarrhea or leakage soon after IPAA will ultimately be found not to have a structural/organic basis, one must not overlook the possibility of a postoperative complication. *Small bowel obstruction* occurs in the first weeks after pouch formation in 6 to 20% of patients. Though pain is the expected symptom of obstruction, increased fecal volumes can be the major complaint.

Anastomotic Leakage

Fortunately, *leakage* at the *pouch-anus anastomosis* is rare, especially when the anastomosis is protected by a diverting ileostomy. Most surgical series report this as less than 10%, though some higher rates are reported. Anastomotic leakage typically causes *pelvic pain and abscess*. Pouch dysfunction is exemplified by painful, incomplete evacuation, and excessive frequency. Demonstration of a leak with a retrograde barium contrast study (pouchogram) is usually diagnostic. Occasionally, a *pouch-vaginal* or *pouch-perineal fistula* may develop in association with anastomotic leakage; this should always raise the question of unrecognized Crohn's disease (CD). However, further investigation should be delayed until after the initial postoperative period. Treatment is *surgical*, and may require intestinal diversion, drainage of an abscess if present, and possibly revision of the pouch.

Defective Sphincteric Continence

Innervation of the internal anal sphincter may be disrupted during the perineal dissection and construction of the pouch-anus anastomosis. Consequently, resting pressures of the internal anal sphincter are usually reduced, at least for 6 to 12 months postoperatively. After this, there is a gradual return of basal anal tone; fortunately, function of the external sphincter, which is usually preserved, helps compensate for any lowering of internal sphincter pressures. Exceptions may be seen in elderly patients and multiparous women whose anal pressures were low before pouch construction. In this situation, defective anal continence can lead to leakage, which may be presented by the patient as excessive bowel motions ("diarrhea") after IPAA. Indeed, even patients who will subsequently develop excellent pouch function may experience soiling, incontinence, and some degree of urgency soon after ileostomy closure.

Physical examination of the sphincter in these patients reveals low resting tone and sometimes low squeeze pressures, findings that can be confirmed by anal manometry if necessary. Effective management involves the judicial use of antidiarrheals such as *loperamide*, 2 to 4 mg 30 minutes before meals, and *fiber supplements* to increase stool consistency. *Biofeedback* may be helpful later, for those patients whose sphincter function returns only slowly or incompletely; retraining of patients to use the external anal sphincter to greater advantage can be helpful. In a minority of IPAA patients, incontinence due to poor sphincter tone persists, and is occasionally sufficient to require *permanent ileostomy*. This is one of the reasons for "pouch failure."

Pouch Outlet Obstruction

In the early postoperative period, before takedown of the diverting ileostomy, a thin web-like stricture often forms at the ileal pouch-anal anastomotic line. After the fecal stream into the pouch is restored, persistence of this stricture obstructs the pouch outlet, leading to incomplete evacuation, somewhat analogous to bladder outlet obstruction in prostatism. The patient will complain of diarrhea due to incomplete emptying of the pouch, resulting in overflow leakage and fecal frequency. Digital examination of the anus demonstrates a narrowing of the upper anal canal. These strictures can usually be dilated easily with the finger or a rubber dilator. In some patients, anastomotic strictures can progress to become chronic, recurrent and fibrotic, and to require regular dilatation.

Residual Inflammatory Bowel Disease ("Cuffitis")

Modern pouch surgery leaves behind only a small cuff of rectal mucosa, of 1 or 2 cm at the most, when a double-stapled anastomosis is formed. No rectal mucosa should remain when the anastomosis is hand sewn in conjunction with a distal rectal mucosectomy. However, in some cases, for example in obese patients when it is difficult to bring the small bowel deep into the pelvis, the surgeon may need to leave behind a more substantial cuff of rectal mucosa to which the pouch is anastomosed. The term "*cuffitis*" has been used to describe persistent inflammatory bowel disease (IBD) in the remnant of rectal mucosa. Most often it occurs in patients who had active colitis before surgery. Symptoms are proportional to the amount of rectal mucosa that remains and to the severity of the inflammation. Patients complain of fecal frequency and urgency and the motions are commonly watery with mucous and blood. Urgency and leakage occur, especially at night. Rarely, if several centimeters of rectum remain, systemic symptoms of malaise, low-grade fever or weight loss may be experienced. Initial treatment, with standard topical anti-inflammatory agents, such as *mesalamine suppositories* or *hydrocortisone enemas*, may be sufficient. Patients who do not respond to locally applied agents, and who require systemic steroids to control cuffitis, will occasionally require a further operation, to remove the inflamed rectal mucosa and to anastomose the pouch to the upper anal canal, if technically feasible.

Acute Pouchitis

IBD of the pouch (pouchitis) is a syndrome defined by clinical, endoscopic and histologic criteria that occurs in UC-IPAA patients (Mahadevan and Sandborn, 2003), and seldom, if ever, affects familial adenomatous polyposis-IPAA patients. Patients complain of fecal frequency, and the motions are commonly loose and watery and may contain mucous and blood. Urgency and leakage, especially at night, are common. In addition, depending on the severity of pouch inflammation, the presence of associated fistulas, CD or concurrent pouch outlet obstruction, pelvic pain may be present. Systemic symptoms of malaise, low-grade fever or weight loss are often present in the more severe cases of pouch inflammation. Physical examination in patients with pouch inflammation is often normal. However, individuals with marked inflammation of the pouch from any cause may have the general features of patients with IBD, with low-grade fever, weight loss, and pallor. CD is suggested by signs of small bowel obstruction, abdominal mass or tenderness, or perineal sepsis.

In most cases, *endoscopy* and *biopsy* of the pouch will be diagnostic. We use flexible upper gut endoscopes to examine ileal pouches, because of their narrower caliber and superior flexibility compared to sigmoidoscopes. It must be recognized that even in a healthy pouch, the ileal mucosa undergoes metaplasia to a more colonic type; accordingly, normal ileum is not seen endoscopically or histologically. The presence of edema, erythema, mucous exudates, and ulceration suggest pouch inflammation. If endoscopic changes are confined to the pouch and do not extend into the prepouch ileum, pouchitis is the likely diagnosis. However, if aphthous or deep ulcerations and other mucosal abnormalities extend proximal from the pouch, or are seen solely in the prepouch ileum, CD is more likely. Occasionally, a linear series of shallow ulcerations will be observed extending along the divided pouch septum. This appearance is suggestive of pouch ischemia, a complication that may occur if the mesenteric vessels have been stretched too deeply into the pelvis (de Silva et al, 1991).

Severe microscopic inflammation can be found in a pouch with a relatively normal endoscopic appearance. Thus, biopsy and histological evaluation of the mucosa are essential. An experienced pathologist should be able to distinguish between pouchitis, CD, and mucosal ischemia. Pouchography detects pouch leaks, fistulas and strictures, and thus can be helpful if these complications are suspected, or if pouchitis needs to be differentiated from CD. Almost all cases of acute pouchitis will promptly respond to a course of antibiotics, such as metronidazole 250 to 500 mg 3 times daily or ciprofloxacin 500 mg twice daily for 10 to 14 days. Rarely, cytomegalovirus can infect pouch mucosa leading to chronic inflammation; the diagnosis is suggested by the presence of viral inclusions on histology. Treatment with ganciclovir is reported to be effective.

Excessive Bowel Frequency in Patients with Established Pouches

General Approach

Several large series have reported excellent long term functional outcomes of IPAA for UC; these have been summarized and reviewed (Dean and Dozois, 1997). Ten years after IPAA, incontinence had not occurred during the day in 73% of patients, nor at night in 48% (Meagher et al, 1998). However, many IPAA patients, at some time after construction of the pouch, experience increased bowel frequency, urgency or incontinence, all symptoms that may be presented as "diarrhea" (Table 90-2). Pouchitis is the most common, but not the only, cause of these symptoms. Disorders of the pouch other than pouchitis include disorders of pouch emptying, diseases in the prepouch ileum, and any of the causes of diarrhea that may occur in patients with an intact bowel. In the majority of cases, a correct diagnosis should provide a management strategy that brings about improvement. Ten years after IPAA surgery, pouch failure requiring pouch excision or permanent ileostomy occurs in less than 5% of patients.

TABLE 90-2. Approach to Patients After Ileal Pouch-Anal Anastomosis Who Complain of Excessive Bowel Movements 6 or More Months After Reanastomosis

Cause	Diagnostic Approaches	Treatment
Normal pouch	Exclude pathology Consider unrelated causes of diarrhea Preexisting irritable bowel syndrome Stool culture, microscopy Endoscopy ± pouchogram	Treat intercurrent diseases Reassurance Fiber supplements, antidiarrheals
Defective anal continence	Physical examination Anal manometry	Fiber supplements, antidiarrheals Biofeedback
Pouch outlet obstruction	Physical examination	Dilatation
Cuffitis	Pouchoscopy and biopsy	Mesalamine, steroids
Pouchitis	Pouchoscopy and biopsy	Antibiotics, mesalamine
Crohn's disease	Pouchoscopy and biopsy Pouchogram	Antibiotics, azathioprine, infliximab

Problems with the Outlet

Pouch outlet obstruction, usually due to anastomotic scarring and stricture, leads to incomplete evacuation. Not only will this increase stool frequency, but patients may complain of the need to strain, defecation may be painful, and there may be a recognition that the pouch has not been completely emptied. Incomplete evacuation often results in leakage of liquid stool around retained material in the pouch and the constant desire to defecate. The patient makes repeated and frustrating trips to the toilet. Typically, pouch outlet obstruction may cause a feeling of pelvic fullness or bloating, but systemic symptoms such as weight loss and malaise are absent. Many IPAA patients have mild degrees of anal stenosis, and the index finger should be inserted easily into the pouch through a rather snug anastomosis. Inability to pass the examining finger easily into the pouch, or marked tenderness on attempting to do so, are indicative of an anastomotic stricture.

It is usually possible to pass an endoscope through the stricture; this should be done to exclude a coexistent inflammation of the pouch. Indeed, incomplete emptying is thought to predispose to pouchitis (Mahadevan and Sandborn, 2003). If pouchitis is present, it will deserve treatment. Dilatation of the stricture will relieve pouch outlet obstruction, thereby improving the ease and completeness of defecation. If the stricture is tight or tender, dilatation is best done under general anesthesia. Thereafter, anal dilation can be repeated as needed, possibly with conscious sedation. A small number of patients with tighter and recurrent strictures need very frequent dilation, even once or twice per week. It is our practice to train these individuals to perform self-anal dilatation using a rubber dilator. The need for more definitive surgical treatment of stubborn strictures needs to be a constant consideration of gastroenterologists and surgeons.

Recurrent or Chronic Pouchitis

Defective function of the pouch is probably the commonest reason for excessive bowel frequency in IPAA patients. Pouch inflammation, from pouchitis, unrecognized CD, or infectious causes, often is the cause of a "true diarrhea," (ie, passage of an abnormally high volume of feces). Ten to 20% of IPAA patients experience recurrent episodes of acute pouchitis. Although it is important to confirm the diagnosis of pouchitis with endoscopy and biopsy to exclude other explanations for symptoms, many patients become expert in recognizing stereotypic flares of pouchitis and can be treated without repeated investigations. The majority of patients respond to antibiotic treatment, such as 10 to 14 days therapy with metronidazole 250 mg 3 times daily or ciprofloxacin 500 mg twice daily (Figure 90-1). A minority of patients respond poorly to antibiotics or relapse immediately after discontinuing them and can be categorized as suffering from chronic pouchitis. Overall, this occurs in about 5% UC-IPAA patients. First line therapy usually comprises *maintenance antibiotics*, such as *ciprofloxacin* 500 mg/d. Anecdotal evidence also supports the use of *mesalamine* (oral or as suppositories), *corticosteroids*, *azathioprine (AZA)* or *6-mercaptopurine (6-MP)*, *bismuth*, and *infliximab*. A randomized placebo controlled trial showed that VSL-3, a probiotic cocktail administered daily in an oral dose of 6 g (two packets twice per day), was highly efficacious in maintaining antibiotic-induced remission in patients with chronic pouchitis. VSL-3 is only available in the United States through an Internet Web site, and our limited clinical experience with this compound is disappointing.

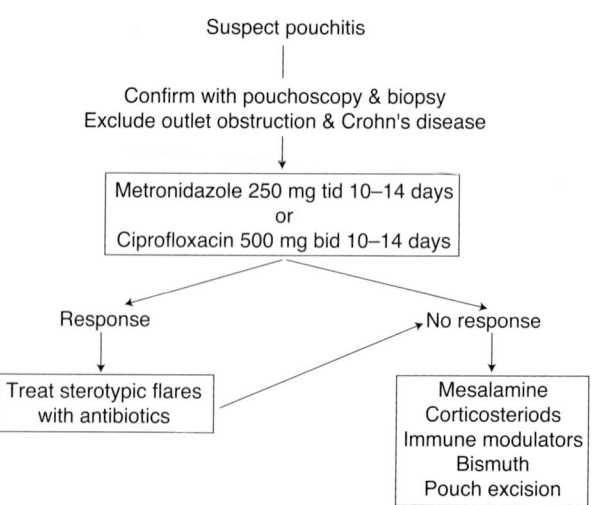

FIGURE 90-1. Management algorithm in ulcerative colitis-ileal pouch-anal anastomosis patients suspected of having pouchitis. bid = twice daily; tid = 3 times daily.

CD

Approximately 5% of IPAA procedures are performed in patients whose primary diagnosis is revised at some point after surgery from UC to CD. Many had their original colectomy for "fulminant colitis." CD may be the cause of chronic pouch and prepouch inflammation and perianal fistulas. Once the diagnosis is confirmed, therapy is no different from that of pelvic and perianal CD in patients still with a rectum. Infected cavities must be drained, obstruction must be excluded, and medical therapy with antibiotics such as metronidazole (250 to 500 mg 3 times daily) or ciprofloxacin (500 mg twice daily) should be begun.* It is our practice to start immunosuppressive therapy with AZA (2 to 2.5 mg/kg/d) or 6-MP (1.5 mg/kg/d) in CD patients whose conditions do not warrant immediate pouch excision. Open-label experience with the tumor necrosis factor alpha antibody (infliximab) for CD of pouches has been published by Ricart and colleagues (1999). A single infusion of infliximab (5 mg/kg) resulted in a rapid and favorable response in most patients.

Despite the use of powerful immunosuppressive medications in patients with pouchitis, CD of the pouch, or cuffitis, a minority of patients will not respond. The resulting chronic inflammation leads to a scarred, noncompliant pouch. In such patients, it may become futile to continue attempts at medical therapy, because the quality of life will clearly be much better after pouch excision and permanent ileostomy.

Irritable Pouch Syndrome

A small minority of IPAA patients will experience symptoms suggestive of pouchitis, but investigations reveal little inflammation and the absence of pouch outlet or other problems. These patients respond poorly to antibiotic therapy and are best considered as having "irritable pouches" (Schmidt et al, 1995). Empiric use of antidiarrheals or antispasmidics and fiber supplements is the most prudent approach.†

---

*Editor's Note: If the dose of metronidazole is less than 1g/d, peripheral neuropathy is rare.

---

†Editor's Note: Some patients give a history of classic irritable bowel syndrome (IBS) as teenagers, years before the onset of UC. If they have an IPAA, the ileum is as spastic as their colon had been as a teenager. Their pouches hold only 90 cc; on average they are only able to expel half of the contents so they experience 10 to 20 bowel movements per day. Some do better with decycloline than with loperamide, which contracts the pouch. I tend to urge against an IPAA in a patient with severe preexisting IBS.

Diarrhea Unrelated to the Pouch

After IPAA, patients are not immune to any of the more than 100 causes of diarrhea to which those with an intact bowel are equally susceptible. However, local symptoms, bleeding, incontinence and urgency tend to focus attention towards a local cause in the pouch. It must be recognized though that increased fecal volumes, from any generalized osmotic or secretory form of diarrhea, will, of necessity, stress pouch function and focus attention on pouch dysfunction, perhaps inappropriately.

Thus, any of the infectious diarrheas must always be considered and excluded in patients with IPAA diarrhea. Moreover, patients lacking a colon are more sensitive to the fluid losses that accompany any common infectious diarrhea which increase fecal volumes. Thus, consideration must always be given to small bowel diseases, such as celiac sprue, lactase deficiency, CD of the proximal bowel, and bacterial overgrowth. If a positive diagnosis of a pouch-related cause cannot be made, etiologies outside the pouch must be sought. Chapter 56, "Dietary-Induced Symptoms," has additional clues.

Supplemental Reading

Dean PA, Dozois RR. Surgical options—ileoanal pouch. In: Allan RN, Rhodes JM, Hanauer SB, et al, editors. Inflammatory bowel diseases, 3rd ed. London: Churchill Livingstone; 1997. p. 761–72.

de Silva HJ, Kettlewell MGW, Mortensen NJ, Jewell DP. Acute inflammation in ileal pouches. Eur J Gastroenterol Hepatol 1991;3:343–9.

Levitt MD, Kuan M. The physiology of ileo-anal pouch function. Am J Surg 1998;176:384–9.

Mahadevan U, Sandborn WJ. Diagnosis and management of pouchitis. Gastroenterology 2003;124:1636–50.

Meagher AP, Farouk R, Dozois RR, et al. J ileal pouch-anal anastomosis for chronic ulcerative colitis: complications and long-term outcome in 1310 patients. Br J Surg 1998;85:800–3.

Metcalf AM, Phillips SF. Ileostomy diarrhea. In: Krejs GJ, editor. Clinics in gastroenterology. London: WB Saunders Company; 1986. p. 705–22.

Ricart E, Panaccione R, Loftus EV, et al. Successful management of Crohn's disease of the ileoanal pouch with infliximab. Gastroenterology 1999;117:429–32.

Schmidt CM, Horton KM, Sitzmann JV, et al. Simple radiographic evaluation of ileo and pouch volume. Dis Colon Rectum 1995;38:203–8.

Stryker SJ, Kelly KA, Phillips SF, et al. Anal and neorectal function after ileal pouch-anal anastomosis. Ann Surg 1986;203:55–61.

Thompson-Fawcett MW, Mortensen NJ, Warren BF. "Cuffitis" and inflammatory changes in the columnar cuff, anal transitional zone, and ileal reservoir after stapled pouch-anal anastomosis. Dis Colon Rectum 1999;42:348–55.

# CHAPTER 91

ANORECTAL DISEASES

STEVEN D. WEXNER, MD, AND GIOVANNA DESILVA, MD

Anal Fissure

Anal fissure can be acute or chronic and is usually located in the midline of the anal canal, most commonly posteriorly. When a fissure is situated off the midline, other conditions, such as Crohn's disease (CD), mucosal ulcerative colitis, syphilis, tuberculosis, or leukemia, should be investigated.

The main goal of treatment is breaking the cycle of hard stool, pain, and reflex spasm. This objective can usually be achieved by increasing dietary fiber using fiber supplements, adequate liquid intake, and possibly stool softeners. Warm baths and topical anesthetics are helpful in providing symptomatic relief. The great majority of patients with acute anal fissure will respond to medical treatment. For patients with chronic anal fissure, several recently developed nonsurgical methods, including nitric oxide and botulinum toxin, are available (Utzig et al, 2003). Calcium channel blockers and α-adrenoceptor antagonists are still at the developmental stage. *Nitric oxide ointment* is used in a concentration of 0.2%, usually tolerable by patients, and applied in the anal canal 2 or 3 times daily for 8 weeks. Transient headache is a major side effect of this treatment, more commonly seen at higher concentrations of the compound.

Botulinum toxin injection is indicated for patients who are unresponsive to or have contraindications for nitric oxide treatment. Two, 0.1 mL doses of diluted toxin are injected beneath the anal fissure with a short, thin needle; injections can be repeated if necessary. There is a risk for minor incontinence, flatus, and soiling with this treatment. *Surgical lateral sphincterotomy* is associated with a greater risk of incontinence and is offered to patients who relapse or fail these newer nonsurgical methods. Sphincterotomy can be performed under local, regional, or general anesthesia as an open or closed procedure and is routinely performed on an outpatient basis.

Anorectal Abscess

Anorectal abscess frequently results from a cryptoglandular infection. Extension may lead to perianal, ischiorectal, intersphincteric, or supralevator abscess. A horseshoe abscess originates from the deep postanal space communicating to the right and left ischiorectal spaces.

The treatment of an anorectal abscess is incision and drainage. With the exception of simple perianal and ischiorectal abscesses, the surgery is performed in the operating room under adequate anesthesia. A cruciate incision is made and the edges of the skin are excised to allow adequate drainage. A *horseshoe abscess* is drained through an incision made between the coccyx and the anus, exposing the deep postanal space. An opening made in the posterior midline and the lower part of the internal sphincter is divided to eradicate the source of the infected gland. Counter incisions are made over each ischiorectal fossa to allow drainage of the anterior extensions of abscess (Figure 91-1).

An *intersphincteric abscess* usually requires evaluation under anesthesia for the diagnosis. Treatment involves unroofing of the abscess cavity by partially dividing the internal sphincter along the length of the abscess cavity. A *supralevator abscess* most often results from a pelvic abscess, but can also result from an upward extension of an intersphincteric or ischiorectal abscess. It is important to determine the source of the abscess, as the surgical approach differs in each case. If the origin is an intersphincteric abscess, it is drained through the rectum in order to avoid a suprasphincteric fistula, as would occur through the ischiorectal fossa. In contrast, if the cause is an upward extension of an ischiorectal abscess, drainage should be through the ischiorectal fossa. Finally, if the abscess originates from the pelvis, drainage can be achieved either through the rectal lumen or by laparotomy. It is our practice *not* to perform a fistulotomy during drainage due to the risk of incontinence as the tissue planes are inflamed and distorted, precluding accurate assessment of sphincter involvement.

Fistula in Ano

Fistulas are classified as intersphincteric, transsphincteric, extrasphincteric, and suprasphincteric. Treatment is generally surgical, except in patients with CD with active proximal intestinal disease. The goal of treatment is to cure the fistula, avoid recurrence, and preserve continence. Therefore, identification of the primary opening and side tracts and division of the least amount of muscle are the key factors for surgical success.

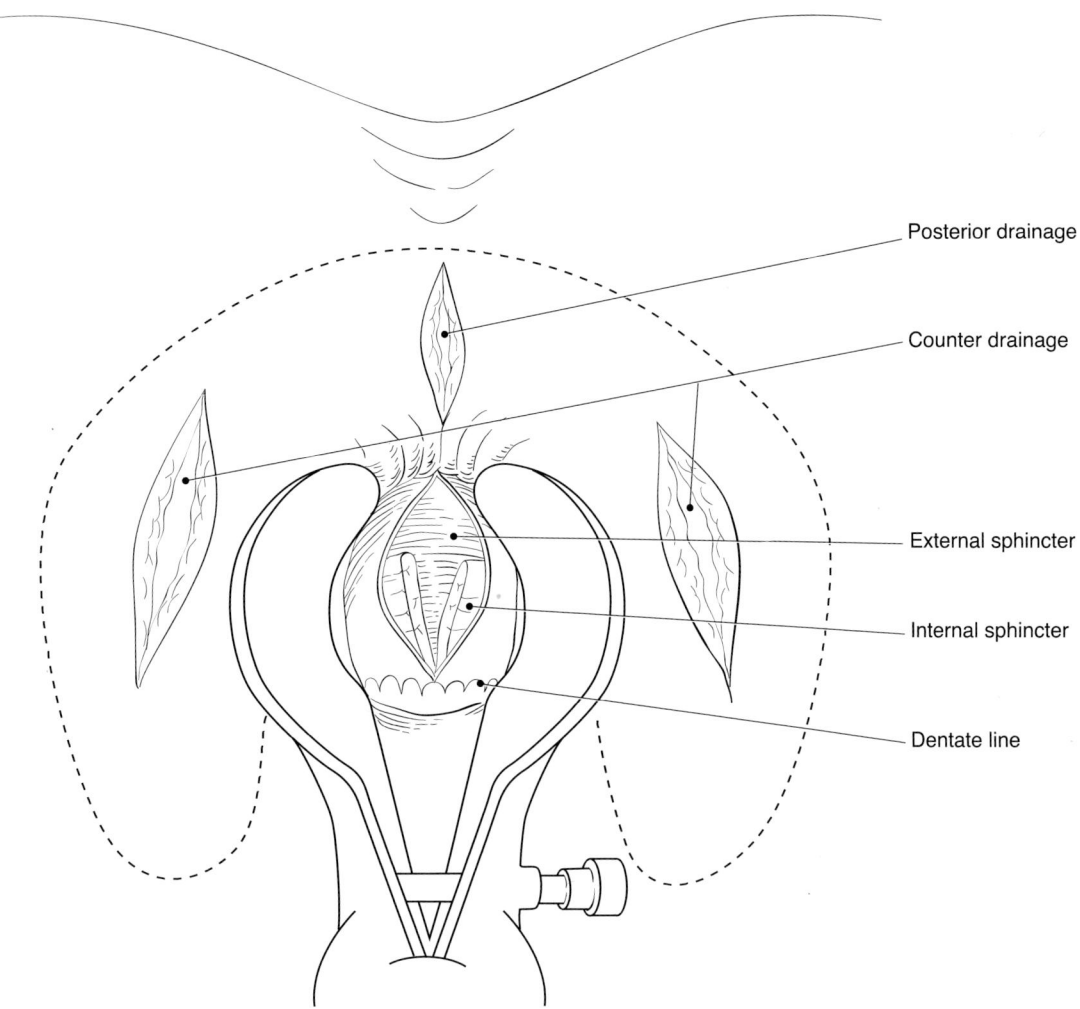

FIGURE 91-1. Drainage of horseshoe abscess. Reprinted from Vasilevsky CA. Fistula in ano and abscess. In: Beck DE, Wexner SD, editors. Fundamentals of anorectal surgery, 2nd ed. London: WB Saunders;1996. p. 156. Reproduced with permission from Elsevier Ltd.

Treatment options include dividing the fistula, seton placement, endorectal advancement flap, and injection of fibrin glue. For simple intersphincteric and low transphincteric fistulas that involve a small portion of the sphincter muscle, a fistulotomy with curettage of the granulation tissue is usually optimal.

For fistulas that involve a significant portion of anal muscle or complex fistulas, the *cutting seton technique* may be used. This seton is a nonabsorbable suture that is placed around the sphincter musculature at the time of surgery and tightened at regular postoperative intervals. It works by slowly cutting through the sphincter allowing the development of fibrosis, which avoids retraction of the muscles at once, as occurs with fistulotomy, and has the advantage of being a safer maneuver, although still associated with a *risk of incontinence.* Consequently any anoderm and anal mucosa between the seton and the sphincter muscle should be divided at the time of seton placement. If the fistula is secondary to CD, a loose (draining) seton is maintained for prolonged periods to establish drainage and prevent abscess recurrence.

The *endorectal advancement flap* is a good option for the treatment of high fistulas with a normal rectal mucosa. It has the advantage of closing the internal sphincter opening without dividing the anal muscle. We recently reported our experience with 106 consecutive procedures performed in 94 patients with complex perianal fistula. At a mean follow-up of 40.3 months, the procedure was successful in 60% of patients (Mizrahi et al, 2002).

Another option for fistula treatment is *fibrin glue,* which can be used alone or in combination with other techniques. It is associated with minimal risk and a moderate success rate. In a previous study from our institution, 33% of the patients, in whom fibrin glue was the only therapy used, were able to avoid more extensive surgery.

There are two chapters on perianal disease in CD (see Chapter 82, "Perianal Disease in Inflammatory Bowel Disease" and Chapter 83, "Dysplasia Surveillance Program").

Anal Neoplasm

Evaluation including digital *rectal examination, colonoscopy, endorectal ultrasound, computed tomography,* and *examination of inguinal lymph nodes* is performed to evaluate the nodal and systemic spread of the disease. The great majority of anal tumors consist of *squamous cell carcinoma.* Our management consists of a modified version of Nigro's protocol with *combined chemoradiation therapy* (Beck and Wexner, 1996) Radiation entails 30 to 48 Gy given over 4 weeks plus administration of IV 5- fluorouracil (1,000 mg/m^2/d) on days 1 to 5 and days 31 to 35 and mitomycin C (15 mg/m^2) on day 1. After completion of chemoradiation, patients are closely monitored with digital examination, proctoscopy, and biopsies of tissue from any suspicious areas. Patients with persistent or recurrent disease may be recommended to undergo *salvage chemotherapy* with *cisplatin* with or without *radiation.* However, *abdominoperineal resection* is still occasionally indicated. *Adenocarcinoma* of the *anal canal* may arise from a chronic fistula. Because of the high recurrence rates despite radical surgery, we have also used combined modality therapy for these tumors.

Anorectal melanoma is associated with a very poor prognosis. The treatment is *surgical* as these tumors are resistant to chemoradiation therapy. The size and depth of the tumor is the strongest determinant of outcome. If local control can be obtained, or in the case of advanced disease, *wide local excision* is performed. *Abdominoperineal resection* is reserved for patients in whom local control is not possible by wide local excision or for salvage local control in selected patients with an isolated local recurrence. However, in the vast majority of these patients local excision is the appropriate therapy as abdominoperineal resection does not appear to confer any additional advantages related to recurrence or survival.

Bowen's Disease

Bowen's disease is a rare, *potentially malignant intraepithelial squamous cell carcinoma* (carcinoma in situ). If the lesion is visible, biopsy and histopathologic evaluation is required to distinguish it from other perianal dermatoses. Once the diagnosis is made, we perform "*anal mapping,*" to assess the extent of the disease and to ensure excision of the lesion with negative microscopic margins. The "anal mapping" technique consists of biopsies taken at 1 cm from the edge of the lesion and in all four quadrants of the perineum. Biopsies are taken at the dentate line, anal verge, and the perineum. In the absence of invasive cancer, a wide local excision is performed. Small defects are primarily closed, while large wounds are covered by split thickness or rotational or advancement flaps or left to heal by secondary intention. In the presence of invasive carcinoma, a more aggressive approach such as abdominoperineal resection or combined chemoradiation therapy is indicated. Microscopic disease serendipitously found in hemorrhoidectomy specimens is conservatively treated with close follow up. Current controversy surrounds the treatment of Bowen's disease. Recent data suggest that areas of anal intraepithelial neoplasia can usually be evaluated. If this conservative approach is ultimately proven sufficient, then the disfiguring excisional procedure will be avoided.

Paget's Disease

Paget's disease is a *potentially malignant* lesion consisting of *intraepithelial adenocarcinoma.* Association with *synchronous visceral carcinomas* is stronger for Paget's than for Bowen's disease, and, therefore, appropriate evaluation to exclude malignancies is recommended. Diagnosis and management is similar to that for Bowen's disease. Patients are closely monitored and a biopsy of any suspicious lesion is performed; local recurrence is treated with repeat wide local excision.

Rectal Prolapse

Rectal prolapse is a full thickness protrusion of the rectum through the anal sphincters. The treatment is surgical repair; whether a perineal or a transabdominal repair is indicated depends mainly on the patient's medical condition (Figure 91-2). The laparoscopic technique consists of mobilization of the rectum in the presacral space to the levator ani and direct suture of the lateral rectal attachments to the presacral fascia. Because division of the lateral stalks decrease the recurrence rate but increase postoperative constipation, we perform a full posterior and anterior mobilization but only divide the upper half of the lateral stalks. Other fixation procedures which use mesh to fix the rectum to the presacral fascia have been advocated; however, we prefer to avoid using foreign material in the pelvis. The abdominal approach has lower recurrence rates with slightly higher morbidity compared with the perineal approach. Regarding the perineal techniques, in a previous report from our institution comparing Delorme procedure and perineal rectosigmoidectomy with and without levatorplasty, the recurrence rate was statistically significantly different at 27.5%, 12.5% and 4%, respectively (Agachan et al, 1997).

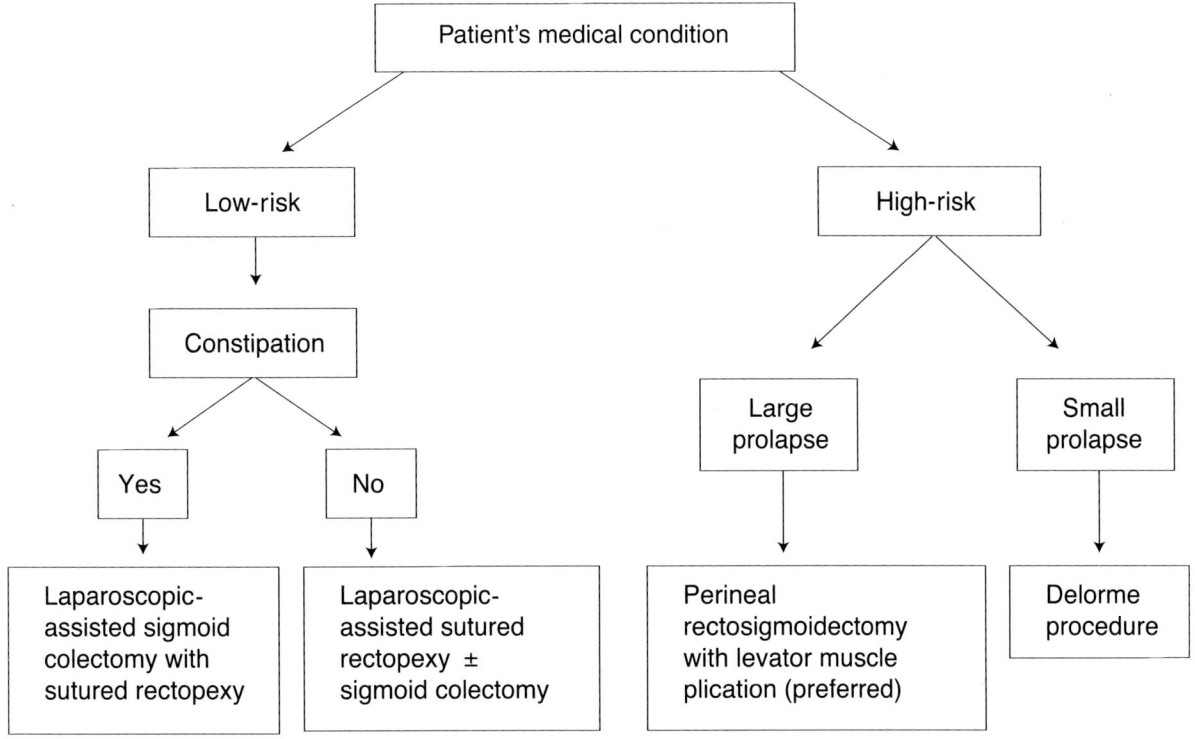

FIGURE 91-2: Suggested algorithm for treatment of rectal prolapse.

Hidradenitis Suppurativa

Treatment of perianal hidradenitis is tailored to the severity and chronicity of the presenting disease. *Uncomplicated disease* is treated by conservative measures, including warm sitz baths, topical cleansing agents to improve hygiene, and avoidance of tight fitting garments. A broad spectrum antibiotic, such as oral erythromycin or topical clindamycin, is added if *cellulitis* is present and any localized infections are drained. For limited disease *local excision* with primary closure should be performed. Unroofing is reserved for patients with chronic but mild perineal disease. This technique involves probing and exploring all sinus tracts and fistulas, completely removing the roof of all tracts, curetting the tract, and leaving the floor intact to aid in closure by secondary infection. This method has the disadvantage of developing *squamous cell carcinoma* since the disease is left in situ. Once the disease process has become *chronic* and *extensive, wide excision* is performed removing the affected area of skin 1 to 2 cm beyond visible evidence of disease to minimize recurrence. The area can be *mapped* with methylene blue solution into the sinus tract to define the extent of disease. If the wound is small, it can be primarily closed or treated with skin flaps. Large defects can be closed by secondary intention or by split thickness skin grafting. Despite aggressive surgical therapy, *high recurrence rates* can be anticipated. Association with *CD* and *smoking* should be recognized. Also, because the disease can be multifocal, the groins and axillae should be examined and treated as necessary.

Anal Stenosis

The treatment of anal stenosis depends on its position in the anal canal and the severity of the stenosis. High anal strictures that are entirely covered by mucosa are more difficult to treat than low anal strictures at the level of the anoderm.

Mild stenosis with minimal symptoms can usually be managed with dietary modifications and "bulking" agents, with the intention of naturally dilating the anal canal. *Self-dilation* using a Hegar's dilator may result in hematoma formation and further fibrosis. Therefore, we do not recommend this method, except possibly in some patients with strictures secondary to inflammatory bowel disease. Patients who fail conservative management and have satisfactory sphincter pressures may be treated by *surgical sphincterotomy*. However, this technique does not treat the *ectropion*, which is a protrusion of mucosa onto the anoderm that may be associated with the stenosis. There is a separate chapter on dilations of intestinal and colonic strictures (see Chaper 86, "Acute Colonic Pseudo-Obstruction").

Patients with *moderate to severe stenosis* are treated with advancement flap procedures, which replace the fibrous tissue with elastic compliant neoanoderm. We prefer to use the house shape flap (Figure 91-3). The advantage of this flap over other described flaps (V-Y, Y-V) is that it has a broader base allowing advancement of maximal skin to the stenosis without tension on the flap. This technique consists of performing an incision in the stenotic area and advancing the mobilized flap of skin in that area. The edges of the flap are then sutured at the level of the stenosis. Either the flap may be unilateral or bilateral.

For patients who may require excision of a large amount of skin, such as patients with Bowen's or Paget's disease, the S-plasty is a good option. The defect is covered by a double rotational flap, outlined by a large "S" with the anal canal in the center (Figure 91-4).

Sexually Transmitted Diseases

Gonorrhea

Gonorrhea is caused by *Neisseria gonorrhea*, affecting primarily the rectum, leading to *severe proctitis* with a *yellow mucopurulent discharge*. The diagnosis is confirmed by a *swab* and *culturing* of the rectal discharge using Thayer–Martin medium. The treatment is instituted empirically with 4.8 million units of intramuscular aqueous procaine *penicillin* G and 1 g oral *probenecid*. Due to the high penicillin resistance, a single dose of 250 mg intramuscular *ceftriaxone* (Rocephin) followed by 100 mg oral *doxycycline* bid for 7 days may be used as a first choice. Recurrence rates may be high (up to 35%), therefore, the patient is instructed to return for follow-up for smears and cultures to confirm remission. Because patients with gonorrhea may have *associated chlamydial infection*, treatment for chlamydia is instituted as well.

Chlamydia trachomatis

Chlamydia infection is caused by *Chlamydia trachomatis*. The organism can cause *proctitis similar to that of CD*. Untreated disease may become *ulcerated* causing *fistulas, abscesses*, or *rectal stricture*, which may be misdiagnosed as adenocarcinoma. *Diagnosis* is usually made by *serology*. Treatment consists of oral *tetracycline* or *erythromycin*, 500 mg 4 times a day for 3 weeks. Rectal strictures are primarily treated medically; in case of failure, surgical resection with coloanal anastomosis may be required.

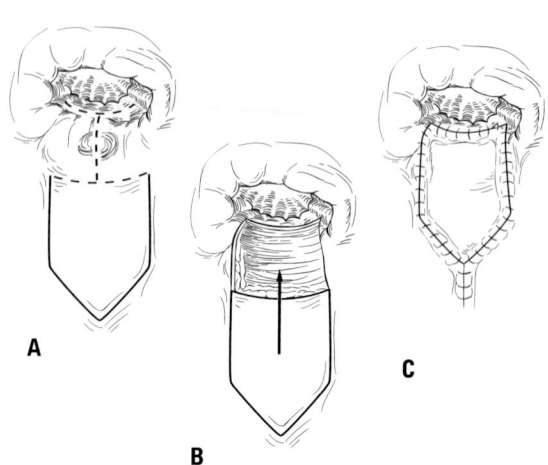

FIGURE 91-3. House shape (advancement) flap: *A*, House shaped flap is created; *B*, the flap is advanced into the anal canal; and *C*, sutured in place. Reprinted from Fundamentals of Anorectal Surgery, 2nd Edition, Wexner et al, Fistula in ano and anal stenosis (Fig 14.12, page 221). Reproduced with permission from Elsevier Ltd.

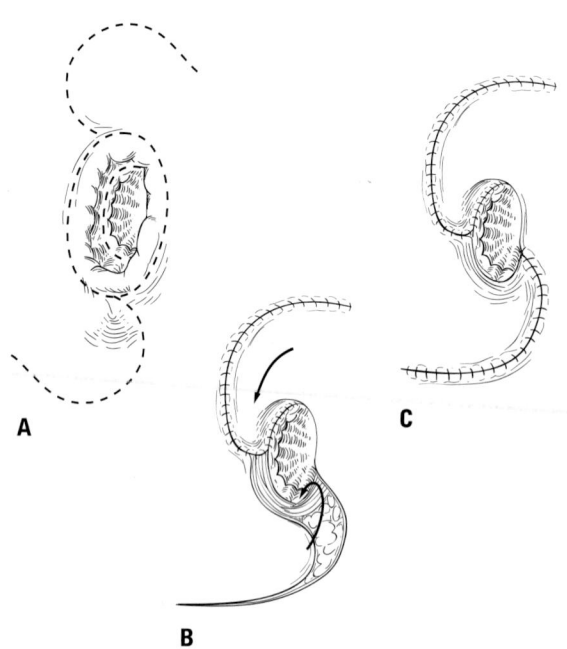

FIGURE 91-4: S-plasty. *A*, Perianal skin lesion requiring removal of large skin area; *B*, area of perianal skin excised, lateral curves incised into buttocks; *C*, curves of skin advanced into perianal defect and secured laterally to produce S-shaped closure of rotated flaps. Reprinted from Fundamentals of Anorectal Surgery, 2nd Edition, Wexner et al, Fistula in ano and anal stenosis (Fig 14.13, page 221). Reproduced with permission from Elsevier Ltd.

Herpes

Herpetic infection is confirmed by *culture* of suspicious *vesicles*. Management of acute symptoms includes analgesics, sitz baths, and stool softeners. Oral *acyclovir* (Zocyrax), 200 to 400 mg 5 times a day for 10 days is prescribed to shorten the duration of pain, viral shedding, and systemic symptoms in primary herpes.

Syphilis

Primary anal syphilis can manifest as a *painless fissure*. If left untreated it can progress to *secondary syphilis* manifested in the perianal area as *condyloma latum*, multiple raised warty lesions that coalesce. *Tertiary syphilis* can occur at more than 1 year following primary infection, manifesting as neurologic, cardiovascular, renal, hepatic, mucosal, and ocular symptoms. Once the diagnosis is considered, a biopsy is performed on the suspicious ulcer and the tissue is evaluated under *darkfield microscopy* and with *serologic testing*. Therapy consists of a 2.4 million units intramuscular *benzathine penicillin* injection. In patients allergic to penicillin, doxycycline may be used.

Condylomata Acuminata

The management of condylomata acuminata depends on the extent and location of the lesions. Treatment options include destructive therapy (podophyllin, trichloroacetic acid, bichloroacetic acid, electrocautery, and laser surgery), excisional therapy, and immunotherapy. We prefer *bichloroacetic acid* 89 to 90%, a caustic agent that, unlike podophyllin, can be used on the perineum and inside the anal canal, has no systemic toxicity, and does not cause the histological changes resembling carcinoma in situ, which can occur after podophyllin application. Application can be done at 7 to 10 day intervals. *Surgical excision* has the immediate advantage of reliably eliminating warts and allowing tissue collection for histopathologic analysis. However, it is associated with significant pain, potential stricture formation, and cost for the anesthesia. Thus, topical therapy is preferred unless there is extensive condyloma. *Immunotherapy* is reserved for patients with recurrent warts.

Pruritus Ani

Pruritus ani is a difficult condition to treat. A careful history and physical examination should be performed to exclude secondary causes, such as diseases of the anorectum, systemic diseases, diarrheal states, and dermatologic conditions, in which case appropriate therapy is instituted. The majority of cases, however, are idiopathic and there is no panacea treatment for this condition. First, it is important to *reassure* these patients that they do not have a cancer; *avoidance of scratching* is essential and is emphasized in order to break the scratch-itching-scratch cycle. *Clothing* is discussed and tight fitting pants or undergarments should be avoided, and all possible *irritants* to the perianal area, such as harsh toilet papers, soaps, creams, and ointments, should be discontinued. *Foods* and *beverages* such as tomatoes, spicy foods, nuts, coffee (regular or decaffeinated), milk products, tea, beer, wine, and chocolate can cause pruritus and the patient is instructed to *eliminate* each of these products for a 1 week duration to help determine if any are causative factors. It is extremely important that the *perianal skin* be kept *clean* and *dry*. Patients are instructed to clean the perianal area gently but thoroughly after each bowel movement with water or a nonalcoholic towelette and dry it with a hair dryer at a cool setting or by dabbing with a soft cotton cloth. Bulking agents are added to regulate bowel habits and minimize incomplete evacuation and soiling. Warm sitz baths for 20 minutes may also provide some relief. *Short term hydrocortisone cream* 0.5 to 1% can be used in resistant cases.

Supplemental Reading

Agachan F, Reissman P, Pfeifer J, et al. Comparison of three perineal procedures for the treatment of rectal prolapse. South Med J 1997;90:925–32.

Beck ED, Wexner SD. Anal neoplasms. In: Beck DE, Wexner SD, editors. Fundamentals of anorectal surgery. 2nd ed. London: WB Saunders; 1996. p. 261–77.

Fleshman JW. Fissure in ano and anal stenosis. In: Beck DE, Wexner SD, editors. Fundamentals of anorectal surgery, 2nd ed. London: WB Saunders; 1996. p. 221.

Mizrahi N, Wexner SD, Da Silva GM, et al. Endorectal advancement flap: are there predictors of failure? Dis Colon Rectum 2002;45:1616–21.

Utzig MJ, Kroesen AJ, Buhr HJ. Concepts in pathogenesis and treatment of chronic anal fissure—a review of the literature. Am J Gastroenterol 2003;98:968–74.

Vasilevsky CA. Fistula in ano and abscess. In: Beck DE, Wexner SD, editors. Fundamentals of anorectal surgery, 2nd ed. London: WB Saunders; 1996. p. 156.

Zmora O, Mizrahi N, Rotholtz N, et al. Fibrin glue sealing in the treatment of perineal fistulas. Dis Colon Rectum 2003;46:584–9.

CHAPTER 92

Hemorrhoids

Nir Wasserberg, MD, and Howard S. Kaufman, MD

Hemorrhoidal disease is a very common medical disturbance, equally distributed among males and females. Incidence peaks at middle age, and declines after the age of 65 years. Because many patients attribute anorectal symptoms to hemorrhoids, the precise occurrence of hemorrhoidal disease is difficult to compute. The probable prevalence of this condition as estimated by questionnaires is between 4 to 40%, with approximately 1,100 medical office visits per 100,000 persons annually (Sardinha and Corman, 2002).

Anatomy and Physiology

Hemorrhoids are cushions of vascular tissue that are present from birth and are therefore considered normal anatomy. Internal hemorrhoids arise from the superior hemorrhoidal vascular plexus cephalad to the dentate line and are covered by mucosa. External hemorrhoids are dilations of the inferior hemorrhoidal plexus. Located below the dentate line, they are covered with anoderm and perianal skin. Because these plexuses communicate, a combination of external and internal hemorrhoid (mixed hemorrhoids, Figure 92-1) is often seen.

There are three major hemorrhoidal cushions, which appear in the left lateral, right anterior, and right posterior positions; however, intervening minor hemorrhoidal complexes may obscure this order. Although the exact role of hemorrhoidal cushions has yet to be defined, it is generally accepted that these vascular cushions contribute to continence by partially occluding the anus. Additionally, they may protect the anal canal during defecation.

Pathophysiology

Many theories have been proposed to describe the mechanism by which hemorrhoids protrude and become symptomatic, causing bleeding, soiling, pruritus, difficulty with hygiene, and occasional pain (Loder et al, 1994). Hemorrhoids were once believed to be varicosities of the hemorrhoidal veins induced by portal hypertension. Although portal hypertension may contribute to the development of anorectal varices, hemorrhoids may form independently and distinctively to the degree of portal hypertension. Another popular explanation is that hemorrhoids are occluded veins induced by congestion and vascular hyperplasia. However, the most widely accepted theory suggests that pathologic slippage of the anal canal lining is induced by attenuation of the muscular fibers anchoring the vascular cushions caused by continued downward pressure during defecation. This process results in sliding, congestion, bleeding, and eventual prolapse of the hemorrhoids. Contributing factors include chronic straining, aging, increased intra-abdominal pressure, and absence of sinusoidal valves. Elevated anal resting pressures and ultraslow waves are associated physiological changes; however, the importance of these findings is unclear and may only represent secondary phenomena.

Diagnosis

The diagnosis of hemorrhoidal disease is based upon elucidating a proper history and performing a physical examination. Patients usually complain of blood appearing on the toilet tissue and/or in the toilet bowl after defecation. In

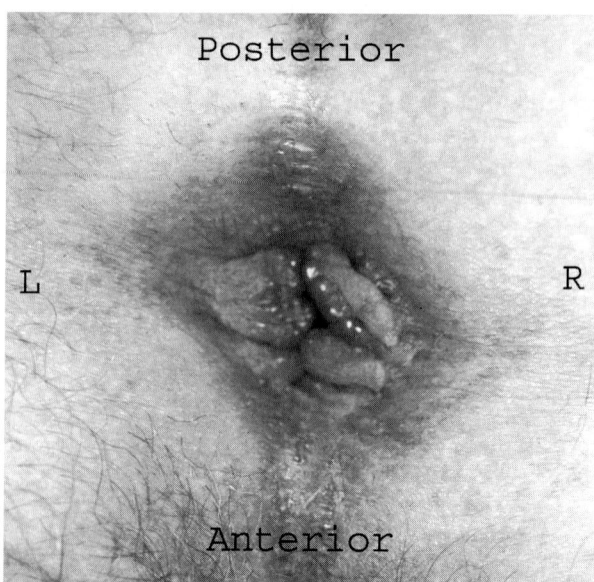

FIGURE 92-1. Patient in prone position with mixed hemorrhoids (both internal and external components) in classic locations in the left lateral, right posterior, and right anterior positions.

some patients, chronic hemorrhoidal bleeding may cause asymptomatic or even symptomatic anemia. Patients may complain of tissue protrusion, mucus discharge, itching, perianal hygiene difficulties, and incomplete evacuation. Constipation is common but not secondary to hemorrhoids. Pain is uncommon and is usually associated with complicated thrombosed or ulcerated hemorrhoids. Other anorectal pathologies such as anal fissures, fistulas, skin tags, inflammatory bowel disease (IBD), tumor, and rectal prolapse should be included in the differential diagnosis.

The patient should be thoroughly examined in the left lateral decubitus position with a step-by-step explanation provided to the patient of what will occur during the examination. Digital examination should be gently performed after inspection and palpation of the perianal region for masses and tenderness. Abnormalities should be anatomically described and recorded (ie, left lateral, right posterior, etc) with particular attention to thrombosis, ulceration, sites of drainage, and/or any signs of necrosis. The examination should be completed by anoscopy and by rigid or, preferably, flexible sigmoidoscopy. Full colonoscopy is indicated to rule out any other proximal pathology in patients > 50 years of age or younger, if risk factors for colorectal carcinoma exist or if bleeding persists after treatment of hemorrhoids. Other anorectal physiology tests have no use, thus far, in the diagnosis of hemorrhoidal disease.

Classification

Hemorrhoids are classified by location as *internal*, *external* or *mixed* in relation to the dentate line, and by the degree of *prolapse*. *External* hemorrhoids are located below the dentate line, are covered by squamous mucosa, and are painful when thrombosis occurs. *Internal* hemorrhoids are located above the dentate line and may prolapse, thrombose, or bleed. The degree of *prolapse* is staged as follows:
1. Cushions bulge into the lumen and may bleed during defecation but do not prolapse
2. Cushions prolapse during defecation or straining but reduce spontaneously
3. Cushions prolapse outside the anal canal and may be manually reduced
4 Irreducible piles

Treatment

Management of hemorrhoidal disease is dictated by symptoms, location (external versus internal versus mixed), the degree of prolapse, and the length of time from presentation (for thrombosed external hemorrhoids). Therapy should be tailored appropriately to relieve symptoms and to uphold remission (The Standards Task Force, 1993). Aside from hemorrhoidectomy, most types of therapy can be performed in a medical office setting.

Certain practical guidelines should be applied regardless of the hemorrhoidal type or stage. Patients should be instructed on proper bowel habits including quick response to defecation urge and avoidance of unnecessary prolonged toilet time. Proper perianal hygiene may reduce irritation and itching. Patients should be instructed to use moistened toilet paper (not recycled or perfumed) or wipes, and frequent sitz baths are recommended, particularly following a bowel movement.

Dietary high fiber supplements (20 to 30 g/d) with or without additional bulking agents, such as psyllium, are recommended to reduce the need to apply increasing downward pressure during defecation. Fiber supplements have been suggested to reduce bleeding and pain during defecation, however, the data are inconsistent.

Prescription and nonprescription topical agents are plentiful and include creams, suppositories, and ointments. These products may contain astringents, analgesics, and steroidal and nonsteroidal elements that function as anti-inflammatory, local vasoconstrictors and anesthetic mediators to relieve local symptoms. Allergic reactions to anesthetic preparations have been reported. Other than the potential risk of developing contact dermatitis after long term use of topical steroids, topical substances are generally considered safe. Despite the widespread use of these products, there have been no clinical trials to confirm their therapeutic value.

Management of External Hemorrhoids

Patients who present with acutely thrombosed external hemorrhoids will typically complain of an intensely painful anal mass. Inspection of the perianal skin reveals the diagnosis with a swollen, tense external hemorrhoid. If such a lesion is not present, anal fissure or perianal abscess must be ruled out.

Excision is recommended for a thrombosed hemorrhoid manifested with intense pain if duration is within 48 hours of onset, or if ulceration or rupture occurs. If pain is improving, symptomatic therapy with sitz baths, bulking agents, and analgesics is preferred. Excision may be performed in the office using local anesthetic. The wound is left open to heal by secondary intention. Larger, more broadly based thromboses may be managed by incision and evacuation of the clot to avoid creation of a large skin defect.

Management of Internal and Mixed Hemorrhoids

Nonsurgical Treatment

Most patients visiting a physician have already tried some form of conservative therapy and come for medical attention because of persistent symptoms. A variety of office-based therapies are available, and common to these nonoperative procedures is the aim of abolishing the underlying pathophysiologic mechanism of advanced hemorrhoidal disease. By promoting tissue fibrosis in various ways, the vascular cushions become fixed to the underlying muscular tissue.

Injection Sclerotherapy

Injection sclerotherapy has been used for hemorrhoidal disease treatment for over 100 years. Indicated to treat bleeding first, second, or early third degree internal hemorrhoids, a small amount of a sclerosing agent is injected above the dentate line. Five percent *phenol* in vegetable oil has been traditionally used, but other agents such as *quinine*, *urea hydrochloride*, and *sodium morrhuate*, are available. It is a straightforward, quick, painless, and inexpensive method, with success reported in up to 75% of patients. Although complications of pelvic sepsis and perianal necrosis have been reported, sloughing of the overlying mucosa, local infections, and allergic reactions to the injected material are more commonly described side effects.

Rubber Band Ligation

Rubber band ligation is probably the most commonly used nonoperative modality to treat internal hemorrhoids. It is generally a safe, simple and cost effective procedure indicated for second or third degree hemorrhoidal disease. An elastic rubber band is applied anoscopically or endoscopically by means of a special introducer to the tissue just above or at the base of a symptomatic pile. Care must be taken to apply the band above the dentate line, otherwise severe pain will ensue, and the band will need to be removed. Rubber band ligation induces necrosis and slough of the strangulated mucosa. Fibrosis occurs, and the remaining cushion becomes fixed to the underlying tissue. Patients should be informed to expect *delayed rectal bleeding* in about 7 to 10 days after the procedure.

Treatment of more than one hemorrhoidal group per session is the subject of continued debate. Proponents of multiple banding at a single session cite a low completion rate and quicker total treatment time with less office visits and more rapid resolution of symptoms (Armstrong, 2003). Alternatively, those who believe in banding only one group per visit avoid multiple bands because of the potential for increased discomfort, potential for obstruction, and an increased risk of septic complications. Up to *80% of patients will benefit* from rubber band ligation. The *recurrence rate is between 15 to 20%*, with < 2% incidence of *minor complications* such as anal pain and bleeding. Rare cases of pelvic sepsis have been reported.

Thermal Injury

Alternative methods of treatment use different energy sources to induce hemorrhoidal fixation by way of thermal injury. These techniques include *electrocoagulation, heater probes, laser photocoagulation*, and infrared photocoagulation (IRC). *IRC* uses an infrared source to generate high temperature to induce submucosal tissue destruction. This technique is uncomplicated, easy to perform, and mild with good results and low morbidity. However, the expense of this equipment for office-based therapy has diminished its use. *Cyrotherapy* produces tissue destruction by a rapid cellular freezing and thawing. Postprocedural pain, slow healing and risk for internal sphincter damage have led most surgeons to abandon this method.

There are no good prospective randomized control studies that compare the various fixation modalities, and existing trials do not demonstrate superiority of any particular method. In a meta-analysis comparing injection sclerotherapy, IRC, and rubber band ligation, injection sclerotherapy was found to be somewhat less efficient than the other forms of therapy.[5] In the absence of randomized trials, and because treatment methods appear equally effective, the technique chosen for each patient should be customized to the problem and to the experience of the treating surgeon or physician. Regardless of the solution offered, patients should be advised to continue following general recommendations, such as avoiding straining and maintaining fiber use. Patient follow-up should continue for treatment effectiveness and to complete the colon evaluation as described above.

Strangulated Prolapsed Internal Hemorrhoids

Strangulated prolapsed internal hemorrhoids are often edematous and thrombosed due to a compromised venous return. Initial management is usually nonoperative. If the piles are not gangrenous, a perineal field block may be performed to aid in manual reduction. Application of *table sugar (sucrose)* to prolapsed hemorrhoids acts as a desiccant to absorb fluid and reduce hemorrhoidal edema. If successful in reducing incarcerated piles, less morbid treatment may then be performed more electively. Severe pain accompanied by a foul smelling discharge usually implies the presence of gangrene. Under these conditions, urgent hemorrhoidectomy is indicated.

Special situations deserve mention. *Pregnant* women frequently endure hemorrhoidal disease. Conservative treatment is recommended, because symptoms usually subside after delivery. Nonsurgical treatment is also advised for *immunocompromised patients* and/or in patients suffering from *IBD*. Perianal procedures may result in infection and delayed wound healing in these patients.

Surgical Treatment

Indications for surgical hemorrhoidectomy include advanced third or fourth degree piles, mixed hemorrhoids, extensive thrombosis, ulceration, and gangrene. The choice of surgical procedure depends upon the patient's condition, and surgeon and patient preferences. Similarly, anesthetic choices include local anesthesia plus monitored sedation, regional techniques, and general anesthesia. Traditionally, regional training and culture have influenced the choice of operation. Most surgeons in the United States practice the *closed technique*, or *Ferguson hemorrhoidectomy*, where following hemorrhoidal excision, the rectal mucosa and anoderm are closed with an absorbable radial suture line beginning at the apex of each hemorrhoidal complex. Recurrence rates are < 2%. Scissors, *electrocoutery*, *laser*, and *scalpel* may be used; however, none have been proven to be superior over other means of excision. Hemorrhoidectomy using advanced technologies such as *harmonic scalpel* and *ligasure* have been reported to have fewer complications and a quicker return to daily living, however, further evaluations are indicated.

Alternatively, surgeons in the United Kingdom, Europe, and many parts of Asia favor the *open hemorrhoidectomy* technique described by Milligan and Morgan. After excision of the hemorrhoidal complex(es) with overlying skin and rectal mucosa and ligation of the base(s) of the pile(s), surgical wounds are left open to heal by secondary intention. An open wound minimizes the risk for infection, but a longer convalescence period and considerable discomfort may result (Senagore, 2002). This technique is advised in the presence of gangrene where there is a greater risk for infection, or when surgical judgment suggests that closure may be too tight or promotes stricture formation.

Procedure for Prolase and Hemorrhoids

Recently, an alternative technique has been developed and tested that is associated with markedly reduced postoperative pain (Sutherland et al, 2002). The procedure for prolapse and hemorrhoids (PPH), or *stapled hemorrhoidectomy*, employs a circular stapler with a hollow head to *excise a cuff of tissue* at the most superior aspect of hemorrhoidal complexes and create a superficial end-to-end anastomosis (Figure 92-2). During this procedure, a submucosal pursestring is placed 4 cm above the dentate line and is secured to the post of the anvil of the stapler. The excess tissue is pulled into the hollow head of the stapler as the stapler is closed. As the stapler is fired, a circumferential cuff of tissue is excised, and the superficial anastomosis is created. In effect an *anopexy* is performed which lifts the prolapsed tissue into the anal canal. Randomized trials have reported significantly lower pain scores when compared to conventional hemorrhoidectomy procedures. Although higher instrument costs may deter widespread acceptance of the PPH, less pain, a shorter convalescence, and earlier return to normal activity should be considered in the choice of surgical therapy.

Conclusions

Hemorrhoids are a common condition with a variety of presenting symptoms. Rectal bleeding should not be attrib-

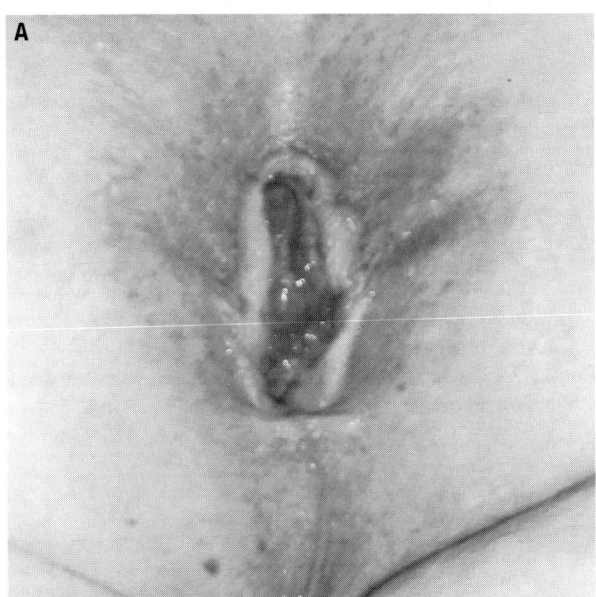
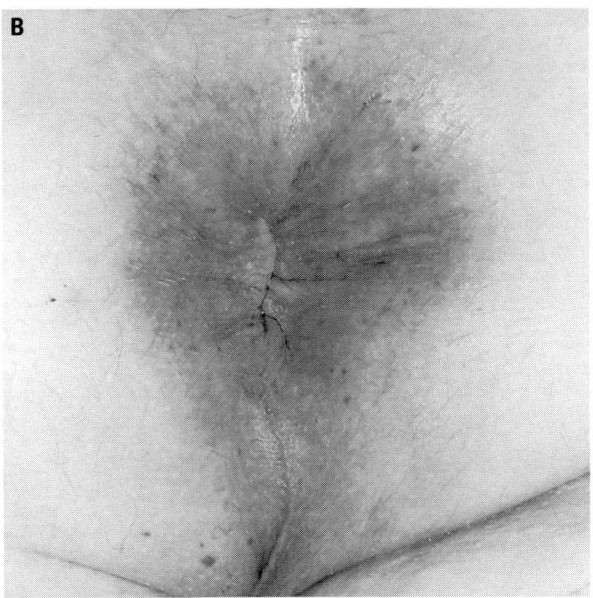
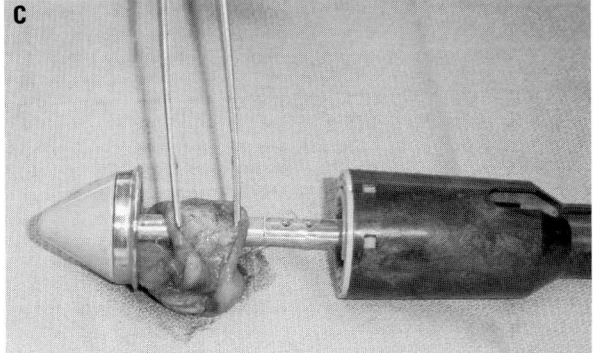

FIGURE 92-2. Fourth degree (irreducible) hemorrhoids before (A) and immediately after (B) procedure for prolaspe and hemorrhoids (PPH) has been performed. Circumferential specimen of mucosa and submucosa excised with the PPH stapler (C).

uted to hemorrhoids alone without proper investigations, especially if symptoms persist following therapy. Most early lesions may be treated in the office setting. Advances in stapling devices offer less painful means of surgical management for advanced hemorrhoidal disease.

Supplemental Reading

Armstrong DN. Multiple hemorrhoidal ligation: a prospective, randomized trial evaluating a new technique. Dis Colon Rectum 2003;46:179–86.

Guy RJ, Seow-Choen F. Septic complications after treatment of haemorrhoids. Br J Surg 2003;90:147–56.

Johanson JF. Nonsurgical treatment of hemorrhoids. J Gastrointest Surg 2002;6:290–4.

Johanson JF, Rimm A. Optimal nonsurgical treatment of hemorrhoids: a comparative analysis of infrared coagulation, rubber band ligation, and injection sclerotherapy. Am J Gastroenterol 1992;87:1600–6.

Loder PB, Kamm MA, Nicholls RJ, Phillips RK. Hemorrhoids: pathology, pathophysiology and aetiology. Br J Surg 1994;81:946–54.

Sardinha TC, Corman ML. Hemorrhoids. Surg Clin North Am 2002;82:1153–67.

Senagore AJ. Surgical management of hemorrhoids. J Gastrointest Surg 2002;6:295–8.

Sutherland LM, Burchard AK, Matsuda K, et al. A systematic review of stapled hemorrhoidectomy. Arch Surg 2002;137:1395–406.

The Standards Task Force American Society of Colon and Rectal Surgeons. Practice parameters for the treatment of hemorrhoids. Dis Colon Rectum 1993;36:1118–20.

CHAPTER 93

COLORECTAL POLYP AND CANCER SCREENING

JOHN H. BOND, MD

Separate evidence-based guidelines developed and revised during the past 8 years by the US Preventive Services Task Force, a consortium of medical and surgical gastrointestinal (GI) societies, and by the American Cancer Society, all strongly recommend that physicians screen their patients over the age of 50 years for colorectal cancer (Pigone et al, 2002; Winawer et al, 2003; Smith et al, 2001). The guidelines also recommend that before beginning screening, each patient first should be examined for any *special risks* of colorectal cancer that might indicate the need for more intense examination and surveillance, rather than the use of standard screening meant for asymptomatic, average-risk individuals. If a screening test is positive, appropriate diagnostic evaluation and treatment of detected neoplasia is essential. If screening is negative, repeat screening should be arranged appropriately for the method used. This chapter will include the advantages and disadvantages of current screening options. I will also present my preferred methods to accomplish these objectives and discuss the reasons for their selection from the menu of options contained in the guidelines.

Objectives of Colorectal Cancer Screening

There are two primary objectives of colorectal cancer screening. The first is to *detect* cancers that have already developed while they are *still confined* to the bowel and no lymph node or distant metastases yet have occurred. Studies indicate that the average surgical cure rate for such Dukes A and B cancers (Stage I and II) exceeds 85% (Mandel et al, 1993). Because most of these early, favorable cancers are asymptomatic, they must be detected by screening.

The second major objective of colorectal cancer screening is *prevention*. Studies now indicate that > 95% of colorectal cancers originate in *benign adenomatous polyps* (adenomas) that develop and grow very slowly in the colon over many years before they turn cancerous (Bond, 2000). Detection and resection of premalignant polyps therefore prevent cancer, and this has become an objective of screening that is as important, or perhaps even more important, than just detecting early cancers. Studies, such as the National Polyp Study and the Minnesota Fecal Occult Blood Screening Trial have demonstrated that when screening leads to resection of adenomas before they turn malignant, not only is cancer death prevented, but the incidence of colorectal cancer with its attendant morbidity and treatment costs also is substantially reduced (Winawer et al, 1993; Mandel et al, 2000).

The Advanced Adenoma as the Primary Target of Screening

The prevalence of *small (≤ 1 cm) simple tubular adenomas* in adults over the age of 50 years exceeds 30%. These common small adenomas, however, have a very low malignant potential. Studies indicate that most remain static or actually regress with time, whereas only a few develop the additional acquired genetic changes that make them grow, develop the advanced histologic changes of villous architecture or high grade dysplasia, and turn eventually to cancer. *Advanced adenomas* as defined by the National Polyp Study are those that are ≥ *1 cm in size or contain villous tissue or high grade dysplasia.* These advanced polyps are much less common, but much more likely to progress to cancer if not detected by screening. A large body of recent scientific data indicates that we clinicians should shift our focus away from simply detecting and removing large numbers of small tubular adenomas, toward *strategies that reliably detect most advanced adenomas*. Long term postpolypectomy studies nicely demonstrate the validity of this important concept (Bond, 2000). Follow-up studies from the Mayo Clinic and from St. Mark's Hospital in London show that patients with resection of only one or two small tubular adenomas have no measurable increased risk of developing subsequent colorectal cancer compared with the average population. In contrast, patients with large (≥ 1 cm) or multiple (≥ 3) adenomas, or adenomas with villous changes or high grade dysplasia have a risk of metachronous cancer that is increased 3- to 6-fold. Thus, the *objectives of colorectal cancer screening* are to (1) *detect cancers* that have developed while they are *still confined* to the bowel and surgical cure is very likely or (2) to detect and resect *advanced adenomas* thereby preventing cancer. The choice of a screening option should be guided by how well it accomplishes these two objectives.

Risk Stratification for Colorectal Cancer

Most people are at average risk for colorectal cancer simply because they have reached the age when the prevalence of cancer is sufficient to justify screening. Based on age-incidence curves for this disease, guidelines recommend that screening of the average-risk population (both men and women) begin at the age of 50 years. Reported direct screening colonoscopy experiences in people age 40 to 49 years confirm the very low prevalence of advanced neoplasia in average-risk people under age 50 years of age. Patients with a *personal or family history* of *colorectal cancer* or *adenomas*, or those with long standing *ulcerative colitis (UC)* or *Crohn's colitis* may have a higher risk of colorectal cancer that often begins at an earlier age, and these patients may benefit from special, more intensive examination or screening. Screening recommendations for these high risk groups are clearly outlined in the GI Consortium Guideline (Winawer et al, 2003) and will not be discussed further here. There is a separate chapter on inflammatory bowel disease and cancer (see Chapter 83, "Dysplasia Surveillance Programs").

In order to determine whether a patient is average or above average risk, I recommend taking a careful family and personal history before initiating a screening option. As spelled out in this guideline, risk stratification can quickly be accomplished in just a few minutes by asking each patient the following several questions well in advance of the earliest potential initiation of screening:

1. Has the patient had colorectal cancer or resection of a benign adenomatous polyp?
2. Does the patient have long standing chronic UC or Crohn's colitis that predisposes him or her to colorectal cancer?
3. Has a family member had colorectal cancer or an adenomtous polyp? If so, how many relatives were affected, at what age was the cancer or polyp diagnosed, and were they first-degree relatives (parent, sibling, or child)?

A positive response to any of these questions indicates the need to do a more formal family history or more detailed investigation of the patient's past history to determine if more intense screening or screening at an earlier age is justified according to the guidelines. There are separate chapters on colonic neoplasia and genetic counseling (see Chapter 94, "Colonic Neoplasia: Genetic Counselling"), and colorectal polyps and polyposis syndrome (see Chapter 95, "Colorectal Polyps and Polyposis Syndromes").

Guideline Options for Screening

Unlike screening for other major malignancies (ie, breast, cervix, and prostate) where a single screening test usually is recommended, the colorectal cancer screening guidelines present a menu of five different options, any one of which is considered satisfactory. These options include the following:

1. Annual screening with fecal occult blood tests (FOBT)
2. Flexible sigmoidoscopy screening every 5 years
3. The combination of annual FOBTs and flexible sigmoidoscopy every 5 years
4. Double-contrast barium enema (DCBE) every 5 years
5. Direct colonoscopy screening every 10 years

As discussed below, the guidelines emphasize that each of these five options has advantages and limitations that should be presented to the patient. Then, in a "shared decision process" the patient should be given an opportunity to choose their own preference as to how they wish to be screened. Proponents of screening stress that "the only unacceptable option is to do no screening" and "the best screening option may be the one that the patient actually will agree to do."

Advantages and Limitations of the Five Screening Options

FOBT

The *FOBT* is the most intensively studied of the different screening options and is the only method that has been shown to be efficacious in randomized, controlled trials. The Minnesota FOBT Trial demonstrated a *reduction in colorectal cancer mortality* of 33.4% and 21%, respectively, for annual and biennial FOBT screening followed by colonoscopy for anyone with a positive screening test (Bond, 2002). When the data were analyzed just for those who complied with all recommended screening, annual FOBT screening resulted in *a 45% colorectal cancer mortality reduction*. This is an important number because it is the benefit that clinicians can inform their patients to expect if they comply with recommended screening. Further follow-up in the Minnesota Trial also demonstrated a significant reduction in colorectal cancer incidence in those screened annually, presumably as the result of detection and resection of advanced adenomatous polyps. Although FOBT screening has been disparaged by many proponents of alternative methods, it does have a number of proven advantages. A program of *annual screening*, using a reasonably sensitive FOBT (ie, HemoccultSensa guaiac cards [Beckman-Coulter, Palo Alto, CA] or one of the newer immunochemical FOBTs) followed by colonoscopy for a positive result, detects most colorectal cancers and many advanced adenomas. Screening reduces both colorectal cancer mortality and incidence and is feasible, widely available, and generally acceptable to patients. Furthermore, this option of screening has a very low upfront cost. Disadvantages of FOBT screening include low sensitivity for polyps, especially smaller ones, and a relatively high false-positivity rate for advanced neoplasia. In addition, to be effective, relatively frequent screening is required.

Flexible Sigmoidoscopy

Flexible sigmoidoscopy screening also has a number of important advantages. It detects most colorectal cancers and many advanced adenomas. An analysis from the Veterans Affairs Multicenter Colonoscopy Screening Study indicated that a single screening flexible sigmoidoscopy would detect about 70 to 80% of all advanced colorectal neoplasia, provided that those who have a left-sided neoplasm detected undergo subsequent full colonoscopy (Lieberman and Weiss, 2001). Flexible sigmoidoscopy can be performed by trained, experienced examiners accurately, safely, and quickly following a simple bowel preparation. The procedure is generally well tolerated by patients, and has been shown in cohort and case-control studies to *reduce mortality from colorectal cancer* within its reach by 60 to 80%. These studies also indicate that the protective effect of a single examination lasts for 5 to 9 years; therefore, infrequent screening is possible.

Combination FOBT Plus Flexible Sigmoidoscopy

The combination of annual FOBT screening plus flexible sigmoidoscopy every 5 years largely corrects the limitations of doing either method of screening alone. The FOBT misses many polyps and has been shown to be relatively insensitive for distal rectosigmoid cancers. When performed *annually*, however, it will detect most colorectal cancers before they become incurable. The flexible sigmoidoscopy is highly accurate in the high risk left colon, but will *miss up to 30% of proximal advanced neoplasia* in patients who do not have a synchronous distal polyp or cancer.

Barium Enema

Screening DCBE, although included in the menu of guideline options, is not used much for screening in the United States and has not been directly studied for this purpose. Furthermore, DCBE recently has been shown to be relatively insensitive for detecting advanced neoplasia. A retrospective study by Rex and colleagues (1997) showed that about 15% of colorectal cancers are missed by barium enema examination. The National Polyp Study performed back-to-back DCBE and colonoscopy on 580 patients undergoing postpolypectomy surveillance and showed that the sensitivity of this method for detecting large polyps (≥ 1 cm) was only 48% (Winawer et al, 2000). For these reasons, when this method is used for screening, the guidelines recommend a *screening interval of 5 years*.

Three-Dimensional Virtual Colonscopy

A recent *New England Journal of Medicine* editorial suggested that three-dimensional computed tomography (CT) scanning and reconstruction may be a consideration for screening in the near future. The article by Pickhardt and colleagues (2003) described 1233 asymptomatic adults who underwent a new sophisticated 3-dimensional virtual colonoscopy and same-day conventional colonoscopy. More than 97% were at average risk for colorectal neoplasmia. The sensitivity and specificity of virtual colonoscopy for adenomatous polyps was comparable to standard colonoscopy, 94% and 96% respectively for adenomatous polyps > 10 mm on virtual colonoscopy. The sensitivity for polyps at least 6 mm was 88.7%. Only two cancers were found, both on virtual colonoscopy, and only one was found on standard colonoscopy until results of the virtual colonoscopy were revealed. Although this study should be repeated to verify the results, its findings appear to be a breakthrough in the use of virtual three-dimensional colonoscopy. As the editorial asks: Is it ready for prime time?

Colonscopy Screening

Increasingly in the United States, direct *colonoscopy screening* has become the overwhelming preference of gastroenterologists and many others. In the broad area of preventive screening, this option is somewhat of a perturbation of the classic definition of a screening test. Instead of performing a simple, acceptable, inexpensive and indirect test to identify those in the healthy at-risk population who might benefit from further examination, we are substituting upfront a highly definitive, complex, expensive and somewhat invasive, diagnostic and therapeutic method. Direct screening colonoscopy, however, is now being increasingly championed by physician and patient groups because it detects almost all cancers and advanced adenomas, and it allows for resection of most polyps during a single sitting. Thus it is the most effective way of achieving both the major goals of colorectal cancer screening—cancer prevention through polypectomy and reduced mortality through the detection of early cancers. Because of colonoscopy's great accuracy and the relatively long natural history of the adenoma-carcinoma sequence, *infrequent screening (every 10 years)* is possible. The VA Multicenter Colonoscopy Screening Study demonstrated that, when performed by well-trained experienced colonoscopists, colonoscopy screening is feasible and very safe (Nelson et al, 2002).

Although there are no randomized controlled trials of screening colonoscopy, compelling indirect evidence suggests that this approach is very effective at reducing both the incidence and mortality of colorectal cancer. For example, colonoscopy and polypectomy in the National Polyp Study cohort reduced colorectal cancer incidence by up to 90%; there are a number of supportive case-control studies of both flexible sigmoidoscopy and colonoscopy, and the FOBT trials effected their demonstrated reduction of cancer incidence and mortality by doing colonoscopy on those with a positive screen. Limitations of direct screening colonoscopy that have not yet been satisfactorily addressed include questions of risk, cost, patient acceptability, and capacity. Conscious sedation usually is required with its attendant risk, cost, and inconvenience. A screen requires the better part of 2 days to complete the bowel purging preparation, the examination, and recovery. Although screening colonoscopy has been shown to be safe when performed by experienced physicians, I still have concerns about both the accuracy and risk of this option when it is carried out in increasing numbers by less experienced examiners. Last, the great demand for screening colonoscopy already shows signs of overwhelming the capacity to perform these additional examinations. In some parts of the country, long waiting times to have a screening colonoscopy may be diminishing the attractiveness or practicality of this option.

My Preference for Screening the Average-Risk Population

Although ideal, due to time constraints and other issues, it is not feasible for each physician to present to every patient the advantages and disadvantages of five screening options. Rather, I believe that each individual health care delivery system (large and small) needs to evaluate its resources and capacity to screen, and then choose one or two options for its patients. Due to limited colonoscopy capacity in my institution, my current screening practice is still a program of annual FOBTs plus flexible sigmoidoscopy every 5 years. Colonoscopy is performed, of course, whenever there is a positive screen, a patient has signs or symptoms possibly due to colorectal cancer, or a patient is identified as being above-average risk. It is my opinion that neither FOBT alone or flexible sigmoidoscopy alone is a satisfactory way to screen because of their appreciable miss rates for advanced neoplasia. Because of its low sensitivity and specificity, I would not consider DCBE as an acceptable screening option.

If resources and capacity exist, my preference for colorectal cancer screening is direct colonoscopy performed by a well-trained, experienced endoscopist. Colonoscopy clearly is the only screening method capable of fulfilling most of the criteria of an ideal screening test.* It is feasible, acceptable and safe, and it accurately detects almost all cancers and advanced adenomas. It allows for biopsy of suspicious lesions and immediate resection of advanced adenomas throughout the colon, all at a single sitting with a single bowel cleansing preparation. Although relatively expensive, it is cost effective and infrequent screening is possible (Wagner et al, 1996). Anyone who undergoes direct colonoscopy screening as recommended by the guidelines should have a very low chance of developing or dying from colorectal cancer, the second most common cancer killer of Americans.

---

*Editor's Note: Virtual colonoscopy, three-dimensional CT scan reconstructions are being used for patients in whom a complete colonoscopy is not possible. As the techniques improve, this procedure may assume a role in colorectal cancer screening.

Supplemental Reading

Bond JH. Clinical evidence for the adenoma-carcinoma sequence, and the management of patients with colorectal adenomas. Semin Gastrointest Dis 2000;11:176–84.

Bond JH. Fecal occult blood test screening for colorectal cancer. Gastrointest Clin N Am 2002;12:11–22.

Bond JH, for the Practice Parameters Committee of the American College of Gastroenterology. Polyp guideline: diagnosis, treatment, and surveillance for patients with colorectal polyps. Am J Gastroenterol 2000;95:3053–63.

Lieberman DA, Weiss, DG, for the VA Cooperative Study Group 380. One-time screening for colorectal cancer with combined fecal occult blood testing and examination of the distal colon. N Engl J Med 2001;345:555–60.

Mandel JS, Bond JH, Church TR, et al. Reducing mortality from colorectal cancer by screening for fecal occult blood. N Engl J Med 1993;328:1365–71.

Mandel JS, Church TR, Ederer F, Bond JH. The effect of fecal occult-blood screening on the incidence of colorectal cancer. N Engl J Med 2000:343:1603–7.

Nelson DB, McQuaid KR, Bond JH, et al. Procedural success and complications of large-scale screening colonoscopy. Gastrointest Endosc 2002;55:307–14.

Pickhardt PJ, Choi R, Hwang I, et al. Computed tomographic virtual colonoscopy to screen for colorectal neoplasia in asymptomatic adults. N Engl J Med 2003;349:2191–200.

Pigone M, Rich M, Teutsch SM, et al. Screening for colorectal cancer in adults at average risk: summary of the evidence for the U.S. Preventive Services Task Force. Ann Intern Med 2002;137:132–41.

Rex, DK, Rahmani EY, Haseman JH, et al. Relative sensitivity of colonoscopy and barium enema for detection of colorectal cancer in clinical practice. Gastroenterol 1997;112:17–23.

Smith RA, von Eschenbach AC, Wender R et al. American Cancer Society guidelines for the early detection of cancer: update of early detection guidelines for prostate, colorectal, and endometrial cancers. CA Cancer J Clin 2001;51:38–75.

Wagner J, Tunis S, Brown M, et al. The cost effectiveness of colorectal cancer screening in average risk adults. In: Young G, Rozen P, Levin B, editors. Prevention and early detection of colorectal cancer. Philadelphia: WB Saunders; 1996. p. 321–56.

Winawer SJ, Fletcher RH, Rex D, et al. Colorectal cancer screening and surveillance: clinical guidelines and rationale based on new evidence. Gastroenterol 2003;124:544–60.

Winawer SJ, Stewart ET, Zauber AG, et al. A comparison of colonoscopy and double-contrast barium enema for surveillance after polypectomy. N Engl J Med 2000;342:1766–72.

Winawer SJ, Zauber AG, Ho MN, et al. Prevention of colorectal cancer by colonoscopic polypectomy: The National Polyp Study Workgroup. N Engl J Med 1993;329:1977–81.

CHAPTER 94

Colonic Neoplasia: Genetic Counseling

Jennifer E. Axilbund, MS, CGC, and Francis M. Giardiello, MD

Approximately 5 to 10% of colorectal cancer (CRC) is hereditary in origin, with linkage to a specific gene mutation. Moreover, some hereditary syndromes have an 80 to 100% lifetime risk for CRC, whereas others carry a 10 to 20% chance. Colorectal tumors are largely preventable through regular endoscopic evaluation, and some at-risk individuals require annual screening. However, there are also known risks and costs associated with repeated endoscopy. Furthermore, depending upon the specific syndrome, screening may be recommended as early as the age of 10 to 12 years, and some require prophylactic colectomy. Therefore, the key is to differentiate those individuals who would benefit from increased and/or earlier surveillance from those who would not. With the discovery of hereditary CRC genes, genetic testing, with accompanying management recommendations, has become the standard of care in some syndromes.

Appropriate Use of Genetic Testing

Most CRC are sporadic (ie, not inherited). Consequently, genetic testing is not appropriate for most patients or for general population screening. However, genetic testing is deemed appropriate when the following three criteria are met: (1) *family history is suspicious* for a hereditary syndrome, (2) the *genetic test result is interpretable,* and (3) the genetic test *result will influence medical management* of the patient or the patient's family members, or is *integral to reproductive decision making.*

Several professional organizations have policy statements regarding genetic testing for CRC susceptibility, including the American Society of Clinical Oncology (ASCO) and the American Gastroenterological Association (AGA). In addition to supporting the three criteria above, ASCO defines 12 basic elements of informed consent, and emphasizes the need for pretest and posttest genetic counseling from a qualified health care professional. The AGA guidelines reiterate the need for pretest and posttest genetic counseling and written informed consent, and outline appropriate indications for hereditary CRC predisposition testing.

Genetic counseling is best conducted by professionally trained genetic counselors. These health care providers typically have a masters-level graduate degree in genetics, with emphasis on the effect of a genetic diagnosis in a person or family. There are approximately 1,800 genetic counselors in the United States, and most are certified by the American Board of Genetic Counseling. Genetic counselors work closely with physicians of various disciplines, providing services in prenatal, pediatric, metabolic, and cancer clinics, among others. The National Society of Genetic Counselors maintains a directory of genetic counselors categorized by state, institution, and area of specialty (http://www.nsgc.org).

Features of Hereditary Cancer

The following list contains features suggestive of hereditary cancer, including hereditary CRC:
- Cancer diagnosed at a younger age than seen in the general population (< 50 years)
- The same cancer diagnosed in two or more blood relatives in the same lineage
- One individual with two separate primary cancers
- Clustering of different cancers known to be associated with a hereditary syndrome (eg, colorectal and endometrial)
- The presence of noncancerous features associated with a hereditary cancer syndrome
- Greater than 10 colorectal polyps

The Genetic Counseling Process

1. Risk Assessment: Risk assessment has three major components. The first is to construct a pedigree to view the cancer pattern in the family. The second is to obtain medical records, including endoscopy, surgical, and pathology reports, from the patient and as many affected family members as possible. The third is to develop an overall assessment of the family, attempting to recognize a hereditary cancer syndrome.
2. Patient Education: Genetic counseling includes education of the patient regarding basic genetic concepts, inheritance patterns, and features of hereditary cancer. It also entails a discussion of the differential diagnosis, describing the features of each disorder that are, and are not, consistent with the patient's history. A physical

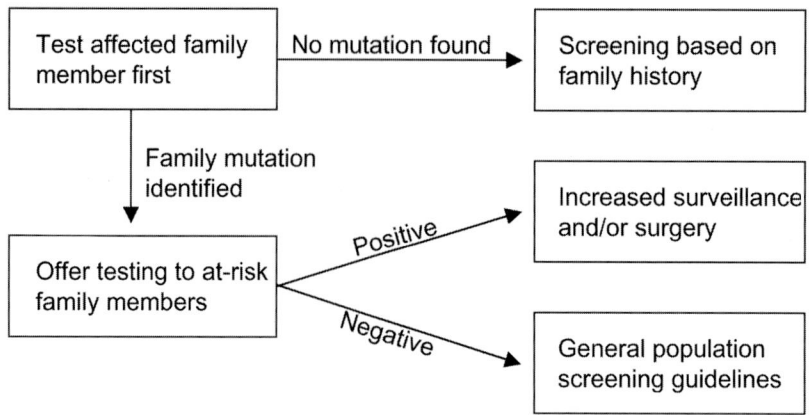

FIGURE 94-1. Flowchart for use of genetic testing to determine screening of at-risk individuals.

examination may be performed to look for stigmata of a hereditary syndrome, and medical management recommendations are provided.

3. Genetic Testing Strategy: Genetic testing is usually most informative when it begins with an individual affected with the cancer of interest, since most genetic tests are not 100% sensitive (Figure 94-1). By testing the affected person first, he or she serves as a "control" for genetic testing in the family. If a positive result is obtained, then the family mutation is known and definitive test information can be given to at-risk family members. If no mutation is found in an affected family member, the result is considered to be inconclusive and genetic testing of at-risk relatives is not usually feasible.

4. Cost and Insurance Coverage: Full gene sequencing is the gold standard for genetic testing, and the expense depends upon the gene analyzed. Gene sequencing for the first family member typically costs between $1,000 and $2,500. Once a mutation is identified, other family members are tested for only the specific mutation. Such targeted analysis usually costs $150 to $400. Many insurance companies cover at least a portion of the cost of genetic testing if the family history is reasonably suggestive of a hereditary syndrome. However, patients should consider obtaining insurance authorization prior to testing. This often requires a letter of medical necessity from the requesting health care provider, accompanied by diagnostic and testing codes.

5. Psychosocial Issues: A variety of emotions surround genetic testing. Patients who test positive may experience fear, depression, anger, pessimism, or shock, and some feel guilt for potentially passing the mutation to offspring. Others express relief that the cause of their cancer was identified, or that cancer risk is better defined. Patients who test negative often experience relief and happiness. However, some feel guilty for having been spared ("survivor guilt"), whereas others express disbelief. The most common reaction from patients who receive inconclusive test results is disappointment, though some are falsely reassured because a definitive mutation was not detected. Importantly, *genetic testing potentially affects an entire family*, and could have positive or negative effects on familial relationships.

6. Genetic Discrimination:* Genetic discrimination may occur with health, life, or disability insurance, or in the workplace. Currently, the Health Insurance Portability and Accountability Act (HIPAA) protects patients who have health insurance through group plans. However, there is no federal legislation offering protection for health insurance purchased in the individual market, or for life and disability coverage.

7. Informed Consent: Before testing, the risks, benefits and limitations of the test must be thoroughly discussed with the patient. This includes potential implications of a positive, negative, or inconclusive test result, as well as alternatives to genetic testing. Written informed consent is obtained from adults, and assent is obtained from children.

8. Follow Up: A written summary of the consultation is sent to the patient and the referring provider. Other follow-up responsibilities may include identification of support resources, coordination of genetic counseling for family members, and patient enrollment in a research registry. If genetic testing is performed, disclosure of genetic test results is performed in person, paying particular attention to medical and psychosocial implications.

---

*Editor's Note: Concern over genetic discrimination is still an important issue to some patients that requires personal discussion.

TABLE 94-1. Hereditary Colorectal Cancer Syndromes: Clinical Characteristics and Genetic Features

Disease	Inheritance Pattern	Gene	Malignancies (% Lifetime Risk)	Colorectal Cancer Dx (Average Age)	Noncancerous Features
HNPCC	AD	MLH1, MSH2, MSH6, PMS1, PMS2	Endometrial (40%), ovarian (10%), small bowel, stomach, urinary tract, biliary tract (all < 10%), glioblastoma (Turcot Variant, < 1%), sebaceous carcinoma (Muir-Torre variant, < 1%)	Mid-40s	Sebaceous adenomas (Muir-Torre variant), café-au-lait spots, keratoacanthomas
FAP	AD (20-30% of cases are de novo)		Colorectal (100%), duodenal (4 to 12%), thyroid (2%), pancreas (1 to 2%), hepatoblastoma (1% age 0 to 7 years), medulloblastoma (Turcot variant, < 1%)	Late 30s (adenomas diagnosed in adolescence)	> 100 colorectal adenomas (100%), upper tract adenomas (50 to 90%), fundic gland polyps (50%), osteomas, dental abnormalities, desmoid tumors (10%), epidermoid cysts, CHRPEs, angiofibroma
	AR	MYH			
AFAP	AD (20 to 30% of cases are de novo)	APC	Colorectal (95 to 100%), duodenal, thyroid, pancreas, hepatoblastoma (1% age 0 to 7 years), medulloblastoma (Turcot variant, < 1%)	Early to Mid-50s (Adenomas diagnosed mid-40s)	< 100 colorectal adenomas, epidermoid cysts, osteomas, CHRPEs (rare), angiofibroma, desmoid tumors (rare), fundic gland polyps, upper tract adenomas, dental abnormalities
	AR	MYH			
I1307K Mutation (Ashkenazi Jewish Population)	AD	APC	Colorectal (10 to 20%)	Late 50s	< 10 adenomas
PJS	AD (50% of cases are de novo)	STK-11	Breast (54%), colorectal (39%), pancreas (36%), stomach (29%), ovarian (sex cord; 21%), lung (15%), small bowel (13%), cervical (10%), testicular (Sertoli cell, 9%), endometrial (9%)	Mid-40s	Melanin pigmentation (lips, buccal, eyelids, fingers, toes), GI hamartomas, small bowel intussusception
JPS	AD (25% of cases are de novo)	BMPR1A SMAD4	Colorectal, small bowel (9 to 50%), stomach	85% have polyps by 20 years	Colorectal hamartomas (98%), upper tract hamartomas (2 to 13%) arteriovenous malformations, hemorrhagic telangiectasias

AD = autosomal dominant; AFAP = attenuated familial adenomatous polyposis; AR = autosomal recessive; FAP = familial adenomatous polyposis; HNPCC = hereditary nonpolyposis colorectal cancer; JPS = juvenile polyposis; PJS = Peutz-Jeghers syndrome.

Hereditary CRC Syndromes

To date, six hereditary syndromes are known to strongly predispose to CRC. The clinical characteristics and genetic features of each are outlined in Table 94-1. This section will overview genetic testing for each syndrome, and discusses the potential effects of testing on medical management within a family. Management of colorectal polyps and polyposis syndromes is discussed in the next chapter (see Chapter 95, "Colorectal Polyps and Polyposis Syndromes").

Hereditary Nonpolyposis CRC

Families that meet the Amsterdam criteria have a clinical diagnosis of hereditary nonpolyposis colorectal cancer (HNPCC) (Table 94-2). Testing of an affected family member begins with germline analysis of *MLH1* and *MSH2*; mutations in these genes account for 90% of mutations detected in this disorder. Starting with germline testing is often appropriate for individuals meeting one of the first three Bethesda criteria (Table 94-3). Approximately 60% of Amsterdam-positive families will have a mutation in one of these two genes. If no mutation is found in *MLH1* and *MSH2*, testing of *MSH6* may be beneficial. No commercial testing for *PMS1* or *PMS2* exists. For individuals with HNPCC by clinical criteria or genetic analysis, annual colonoscopy begins at age 25 years, or 5 to 10 years before the earliest CRC diagnosis in the family, whichever is younger. Women should have annual transvaginal ultrasound with consideration of endometrial biopsy and/or serum CA-125. If a family HNPCC mutation is identified, any biological relatives who have this mutation should

TABLE 94-2. Amsterdam Criteria: Families That Meet All Criteria Have a Clinical Diagnosis of Hereditary Nonpolyposis Colorectal Cancer

Three relatives with colorectal cancer (one a first-degree relative of the other two)
Two or more generations of colorectal cancer
One or more cases of colorectal cancer diagnosed before age 50 years
Familial adenomatous polyposis is excluded

TABLE 94-3. Bethesda Criteria: Individuals That Meet One or More Criteria are Suspicious for HNPCC

1. Individuals with cancer in families that fulfill the Amsterdam criteria
2. Individuals with two HNPCC-related cancers, including synchronous and metachronous colorectal cancers or associated extracolonic cancers
3. Individuals with colorectal cancer and a first-degree relative with colorectal cancer and/or HNPCC-related extracolonic cancer and/or adenoma; one of the cancers diagnosed under age 45 years and the adenoma diagnosed under age 40 years
4. Individuals with colorectal cancer or endometrial cancer diagnosed under age 40 years
5. Individuals with right-sided colorectal cancer with an undifferentiated pattern (solid/cribiform) on histopathology diagnosed under age 45 years
6. Individuals with signet-ring cell-type colorectal cancer diagnosed under age 45 years
7. Individuals with adenomas diagnosed under age 40 years

HNPCC = hereditary nonpolyposis colorectal cancer.

undergo surveillance as described above. Those relatives without the family mutation are unaffected and can follow general population screening guidelines. If genetic testing is inconclusive (no mutation is detected in an affected person *or* no affected person has undergone genetic testing), screening is based on family history.

Individuals that meet one or more of the Bethesda criteria are suspicious for HNPCC. Colorectal tumors from such individuals should be analyzed for microsatellite instability (MSI) at the five National Cancer Institute recommended marker sites. If the tumor is MSI-positive at two or more markers (MSI-High), germline testing of the individual is recommended, and screening intervals are determined as above. If the tumor is MSI-low or MSI-negative, HNPCC is less likely, and screening is based on family history.

Familial Adenomatous Polyposis

This syndrome involves the development of hundreds to thousands of colorectal adenomas. Full genetic sequencing will detect pathogenic mutations in 80 to 90% of affected individuals. For individuals with familial adenomatous polyposis (FAP) by clinical criteria or genetic analysis, annual or semi-annual flexible *sigmoidoscopy* should begin at *age 10 to 12 years.* Once polyps are discovered, *prophylactic colectomy* is usually required. If the rectum is retained, semiannual endoscopy is advised. Upper endoscopy is recommended every 1 to 4 years. If a family FAP mutation is identified, any biological relatives who have this mutation should undergo surveillance and/or surgery as described above. Those relatives without the family mutation are unaffected and can follow general population screening guidelines. However, it is recommended that they each undergo flexible sigmoidoscopy once at age 25 years as a safeguard. If genetic testing is inconclusive (no mutation is detected in an affected person *or* no affected person has undergone genetic testing), the individual should be screened as though affected.

Attenuated FAP

Individuals with AFAP develop dozens of colorectal adenomas at later ages and in smaller numbers than with classic FAP. Full sequencing of the APC gene will detect a pathogenic mutation in < 80% of individuals with an attenuated phenotype. For family members shown to have AFAP by clinical criteria or genetic analysis, annual colonoscopy should begin at age 12 years. Once polyps are numerous, large, or colonic surveillance is not otherwise feasible, prophylactic colectomy is usually required. If the rectum is retained, annual endoscopy is advised. Upper endoscopy is recommended every 1 to 4 years. If a family FAP mutation is identified, any biological relatives who have this mutation should undergo surveillance and/or surgery as described above. Those relatives without the family mutation are unaffected and can follow general population screening guidelines. However, it is recommended that they each undergo colonoscopy once at age 25 years as a safeguard. If genetic testing is inconclusive (no mutation is detected in an affected person *or* no affected person has undergone genetic testing), the individual should be screened as though affected.

APC I1307K

The I1307K mutation in the *APC* gene is present in 6% of the general Ashkenazi Jewish population, and in 10 to 15% of Ashkenazi Jews with CRC. Unlike other *APC* mutations, I1307K does not predispose to polyposis. Testing for the mutation is site-specific, with > 99% accuracy. For individuals with this mutation, biennial colonoscopy should begin at age 35 years, or 5 to 10 years before the earliest CRC diagnosis in the family, whichever is younger. If the tested individual does not have this mutation, and an affected family member has previously tested positive for this mutation, screening should follow general population screening guidelines. If the tested individual does not have this mutation, and no affected family member has been tested screening is based on family history.

Peutz-Jeghers Syndrome

Diagnosis of Peutz-Jeghers syndrome (PJS) requires the presence of histologically verified PJS polyps in the gastrointestinal (GI) tract and at least two of the following: (1) small bowel polyps, (2) melanin pigmentation, and/or (3) a family history of PJS. As many as half of all PJS cases are thought to be de novo. Therefore, genetic testing should begin with an affected individual. Full sequencing of the *STK*-11 gene detects 30 to 70% of pathogenic mutations in sporadic cases and 70% in familial cases. For individuals with PJS by clinical criteria or by genetic analysis, biennial colonoscopy, upper endoscopy, and small bowel series, should begin at age 12 years. At age 18 years, affected females should begin annual gynecologic exams with transvaginal ultrasound and CA-125. At age 25 years, affected patients should begin computed tomography scans or endoscopic ultrasound every 1 to 2 years, and females should undergo yearly clinical breast examination with mammography. If a family PJS mutation is identified, any biological relatives who have this mutation should undergo surveillance as described above. Those relatives without the family mutation are unaffected and can follow general population screening guidelines. If genetic testing is inconclusive (no mutation is detected in an affected person *or* no affected person has undergone genetic testing), the individual should be screened as though affected.

Juvenile Polyposis

Diagnostic clinical criteria for juvenile polyposis (JPS) include more than five colorectal juvenile polyps *or* multiple juvenile polyps throughout the GI tract *or* any number of juvenile polyps plus a family history of JP. Approximately 25% of cases are de novo mutations without a family history. Therefore, genetic testing should begin with an affected individual. Mutations of the *BMPR1A* gene are found in 25%, and of the *SMAD4* gene in 20%, of cases. Testing of the two genes via full sequencing may be sequential or concurrent. For family members with JPS by clinical criteria or genetic analysis, surveillance should begin at age 15 years (or at symptom onset, whichever is earlier) and should include complete blood count, colonoscopy and upper endoscopy every 3 years. Colectomy is recommended if the number of polyps becomes unmanageable via colonoscopic removal. If a family JPS mutation is identified, any biological relatives who have this mutation should undergo surveillance as described above. Those relatives without the family mutation are unaffected and can follow general population screening guidelines. If genetic testing is inconclusive (no mutation is detected in an affected person *or* no affected person has undergone genetic testing), the individual should be screened as though affected.

Future Directions

A number of genes responsible for hereditary CRC predisposition have been identified, and genetic testing has been implemented in a variety of settings to influence medical management. However, likely 10 to 30% of CRC is familial, caused by the interaction of lower penetrance genes with environmental factors. Investigation continues to identify such genes through family studies. Although the currently known syndromes are autosomal dominant, future discoveries may be recessive. Recently, mutations of the *MYH1* gene, a base excision repair gene, appear to be associated with the autosomal recessive development of multiple colorectal adenomas, similar to the colonic manifestations of attenuated FAP and/or FAP. Commercial testing for mutations in this gene is currently unavailable.

Supplemental Reading

American Gastroenterology Association Medical Position Statement: Hereditary colorectal cancer and genetic testing. Gastroenterol 2001;121:195–7.

American Society of Clinical Oncology Policy Statement Update. Genetic testing for cancer susceptibility. J Clin Oncol 2003;21:2397–406.

Sollenberger JE, Griffin CA. Genetic testing and counseling. In: Barker LR, Burton JR, Zieve PD, editors. Principles of ambulatory medicine. 6th ed. Philadelphia, PA: Lippincott Williams and Wilkins; 2003. p. 217–24.

Trimbath JD, Giardiello FM. Genetic testing and counseling for hereditary colorectal cancer. Aliment Pharmacol Ther 2002;16:1843–57.

CHAPTER 95

Colorectal Polyps and Polyposis Syndromes

ROBERT F. WONG, MD, AND RANDALL W. BURT, MD

Colorectal Polyps

Colorectal polyps are a common finding during any diagnostic or screening evaluation of the colon. Polyps can be broadly classified into neoplastic (adenomatous) or nonneoplastic. The latter category of polyps includes hamartomas, hyperplastic polyps, mucosal polyps, lymphoid hyperplasia, and inflammatory polyps. These are usually considered benign with minimal to no risk of progression to cancer. Distinguishing between these subgroups based on endoscopic or radiographic features is not reliable and requires histologic evaluation. Furthermore, clinical insignificance cannot be entirely applied to nonneoplastic polyps. Many of the polyposis syndromes (see below) are associated with polyps of nonneoplastic histology. Cleary, these syndromes need to be clinically recognized because of the associated risk of colon cancer as well as malignancies in other gastrointestinal (GI) sites and extra-intestinal organs. When to suspect a polyposis syndrome depends on the number and distribution of polyps, other clinical features compatible with a syndrome, and familial clustering of cancers as discussed in later sections.

Adenomas are the most common colorectal polyp accounting for up to 75% of polyps. Overall prevalence of adenomas in the United States is about 40 to 50% (Young and Macrae, 2003). Large adenomas tend to be found more frequently in the distal colon; this distribution parallels that of colorectal cancers (CRCs). Several lines of evidence suggest an adenoma-to-carcinoma sequence. This includes not only epidemiologic evidence, but also molecular and morphologic studies that correlate histologic progression of polyps with accumulation of genetic mutations in certain genes. Furthermore, family studies have shown clustering of adenomas and CRCs. About 30% of adenomas appear to have a hereditary basis. A family history of colon adenomas and/or CRC increases an individual's risk of colon cancer (Johns and Houlston, 2001). One of the best characterized hereditary CRC syndromes, familial adenomatous polyposis (FAP) (see below), is associated with thousands of colonic adenomas and a subsequent 100% lifetime risk of CRC.

Because of the association with colon cancer, treatment of adenomas and future surveillance for recurrent adenomas are central aspects of colon cancer prevention. Strong evidence exists that removal of adenomas is associated with a decreased incidence of subsequent advanced adenomas and colorectal carcinoma (Winawer et al, 1993). Therefore, after diagnosis and removal of adenomas, a major question is when and how often to repeat endoscopic surveillance to remove recurrent polyps. Surveillance can discover new adenomas as well as adenomas that were potentially missed on prior colonoscopy. The National Polyp Study showed that the incidence of advanced neoplasia (polyps at least 1 cm in size, or with high grade dysplasia or invasive cancer) with postpolypectomy surveillance at 1 and 3 years was the same as those who underwent surveillance at 3 years only (Winawer et al, 1993). Thus, 3-year follow-up is recommended after the discovery and removal of advanced adenomas. Predictors of adenoma recurrence include multiple adenomas (at least 3), villous architecture, large adenomas, and age (Winawer et al, 1993; Van Stolk et al, 1998).

Several groups have published surveillance strategies. A panel of experts in several fields, including gastroenterology, surgery, and oncology, combined with representatives form the US Multisociety Task Force on Colorectal Cancer, collectively called the Gastroenterology Consortium Panel, recently published recommendations for adenoma surveillance (Winawer et al, 2003). Patients with advanced (≥ 1 cm, villous architecture or high-grade dysplasia) or multiple adenomas (≥ 3) should undergo surveillance colonoscopy in 3 years. Those with 1 or 2 small (< 1cm) tubular adenomas should have a follow-up colonoscopy in 5 years. If the first 3-year follow-up colonoscopy shows no polyps or only 1 to 2 small adenomas are found, then repeat colonoscopy can be extended to 5 years. Although these guidelines provide reasonable timeframes for surveillance, modifications to the intervals should be considered in certain clinical situations, taking into account the number and degree of individual risk factors. Colonoscopy is the recommended surveillance strategy as double-contrast barium enema has been shown to be less effective (Winawer et al, 2000).

Polyposis Syndromes

The GI polyposis syndromes are a group of heterogeneous disorders typified by numerous GI polyps that can be encountered throughout the GI tract. Many of these syndromes have known associated genetic mutations that allow for specific genetic testing to confirm a suspected diagnosis. There is a separate chapter on colonic neoplasia and genetic counseling (see Chapter 94, "Colonic Neoplasia: Genetic Counseling"). The best known and characterized of these syndromes is FAP, however, the clinician must be aware of several other syndromes. Diseases, such as Cowden syndrome, can have a subtle presentation and only recognized by astute observation. The polyposis syndromes are important to correctly identify and diagnose for several reasons. First, patients are at increased risk not only for CRC, but also for several other GI cancers and even extra-GI cancers. Second, because of the high associated cancer risks, certain cancer surveillance recommendations and prophylactic therapies apply to this population of patients. Finally, the hereditary nature of most of these disorders allows for presymptomatic diagnosis in other family members.

Management of patients with polyposis often involves a multidisciplinary approach secondary to the complexity of management decisions. We frequently consult and involve several other specialties in addition to gastroenterology and genetic counseling, including surgery, gynecology, and dermatology.

Although several other polyposis conditions exist, including Cronkite-Canada syndrome, lymphomatous polyposis, nodular lymphoid hyperplasia, and lipomatous polyposis, these are beyond the scope of this chapter and will not be discussed.

FAP

The striking number of adenomatous polyps that often carpet the colon and the 100% lifetime risk of CRC characterize FAP. The average age of colorectal polyp formation is 16 years and of CRC is 39 years (Burt and Jacoby, 2003). The *adenomatous polyposis coli (APC)* gene is mutated in FAP, and patients inherit the disease in an autosomal dominant fashion, though about one-third of patients have no known family history and presumably are new mutation carriers. The frequency of FAP in the general population is about 2 to 3 in every 100,000 persons; the disease accounts for < 1% of all CRCs.

The diagnosis of classical FAP is often clinically apparent due to the profound phenotype these patients have. The number of colonic polyps in FAP can vary from family to family and even within families, although, typically, the numbers are in the thousands in fully expressed disease (Burt and Jacoby, 2003). The polyps are characteristically adenomatous and are usually small (< 1cm). In the upper GI tract, polyps can line the entire stomach. Polyps in the corpus and fundus are usually fundic gland polyps, though adenomatous polyps can arise in these locations as well. Polyps in the antrum tend to be adenomatous and, therefore, deserve special attention. Duodenal polyps are usually adenomatous and have a predilection for the duodenal papilla. As a consequence, cancers on or around the papilla are the most frequent GI cancers in FAP patients who have had a colectomy. Polyps in other areas of the small bowel (SB) are less frequent, but are known to occur in FAP and exhibit an associated risk of SB cancer.

Besides GI manifestations, patients with FAP have several other clinical findings. These include benign growths with little clinical significance, such as osteomas (bony cysts found usually in the mandible, skull), abnormal dentition, congenital hypertrophy of the retinal epithelium and several skin findings, especially epidermoid cysts and fibromas. Other extra-intestinal manifestations, however, can have more important clinical implications. Desmoid tumors are benign growths of fibrous tissue that can occur intra-abdominally or extra-abdominally. Though not invasive, desmoid tumors can enlarge and impinge on adjacent structures, such as bowel, vasculature, and nerves, causing a high degree of morbidity. The phenotype of FAP varies in different families and has been associated with the different mutation locations within the *APC* gene. Associated malignancies besides colon cancer (although all exhibit < a 2% lifetime risk), include SB cancer, stomach cancer, pancreatic cancer, thyroid cancer, hepatoblastoma (mostly in children), brain cancer, adrenal carcinomas, and, rarely, biliary tract cancers.

Variants of FAP include Gardner's syndrome, Turcot's syndrome (TS) and attenuated adenomatous polyposis coli (AAPC). The former is associated with several extra-intestinal growths, such as desmoids, fibromas, and osteomas. TS is associated with FAP together with central nervous system tumors in about two-thirds of families. Interestingly, the other one-third have hereditary non-polyposis CRC. AAPC will be described later.

Management of patients with FAP focuses on several important clinical decisions, including treatment options and cancer surveillance. Though colectomy is indicated as prophylaxis to prevent the otherwise inevitable development of CRC, the age to perform the surgery and what surgery to perform can be potential issues. We usually wait until patients are postadolescence before performing colectomy as the psychosocial impact tends to be less significant at later ages although sometimes polyp severity requires earlier surgery. Surgical options include total colectomy with ileal pouch-anal anastomosis (IPAA) and subtotal colectomy. The latter procedure leaves a rectal remnant that requires periodic endoscopic examinations and polyp ablation. Total colectomy with IPAA removes the rectal mucosa, though there is potential to develop ileal polyps (usually lymphoid hyperplasia, but sometimes adenomas) warranting periodic surveillance of the terminal ileum.

Duodenal polyps can pose therapeutic challenges to the endoscopist and surgeon. Smaller ampullary tumors can be managed endoscopically with papillectomy. However, larger lesions need to be removed surgically. Gastric polyps

(Figure 95-1) are usually fundic gland polyps, but some can be adenomatous and require removal. We usually remove larger polyps (> 1 cm), antral polyps or polyps that appear endoscopically unique from the other polyps, including those that are reddish in appearance (Figure 95-2).

Medical management has a potential role in controlling adenomas. Nonsteroidal anti-inflammatory drugs and selective cyclooxygenase-2 inhibitors have both been shown to reduce the number of colorectal polyps in patients with FAP (Giardiello et al, 1993; Steinbach et al, 2000) and may be used to assist in management in patients who have a remaining rectum.

Because patients with FAP are at higher risk for several malignancies, regular surveillance for malignancy is recommended and is important not to overlook. Tables 95-1 and 95-2 outline the suggested surveillance strategies and intervals for each of the potential malignancies in FAP (McGarrity et al, 2000).

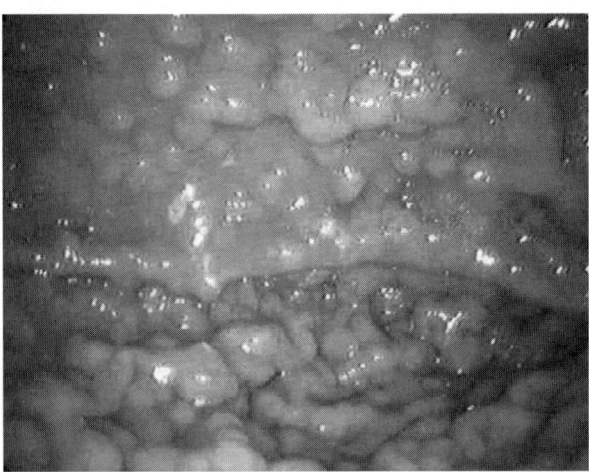

FIGURE 95-1. Carpeting of polyps in the stomach of a patient with familial adenomatous polyposis. The vast majority of these are fundic gland polyps.

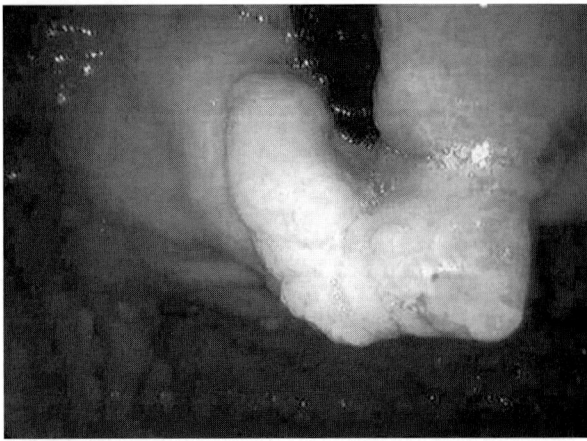

FIGURE 95-2. A large sessile tubulovillous adenoma beneath the gastroesophageal junction in a patient with familial adenomatous polyposis.

AAPC (Also Attenuated FAP)

Unlike FAP, the clinical presentation in AAPC can be less striking and the diagnosis more difficult without genetic testing. AAPC also is due to a mutation in the *APC* gene, but typically more on the extreme 3′ and 5′ ends of the gene or in exon 9 (Burt and Jacoby, 2003). As the name implies, patients present with fewer polyps and at a later age; both in terms of polyps and cancers. Whereas 100 colon polyps are usually required to make the diagnosis of FAP, polyp numbers in AAPC can range from 5 to 100 (average 30), and the numbers can vary amongst individuals within the same family. The polyps tend to be more proximal colonic, which is important to remember when considering endoscopic screening of at-risk individuals for the disease. A high index of suspicion is needed to make the diagnosis and AAPC should be suspected when patients present with multiple polyps at a young age, especially with a compatible family history. An important observation is that the manifestations in the upper GI tract tend not to be attenuated and can assist in confirming a clinical suspicion.

Our management of patients with AAPC differs significantly with classical FAP in certain regards. First of all, the indication for colectomy is not as universal. Many patients can be managed endoscopically with periodic colonoscopy and polypectomies (see Tables 95-1 and 95-2). Colectomy

TABLE 95-1. Risk and Surveillance Recommendations for the Polyposis Syndromes

Syndrome	Lifetime Risk of Colon Cancer	Screening Recommendations
Familial adenomatous polypopsis gene carrier*	Near 100%	Sigmoidoscopy annually, beginning at 10 to 12 years[†]
Peutz-Jeghers syndrome	2 to 13%[‡]	Colonoscopy, beginning with symptoms, or in late teens, if no symptoms occur. Interval determined by number of polyps but a least every 3 years once begun.
Juvenile polyposis	May be as high as 50%	Colonoscopy, beginning with symptoms or in early teens if no symptoms occur. Interval determined by number of polyps but at least every 3 years once begun.
Cowden syndrome	Little, if any	No recommendations give

Reprinted from Burt RW, 2000, with permission from the American Gastroenterological Association.
*Includes the subcategories of familial adenomatous polyposis, Gardner syndrome, Turcot syndrome, and attenuated adenomatous polyposis (AAPC).
[†]In AAPC colonoscopy should be used instead of sigmoidoscopy because of the preponderance of proximal colonic adenomas. Colonoscopy screening in AAPC should probably begin in the late teens or early 20s.
[‡]Risk estimates are for all gastrointestinal malignancies, including colon.

TABLE 95-2. Risks and Surveillance Recommendations for Extra-Colonic Cancers in the Polyposis Syndromes

Syndrome	Lifetime Risk*	Screening Recommendations
Familial adenomatous polyposis		
Duodenal or peri-ampullary cancer	5 to 12%	Upper GI endoscopy (including side-viewing exam) every 1 to 3 years, start at age 20 to 25 years
Pancreatic cancer	About 2%	Possibly periodic abdominal ultrasound after age 20 years
Thyroid cancer	About 2%	Annual thyroid examination, start age 10 to 12 years
Gastric cancer	About 0.5%	Same as for duodenal
CNS cancer, usually cerebellar medulobastoma (Turcot syndrome)	< 1% but RR[‡] = 92	Annual physical examination, possible periodic heat CT in affected families
Hepatoblastoma	1.6% of children < 5 years of age	Possibly liver palpation, hepatic ultrasound, α-fetoprotein, annually, during first decade of life
Small bowel cancer	1 to 4%	No recommendations given
Peutz-Jeghers Syndrome		
Stomach, duodenum	2 to 13%[†]	Upper GI endoscopy every 2 years, start at age 10 years
Small bowel	[‡]RR = 13	Annual hemoglobin, small bowel radiography every 2 years, both start at age 10 years[§]
Breast cancer	[‡]RR = 8.8	Annual breast exam and mammography every 2 to 3 years, both start at age 25 years
Pancreatic cancer	[‡]RR = 100	Endoscopic or abdominal ultrasound every 1 to 2 years, start at age 30 years
Uterine	[‡]RR = 8.0	Annual pelvic exam with pap smear and annual pelvic ultrasound, both start at age 20 years
Ovarian cancer	[‡]RR = 13	
Adenoma malignum (cervix)	Rare	
SCTAT tumors (females), in almost all women with PJS	20% become malignant	
Sertoli cell tumor (males), unusual	10 to 20% become malignant	Annual testicular exam, start at age 10 years; testicular ultrasound if feminizing features occur
Juvenile Polyposis		
Gastric and duodenal cancer	Rare	Upper GI endoscopy every three years, start in early teens (mainly to avoid complications of benign polyps)
Cowden Syndrome		
Thyroid cancer	3 to 10%	Annual thyroid exam, start in teens
Breast cancer	25 to 50%	Annual breast exam, start age 25 years; annual mammography, start age 30 years
Uterine and Ovarian	Possible increase	No recommendations given

Reprinted from Burt RW, 2000, with permission from the American Gastroenterological Association.
CNS = central nervous system; CT = computed tomography; GI = gastrointestinal; PJS = Peutz-Jeghers syndrome; RR = relative risk; SCTAT = sex cord tumor with annular tubules.
*Some studies give a risk to age 70 years.
[†]Risk for all GI tumors.
[‡]Relative risk, rather than lifetime risk given for this tumor.
[§]Interval may be lengthened if polyps not found, to avoid excess irradiation.

may be recommended when the polyp burden is too difficult to manage endoscopically or when high grade, larger or cancerous lesions arise. Subtotal colectomy is usually a reasonable option given the proximal nature of the polyps. Another important distinction is cancer surveillance. Although the upper GI tract tends to have a similar phenotype to FAP and warrants the same endoscopic surveillance and management as FAP, other malignancies may not be more common than the general population and routine surveillance for other cancers may not be necessary.

Peutz-Jeghers Syndrome

Peutz-Jeghers syndrome (PJS) is another polyposis syndrome with associated malignancy risk, not only in the colon, but also in other organs. The classic clinical feature of PJS is the pigmented macules that frequently occur on the lips and buccal mucosa, though they can appear in other areas including the fingertips and perianal region. It is important to realize that these pigmented spots may fade, though the buccal mucosal lesions tend to persist. The syndrome is due to a mutation in the *STK11/LKB1* gene, which can be found in about 50 to 75% of individuals. Importantly, about 50% of patients come from families with histories compatible with PJS, whereas the other patients are presumably new mutation carriers. Genetic testing is available.

Unlike FAP and AAPC, the polyps in PJS are hamartomatous and, therefore, distinguish PJS as a hamartomatous polyposis syndrome. Hamartomas are growths of tissue that can be of endodermal, mesodermal, and/or ectodermal origin, but with an epithelial covering typical of the bowel location where the polyp is found. Hamartomas in PJS histologically appear as a collection of complex glands with normal appearing epithelium and interdigitating muscular bundles. Although patients with PJS at are higher risk for GI cancers, the origin of these cancers is not entirely clear, though they are presumed to arise from the hamartomatous polyps. Hamartomas have been shown to develop foci of adenomatous changes as well as progressing directly to a carcinoma. Distinct adenomas and hamartomas have also been found in the large intestine of PJS patients. Polyps are most frequent in the SB, but can develop anywhere in the GI tract as follows: (1) SB, 96%; (2) colon, 27%; (3) stomach, 24%; and (4) rectum, 24% (McGarrity et al, 2000).

Patients with PJS typically have several potential complications from hamartomatous polyps. Not only is malignant transformation a concern, but the polyps can also ulcerate, bleed, infarct, and intussuscept. After the age of 30 years, malignant complications become the major concern; by the age of 65 years, over 90% of patients will have a malignancy. The most common GI cancers include colon, with a lifetime risk of 39%, pancreatic, with a lifetime risk of 36%, gastric, and SB (Giardiello et al, 2000). Non-GI malignancies include breast (54% lifetime incidence), ovarian (21% lifetime incidence), Sertoli cell tumors (9% lifetime incidence with 10 to 20% becoming malignant), and lung (15% lifetime incidence).

Because of the associated morbidity of large polyps in PJS and the potential malignant transformation, patients with PJS require regular surveillance as outlined in Tables 95-1 and 95-2. The high rate of extra-intestinal cancers also deserves attention with regular examination of potentially involved organs. Specific symptoms require special attention and should lead to an aggressive workup to exclude a malignant cause. Many of the surveillance recommendations in polyposis syndromes are empiric and risk-based rather than evidence-based, as appropriate evidence is difficult to obtain in rare conditions. The role of potentially valuable surveillance methods, such as endoscopic ultrasound for pancreatic cancer for instance, has not been examined in this clinical scenario.

Management of polyps in PJS can be clinically challenging. We recommend regular surveillance for GI tract polyps as outlined in the tables. When polyps are encountered on routine endoscopy, we remove all of them if possible. When the colon polyp burden is too difficult to control endoscopically, then referral for subtotal colectomy should be offered. Polyps in the SB can pose a different challenge. If polyps are particularly large (> 1 cm) or causing symptoms, we recommend removal either endoscopically, if amenable, or surgically. In the latter case, consideration for intraoperative endoscopy should be given.

Juvenile Polyposis

Juvenile polyposis (JP) is another polyposis syndrome inherited as an autosomal dominant disease. Juvenile polyps characterize this disease, though this type of polyp can be found in otherwise normal children. The clinical criteria for the diagnosis of JP include: (1) at least five juvenile polyps in the colorectum, (2) juvenile polyps throughout the GI tract, and (3) any number of juvenile polyps in a person from a family with known JP. The syndrome is due to genetic mutations in *SMAD 4* (15% of families) or *BMP1R* (38% of families). The remainder of clinically diagnosed JP families have unknown genetic mutations. Genetic testing is available for JP. Histologically, the surface mucosa is nondysplastic with abundant lamina propria. There are elongated, benign cystically dilated glands that lack a smooth muscle core. Endoscopically, polyps are usually round, reddish and smooth and often they have a white exudate on their surface (Figure 95-3). On cut surface, the polyps contain cystic spaces filled with mucin. The surface mucosa is nondysplastic with abundant lamina propria. There are elongated, benign cystically dilated glands that lack a smooth muscle core.

Like PJS, polyps can occur throughout the GI tract, but in JP they are most common in the colon. They can bleed, infarct or intussuscept with subsequent obstruction. GI malignancy is believed to arise from juvenile polyps. Lifetime risk of colon cancer has been reported to be as high as 68%. Cancers in other organs, including stomach, duodenum, and the pancreaticobiliary tree, have been associated with JP.

Cancer surveillance is recommended as summarized in Tables 95-1 and 95-2. Polyp management can be done endoscopically, though sometimes surgery is necessary when the polyp burden becomes too high. This applies mainly to colon polyps, but possibly the upper GI tract as well.

Cowden Syndrome

Cowden syndrome (CS), also called multiple hamartoma syndrome, is a syndrome characterized by cutaneous findings, in addition to polyposis, and a significant risk for development of extra-intestinal malignancy. The disease is associated with a mutation in the *PTEN/MMAC1* gene on chromosome 10 that is found in about 80% of patients

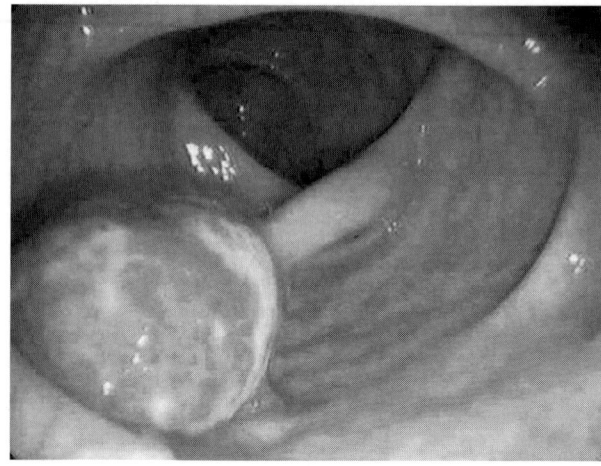

FIGURE 95-3. A typical polyp in juvenile polyposis characterized by a white exudate on the polyp surface.

meeting strict Consortium criteria for the syndrome. Diagnostic criteria have been published (Eng, 2000) and include mucocutaneous lesions (facial trichilemmomas, acral keratoses, papillomatous papules), malignancies (breast, thyroid, and endometrial) and GI findings (hamartomas of the stomach, SB, and colon and glycogen acanthosis in the esophagus) (Figures 95-4 and 95-5). The hamartomas include juvenile polyps, lipomas, and ganglioneuromas. Juvenile polyps are the most common and, characteristically, contain neural elements. Two variants of CS have been described. Bannayan-Riley-Ruvalcaba syndrome is associated with typical CS findings and macrocephaly, delayed psychomotor development, lipomatosis, hemangiomatosis, and pigmented macules of the glans penis. Lhermitte-Duclos disease is characterized by hamartomatous growths in the cerebellum.

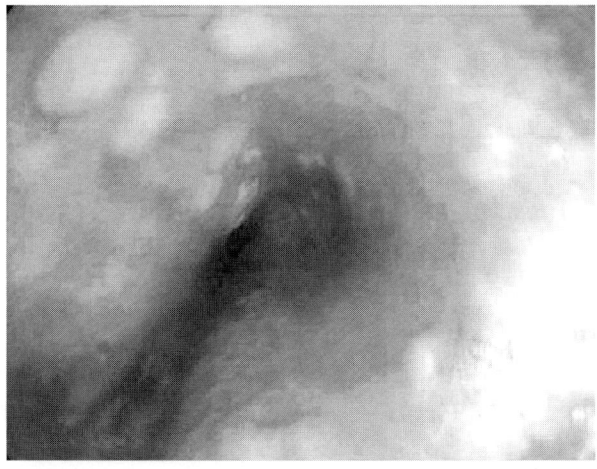

FIGURE 95-4. Glycogen acanthosis, a characteristic finding in the esophagus of a patient with Cowden syndrome.

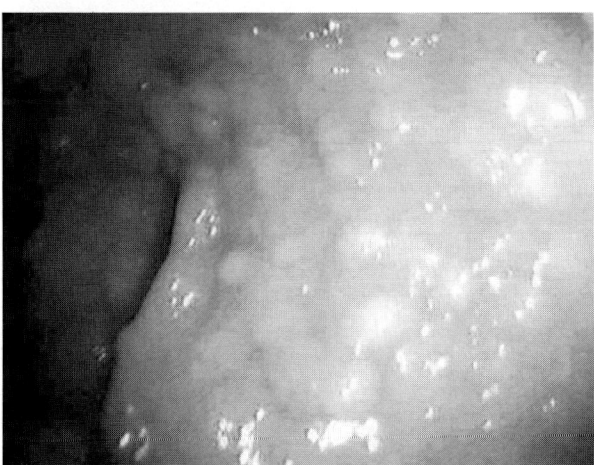

FIGURE 95-5. Multiple sessile polyps in the rectosigmoid colon in a patient with Cowden syndrome.

GI malignancy risk is not well defined in this population, though colon cancer risk appears to be slightly above the general population (9%). Particularly concerning, however, is the lifetime risk of breast cancer (25 to 50%), thyroid cancer (10%), and endometrial cancer (2 to 5%). Although no specific screening recommendations exist for GI cancers, surveillance for extra-intestinal malignancies is recommended and summarized in Tables 95-1 and 95-2. In our institution, we generally perform an initial colonoscopy and continue surveillance depending on the number of polyps.

Hyperplastic Polyposis

Although hyperplastic polyps are a common finding, especially in the distal colon and rectum, hyperplastic polyposis (HP) is a unique clinical entity with a predisposition to develop numerous hyperplastic polyps in all colon segments. Clinical criteria for the diagnosis of HP include (1) at least 5 hyperplastic polyps proximal to the sigmoid colon, 2 of which need to be > 1cm, (2) any number of hyperplastic polyps proximal to the sigmoid colon in an individual with a first-degree relative with HP, and (3) > 30 hyperplastic polyps of any size, but distributed throughout the colon (Burt and Jass, 2000).

HP is not as well characterized as the other polyposis syndromes. Although families have been described with HP, little is known of the hereditary attributes of the disease. There is no available genetic testing for this condition.

Typically, the hyperplastic polyps predominate, however, patients can also have serrated adenomas, pure adenomas, or mixed adenomas and hyperplastic polyps. CRC has been associated with HP, though the lifetime risk is not clear (Leggett et al, 2001).

Because of the risk of colorectal neoplasms, we recommend routine colonoscopic surveillance in these patients with an attempt to control the polyp burden endoscopically. Intervals between colonoscopies vary from individual to individual and are largely determined by polyp burden, presence of adenomas and family history. However, when the polyp burden is difficult to manage, especially in the coexistence of adenomas, we recommend subtotal colectomy.

Summary

Colorectal polyps, including adenomas, are common among the general population and are precursors of CRC. Appropriate screening for colon polyps and subsequent removal results in a decrease in CRC incidence. Identifying those at high risk for the subsequent development of adenomas, especially, advanced adenomas, is important in determining appropriate surveillance strategies.

Differentiating between spontaneous polyps and polyps that develop in the setting of polyposis syndromes has important implications for patient management. The polyposis syndromes have a large spectrum of clinical presentations and often the gastroenterologist is the first to make the diagnosis. After suspecting the diagnosis of a polyposis syndrome, the physician must initiate a management plan that is often multifaceted and complex. Patients should undergo appropriate genetic counseling and testing, regular cancer surveillance and should understand their therapeutic options. The appropriate testing of family members is also an intricate part of management. Although they represent a small fraction of CRC cases, the polyposis syndromes have contributed greatly to our understanding of colorectal tumorigenesis.

Supplemental Reading

Burt RW. Colon cancer screening. Gastroenterology 2000;119:837–53.

Burt RW, Jacoby RF. Polyposis syndromes. In: Yamada T, Alpers DH, Kaplowitz N, et al, editors. Textbook of gastroenterology. Vol 2. 4th ed. Philadelphia: Lippincott Williams & Wilkins; 2003. p. 1914–39.

Burt R, Jass J. Hyperplastic polyposis. In: Hamilton SR, Aaltonen LA, editors. WHO international classification of tumors: pathology and genetics of tumors of the digestive system. 3rd ed. Berlin: Springer-Verlag; 2000. p. 135–6.

Eng C. Will the real Cowden syndrome please stand up: revised diagnostic criteria. J Med Genet 2000;37:828–30.

Giardiello FM, Brensinger JD, Tersmette AC, et al. Very high risk of cancer in familial Peutz-Jeghers syndrome. Gastroenterology 2000;119:1447–53.

Giardiello FM, Hamilton SR, Krush AJ, et al. Treatment of colonic and rectal adenomas with sulindac in familial adenomatous polyposis. N Engl J Med 1993;328:1313–6.

Johns LE, Houlston RS. A systematic review and meta-analysis of familial colorectal cancer risk. Am J Gastroenterol 2001;96:2992–3003.

Leggett BA, Devereaux B, Searle J, Jass J. Hyperplastic polyposis association with colorectal cancer. Am J Surg Pathol 2001;25:177–84.

McGarrity TJ, Kulin HE, Zaino RJ. Peutz-Jeghers syndrome. Am J Gastroenterology 2000;95:596–604.

Steinbach G, Lynch PM, Phillips RK, et al. The effect of celecoxib, a cyclooxygenase-2 inhibitor, in familial adenomatous polyposis. N Engl J Med 2000;342:1946–52.

Van Stolk RU, Beck GJ, Baron JA, et al. Adenoma characteristics at first colonoscopy as predictors of adenoma recurrence and characteristics at follow-up. Gastroenterology 1998;115:13–8.

Winawer S, Fletcher R, Rex D, et al. Colorectal cancer screening and surveillance: clinical guidelines and rationale-update based on evidence. Gastroenterology 2003;124:544–60.

Winawer SJ, Stewart ET, Zauber AG, et al. A comparison of colonoscopy and double-contrast barium enema for surveillance after polypectomy. N Engl J Med 2000;342:1766–72.

Winawer SJ, Zauber AG, Ho MN, et al. Prevention of colorectal cancer by colonoscopic polypectomy. N Engl J Med 1993;329:1977–81.

Winawer SJ, Zauber AG, O'Brien MJ, et al. Randomized comparison of surveillance intervals after colonoscopic removal of newly diagnosed adenomatous polyps. N Engl J Med 1993;328:901–6.

Young GP, Macrae FA. Neoplastic and nonneoplastic polyps of the colon and rectum. In: Yamada T, Alpers DH, Kaplowitz N, et al, editors. Textbook of gastroenterology. Vol 2. 4th ed. Philadelphia: Lippincott Williams & Wilkins; 2003. p. 1883–913.

CHAPTER 96

COLON CANCER

EUGENE KENNEDY, MD, AND MICHAEL A. CHOTI, MD

Colorectal cancer (CRC) is the fourth most common malignancy in the United States with 147,500 new cases in 2003, ranking behind lung, breast, and prostate cancer. With 57,100 deaths, it is the second to lung cancer as the leading cause of cancer related deaths (Jemal et al, 2003). Large bowel cancer can be further divided by the anatomic location of the tumor into colon and rectal cancer. Colon cancers are those that arise within the portion of the large bowel that is within the peritoneal cavity, from the cecum to the peritoneal reflection where the large bowel becomes the rectum. The distinction from rectal cancer, although seemingly somewhat arbitrary, is important to make for several reasons, including the clinical presentation, the operative management, and the type of adjuvant therapy offered. Of all large bowel cancer, the colonic site makes up approximately 70%. Like rectal cancer, colon cancer management requires a multidisciplinary team approach in order to optimize detection, treatment and subsequent surveillance. There is a separate chapter on rectal cancer (see Chapter 98, "Rectal Cancer").

Presentation

Screening for CRC before it becomes clinically apparent has been shown to reduce cancer related mortality. The success of screening programs is one of the reasons cited for the decline in mortality rates from CRCs over the past 20 years. Screening is generally recommended to begin at the age of 50 years, unless risk factors including family history are present. Recommended screening options include colonoscopy every 5 to 10 years, flexible sigmoidoscopy every 5 years, and/or annual fecal occult blood testing (FOBT). Despite these recommendations, only about one-third of Americans have routine fecal occult blood testing and even fewer comply with endoscopic screening (Quinn, 2003). With increased patient and physician awareness, however, screening compliance for CRC has been on the rise in recent years. Yet even today, the majority of patients with colon cancer come to medical attention through symptomatic presentation rather than from screening (Smith et al, 2001) There is a separate chapter on colon cancer screening (see Chapter 93, "Colorectal Polyp and Cancer Screening") and another on genetic counseling (see Chapter 94, "Colonic Neoplasia: Genetic Counseling").

The most common presenting symptoms are abdominal pain, blood per rectum, anemia, constipation, diarrhea, or change in stool character. In contrast to rectal cancer, colon cancer rarely presents with anal pain, tenesmus, or incontinence. The location of the tumor within the colon often dictates the type of symptoms experienced. Right-sided tumors tend to present with anemia or the constitutional symptoms produced by such. Obstruction from right-sided tumors are more commonly in the region of the ileocecal valve. Left-sided tumors are more likely to present with obstruction, largely due to the narrow bowel caliber, circumferential lesions, and firmer stool consistency. Evident blood in the stool and a change in stool caliber are also more commonly seen with distal colon cancer.

Diagnosis

Once cancer is suspected through either screening or symptoms, it is imperative that a thorough evaluation be performed. A complete history and physical examination is necessary to assess comorbid conditions prior to treatment. A detailed family history is important to determine the possibility of a familial or hereditary syndrome. Physical examination is most often unremarkable but can help determine the presence of advanced disease through findings such as hepatomegaly, adenopathy, or an abdominal mass. A complete colonoscopy should be performed, if possible, prior to definitive therapy to confirm the histologic diagnosis and to rule out synchronous polyps or cancers. In addition, colonoscopic tattooing of the index lesion is important when the tumor is small or has been endoscopically excised to facilitate localization of these lesions at the time of operation.

In addition to routine laboratory blood studies, a preoperative serum carcinoembryonic antigen (CEA) measurement is useful in both prognosis and postoperative surveillance. An elevated preoperative CEA is more likely associated with advanced disease and is an independent predictor of poor outcome (Duffy et al, 2003). Although a preoperative CEA level is advocated as a guide to postoperative management, it is important to realize that a normal preoperative CEA should not influence the utility of CEA for postoperative surveillance. Patients with normal levels at presentation, when the disease is clinically localized, often will develop CEA elevation with recurrence. Liver function tests can also be useful as a preoperative indicator of metastatic liver disease.

The role of radiographic studies prior to surgical therapy is controversial. Preoperative computed tomography (CT) of the abdomen can detect evidence of locally advanced or metastatic disease. Up to 25% of patients present with metastatic disease and preoperative identification may result in different initial management. Preoperative CT can help identify patients with advanced disease in which treatment is clearly palliative and thereby help limit the extent of surgery and minimize morbidity. Conversely, the identification of resectable and potentially curable liver metastases prior to the initial colonic resection can allow for the planning of a combined surgical approach or a more careful intraoperative assessment of the liver with intraoperative ultrasonography. Opponents argue that the extent of disease can often be assessed during surgery and the surgical plan should account for multiple possibilities. Many surgeons, however, do obtain an abdominal CT to gain as much information as possible prior to surgery, particularly in those with locally advanced disease or if the CEA is elevated.

Positron emission tomography (PET) or PET–CT is being used with increasing frequency for staging patients with various malignancies. PET has been found to be useful in patients with advanced CRC, primarily to assess chemotherapy response or to stage patients prior to resection of metastases. Current evidence on cost effectiveness currently does not support its routine use in staging patients with primary colon cancer. Perhaps as PET becomes less costly, we may be seeing increased use for primary colon cancer staging in the future.

Staging

Historically, staging systems for colon cancer have evolved over the last century. In the 1930s Dukes originally proposed a system for the classification of large bowel cancer based on depth of tumor wall penetration and nodal status. Subsequent modifications in the 1950s included the Astler-Coller modification based on refinements of the original Dukes classification. Stage A was limited to tumors that involved the mucosa and submucosa only. Stage B1 described tumors penetrating into the muscularis propria but not through it whereas B2 described penetration through the bowel wall and B3 represented invasion of adjacent organs. Stage C were those cancers with nodal involvement with stage C1 describing node positive cancers without transmural disease, C2 those with transmural disease, and C3 those with invasion into adjacent organs. Stage D described distant metastases.

In the last decade, these previous staging systems have largely been supplanted by the TNM staging system (Table 96-1). This system was developed by the American Joint Committee on Cancer (AJCC) in cooperation with the TNM Committee of the International Union Against Cancer (UICC), and is currently accepted as the universal staging system for colon cancer. With this staging system, stage I and II describe tumors without evidence of nodal or distant disease, without or with transmural involvement, respectively. Stage III are those with nodal involvement and stage IV have distant metastatic disease. More recently, the TNM staging system has been modified to include subdivision of stage III into stage IIIA describing tumors without transmural involvement and limited nodal spread, stage IIIB for those with transmural involvement and limited nodal spread, and stage IIIC for those with any degree or wall penetration and significant nodal spread.

Management

The management of colon cancer depends upon the stage at presentation. Patients can be divided into the following two categories: (1) patients with a tumor amenable to resection with curative intent and (2) patients in whom palliation is the goal. In patients with localized and potentially

TABLE 96-1. American Joint Commission on Cancer TNM Staging System for Colon Cancer (6th Edition, 2002)

Primary Tumor (T)
- TX Primary tumor cannot be assessed
- T0 No evidence of primary tumor
- Tis Carcinoma in situ: intraepithelial or invasion of lamina propria*
- T1 Tumor invades submucosa
- T2 Tumor invades muscularis propria
- T3 Tumor invades through the muscularis propria into the subserosa, or into nonperitonealized pericolic or perirectal tissues
- T4 Tumor directly invades other organs or structures, and/or perforates visceral peritoneum**

Regional Lymph Nodes (N)
- NX Regional lymph nodes cannot be assessed
- N0 No regional lymph node metastasis
- N1 Metastasis in 1 to 3 regional lymph nodes
- N2 Metastasis in 4 or more regional lymph nodes

Distant Metastasis (M)
- MX Distant metastasis cannot be assessed
- M0 No distant metastasis
- M1 Distant metastasis

Stage Grouping

	AJCC/UICC			Dukes
Stage 0	Tis	N0	M0	—
Stage I	T1	N0	M0	A
	T2	N0	M0	—
Stage IIA	T3	N0	M0	B
Stage IIB	T4	N0	M0	B
Stage IIIA	T1–2	N1	M0	C
Stage IIIB	T3–4	N1	M0	C
Stage IIIC	Any T	N2	M0	C
Stage IV	Any T	Any N	M1	—

AJCC = American Joint Committee on Cancer; UICC = International Union Against Cancer.

curable disease, surgical resection is generally the primary and initial therapy, followed by adjuvant chemotherapy in some cases. When patients present with advanced disease, chemotherapy is often the first line of therapy and palliative resection is reserved for cases of locally symptomatic disease.

Colon Resection

The goals of surgical therapy with curative intent are to achieve complete removal of the primary cancer with adequate tumor free margins, an anatomically complete lymphadenectomy of the draining lymph nodes, en bloc resection of any involved adjacent organs, and avoidance of contamination of the surgical field with tumor cells. Between 80 to 90% of patients are appropriate candidates at presentation for an attempt at curative resection. The extent of colonic resection is determined by the vascular pedicles in order to achieve an adequate regional lymphadenectomy. Often this requires resection of a larger segment of bowel beyond that necessary simply to obtain negative margins. Histologic studies suggest that tumor rarely spreads submucosally > 1 cm from the edge of the grossly involved colon. This should be considered only in cases of rectal cancer in which the distal margin may dictate the opportunity for sphincter preservation. In the case of colon cancer resection, in most cases, at least a 5 cm bowel margin should be achieved.

The pericolic and intermediate draining lymph nodes are removed as part of a curative resection. Regional nodes are located along the course of the major vessels supplying the colon, along the vascular arcades of the marginal artery; and adjacent to the colon along the mesocolic border. Resection of intermediate and pericolic nodes requires ligation and division of the main vascular trunks to the affected colon segment. In tumors that are located between vascular pedicles (eg, hepatic or splenic flexures), extended colectomy is performed to remove nodes along both associated vascular pedicles. More extensive colonic resections, including subtotal or total colectomy, are typically reserved for those patients with multiple tumors or in cases where a prophylactic component is being performed for those at risk for metachronous disease.

All operations with curative intent must include a through exploration of the abdominal cavity for evidence of metastatic disease. Peritoneal surfaces, omentum, and paraaortic nodes should be grossly assessed. Particular attention should be paid to the liver, the most common site for metastatic disease. Visualization and careful manual palpation of all segments of the liver should be conducted, including the periportal nodal region. *Intraoperative ultrasound (IOUS)* can be used in some cases to more carefully assess the liver. In cases in which liver metastases are known to be present based on preoperative imaging, IOUS should be considered to assess potential resectability of the hepatic metastases.

Tumors of the cecum and ascending colon are typically managed with a *right hemicolectomy* (Figure 96-1A). This involves resection of the terminal ileum, cecum, and ascending colon including the hepatic flexure. High ligation of the ileocolic and right colic vessels provides for an adequate lymphadenectomy. Tumors of the transverse colon are often managed with a *transverse colectomy*, including the middle colic and lymphatics. *Left hemicolectomy* (Figure 96-1B) is performed for tumors arising in and descending colon and includes ligation of the left colic artery. The splenic flexure is mobilized and the transverse colon is anastomosed to the proximal rectum. For sigmoid cancers, either a left hemicolectomy or a *sigmoid colectomy* (Figure 96-1C) can be performed. When performing the bowel anastomosis, various methods can be used, including hand-sewn or stapling techniques.

Laparoscopic Colectomy

The widespread application of laparoscopic approaches to common general surgical operations has changed abdominal surgery. This technology has also been applied to resections of the colon. When compared with other commonly performed laparoscopic procedures, such as cholecystectomy, laparoscopic colon resection is technically more chal-

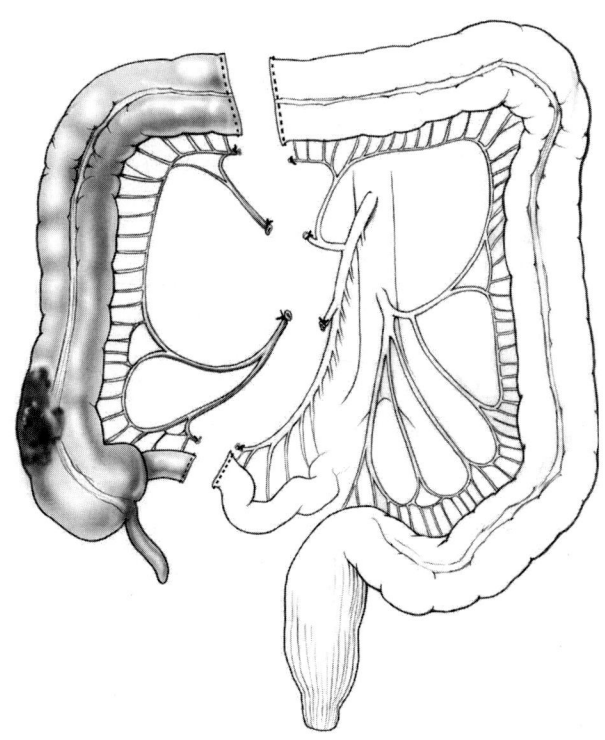

FIGURE 96-1A. Right hemicolectomy.

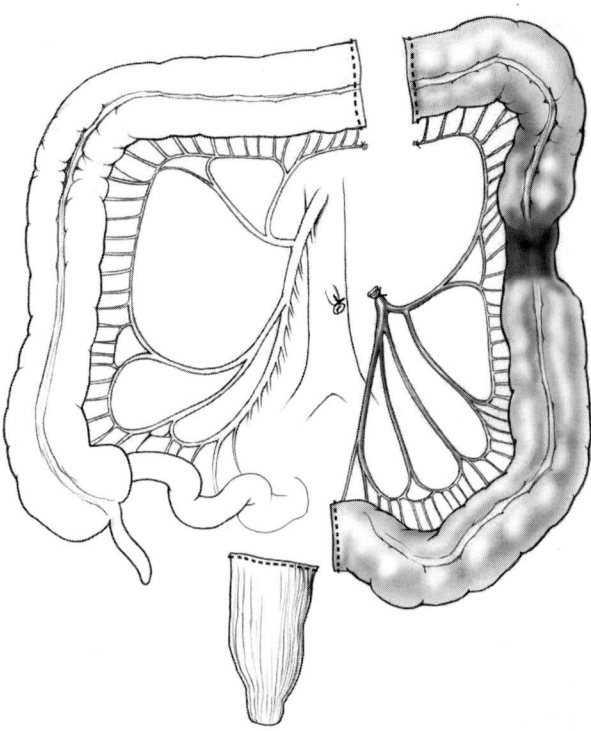

FIGURE 96-1B. Left hemicolectomy.

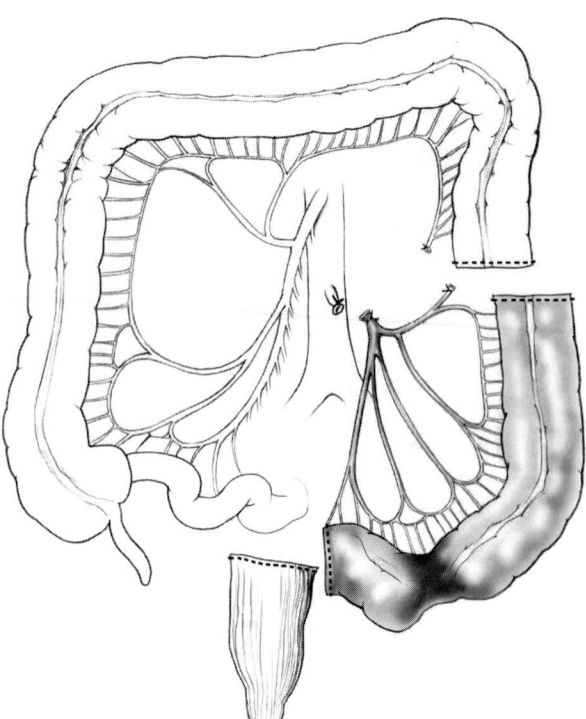

FIGURE 96-1C. Sigmoid colectomy. Illustrations by Corinne Sandone from Cameron JL. Current surgical therapy, 7th ed. St. Louis: Mosby; 2001.

lenging because of necessary mobilization and the anastomosis that must be performed. Concerns about this approach include difficulty localizing small lesions because of the lack of the ability to palpate the colon. Preoperative colonoscopic tattooing of the lesion, as well as the ability to perform intraoperative colonoscopy, aids in finding these small lesions. Early experience with this technique also raised concerns about the oncologic adequacy of the laparoscopic approach (Wexner and Cohen, 1995). Resections with curative intent must adhere to oncologic principles. Laparoscopic colectomy must maintain adequate margins as well as a proper lymphadenectomy. Thus far, studies have shown these concerns to be unfounded. The data has shown that margins and numbers of lymph nodes harvested are comparable to open techniques (Korolija et al, 2003). The advantages of the laparoscopic approach, however, are less evident than with other laparoscopic operations. Laparoscopic colon resection tends to take longer to perform, requires expensive operative equipment, and still requires an incision. Studies to date have shown reduction in hospital length of stay, pain, and morbidity, but no difference in mortality when compared to open colectomy. Only a small fraction of colon resections are currently performed laparoscopically.

Lymphadenectomy and Sentinel Lymph Node Mapping

Mapping of the *sentinel lymph nodes* is a technique that has proved successful in improving nodal staging in various malignancies, including melanoma and breast cancer. Identifying and assessing the initial node to which a tumor would spread could increase nodal staging accuracy. Some centers have begun applying sentinel lymph node mapping for colon cancer. With this technique, the colon tumor is typically injected with vital dye or fluorescein during surgery and the nodes are assessed minutes later. It can be performed either in vivo or ex vivo immediately following resection. The sentinel nodes are identified and analyzed separately, often using more complete histologic evaluation than what could be done for all the nodes in the specimen. Several studies have shown an increased sensitivity with this technique at detecting otherwise occult nodal involvement, which than may identify those at increased risk for recurrence (Bendavid et al, 2002; Paramo et al, 2002). The principal advantage of sentinel lymphatic mapping for melanoma and breast cancer, however, is the ability to remove only the sentinel node, sparing the additional morbidity of a formal lymph node dissection. When applied to colon cancer staging, because the vascular pedicles primarily determine the length of colon resected, the ability to find a single node is unlikely to change the extent of lymphadenectomy. Moreover, returning to perform an adequate lymphadenectomy when nodes are found to be positive would require an additional major abdominal surgery with associated morbidity. For these reasons, sentinel lymph node mapping for colon cancer remains *investigational*. Further studies are needed to determine if this potentially promising technique will provide sufficient benefit to become clinically useful for colon cancer.

Management of Obstructing or Perforated Colon Cancer

The management of obstructing or perforated colon cancer presents unique considerations. When patients present with urgent evidence of obstruction without the opportunity to prepare the bowel, they must be expediently resuscitated and undergo immediate surgical exploration. If the obstruction is due to a proximal lesion near the ileocecal valve, a right hemicolectomy with primary anastomosis may be performed safely in most cases, even with an unprepared colon. More distal obstructions are problematic because the proximal colon is dilated and typically full of stool. Once the involved segment of colon is resected, on-table lavage can be performed. This involves mobilization of the colon, attachment of large bore sterile tubing to drain the effluent, and instillation of a large volume of warm saline through a catheter placed through an appendicostomy or the terminal ileum. The distal segment of bowel can be washed out from below. This technique can allow for a primary anastomosis in some cases provided the bowel is not dilated and appears relatively healthy.

Perforations at the tumor site can present either as locally contained abscesses or as free perforation with peritonitis. In addition, obstructing tumors can result in colonic perforation, typically proximal to the tumor or at the cecum. In the case of contained perforations, abscesses can be drained percutaneously with subsequent investigations and elective surgical management. Free perforation with peritonitis is a surgical emergency that necessitates rapid resuscitation and operation. In the setting of gross fecal contamination, resection of the tumor and perforation are performed when possible with a proximal colostomy or ileostomy (Hartmann's procedure). In some cases, a primary anastomosis can be performed with a protecting proximal ostomy. An unprotected anastomosis without diversion is ill advised in these unstable patients.

Adjuvant Therapy

Despite apparently curative resections, many CRC patients develop recurrence of their disease. Among lymph node positive patients, 30 to 70% will develop recurrence and eventually die from recurrent disease. The goal of adjuvant therapy is to provide additional treatment to those patients most likely to recur while avoiding overtreatment in those with only a modest chance of benefit. Current standard recommendations are that all medically appropriate patients who are node positive (stage III disease) receive adjuvant chemotherapy. There is also a trend towards treating some stage II patients, particularly those with other poor prognostic features. The chemotherapeutic regimens most often are fluorpyrimadine-based, including 5-fluorouracil and leucovorin. Newer agents that have shown benefit in advanced CRC, including irinotecan and oxaliplatin, are currently being studied in the adjuvant setting. Unlike with rectal cancer, adjuvant radiation therapy for colon cancer is rarely indicated. The next chapter is on adjuvant and chemotherapy (see Chapter 97, "Colorectal Carcinoma"). There is also a chapter on abdominal radiation (see Chapter 100, "Abdominal Radiation").

Follow-Up

Following patients after treatment for colon cancer serves several functions. First, surveillance attempts to identify recurrent disease at a stage potentially resectable for cure. Secondly, following patients with colonoscopy can identify metachronous polyps or cancers at an early stage. Finally, surveillance serves to reassure the patient. A balance must be struck between accomplishing the above goals and providing care that has minimal morbidity and is cost effective. Based on available data, guidelines for follow-up have been developed, including by the National Comprehensive Cancer Network (NCCN) (Engstrom et al, 2003). Patients with T2 or greater tumors should be followed with history and physical examination and a CEA level every 3 months for the first 2 years after treatment and then every 6 months for the next 3 years. If a rising CEA is identified, further testing should be performed, including imaging studies and colonoscopy. CT scan is the most frequently used imaging modality. If negative with a continuing rise of the CEA, PET imaging should be considered. In addition, PET can be useful in cases where resection of metastatic disease is being considered to rule out more extensive disease. In cases where the primary tumor is of early stage (Tis, T1) or where the patient may not be a candidate for aggressive treatment of recurrent disease, follow-up testing can be more limited. There is a separate chapter on metastatic cancer of the liver (see Chapter 129, "Metastatic Cancer of the Liver").

Colonoscopy should be performed at 1 year postoperatively, or within 6 months, if a complete colonoscopy was not possible preoperatively due to obstruction or perforation. If the postoperative colonoscopy is free of polyps, repeat surveillance every 3 years is generally recommended. In patients where adenomas are found or if a hereditary syndrome is present, annual colonoscopy should be considered.

Chemo prevention of colorectal adenomas is discussed in the February 3, 2004 issue of the *Annals of Internal*

Medicine, Chan, et al. 140:157–66, in an editoral by Sandler, and in the chapter on colonic polyps (see Chapter 95, "Colorectal Polyps and Polyposis Syndromes").

Supplemental Reading

AJCC Cancer staging manual, 6th Ed. New York: Springer-Verlag; 2002.

Bendavid Y, Latulippe JF, Younan RJ, et al. Phase I study on sentinel lymph node mapping in colon cancer: a preliminary report. J Surg Oncol 2002;79:81–4.

Clinical Outcomes of Surgical Therapy Study Group. A comparison of laparoscopically assisted and open colectomy for colon cancer. N Engl K Med 2004;350(20):2050–9.

Duffy MJ, van Dalen A, Haglund C, et al. Clinical utility of biochemical markers in colorectal cancer: European Group on Tumour Markers (EGTM) Guidelines. Eur J Cancer 2003;39:718–27.

Engstrom PF, Benson AB, Saltz L. National Comprehensive Cancer Network Clinical Practice Guidelines in Oncology Colon Cancer Version 2;2003.

Jemal A, Murray T, Samuels A, et al. Cancer statistics, 2003. CA Cancer J Clin 2003;53:5–26.

Korolija D, Tadic S, Simic D. Extent of oncological resection in laparoscopic vs. open colorectal surgery: meta-analysis. Langenbecks Arch Surg 2003;387:366–71.

Paramo JC, Summerall J, Poppiti R, Mesko TW. Validation of sentinel node mapping in patients with colon cancer. Ann Surg Oncol 2002;9:550–4.

Quinn MJ. Cancer trends in the United States—a view from Europe. J Natl Cancer Inst 2003;95:1258–61.

Smith RA, von Eschenbach AC, Wender R, et al. American Cancer Society Guidelines for the Early Detection of Cancer: Update of Early Detection Guidelines for Prostate, Colorectal, and Endometrial Cancers. Also: Update 2001—Testing for Early Lung Cancer Detection. CA Cancer J Clin 2001;51:38–75.

Wexner SD, Cohen SM. Port site metastases after laparoscopic colorectal surgery for cure of malignancy. Br J Surg 1995;82:295–8.

CHAPTER 97

Colorectal Carcinoma: Adjuvant and Chemotherapy

Sharlene Gill, MD, and Richard M. Goldberg, MD

Chemotherapy for colorectal cancer (CRC) is typically applied in the following two clinical settings: (1) for the *adjuvant* management of curatively *resected* early-stage disease and (2) for the primary management of *unresectable distant metastases*. Until the early 1990s, options for chemotherapy were essentially limited to *5-fluorouracil* (5-FU). Recent exciting advances have resulted in the integration of new agents, including *oxaliplatin* and *irinotecan*, for the treatment of patients with advanced disease with consequent significant improvements in survival benefit. Although *5-FU* remains the mainstay of treatment for *adjuvant therapy*, efforts to evaluate the role of *oxaliplatin* and *irinotecan* in this setting are already underway. In this chapter, current standards of chemotherapy management for CRC will be reviewed. There are separate chapters on colon cancer (see Chapter 96, "Colon Cancer"), rectal cancer (see Chapter 98, "Curative Intent Management of Rectal Cancer"), rectal cancer palliation (see Chapter 99, "Palliative Therapy for Rectal Cancer") and abdominal radiation (see Chapter 100, "Abdominal Radiation").

Primary Chemotherapy for Advanced CRCs

5-FU

Developed in 1957, 5-FU represents one of the earliest examples of a rationally designed drug, and now, almost five decades later, it still remains the base of almost all CRC chemotherapy regimens. Following metabolic activation to 5-fluoro-2´-deoxyuridylate (FdUMP), this fluorinated pyrimidine combines with methylenetetrahydrofolate (CH_2FH_4) to form a ternary complex with thymidylate synthase (TS) thus interfering with DNA synthesis by inhibiting the conversion of deoxyuridylate to thymidylate. Additional mechanisms of action include direct incorporation into ribonucleic acid (RNA) to interfere with RNA transcription and, to a lesser extent, direct incorporation into deoxyribonucleic acid (DNA).

Adverse Effects

Hematologic effects and gastrointestinal (GI) mucosal toxicity are the common *dose-limiting toxicities* of 5-FU. Severe *diarrhea* (≥ grade 3 as defined by the National Cancer Institute Common Toxicity Criteria) will be experienced by 30% of patients, and grade 3 *stomatitis* can be anticipated in 15 to 20% of patients. The risk of nausea and vomiting is low.

Combination Therapy

With response rates of < 10 to 15%, the single agent activity of 5-FU is modest (Advanced Colorectal Cancer Meta-Analysis Project, 1992) but can be enhanced by the addition of *leucovorin calcium* (LV, also known as *folinic acid*) which increases the stability of the FdUMP-TS-CH_2FH_4 ternary complex (Danenberg and Danenberg, 1978). In a meta-analysis using 2,751 patients with advanced CRC from 18 randomized trials comparing 5-FU/LV to 5-FU alone, the addition of LV conferred a doubling in response rates (23% vs 12%, $p < .0001$) with a small but statistically significant improvement in 1 year survival (48% vs 43%, $p = .003$) (Piedbois et al, 2003). In addition to biochemical modulation with LV, differences in activity and toxicity are also observed between infusional and bolus administration schedules of 5-FU. The two commonly used bolus regimens of biomodulated 5-FU are as follows:

1. The Mayo/NCCTG regimen: 5-FU 425 mg/m²/d and LV 20 mg/m²/d administered for 5 consecutive days repeated every 4 weeks for 2 cycles then every 5 weeks thereafter.
2. The Roswell Park regimen: 5-FU 500 mg/m² and high dose LV 500 mg/m² administered weekly for 6 consecutive weeks and repeated every 8 weeks.

A pooled analysis of 1,219 patients from 6 trials comparing continuous infusion to bolus administration of 5-FU in patients with advanced CRC reported higher response rates (22% vs 14%, $p = .0002$) and a modest improvement in survival (median 12.1 months vs 11.3 months, $p = .04$) in patients assigned to *continuous infusion* 5-FU (Meta-analysis Group in Cancer, 1998).

The Mayo/NCCTG bolus schedule was compared with a 48 hour high dose biomodulated infusion schedule administered every 2 weeks (LV5-FU2) in a French study with 433 patients. LV5-FU2 was associated with higher response rates (32.6% vs 14.4%, $p = .0004$), longer progression-free survival (27.6 weeks vs 22 weeks, $p = .0012$) and a trend towards improved overall survival (62 weeks vs 56.8 weeks, $p = .067$). The LV5-FU2 arm also had less neutropenia, diarrhea, and mucositis (de Gramont et al, 1997). Reluctance to widely adopt infusional 5-FU as a standard regimen, particularly in North America, has been based on concerns of patient inconvenience and the risk of catheter-related complications.

Capecitabine

Oral fluoropyrimidines offer a more convenient alternative to continuous infusion 5-FU. 5-FU has been unsuitable for oral delivery due to its poor bioavailability and rapid catabolic clearance by dihydropyrimidine dehydrogenase. Capecitabine is an oral 5-FU prodrug that is well absorbed by the GI tract and undergoes a three-step enzymatic conversion to active 5-FU. Two randomized trials of first line twice-daily oral capecitabine with bolus 5-FU/LV in patients with advanced CRC have reported equivalent survival efficacy with a more favorable toxicity profile for capecitabine (Hoff et al, 2001; Van Cutsem et al, 2000). Capecitabine thus represents a reasonable option for patients who would be candidates for treatment with 5-FU/LV alone.

Irinotecan

Irinotecan (also known as CPT-11) is a semisynthetic derivative of the natural alkaloid camptothecin which antagonizes the activity of topoisomerase I. Topoisomerase I plays a key role in replication by relaxing the supercoiled DNA helix with reversible and transient single stranded DNA breaks. Following conversion to irinotecan's active metabolite, SN-38, these transient breaks are stabilized resulting in replication arrest and apoptosis. The major toxicity of irinotecan is delayed onset diarrhea. An acute cholinergic syndrome characterized by diaphoresis, salivation, lacrimation, abdominal cramps, and bradycardia, may be observed during administration and typically responds to atropine (Takasuna et al, 1996). When compared to infusional 5-FU in patients who progressed on first line bolus 5-FU, irinotecan resulted in an improved overall survival and time to progression (4.2 vs 3.9 months, $p = .030$) (Rougier et al, 1997). A second study by Cunningham and colleagues (1998) showed an improved overall survival of 9.2 vs 6.5 months ($p = .0001$) with irinotecan vs best supportive care alone. Two subsequent studies established the combination of irinotecan with 5-FU/LV as an important combination for patients with advanced CRC (Table 97-1). Concerns regarding toxicity with the weekly schedule of irinotecan and bolus 5-FU/LV (IFL) were raised due to an unexpected number of early deaths in two cooperative group studies involving IFL (Rothenberg et al, 2001). The majority of deaths were attributed to GI toxicities or thromboembolic events, prompting recommendations for close clinical monitoring and early supportive intervention for patients treated with IFL.

Oxaliplatin

Oxaliplatin is a third generation platinum with a 1,2 diaminocyclohexane carrier ligand that forms DNA adducts and secondary strand breaks. It has a distinctive *neurotoxicity profile,* which includes an acute cold-induced sensory neuropathy characterized by dysesthesias and paresthesias during or soon after the infusion and a delayed onset dose-dependent neuropathy occurring hours to days after treatment. The latter typically occurs in 10 to 15% of patients after a cumulative dose of 780 to 850 mg/m^2, with at least partial reversibility in 75% of patients within 3 to 5 months of treatment discontinuation. In a randomized trial comparing infusional 5-FU/LV (LV5FU2), single-agent oxaliplatin and the combination (FOLFOX) in 459 patients with recurrence following IFL, treatment with FOLFOX yielded higher response rates (9.9% vs 1.3% oxaliplatin vs 0% LV5FU2) and a longer time to progression (4.6 months vs 1.6 months vs 2.7 months) (Rothenberg et al, 2003). A survival advantage for first line FOLFOX has been established in a three-arm NCCTG-led intergroup trial (N9741) of

TABLE 97-1. Phase III Trials of Irinotecan Combined with 5-Fluorouracil and Leucovorin

Study	0038[31]		0038[31]	
	5-FU/LV Bolus	Irinotecan + Bolus 5-FU/LV*	5-FU/LV Infusional	Irinotecan + Infusional 5-FU/LV
Number of patients	221	222	188	199
Response rate	21%	39% ($p < .001$)	22%	35% ($p < .005$)
Median TTP†	4.3 mo	7.0 mo ($p = .004$)	4.4 mo	6.7 mo ($p < .001$)
Grade 3 or greater‡ toxicity	—	—	—	—
Diarrhea	13%	23%	6%	14%
Vomiting	4%	10%	2%	4%
Febrile neutropenia	15%	7%	1%	3%
Neutropenia	67%	54%	14%	46%

*IFL (irinotecan and bolus 5-fluorouracil/leucovorin).
†Time to progression.
‡National Cancer Institute Common Toxicity Criteria.

patients with advanced CRC randomly assigned to bolus IFL, FOLFOX, or a combination of irinotecan plus oxaliplatin (IROX) (Goldberg et al, 2004). As presented in Table 97-2, FOLFOX was associated with improved response rates, a longer time to progression and a longer median survival when compared to IFL and IROX.

In an analysis of randomized trials, a linear association between a prolonged median survival and the successive availability of 5-FU, irinotecan and oxaliplatin was seen with *median survivals* approaching a previously unheard of *21.4 months*, hence emphasizing the need for access to all three active agents in order to significantly impact the survival of patients with advanced CRC (Grothey et al, 2004). In addition, based on case series and phase II data, there now exists the hope of altering the natural history for selected patients with unresectable disease by *downstaging liver-limited metastases* with primary chemotherapy and rendering them amenable to a potentially curative resection (Giacchetti et al, 1999; Alberts et al, 2003).

Given the number of options currently available, patients with advanced CRC warrant an early referral to medical oncology for discussion. At present, either oxaliplatin or irinotecan in combination with 5-FU/LV (preferably as an infusional regimen) represent reasonable strategies for first line primary chemotherapy in good performance status patients with unresectable metastatic CRC. The choice of regimen can be somewhat tailored by the differences in toxicity profiles for oxaliplatin and irinotecan. Capecitabine may be offered to patients not suitable for combination therapy.

Regional Chemotherapy

The rationale for regional chemotherapy by hepatic arterial infusion (HAI) is based upon the recognition that the liver is the most likely site of distant metastases for CRC and it has a *unique dual blood supply*, with the hepatic vein serving as the primary source of vascularization for the normal parenchyma while the *hepatic artery supplies tumor*. Fluorodeoxyuridine (FUDR) is the preferred agent for HAI delivery. When delivered by HAI, > 90% of FUDR is extracted by the liver on first pass with an estimated 100- to 400-fold increase in hepatic exposure when compared to intravenous administration (Ensminger, 2002). A meta-analysis including 654 patients with unresectable hepatic metastases enrolled in 7 randomized trials comparing HAI to systemic 5-FU therapy did show greater tumor response rates with HAI (41% vs 14%, $p < .001$). However there was no significant survival advantage (16 months vs 12.2 months, $p = .14$) (Meta-Analysis Group in Cancer, 1996). Kerr and colleagues (2003) randomized 209 patients to systemic therapy (LV5FU2) or HAI with 5-FU/LV with no observed differences in progression-free survival or overall survival (14.7 months vs 14.8 months, $p = .79$). More recently, 117 patients with liver-limited unresectable metastases were randomized to bolus 5-FU/LV or HAI with FUDR by Kemeny and colleagues (2003). Response rates (51% vs 24%, $p = .009$) and survival (22.7 months vs 19.8 months, $p = .027$) favored HAI although time to extrahepatic progression was significantly shorter (7.8 months vs 23 months $p = .0007$). *With the availability of more efficacious systemic multiagent chemotherapy regimens, the clinical utility of HAI in unresectable advanced CRC remains limited.*

TABLE 97-2. Results from N9741

	IFL* (control)	FOLFOX†	CPT11+OXAL‡ (IROX)
Number of patients	264	267	264
Response rate	31%	45% ($p = .002$)	34% ($p = .03$)
Median time to progression	6.9 mo	8.7 mo ($p = .0014$)	6.5 mo ($p =$ NS)
Median survival	14.8 mo	19.5 mo ($p = .0001$)	17.4 mo ($p = .09$)
1 year survival	59%	72%	67%
Grade 3 or greater toxicity	–	–	–
Paresthesias	3%	18%§	7%
Diarrhea	28%	12%§	24%
Vomiting	14%	3%§	22%
Febrile neutropenia	15%	4%§	11%
Neutropenia	39%	47%?	35%

IROX = irinotecan and oxaliplatin.
FOLFOX = 5-fluorouracil/leucovorin and oxaliplatin.
IFL = irinotecan and bolus 5-fluorouracil/leucovorin.
OXAL = oxaliplatin.
*24% of patients received oxaliplatin on progression.
†60% of patients received irinotecan on progression.
‡50% of patients received 5-fluorouracil on progression.

Adjuvant Chemotherapy for CRC

Although surgery remains the primary curative modality for localized disease, the presence of micrometastases will be responsible for disease relapse in a significant proportion of patients. *Six months of 5-FU/LV* remains the current standard of care for *adjuvant therapy* following resection of *high risk localized CRC*, credited with a *one-third decrease* in the risk of *disease recurrence and death* (Macdonald and Astrow, 2001). For patients with *node-positive colon cancer*, this translates into an overall *absolute 5-year survival improvement* from approximately 50% to 60 to 65%, as was observed in Intergroup 0035, the first trial to confirm the efficacy of adjuvant therapy (Table 97-3). In the subsequent Intergroup 0089 randomized trial of 3759 patients with resected high risk stage II (node-negative) or stage III (node-positive) colon cancer, no advantage was observed with 12 months of therapy over 6 months, or with the addition of levamisole (an antihelminthic biomodulator of 5-FU) to LV. As well, no significant survival differences were observed between 6 months of 5-FU/LV delivered by the Mayo regimen or the Roswell Park regimen (Haller et al, 1998). Adjuvant chemotherapy should commence within 3 to 8 weeks following surgery.

TABLE 97-3. Randomized Trials of Postoperative Adjuvant Therapy for Colon Cancer

	Treatment Assignment	Months of Treatment	5-Year Overall Survival
INT 0035	Observation	–	54%
	LEV	12	54%
	5-FU/LEV	12	65%
INT 0089	5-FU/LEV	12	63%
	5-FU/LV-HD	6	65%
	5-FU/LV-LD	6	66%
	5-FU/LV-LD/LEV	6	67%

5-FU = 5-fluorouracil; LEV = levamisole (antihelminthic, for biomodulation); 5-FU/LV-LD = leucovorin, low dose (Mayo regimen); 5-FU/LV-HD = leucovorin, high dose (Roswell Park regimen).

As shown in Table 97-4, the integration of newer agents including *capecitabine, irinotecan* and *oxaliplatin* into adjuvant regimens is currently under active investigation. Efficacy results of the international MOSAIC phase III trial were recently reported with 2,246 patients with resected stage II and III colon cancer randomized to LV5FU2 or FOLFOX bimonthly for 12 cycles. The FOLFOX cohort had a 23% decrease in risk of recurrence with an improved 3-year disease free survival (78% vs 73%). Significant sensory neuropathy was experienced by 12% of FOLFOX patients with resolution seen in all but 1% at 1 year. Overall survival data have not yet matured (Topham et al, 2003).

Although randomized trials have clearly demonstrated the *benefits* of *adjuvant therapy* in *node-positive colon cancer*, the role of chemotherapy following curative resection of node-negative colon cancer is still debated. The debate had been propelled by two conflicting meta-analyses: the NSABP series and IMPACT B2. A pooled analysis of data from the NSABP adjuvant studies with very heterogeneous treatment arms compared the relative efficacy of adjuvant therapy for stage II patients with stage III patients and demonstrated significant proportional reductions in mortality for both stage II and stage III disease, concluding that adjuvant chemotherapy should be considered in all patients

TABLE 97-4. Forthcoming Adjuvant Trials of Interest

Study	Number of Patients	Stage	Treatment Arms*
CALGB C89803	1,264	III	IFL vs RP
NSABP C-07	2,492	II and III	FLOX vs RP
PETACC 3	1,800	III	FOLFIRI vs LV5FU2
ACCORD-02	400	III	FOLFIRI vs LV5FU2
X-ACT	1,956	III	Capecitabine vs Mayo

Capecitabine = 1250 mg/m^2 by mouth 2 times daily for 14/21 days;
FLOX = oxaliplatin every 2 weeks with Roswell Park (RP);
FOLFIRI = irinotecan 180 mg/m^2, LV5-FU2;
*IFL = irinotecan 125 mg/m^2, 5-fluorouracil (5-FU) 500 mg/m^2 + leucovorin (LV) 20 weekly for 4 out of every 6 weeks;
LV5FU2 = 5-FU 400mg/m^2 bolus, 5-FU 600 mg/m^2 continuous venous infusion for 48 h;
Mayo = 5-FU 425 mg/m^2 + LV 20 days 1 to 5 every 4 to 5 weeks;RP = Roswell Park 5-FU 500mg/m^2 + LV 500 weekly for 6/8 wks.

with stage II colon cancer (Mamounas et al, 1999). In a separate IMPACT B2 meta-analysis of stage II patients entered in 5 randomized trials evaluating 5-FU/LV, a significant survival advantage for adjuvant therapy could not be demonstrated with only a modest 2% absolute risk reduction in 5-year survival (82% vs 80%), prompting the IMPACT investigators to conclude that adjuvant therapy should not be routinely offered to all patients with stage II disease. Hopefully, prospective data will help to settle this ongoing controversy. Until then, patients with node-negative disease should be evaluated for discussion about the available data so that they may participate in the decision to receive treatment. Consideration for adjuvant intervention is particularly warranted in those with high risk prognostic features (such as bowel obstruction, tumor adherence, perforation, and poor differentiation). When available, patients should continue to be offered participation in clinical trials.

Rectal Cancer

Although a detailed discussion is beyond the scope of this chapter, it is important to note that *pelvic external beam radiation therapy* is an important component of *adjuvant protocols for stage II and III cancers of the rectum*. This is typically delivered over 5 to 6 weeks to a total dose of 50.4 Gy with concurrent administration of continuous infusion 5-FU, which acts as a radiosensitizer (O'Connell et al, 1994). Several randomized trials have raised questions regarding the appropriate timing, dose and chemoradiation combination, particularly in view of improved surgical outcomes with *total mesorectal excisions*. Regardless of the type of resection, however, these data have been consistent in demonstrating that the contribution of radiation to the benefit of adjuvant therapy in rectal cancer is limited to reducing locoregional relapse with no significant effect on survival. A recent meta-analysis examined pooled data for 6,350 patients in 13 trials of preoperative radiotherapy and 2,157 patients in 8 trials of postoperative radiotherapy. A 37 to 46% decrease in annual risk of local recurrence was seen with the largest reduction in the preoperative radiotherapy studies (Adjuvant, 2001).

Postoperative radiotherapy remains a prevalent practice in North America, but emerging data has led many practitioners to consider *preoperative radiation with or without 5-FU*, particularly if the tumor is low lying or locally advanced.

Monoclonal Antibodies as Therapeutic Agents in CRC

An improved understanding of the molecular pathogenesis of cancer has advanced the development of novel agents designed to target critical cellular pathways. Although several compounds are in early stages of development, the following two agents were recently approved by the U.S. Food and Drug Administration (FDA) for colorectal cancer therapy: (1) bevacizumab and (2) cetuximab. *Bevacizumab* is a recombinant humanized monoclonal antibody against vascular endothelial growth factor. The impressive results of a first line phase III trial in 815 patients with metastatic CRC randomized to IFL vs IFL plus bevacizumab were reported in 2003 (Hurwitz et al, 2003). The combination was associated with improved response rates (45% vs 35%, $p = .0029$), progression-free survival (10.6 months vs 6.2 months, $p < .00001$), and median survival (20.3 months vs 15.6 months, $p = .00003$). The incidence of grade 3 hypertension was higher with bevacizumab (10.9% vs 2.3%), but no significant increases in bleeding or thrombotic events were observed. Bevacizumab is being studied in combination with FOLFOX. *Cetuximab* is a chimeric monoclonal antibody against the epidermal growth factor receptor (EGFR). In a phase II trial of cetuximab in 57 patients with EGFR+ CRC refractory to both 5-FU and irinotecan, objective responses were seen with 6 patients (11%) achieving a partial response (Saltz et al, 2002). This study coupled with other data led to a recent FDA approval of cetuximab for treatment of irintoecan refractory patients with advanced colorectal cancer. First line trials of cetuximab with irinotecan/5-FU/LV are also currently underway.

Summary

Much is rapidly changing in the landscape of the chemotherapeutic management for CRC. Current evidence supports the use of 5-FU/LV in combination with irinotecan or oxaliplatin as primary chemotherapy for reasonable performance status patients with unresectable advanced CRC. Capecitabine represents a more tolerable option for patients who would be candidates for palliative chemotherapy with 5-FU/LV alone. Regional chemotherapy strategies using HAI may be a consideration for selected patients with liver-limited metastatic disease. In the adjuvant setting, 6 months of 5-FU/LV remains the standard recommendation for patients with resected stage III disease and can be considered in select patients with stage II disease. This adjuvant standard may be revised to include combinations with either oxaliplatin or irinotecan pending the final results of several recent trials. Although current chemotherapy practices remain primarily defined by cytotoxic therapies, the future integration of targeted therapies holds the promise of further improving outcomes for patients with CRC.

Supplemental Reading

Anonymous. Adjuvant radiotherapy for rectal cancer: a systematic overview of 8,507 patients from 22 randomised trials. Lancet 2001;358:1291–304.

Advanced Colorectal Cancer Meta-Analysis Project. Modulation of fluorouracil by leucovorin in patients with advanced colorectal cancer: evidence in terms of response rate. J Clin Oncol 1992;10:896–903.

Alberts SR, Donohue JH, Mahoney MR, et al. Liver resection after 5-fluorouracil, leucovorin and oxaliplatin for patients with metastatic colorectal cancer limited to the liver: A North Central Cancer Treatment Group phase II study. Proc Am Soc Clin Oncol 2003;22:263.

Cunningham D, Humblet Y, Siena S, et al. Cetuximab monotherapy and cetuximab plus irinotecan in irinotecan-refractory metastatic colorectal cancer. N Engl J Med. 2004;351:337–45.

Cunningham D, Pyrhonen S, James RD, et al. Randomised trial of irinotecan plus supportive care vs supportive care alone after fluorouracil failure for patients with metastatic colorectal cancer. Lancet 1998;352:1413–8.

Danenberg PV, Danenberg KD. Effect of 5,10-methylenetetrahydrofolate on the dissociation of 5-fluoro-2´-deoxyuridylate from thymidylate synthetase: evidence for an ordered mechanism. Biochemistry 1978;17:4018–24.

de Gramont A, Bosset JF, Milan C, et al, Randomized trial comparing monthly low-dose leucovorin and fluorouracil bolus with bimonthly high-dose leucovorin and fluorouracil bolus plus continuous infusion for advanced colorectal cancer: a French intergroup study. J Clin Oncol 1997;15:808–15.

Douillard JY, Cunningham D, Roth AD, et al. Irinotecan combined with fluorouracil compared with fluorouracil alone as first-line treatment for metastatic colorectal cancer: a multicentre randomised trial. Lancet 2000;355:1041–7.

Ensminger WD. Intrahepatic arterial infusion of chemotherapy: pharmacologic principles. Semin Oncol 2002;29:119–25.

Giacchetti S, Itzhaki M, Gruia G, et al. Long-term survival of patients with unresectable colorectal cancer liver metastases following infusional chemotherapy with 5-fluorouracil, leucovorin, oxaliplatin and surgery. Ann Oncol 1999;10:663–9.

Goldberg RM, Sargent DJ, Morton RF. A randomized controlled trial of fluorouracil plus leucovorin, irinotecan, and oxaliplatin combinations in patients with previously untreated metastatic colorectal cancer. J Clin Oncol 2004;22:23–30.

Grothey A, Sargent DJ, Goldberg RM, Schmoll HJ. Overall survival in advanced colorectal cancer correlates with the proportion of patients treated with 5-fluorouracil/leucovorin, irinotecan, and oxaliplatin. J Clin Oncol 2004;22:1209–14.

Haller DG, Catalano PJ, Macdonald JS, et al. Fluorouracil, leucovorin and levamisole adjuvant therapy for colon cancer: five-year final report of INT-0089. Proc Am Soc Clin Oncol 1998;17:256a.

Hoff PM, Ansari R, Batist G, et al. Comparison of oral capecitabine vs intravenous fluorouracil plus leucovorin as first-line treatment in 605 patients with metastatic colorectal cancer: results of a randomized phase III study. J Clin Oncol 2001;19:2282–92.

Hurwitz HI, Fehrenbacher L, Cartwright T, et al. Bevacizumab (a monoclonal antibody to vascular endothelial growth factor) prolongs survival in first-line colorectal cancer: results of a phasc III trial of bevacizumab in combination with bolus IFL as first line therapy in subjects with metastatic CRC. Proc Am Soc Clin Oncol 2003;22:36–46.

International Multicentre Pooled Analysis of B2 Colon Cancer Trials (IMPACT B2) Investigators. Efficacy of adjuvant fluorouracil and folinic acid in B2 colon cancer. J Clin Oncol 1999;17:1356–63.

Kemeny NE, Niedzwiecki D, Hollis DR, et al. Hepatic arterial infusion vs systemic therapy for hepatic metastases from colorectal cancer: a CALGB randomized trial of efficacy, quality of life, cost effectiveness and molecular markers. Proc Am Soc Clin Oncol 2003;22:252.

Kerr DJ, McArdle CS, Ledermann J, et al. Intrahepatic arterial vs intravenous fluorouracil and folinic acid for colorectal cancer liver metastases: a multicentre randomised trial. Lancet 2003;361:368–73.

Macdonald JS, Astrow AB. Adjuvant therapy of colon cancer. Semin Oncol 2001;28:30–40.

Mamounas E, Wieand S, Wolmark N, et al. Comparative efficacy of adjuvant chemotherapy in patients with Dukes' B vs Dukes' C colon cancer: results from four National Surgical Adjuvant Breast and Bowel Project adjuvant studies (C-01, C-02, C-03, and C-04). J Clin Oncol 1999;17:1349–55.

Meta-Analysis Group in Cancer. Efficacy of intravenous continuous infusion of fluorouracil compared with bolus administration in advanced colorectal cancer. J Clin Oncol 1998;16:301–8.

Meta-Analysis Group in Cancer. Reappraisal of hepatic arterial infusion in the treatment of nonresectable liver metastases from colorectal cancer. J Natl Cancer Inst 1996;88:252–8.

O'Connell MJ, Martenson JA, Wieand HS, et al. Improving adjuvant therapy for rectal cancer by combining protracted-infusion fluorouracil with radiation therapy after curative surgery. N Engl J Med 1994;331:502–7.

Piedbois PS, for the Meta-Analysis Group in Cancer. Survival benefit of 5FU/LV over 5FU bolus in patients with advanced colorectal cancer: an updated meta-analysis based on 2,751 patients. Proc Am Soc Clin Oncol 2003;22:294.

Rothenberg ML, Meropol NJ, Poplin EA, et al. Mortality associated with irinotecan plus bolus fluorouracil/leucovorin: summary findings of an independent panel. J Clin Oncol 2001;19:3801–7.

Rothenberg ML, Oza AM, Bigelow RH, et al. Superiority of oxaliplatin and fluorouracil-leucovorin compared with either therapy alone in patients with progressive colorectal cancer after irinotecan and fluorouracil-leucovorin: interim results of a phase III trial. J Clin Oncol 2003;21:2059–69.

Rougier P, Bugat R, Douillard JY, et al. Phase II study of irinotecan in the treatment of advanced colorectal cancer in chemotherapy-naive patients and patients pretreated with fluorouracil-based chemotherapy. J Clin Oncol 1997;15:251–60.

Saltz LB, Cox JV, Blanke C, et al. Irinotecan plus fluorouracil and leucovorin for metastatic colorectal cancer. Irinotecan Study Group. N Engl J Med 2000;343:905–14.

Saltz L, Meropol NJ, Loehrer PJ, et al. Single agent IMC-C225 (Erbitux) has activity in CPT-11 refractory colorectal cancer (CRC) that expresses the epidermal growth factor receptor (EGFR). Proc Am Soc Clin Oncol 2002;21:127a.

Takasuna K, Hagiwara T, Hirohashi M, et al. Involvement of beta-glucuronidase in intestinal microflora in the intestinal toxicity of the antitumor camptothecin derivative irinotecan hydrochloride (CPT-11) in rats. Cancer Res 1996;56:3752–7.

Topham C, Boni C, Navarro M, et al. Multicenter international randomized study of Oxaliplatin-5FU/LV (folfox) in Stage II and III Colon cancer: final results. Eur J Cancer Suppl 2003;1:S324.

Van Cutsem E, Twelves C, Cassidy J, et al. Oral Capecitabine compared with intravenous fluorouracil plus leucovorin in patients with metastatic colorectal cancer: Results of a large phase III study. J Clin Oncol 2000;19:4097–106.

CHAPTER 98

CURATIVE INTENT MANAGEMENT OF RECTAL CANCER

NANCY N. BAXTER, MD, PHD, AND DAVID A. ROTHENBERGER, MD

Rectal cancer is a common and lethal disease. In the year 2002, there were an estimated 41,000 new cases of rectal cancer in the United States. The management of rectal cancer has changed radically in the past several decades. Formerly, surgery often requiring a permanent colostomy was the only therapy offered to most patients with rectal cancer regardless of stage. Today, therapy is based primarily on stage of disease, and protocols vary from local, outpatient treatment to complex multimodality treatments combining surgery, radiation, and chemotherapy. The rationale of such stage-specific therapy is to optimize cancer control, lessen morbidity, and maintain normal bodily functions. However, the goal of selecting the optimal therapy for an individual with a rectal cancer based on an accurate assessment of the stage of disease, as well as the specific biology of the tumor and tumor-host interaction, remains elusive. Indeed, the optimal management of rectal cancer is more controversial than ever (Rothenberger, 2000).

Preoperative Examination

Pretreatment planning requires that patients have a thorough and detailed preoperative examination (Kwok et al, 2000). Stage of disease and tumor location are the primary determinants of therapy for rectal cancer but patient variables often necessitate modification of standard treatment algorithms.

History

A history of preexisting incontinence or chronic diarrhea may be contraindications to a colo-anal anastomosis because such patients will inevitably have poor function after such an ultralow anastomosis. Patient preferences and special needs that would make colostomy management more difficult (blindness, severe arthritis) should be identified and included in decision-making. Rapid weight loss or pelvic pain are particularly ominous symptoms and should intensify the search for metastatic disease.

Digital Exam

Digital rectal examination for low rectal tumors is essential to define the distal extent, location, mobility, and relationship to the anal sphincter muscles and surrounding structures. Digital rectal examination also allows a simple evaluation of sphincter competence, an important factor in management, particularly of low rectal lesions. Importantly, the exact location of the tumor must be determined as small differences in distance from the anal verge may have a major impact on therapy, particularly the ability to preserve intestinal continuity.

Rigid Proctoscopy

Rigid proctoscopy more accurately determines the level, extent, and quadrant(s) involved by the lesion, than does flexible endoscopy. Rigid proctoscopy also facilitates obtaining large biopsies of the lesion needed to confirm the diagnosis of adenocarcinoma (AC) and to identify any unfavorable histologic features (poorly differentiated, mucinous, or signet ring histology) that may influence choice of therapy. Risk of obstruction is a significant concern and therefore the degree of constriction of the lumen must be assessed.

Colonoscopy

The entire colon should be visualized by *colonoscopy* to rule out synchronous tumors that would influence the planned resection. If an endoscopist elects to remove a rectal lesion by polypectomy under the assumption that it is benign, every effort should be made to remove it in one piece, orient the specimen before fixation and accurately localize the lesion site by *injection of India ink*. These steps are essential to planning therapy if the subsequent pathology reveals an unsuspected AC.

Classification

The American Joint Commission on Cancer bases the classification of rectal cancer on the extent of local and/or distant spread (Table 98-1) (Greene et al, 2002). Preoperative staging is used to direct treatment of rectal cancer.

DISTANT SPREAD

A *chest radiograph* is performed routinely and any suspicious abnormalities should be evaluated preoperatively

TABLE 98-1. TNM Staging of Colorectal Carcinoma

Tumor State (T)	Definition
TX	Cannot be assessed
T0	No evidence of cancer
Tis	Carcinoma in situ
T1	Tumor invades submucosa
T2	Tumor invades muscularis propria
T3	Tumor invades through muscularis propria into subserosa or into nonperitonealized pericolic or perirectal tissues
T4	Tumor directly invades other organs or tissues or perforates the visceral peritoneum of specimen

Nodal Stage (N)	Definition
NX	Regional lymph nodes cannot be assessed
N0	No lymph node metastasis
N1	Metastasis to one to three pericolic or perirectal lymph nodes
N2	Metastasis to four or more pericolic or perirectal lymph nodes
N3	Metastasis to any lymph node along a major named vascular trunk

Distant Metastasis (M)	Definition
MX	Presence of distant metastasis cannot be assessed
M0	No distant metastasis
M1	Distant metastasis present

with a computed tomography (CT) scan of the chest. A *CT scan of the abdomen and pelvis* is also routine, both to rule out the presence of liver metastases and to evaluate the relationship between the rectal tumor and contiguous structures. *Positron emission tomography (PET) scanning* is not routinely recommended for preoperative evaluation but may be useful in select patients, for example in patients with locally advanced disease who are at high risk of occult metastases or in the examination of patients with equivocal lesions on chest or abdominal CT.

Local Staging

Accurate local staging to determine invasion through the rectal wall and the presence or absence of lymph node metastasis guides selection of appropriate therapy. For early stage disease, local therapy may be appropriate, whereas for advanced rectal cancer, neoadjuvant chemoradiation may be indicated. Imaging with *endorectal ultrasound (US)* or *magnetic resonance imaging (MRI)* is recommended for preoperative staging. *Endo-anal coils* may increase the accuracy of MRI. Sensitivity and specificity for depth of invasion are highest for endorectal US, 93% and 78% respectively, although endo-anal coil MRI approaches these values (Kwok et al, 2000). Endorectal US accurately distinguishes T2 from T3 cancers but is less accurate at differentiating T1 from T2 cancers. Endorectal US is less accurate than MRI in the determination of lymph node involvement, with sensitivity and specificity of 71% and 76% versus 82% and 83%, respectively. CT scanning does not have adequate sensitivity or specificity to accurately direct choice of therapy protocol.

Preparation for Surgery

In general, patients with rectal cancer are elderly, and their medical condition should be optimized preoperatively. *Prophylactic antibiotics* and *maintenance of normothermia intraoperatively* have been demonstrated to reduce postoperative morbidity from wound infections. Although mechanical bowel preparation is routinely performed, it is unclear if this has a positive influence on outcome. The presence of malignant disease, prolonged operative time, pelvic surgery, and the positioning requirements of the patient predispose to thromboembolic events. Deep venous thrombosis prophylaxis with *compression stockings* and *pneumatic compression* devices with or without subcutaneous heparin is standard. For people who will require a temporary or permanent stoma, preoperative consultation with an *enterostomal therapy nurse* facilitates proper siting of the stoma, patient education, and acceptance.

Surgical Therapy

The goals of surgical therapy are to remove all disease and maximize the potential for long term survival while minimizing the impact of treatment on quality of life. Surgical therapy for cure may be divided into local approaches and radical approaches. Both approaches may be combined with chemoradiation. With radical approaches, bowel continuity may be restored or the patient may be left with a permanent colostomy.

Local Therapy

Local therapies include snare polypectomy, local excision (wedge resection of the tumor either by endo-anal approach or by transanal endoscopic microsurgery), or endocavitary radiation. There are many advantages of local therapies, including minimal postoperative morbidity and mortality and rapid postoperative recovery. Local therapy minimizes the impact of rectal cancer treatment on long term function and in some cases is the only alternative to permanent colostomy. However, by definition, local therapies leave all lymph node-bearing tissue *in situ*. Thus, the major concern with local therapy is undertreatment. Criteria for lesions appropriate for local therapy with curative intent are evolving and controversial. Today, most experts agree that < 10% of rectal cancers are appropriate for curative intent local therapy.

As screening colonoscopy becomes more commonplace, the diagnosis of invasive cancer in a polyp will undoubtedly be made more often, and appropriate management of such early-stage cancer will become increasingly important. Polypectomy and observation may be appropriate for cancer arising in a polyp if the lesion fits the favorable criteria noted in Table 98-2 (Rothenberger and Garcia-Aguilar, 2002). However, radical resection is generally recommended for less favorable situations as noted in Table 98-3. Similarly, local excision or endocavitary radiation may be appropriate for curative intent treatment of rectal cancers with highly favorable features, that is, T1, small (< 3 to 4 cm in diameter), exophytic lesions with favorable histology (moderate or well-differentiated, nonmucinous, nonsignet cell with no lymphovascular or neural invasion), involving less than one-third of the circumference of the rectum, and located such that local therapy is technically feasible and safe. The *local recurrence rate* after local therapy alone even for such favorable lesions is disappointingly high (5 to 18%) and for this reason, some centers have combined local excision with pre- or postoperative chemoradiation (Rothenberger, 2000). Whether this approach will improve outcomes awaits further research. A previously more liberal approach to local excision, with the inclusion of T2 lesions, resulted in an unacceptably high recurrence rate and is not advised. There is general consensus that using local therapy for more advanced or more aggressive disease will expose the patient to an increased rate of recurrence and decreased cancer specific survival. A radical resection should be performed in such patients, unless severe comorbidities preclude a safe operation.

TABLE 98-2. Suggested Criteria for Polypectomy and Observation for Cancer in a Polyp

- Complete excision of lesion
- ≥ 2 mm clear margins
- Well or moderately differentiated
- No lymphovascular invasion
- Haggitt levels 1, 2, or 3 in pedunculated polyps
- Haggitt level 4 (pedunculated or sessile polyp) with Sm_1 invasion

Adapted from Rothenberger and Garcia-Aguilar, 2002.

TABLE 98-3. Suggested Criteria for Radical Colorectal Resection for Cancer in a Polyp

Strong indicators
- Incomplete excision of lesion
- Microscopic cancer at resection margin
- Haggitt level 4 (pedunculated or sessile polyp) with Sm_3 invasion

Relative indicators
- Poorly differentiated
- Lymphovascular invasion
- Excision doubtfully complete
- Haggitt level 4 (pedunculated or sessile polyp) with Sm_2 invasion

Adapted from Rothenberger and Garcia-Aguilar, 2002. Reproduced with permission from Humana Press.

Radical Resection

The majority of patients with operable rectal cancer require a radical proctectomy, as this will minimize the probability of local recurrence and provide accurate staging. The primary goal of radical resection is to remove the rectal tumor and all the adjacent lymph node-bearing tissue (the rectosigmoid mesentery and mesorectum) with clear margins. A secondary goal of radical surgery is to restore bowel continuity providing cure of the rectal cancer is not compromised and that high quality sphincter function can be maintained. All radical resection operations for rectal cancer use an identical *proximal, lateral* and *radial (mesorectal) dissection* technique. Recent emphasis has been placed on the technique of *total mesorectal excision (TME)* in which the mesorectum is sharply mobilized from the presacral space to at least 5 cm beyond the tumor (MacFarlane et al, 1993; Martling et al, 2000). Clear radical margins are obtained by performing a meticulous circumferential pelvic dissection within the endopelvic fascial plane. Appropriately performed TME has decreased local recurrence rates after radical surgery. Management of the distal margin determines whether the proctectomy is sphincter-preserving or sphincter-ablative.

In *an anterior resection (AR)*, the sigmoid, rectum and mesorectum are removed through an abdominal "anterior" approach to the pelvis. ARs may be classified as high, low, or extended-low depending on the extent of rectal mobilization and resection. Intestinal continuity is usually restored after an AR by mobilizing the proximal descending and transverse colon and performing a colorectal or colo-anal anastomosis.

If such an anastomosis is technically impossible or contraindicated, the surgeon can perform an *abdominoperineal resection (APR)*. This operation combines the dissection of an extended low AR to the levator muscles with the perineal dissection of the anus, anal canal, anal sphincters, levators and surrounding fat to allow an *en bloc* removal of the specimen. The operation is completed by closing the perineal wound and constructing a permanent colostomy, generally using the distal decending or proximal sigmoid colon.

A third operative option, the *Hartmann procedure*, is used rarely but may be preferred if the cancer has perforated or spread locally making early recurrence likely, or if the patient has preexisting sphincter dysfunction making a low anastomosis unwise. In this procedure, after completing the AR to remove the rectal cancer, the distal rectum is closed and left *in situ*. An end colostomy is constructed usually from the descending colon.

Choice of Radical Resection

The choice of radical resection in most cases is determined by the level and location of the rectal cancer. Sphincter invasion is a clear indication for APR, whereas proximal rectal cancers can almost always be treated by AR and primary colorectal anastomosis. The challenge is to properly manage rectal cancers located between the two extremes. In general, the more distal the rectal cancer, the greater the technical challenge to perform a reliable anastomosis. Obesity and a narrow pelvis, as noted in most males, add to the technical challenge. In addition, other patient factors, such as preexisting partial incontinence or immobility, must be considered when making the choice of anastomosis versus permanent colostomy. The risk of perioperative anastomotic leakage is significant if an anastomosis is performed within 5 cm of the anal verge after extended low AR and colo-anal anastomosis. Anastomoses involving *irradiated bowel* are especially prone to leakage. In such cases, a *temporary diverting loop ileostomy* is often performed to minimize the risk and consequences of pelvic sepsis. Three months after resection (if the patient's medical status permits), a *water-soluble contrast enema* is performed to establish the soundness of the anastomosis and the diverting loop ileostomy may then be reversed.

Special Considerations

There are special considerations that require modification in evaluation and/or operative approach to rectal cancer.

COLONIC J-POUCH

An ultralow anastomosis to the distal anal canal often results in urgency, frequency, partial incontinence, and clustering of bowel movements. To improve function, we often create a 5-cm *colonic "J" pouch* using descending colon and anastomose the apex of the "J" to the rectal or anal remnant. Forming such a reservoir has been demonstrated to improve function especially in the first year post operation but has the potential disadvantage of interfering with complete evacuation of the rectum.

LAPAROSCOPIC RESECTION

Although laparoscopic resection for colon cancer is gaining acceptance, laparoscopic resection of rectal cancer is in its infancy. The high level of difficulty of the procedure and the need for meticulous mesorectal excision may limit this approach to all but a few expert centers.

EN BLOC RESECTION

Because the pelvis is a fixed and relatively narrow space, rectal cancers may involve contiguous structures. Such T4 tumors may still be cured with surgery and adjuvant therapy, however it is essential that involved organs (or portion thereof) are resected with the rectum in an *en bloc fashion*. Peeling tumor off adjacent organs will almost certainly leave disease behind and predispose to local recurrence. Anterior tumors in women may necessitate a hysterectomy or a posterior vaginectomy. Similarly such tumors may require bladder resection and urinary diversion. With posterior tumors, *en bloc* sacrectomy may occasionally be necessary. Even when such a radical approach is required, if an R0 resection (complete resection, no residual disease) can be performed, a significant number of patients will be long term survivors.

EMERGENT CASES

Approximately 10% of patients with rectal cancer will present emergently, most commonly with increasingly symptomatic obstruction. Rarely, this progresses to a complete *large bowel obstruction* with a risk of intestinal perforation. Large volume lower gastrointestinal bleeding is far less common but can occur. Workup and treatment paradigms must be adjusted in the face of emergency presentation. The first priority must be prevention or treatment of life threatening complications. For patients who present with impending obstruction, an endoscopically or fluoroscopically placed *colonic stent* may temporally relieve the obstruction, allowing the patient to be treated in a more standard elective fashion. There are two chapters on rectal stenting (see Chapter 86, "Acute Colonic Pseudo-Obstruction" and Chapter 99, "Palliative Therapy for Rectal Cancer"). Though useful in rectosigmoid and proximal rectal obstructing cancers, *stenting is not possible in low-lying rectal lesions*. If complete obstruction or perforation has occurred, emergent operative management is almost always necessary to relieve the obstruction and control the peritoneal contamination. If technically safe, the rectal cancer should be resected at the initial operation. However, if the disease is advanced, if adequate treatment would require an APR, or if the patient is unstable, enteric diversion by formation of an ileostomy or colostomy followed by complete postoperative evaluation, consideration of neoadjuvant therapy and subsequent definitive treatment may be the most prudent course.

Adjuvant/Neoadjuvant Therapy

In the United States, chemoradiation is commonly administered to patients with Stage II or III rectal cancer to improve both local control and long term outcomes. Radiation is generally given over a 5-week period, with the total dose in the range of 45 to 54 Gy. Adjuvant radiation may be given preoperatively or postoperatively, and the advantages and disadvantages of both methods are detailed (Table 98-4) (Colorectal Cancer Collaborative Group, 2001). No mature randomized trials have compared preoperative to postoperative radiation. Although several such trials have failed to accrue patients in the United States, a German trial is being conducted and has successfully recruited over 800 patients. Results from this trial should be available in the near future. If radiation is given preoperatively, surgery is *delayed 4 to 6 weeks* after completion of radiation to permit tumor shrinkage. In patients with locally advanced cancers, tumor regression after radiation may allow

TABLE 98-4. Preoperative versus Postoperative Adjuvant Radiation

Timing of Radiation	Advantages	Disadvantages
Preoperative	Theoretical increased efficacy of radiation due to better blood supply to tumor before operation Much of radiated bowel is resected, possible improvement in function Significant tumor shrinkage may facilitate dissection Minimizes risk of radiation injury to small bowel and other viscera Complete response may predict favorable outcome Survival advantage demonstrated in some trials	Surgical delay Increased surgical morbidity and wound complications Some patients over treated as preoperative staging is imperfect
Postoperative	Pathologic evaluation of specimen determines staging, only appropriate patients treated No delay to surgery Not operating in a radiated field	Radiation delayed if problems with wound healing Residual tumor may be relatively ischemic postoperatively Pelvic adhesions may increase chance of small bowel irradiation Survival advantage has not been demonstrated Possibly worse functional outcome

complete excision. Chemotherapy is often given with the radiation as there is some limited evidence that the combination enhances tumor response. There is a separate chapter on radiation (see Chapter 100, "Abdominal Radiation") and on adjuvant chemotherapy (see Chapter 97, "Colorectal Carcinoma").

The rationale for the standard American approach is based on the results of numerous trials clearly showing that pre- or postoperative radiation lowers the risk of local recurrence of rectal cancer compared to the local recurrence risk for those undergoing radical surgery alone. In most of these studies, however, there was a high rate of local recurrence in the control arms indicating that surgical management may not have been optimal. Several European centers now question the need for perioperative radiation therapy and suggest that appropriately performed radical surgery alone following the principles of TME will achieve similarly low local recurrence rates without the associated morbidity of radiation. However, even with TME, the risk of local recurrence may be reduced further with radiation. After a 2-year follow-up in a recent randomized trial comparing preoperative radiation plus TME with TME surgery alone, the rate of local recurrence in radiated patients was lower than nonirradiated patients (2% versus 8%) (Kapiteijn et al, 2001).

Surveillance

Rectal cancer patients are at significant risk of developing metachronous colorectal cancers; thus, colonoscopy to remove metachronous benign polyps should be performed 1 year after initial diagnosis and, if normal, repeated 3 years later. Almost all patients regardless of age and comorbidities can safely tolerate such surveillance.

In general, aggressive follow up to detect recurrent cancer after curative intent therapy is restricted to patients who would tolerate a major reoperation to resect a local (pelvic) or distant (liver, lung, or abdominal) recurrence. Frequent surveillance with digital rectal examination, proctoscopy, and endorectal US may detect pelvic recurrences when still amenable to radical excision. Surveillance with regular performance of carcinoembryonic antigen (CEA) and/or CT imaging may detect metastatic disease when still amenable to resection. Although evidence for the effectiveness of such intensive follow up is weak, there is a general consensus among colorectal surgeons and a recent meta-analysis that supports using this approach (Berman et al, 2000).

Any patient who has symptoms or abnormal findings on clinical examination that suggest recurrence deserves a workup. If curative-intent reoperation is not feasible or safe, palliative therapy can be instituted. There is a separate chapter on palliative therapy for rectal cancer (see Chapter 99, "Palliative Therapy for Rectal Cancer").

Outcomes

Mortality following radical surgery for rectal cancer ranges from 2 to 5% and major *morbidity is common*. There is a particularly high rate of perineal wound complications in patients undergoing preoperative radiation and APR. In addition, for those with permanent colostomy, there is a high lifetime rate of symptomatic peristomal hernia. Urinary and sexual dysfunction is significant, particularly in older males. Poor function may occur after restoration of intestinal continuity, particularly when a very distal rectal resection is required. The proximal colon is often noncompliant and cannot compensate for the loss of the reservoir function of the rectum. Radiation may also have a negative effect on the compliance of the remaining distal rectum and on sphincter function. Some will experience such life-altering incontinence that ultimately a colostomy is constructed to improve quality of life.

Local recurrence is a significant problem after resection of rectal cancer. Disturbing differences in outcome between different surgeons and different centers have been found in terms of local recurrence, survival, and rate of permanent colostomy. Adherence to TME can result in significant reduction in local recurrence, improvement in survival and reduction in the permanent colostomy rate. The average rate of local recurrence after radical resection of rectal cancer in the past was as high as 30% but should be < 10% in the TME era. Local recurrence rates will be higher in patients with more aggressive disease, especially if the cancer is located in the distal rectum, regardless of the treatment protocol. Neoadjuvant therapy with chemoradiation may further decrease local recurrence rates.

The *surgeon* is clearly an important *prognostic variable* in the treatment of rectal cancer. Hospital procedure volume, surgeon procedure volume and surgical specialty have been found by many studies to affect outcome in terms of local recurrence, colostomy rates, and long term survival (Hodgson et al, 2003; Schrag et al, 2002). Higher volumes and increased specialization appear to be associated with better outcomes. Although not surprising, this volume–outcome relationship may have future implications in terms of regionalization of care.

Conclusions

Although treatment of rectal cancer continues to improve, we have much to learn. A multimodality approach is essential to improve local recurrence rates and increase long term survival, and the surgeon is a particularly important prognostic variable. With optimal preoperative staging, surgical treatment, and adjuvant therapy, we can maximize the potential for long term cure while preserving quality of life for our patients. Our current therapy strategy for resectable rectal cancer is outlined in Table 98-5.

Supplemental Reading

Berman JM, Cheung RJ, Weinberg DS. Surveillance after colorectal cancer resection. Lancet 2000;355:395–9.

Colorectal Cancer Collaborative Group. Adjuvant radiotherapy for rectal cancer: a systematic overview of 8,507 patients from 22 randomized trials. Lancet 2001;358:1291–304.

Greene FL, Page DJ, Fleming, et al. AJCC cancer staging manual, 6th ed. New York: Springer-Verlag; 2002.

Hodgson DC, Zhang W, Zaslavsky AM, et al. Relation of hospital volume to colostomy rates and survival for patients with rectal cancer. J Natl Cancer Inst 2003;95:708–16.

Kapiteijn E, Marijnen CA, Nagtegaal ID, et al. Preoperative radiotherapy combined with total mesorectal excision for resectable rectal cancer. N Engl J Med 2001;345:638–46.

Kwok H, Bissett IP, Hill GL. Preoperative staging of rectal cancer. Int J Colorectal Dis 2000;15:9–20.

MacFarlane JK, Ryall RD, Heald RJ. Mesorectal excision for rectal cancer. Lancet 1993;341:457–60.

Martling AL, Holm T, Rutqvist LE, et al. Effect of a surgical training programme on outcome of rectal cancer in the County of Stockholm. Stockholm Colorectal Cancer Study Group, Basingstoke Bowel Cancer Research Project. Lancet 2000;356:93–6.

Rothenberger DA, Garcia-Aguilar J. Management of cancer in a polyp. In: Saltz L, editor. Colorectal cancer: multimodality management. Totawa (NJ): Humana Press; 2002. p. 325–35.

Rothenberger DA. Guest Ed. Colorectal cancer. Surg Oncol Clin N Am 2000;9:643–878.

Schrag D, Panageas KS, Riedel E, et al. Hospital and surgeon procedure volume as predictors of outcome following rectal cancer resection. Ann Surg 2002;236:583–92.

TABLE 98-5. Therapy Strategy for Rectal Cancer

Pretreatment Stage		Preferred Treatment	Alternative Treatment
Stage 0	Tis N0 M0	Local therapy if technically feasible (prefer excision to ablation to obtain pathologic confirmation of T stage)	Radical resection (APR rarely indicated for noninvasive lesion) if local therapy not feasible or safe
Stage I	T1 N0 M0 (favorable features)	Local therapy for distal ⅓ lesions or patients with severe comorbidity; radical resection for proximal lesions	Radical resection
	T1 N0 M0 (unfavorable features)	Radical resection	Local therapy plus chemoradiation
	T2 N0 M0	Radical resection	Local therapy plus chemoradiation
Stage II	T3 N0 M0	Preoperative chemoradiation, radical resection and adjuvant chemotherapy	Radical resection, postoperative chemoradiation plus adjuvant chemotherapy if pathology appropriate. Some early lesions may not require adjuvant Rx.
	T4 N0 M0	Preoperative chemoradiation, radical resection with en bloc resection of involved organs plus adjuvant chemotherapy	Radical resection, postoperative chemoradiation plus adjuvant chemotherapy.
Stage III	T any N+ M0	Preoperative chemoradiation, radical resection plus adjuvant chemotherapy	Radical resection, postoperative chemoradiation plus adjuvant chemotherapy.

APR = abdominoperineal resection; Rx = treatment.

CHAPTER 99

Palliative Therapy for Rectal Cancer

Jeffrey R. Avansino, MD, and Matthias Stelzner, MD

Annually in the United States, it is estimated that there are approximately 42,000 new cases of rectal cancer. In most series, approximately 80% of patients undergo resections with curative intent with the remaining 20% requiring palliation. Of the 80% that receive resections with curative intent, approximately 40% will develop a recurrence (Jemal et al, 2003). The majority of these patients will not be eligible for further resections with curative intent. Thus palliation of rectal cancer is a major health issue. This chapter will focus on both invasive and noninvasive palliative modalities in rectal cancer that are currently available and the clinical scenarios in which they are most frequently used.

Indications for Palliation

Palliative therapy is indicated for all patients with incurable rectal cancer. It may be operative or nonoperative. Rectal cancer may be deemed incurable for a variety of reasons. Patients may have advanced or recurrent locoregional disease or distant metastasis. Significant comorbidities may preclude chemo- or radiation therapy or a surgical resection in patients with technically resectable cancer. Patients who are limited to a bed-to-chair existence should not receive surgical treatment or chemotherapy.

In some cases, the patient with a resectable primary lesion will decline the extent and consequences of radical surgery (eg, if it is likely to result in the formation of a permanent colostomy). Finally, a few patients decline surgery even if the cancer is technically resectable and a need for a colostomy is not anticipated.

Goals of Palliation

Patients requiring palliation for rectal cancer are a heterogeneous population with a wide spectrum of clinical presentations ranging from a microscopic focus of local tumor with distant metastases causing no symptoms to a large tumor causing major symptoms. The primary goals of palliative therapy are to maximize the quality of remaining life by controlling symptoms and preserving normal bodily functions, and helping the patient and their family and friends to develop realistic expectations about their impending death from the incurable cancer. This begins with a multidisciplinary approach to each individual patient involving physicians, nurses, social workers, and spiritual counselors.

Although physicians often estimate their patients' life expectancies accurately, many times the patients themselves overestimate their survival probabilities and these inaccurate impressions will influence their treatment choices (Weeks et al, 1998). They will then be more likely to choose more aggressive therapy regimens and this can decrease their quality of life without any survival benefit. It is therefore of paramount importance that the team communicates a clear and accurate message to the patient regarding prognosis and treatment options. This information should be based on a thorough evaluation of the patient's general health and an accurate staging of cancer. Treatment should focus on prevention and management of symptoms and pain with the main focus on improving the patient's quality of life.

Clinical Evaluation

After the initial diagnosis of rectal cancer is made, further workup should determine if the patient is a candidate for different palliative therapy regimens and what aspect of the patient's disease is likely to cause symptoms. This diagnostic workup is initially based on physical findings and symptoms. If these first data suggest the presence of advanced disease, then further workup should be minimized. In other words, patients who have clear evidence for disseminated rectal cancer or who are in frail health often do not require further computed tomography (CT) or magnetic resonance imaging (MRI) scans. In every case of incurable rectal cancer, the extent of the workup must assure that the potential treatment morbidity is justified by the anticipated outcome. In patients who are candidates for surgery, a CT of the abdomen/pelvis is performed to determine resectability and extent of abdominal metastases. Endorectal ultrasound or pelvic MRI can be used if findings on CT are unable to determine resectability. If the rectal cancer appears resectable, then CT of the upper abdomen and chest and positron emission tomography scanning are done to exclude distant metastases. In addition, diagnostic laparoscopy can be used to identify widespread disease prior to laparotomy in patients with an otherwise negative workup. Despite recent advances in imaging technologies and intensive investigations, the surgeon often finds that the preoperative workup underestimated the full extent of the disease. The true extent of local involvement and distant spread, and thus the need for palliative treatment, only become evident at examination of the abdomen in the operating room.

Invasive Therapy

Surgery

Surgical therapy is the principal modality used for treatment of rectal cancer with curative intent. Yet it is only one of many modalities used in palliative therapy. Although many options are available for the palliation of cancer of the intra-abdominal colon, such as abdominal colectomy, segmental resection, internal bypass, or fecal diversions, surgical palliation of rectal cancer is technically more difficult and options are more limited. This is due to the anatomic restrictions of the pelvis and the fact that there is more commonly fixation of the tumor to major structures like the iliac vessels, prostate, bladder, or nerve roots. Operative palliative therapy is indicated in patients that are able to tolerate surgery and with the intent of providing relief or improvement of symptoms while maintaining normal function. *Indications* include bowel obstruction, perforation of the rectum, formation of rectal fistulas to the vagina, bladder or prostate, bleeding, pain, and local obstructions of the urinary system. Surgical resection should be avoided in patients with extensive pelvic disease. This includes patients with invasion of the pelvic sidewall or of the sacrum above S2, bilateral ureteral obstruction, lymphedema, and encasement of major vascular structures, extensive nodal disease and distant metastases. Surgery is also not a good modality in most patients with a life expectancy < 3 to 6 months. Surgical options include tumor resection and fecal diversion by way of a colostomy. The best option is dictated by the clinical scenario with the intent of minimizing morbidity while obtaining optimal quality of life.

Colostomy

Fecal diversion is most often achieved by creating a sigmoid colostomy. This is probably the most common surgical therapy for palliation of unresectable rectal cancer. Formation of such a colostomy used to require a limited open laparotomy. However, now palliative stomas are commonly created *laparoscopically* to minimize the impact on the patient's quality of life. Whether laparoscopic creation of such colostomies is superior to the open method is still unproven. In most cases, an end colostomy with mucus fistula is preferred to a loop colostomy because it results in complete fecal diversion and avoids stoma recession, which would make stoma management more difficult. A transverse colostomy is a lesser alternative but can be used in patients who require an operation with minimal negative physiologic impact. In patients with mid and low rectal cancers, colostomies are increasingly being replaced with *endoscopic stenting* and by conventional *transanal debulking* (eg, by *transanal endoscopic excision*). These procedures can be carried out with less morbidity compared to transabdominal palliative procedures. However, formal randomized studies comparing colostomies with other invasive treatment options are scant.

Resections

In patients with an incurable condition but technically resectable local disease, an anterior resection with primary anastomosis can be considered if the distal rectal remnant is > 4 cm. Ultralow anterior resections with coloanal anastomoses require temporary colostomies. They often lead to temporary continence problems after colostomy takedown that can persist for a few weeks or months. These operations are not a good option for palliation. An *extended low Hartmann operation* leaving a minimal distal rectal stump is an excellent alternative if the patient is willing to accept a permanent colostomy because it completely eliminates the risk of anastomotic leakage. Also, if the patient has received previous pelvic irradiation or has poor anal sphincter function, a colostomy would be the preferred surgical palliative therapy. However, if the tumor involves the low rectum or the sphincter complex, an abdominal-peritoneal resection is optimal. A pelvic exenteration is rarely performed for rectal cancer because of an associated high morbidity, which in turn negatively affects the patient's quality of life. However, limited involvement of the vagina or the uterus is not a contraindication and many surgeons will include a posterior vaginectomy or hysterectomy as part of the procedure if necessary. In contrast, few surgeons will extend their resection to include the bladder or prostate.

Rectal Stenting

Self-expanding metal stents are becoming a more widely accepted alternative to surgical palliation in patients with incurable rectal cancer that have extensive locoregional or metastatic disease, comorbidities precluding surgery, or recurrent disease after resection. Successful palliation with stenting has been achieved in approximately 90% of patients while avoiding a colostomy. These stents provide good long term resolution of obstruction that exceeds 1 year in some studies and have acceptable complication rates. Migration of stents is the most common issue and rates have been reported as < 15% (Fernandez et al, 1999; Baron, 2001). Migration rates appear to be higher with covered stents, which have been successfully used in palliation of rectovaginal or rectovesical fistulas resulting from the rectal cancer. Patients with stents placed too distally may experience tenesmus, rectal pain, and fecal incontinence. Stent occlusion resulting from tumor ingrowth can be treated with argon beam coagulation, laser, or restenting. The relationship of stents and radiotherapy and chemotherapy has not been clearly defined. However, a few patients with stents have been reported to have undergone successful subsequent radiation therapy. There is a separate chapter on intestinal and colonic strictures (see Chapter 85, "Intestinal and Colonic Strictures").

Other Endoscopic Methods

Expandable metal stents have largely replaced older forms of endoscopic palliation of obstructive rectal cancer. Laser ablation is still a useful therapy for some patients, especially those with rectal bleeding. Quality of life can also be improved in those patients with symptoms of diarrhea, mucus discharge, tenesmus, and obstruction. Palliation of obstructive symptoms is usually obtained after 2 to 5 sessions in 80 to 90% of patients (McGowan et al, 1989). Typically, however, palliation is not long lasting and symptoms often recur within 6 months requiring further sessions. Laser ablation is not effective in the treatment of *pain* or in patients with tumor involvement of the anal canal or sphincter. Complications of laser therapy occur in 5 to 15% of patients and are mostly minor; however, perforation, sepsis, and death have been reported (Gevers et al, 2000).

Argon plasma coagulation is a cost effective alternative to laser therapy for control of *bleeding*, but is not very useful in patients with obstruction. However, comparative studies testing the role of argon beam coagulation against other therapeutic measures are lacking (Canard et al, 2001). *Injection therapy* including alcohol or sclerosing agents has the advantage of low cost and simplicity of technique, but typically requires multiple treatment sessions (Marini et al, 1990). Photodynamic therapy, electrotherapy, and cryotherapy should no longer be used due to their high complication rates or side effects.

Chemotherapy and Radiation Therapy

Chemotherapy and radiation therapy are important instruments in the palliation of incurable rectal cancer and are generally indicated in patients with unresectable local disease that present with nerve pain, ureteral obstruction, and extensive pelvic sidewall involvement with compression of adjacent structures resulting in lymphedema or deep venous thrombosis. These modalities are also used in patients with an incurable condition but technically resectable local disease to enable down staging of the locoregional disease and slow distal progression.

Tumors that are *asymptomatic* or *minimally symptomatic* are at low risk of obstruction and can be treated with *chemotherapy or combination chemoradiation* therapy. In lesions that are *obstructing or near obstructing, mechanical palliation* is required in the form of surgery or endorectal stenting before the initiation of chemotherapy. However, although formerly many experts advised that every patient with a large resectable rectal cancer should be operated on, almost irrespective of the extent of metastatic disease to prevent obstruction, this recommendation had to be modified in more recent years. As a rule, tumors that are unlikely to obstruct in an 8 to 10-week period will not require palliative mechanical management before initiation of chemotherapy. The efficacy of chemotherapy is typically assessed at 6 to 8 weeks into treatment. If tumor regression is demonstrated, the risk of obstruction will be substantially decreased. Combination chemotherapy and radiation therapy is dependent upon the extent of the metastatic disease and the primary rectal cancer. Patients should be considered for pelvic radiation therapy if they have small asymptomatic distant metastases and a large rectal primary. The decision to administer radiation therapy should be made by an experienced multidisciplinary treatment team because the addition of radiation limits the chemotherapeutic regimen due to toxicity. Also, patients with recurrence after radiation therapy are limited to diverting surgery, stenting, and systemic chemotherapy, because of the limited tolerance of normal tissues to further radiation.

Radiation therapy alone has definite benefits in relieving symptoms. Pain and bleeding can be treated with low dose radiation therapy in about 75% of patients; however, palliation is often of short duration and is expected to last only about 3 to 9 months. Radiation therapy is thus most useful to patients with advanced disease and short life expectancy. By itself, it offers no survival benefit. A positive effect on long term survival can only be attained with the addition of chemotherapy. External beam and intraoperative radiation therapy combined with surgery has been attempted to improve palliation in patients with locally recurrent rectal cancer. Available evidence suggests that this is most beneficial in patients with negative margins at resection (Lindel et al, 2001). There are separate chapters on rectal cancer (see Chapter 98, "Curative Intent Management of Rectal Cancer"), abdominal radiation (see Chapter 100, "Abdominal Radiation") and on colorectal cancer: adjuvant and chemotherapy (see Chapter 97, "Colorectal Carcinoma").

Other Noninvasive Therapies

If patients have comorbidities rendering them intolerant to chemotherapy and radiation therapy or surgery, they should be provided comfort care only. Comfort care should also be extended to patients with multiple peritoneal metastases, metastases that are fixed or invading vital structures that are not amenable to safe resection or multiple metastases to other organs. Comfort care should include rigorous state-of-the-art pain control and spiritual support. Parenteral fluids may provide some additional comfort. In contrast, total parenteral nutrition or enteral tube feedings have not been shown to be of benefit in the comfort care cancer patient and should not be used.

Summary

Palliative therapy of rectal cancer is a highly individualized process for each patient involving a multidisciplinary care team. The goal is to enhance the quality of life by minimizing symptoms, maintaining normal function, and helping the patient and their support network to maintain realistic expectations without eliminating hope. Studies should be limited and be used to assist in decisions regarding palliative therapy. Both invasive and noninvasive therapy modalities exist to palliate patients with incurable rectal cancer. Inadequate data concerning decision pathways should prompt further studies that examine and compare the different therapies.

Supplemental Reading

Baron TH. Expandable metal stents for the treatment of cancerous obstruction of the gastrointestinal tract. N Engl J Med 2001;344:1681–7.

Canard JM, Vedrenne B. Clinical application of argon plasma coagulation in gastrointestinal endoscopy: has the time come to replace the laser? Endoscopy 2001;33:353–7.

Fernandez Lobato R, Pinto I, Paul L, et al. Self-expanding prostheses as a palliative method in treating advanced colorectal cancer. Int Surg 1999;84:59–62.

Gevers AM, Macken E, Hiele M, Rutgeerts P. Endoscopic laser therapy for palliation of patients with distal colorectal carcinoma: analysis of factors influencing long-term outcome. Gastrointest Endosc 2000;51:580–5.

Jemal A, Murray T, Samuels A, et al. Cancer statistics, 2003. CA Cancer J Clin 2003;53:5–26.

Lindel K, Willett CG, Shellito PC, et al. Intraoperative radiation therapy for locally advanced recurrent rectal or rectosigmoid cancer. Radiother Oncol 2001;58:83–7.

Marini E, Frigo F, Cavarzere L, et al. Palliative treatment of carcinoma of the rectum by endoscopic injection of polidocanol. Endoscopy 1990;22:171–3.

McGowan I, Barr H, Krasner N. Palliative laser therapy for inoperable rectal cancer–does it work? A prospective study of quality of life. Cancer 1989;63:967–9.

Weeks JC, Cook EF, O'Day SJ, et al. Relationship between cancer patients' predictions of prognosis and their treatment preferences. JAMA 1998;279:1709–14.

CHAPTER 100

Abdominal Radiation

Michael A. Hughes, MD, MS, and Ross A. Abrams, MD

Basic Paradigms of Oncologic Management

The role of radiation therapy is well established in the management of gastrointestinal (GI) malignancies in some anatomical sites and is evolving in others. With the exception of various GI presentations of lymphoma, localized presentations of anal cancer, and selected patients with esophageal and rectal cancer, most GI malignancies will require surgical resection to negative margins to have a meaningful chance of cure. For many apparently localized presentations, surgery alone proves to be insufficient to effect cure, particularly for more advanced lesions (stage T3 or T4) or extensive lymph node involvement. In such settings, the use of radiotherapy naturally combines with surgery, given preoperatively or postoperatively. In both preoperative and postoperative settings, radiotherapy has long been combined with chemotherapeutic agents that have been shown to enhance radiotherapeutic efficacy (radiosensitization).

Therapeutic Intent

The most critical decision in treatment selection is to determine the intent of the treatment to be administered. The therapeutic intent may be curative or palliative. Curative intent treatment is administered with expectation that there is some chance (high or low, but not zero) that the patient's tumor will be permanently controlled. Curatively, organ preservation may involve surgery for biopsies or limited local resection, followed by chemotherapy and/or radiation. If organ-preserving surgery is not an option and the organ must be removed, radiation is commonly used postoperatively to kill remaining tumor cells in the surgical bed or adjacent lymph node regions.

Palliative therapy is aimed at symptom relief, ideally for the expected duration of survival. Palliation of pain, GI obstruction, or bleeding may be achieved by a short course of radiotherapy. There are several sources of pain caused by GI malignancy, including: (1) organ capsular distention, (2) tumor infiltration of nerves, (3) GI tract obstruction, and (4) extension into vertebral bodies or ribs. Radiation is generally used along with appropriate narcotics and/or surgical interventions, such as stenting, surgical bypass, or celiac block. Pain relief from a nonobstructive source may take days to weeks, but is enduring. Pain from obstruction is often not well palliated by radiation alone, and relief may take weeks, if it occurs at all.

Bleeding due to diffuse mucosal infiltration of the tumor may also be palliated by radiation. The patient must be in relatively stable condition, and the site of bleeding must be localized such that a radiotherapy port can be placed with confidence. Patients with unlocalizable or severe bleeding are not suitable candidates. Control of bleeding can often be achieved with only one or a few treatments.

Radiation Modalities

Radiation itself may be delivered in a number of ways, broadly categorized as external beam or brachytherapy (Table 100-1). For GI malignancies, external beam radiation using photons (energy) produced by a linear accelerator is most common. The volume receiving radiation is delineated during treatment planning. Radiographic films or computed tomography scans are used to define the tumor, lymph nodes, surgical bed, and normal tissues. Radiation can then be precisely and accurately delivered to the tumor and minimized to the surrounding normal tissue. Advances in computer software now allow for 3-dimensional representations of tissues and radiation dose distributions to be modeled and modified. Brachytherapy, a procedure where radioactive sources are placed very near the treatment area, is less common but is useful under certain conditions. Instillation of radioactive isotopes into the abdominal cavity is rarely used.

TABLE 100-1. Radiation Therapy Modalities of Gastrointestinal Tumors

External Beam
    Energy
        Photons
    Particulate
        Protons, Neutrons, Electrons, Alpha
Brachytherapy
    Catheters
    Seeds
    Liquid intraperitoneal

Radiation "works" primarily by damaging DNA through the creation of free radicals. Cells may be killed directly, or die during mitosis when severely damaged DNA is unable to replicate. A differential effect on tumor versus normal tissue is achieved due mainly to better DNA repair mechanisms in the normal tissue. Radiation is often fractionated (given in many small doses) to take advantage of these differences in repair and to overcome tumor hypoxia. Hypoxia is common in malignant tissues and causes relative radioresistance, but decreases quickly as cells are killed following each treatment. Although the organ of origin of the malignancy is important, the cell type of origin also plays a role in the management of the patient. Most tumors of the GI tract are adenocarcinomas (ACs), but there are many other malignancies, including squamous cell carcinomas, lymphomas, and GI stromal tumors. Different cell types have different responsiveness to radiation or chemotherapy. The *standard unit of radiation dose* is now the "*Gray*," which in the J/kg/s system of measurements is equivalent to 1 J of energy absorbed into 1 kg of mass. Earlier units of radiation included the "Roentgen," which is a measure of the number of ionizations produced in air by a radiation beam (and is not a suitable unit for radiotherapy dose consideration), and the "Rad" (an acronym for "radiation absorbed dose"), which is equivalent to 100 erg of energy absorbed into 1 g of mass. It is convenient that *1 rad is equal to 0.01 gray* (a "Centigray").

Treatment Sequence

The sequence of treatments may be important (Table 100-2). For example, should radiation be given before (neoadjuvant), during (intraoperative), or after (adjuvant) surgery? Each has both theoretical and practical advantages and disadvantages. Neoadjuvant therapy may change a previously unresectable tumor into a resectable one, or reduce the extent of surgery necessary. However, it also may obscure tissue planes or confuse surgical pathologic staging information. Intraoperative radiation allows normal tissues to be moved out of the treatment field, but is technically demanding, requires special equipment, and can be given in only one fraction. After surgery, adjuvant radiation can be directed to areas of histologically proven disease. However, tissue may be hypoxic due to disruption of the blood supply, decreasing the oxygen available to become free radicals.

The sequencing of radiation and chemotherapy is also important. Should radiation be given before, during, or after chemotherapy? Again, there are theoretical advantages to each. The answer depends on the site and stage of disease, the therapeutic goal, and the degree of morbidity that can be tolerated and justified, because the sequence impacts not only on efficacy of treatment but on side effects (intensity), as well. With esophageal squamous and AC being treated preoperatively, chemotherapy and radiotherapy are given concurrently (Forastiere et al, 1997).

Side Effects of Radiation

The side effects of abdominal radiation are divided into short term (during and just after treatment) and long term (months to years later). A major consideration in treatment planning for radiation therapy is the minimization of these side effects, particularly long term effects. Common short-term reactions include skin irritation, fatigue, dysphagia or odynophagia, nausea, weight loss, diarrhea, and anoproctitis (depending upon the region irradiated). Long term effects are less common and are more specific to the exact area treated. Acute side effects occur (are increased) in proportion to the volume irradiated, the amount of daily treatment, the frequency of treatments, and in the presence of concurrent chemotherapy. Late side effects relate mostly to the amount of an organ irradiated, the fraction size used each day, and the total radiation dose, as well as the nature of the organ in question. For upper GI malignancies, portions of the liver, or one or both kidneys, may have reduced function (Table 100-3). In 5% or less of patients, there may be chronic diarrhea or intestinal damage requiring surgery. Late effects typically occur 6 months to 2 years after radiation treatment, but may be seen earlier or later.

Ten to 20 years after radiation, radiation induced second malignancy may occur within or adjacent to radiated volumes. This is more likely in patients irradiated as children, patients with specific heritable syndromes, and

TABLE 100-2. Preoperative versus Postoperative Radiation Therapy

	Preoperative Radiation	Postoperative Radiation
Advantages		
	Decreased tumor seeding	Tailored treatment fields to proven cancer sites
	Convert unresectable to respectable	Complete surgical staging
	No compromise of vascular supply	Complete surgical pathology
Disadvantages		
	Incomplete surgical pathology	Surgically altered anatomy
	Incomplete surgical staging	Treatment of hypoxic tissue
	Delay of surgery	
	Increased wound complications	

TABLE 100-3. Typical Normal Organ Tolerances for Radiotherapy Late Effects*

Organ	Dose (cGy) (large volumes and/or circumferential)	Clinical Syndrome
Esophagus	> 6000	Dysphagia, stricture, ulceration, bleeding
Stomach	> 4500 to 5000	Bleeding, ulceration
Small bowel	> 4500 to 5400	Bleeding, ulceration, fibrosis, obstruction
Colon	> 5500 to 6000	Bleeding, ulceration, fibrosis, obstruction
Liver	> 2500 to 3000	Radiation hepatopathy: hepatomegaly, striking elevations of alkaline phosphatase, central veins thrombosed, jaundice, organ failure
Kidney	> 2000	Decreased function with elevated creatinine

cGy = centiGray = 1 rad = 0.01 Gray.
*Radiotherapy complications are dose, volume, and fraction size dependent. Stated doses are threshold doses for 5 to 10% risk for large volume organ irradiation given at 180 to 200 cGy daily. Small volumes of organs can often be taken to higher doses without apparent consequence.

patients with Hodgkin's disease at the time of irradiation. Although secondary malignancy is a serious effect, the benefit of therapy for a known cancer far outweighs the risk of a potential second neoplasm.

Role of Radiation by Site

Esophagus

Cancer of the esophagus is a highly lethal disease, with 5-year survival of 28% for localized disease, 12% for regional disease, and only 2% for metastatic disease. This is due, in part, to the propensity for early metastatic spread of the disease. Surgery alone has been the historic standard of care for esophageal cancer (EC), but has had poor outcomes. Recent studies of nonmetastatic EC suggest that preoperative chemoradiotherapy provides a survival benefit and improves local control compared to surgery alone (Forastiere et al, 1997; Herskovic et al, 1992). There is a separate chapter on esophageal cancer (Chapter 21, "Cancer of the Esophagus"). The role of adjuvant radiotherapy is not well studied. The optimal chemotherapy regimen is unclear, but multiagent chemotherapy appears to be better than single agent cisplatin (Forastiere et al, 1997). The optimal dose fractionation schedule of radiation for concurrent chemoradiotherapy regimens remains to be determined. Three dimensional, conformal treatment planning techniques should be used to minimize toxicities to critical adjacent organs, such as the spinal cord, heart, and lung. The standard dose of radiation for patients treated with concurrent 5-fluorouracil (5-FU) and cisplatin is 50.4 Gy given over 5 to 6 weeks.

Locally unresectable, nonmetastatic esophageal cancer is incurable in the majority of patients. There is a separate chapter (Chapter 22, "Palliation of Esophageal Cancer") on EC. Combined chemoradiotherapy offers only a small chance of sustained disease control and long term survival. However, a majority of patients achieve sustained relief of dysphagia. Combined chemoradiotherapy is generally recommended for patients who are able to tolerate this therapy. The use of a brachytherapy boost may provide additional benefit. However, the optimal use of brachytherapy is not clearly defined.

Stomach

Patients who have undergone a potentially curative resection for carcinoma of the stomach should be considered for adjuvant chemoradiotherapy. A large multicenter trial clearly demonstrated a survival benefit for adjuvant treatment and established the standard of care (Macdonald et al, 2001). Specifically, the current standard protocol consists of 5-FU and leucovorin along with radiation therapy to 45 Gy. There is a separate chapter on gastric cancer (GC) management (Chapter 34, "Gastric Cancer").

When surgery is not possible, radiation therapy also can be useful in the palliative management of GC. Radiation can assist in shrinking tumors, controlling pain, and decreasing bleeding. There is currently insufficient evidence from randomized trials to support neoadjuvant chemoradiotherapy or immunotherapy, either alone or in combination, outside of a clinical trial.

Liver/Intrahepatic Bile Ducts

Surgery is the only potentially curative treatment for primary hepatic malignancies. The radiation dose required for meaningful antineoplastic effect on unresected tumor of the liver is much higher (~50 Gy) than the tolerance to radiation of the whole liver (~30 Gy). However, recent technical improvements, such as 3-dimensional conformal radiation, inverse treatment planning methods, and accounting for respiratory movement (respiratory gating) may allow potentially tumoricidal doses to be delivered with acceptable risk.

Pancreas

The surgical management of periampullary pancreatic cancer (PC) has improved dramatically in the last decade, decreased operative mortality to < 5%, and decreased hospital stays to approximately 14 days. However, the overall 5-year survival is less than 5%. Most patients still have recurrence of their tumors after surgery, spurring interest in adjuvant therapies. Several randomized trials are currently ongoing and exploring various chemoradiotherapy regimens. At our institution, we have found that patients fare better with adjuvant chemoradiotherapy and, therefore, it is routinely offered (Willet et al, 2003). Our radiation doses are from 50 to 54 Gy, along with concurrent 5-FU based chemotherapy. There is a separate chapter on PC therapy (Chapter 142, "Pancreatic Cancer Therapy").

For locally advanced, unresectable carcinoma of the pancreas, combined chemoradiotherapy is recommended for palliation in suitable patients. Radiation to 50.4 Gy combined with 5-FU is most commonly used. Radiation combined with other chemotherapeutic agents (such as gemcitabine or paclitaxel) is being investigated.

Gallbladder

Surgical management is the only potentially curative treatment for cancer of the gallbladder. Local recurrence is the most common mode of treatment failure after surgery. No randomized controlled trials of adjuvant radiation therapy or chemoradiotherapy have been performed. Several retrospective reports show encouraging results for local control and survival with intraoperative or postoperative radiation, with or without chemotherapy. The use of adjuvant chemoradiotherapy is relatively common is the United States. Generally, the treatment regimen is external beam radiation to 45 to 54 Gy with concomitant 5-FU chemotherapy.

For advanced, unresectable disease, palliation should focus on relief of pain, jaundice, and bowel obstruction, along with prolongation of life. Surgical bypass by open or percutaneous/endoscopic procedure may be considered. The role of radiation or chemoradiotherapy in this setting is unclear given the limited median survival in patients with advanced disease (< 6 months). There are two chapters on endoscopic management of bile duct obstructions and strictures (Chapter 133, "Biliary Strictures and Neoplasms" and Chapter 134, "Endoscopic Management of Bile Duct Obstruction and Sphincter of Oddi Dysfunction").

Small Bowel

Due to the rarity of small bowel carcinomas, no prospective studies have been performed. ACs of the small bowel are treated surgically with wide segmental resection. Adjuvant therapy for small bowel cancer has not been well studied. However, patients with close or positive margins involving the retroperitoneum may be considered for treatment with combined chemoradiation. Neoadjuvant chemoradiotherapy radiation therapy to 50 Gy with concurrent 5-FU and mitomycin has been studied in only a very small number of patients but shows some promise. The role of chemotherapy alone for small intestine ACs remains undefined.

Colon

Surgical resection is the cornerstone of potentially curative therapy for colon cancer. Current evidence is inconclusive regarding whether adding radiation therapy to chemotherapy postoperatively enhances survival in patients with colon cancer, even for those who are at increased risk for local recurrence (Willett et al, 1999). Patients at high risk for local recurrence include those with perforation or invasion of other adjacent organs. For these patients, adjuvant radiation should be considered on a case-by-case basis. There is a separate chapter on colon cancer management (Chapter 96, "Colon Cancer") as well as a chapter on chemotherapy (Chapter 97, "Colorectal Carcinoma").

Rectum

Surgical resection is the foundation of potentially curative therapy. However, surgery alone is curative only for early stage patients. The site of first failure in patients with rectal cancer is equally distributed locally and distantly. Local recurrence is due mainly to difficulty in obtaining adequate tumor-free radial resection margins. Randomized trials suggest that there is a local control and a survival advantage for patients receiving adjuvant chemoradiotherapy, particularly for patients with a high risk for recurrence (stage II and stage III) (GI Tumor Study Group, 1985; Colorectal Cancer Collaborative Group, 2001). Radiation therapy to a total dose of 45 to 50.4 Gy is combined with infusional 5-FU-based chemotherapy regimens. There is a separate chapter on rectal cancer (Chapter 98, "Curative Intent Management of Rectal Cancer").

For unresectable rectal carcinomas, preoperative radiation with concurrent chemotherapy prior to planned resection is recommended. This permits a sphincter-preserving low anterior resection to be performed rather than an abdominoperineal resection, which entails a permanent colostomy and a higher incidence of genitourinary and sexual dysfunction. Preoperative radiation does not appear to increase the complication rate from surgical resection. The following chapter is devoted to the palliation of rectal cancer (Chapter 99, "Palliative Therapy for Rectal Cancer").

Supplemental Reading

Colorectal Cancer Collaborative Group. Adjuvant radiotherapy for rectal cancer: a systematic overview of 8,507 patients from 22 randomised trials. Lancet 2001;358:1291–304.

Devita V, Hellman S, Rosenberg S, editors. Cancer: principles and practice of oncology. 6th ed. Lippincott Williams and Wilkens; 2001.

Gastrointestinal Tumor Study Group. Prolongation of the disease-free interval in surgically treated rectal carcinoma. N Engl J Med 1985;312:1465–72.

Gunderson L, Tepper J, editors. Clinical radiation oncology. 1st ed. Church Livingstone; 2000.

Forastiere AA, Heitmiller RF, Lee DJ, et al. Intensive chemoradiation followed by esophagectomy for squamous cell and adenocarcinoma of the esophagus. Cancer J Sci Am 1997;3:144–52.

Herskovic A, Martz K, al-Sarraf M, et al. Combined chemotherapy and radiotherapy compared with radiotherapy alone in patients with cancer of the esophagus. N Engl J Med 1992;326:1593–8.

Jemal A, Murray T, Samuels A, et al. Cancer statistics, 2003. CA Cancer J Clin 2003;53:5–26.

Macdonald JS, Smalley SR, Benedetti J, et al. Chemoradiotherapy after surgery compared with surgery alone for adenocarcinoma of the stomach or gastroesophageal junction. N Engl J Med 2001;345:725–30.

Willett CG, Goldberg S, Shellito PC, et al. Does postoperative irradiation play a role in the adjuvant therapy of stage T4 colon cancer? Cancer J Sci Am 1999;5:242–7.

Willett CG, Safran H, Abrams RA, et al. Clinical research in pancreatic cancer: The Radiation Therapy Oncology Group trials. Int J Radiat Oncol Biol Phys 2003;56(4Suppl):31–7.

CHAPTER 101

Lower Gastrointestinal Bleeding

Carlos G. Micames, MD, Michael F. Byrne, MD, and John Baillie, MB, ChB, FRCP

Lower gastrointestinal (GI) bleeding is a frequently encountered problem, accounting for 24% of all GI bleeding events. It is sometimes defined as hemorrhage arising distal to the ligament of Treitz, which includes both small bowel and colonic sources. However, the vast majority of cases originate from the colon. Although diagnostic methods for localizing bleeding have dramatically improved during the past 20 years, they are not universally successful or reliable. In fact, as many as 8 to 12% of patients fail to have the precise origin and location of bleeding identified despite an exhaustive diagnostic examination. Bleeding can be occult, slow, moderate, or severe and life threatening. This chapter will focus on clinical presentation, etiology, diagnosis, and treatment of severe colonic bleeding. There is a separate chapter on occult bleeding that concentrates on the small bowel.

Clinical Presentation and Etiology

Lower GI bleeding usually presents as hematochezia, or passage of maroon or bright red blood or blood clots per rectum. This is different from upper GI bleeding, which usually presents with hematemesis and/or melena. Although helpful, these distinctions are not absolute. In up to 11% of patients with hematochezia, the culprit lesion is identified in the upper GI tract. Conversely, 19% of patients with lower GI bleeding can present with melena. Overall, the acuity and severity of lower GI bleeding is less than upper GI bleeding. According to a survey of members of the American College of Gastroenterology (ACG), patients with lower GI bleeding were less likely to present to the physician with shock or orthostasis compared with patients with upper GI bleeding (19% versus 35%, respectively) and less likely to require blood transfusions (36% versus 64%, respectively). Lower GI bleeding is self-limiting in approximately 80% of cases, although intermittent bleeding episodes do occur. The incidence of lower GI bleeding, as well as its morbidity and mortality, increases with age due to the higher rate of comorbid conditions and use of medications. The reported mortality rate varies between 2.0 to 3.6%.

The causes of lower GI hemorrhage vary depending on the age of the patient and the severity of the bleeding. In patients under the age of 50 years, the most common causes are *infectious colitis, anorectal disease*, and *inflammatory bowel disease (IBD)*. In older patients, significant hematochezia is usually due to *diverticulosis, angiodysplasia, neoplasia*, or *ischemia* (Table 101-1).

Diverticulosis

Diverticulosis is a common colonic condition in elderly patients of the Western world, with a prevalence of 37 to 45%. Although diverticula more commonly occur on the left side of the colon, bleeding usually originates from right-sided lesions. It is estimated that hemorrhage occurs in 3 to 5% of all patients with diverticulosis. Due to the high prevalence in the general population, and particularly the elderly, it is the most common cause of lower GI bleeding, accounting for over 30% of cases. Diverticular bleeding usually presents as painless, large-volume hematochezia of abrupt onset; bleeding ceases spontaneously in up to 90% of patients. Rebleeding occurs 22 to 38% of the time, and the likelihood of a third bleeding episode in such

TABLE 101-1. Etiology of Colonic Bleeding

Diverticulosis
Angiodysplasia
Cancer/Polyps
Inflammatory bowel disease
Radiation proctocolitis
Infectious colitis
Ischemic colitis
Anorectal disease
   Hemorrhoids
   Anal fissures
   Rectal ulcers
   Fistula in ano
Rare Causes
   Portal hypertensive colopathy
   Small bowel varices
   Colonic and rectal varices
   Endometriosis
   Dieulafoy's lesion of the colon
   NSAID-induced colonic ulcers
   Vasculitis
   Aortocolonic fistula
   Acute graft-versus-host disease

NSAID = nonsteroidal anti-inflammatory.

patients is approximately 50%. This has led some experts to recommend surgical resection of the involved section of colon after a second bleeding event.

Angiodysplasia

Angiodysplasia (or vascular ectasias) occur throughout the whole GI tract, particularly in the right colon. They are responsible for 3 to 12% of cases of lower GI bleeding. They are flat, red lesions (2 to 10 mm) with ectatic peripheral vessels radiating from a central vessel, and are most common in patients over 70 years old and those with chronic renal failure. Synchronous angiodysplasia occurs in different segments of the GI tract in about 20% of cases. Thus, to establish that a specific lesion is the source of GI blood loss it needs to be identified while it is actively bleeding.

IBD

IBD is a common source of lower GI bleeding, usually presenting with diarrhea and variable amounts of hematochezia. Although the risk of life threatening hemorrhage is low, it does occur and occasionally mandates emergency surgery. It is estimated that 6% of patients with either Crohn's disease (CD) or ulcerative colitis experience severe lower GI bleeding. Brisk hematochezia can occur with deep ulceration in the absence of diarrhea in CD.

Infectious Colitis

Infectious colitis can present with frequent bloody, small volume stools, often associated with fever, abdominal cramps, tenesmus, and rectal urgency. Although the commonest infectious cause of bloody diarrhea in adults in the West is *Campylobacter*, pseudomembranous colitis, caused by *Clostridium difficile*, is one of the most common nosocomial infections; it is usually seen during or following antibiotic administration. Its clinical presentation ranges from mild diarrhea to severe colitis and hematochezia. Patients infected with Shiga toxin-producing *Escherichia coli* (particularly serotype O157:H7) present with acute onset of bloody diarrhea, especially without fever, and with the hemolytic-uremic syndrome. In immunocompromised hosts, most episodes of lower GI bleeding are associated with opportunistic infection, such as cytomegalovirus colitis.

Radiation Proctocolitis

Patients with a past history of radiation therapy for prostate cancer or gynecologic malignancy can have lower GI bleeding as either an early or late complication of radiation damage. Acute radiation proctocolitis usually presents as transient diarrhea, tenesmus, and mucoid or bloody discharge per rectum. These signs and symptoms are usually resolved within days or weeks without specific therapy. Chronic radiation injury is an ischemic process, usually beginning 2 to 3 months after treatment has ended. Hemorrhage is the most common feature, ranging from occasional mild spotting to passing blood clots with every bowel movement.

Ischemic Colitis

Ischemic colitis is usually seen in older patients, most of whom have atherosclerotic disease. The segments of colon most susceptible to ischemic injury are so-called "watershed" areas between the major mesenteric arteries, such as the splenic flexure, descending colon, and sigmoid colon. Physiologic factors such as low perfusion pressure (eg, from hypotension, tachydysrhythmia), decreased colonic perfusion secondary to altered colonic motility, and sustained mesenteric vasospasm predispose patients to colonic ischemia. Ischemic colitis usually presents as abrupt, crampy abdominal pain, most often located in the left lower quadrant. This pain is often accompanied by the sudden urge to defecate and the passage of bright red blood or dark clots. It accounts for 3 to 9% of cases of lower GI bleeding and usually is self-limiting. There is a separate chapter on ischemic bowel disease (see Chapter 70, "Mesenteric Vascular Ischemia").

Neoplasia

Benign adenomatous polyps and adenocarcinoma of the colon and rectum are associated with chronic occult blood loss or intermittent hematochezia. Up to 10% of cases with severe lower GI bleeding in the elderly are related to benign or malignant neoplasia. These lesions often bleed from erosions or ulcers on the surface. Colonic bleeding can occur following endoscopic removal of polyps, with a reported incidence of 0.2%. Hemorrhage may be immediate, as a result of incomplete coagulation of the polyp stalk, or delayed up to 15 days, from sloughing of the eschar or erosion of a polypectomy ulcer. Elderly patients seem to be most prone to this complication. Although several studies have shown that endoscopic procedures can be performed safely in patients taking aspirin and other nonsteroidal anti-inflammatory drugs (NSAIDs) without an increased risk of bleeding complications, some experts still recommend avoiding these medications for 7 days before and 7 to 10 days after polypectomy.

Hemorrhoids, Anal Fissures, and Rectal Ulcers

The anorectum is a frequent source of significant lower GI bleeding. It frequently manifests with small amounts of bright red blood noted on the toilet paper, coating the stool, or dripping into the toilet bowl. Many causes of anorectal bleeding, such as hemorrhoids and fissures, are recurrent. Constipation occasionally causes stercoral ulcers due to fecal impaction or the solitary rectal ulcer syndrome from mucosal trauma, rectal prolapse, or direct digital trauma to aid evacuation, which can lead to anorectal hemorrhage. In patients with portal hypertension, rectal varices can cause life threatening hemorrhage which often requires rectal packing or even emergent surgery to control. The finding of very prominent hemorrhoids should always prompt the question: "Does this patient have portal hypertension?" There is a separate chapter on hemorrhoids (see Chapter 92, "Hemorrhoids").

Rare Causes of Colonic Bleeding

Uncommon causes of acute lower intestinal bleeding include portal hypertensive colopathy and colonic varices, endometriosis, Dieulafoy's lesion of the colon, NSAID-induced ulcers of the colon, vasculitic ischemia, acute graft-versus-host disease, and aortocolonic fistula formation following aortic graft surgery.

Diagnosis and Initial Management

In all patients with lower GI bleeding, fluid resuscitation and correction of coagulopathy or thrombocytopenia take precedence over diagnostic or therapeutic procedures. Nasogastric (NG) lavage is performed looking for fresh blood, clots, or "coffee grounds" suggestive of an upper GI source. The absence of blood on NG lavage does not exclude upper GI bleeding, unless bile is obtained. Evaluation of the anorectum should include digital rectal exam and anoscopy. The latter will allow identification of internal hemorrhoids, fissures, or fistulas. After this point, the decision between further diagnostic studies will depend on the severity of bleeding, overall condition of the patient and comorbid diseases, and the availability of each diagnostic tool in a specific hospital. Available options include colonoscopy, tagged red blood cell (RBC) scan, and

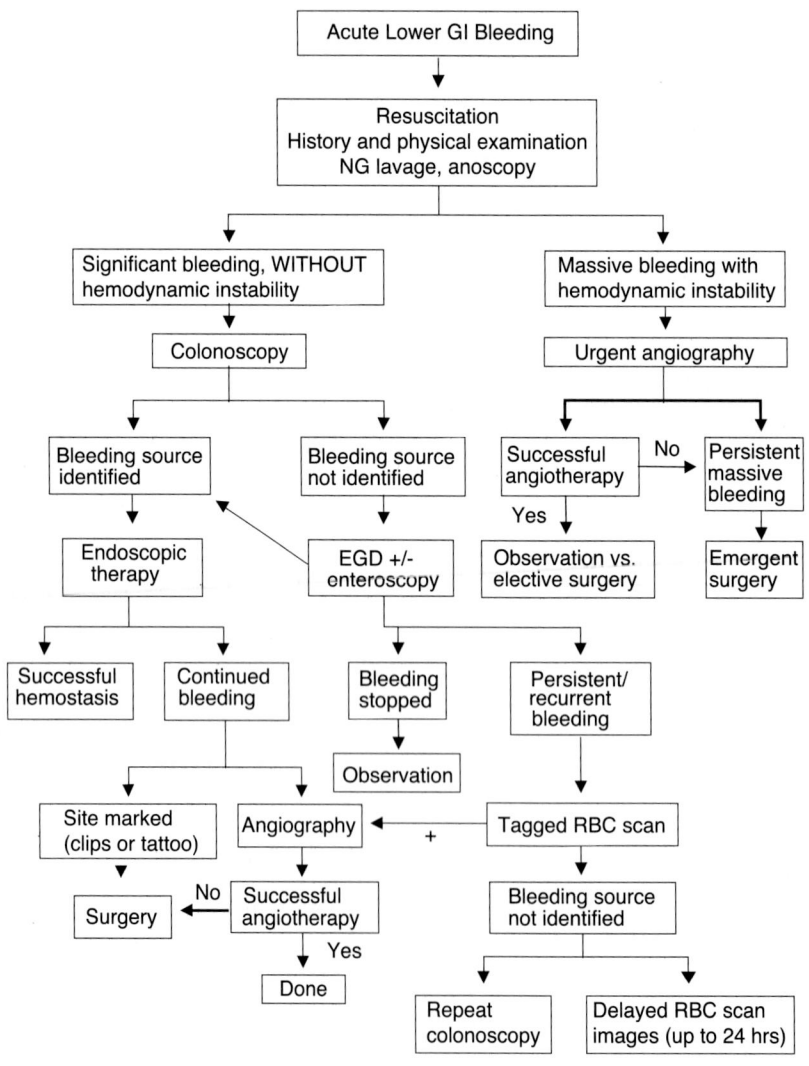

FIGURE 101-1. Algorithm for the management of lower gastrointestinal bleeding. EGD = Esophagogastroduodenoscopy; NG = nasogastric; RBC = red blood cells.

angiography. Contrast radiology (barium enema) has been shown in multiple studies to have a low diagnostic yield for localizing a colonic bleeding source, and interferes with subsequent attempts to perform colonoscopy and angiography. Barium enema it is not recommended as part of the evaluation of acute lower GI bleeding. Capsule endoscopy is a recent option for evaluating recurrent acute hemorrhage of possible small bowel origin. This is discussed in the chapter on occult bleeding (see Chapter 59, "Obscure Gastrointestinal Bleedings").

Colonoscopy

Colonoscopy can be both diagnostic and therapeutic. Studies have shown that it is a safe and accurate test early in the course of acute lower GI bleeding. Urgent colonoscopy is usually done within 6 to 24 hours of admission after a rapid colonic lavage using 4 to 8 L of a polyethylene glycol solution given orally or via NG tube over 3 to 5 hours until the rectal effluent is clear. There is ample evidence that a colonic purge is safe and will not reactivate or increase the rate of bleeding. The likelihood of finding a bleeding source is increased by performing urgent colonoscopy. The yield increases if the colonoscopy is performed while the patient is actively bleeding. The patient should be adequately resuscitated prior to performing urgent colonoscopy so that he or she can tolerate bowel purge and conscious sedation. As with peptic ulcer disease, criteria have been used to identify a colonic bleeding site. These include the finding of active bleeding, a nonbleeding visible vessel or an adherent clot, in conjunction with a diverticulum or angiodysplasia. Although these findings have been associated with increased bleeding severity in several studies, they lack validation. If colonoscopy does not reveal a bleeding source, an upper GI endoscopy is performed immediately. Colonoscopy can also be useful in localizing the bleeding source to the small bowel when fresh blood is seen in the terminal ileum, but not in the colon, and upper GI endoscopy is negative.

Enteroscopy and Capsule Endoscopy

Endoscopy of the small bowel has always been problematic due to the technical problems associated with long endoscopes. Standard "push" endoscopes rarely advance beyond the mid-jejunum. "Sonde" enteroscopes are designed to view the entire small bowel; a very long, thin endoscope with a balloon on the tip advances down the small bowel by peristalsis, aided by patient positioning and a prokinetic agent (eg, metoclopramide). Unfortunately, the Sonde procedure is time consuming (typically 6 to 8 hours), uncomfortable for the patient (cramps) and has a yield of only 30% for pathology, even in the best hands. Recently, remote sensing endoscopy—so-called "capsule endoscopy"—has provided an easier and more sensitive way to look at the small bowel. Data on capsule endoscopy in the setting of recurrent severe lower GI bleeding are limited, but this technique has "picked up" previously unsuspected pathology, such as small bowel varices. Although mainly used to look for causes of chronic occult GI blood loss, capsule endoscopy may have a role in examining patients who present with repeated hematochezia without a likely colonic source. This is discussed in the chapter on occult bleeding (see Chapter 59).

Nuclear Bleeding Scans

Technetium Tc^{99m}-labeled RBC scans can detect intestinal bleeding rates as low as 0.1 mL/min. After the infusion of radiotracer, patients are imaged for 1 to 2 hours initially. If the initial scan is negative, they can be rescanned without reinjection for up to 24 hours. In patients with lower GI bleeding, only 45% will have a positive tagged RBC scan. The chances of obtaining a positive scan are increased if the patient is actively bleeding, as evidenced by hematochezia, at the time of the test. Neither hemodynamic compromise nor the number of units of blood transfused has been shown to predict a positive tagged RBC scan. The timing at which the study becomes positive, immediate, or delayed is an important factor in predicting the accuracy of the scan. Patients in whom the radionuclide spot is seen *immediately* after scanning had bleeding *confirmed* with *angiogram* in 61% of cases, compared with only 7% of cases in which the spot developed later during the scan. The accuracy of localizing the bleeding site is also higher when identified during images obtained *within 2 hours* of performing the radionuclide injection. Late positive scans (after 6 hours) may represent blood that has moved down the GI tract by peristalsis and are only useful in providing evidence that intermittent bleeding continues. Thus, confirmation of tagged RBC scan localization by angiography or another diagnostic modality must be performed prior to undergoing surgery. Due to its noninvasive nature and its lower threshold for detecting intestinal bleeding, this technique is routinely performed as a screening test before angiography, because *patients with a negative tagged RBC scan are unlikely to have a positive angiogram*. A limitation of this approach is that the *delay* in getting angiography may allow the bleeding to spontaneously cease, eliminating the opportunity to definitely localize the bleeding source and potentially intervene.

Angiography

Selective mesenteric angiography should be reserved for patients with massive, ongoing lower GI bleeding when colonoscopy is not feasible, or with recurrent hematochezia when colonoscopy did not reveal a source. Angiography is able to detect small and large bowel bleeds at a rate greater than 0.5 mL/min. In patients with severe lower GI bleeding, angiography was able to detect hemorrhage, as evidenced by extravasation of contrast, in 47% of the cases. As with nuclear scans, the positivity rate can be as high as 61 to 72% if performed on patients with active bleeding, defined as requiring a blood transfusion, causing hemodynamic compromise, or with an immediately positive tagged RBC scan. Once a source of bleeding is identified, angiographic techniques (discussed later in this chapter) or surgery can be performed. Significant complications associated with angiography include hematomas, contrast reactions, renal failure, femoral artery thrombosis, and mesenteric vessel laceration.

Treatment

In most cases, lower GI bleeding ceases spontaneously. In those with persistent or recurrent hematochezia, the management will involve colonoscopic, angiographic, or surgical intervention, or a combination of these techniques. Ideally any therapeutic procedure should be performed once the patient is adequately volume resuscitated and coagulopathy or thrombocytopenia is corrected. However, in some cases, particularly in the elderly, hemodynamic stability may not be reached due to persistent GI hemorrhage or decompensation of other comorbid diseases (ie, heart failure, chronic renal disease); these patients may thus require an emergent therapeutic intervention.

Endoscopic Therapy

Endoscopic therapy is increasingly used for lower GI bleeding, although less commonly than for upper GI bleeding (27% compared to 51%, respectively), based on a recent ACG survey. In patients with diverticular bleeding, therapeutic options for high risk lesions (active bleeding, visible vessel) that can be delivered through the colonoscope include thermal contact modalities, such as heater probe or bipolar/multipolar coagulation, or epinephrine injection, which may be used independently or in conjunction. The use of metallic clips for treating diverticular hemorrhage has also been reported. An initial study looking at the impact of endoscopic intervention on diverticular bleeding found that none of the patients treated endoscopically had persistent or recurrent bleeding, or required surgery, compared with 35% in the group treated conservatively (Jensen et al, 2000). A recent randomized, controlled trial performed at our institution revealed that urgent colonoscopy identified a definite bleeding source in 42% of cases of lower GI bleeding compared to 8% with tagged RBC scan followed by angiography. The rates of rebleeding for patients who underwent urgent colonoscopy versus those who underwent radiologic intervention were 16% and 14%, respectively, after a mean follow-up of approximately 5 years. However, this difference did not reach statistical significance. There was no difference in mortality, hospital stay, or need for surgery between both groups (Green et al, 2003).

Bleeding caused by *angiodysplasia* can be treated with thermal modalities, injection or noncontact modalities, such as argon plasma coagulation (APC). These lesions are usually found in the cecum and right colon. The use of low power settings with thermal modalities is recommended (10 to 15 J with heater probe; 10 to 15 W, 1 s pulses with bipolar probe) to reduce the risk of perforation. To reduce risk of bleeding during cautery, large lesions should be initially treated around the circumference to obliterate feeder vessels before the center of the lesion is treated. Endoscopic cautery techniques are effective in controlling *radiation-induced rectal bleeding*. Thermal contact modalities are effective in decreasing bleeding episodes. Lasers, including Nd:YAG and argon, have been used successfully for treating telangiectasias in radiation proctitis. Usually, one to three sessions are required. APC is also used and has several advantages over laser, including a more superficial burn, portability, and lower risk of transmural necrosis, stricture formation, and perforation.

Postpolypectomy bleeding can occur immediately or weeks after the procedure. Early rebleeding can be treated by compressing the remaining polyp stalk with a metal snare, detachable plastic snares, or metallic clips. Delayed bleeding can be managed conservatively in the majority of patients. Endoscopic therapy is a safe and effective option in patients with persistent bleeding. Angiotherapy or surgery is usually not required.

Angiotherapy

Once the bleeding site is localized during diagnostic mesenteric angiography, intra-arterial injection of a vasoconstrictor agent can be administered. *Vasopressin* causes reliable arteriolar vasoconstriction and bowel wall contraction resulting in a reduction of blood flow. It successfully controls lower GI bleeding in 62 to 100% of cases, but rebleeding occurs commonly (16 to 50% of the time). Its main limitation is the considerable rate of associated complications, ranging from fluid retention and transient arrhythmias in about 40%, to pulmonary edema and myocardial ischemia in about 15% of interventions.

Selective *transcatheter embolization* is an option for control of hemorrhage when vasopressin fails or in patients with relative contraindications to the use of vasopressin, such as coronary artery disease and peripheral vascular disease. Embolic agents used include gelatin-sponge, coil springs, or polyvinyl alcohols. It is highly effective for control of bleeding (71 to100%), with a low rebleeding rate ranging from of 0% to 12%. Its widespread use has been limited due to the risk of intestinal infarction, reported in up to 20% of cases during initial studies. However, advances in catheter and guidewire design have allowed superselective catheterization and embolization of small, peripheral arteries, significantly reducing complication rates.

Surgery

Emergency surgery for acute lower GI bleeding is usually reserved for patients who have failed medical, colonoscopic, or angiographic intervention. Surgery is usually indicated if there is ongoing bleeding requiring greater than 4 units of packed red blood cells within 24 hours. Recurrent bleeding, especially diverticular, is also considered by some an indication for resection. Accurate localization of the bleeding site by angiography or colonoscopy is required for segmental resection to be performed. If continued hemorrhage and hemodynamic instability mandate an operation before the bleeding site is identified, intraoperative enteroscopy or colonoscopy should be performed to try to localize the site. Subtotal colectomy is reserved for patients who continue to bleed without identification of the bleeding site. It is associated with a significantly higher morbidity and mortality than limited resections. Blind segmental colectomies should never be performed because they carry similar mortality and morbidity as subtotal colectomy, but a much higher rebleeding rate of up to 54%.

Summary

There are several etiologies of lower GI bleeding, *diverticulosis* being the most common. *Colonoscopy* has become the initial test of choice in lower GI bleeding both for diagnosis and therapy. Mesenteric angiography is usually reserved for patients with massive bleeding, when poor visibility will limit the yield of endoscopy, or with ongoing hemorrhage. As with colonoscopy, angiography can serve both diagnostic and therapeutic purposes. Both interventions are equivalent in controlling hemorrhage, rebleeding rate, mortality, and length of hospital stay. Surgery is an option when other methods fail or for definitive treatment of recurrent hemorrhage. Every attempt should be made to localize the site and limit the extent of resection to reduce the morbidity and mortality associated with the operation.

Supplemental Reading

Bloomfield RS, Rockey DC, Shetzline MA. Endoscopic therapy of acute diverticular hemorrhage. Am J Gastroenterol 2001;96:2367–72.

Green B, Rockey DC, Portwood PR, et al. Urgent colonoscopy for evaluation and management of acute lower gastrointestinal hemorrhage: a randomized controlled trial. Gastroenterology 2003;124:A140.

Jensen DM, Machicado GA, Jutabha R, Kovacs TOG. Urgent colonoscopy for the diagnosis and treatment of severe diverticular hemorrhage. N Engl J Med 2000;342:78–82.

Lefkovitz Z, Cappell MS, Lookstein R, et al. Radiologic diagnosis and treatment of gastrointestinal hemorrhage and ischemia. Med Clin North Am 2002;86:1357–99.

Stollman NH, Raskin JB. Diagnosis and management of diverticular disease of the colon in adults. Am J Gastroenterol 1999;94:3110–21.

Strate LL, Orav J, Sapna S. Early predictors of severity in acute lower intestinal tract bleeding. Arch Intern Med 2003;163:838–43.

Vernava AM, Moore BA, Longo WE, et al. Lower gastrointestinal bleeding. Dis Colon Rectum 1997;40:846–58.

Zuccaro G. Management of the adult patient with acute lower gastrointestinal bleeding. Am J Gastroenterol 1998;93:1202–8.

Zuckerman GR, Prakash C. Acute lower intestinal bleeding, Part I. Gastrointest Endosc 1998;48:606–17.

Zuckerman GR, Prakash C. Acute lower intestinal bleeding, Part II. Gastrointest Endosc 1999;49:228–38.

CHAPTER 102

Transcatheter Management of Upper and Lower Gastrointestinal Tract Bleeding

Anthony C. Venbrux, MD, Elizabeth A. Ignacio, MD, Amy P. Soltes, RN, MSN, ACNP-BC, and Albert K. Chun, MD

Gastrointestinal (GI) bleeding is a potentially life threatening condition necessitating immediate medical attention. The goal of the physician is to examine, stabilize, and treat the patient with GI bleeding. Once stabilized, patients are generally admitted to the intensive care unit (ICU) for hemodynamic monitoring and further workup. If the patient cannot be stabilized medically, the interventional radiologist and surgeon are consulted. The location and severity of GI bleeding dictates therapy.

Upper GI Bleeding

If stable, upper GI endoscopy or colonoscopy is performed based on the patient's history. If the patient is not a surgical candidate due to underlying medical conditions, such as chronic obstructive pulmonary disease or severe cardiac disease, the radiologist is frequently asked to perform arteriography and transcatheter embolotherapy in the upper GI tract. The precise site of bleeding can usually be determined by angiography. A site of contrast extravasation on the delayed images obtained during the arteriogram determines the next course of action.

Lower GI Bleeding

Historically, transcatheter embolotherapy was not performed in the lower GI tract because of the risk of small or large bowel infarction. However, this practice has rapidly changed as super-selective catheters/guide wires may now be used to precisely deploy temporary or permanent embolic agents to stop bleeding in the lower GI tract (Sebrechts and Bookstein, 1988). Prior to development of microcatheters, a lower GI bleeding site was treated with a vasoconstricting drug such as vasopressin (Athanasoulis et al, 1982). Vasopressin is still occasionally used if super-selective catheterization of lower GI tract vessels is not technically possible (Table 102-1). However, this may prove risky in patients with coronary artery disease, hypertension, serum electrolyte disorders, and other medical conditions.

TABLE 102-1. Gastrointestinal Bleeding: Vasopressin

The step-by step procedure for Vasopressin infusion is as follows:
1. Selective arteriogram shows extravasation
2. Mixture of vasopressin solution is prepared; 100 U vasopressin is mixed with 500 mL of normal saline or 5% dextrose, giving a concentration of 0.2 U/mL. Alternatively, 200 U vasopressin may be mixed in 500 mL of solution for a concentration of 0.4 U/mL
3. Infusion is delivered with a constant arterial infusion pump at the rate of 30 to 60 mL/hr, depending on the dose rate to be delivered.
4. Infusion of vasopressin is initiated at 0.2 U/min for 20 minutes.
5. After 20 minutes of infusion, a repeat arteriogram is performed. The images are assessed for the presence of extravasation and for evidence of excessive constriction of mesenteric arterial branches. If constriction is excessive, the dose rate is reduced by half and the arteriogram is repeated 20 minutes later. If there is no extravasation, the catheter is secured in the groin, and the patient is transferred to the ICU with the infusion continuing. If extravasation is still present after 20 minutes of infusion, the infusion dose rate is doubled to 0.4 U/min, and a repeat arteriogram is performed 20 minutes later.
6. If bleeding is not controlled after infusion of 0.4 U/min, no further increasing in the dose rate is beneficial, and alternative methods for controlling bleeding should be considered.
7. Once the initial infusion dose rate has been established and control of bleeding confirmed, a usual infusion regime is as follows:
    Vasopressin at 0.2 U/min for 24 hours
    Vasopressin at 0.1 U/min for 24 hours
    Infusion is discontinued if no clinical evidence of further bleeding
    If the initial infusion dose rate is 0.4 U/min, the regime is as follows:
    Vasopressin at 0.4 U/min for 6 to 8 hours
    Vasopressin at 0.3 U/min for 16 hours
    Vasopressin at 0.2 U/min for 16 hours
    Vasopressin at 0.1 U/min for 16 hours
    Infusion is discontinued if no clinical evidence of further bleeding

Reprinted with permission from Athanasoulis et al, 1982.
ICU = intensive care unit.
Authors Technical Addendum To Vasopressin Therapy: After vasopressin has been tapered, an approximate 6- to 8-hour infusion of saline through the indwelling catheter is indicated. Thus, if the patient rebleeds, the catheter is already in place and the vasopressin may be restarted. At this point an alternate therapy should be considered (eg, surgery, super-selective catheterization and embolization, or a repeat course of vasopressin therapy).

Chapter Objectives

1. To briefly review vascular anatomy of the GI tract (ie, normal and variant anatomy)
2. To correlate upper and lower GI tract bleeding sites to specific anatomic vascular territories
3. To review the percutaneous transcatheter techniques used to manage patients with upper and lower GI hemorrhage

We will attempt to simplify the procedures and to briefly discuss indications, methods of treatment, embolic materials, complications, contraindications, and technical points.

Vascular Anatomy of the Upper GI Tract

During fluoroscopy, one notes that the celiac axis arises from the ventral surface of the aorta at the level between the lower half of the T12 vertebral body and the level of the T12 to L1 disc space. The celiac axis generally has the following three major branches: (1) the left gastric artery; (2) the common hepatic artery; and (3) the splenic artery (Reuter et al, 1986). There are several important variants in arterial anatomy and "textbook anatomy" is frequently not found. Knowledge of arterial anatomy is essential so that serious complications can be avoided during embolization procedures.

The arterial variants commonly found in the upper GI tract include the following:

1. The splenic artery may arise as a separate trunk from the aorta
2. The left gastric artery may arise directly from the aorta rather than from the celiac axis
3. Hepatic arterial blood supply is frequently variable

Normally, the right and left hepatic arterial blood supply arises from the proper hepatic artery. The proper hepatic artery is a short trunk that is found just distal to the point where the gastroduodenal artery (GDA) arises from the common hepatic artery. The left hepatic arterial blood supply may arise from the left gastric artery rather than from the proper hepatic artery. This is known as a "replaced" left hepatic artery. Similarly, the right hepatic artery may originate from the proximal aspect of the superior mesenteric artery (SMA). This is known as a "replaced" right hepatic artery. When a portion of the right or left hepatic arterial blood supply arises from the proper hepatic and the remainder arises from either the left gastric (in the case of left hepatic blood supply) or from the SMA (in the case of right hepatic arterial blood supply), the terms "accessory replaced" are used. Thus, a patient with left hepatic arterial blood supply arising in part from the proper hepatic artery (eg, a vessel supplying the medial segment of the left lobe) and from the left gastric artery (eg, supplying the lateral segment of the left lobe) has a so called "accessory replaced" left hepatic artery arising from the left gastric artery. Similarly, an "accessory replaced" right hepatic arterial blood supply may be seen. In the latter case, a portion of right hepatic arterial blood supply arises from the SMA and the remainder from the proper hepatic artery. The vessel arising from the SMA is an "accessory replaced" right hepatic artery. It is important to recognize right and left hepatic artery anatomic variants and to be aware that such variants are extremely common. There are numerous other variants including a "replaced common hepatic artery" to the SMA, etc.

The gastroesophageal junction is supplied primarily by small vessels arising from the left gastric artery. The fundus and a portion of the body of the stomach are also supplied by the left gastric arterial branches. Important arterial anastomoses exist between the left gastric artery and the spleen (ie, short gastric arteries). Terminal branches of the left gastric artery anastomose with the right gastric artery forming an arcade along the lesser curvature of the stomach. The right gastric artery generally arises at the bifurcation of the proper hepatic and gastroduodenal arteries. Variant anatomy may also be found at this location and the right gastric artery may arise from the common hepatic artery, etc. The right gastric artery is frequently not visualized during routine celiac arteriography.

The GDA supplies a portion of the stomach, the duodenum, and the pancreas. A rich anastomotic arcade is found between the pancreaticoduodenal blood supply arising from the GDA and the SMA via the inferior pancreaticoduodenal artery. The inferior pancreaticoduodenal artery arises from the proximal SMA and forms an anastomosis with the posterior and anterior pancreaticoduodenal arteries, the latter arising from the GDA. The terminal branch of the GDA is the right gastroepiploic artery. Similar to the right gastric/left gastric arterial arcade, the right gastroepiploic artery has a rich anastomotic network (arcade) with the left gastroepiploic artery along the greater curvature of the stomach. The left gastroepiploic artery is the terminal branch of the splenic artery.

ESOPHAGEAL VARICES

Life threatening hemorrhage from esophageal varices may result in patients with advanced liver disease and portal hypertension (see Chapter 117). The use of somatostatin in combination with other types of medical therapy has also been shown to be effective. Treatment of esophageal variceal hemorrhage is generally performed using endoscopic banding coupled with aggressive therapy, the latter to include use of drugs to lower portal pressure, occasionally balloon tamponade (eg, Blakemore tube), surgical decompressive portosystemic shunts (eg, mesocaval shunt, distal splenorenal [ie, Warren shunt]), and, recently, the transjugular intrahepatic portosystemic shunt (Zemel et al, 1991; Rosemurgy and Zervos, 2003). Systemic vasopressin (ie, given intravenously) has been used to control esophageal variceal bleeding. Gastric and ileal varices may also be treated using transcatheter techniques (Kiyosue et al, 2003; Kobayashi et al, 2001).

Transcatheter Embolotherapy in the Upper GI Tract

Indications

In general, transcatheter embolotherapy in the upper GI tract is indicated in a patient who (1) is actively bleeding and not a good surgical candidate, (2) is a surgical candidate but refuses an operation, or (3) requires stabilization prior to surgery. "Emergency" surgery, if still required after embolization, may then become "elective." Whether or not emergency surgery is required necessitates an active dialogue between all physicians caring for the patient. Transcatheter embolotherapy may be used in patients with various sources of upper GI bleeding (Table 102-2).

Postgastric Surgery

As mentioned earlier, present clinical and past surgical and medical histories are important. If a patient has had a prior Bilroth surgical procedure for ulcer disease, the normal arterial arcades (collateral blood supply) of the upper GI tract may be disrupted. Such collateral vessels may have been ligated during surgery. Transcatheter embolotherapy in such patients must be performed with caution because there is a greater risk of GI tract infarction. If embolotherapy must be performed, super-selective catheterization must be used. In the event of bowel infarction, the patient will require surgery.

Various options and their potential duration of "function" are shown in Table 102-3.

Technique

The goal of embolotherapy is to use larger particles to occlude vessels at bleeding sites. From a femoral approach, a selective catheter (such as a Cobra catheter) is directed over a guide wire into the celiac trunk. The catheter is advanced into a specific vessel (eg, the GDA). With the catheter tip precisely placed in the vessel to be embolized, occlusion of the vessel in the upper GI tract is generally accomplished using embolic spring coils or Gelfoam. As listed in Table 102-3, embolic spring coils (eg, stainless steel Gianturco coils, platinum "Nester" and "Tornado" coils, Cook, Inc., Bloomington, IN) are permanent embolic

TABLE 102-2. Use of Transcatheter Embolotherapy in Upper Gastrointestinal Bleeding

1. Ulcer disease
2. Gastritis (especially gastritis involving the fundus and upper portions of the stomach)
3. Trauma
4. Mallory-Weiss tear
5. Neoplastic disease
6. Patients with a coagulopathy that cannot be corrected.

TABLE 102-3. Embolic Materials

1. Embolic spring coils (Gianturco, "Nester," "Tornado" coils; Cook, Inc, Bloomington, IN), stainless steel or platinum coils with embedded Dacron fibers, permanent
2. Gelfoam (The Upjohn Company, Kalamazoo, MI) or Surgifoam (Ethicon, Johnson and Johnson, Somerville, NJ), protein foam that is cut into small cubes or "torpedoes," or made into a "slurry" or "pudding," temporary and lasting 2 to 4 weeks
3. Clot, temporary (usually lasting only hours).
4. Particulate polyvinyl alcohol (PVA) (Angiodynamics PVA Plus, Surgical Corporation, El Dorado Hills, CA; Cook, Inc., Bloomington, IN; Ivalon, (Interventional Therapeutics Corp, South San Francisco, CA; Unipoint Industries, Inc, High Point, NC), permanent
5. Embospheres (Biosphere Medical, Rockland, MA), permanent
6. Polymerizing tissue, "glues" (eg, n-butyl cyanoacrylate), (TruFill, Cordis Neurovascular, Johnson and Johnson, Miami, FL), permanent
7. Detachable balloons, permanent. Detachable balloons require placement of a guiding catheter. The balloons may be "floated" to the site of bleeding and used to "bridge" the site

agents; Gelfoam (Upjohn Co., Kalamazoo, MI) is temporary. Gelfoam is occlusive for several weeks and vessels so treated are subject to recanalization. Particulate ("solid") polyvinyl alcohol (ie, polyvinyl alcohol [PVA] or Ivalon), is another permanent embolic material, which may be used. However, Gelfoam powder or extremely small (ie, "dust like") PVA should not be used because of the risk of tissue infarction. Because of the risk of tissue necrosis, alcohol should also not be used to embolize vessels in the GI tract.

Vasoconstrictor

Occasionally a pharmacologic vasoconstrictor such as vasopressin may be infused directly through the catheter into the vascular territory. This method may be useful in patients who have had collaterals disrupted by prior GI surgery. (Please see the later section on the use of vasopressin in patients with lower GI hemorrhage).

Specific Sites

Patients with the following bleeding sites may be treated with transcatheter embolotherapy in the listed vascular distribution:

1. Bleeding peptic ulcer: embolization of the GDA
2. Gastritis: embolization of the left gastric artery or direct intra-arterial infusion of vasopressin into the left gastric artery
3. Trauma: embolization of the injured vessel
4. Mallory-Weiss tear: embolization of the left gastric artery.

Bridging a Bleeding Site

Perhaps the easiest and most rapid transcatheter technique for occluding blood flow is the use of Gelfoam or coils. *It is important to "bridge" a bleeding site so that collateral flow does not cause rebleeding.* For example, if the patient has peptic ulcer disease and a bleeding duodenal ulcer, and the GDA is embolized proximally, the patient may stop bleeding for a period of time and then rebleed several hours later. This may be due to reconstitution of blood flow through the GDA via the left and right gastroepiploic arteries along the greater curvature of the stomach. In this example, blood flows through the splenic artery, through the left gastroepiploic artery, retrograde through the right gastroepiploic artery and then into the GDA. Another pathway for reconstitution of GDA blood flow is via the inferior pancreaticoduodenal artery blood (from the SMA) with flow through the pancreaticoduodenal arteries to the GDA and to the site of hemorrhage. Several other collateral pathways may also contribute. It is therefore important to begin embolization *distal to the bleeding site* (if technically possible) and to occlude across the bleeding site, thereby reducing the chance of collateral blood flow causing recurrent hemorrhage.

Complications of Upper GI Tract Embolization

In general, the most significant complication of embolotherapy is that of organ *infarction*, or inadvertent embolization of other "nontarget" organs (eg, spleen). This occurs in 1 to 4% of cases. Fortunately, the "nontarget" organ embolization is usually well tolerated (eg, a small coil inadvertently enters a hepatic artery branch during GDA embolization). Infrequently, "nontarget" organ embolizations can be destructive (eg, loss of a coil in the hepatic artery during GDA embolization in the setting where the patient has portal vein thrombosis).

If vasopressin is used, bowel ischemia, bowel infarction, angina, serious catheter entry site, or systemic (ie, drug induced) complications, may occur. Examples of the latter include cerebral edema and electrolyte imbalances.

Lower GI Bleeding

Role of Nuclear Medicine Bleeding Scan

Unlike the upper GI tract where a nuclear medicine study is generally not helpful, a ^{99m}Technetium (^{99m}Tc) - labeled "tagged" red blood cell (RBC) study may be useful in helping to localize a bleeding site in the lower GI tract. One of the advantages of a ^{99m}Tc - labeled RBC study is that the patient may be scanned at intervals, thereby increasing the likelihood of detecting the bleeding site. A "single pass" Technetium-labeled sulfur colloid radionuclide study may be useful if the patient is actively bleeding but interval scanning is not possible. In those patients who are debilitated with renal insufficiency, assistance in localizing the bleeding site is useful so that the angiographic exam may be "tailored" and the quantity of contrast reduced. Colonoscopy likewise may prove useful but often patients with a lower GI hemorrhage present emergently and the colon is not clean (ie, prepped). The nuclear medicine "bleeding scan" is more sensitive than angiography in detecting lower GI tract hemorrhage, but less anatomically specific. It is generally stated that the nuclear medicine scan (in ideal situations) will detect a lower GI bleed rate as low as 0.1 cc/min; whereas angiography requires a bleeding rate of 1 cc/min (ie, IDX greater). There is a separate chapter on lower GI bleeding (see Chapter 101).

Anatomy of the Lower GI System

The SMA and inferior mesenteric artery (IMA) are the primary visceral trunks responsible for lower GI bleeding (Defreyne et al, 2003). The SMA is located caudal to the celiac axis (ie, immediately inferior to the celiac axis or usually within 2 cm). The SMA supplies a portion of the duodenum and pancreas (via the inferior pancreaticoduodenal arcade), the entire small bowel, the appendix, ascending colon, and approximately two-thirds to three-fourths of the transverse colon. The IMA arises from the ventral surface of the aorta between the levels of L2 to L4, most commonly at the L3 to L4 disc space level. The IMA supplies the distal most transverse colon, the descending and sigmoid colon, and the rectum. A rich collateral blood supply is found between the SMA and IMA via the middle colic (from the SMA) and the left colic (from the IMA). Another rich collateral network is found between the IMA (superior hemorrhoidal branches) and the internal iliac artery branches. Additional collateral supply is provided by the marginal artery of Drummond and the intra-arterial "bridge" between the left colic artery and middle colic artery called the arc of Riolan. In general, embolization in the SMA/IMA distribution is only performed if superselective catheterization can be achieved. This is further discussed below.

Transcatheter Therapy in the Patient With a Lower GI Hemorrhage

Indications

The indications for transcatheter embolotherapy in a patient with lower GI tract bleeding are similar to those for the patient with upper GI tract bleeding, including (1) the patient is actively bleeding and a poor surgical candidate, (2) the patient is deemed an appropriate surgical candidate but refuses surgery, or (3) the patient requires preoperative stabilization, thereby converting the "emergency" operation to an "elective" procedure. Diseases amenable to transcatheter embolotherapy are listed in Table 102-4.

TABLE 102-4. Diseases Amenable To Transcatheter Embolotherapy

1. A bleeding colonic diverticulum (Evangelista and Hallisey, 2000)
2. Trauma
3. Inflammatory bowel disease (eg, a specific bleeding site in a patient with Crohn's disease or occasionally ulcerative colitis) (Mallant-Hent et al, 2003)
4. Neoplastic disease (Spinosa et al, 1998)
5. Meckel's diverticulum
6. A ruptured aneurysm of the lower GI tract
7. Vascular malformations (focal) (Yoon et al, 2002)
8. Patients with a coagulopathy that cannot be corrected
9. Severe hemorrhoidal bleeding

Transcatheter Embolotherapy in the Lower GI Tract

If stable, a patient with lower GI bleeding should ideally undergo colonoscopy. As mentioned earlier, an nuclear medicine study may prove useful if colonoscopy is negative or indeterminate. The ^{99m}Tc tagged RBC study may help localize the bleeding site (ie, SMA versus IMA vascular territory) (Bentley and Richardson, 1991). The IMA injection is generally performed first during arteriography of the lower GI tract, because as contrast is excreted by the kidneys, the bladder becomes opacified. This opacification may obscure a sigmoid colon or rectal bleeding site. If the tagged RBC study indicates that the patient has a left colon/rectal bleed, an inferior mesenteric arteriogram is performed, generally using a Simmons I (ie, "shepherd's crook") catheter. Once formed, the catheter is used to selectively catheterize the proximal aspect of the IMA trunk. This catheterization technique requires forming the Simmons catheter into a hook configuration prior to engaging the vessel (ie, over the aortic bifurcation or in the aortic arch/descending thoracic aorta).

If the bleeding site is identified in the descending colon, super-selective catheterization is attempted (ie, advancing a microcatheter through the diagnostic catheter), followed by embolization of the bleeding site with microcolis or tiny particles (Nicholson et al, 1998; Cynamon et al, 2003; Bandi et al, 2001). Vasopressin may also be used and is generally infused directly into the IMA trunk (see Table 102-1 for preparation and infusions rates of vasopressin). The use of vasopressin does not require super-selective catheterization to deliver the drug. Instead, the Simmons I catheter may be directed so the catheter tip is engaged in the proximal aspect of the main trunk of the IMA. The technique is similar for the SMA (ie, vasopressin is infused into the main trunk of the SMA, rather than through a super-selective catheter). Vasopressin is then infused according to the scheduled outlined in Table 102-1 (Darcy, 2003).

Lower GI bleeding from the rectum has been treated with transcatheter Gelfoam embolization via super-selective catheterization of the distal most branches of the superior hemorrhoidal artery arising from the IMA. Reports using larger particles or Gelfoam delivered superselectively to stop small bowel and colonic bleeding have appeared in the literature. This has been shown to be safe and effective in experienced hands.

Vasopressin is not without risk (see Complications). Once vasopressin therapy has been initiated, the drug is tapered slowly. It is important that a 20-minute follow-up arteriogram be performed after initiation of vasopressin therapy. If there is excessive "pruning" of SMA or IMA vessels, bowel infarction may occur. Therefore, the vasopressin dosage must be reduced initially by half the amount or discontinued for a period of time, then restarted at a lower dosage. Patients will normally complain of mild abdominal cramping at the start of vasopressin therapy. However, unrelenting and continuous severe cramping necessitates a decrease in the vasopressin dosage because of the risk of bowel ischemia/infarction.

To reemphasize, in the SMA or IMA vascular distributions, transcatheter embolotherapy may be performed if the site of bleeding can be reached using super-selective catheterization techniques. Unlike the upper GI tract, embolization in the lower GI tract is "less forgiving." The microcatheter tip must be positioned as close as possible to the site of hemorrhage (eg, to the level of a single arterial branch at the level of the vasa recta). If possible, the marginal artery of Drummond should be preserved. If super-selective catheterization is not possible, alternative therapies to stop bleeding using vasopression, endoscopy, or surgery must be considered.

As an alternative to the use of iodinated contrast (eg, in patients with renal dysfunction), limited use of Gadolinium may prove helpful. Such magnetic resonance imaging contrast agents are injected intra-arterially and are only useful if digital subtraction arteriography is used (ie, computer-based imaging). In the authors' experience, the image quality and anatomic detail is not as good with Gadolinium as compared to the use of iodinated contrast agents. Intra-arterial injection of Gadolinium is considered "off-label" (ie, not FDA approved). If the cause of GI bleeding (upper or lower) is obscure, arteriography may identify a structural abnormality and should be performed as part of the comprehensive evaluation when other diagnostic tests (endoscopy, nuclear medicine, etc, are negative) (Rollins et al, 1991).

Provocative Testing

In the patient who is intermittently bleeding and in whom endoscopic and transcatheter techniques have failed to localize the site, the use of "provocative" measures to induce bleeding is controversial. The use of heparin, pharmacologic vasodilators and thrombolytic agents is not without considerable risk. Though described in the literature (Ryan et al, 2001), the authors of this chapter reserve this technique as a "last resort" (eg, in the patient who is "transfusion dependent" despite multiple extensive endoscopic and radiographic evaluations).

Complications

Complications of transcatheter therapy in both the upper and lower GI tract are listed in Table 102-5.

Contraindications to Transcatheter Therapy in The Patient with Upper and Lower GI Tract Hemorrhage

Contraindications are relative. A contrast allergy risk must be considered in any patient with a more generalized allergic history (eg, hives). In a patient with a strong allergic history to contrast (ie, anaphylaxis) and a life threatening GI hemorrhage, the arteriographic studies are usually performed with anesthesia backup.

General Technical Notes: Upper and Lower GI Bleeding

In the case of a patient with lower GI bleeding, if the IMA and SMA arteriograms fail to identify a bleeding site, a celiac arteriogram should be performed. Rarely, the middle colic artery (normally arising from the SMA) may have an anomalous origin from the celiac axis arterial distribution. Therefore, a transverse colonic bleeding site would not be detected in such a patient if only the IMA and SMA arteriograms were performed.

Occasionally, "prophylactic" embolization may be necessary in the upper GI tract (eg, endoscopy reveals a bleeding Mallory-Weiss tear). The patient may not be acutely bleeding at the time of the angiographic study; however, the clinical history and endoscopic findings strongly suggest the site.

Vasopressin is delivered intra-arterially with an infusion pump according to the directions outlined in Table 102-1. A vascular sheath is generally placed in the common femoral artery to maintain arterial access for extended periods of time (ie, 24 to 48 hours). The sidearm of the sheath is connected to a standard flush solution (usually with a low dose of heparin to reduce thrombus formation around the sheath).

In general, for digital subtraction arteriography, the rate of injection of contrast (diluted 50% with saline) for the celiac and SMA is 6 to 8 cc per second for a volume of 30 to 50 cc. The IMA injection is generally 4 cc per second for a volume of approximately 25 cc. The imaging sequence is 1 image per second for approximately 8 seconds followed by 1 image every other second for a total run of approximately 20 images. This imaging sequence insures arterial, venous and delayed images to look for "pooling" or "puddling" of contrast at the bleeding site (ie, contrast extravasation).

Technical Pitfalls and Hints

Occasionally, during a GI bleed, contrast may "track" in between the bowel mucosal folds creating a "pseudo-vein sign." If one sees a linear or gently curved "abdominal vessel" during an arteriogram that has the angiographic appearance of a vein (or follows the course of mucosal folds), be suspicious for a site of bleeding. In a brisk bleed, extravasated contrast may also track along the dependent region of a hollow viscus.

It is useful to place an angiographic sheath in the common femoral artery. The sheath can be flushed with heparinized saline and kept in place while the patient is in the ICU. In the event of GI tract rebleeding, percutaneous access is already present.

During infusion of vasopressin (which may last 1 to 2 days), it is useful to cover the percutaneous puncture site with a sterile adhesive clear dressing. (The clear dressing allows the nurses and physicians to clinically evaluate the region for possible groin hematoma formation).

Intravenous antibiotics are generally administered during transcatheter procedures (ie, vasopressin infusions or embolotherapy).

Conclusion

The nonsurgical (ie, transcatheter approach) to the treatment of patients with upper and lower GI bleeding requires knowledge of anatomy and angiographic techniques. Monitoring of patients in an ICU is mandatory. Transcatheter embolotherapy or infusion of vasopressin may prove life saving in patients who are poor surgical candidates, or in patients who refuse surgery or require stabilization. Therapy using transcatheter techniques is often definitive. The use of embolotherapy, as apposed to infusion of vasopressin, is felt to have a more durable clinical result (ie, less chance of rebleeding). Use of vasopressin is not without risk and the trend is to employ super-selective catheterization techniques to treat patients with upper and lower GI tract bleeding.

TABLE 102-5. Complications of Transcatheter Therapy in the Upper and Lower GI Tract

1. Complications of transcatheter embolotherapy include bowel infarction or ischemia. However, the risk–benefit ratio must be considered even in patients who have undergone prior GI surgery or bowel resection. Nontarget organ infarction is the major complication of transcatheter embolotherapy.
2. Complications of intra-arterial vasopression include the following:
    a. Cardiovascular (arrhythmias, myocardial infarction, hypertension)
    b. Metabolic (cerebral edema and electrolyte disturbances)
    c. Catheter related complications (eg, sepsis from indwelling catheters; pseudoaneurysm formation at the site of percutaneous puncture of the common femoral artery; thrombosis; or distal embolization).
    d. Visceral arterial complications to include bowel infarction and ischemia.
    e. Peripheral vascular complications due to the vasoconstrictive effects of vasopressin (eg, digit ischemia).

GI = Gastrointestinal.

Supplemental Reading

Aina R, Oliva VL, Therasse E, et al. Arterial embolotherapy for upper gastrointestinal hemorrhage: outcome assessment. J Vasc Interv Radiol 2001;12:195–200.

Athanasoulis CA, et al. Interventional radiology. Philadelphia: WB Saunders; 1982. p. 55–156.

Bandi R, Shetty PC, Sharma RP, et al. Super-selective arterial embolization for the treatment of lower gastrointestinal hemorrhage. J Vasc Interv Radiol 2001;12:1399–405.

Bentley DE, Richardson JD. The role of tagged red blood cell imaging in the localization of gastrointestinal bleeding. Arch Surg 1991;126:821–5.

Cynamon J, Atar E, Steiner A, et al. Catheter-induced vasospasm in the treatment of acute lower gastrointestinal bleeding. J Vasc Interv Radiol 2003;14:211–6.

Darcy M. Treatment of lower gastrointestinal bleeding: vasopressin infusion versus embolization. J Vasc Interv Radiol 2003; 14:535–43.

Defreyne L, Uder M, Vanlangenhove P, et al. Angiography for acute lower gastrointestinal hemorrhage: efficiency of cut film compared with digital subtraction techniques. J Vasc Interv Radiol 2003;14:313–22.

De Wispelaere JF, De Ronde T, Trigaux JP, et al. Duodenal ulcer hemorrhage treated by embolization: results in 28 patients. Acta Gastroenterol Belg 2002;65:6–11.

Evangelista PT, Hallisey MJ. Transcatheter embolization for acute lower gastroeintestinal hemorrhage. J Vasc Interv Radiol 2000;11:601–6.

Hastings GS. Angiographic localization and transcatheter treatment of gastrointestinal bleeding. Radiographics 2000;20:1160–8.

Hvizda JL, Wood BJ. Selective transcatheter platelet infusion for gastrointestinal bleeding after failed embolization with resistant thrombocytopenia. J Vasc Interv Radiol 2001;12:549–50.

Kiyosue H, Mori H, Matsumoto S, et al. Transcatheter obliteration of gastric varices: Part 1. Anatomic classification. Radiographics 2003;23:911–20.

Kiyosue H, Mori H, Matsumoto S, et al. Transcatheter obliteration of gastric varices: Part 2. Strategy and technique: based on hemodynamic features. Radiographics 2003;23:921–37.

Kobayashi K, Yamaguchi J, Mizoe A, et al. Successful treatment of bleeding due to ileal varices in a patient with hepatocellular carcinoma. Eur J Gastroenterol Hepatol 2001;13:63–6.

Lake JR. A hepatologist's view of TIPS-who needs it and when? Presented at Interventional Hepatobiliary Radiology: Percutaneous Portocaval Shunts, Biliary Stents, Tumor Chemoembolization Lithotripsy. Syllabus; 1992 June 4–6; San Francisco (CA): University of California School of Medicine; 1992. p. 170–7.

Lefkovitz Z, Cappell MS, Lookstein R, et al. Radiologic diagnosis and treatment of gastrointestinal hemorrhage and ischemia. Med Clin North Am 2002;86:1357–99.

Lewis MB, Lewis JH, Marshall H, Lossef SV. Massive hemorrhage complicating percutaneous endoscopic gastrostomy: treatment by means of transcatheter embolization of the right and left gastroepiploic arteries. J Vasc Interv Radiol 1999;10:319–23.

Mallant-Hent RCh, van Bodegraven AA, Meuwissen SG, Manoliu RA. Alternative approach to massive gastrointestinal bleeding in ulcerative colitis: highly selective transcatheter embolization. Eur J Gastroenterol Hepatol 2003;15:189–93.

Nicholson AA, Ettles DF, Hartley JE, et al. Transcatheter coil embolotherapy: a safe and effective option for major colonic hemorrhage. Gut 1998;43:79–84.

Patel TH, Cordts PR, Abcarian P, Sawyer MA. Will transcatheter embolotherapy replace surgery in the treatment of gastrointestinal bleeding? Curr Surg 2001;58:323–7.

Reuter SR, et al. Gastrointestinal angiography. 3rd ed. Philadelphia: WB Saunders; 1986. p. 282–338.

Richter GM, Noelge G, Palmaz JC, Roessle M. The transjugular intrahepatic portosystemic stent-shunt (TIPPS): results of a pilot study. Cardiocasc Intervent Radiolo 1990;13:200–7.

Rollins ES, Picus D, Hicks ME, et al. Angiography is useful in detecting the source of chronic gastrointestinal bleeding of obscure origin. AJR 1991;156:385–8.

Rosch J, Hanafess WN, Snow H. Transjugular portal venography and radiologic portacaval shunt: an experimental study. Radiology 1969;92:112–4.

Rosemurgy AS, Zervos EE. Management of variceal hemorrhage. Curr Probl Surg 2003;40:263–343.

Ryan JM, Key SM, Dumbleton SA, Smith TP. Nonlocalized lower gastrointestinal bleeding: provocative bleeding studies with intraarterial tPA, heparin, and tolazoline. J Vasc Interv Radiol 2001;12:1273–7.

Schenker MP, Duszak R Jr, Soulen MC, et al. Upper gastrointestinal hemorrhage and transcatheter embolotherapy: clinical and technical factors impacting success and survival. J Vasc Interv Radiol 2001;12:1263–71.

Sebrechts C, Bookstein JJ. Embolization in the management of lower gastrointestinal hemorrhage, seminars in interventional radiology. Vol 5. New York: Theime Medical Publishers, Inc; 1988. p. 39–48.

Spinosa DJ, Angle JF, McGraw JK, et al. Transcatheter treatment of life-threatening lower gastrointestinal bleeding due to advance pelvic malignancy. Cardiovasc Intervent Radiol 1998;21:503–5.

Srivastava DN, Gandhi D, Julka PK, Tandon RK. Gastrointestinal hemorrhage in hepatocellular carcinoma: management with transhepatic arterioembolization. Abdom Imaging 2002;25:380–4.

Yoon W, Kim JK, Kim HK, et al. Acute small bowel hemorrhage in three patients with end-stage renal disease: diagnosis and management by angiographic intervention. Cardiovasc Intervent Radiol 2002;25:133–6.

Zemel G, Katzen BT, Becker GJ, et al. Percutaneous transjuguluar portosystemic shunt. JAMA 1991;266:390–3.

CHAPTER 103

Diverticular Disease of the Colon

James W. Thiele, MD, and Ira J. Kodner, MD

Background

Diverticulosis of the colon is a relatively common condition in Western countries. The incidence of this condition increases with age and with the physiologic changes in the colon associated with a low fiber diet. Colonic diverticula consist of protrusions of the mucosa alone through the muscular layer of the colon wall. Since they lack a muscular coat and thus do not include all of the layers of the colon wall, they are considered "false" diverticula. Diverticulosis is a condition that implies only the presence of diverticula in the colon. Although a clinical syndrome often indistinguishable from the irritable bowel syndrome (IBS) consisting of intermittent left lower quadrant pain and cramping without sepsis may occur, this condition rarely requires operative intervention in the absence of bleeding. In contrast, the term diverticulitis describes the inflammation and infectious process that results from perforation of a diverticula. Symptoms can be local or diffuse, and the management of the acute condition relies on numerous factors.

Etiology

Diverticular disease and its complications were rare prior to the early twentieth century. It was only after 1920 that the condition was more commonly observed in Western countries, and many authors have postulated that such a dramatic change was likely due to dietary changes. In the later part of the nineteenth century, the grist mills that ground wheat into whole meal flour were replaced by more efficient roller mills that produced very pure white flour that lacked the fiber content of whole meal flour. In addition, improvements in refrigeration and food preservation led to an increase in fat, sugar, and protein intake. The overall result was a relatively dramatic decrease in dietary fiber. A high fiber diet produces a bulky stool that is more easily advanced by the peristaltic action of the colon. Constipated stools resulting from a lack of dietary fiber require more vigorous colonic contractions to be propelled through the colon. The ultimate result is increased collagen, elastin, and reticular tissue formation causing thickening of the colon wall. Thickening of the colon wall ultimately reduces the lumen and, according to the law of Laplace, subsequently raises intralumenal pressure causing the outward propulsive force that results in diverticula formation. This entire process is most prominent in the sigmoid colon because it is anatomically the narrowest portion. Subsequently, the sigmoid colon is also the most common site of diverticular formation.

Age is also a factor in development of diverticular disease. Not only does it take years of exposure to a low fiber diet for the above-mentioned changes to take place, but it has also been shown that the tensile strength and elasticity of the colon both decrease with age. Although diverticular disease is the most common pathologic condition affecting the colon, it is rare before the age of 30 years. However, it is estimated that diverticulosis affects as many as 40% of Americans over the age of 50 years and 75% of those over age 80 years.

Complications

Spasm

The changes in the wall of the colon seen with diverticulosis can result in a syndrome of intermittent abdominal pain and spasm that mimics *IBS*. Symptoms are generally mild and are not associated with fever or signs of sepsis. Treatment is usually conservative and includes measures such as a high fiber diet and pharmacologic agents aimed at decreasing colon spasm, such as hyoscyamine. Symptoms are usually self-limited but may recur with some degree of regularity. Many patients with presumed recurrent "diverticulitis" may actually be suffering from intermittent spasm associated with diverticulosis. An antibiotic regimen is often started without radiographic confirmation of true diverticulitis, and in patients with spasm alone, it is simply the tincture of time, not antibiotic therapy, which has improved their condition. This fact is important to remember because true recurrent diverticulitis may warrant surgical intervention whereas the treatment of pain associated with spasm alone rarely does.

Bleeding

One of the weakest areas in the muscular wall of the colon, and thus a common site of diverticular formation, is the point at which perforating mesenteric arterial vessels penetrate. Because of the close association of the diverticula to the adjacent artery, erosion can occur resulting in significant blood loss. Despite the fact that only a thin membrane of mucosa separates the lumen of the colon from the peritoneal cavity within the diverticulum, bleeding is virtually always into the colon rather than the peritoneal cavity. Blood is a cathartic and moves quickly through the colon. Thus, brisk bleeding in the colon is usually evident relatively soon after it starts and presents as the passage of large amounts of bright red blood per rectum. It is important to differentiate diverticular bleeding from that of other sources of colonic bleeding and from upper gastrointestinal (GI) bleeding. There is a separate chapter on lower GI bleeding (see Chapter 101, "Lower Gastrointestinal Bleeding"). Acute lower GI bleeding most often occurs in patients older than 60 years, and although medical management combined with colonoscopy and interventional radiology is most often effective in controlling the blood loss, surgical intervention is necessary in 10 to 25% of patients.

Infection

Simple

Most patients who present with acute diverticulitis complain of acute onset left lower quadrant abdominal pain. Fever is often present as well and the patient may report bowel changes such as diarrhea or constipation. Bleeding is not generally associated with acute infection, and although patients may report association with a particular type of food, diet is generally not a contributing factor. Diagnostic studies should be aimed at both demonstrating the presence of inflammation as well as ruling out complications such as abscess, fistula, or free perforation. Computed tomography (CT) scan is probably the single best test in the setting of presumed acute inflammation because it reliably detects the location of inflammation and also detects any associated abscess that may be present. Fistulas may also be demonstrated if air is seen in adjacent structures such as the urinary bladder. Colonoscopy and contrast enema studies are less desirable in the acute setting as they carry the risk of extravasation of contrast or air via the involved diverticulum

The presence of diverticulitis alone implies perforation of a diverticulum at some level. Most cases are mild and associated with microperforation of a diverticulum that allows intralumenal bacteria to escape and incite a pericolonic inflammatory process. In general, the treatment of acute diverticulitis not associated with abscess, stricture, fistula, or free perforation is *broad spectrum antibiotic* coverage with or without diet alterations. Seventy percent or more of patients who have recovered from an uncomplicated episode of diverticulitis will have no further problems in their lifetime. However, after a *second uncomplicated attack*, the odds of further episodes are > 50%. Recurrent episodes of radiographically documented diverticulitis, especially in young patients, are an indication for elective surgical resection of the involved segment.

Complicated

Diverticulitis is considered complicated when the disease process is associated with abscess, fistula to and adjacent an organ, stricture, or free perforation into the peritoneal cavity. As with uncomplicated disease, the best initial diagnostic test is a CT scan in any patient suspected of having complicated disease. Depending on the type of complication present, patients may present with symptoms similar to uncomplicated disease, or they may present in distress with signs of an acute abdomen. Patients with stricture formation may have few acute symptoms as the complication generally develops slowly over time. They will however likely describe a history of multiple episodes of acute diverticulitis. If stricture is suspected and the patient lacks acute symptoms, colonoscopy or a contrast study is indicated to further evaluate the diseased segment as well as the more proximal colon. Similarly, patients with fistulas to pelvic organs may have few acute symptoms but are likely to report problems such as recurrent urinary tract infection, vaginal discharge, or pneumaturia. Colonoscopy is not likely to be helpful, and contrast studies may or may not demonstrate the fistula tract (Figure 103-1). If a fistula to the bladder is suspected but cannot be definitely demonstrated on contrast study, oral administration of 30 cc of activated charcoal can be helpful. Urinalysis performed daily should yield charcoal crystals on examination if a fistula is present. In the absence of acute symptoms, patients with stricture or fistula can often be treated electively and do not need urgent hospital admission.

In contrast, patients who present with abscess formation or free intraperitoneal perforation are often acutely ill and require hospitalization and, *occasionally,* urgent operative intervention. In the past most patients who presented with abscess or perforation were treated with urgent resection of the diseased segment and diversion via either a colostomy or ileostomy. Recent advances in *interventional radiology* and the aggressive use of *total parenteral nutrition (TPN)* and *intravenous (IV) antibiotics* have changed the approach to many of these patients, allowing for an *elective resection* with avoidance of a diverting ostomy.

Treatment of Diverticular Disease

Bleeding

Management of acute lower GI bleeding from diverticular disease should start with resuscitation of the patient followed by identification of the bleeding site. Most patients either stop bleeding spontaneously, or respond to medical or less invasive measures. However, almost a quarter of these patients will require surgical intervention for treatment of their disease.

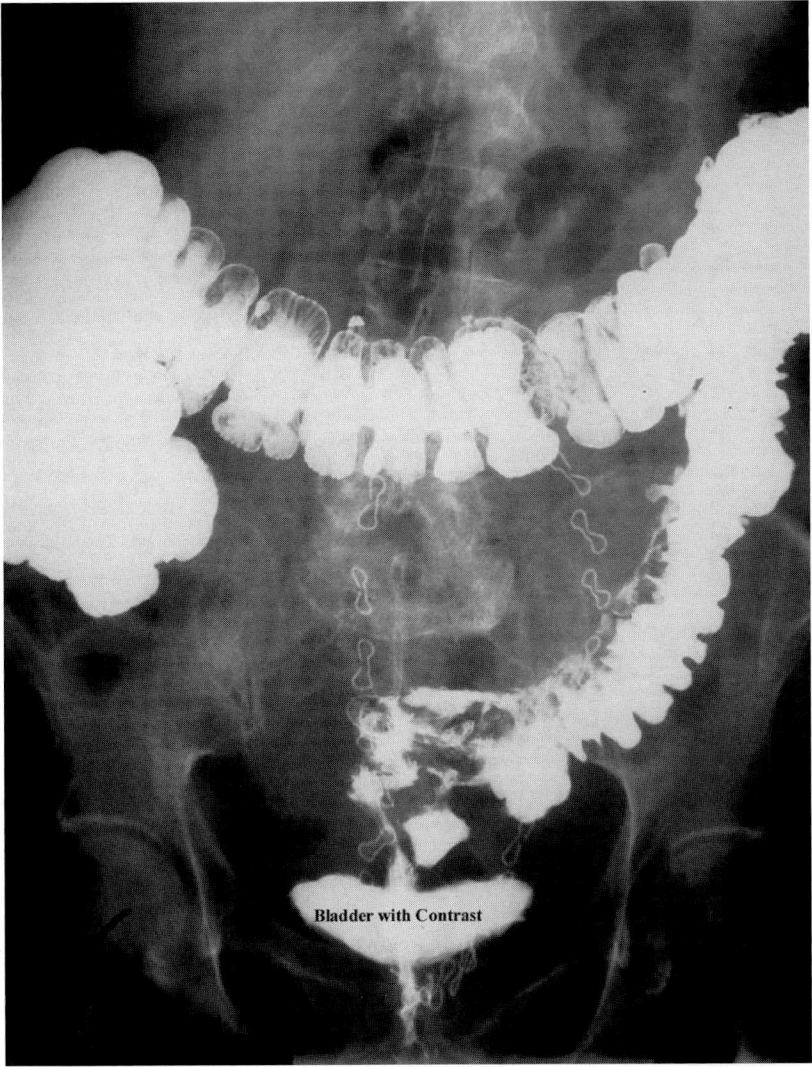

FIGURE 103-1. Contrast enema demonstration filling of the bladder due to a colovesicle fistula.

The steps in identification and treatment of a suspected colonic diverticular bleed are relatively straight-forward (Figure 103-2). It is important that after a nasogastric tube is placed that bilious aspirate devoid of blood is demonstrated. Clear fluid without bile may represent only stomach contents and brisk duodenal bleeding could still be present. Once an upper GI bleed has been ruled out, proctoscopy can be easily performed at the bedside. This will allow evaluation of the distal 15 to 18 cm and effectively rule out that site as a source of bleeding. This is important should an emergent operation be needed without a definite site identified, as will be discussed later.

A tagged red blood cell scan is generally seen as the best initial study in determining the site of GI bleeding. In addition to being the least invasive test, it also has no detrimental affect on renal function. This is an important advantage as many patients with brisk GI bleeding are severely hypovolemic and present with an elevated creatinine. Although a nuclear scan is the least accurate in determining the specific site of bleeding, it generally does provide enough information to allow for a segmental resection if needed. It also is helpful in determining if the bleeding is originating from the superior or inferior mesenteric artery distribution. This will allow for selective catheterization of the appropriate vessel should arteriography be necessary, thus limiting IV dye load to the patient.

If bleeding continues and the patient is stable, the next step in treatment is arterial catheterization of the appropriate vessel. This will not only provide information about the specific site of bleeding (Figure 103-3), but will also allow for the infusion of vasopressin or selective embolization to control bleeding. The preceding chapter is on therapeutic radiologic approaches (see Chapter 102, "Transcatheter Management of Upper and Lower Gastrointestinal Bleeding"). If bleeding either

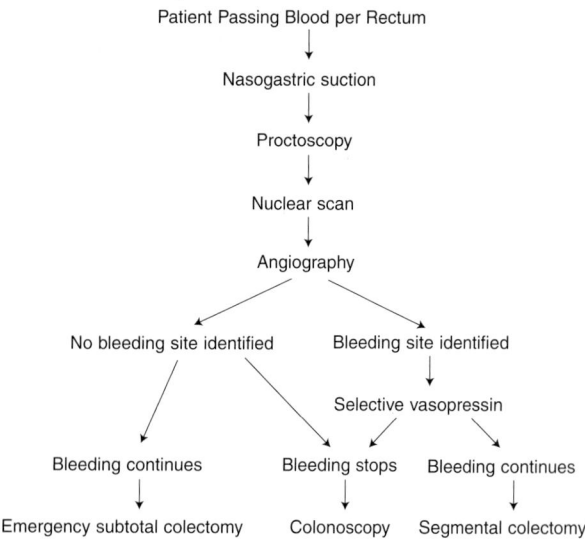

FIGURE 103-2. Evaluation and treatment of lower gastrointestinal bleeding. Reprinted with permission from Kodner IJ, et al, 1993.

stops spontaneously or can be controlled with angiographic techniques but the actual diagnosis (ie, diverticular bleed, arteriovenous malformation [AVM], cancer, etc.) is in question, elective colonoscopy after bowel preparation is indicated. Some causes of bleeding, such as AVMs, can be treated with cauterization whereas cancers or polyps can be biopsied or removed.

Some clinicians advocate the use of "emergent colonoscopy" in the setting of acute hemorrhage as a single procedure for both diagnosis and treatment. Orally administered lavage permits adequate colon preparation within 2 hours. An experienced colonoscopist can reach the cecum in 90% of cases, and modalities such as electrocoagulation, photocoagulation, or heater probe can be used to address bleeding sites via the colonoscope. There is a separate chapter on lower GI bleeding (see Chapter 101, "Lower Gastrointestinal Bleeding"). Despite the success rate of emergent colonoscopy, we still feel that the approach outlined in figure Figure 103-2 is the best in treating patients with continuing lower gastrointestinal GI bleeding with known diverticular and no other known disease.

Indications for surgical intervention in the treatment of lower GI bleeding include (1) the need for transfusion of more than 4 units of packed red blood cells in a 24-hour period to maintain adequate hematocrit levels, (2) any patient who rebleeds during the same hospitalization, and (3) hemodynamic instability despite resuscitation efforts. In the event that the bleeding site had been demonstrated by nuclear scan, angiography, or colonoscopy, *segmental colon resection* is the procedure of choice. Right-sided lesions can be treated with resection and primary anastomosis even without formal preoperative bowel preparation whereas left sided lesions have traditionally required resection and diverting colostomy. Recently, several authors have advocated *intraoperative colonic lavage* as a method of

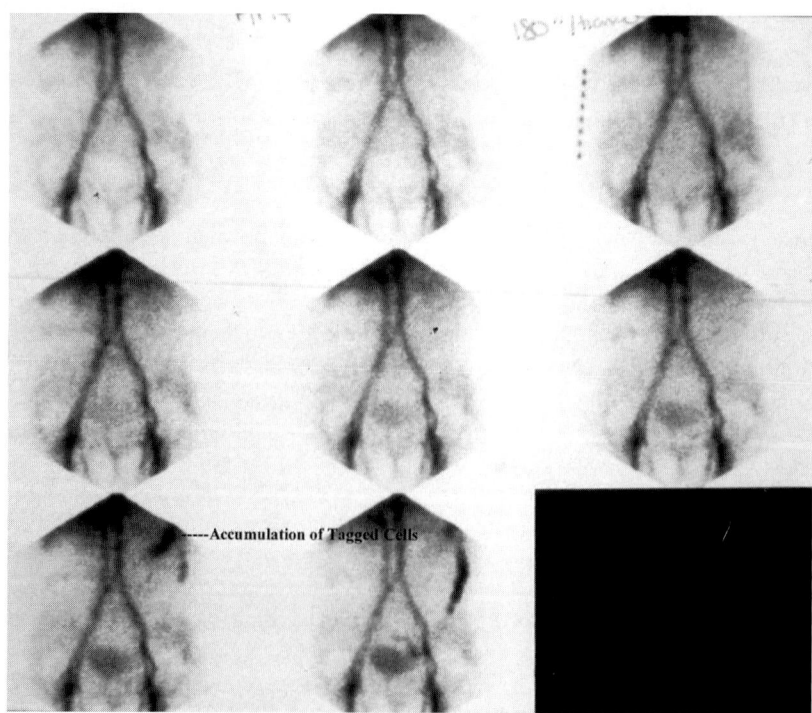

FIGURE 103-3. Bleeding scan showing accumulation of tagged cells in the area of the splenic flexure on the final two images.

mechanical bowel cleansing and subsequent primary anastomosis for left-sided lesions without preoperative bowel preparation. Although success rates are good with this approach, we still feel that unstable patients should undergo resection and diversion, either with an end colostomy or with primary anastomosis and a diverting loop ileostomy.

If a definitive bleeding site has not been located on any preoperative testing then the procedure of choice is a *total abdominal colectomy* with ileorectal anastomosis. As long as the rectum is devoid of solid stool, an anastomosis can be safely performed even in the absence of preoperative bowel preparation. The anastomosis should be at the level of the sacral promontory and special care should be taken to preserve the superior rectal artery in ensure adequate blood supply to the anastomosis. Most patients generally tolerate this procedure very well and fears of postoperative diarrhea are as a whole unwarranted. Although several loose bowel movements per day are to be expected, continence is generally not a problem because the rectum is left entirely intact. Those patients who do complain of incapacitating diarrhea generally respond well to antimotility agents such as Immodium or Lomitil.

Diverticulitis

Simple

The treatment of uncomplicated diverticulitis is relatively straight-forward in most cases. Patients usually respond to broad spectrum antibiotics (*ciprofloxocin* 500 mg twice daily combined with *metronidazole* 500 mg 4 times daily) given orally in an outpatient setting. Many practitioners choose to also limit the patient's diet during the first 48 to 72 hours of treatment depending on the severity of symptoms. Diet alterations may include keeping the patient on liquids, with or without high calorie supplements such as Ensure, or simply a low residue diet devoid of fiber. Pain control is important, especially if the patient is ill enough to be admitted to the hospital. If patients respond clinically in the first 48 to 72 hours with significant resolution of symptoms, they are generally transitioned back to a regular diet and eventually to a high fiber diet.

Patients who do not respond to conservative management as an outpatient should be considered for inpatient treatment with *IV antibiotics* and possibly more severe diet restrictions with the addition of *parenteral nutrition*. Morphine should be *avoided* as it has the side effect of increasing colonic intralumenal pressure, which can actually worsen the inflammatory process. *Meperidine* or *Toradol* are better choices for analgesia in patients with acute diverticulitis. Repeat CT imaging should also be considered as a lack of resolution of symptoms may indicate a complication, such as abscess or free perforation, that needs to be addressed. Failure to resolve an acute, uncomplicated episode of diverticulitis is an indication for elective resection. However, in our experience it is unusual for patients to fail to respond to aggressive treatment with IV antibiotics and complete bowel rest with the addition of TPN in the absence of complicated disease.

After resolution of the acute inflammatory process, the colon should be imaged to rule out the possibility of cancer and to evaluate the extent of disease. Colonoscopy is probably the best test, especially in patients over 50 years of age who have never been screened for colon cancer. Barium enema may suffice in younger patients, although the presence of any mucosal abnormalities would necessitate an endoscopic study for further examination and biopsy if appropriate.

Complicated

Any complication associated with diverticulitis is an indication for resection of the diseased segment, although the goal should be to approach the procedure in an elective setting after complete bowel prep and proper medical clearance of the patient. If managed properly most patients with complicated diverticulitis, even those with free perforation, can be treated with a single stage procedure that avoids colostomy.

Patients who present with stricture or fistula associated with diverticular disease often do not have signs and symptoms of acute inflammation or active diverticulitis. *Stricture* is usually the result of recurrent episodes of acute inflammation resulting in thickening and fibrosis of the wall of the colon. Most patients present with signs of partial colonic obstruction that can be documented by both CT or water soluble contrast enema. Patients who develop *colonic fistulas* as a result of diverticular disease can present with a variety of complaints depending on the site of the fistula. Air in the urine (pneumaturia) or stool in the urine (fecaluria) are common complaints of patients who present with a colovesical fistula, and, although these are relatively benign complaints, urosepsis can also develop as a result of chronic contamination of the urinary tract. Female patients may complain of vaginal discharge if a colovaginal fistula is present, and weight loss with chronic diarrhea can be the result of a functional intestinal bypass if a proximal enterocolonic fistula is present. Demonstration of the fistula tract on contrast studies may not always be successful, even with an obvious clinically symptomatic fistula.

Treatment of both stricture and fistula consists of *elective resection* of the diseased colonic segment with primary anastomosis. Due to the often chronic nature of these complications, diet alterations and long term antibiotic therapy are often not needed in the preoperative period. However, if the fistula or stricture is associated with acute inflammation, TPN, bowel rest, and antibiotics are indicated prior to surgery. Management of the affected secondary organ in fistula disease can vary depending on the size of the fistula. Small defects in the bladder or vagina can be closed primarily if there is minimal surrounding inflammation. Placement of a drain in the area is suggested and if the bladder is repaired primarily, an indwelling foley catheter should be left in place for 5 to 7 days. Placement of ureteral stents is recommended when approaching any case of complicated diverticular disease to aid in identification of the ureters and to ensure that if ureteral damage occurs it will be identified. Colonic stenting has no place in the long term treatment of stricture secondary to diverticular disease but may be used as a temporizing measure to allow for mechanical preparation prior to elective colon resection.

Patients who present with *abscess* or *free perforation* as a result of diverticular disease are generally more acutely ill and have signs and symptoms of acute diverticulitis. Localized abdominal pain may progress to more diffuse peritoneal signs with unstable vital signs if free perforation is present. Abscess should be suspected if patients fail to respond to appropriate therapy for presumed uncomplicated diverticulitis. The ultimate goal in treatment of colonic perforation and abscess is resection of the affected segment. In the past this was accomplished with a two or three stage procedure that involved temporary diversion of the fecal stream. However, the advent of radiologic techniques for drainage of abscess and more aggressive preoperative and operative management of these patients, the treatment of perforation and abscess associated with diverticular disease has certainly been in evolution.

The current approach to an abscess associated with diverticular disease is generally *antibiotics*, *bowel rest*, and *drainage* of larger abscesses via *interventional radiologic techniques*. After an abscess is diagnosed by CT scan patients are made NPO and started on appropriate IV antibiotic therapy. Small abscesses (< 4cm) will often resolve with this approach alone and after 5 to 7 days of therapy, patients should be re-evaluated with a second CT scan to ensure resolution. Persistent abscesses my require drainage, whereas those that are resolving will likely continue to do so with continued medical management alone. Larger abscesses (> 4 cm) should be drained early in the course of treatment, as they are unlikely to resolve with medical therapy alone. The length of time needed for bowel rest will vary from case to case but if patients are improving after 5 to 7 days of bowel rest and IV antibiotics, they can usually be transitioned to a liquid diet with high calorie shake supplements and oral antibiotics. Timing of elective resection will vary but should be delayed until complete resolution of the abscess, and significant improvement of the surrounding inflammatory process can be documented a soft, nontender abdomen on physical examination is reassuring. Colonoscopy should also be considered prior to elective resection in those patients who have not had a full colonic evaluation in the past 12 months.

Free intraperitoneal perforation of the colon associated with *acute diverticulitis* has generally been treated with *emergent resection* of the colon with *diversion* of the fecal stream (Hartmann's procedure, Figure 103-4). This approach has been met with a great deal of success with respect to patient survival. However, it does result in a colostomy and the need for a second major abdominal procedure in order to restore intestinal continuity. We have recently been approaching this situation differently in an attempt to manage free perforation associated with acute diverticulitis with a *single stage procedure* that can be performed electively and avoids colostomy. Most patients who present with free intraperitoneal air associated with acute diverticulitis are stable and despite the free perforation have only localized peritoneal signs. Many of these patients are noted to have free air only because of improvements in diagnostic techniques such as CT scanning. It is our belief that in most of these patients the area of perforation has already been sealed secondary to surrounding inflammation and that the only treatment required is *strict bowel rest* and *antibiotic therapy* in the initial stages of presentation. Most of these patients can then be converted from an emergent surgical setting to an elective setting without the need for a colostomy. Certainly, patients with *feculent peritonitis* (grade 4 perforation, Figure 103-5) or those that are unstable are not candidates for this approach. However, those that are candidates can be managed by following the

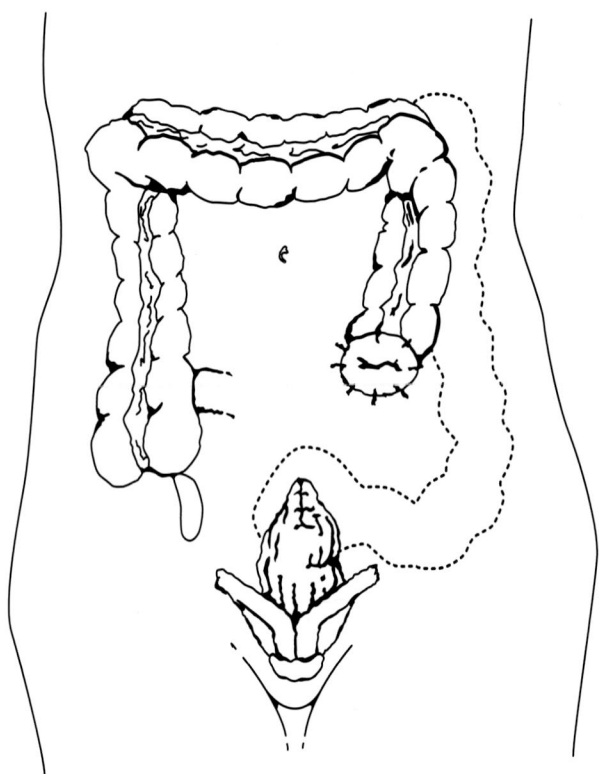

FIGURE 103-4. Hartmann resection. Reprinted with permission from Kodner IJ et al, 1993.

Perforated Diverticulitis CT Grading System

- <u>Grade 1</u> Localized free air (peri-colonic) without abscess

- <u>Grade 2</u> Small (< 2 cm) collections of distant free air OR small (< 4 cm) abscess

- <u>Grade 3</u> Larger (> 2 cm) collections of distant free air OR large (> 4 cm) abscess

- <u>Grade 4</u> Free air with non-loculated free fluid in the peritoneal cavity (feculent peritonitis)

FIGURE 103-5. Computed tomography (CT) grading system for perforated diverticulitis.

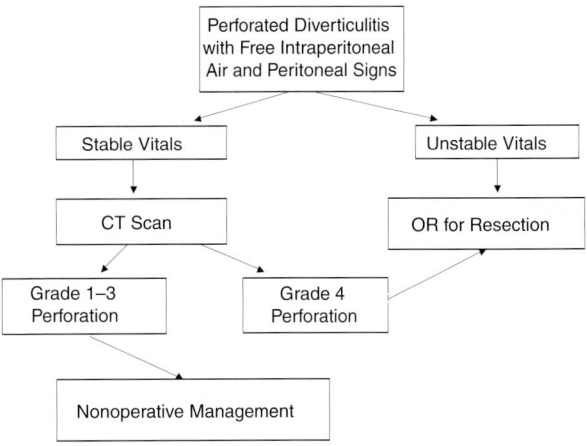

algorithm outlined in Figure 103-6. It should be stressed that if at any point in the algorithm the patient becomes unstable or is not responding appropriately to therapy, this approach should be abandoned and the patient should be taken to the operating room for a Hartmann's procedure. If conversion of a case of free perforation to an elective procedure is successful, as mentioned with the treatment of abscess disease, the patient should have colonic clearance preoperatively and consideration should be given to placement of *ureteral stents* preoperatively.

The exact management must be determined by not only the presence of either recurrent or complicated disease but also by the overall health and living situation of the patient. For example, a very young man with a single episode of severe inflammation requiring hospitalization should be considered for an elective resection after the acute episode resolves due to the high likelihood of future problems in his lifetime. Likewise, a frail elderly person who lives in a remote area and had cardiac instability after one episode of an acute diverticular bleeding should also be considered for elective resection if it is felt that the risk of complication from future bleeding is greater than the risk of surgery. Because of the increasing numbers of planned immune suppression (ie, organ transplantation) patients who are at increased risk from the ravages of colonic diverticular perforation, *elective colonic resection* is often advocated prior to the initiation of the compromised state.

The indications for surgery are further confused by notoriously variable data. Results of resection after one relatively minor episode of inflammation will obviously be superior to those where the indication for resection is either serious septic complications or life threatening bleeding. It is important that the ultimate decision to proceed with elective resection for diverticular disease be one made by both the physician and informed patient who knows the options for operative and nonoperative management and the risks and benefits of each approach.

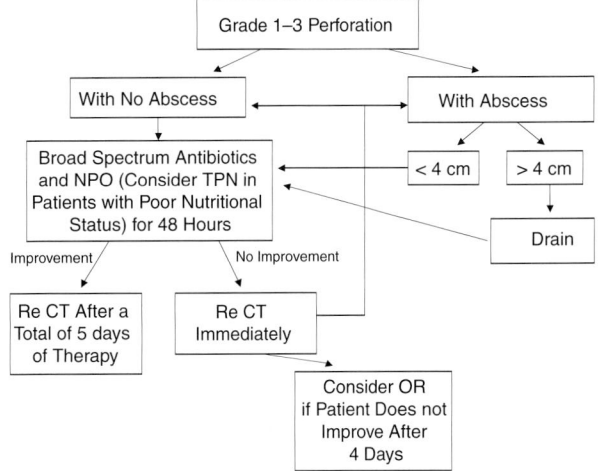

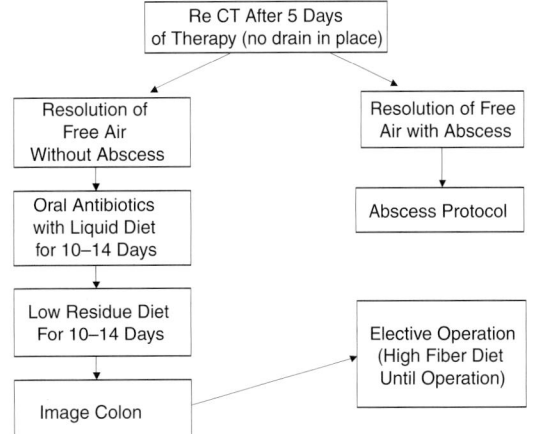

FIGURE 103-6. Algorithm for managing diverticulitis with free perforation. CT = computed tomography; NPO = nothing by mouth; OR = operating room; TPN = total parenteral nutrition.

Supplemental Reading

Kodner IJ, Fry RD, Fleshman JW, Birnbaum EH. Colon rectum and anus. In: Schwartz SI, editor. Principles of surgery. 6th ed. New York: McGraw-Hill; 1993. p. 1209.

CHAPTER 104

Laboratory Evaluation and Liver Biopsy Assessment in Liver Disease

F. Fred Poordad, MD

The appropriate use and understanding of serum liver biochemical tests has been a source of some confusion for health care providers at all levels. There have been changes in nomenclature for some of the enzymes, adding to the confusion. More importantly, the relative usefulness of the serum tests varies by disease state, and this perhaps leads to the greatest misunderstanding of how best to use these tests. Because the liver has such diverse functions, assessing injury requires the use of multiple tests in combination, with no single test or panel being sufficient to assess liver dysfunction or disease.

The liver biopsy has evolved recently in both technique and application. Until the percutaneous biopsy technique was adopted for routine use, liver biopsy was considered a major undertaking that was performed surgically, usually via laparoscopy. It was an inpatient procedure requiring at least a 24-hour stay. Now, percutaneous biopsies are routinely performed with a variety of needles and techniques and have evolved from being an inpatient procedure to an outpatient procedure often performed with only local anesthesia. The appropriate use and timing of liver biopsies for some liver disorders is well established, but for others like hepatitis C (HC), there is no consensus about how it should best be used. In addition, there have been noninvasive assays recently developed to complement the liver biopsy and perhaps in the future supplant it.

This chapter describes the various patterns of liver enzyme abnormalities and how they correlate with hepatic disorders. It also addresses the techniques of liver biopsy and its applications.

Liver Enzymes

There are multiple biochemical tests commonly referred to as liver enzymes, but for the purposes of this chapter we will discuss only those that are readily available and used in routine clinical practice. Biochemical liver tests can be summarized as those that reflect injury and those that reflect synthetic or excretory function. This text will refer to liver function tests (LFTs) as those tests that reflect the latter, and will not refer to the enzymes that generally reflect injury, the aminotransferases. The most commonly used liver tests are bilirubin, alkaline phosphatase, and the aminotransferases. Other less commonly used but useful tests are γ-glutamyl transpeptidase (GGT), 5′-nucleotidase (5′NT), albumin, and prothrombin time (PT). Aminotransferase tests are for aspartate aminotransferase (AST), formerly serum glutamic oxaloacetic transaminase, and alanine aminotransferase (ALT), formerly serum glutamic pyruvic transaminase, both of which participate in hepatic gluconeogenesis. Leakage of these enzymes into serum occurs with hepatocyte injury and death. Whereas ALT is quite liver specific, AST is not and is also commonly found in skeletal and cardiac muscle tissue. A more complete description of each is given in Tables 104-1 and 104-2.

The aminotransferases are generally reflective of parenchymal liver injury, such as that seen with viral hepatitis, medication or toxin-induced injury, autoimmune hepatitis, and several infiltrative disorders, such as hemochromatosis, Wilson's disease, α-1-antitrypsin deficiency, and fatty liver disease. Of course, in some of these conditions, alkaline phosphatase and GGT can be elevated to some extent as well, but bilirubin is not elevated unless there is obstruction to bile flow or significant liver dysfunction or injury.

Alkaline phosphatase is a ubiquitous enzyme often elevated in disorders of the biliary tract, but can also be mildly elevated in various liver diseases primarily involving the parenchyma, possibly as a result of injury to small bile ducts. It can also be elevated as a result of normal physiology in pregnancy and childhood, and in pathologic bone conditions. Interestingly, alkaline phosphatase does not always rise immediately with bile duct obstruction. Elevations are not simply a "backwash" of the enzyme into the serum, but rather require upregulation of messenger ribonucleic acid for increased production of alkaline phosphatase in response to bile duct epithelial injury.

GGT is an ubiquitous enzyme found in many organs including brain, intestine, heart, kidney, and the liver, but importantly not found in bone. Hence, its elevation suggests alkaline phosphatase elevation is not of bone origin. A more specific, but rarely used test is for 5′NT, which is also found in several organs but only released into plasma by the liver when injured. Hence, its elevation is very specific to the liver.

Bilirubin can be elevated for a myriad of reasons, some attributable to liver excretory dysfunction or significant

TABLE 104-1. Enzymes Reflecting Liver Injury

Lab Test	Physiologic Function	Source	Commonly Associated Liver Abnormalities	Of Note	Pitfalls
AST	Catalyzes transfer of aminogroup from aspartic acid to ketoglutaric acid to produce oxaloacetic acid	Liver, heart, kidney, pancreas, brain, RBC, WBC	Viral hepatitis, alcohol liver injury, ischemichepatic injury, drug induced hepatitis, fatty liver disease, Wilson's disease, celiac disease, α-1-Antitrypsin deficiency	AST/ALT ratio > 2 typically due to alcohol injury. AST/ALT > 1 also seen in cirrhosis. ALT rarely > 300 U/L in chronic conditions.	May be normal viral hepatitis or with advancing fibrosis. Falsely low with dialysis. Poor correlation with degree of liver necrosis in acute setting.
ALT	Catalyzes transfer of amino group from alanine acid to ketoglutaric acid to ketoglutaric produce pyruvic acid	Liver			
LDH	Catalyzes interconversion of lactate and pyruvate	Heart, liver, kidney, muscle, brain, blood cells, lungs, necrotic conditions, infiltrative disorders, hemolysis, muscle injury, malignancies	Several isoenzymes which can be measured. Poor specificity for liver disease, and not useful overall.		

ALT = alanine aminotransferase; AST = aspartate aminotransferase; LDH = lactate dehydrogenase; RBC = red blood cells; WBC = white blood cells.

liver injury, and at other times, not related to the liver at all. The most important reasons for bilirubin elevation are obstructive disorders of bile flow and hepatic dysfunction, which may be mild or indicative of liver failure. The latter is generally accompanied by other signs, including cognitive and psychomotor dysfunction and coagulation disorders. Liver related disorders such as congenital hyperbilirubinemias (Tables 104-2 and 104-3) are characterized by bilirubin abnormalities due to enzyme deficiencies but are not reflective of liver failure or synthetic dysfunction per se.

A general scheme of the proper workup and diagnosis of disorders associated with patterns of liver disease is outlined in Figure 104-1. Although this is simplified, it does reflect the thought process one should have when assessing elevated enzymes. The old axiom of rechecking abnormal enzymes to confirm chronicity holds true, but enzymes are rarely spuriously elevated without some underlying pathology, even if the pathology is transient, such as idiosyncratic medication-induced injury. Occasionally enzymes may be elevated with systemic disease and not reflect underlying liver disease, but these situations are generally understood because of other

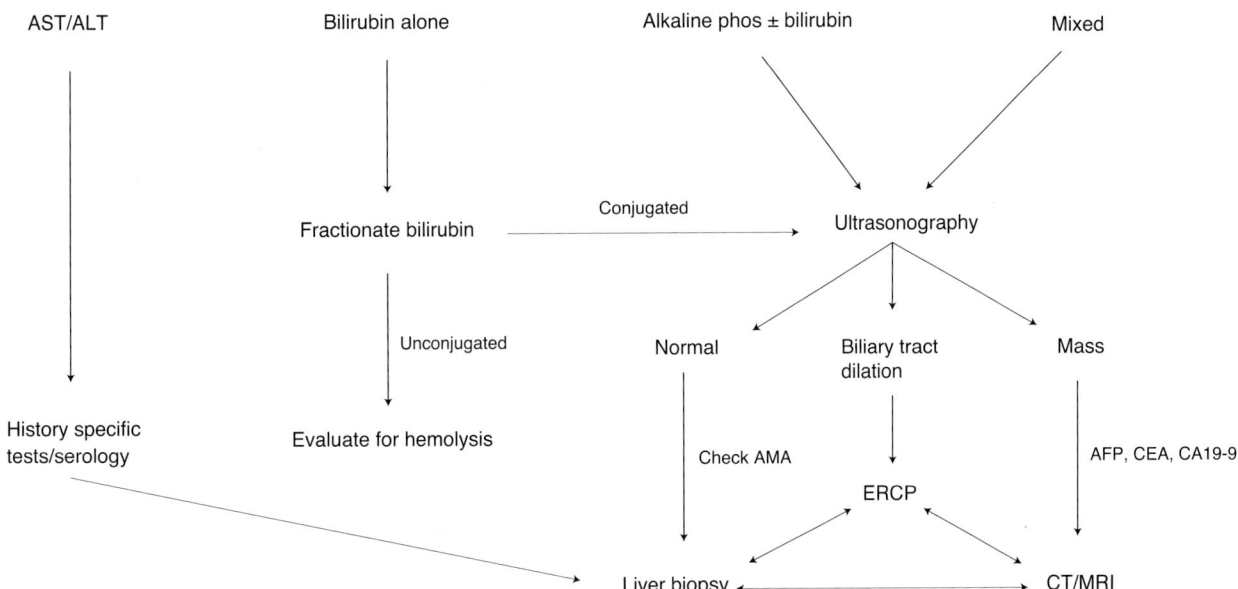

FIGURE 104-1. A general scheme of the proper workup and diagnosis of disorders associated with patterns of liver disease. ALT = alanine aminotransferase; AST = aspartate aminotransferase; CA = cancer antigen; CEA = carcinoembryonic antigen; CT = computed tomography; ERCP = endoscopic retrograde cholangiography; MRI = magnetic resonance imaging.

TABLE 104-2. Liver Tests Reflecting Cholestasis and Biliary Tract Disorders

Laboratory Test	Physiologic Function	Source	Commonly Associated Liver Abnormalities	Of Note	Pitfalls
Bilirubin, conjugated	Bilirubin glucoronide, results from conjugation of bilirubin in the liver. Water soluble.	Liver	Liver necrosis, PBC/PSC, cirrhosis, intrahepatic cholestasis due to drugs or genetic abnormality, sepsis, biliary tract obstruction	Prognostically useful in alcohol liver disease, PSC, PBC; Renally excreted, so rarely > 30 mg/dL with normal renal function	Value of conjugated bilirubin may be overestimated with diazo method of measurement; Often elevated in sepsis or postoperative situations in setting of no liver disease
Bilirubin, unconjugated	Organic anion from hemoglobin degradation. Lipid soluble.	RBC breakdown Defects in hepatic conjugation or uptake	Hemolysis Physiologic jaundice of newborn Inherited defects of bilirubin uptake	Sustained hemolysis will not result in value > 5 mg/dL in setting of normal liver function	
Alkaline hosphatase	Group of glycoprotein isoenzymes that catalyze hydrolysis of phosphate esters	Liver, bone, kidney, intestines, placenta, cancers, WBCs	Cholestatic liver diseases Obstruction of bile flow Infiltrative disorders of liver Malignancies	Coded by four genes Immunologically distinct Found on plasma membranes Elevations due primarily to increased synthesis in obstructive liver disease, not impaired excretion in bile	Multiple sources; Exact physiologic function not clear; Degree of elevation often does not correlate with clinical finding
GGT	Catalyzes transfer of γ-glutamyl groups of peptides to other amino acids	Liver, spleen, kidney, brain, heart, lung, pancreas, seminal vesicles	Cholestatic liver disease, alcohol injury, biliary tract disease	Membrane associated and found in biliary tree; Catalyzes metabolism of glutathione conjugates with some xenobiotics	Found in many tissues Sometimes not elevated with alkaline phosphatase in liver disease Elevated with alcohol use in some patients and with certain medications
5′NT	Catalyzes hydrolysis of nucleotides by releasing phosphate from pentose ring	Liver, intestines, brain, heart, vascular tissue, pancreas	Cholestatic disease where alkaline phosphatase is elevated	Physiologic significance not known; Although found in several tissues, only released from plasma membranes of hepatobiliary tissue with injury	Not readily available through all laboratories

GGT = γ-glutamyl transpeptidases; 5′NT = 5′ nucleotidase; PBC = primary biliary cirrhosis; PSC = primary sclerosing cholangitis; RBC = red blood cell; WBC = white blood cells.

TABLE 104-3. Liver Disorders and Associated Laboratory Test Abnormalities

Conjugated Bilirubin	Unconjugated Bilirubin	Alkaline Phosphatase	GGT	Aminotransferase
Hepatitis, cirrhosis, biliary tract obstruction, Dubin-Johnson syndrome, Rotor's syndrome, intrahepatic cholestasis	Hemolysis, physiologic jaundice of newborn, Gilbert's syndrome, Crigler-Najjar syndromes, medications	Physiologic (pregnancy, childhood), biliary tract disease, infiltrative disease, malignancy, bone disorders	Hepatobiliary disorders, pancreatitis, alcohol, renal disease, medications	Viral hepatitis, medications, herbs/supplements, alcohol, autoimmune hepatitis, hemochromatosis, wilson disease, α-1-antitrypsin deficiency, endocrinologic disorders, celiac disease

GGT = γ-glutamyl transpeptidases.

circumstances. In other words, enzymes should be evaluated in conjunction with a careful history and examination of the patient, the information from which is invaluable to making sense of the enzyme abnormalities. For example, in a patient with elevated aminotransferases and a history of intravenous drug use, HC is a common finding. Rechecking the enzymes several months later to see if the abnormality persists is not necessary prior to checking viral hepatitis serologies, because the risk factor for enzyme elevation has been assessed. Likewise, in an individual with newly elevated enzymes soon after beginning therapy with a known potential hepatotoxin, such as a nonsteroidal anti-inflammatory drug (NSAID) or lipid-lowering agent, the diagnosis becomes slanted in favor of drug hepatotoxicity.

Interpretation of Abnormal Liver Enzymes

Although the patterns of liver enzyme elevations are not always consistent between patients with similar disease states, there are some general rules that can be applied to interpreting enzymes. Aminotransferase elevations are typically seen with hepatocellular injury and often occur in the setting of normal or near normal bilirubin and alkaline phosphatase. In almost all liver diseases except those that are alcohol related, the ratio of AST/ALT is less than one, until cirrhosis develops when there is often a reversal of this ratio.

The most common cause of ALT elevation is drug-induced toxicity, which is generally mild and transient. Continued use of the offending agent will often lead to persistent ALT elevations, but values generally remain below 300 U/L. Common offending agents include NSAIDs, antibiotics, statin compounds, antiseizure medications, antiretrovirals for human immunodeficiency virus, and isoniazid. Serial enzyme assessment is necessary when patients are consuming these agents. Herbal and complementary medicine hepatotoxicity is increasingly being recognized and will also require further study to assess how to follow patients on these drugs.

Chronic viral infections, such as hepatitis B (HB) or HC, and fatty liver disease are the most common causes of persistently elevated enzymes. Again, enzymes rarely rise above 300 U/L in these settings. HC is the most common chronic hepatotropic infection in Western countries, is asymptomatic, and ALT can range from normal to 10-fold above normal values. HB affects 400 million worldwide and can also present with a spectrum of aminotransferase abnormalities ranging from normal levels to the thousands (U/L). Nonalcoholic fatty liver disease is increasingly recognized even in those without the classic risk factors of obesity and diabetes mellitus. Steatosis may develop from medication use, including *corticosteroids, amiodarone,* and *tamoxifen*. There is more evidence lately that steatosis may not cause significant enzyme elevations. The typical pattern of enzyme elevation is AST/ALT ratio of less than one, with numbers sometimes as high as fivefold the upper limit of normal. Unfortunately, there is no relationship between liver enzymes and degree of steatosis, or even the presence of inflammation, or nonalcoholic steatohepatitis (NASH), which is thought to be the more aggressive variant of this condition. Liver biopsy is necessary to confirm the diagnosis of NASH, though imaging may be suggestive of steatosis.

Alcohol-related liver injury is still a common phenomenon, and clinical examination requires diligence in history taking. An AST/ALT ratio of greater than two is often, but not always, seen in the setting of acute injury. GGT may also be greater than twice the normal. These values are generally below 300 U/L, except in the setting of concurrent *acetaminophen* toxicity, when the values may be in the thousands.

Autoimmune hepatitis is another cause of ALT elevation. In some cases, it presents with significant enzyme elevations, with or without jaundice. With corticosteroid therapy, enzymes typically normalize within weeks or months. Wilson's disease can cause ALT elevations, but is relatively rare and seen almost exclusively in patients under the age of 40 years. Iron overloaded states, the most important of which is hereditary hemochromatosis, can also elevate aminotransferases, and most commonly presents in the fifth or sixth decades of life. Figure 104-2 outlines the evaluation of persistently elevated ALT.

There are generally only the three following conditions where very high aminotransferase levels (ie, > 2000 IU) are seen: (1) ischemic liver injury, (2) acute viral hepatitis, and (3) drug-induced hepatotoxicity. Hepatitis A and HB, and in some countries E, are the viruses most likely to cause very high enzyme elevations, but all more commonly present without jaundice and generally are not symptomatic in immune competent adults.

Alkaline phosphatase elevation as an isolated finding should first be confirmed to be of hepatic origin by evaluating GGT or 5'NT. Once this has been confirmed, the next step is ultrasound or computed tomography scan to assess for biliary tree dilatation or infiltrative process. If the biliary tree is dilated, the next step is endoscopic retrograde cholangiography (ERCP). Although a percutaneous transhepatic cholangiogram can also be performed, the ERCP is the preferred diagnostic test in most scenarios due to relatively lower morbidity and ability to perform therapeutic measures more easily. If the biliary tree is normal, then a liver biopsy to assess for infiltrative disease or small bile duct disease states such as primary biliary cirrhosis (PBC) may be more appropriate. Occasionally, infiltrative disorders or systemic infections will result in profoundly high alkaline phosphatase levels. In fulminant Wilson's disease, alkaline phosphatase levels may be disproportionately low. Often, more than one diagnostic test is necessary to make the diagnosis with alkaline phosphatase elevations (see Figure 104-2). Although a space-occupying lesion in the liver may cause one or more enzyme abnormalities, often the enzymes are normal or minimally elevated.

Isolated hyperbilirubinemia is generally not due to obstructive biliary disease, yet ERCP is often performed in this setting in clinical practice. The lack of alkaline phosphatase or GGT elevation is an indicator that a disproportionate rise in bilirubin is not likely due to obstructive biliary tract disease. If the fractionated form of bilirubin is predominantly unconjugated, then extrahepatic sources such as hemolysis must be considered. Another clinically challenging scenario is distinguishing intrahepatic cholestasis from biliary tract obstruction. Again, a multitude of laboratory and imaging studies is usually required to assess this, because the bilirubin and alkaline phosphatase with GGT are elevated in both conditions. One must keep in mind that biliary tract disease or obstruction will generally have imaging consistent with this, unless it is an acute presentation, in

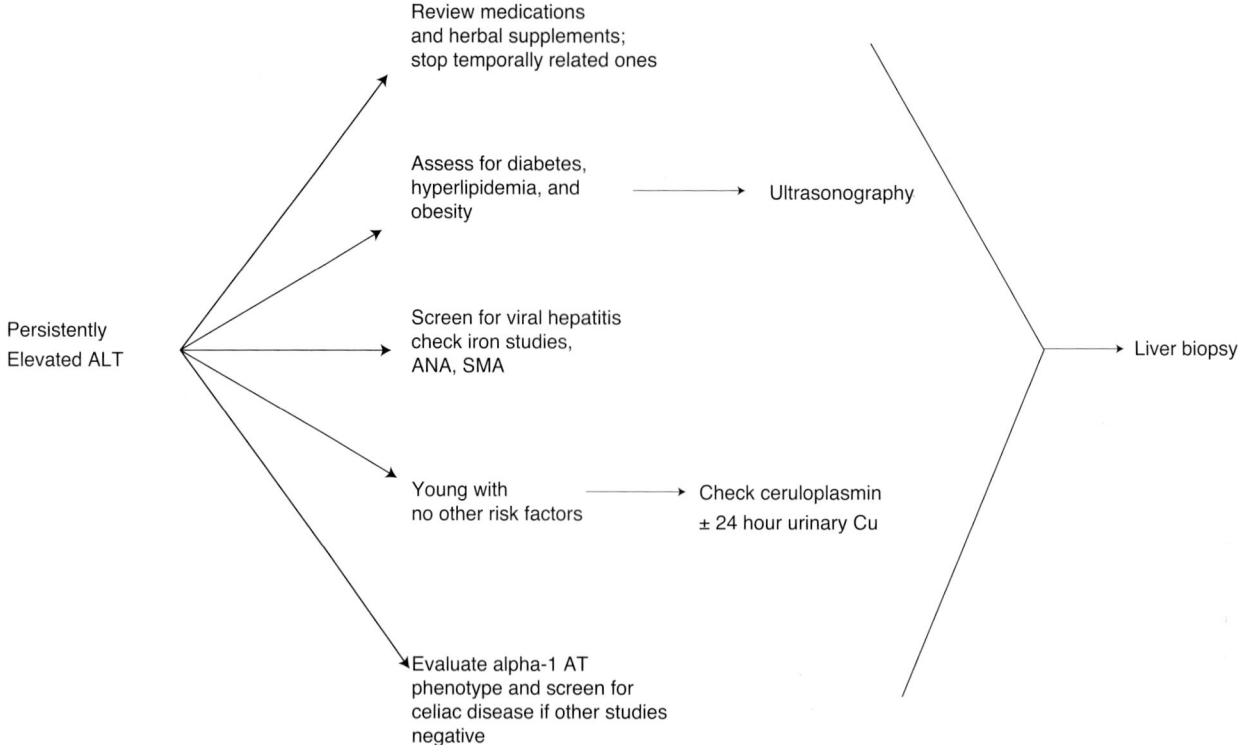

FIGURE 104-2. Algorithm to evaluate persistently elevated alanine aminotransferase (ALT). ANA = antinuclear antibody; AT = α-1-antitrypsin; Cu = copper; SMA = smooth muscle antibody.

which case imaging may not reflect changes such as dilated bile ducts. Ultrasound is the most reasonable first line examination, because it can reliably assess for bile duct dilatation. If present, then ERCP can be performed. Cholangiography often is performed early in the examination process in spite of other imaging tests not supporting the diagnosis of biliary tract obstruction. If there is no evidence of bile duct dilatations, ERCP rarely reveals an abnormality. Liver biopsy in those settings should be the initial diagnostic test.

Tests of Hepatic Function

The true LFTs reflect the synthetic capacity of the liver. Although conjugation and excretion of bilirubin is one such test, there are other variables that affect bilirubin levels, including the rate of production outside of the liver. Bile acids measured in the serum can be a useful tool to measure hepatic function. Because the pool of bile acids is much greater than bilirubin and enterohepatic cycling occurs, any change in the serum values will reflect even small changes in hepatic function. The main difficulty in establishing clinical utility for serum bile acids has been the lack of a true advantage in diagnostic capabilities over standard liver tests. The use of postprandial serum bile acid measurements is cumbersome requiring multiple blood draws, and is affected by changes in portal venous blood flow in the setting of portal hypertension. Hence, although the sensitivities of serum bile acids are high in detecting liver disease, there is no real advantage to routine clinical use.

PT is a very useful marker of hepatic function, and in acute liver failure it can impart prognostic information. Coagulation factors made in the liver include I, II, V, VII, IX, and X. Notably, factor VIII is not made in the liver and can be used to distinguish disseminated intravascular coagulation from liver related abnormalities in bleeding parameters, though this is rarely a clinical dilemma. More importantly, since factor V production is not dependent on vitamin K presence, measurement can be used to distinguish vitamin K deficiency as a cause of prolonged PT from liver disease-related causes. Vitamin K dependent factors are II, VII, IX, and X. Although prolonged PT is not specific for liver diseases, the other causes of prolonged PT, such as consumptive coagulapathy, vitamin K deficiency states, or medication-related causes, are generally simple to rule out. Hence, PT becomes a critical test for liver synthetic function. In fact, the international normalization ratio (INR) is now one of three tests used in the current liver cadaveric organ allocation scheme which uses a logarithmic calculation (model for end-stage liver disease) to categorize patients into 1 of 34 levels of illness and prioritizes their medical need for a transplant. The other two values used in the assessment are total bilirubin and creatinine.

Albumin is synthesized in the liver at a rate of 10 to 15 g daily with a pool of roughly 500 g. Although not useful as a marker of acute liver disease, it is very useful as an indicator of chronic liver disease, and is used in the Child-Turcotte-Pugh scoring systems. Because levels of albumin are depressed in malnourished states, nephrotic syndromes, and protein losing enteropathies, its clinical utility should be assessed in the setting of other tests of synthetic liver function.

Lipid and lipoprotein synthesis occurs in the liver, and levels of various lipid molecules change with both acute and chronic liver disease. For example, in cholestatic forms of liver disease, cholesterol levels rise, whereas in acute liver injury, plasma triglycerides are often elevated. In advanced liver disease, cholesterol levels are frequently low. Unfortunately, because of individual differences in these lipid values, as well as their dependence on nutritional status, there is no reliable way to use them to assess hepatic function.

Finally, several quantitative hepatic function assessments have been developed and remain experimental for the most part. These include the indocyanine green clearance test, aminopyrine breath test, antipyrine clearance, and caffeine clearance among others. None of these have any proven utility over standard tests in clinical practice, and they are difficult to perform compared to serum blood tests.

Liver Biopsy

Percutaneous liver biopsy is one of the most widely used procedures in hepatology today. Although there are some limitations to the procedure and histologic analysis, there is still no reliable noninvasive alternative. The primary purpose of a biopsy is to confirm the suspected diagnosis, and to quantify the extent of hepatic damage that has occurred. In addition to these indications, occasionally a systemic disease diagnosis is made through liver biopsy. For example, tuberculosis and sarcoidosis are occasionally first diagnosed through histologic assessment and culture of the liver tissue. Likewise, the diagnosis of amyloidosis is often made by liver biopsy. It is still the only definitive way to diagnosis hemochromatosis and fatty liver disease. Medication-induced hepatotoxicity can only be confirmed through liver biopsy, though it may be suspected based on history and enzyme abnormalities.

There are few true contraindications to liver biopsy. Significant coagulopathy with INR > 1.5, platelet count < 60,000, or prolonged PTT should all be corrected prior to percutaneous biopsy. Relative contraindications include ascites, large hemangiomas, and intra-abdominal infections. Patient compliance is critically important, and those not willing to cooperate cannot undergo biopsy. In these scenarios, alternative methods such as transvenous routes can be used to obtain tissue.

The technique and instrumentation used for biopsy is one that has continued to evolve over time. Most centers now use disposable needles or guns to reduce costs and accommodate the larger numbers of biopsies being performed. The most commonly practiced technique is outpatient percutaneous biopsy, with or without conscious sedation, followed by an observation and monitoring period of 2 to 6 hours before discharging the patient. Prebiopsy ultrasound has been advocated as a reasonable safety measure to prevent inadvertent puncture of the gallbladder or large intrahepatic blood vessels.

Complications of biopsies include pain, perforation of the gallbladder, colon, kidney or lung, intraabdominal bleeding, infection, pneumothorax, and vasovagal responses. Rarely, an intrahepatic arteriovenous fistula or hemobilia can occur. These generally resolve spontaneously with conservative management. Significant postbiopsy bleeding is evident by hemodynamic changes and pain. Subclinical bleeding when evaluated by imaging is not uncommon, but is of no clinical significance. The incidence of significant bleeding varies by patient population, but in a large cohort of over 9,000 patients undergoing a percutaneous liver biopsy procedure over 20 years at the Mayo clinic, only 0.24% had bleeding, with 0.11% having fatal bleeding. In a more recent evaluation of bleeding risk factors, biopsy-related bleeding occurred in 1.6% of 629 patients that had liver biopsies. Biopsy-related mortality was surprisingly high at 0.48%, but this was found to be the case in those with mycobacterial infections, thrombocytopenia, recent heparin administration, and advanced cirrhosis. In another recent review of 861 biopsies, the overall incidence of significant complication, including bleeding, pneumothorax, and severe hypotension was 1.4%. The majority of these occurred again in the setting of cirrhosis. A gelfoam plug can be used in settings of mild coagulopathy or ascites with apparent reasonable safety, but is not widely practiced. In settings where a percutaneous biopsy is deemed unsafe, a transvenous, typically transjugular biopsy can be performed by an interventional radiologist. This procedure was recently analyzed at a single center. Over an 80-month period, 371 patients had 410 attempted biopsies, with a mean of 3.4 needle passes per procedure. A tissue diagnosis was achieved in 98%, with 6 samples being too small to analyze. There were 10 (2.4%) complications, including 3 intraperitoneal bleeds and 1 death. Overall, it is a safe procedure if performed in a center with a high level of experience and expertise.

The ability to assess histologic aspects of liver disease has been a vital tool in our understanding of the natural history and pathogenesis of many disorders. Although accurate and reproducible, biopsy sampling error does exist, and has been shown to be as high as 30% in terms of minor differences in inflammation and fibrosis. This is also partially determined by the size of the core of tissue obtained and the number of portal tracts seen in the specimen. Still, it is considered the gold standard, and to date, there are no alternative markers of inflammation or fibrosis that have gained widespread use. There are commercially available test kits of fibrosis currently available on the market for use in viral hepatitis, including: (1) *FibroSpect* (Prometheus Labs, San Diego) and (2) *FibroTest* (BioPredictive, France; FibroSURE, LabCorp, USA). However, the limitation with both is a lack of optimal sensitivity when little fibrosis is present. Further testing and modification is necessary before these modalities can replace liver biopsies. Their current utility is predominantly in a research setting or in clinical practice where liver biopsies cannot be done.

Summary

The combined use of serum biochemical markers and liver biopsies with various imaging tests has become the standard for evaluating liver disease. All of these, in combination with careful history and patient examination, allow the clinician to derive a diagnosis in most cases. The ongoing development of noninvasive markers of inflammation, steatosis, and fibrosis will continue to change the landscape of how liver disease is evaluated and managed. New imaging modalities, such a magnetic resonance spectroscopy, may also broaden the armamentarium of tests, particularly for common disorders such as fatty liver disease. Further prospective testing of these markers will be needed before they can be adopted into routine clinical practice.

Supplemental Reading

Abdi W, Millan JC, Mezey E. Sampling variability on percutaneous liver biopsy. Arch Inten Med 1979;139:667–9.

Clark JM, Brancati FL, Diehl AM. The prevalence and etiology of elevated aminotransferase levels in the United States. Am J Gastroenterol 2003;98:960–7.

Fang MH, Ginsberg AL, Dobbins WO. Marked elevation in serum alkaline phosphatase activity as a manifestation of systemic infection. Gastroenterology 1980;78:592.

Freeman RB Jr. MELD/PELD: one year later. Transplant Proc 2003;35:2425–7.

Jalan R, Hayes PC. Review article: quantitative tests of liver function. Aliment Pharmacol Ther 1995;9:263.

Kamphuisen PW, Wiersma TG, Mulder CJ, De Vries RA. Plugged-perctaneous liver biopsy in patients with impaired coagulation and ascites. Pathophysiol Haemost Thromb 2002;32:190–3.

Lee WM. Drug induced hepatotoxicity. N Engl J Med 2003;349:474–85.

Mammen EF. Coagulation defects in liver disease. Med Clin North Am 1994;78:545–54.

Regev A, Berho M, Jeffers L, et al. Sampling error and intraobserver variation in liver biopsy in patients with chronic HCV infection. Am Coll Gastroenterol 2002;97:2614–8.

Rossi E, Adams L, Prins A, et al. Validation of the FibroTest biochemical markers score in assessing liver fibrosis in hepatitis C patients. Clin Chem 2003;49:450–4.

Smith TP, Prsson TL, Heneghan MA, Ryan JM. Transjugular biopsy of the liver in pediatric and adult patients using an 18-gauge automated core biopsy needle: a restospective review of 410 consecutive procedures. AJR Am J Roentgenol 2003;180;167–72.

Terjung B, Lemnitzer I, Dumoulin FL, et al. Bleeding complications after percutaneous liver biopsy: an analysis of risk factors. Digestion 2003;67:138–45.

Wawrzynowicz-Syczewska M, Kruszewski T, Boron-Kaczmarska A. Complications of percutaneous liver biopsy. Rom J Gastroenterol 2002;11:105–7.

Williams AL, Hoofnage JH. Ratio of serum aspartate to alanine aminotransferase in chronic hepatitis. Relationship to cirrhosis. Gastroenterology 1988;95:734–9.

Willson RA, Clayson KH, Leon S. Unmeasurable serum alkaline phosphatase activity in Wilson's Disease associated with fulminant hepatic failure and hemolysis. Hepatotolgy 1987;7:613–5.

CHAPTER 105

ACUTE HEPATITIS: MANAGEMENT AND PREVENTION

MARIA H. SJOGREN, MD, MPH

Acute viral hepatitis has generally been of minimal medical interest because it has been viewed as a mild illness where observation and supportive therapy have been the expected management. However, with the advent of safe and effective vaccines and effective medical therapies, the concept of management of acute hepatitis is changing. In addition, variations in epidemiology and an increase in costs associated with liver transplants are compelling clinicians and regulators to have a more comprehensive approach and to prevent or treat early in an attempt to prevent complications of chronic liver disease. The purpose of this chapter is to review the current status of management and prevention of hepatitis A, hepatitis B, hepatitis C, hepatitis D, and hepatitis E.

Acute Hepatitis A

Once acute hepatitis A is diagnosed, the management of the patient is mainly supportive. There is no specific therapy to accelerate the recovery. In very young patients, acute hepatitis A is a benign disease. It is a reportable infectious disease in the United States with a rate of infection of 4 in 100,000 habitants. The seroepidemiology of the infection is rapidly changing, particularly in the developing world, with increasing portions of the population escaping childhood infection, rendering increasing number of adults susceptible to the infection. Hospitalization rates vary but have been reported as high as 15% in recent outbreaks. Current publications on hospitalized patients due to fulminant hepatic failure cite hepatitis A as a frequent cause of liver failure requiring liver transplant. A 1998 scientific report described the clinical outcome of 256 individuals hospitalized with acute hepatitis A. On admission, 89% had prolonged nausea or vomiting, 26% had a prothrombin time prolonged (> 3 seconds), 39 patients had serious complications (19 were hepatobiliary in nature and 20 were extrahepatic complications), and 5 (2%) died. The age of the individuals played a major role when rates of complications were analyzed. Twenty-five percent of patients aged 40 years or older compared with 11% of patients under 40 years of age had at least one complication ($p = .014$). Recently, a major outbreak in the United States reported in Georgia, Tennessee and Pennsylvania during September to November 2003 underscored the susceptibility of the population to acute hepatitis A. In this outbreak, more than 600 cases were diagnosed and 3 patients died (at least 1 was under 40 years of age). The outbreak is still being studied, but early reports have attributed it to contamination of green onions.

In addition to the severity of symptoms, some patients may develop unusual clinical presentations following acute infection with hepatitis A, including prolonged cholestasis, relapsing hepatitis, or acute liver failure syndrome (ALF). ALF may occur in previously healthy subjects. During the last two decades, it has been appreciated that certain populations are at high risk for developing increased morbidity and ALF due to hepatitis A infection, including older individuals (> 40 years of age) and subjects with chronic liver disease. An acute episode of hepatitis A in patients with underlying chronic liver disease may cause exacerbation of the chronic liver disease with increased morbidity and accelerated mortality. A liver transplant is a lifesaving intervention for subjects who do not recover from ALF. A recent communication suggested that the finding of a detectable immunoglobulin (Ig)M antibody against hepatitis A and undetectable or low titer HAV ribonucleic acid (RNA) in patients with ALF might signal an ominous prognosis and warrant consideration of early referral for a liver transplant.

Prevention of Hepatitis A

In the United States, hepatitis A is a preventable infection through the use of either of two vaccines that are commercially available, *VAQTA*, manufactured by Merck, Sharp, and Dohme (West Point, Pennsylvania), and *HAVRIX*, manufactured by SmithKline Beecham Biologicals (Rixensart, Belgium). Table 105-1 depicts the principal characteristics and doses for both commercially available vaccines.

Although hepatitis A vaccine is the first line of preventive therapy, administration of *serum IgG* is still of value to prevent hepatitis A infection in certain circumstances. *Immunoglobulins* may be used to provide short term protection in persons who require immediate immunity and in children too young to receive the vaccine; it should be administered to unvaccinated household members of an

TABLE 105-1. Characteristics of Commercially Available Hepatitis A Vaccines

Type	VAQTA	HAVRIX
HAV strain	Inactivated vaccine	Inactived vaccine
Cell culture	Cultured in MRC-5 cells	Cultured in MRC-5 cells
Adjuvant	Aluminum hydroxide	Aluminum hydroxide
Route	Intramuscular	Intramuscular
Adult doses	2 doses 1 mL (50 U) at 0 and 6 months	1 mL (1440 U) at 0 and 6 to 12 months
Pediatric doses (2 to 17 years)	0.5 mL (25 U) at 0 and 6 to 18 months	0.5 mL (720 U) at 0 and 6 to 12 months

HAV = hepatitis A virus; MRC = (confidential initials) = human diploid fibroblast from fetal lung.

acute case of hepatitis A, if uninfected individuals seek attention within 2 weeks of exposure. The recommended dose of IgG for adults is 0.02 mL/kg when the period of exposure will not exceed 3 months. If the period of exposure is prolonged (for example staff deployed to endemic areas who cannot be immunized against hepatitis A virus [HAV]) the recommended immunoglobulin dose is 0.06 mL/kg every 5 months. IgG affords excellent prophylaxis but is impractical because protection lasts only a few months. Although considered safe, it may cause fever, myalgias, and considerable pain at injection sites.

In the United States, vaccination policy does not recommend the vaccine for universal use but rather for individuals in high risk groups such as travelers to countries with high endemicity for HAV infection, military personnel, persons with chronic liver disease of any etiology, homosexually active men, users of illicit drugs, residents of communities experiencing a hepatitis A outbreak, persons with clotting factor disorders, certain institutional workers, employees of child daycare centers, laboratory workers who handle live HAV, and handlers of primates that may harbor HAV. In addition, consideration for vaccination is recommended for children and adolescents living in states with historically elevated rates of hepatitis A, including Alaska (cyclic epidemics), Arizona, California, Idaho, Nevada, New Mexico, Oklahoma, Oregon, South Dakota, Utah, Washington, Arkansas, Colorado, Missouri, Montana, Texas, and Wyoming.

Side effects of the vaccine found in 1 to 10% of immunized individuals are local reactions at injection site, such as induration, redness, and swelling; systemic reactions, such as fatigue, fever, or malaise; anorexia; and nausea. Less than 1% may experience hematoma at injection site, pruritus, skin rash, pharyngitis, upper respiratory tract infections, abdominal pain, diarrhea, vomiting, arthralgia, myalgia, lymphadenopathy, insomnia, photophobia, and vertigo. Vaccines should not be administered to persons with a history of hypersensitivity reaction to alum or, for HAVRIX, reaction to the preservative 2-phenoxyethanol. The safety of hepatitis A vaccine during pregnancy has not been determined.

Acute Hepatitis B

Acute hepatitis B carries the possibility of becoming a chronic infection in 1 to 5% of susceptible adults and > 90% of neonates born to HBV-carrier mothers if the neonate does not receive prophylaxis at birth (Table 105-2).

If the infection does not become chronic, it is benign in the majority of infected individuals, although some develop acute liver failure. The contribution of hepatitis B to the development of ALF has traditionally been larger than hepatitis A. In early studies in US populations, hepatitis B accounted for 18 to 34% of the ALF cases, whereas hepatitis A was a rare contributor of ALF in the United States. The decline of viral hepatitis as a cause of ALF is mainly due to the control of hepatitis B virus (HBV) infection through preventive measures that include education and general immunization. In the 1970s the rate of HBV in ALF cases was reported as 34%, in the 1980s it was reported as 19%, in the 1990s as 10%, and in recent years it dropped off to 7%.

As in acute hepatitis A, there is no specific therapy to accelerate the recovery. Once chronic hepatitis B develops, it requires antiviral therapy to stop the progression of liver disease or infrequently eradicate the infection. Most experts accept the persistence of HB antigens in the blood for 6 months or longer after initial diagnosis as a chronic infection.

Prevention of Hepatitis B

The hepatitis B vaccine was first licensed in the United States in 1981 and is recommended for both pre- and postexposure prophylaxis. *Hyperimmune globulin (HBIG)* is a passive immunization that provides temporary protection and is indicated in certain postexposure situations. HBIG contains high concentrations of HB antigens, whereas regular *immunoglobulin* (like the one used for hepatitis A passive immunization) is prepared from plasma with varying concentrations of HB antigens. In the United States, HBIG has an HB antigen titer > 1:100,000 by radioimmunoassay.

TABLE 105-2. Passive and Active Immunization of Subjects at Immediate Risk of Developing Acute Hepatitis B Virus Infection

	HBIG		Vaccine	
Exposure	Dose	Timing	Dose	Timing
Perinatal	0.5 mL IM	Within 12 hours of birth	0.5 mL at birth	Within 12 hours of birth; repeat at 1 and 6 months
Sexual	0.6 mL/kg IM	Single dose within 14 days of sexual contact	See Table 105-3	Start immunization at once (concurrent with HBIG)

HBIG = hyperimmune globulin; IM = intramuscular.

If a subject is exposed to HBV and was not previously immunized, a combination of HBIG and HB vaccine are recommended as depicted in Table 105-2.

Two vaccines are available in the United States. For practical purposes, they are comparable in immunogenicity and efficacy rates, although the preparations are different. *Recombivax-HB*, manufactured by Merck Sharp & Dohme (West Point, PA) became available in 1989. It is a noninfectious, nonglycosylated HB antigen vaccine, subtype adw, made by recombinant deoxyribonucleic acid (DNA) technology. Yeast cells (*Saccharomyces cerevisiae*) expressing the HB antigen gene are cultured, collected by centrifugation, and broken by homogenization with glass beads. HB antigen particles are purified and absorbed in aluminum hydroxide. Each milliliter has 10 mg of HB antigens.

Engerix-B, manufactured by SmithKline Beecham Biologicals (Rixensart, Belgium), is a noninfectious recombinant DNA vaccine. It contains purified HB antigens obtained by culturing genetically engineered *S. cerevisiae* cells, which carry the surface antigen gene of HBV. This surface antigen is purified from the cells and adsorbed on aluminum hydroxide. Each milliliter has 20 mg of HB antigens. Immunization schedules for adults and children are depicted in Table 105-3. After immunization is complete, booster doses are not recommended for healthy adults or children. For immunocompromised patients (eg, hemodialysis patients), a booster dose should be administered when anti-HBV levels drop to 10 mIU/mL or less. This recommendation can be extended to individuals who are at significant risk of infection with HBV (ie, surgeons, dentists, phlebotomists, etc). Subjects who do not respond to a first series of immunization should be immunized again with a complete series. The persistence of antibody directly correlates with the peak level achieved after the third dose. Follow up of adults who were immunized with plasma-derived hepatitis B vaccine demonstrated that the antibody levels had fallen to undetectable or very low levels in 30 to 50% of recipients. Long-term studies of adults and children indicate that protection lasts at least 9 years, despite loss of HB antigens in serum. After 9 years of follow-up, HB antigens loss ranged from 13 to 60% in a group of homosexual men and Native Alaskans, two groups at high risk of infection. However, vaccine recipients were virtually 100% protected from clinical illness, despite the absence of booster immunization. Among people without detectable HB antigens, some breakthrough infections have been noted in later years based on the detection of hepatitis B core antibody. However, clinical illness did not occur, and HB antigens were not detected. The infection was assumed to be without consequence and to have bestowed permanent immunity.

It is possible to immunize people simultaneously against hepatitis A and hepatitis B. To date, several millions of subjects have received a combined product of both vaccines (*Twinrix* [SmithKline Beecham Biologicals], which is commercially available in the United States, Europe, South America, etc). The vaccine elicits antibodies to HAV and HBV in close to a 100% of immunized subjects. The combined vaccine appears to be safe, well tolerated, and highly immunogenic. The safety profile is similar to the HAV or HBV individual vaccines.

Acute Hepatitis C

Unlike HBV, acute hepatitis C frequently progresses to chronic infection in approximately 80% of infected individuals when acquired as a result of blood transfusion. Early therapy had been advocated for acute hepatitis C because of its propensity to develop into a chronic infection. However, recent reports show that hepatitis C acquired through nontransfusional factors, such as intravenous contamination or sporadic hepatitis C may become chronic with lesser frequency in 40 to 50% of the cases. The new epidemiological data have important implications on the timing of therapy and is discussed further below.

Prevention and Treatment of Acute Hepatitis C

There are no vaccines available to prevent acute hepatitis C. The only way to effectively prevent it is to eliminate exposure to risk factors. No firm recommendation can be made for postexposure prophylaxis for hepatitis C. Study results are equivocal. Some experts recommend administration of *Ig* (0.06 mg/kg) after a bonafide percutaneous

TABLE 105-3. Immunization Schedule for Hepatitis B Vaccine in Adults and Children

Group	Formulation	Initial	Month 1	Month 6
Recombivax-HB Vaccine				
Birth to 10 years	Pediatric dose: 0.5 mL	0.5 mL	0.5 mL	0.5 mL
Adults and older children	Adult dose: 10 mg/1.0 mL	1.0 mL	1.0 mL	1.0 mL
Dialysis patients	Special dose: 40 mg/1.0 mL	1.0 mL	1.0 mL	1.0 mL
Engerix-B Vaccine				
Birth to 10 years	Pediatric dose: 10 mg/0.5 mL	0.5 mL	0.5 mL	0.5 mL
Adults and older children	Adult dose: 20 mg/1.0 mL	1.0 mL	1.0 mL	1.0 mL
After needlestick injury	20 mg/1.0 mL	1.0 mL at 0, 1, and 2 months		
Hemodialysis patients	40 mg/2.0 mL	2.0 mL at 0, 1, 2, and 6 months		

HB = hepatitis B.

exposure. The immunoglobulin should be administered as soon as possible. However, work in animal models (chimpanzees) has shown a lack of protectiveness when animals that received prophylaxis with immunoglobulin were challenged with HCV. Moreover, available data show that in humans the neutralizing antibody evoked after infection with HCV is short lived and does not protect against reinfection. Passive immunoprophylaxis for hepatitis C appears to be inefficient. To date, there is no effective vaccine against HCV infection, possibly because of the extensive genetic and antigenic diversity among HCV strains, the absence of natural immunity after infection, and the lack of tissue culture system or small animal models.

Therapy for acute hepatitis C was successfully reported in 2001 when 42 of 43 German patients (98%) had undetectable HCV RNA in serum and normal alanine aminotransferase following monotherapy with *interferon* α-2b for 24 weeks. A recent study where some patients were untreated and others received *interferon* or *interferon and ribavirin* showed 80% of sustained viral response after therapy, but surprisingly 52% of patients who were not treated recovered spontaneously. Table 105-4 depicts the salient facts of these two studies. Based on this information it would be prudent to state that we should not rush to treat patients with acute hepatitis but rather allow at least 90 days of observation from suspected date of infection; if the HC RNA is still detectable, embarking in a 6 month trial of monotherapy with interferon would be advisable. The use of *pegylated interferon* is warranted, but it appears that *ribavirin* does not add benefit when treating acute hepatitis and should not be used. Patients ought to be reexamined at 6 months following the disappearance of HCV RNA in serum to ensure that the viral eradication is sustained. If HCV RNA should persist or reappear, subjects need to undergo therapy for established chronic hepatitis C infection. A word of caution is that none of these studies treated patients who received contaminated blood transfusion; it is likely that subjects infected through blood products may need therapy soon after acute hepatitis C is diagnosed because of the high propensity to develop chronic hepatitis C. For patients being observed for spontaneous clearance, the rapid decline of viral load may be of help in guiding the need to institute therapy; if the HCV RNA does not decline promptly during the first 3 months, the likelihood of established chronic hepatitis C is high. Therapy during pregnancy is not warranted.

Acute Delta Hepatitis

Acute delta hepatitis can occur simultaneously with acute hepatitis B (co-infection) or occur in a patient who has an established chronic hepatitis B infection (superinfection). The coinfection is usually self-limited and does not require therapy. The superinfection tends to produce a severe acute attack, in many cases fulminant. Survivors of the acute delta hepatitis have an accelerated path towards cirrhosis and require therapy. Treatment is disappointing; high doses of interferon do not eradicate the virus except in rare occasions. Nucleoside analogues like *lamivudine* have been ineffective in controlling delta hepatitis. Prevention of hepatitis B is important because delta hepatitis cannot survive in the absence of HBV infection. Delta hepatitis infection is rapidly declining because of universal vaccination against hepatitis B.

Acute Hepatitis E

Outbreaks of acute hepatitis E have been reported in Mexico, India, Pakistan, Nepal, Afghanistan, and other countries, but not in the United States. However, sporadic cases of acute HEV have been reported in the United States. The acute infection resembles acute hepatitis A and it is distinguished from it only with appropriate serological tests. Most cases have a benign clinical course and require only supportive therapy. However, fulminant cases and mortality have been described during epidemics. Pregnant women appear to be at higher risk of fulminant hepatitis E compared to nonpregnant women or men. Passive immunization is not available for hepatitis E and no specific therapy exists; interferon-based therapy has not been tried. Prevention is best done by better sanitation and water purification. An experimental vaccine has been prepared, phase II studies are promising and there is hope that a phase III study will show acceptable safety and efficacy.

TABLE 105-4. Characteristics of Two Studies Describing Therapy of Acute Hepatitis C

Study reference #8 Risk factors: IVDA, needle-stick injury, medical procedures or sexual contact with infected person(s).

Therapy: On average 89 days from infection to start of therapy. Therapy consisted of 5 million units IFN α-2b/day for 4 weeks followed with IFN doses TIW for 20 weeks, sustained viral response observed in 42/43 (97%). No control group.

Comments: Risk factors did not include blood transfusion, 61% infected with genotype 1.

Study reference #9 Risk factors: IVDA, needle-stick, medical procedures or sexual contact with HCV-infected person(s).

Therapy: On average 90 days from infection to start of therapy. Two groups: one received no therapy, the other received a variety of treatments: IFN monotherapy, IFN in combination with ribavirin or pegylated IFN α-2a. On average treatment was given for 5.7 months, sustained viral response observed in 21 of 26 (81%) treated patients, but 24 of 46 (52%) untreated subjects cleared spontaneously.

Comments: Risk factors did not include blood transfusion, 60% were infected with genotype 1.

HCV = hepatitis C virus; IFN = interferon; IVDA = intravenous drug abuse; TIW = three times weekly.

Supplemental Reading

Acute Hepatic Failure Study Group. Rakela J, Mosley JW, Edwards VM, et al. A double-blinded, randomized trial of hydrocortisone in acute hepatic failure. Dig Dis Sci 1991;36:1223–8.

Gerlach T, Diepolder H, Zachoval R, et al. Acute hepatitis C: high rate of both spontaneous and treatment-induced viral clearance. Gastroenterology 2003;125:80–8.

Hofer H, Watkins-Riedel T, Janata O, et al. Spontaneous viral clearance in patients with acute hepatitis C can be predicted by repeated measurements of serum viral load. Hepatology 2003;37:60–4.

Jaeckel E, Cornberg M, Wedemeyer H, et al. Treatment of acute hepatitis C with interferon alfa 2b. N Engl J Med 2001;345:1452–7.

Prevention of hepatitis A through active or passive immunization: recommendations of the Advisory Committee on Immunization Practices (ACIP). MMWR Recomm Rep 1999:48:1–37.

Rakela J, Lange SM, Ludwig J, Baldus WP. Fulminant hepatitis: Mayo Clinic experience with 34 cases. Mayo Clin Proc 1985;60:289–92.

Rezende G, Roque Afonso AM, Samuel D, et al. Viral and clinical factors associated with the fulminant course of hepatitis A infection. Hepatology 2003;38:613–8.

Schiodt FV, Atillasoy E, Shakill AO, et al. Etiology and outcome for 295 patients with acute liver failure in the United States. Liver Transpl Surg 1999;5:29–34.

Summary of Notifiable Diseases United States 2001. MMWR 2001;50:1–108.

Willner IR, Mark DU, Howard SC, et al. Serious hepatitis A: an analysis of patients hospitalized during an urban epidemic in the United States. Ann Intern Med 1998;128:111–4.

CHAPTER 106

Chronic Hepatitis B

Averell H. Sherker, MD, FRCP(C)

Hepatitis B (HB) is among the most common chronic viral infections of humans. It is estimated that 350 million people—more than 5% of the world's population—are chronically infected with hepatitis B virus (HBV). Among these, approximately 1.25 million HBV carriers are in the United States. These carriers remain at significant risk for the development of cirrhosis, liver failure, and hepatocellular carcinoma (HCC) throughout their lives, and 10 to 25% will die as a result of their infection.

Viral Characteristics

HBV is a member of the hepadnavirus (*hepatotrophic deoxyribonucleic acid [DNA] virus*) family. This family of viruses is characterized by a compact, partially double stranded DNA genome, which replicates via a ribonucleic acid intermediate. The viral genome encodes a polymerase with reverse transcriptase activity and has an organization analogous to that of the retroviruses. Although the retroviruses must integrate their genetic material into the host genome in order to replicate, HBV does not require integration. However, integrations do occur, albeit randomly and with frequent deletions and rearrangements, into the DNA of the host liver cells. It is believed that these genetic integrations play an important role in the generation of liver cancers.

HBV consists of an outer envelope made up of HB surface antigen (HBsAg) and a nucleocapsid or core made up of HB core antigen, which surrounds the DNA genome and DNA polymerase enzyme. Additionally, the virus encodes a soluble protein called 'e' antigen (HBeAg), which generally circulates in the blood when the virus is actively replicating in the liver. The role of HBeAg is not fully understood and even viruses in which this gene has mutated and is not expressed are still capable of replication.

Routes of Infection and Natural History of Infection with HBV

HBV is transmitted by perinatal, parenteral, and venereal exposure. Close person-to-person contact can also be responsible for transmission of infection, especially within households and between young children. HBV is endemic in certain geographic regions, including Asia, the South Pacific region, the Middle East, and Sub-Saharan Africa, as well as in the indigenous population of Alaska and the Arctic. In Western countries, HBV is most common among immigrants from endemic areas, injection drug users, hemodialysis patients, men who have sex with men, and promiscuous heterosexuals. The risk of chronic infection relates largely to the age at exposure. Most adults and adolescents infected will experience an acute infection, which is generally symptomatic but may be subclinical.

Acute infection is characterized by presence of HBsAg in the blood. Recovery is heralded by the loss of HBsAg and generation of antibody to HBsAg (HBsAb). A small proportion of these individuals—probably less than 5%—will go on to establish chronic infections, defined as HBsAg persisting beyond 6 months. In newborns and infants infected by their mothers, infection is rarely diagnosed clinically, but over 90% will develop chronicity. Rates of chronicity in those infected as children are intermediate between these rates. Additionally, immunosuppressed individuals are at high risk for developing chronic HBV infection.

Chronic HBV infection has several different phases, characterized by different levels of viral replication and liver inflammation. Following acute infection, those patients in whom persistent infection is established will enter a relatively quiescent phase of *immunotolerance*. In this phase, liver enzymes are typically normal or modestly increased and the liver biopsy demonstrates minimal necroinflammatory activity. HBV DNA levels tend to be high.

After a variable period of time—often decades in perinatally infected individuals—the immune system becomes activated against the virus, triggering necrosis of infected hepatocytes. Serum aminotransferases are elevated and the liver biopsy reflects ongoing chronic hepatitis, which may be quite severe. HBV DNA levels begin to decrease. During this *inflammatory* phase, liver damage is most likely to occur.

If the immune system is successful in halting viral replication, the patient may enter an *inactive* phase where liver enzymes normalize and HBV DNA either becomes undetectable or is detectable only by sensitive polymerase chain reaction techniques. In this phase, HBeAg is lost, and antibody to HBeAg (HBeAb) develops. Although still at risk for development of HCC and progressive liver dysfunction, patients in the inactive phase of infection have a much improved prognosis (Niederau et al, 1996). Most commonly, patients who achieve the inactive phase of HBV infection remain in that phase, but sometimes, viral replication reactivates. As well, there are some patients who "flip-flop" between active viral replication and inactivity. These patients appear to be at high risk for rapidly progressive liver fibrosis. Among patients who stably convert from HBeAg to HBeAb, some may eventually seroconvert from HBsAg to HBsAb, at an annual rate of approximately 5%.

In a variant form of chronic HBV infection, patients may have high levels of HBV DNA, elevated aminotransferases and necroinflammatory activity on liver biopsy despite the absence of HBeAg, and presence of HBeAb. In most cases, these patients are infected with an HBV strain with a genome that has mutated in the so-called "precore" region. This variant is responsible for many, if not most, chronic HBV infections in the Mediterranean region and Asia, and is being increasingly recognized in North America. Patients infected with precore mutant strains of HBV are more likely to have serum aminotransferases that fluctuate between normal and abnormal, and are less likely to experience a sustained viral response to antiviral therapy.

Diagnosis

High risk populations for HBV infection (as discussed earlier), as well as their sexual and family contacts and all pregnant women, should be screened for HBV infection with HBsAg.

The newly diagnosed patient with HB should undergo a full medical history and physical examination. Emphasis should be placed on trying to identify risk factors for HBV infection and coinfection with hepatitis C virus (HCV) and human immunodeficiency virus (HIV). Factors such as alcohol use, which may aggravate liver disease, should be identified. Family history of HB and HCC should be sought and sexual contacts and household members at risk for infection should be identified for screening and appropriate HBV vaccination.

Initial examinations of a patient with chronic HBV infection should include tests that evaluate liver inflammation, liver function, and viral replication. Serum aminotransferases give a crude indication of ongoing liver injury or inflammation. Bilirubin, albumin and prothrombin time (PT) reflect hepatic synthetic function, although they will generally remain normal until there is a critical loss of hepatic function. As previously discussed, testing for HBeAg, HBeAb and HBV DNA are essential in evaluating the replicative state of the virus. In patients with identified risk factors, HCV and HIV antibody tests should be ordered.

Role of Liver Biopsy

The decision to perform a liver biopsy in a patient with chronic HBV infection is controversial and different practitioners will have different opinions. In patients with increased serum transaminases, positive HBeAg, and significant HBV DNA concentration, many are comfortable offering antiviral treatment without a biopsy. When HBV DNA is positive with normal aminotransferases or negative HBeAg and positive HBeAb (presumed precore mutant virus infection), I find liver biopsy extremely helpful in selecting those patients who would be most likely to benefit from treatment.

Management

Protection Against Other Liver Diseases

Patients with chronic HBV infection should be counseled to minimize alcohol use, although the "safe" level of consumption has not been defined. It is important that patients be advised to have household and sexual contacts tested for both HBsAg and HBsAb to identify both those who are infected and require further examination, and those who are susceptible to infection. Until HBsAb is documented in sexual partners, either via natural infection or vaccination, safe sex techniques must be employed. Hepatitis A (HA) vaccination is advised in all patients with chronic liver disease. Generally, screening for HA antibody is not cost effective before vaccination but may be in selected patients with a high likelihood of prior HA infection, such as those born in developing countries.

Surveillance for HCC

Patients with chronic HBV have an increased lifetime risk for the development of HCC. In a study of middle-aged males in Taiwan, HBsAg positivity was associated with a greater than 200-fold excess risk of death from HCC, with approximately half the deaths in that group being due to liver cancer or liver failure (Beasley et al, 1981). Given that liver cancers have a median doubling time of 4 months, that they are commonly encapsidated and metastasize late, and that the liver is a large organ with marked functional reserve, HCCs may have a lengthly asymptomatic phase. Tumors that are discovered in this preclinical phase, especially if they are less than 5 cm in diameter, may be successfully treated with resection, ablative therapy, or liver transplant. Thus, it is rational to screen those at significant risk for HCC periodically using an imaging study and the tumor marker, alpha-fetoprotein (AFP). As the goal is to discover small HCCs at a stage when they can be cured, the frequency of screening should be dictated by the biology of the tumor and not the perceived risk of HCC in the individual patient. Once the decision is made to screen, the protocol used should be standard. I screen using AFP and liver ultrasound every 6 months, generally starting at the age of 35 years. Patients at highest risk of HCC, including those with cirrhosis, a family history of HCC or birth in sub-Saharan Africa should be screened from the age of diagnosis.

Treatment

The primary goal of HBV treatment is to convert active replicative infection to the inactive nonreplicative state. If this state is achieved and sustained, the risk of liver-related morbidity and mortality is significantly reduced. The following three treatments are currently FDA-approved therapies for HBV: (1) *interferon-α*, (2) *lamivudine*, and (3) *adefovir dipivoxil*. Several other agents are in late-stage clinical study.

INTERFERON-BASED TREATMENTS

Interferons are both antiviral and immunostimulatory. It is believed that the dominant beneficial effect of interferon-α in chronic HBV infection is due to immunostimulation. In fact, when *interferon* is effective in HBV infection it induces a heightened immune response against infected hepatocytes resulting in more marked liver inflammation and increased serum aminotransferases. If the inflammatory reaction is sufficiently vigorous, it may result in conversion from an active replicative infection to an inactive infection.

Interferon-α is given by subcutaneous injection and most patients can be taught to self-administer the drug. The usual dose in chronic HBV infection is 5 MU daily or 10 MU thrice weekly for a duration of 16 weeks. I find that the daily dosing schedule is usually better tolerated by patients. Interferon almost always causes flu-like symptoms, which may vary from mild to debilitating. Usually these symptoms improve after the first few weeks of treatment despite continued therapy. *Interferon* is myelosuppressive and patients must be monitored for neutropenia and thrombocytopenia. Autoimmune disorders can be exacerbated or unmasked by interferon and the treatment is generally contraindicated in patients with autoimmune diseases with the exception of stable hypothyroidism. Depression may occur, especially in patients with a prior history. This treatment should not be used in patients with a history of major depression, suicidal attempts or ideation, or major affective disorders. As effective treatment triggers an exacerbation of hepatitis, interferon should not be used in patients with decompensated liver disease (Child's class B or C) since they may not have the hepatic reserve required to survive the disease flare.

A widely quoted meta-analysis of 15 HBV interferon-α studies has shown that approximately one-third of patients who begin treatment HBeAg and HBV DNA positive will lose these markers, (Wong et al, 1993) although the response may be delayed until up to 6 months after completing therapy. When HBeAg clearance is induced by *interferon-α*, liver histology improves and it is rare for viral replication to reactivate. Patients most likely to respond to *interferon* therapy have increased serum aminotransferases, relatively low HBV DNA levels, and a history of acute hepatitis (as opposed to subclinical or perinatal infection).

With HBeAg negative, HBV DNA positive infection, HBV DNA loss may occur during or following *interferon-α* therapy. Unfortunately, in most of these cases viral replication reactivates some time after treatment is stopped. There is data to suggest that patients with presumed precore mutant virus HBV infection may have a better sustained viral response rate when treated for 12 or more months with *interferon-α*.

Two *PEGylated formulations* of *interferon-α* have recently been approved for the treatment of chronic HCV infection. These agents have the advantage of a prolonged duration of action and once weekly administration. Studies are ongoing to determine the efficacy of these agents in chronic HBV infection. It is not yet known what the appropriate dose and treatment duration will be with these *PEGylated interferons*.

LAMIVUDINE

Lamivudine is an orally administered nucleoside, which integrates into the elongating DNA chains of replicating HBV, thus terminating viral replication. This agent has been shown to be highly efficacious in reducing HBV DNA when given at a dose of 100 mg/d. After 3 years of continuous treatment with *lamivudine*, approximately one-third of patients who were originally HBeAg positive will have converted to HBeAb. It appears that seroconversions induced by *lamivudine* are less durable than those induced by interferon, as a significant proportion of patients will reactivate replication if and when *lamivudine* is stopped. Patients with presumed precore mutant HBeAg-negative chronic HBV infection respond to *lamivudine* therapy but in the vast majority of cases, viral replication resumes after drug is withdrawn. As with interferon-α, high pretreatment aminotransferases are predictive of a good response to lamivudine treatment. Although *lamivudine* is extremely well tolerated, the major problem in its use is its propensity to select for resistant escape mutants. The most common mutant affects the YMDD motif of the DNA polymerase and allows the virus to replicate despite continued exposure to *lamivudine*. Although some studies suggest that this mutated virus is less harmful than the wild-type virus, this finding has not been consistent. About 15% of chronic HB patients develop resistance to *lamivudine* after 1 year of treatment and this increases to approximately 50% at 3 years.

ADEFOVIR DIPIVOXIL

The most recent therapy approved for the treatment of chronic HB is *adefovir dipivoxil*. This nucleotide analog has been shown to be effective in both HBeAg positive and negative chronic HBV infection. *Adefovir dipivoxil* is effective against HBV infections that have acquired resistance to *lamivudine*. The usual dose is 10 mg/d but it must be adjusted for renal impairment. The major adverse effect of *adefovir dipivoxil* is nephrotoxicity. To date, resistance to *adefovir dipivoxil* has been exceedingly rare although there are few patients who have been treated with this agent beyond 2 years.

A number of other agents are in development for chronic HBV infection including *entecavir* and *emtricitabine* (FTC).

SELECTING PATIENTS FOR THERAPY

With several different treatments available, there are options when it comes to the management of patients with chronic HBV infection. Treatment should only be considered in patients with actively replicating infection as indicated by significant serum levels of HBV DNA. Because none of the available therapies is likely to be effective in the immunotolerant phase of infection, patients with persistently normal aminotransferases should generally be followed conservatively and considered for treatment only when and if their liver enzymes become abnormal. However, patients with normal enzymes may be considered for therapy if their liver biopsies demonstrate moderate to severe hepatitis.

Once the decision is made to treat chronic HBV, an appropriate therapy must be chosen. Although not tested head-to-head, the efficacy of *interferon-α* and the oral nucleoside/nucleotide agents appears to be similar. *Interferon-α* must be administered by injection and may be associated with significant side effects. It does, however, have the advantage of a finite course of therapy, whereas the oral agents must be given long term and possibly indefinitely. Although safe and generally well tolerated, the major downside of the oral agents is the induction of resistant escape mutants. This appears to be a larger problem with *lamivudine* than *adefovir dipivoxal*, although longer term data is awaited.

RECOMMENDED TREATMENT PLAN

I believe that it is acceptable to use any of these three agents as first line therapy in chronic HBV infection, depending on physician and patient preference. In the patient with HBeAg positive HBV infection, especially if serum aminotransferases are more than twice normal, I prefer to use a standard 16-week course of *interferon-α* initially. However, many patients have contraindications to the use of *interferon-α* related to psychiatric conditions and autoimmunity. Furthermore, many patients are unwilling or unable to tolerate the side effects of *interferon-α* injections. Because of the potential for life threatening liver failure, patients with decompensated liver disease should not be treated with *interferon-α*. Patients who fail to clear HBV DNA and seroconvert HBeAg to HBeAb within 6 months of completing *interferon-α* therapy can be considered for alternate therapy.

The oral nucleoside/nucleotide drugs, *lamivudine* and *adefovir dipivoxil* are easily administered, well tolerated, and can be safely used in patients with hepatic decompensation. Their major limitation relates to the requirement for long term treatment, without clear cut parameters to stop the medications. In those patients who experience an HBeAg to HBeAb seroconversion on therapy, one can consider stopping treatment after a minimum of 3 months of "consolidation therapy." However, even after this extension of therapy, there is potential for reactivation of viral replication after medication is withdrawn. The longer treatment is continued, the greater the potential for emergence of resistant escape mutants. For these reasons, I prefer to limit the use of these agents to those patients at significant risk of progressive liver disease, so I generally advise a staging liver biopsy before initiating these drugs.

Although *lamivudine* is less expensive than *adefovir dipivoxil*, it appears to be associated with a higher rate of emergence of resistant mutants—at least in the short to medium term. I am concerned that resistance to *adefovir dipivoxil* may become more significant as we accrue more experience with the long term use of this agent. Because the resistant strains selected by each of the two drugs retain sensitivity to the other agent, it may be rational to use combination therapy in a manner analogous to the strategy used to treat HIV infection. It is anticipated that additional antiviral drugs will become available over the next few years. An initial study of combination therapy using *interferon-α* and *lamivudine* failed to show significant benefit. However, this strategy is being revisited in ongoing studies using PEGylated interferon and oral antivirals. Sequential use of nucleoside/nucleotide drugs following the emergence of resistance may be expected to generate multiply resistant strains. This is of particular consequence in the patient who will ultimately require a liver transplant, as recurrent HBV infection is frequently fatal when effective antiviral strategies are not available. Those patients with decompensated liver disease are best treated in concert with a liver transplant program.

DIFFICULT TREATMENT ISSUES

The patient with HBeAg negative, HBV DNA positive infection poses particular issues. If *interferon-α* is used, treatment should be prolonged for at least 12 months, although many patients will have difficulty tolerating interferon for such long periods of time. If oral antivirals are used, there are no parameters to guide us in stopping therapy. I only treat patients with presumed precore mutant virus infection if they have significant hepatic fibrosis, and explain to patients that treatment will be open-ended and likely lifelong.

The treatment of chronic HBV infection is challenging and constantly evolving. With novel therapeutics and treatment strategies being developed, the approach to managing these patients will undoubtedly change in the years to come.

Supplemental Reading

Beasley RP, Hwang LY, Lin CC, Chien CS. Hepatocellular carcinoma and hepatitis B virus. A prospective study of 22,707 men in Taiwan. Lancet 1981;2:8256.

Dienstag JL, Schiff ER, Wright TL, et al. Lamivudine as initial treatment for chronic hepatitis B in the United States. N Engl J Med 1999;341:1256–63.

Hadziyzniss SJ, Tassopoulos NC, Heathcote, EJ, et al. Adefovir dipivoxil for the treatment of hepatitis B E antigen-negative chronic hepatitis B. N Engl J Med 2003;348:800–7.

Leung NW, Lai CL, Chang TT, et al. Extended lamivudine treatment in patients with chronic hepatitis B enhances hepatitis B e antigen seroconversion rates: results after 3 years of therapy. Hepatology 2001;33:1527–32.

Marcellin P, Chang TT, Lim SG, et al. Adefovir dipivoxil for the treatment of hepatitis B e antigen-positive chronic hepatitis B. N Engl J Med 2003;348:808–16.

Niederau C, Heintges T, Lange S, et al. Long-term follow-up of HbeAg-positive patients treated with interferon alfa for chronic hepatitis B. N Engl J Med 1996;334:1422–7.

Wong DK, Cheung AM, O'Rourke K, et al. Effect of alpha-interferon treatment in patients with hepatitis B e antigen-positive chronic hepatitis B. A meta-analysis. Ann Intern Med 1993;119:312–23.

CHAPTER 107

CHRONIC HEPATITIS C

Rudra Rai, MD

Hepatitis C virus (HCV) is a single stranded RNA virus of the *Hepacivirus* genus in the Flaviviridae family. Discovered in 1990 as a causative agent for posttransfusion non-A, non-B hepatitis, it is now known to infect 1.8% of the US population (between 4 to 5 million seropositive individuals). Recent studies performed on serum samples from 21,241 persons 6 years of age or older who participated in the third National Health and Nutrition Examination Survey, conducted during 1988 through to 1994, estimated the number of patients with active HCV infection to be roughly 2.7 million people in the United States. This prevalence has remained stable through the past decade. Worldwide, estimates suggest that there are approximately 170 to 200 million people with HCV infection.

There are approximately 30,000 new cases of acute HCV infection diagnosed each year in the United States. However, the incidence of new infections has declined dramatically over the past decade with improved safety of the blood supply and recognition of potential risk factors. The predominant mode of transmission of HCV has shifted from posttransfusion-associated hepatitis to injection drug use. Other modes of transmission include nosocomial (eg, in hemodialysis units), intranasal cocaine use, tattoos, body piercing, sexual transmission, and perinatal exposure.

Natural History

In most individuals with chronic HC infection there will be biochemical and histological evidence of chronic hepatitis, in addition to circulating HCV ribonucleic acid (RNA). Among the 14 to 46% of acutely infected patients who recover, many will retain HCV antibodies for several years, whereas others will have no serologic markers of HCV infection on extended observation. In a smaller group (approximately 27%), viremia is persistent (or possibly intermittent) but serum alanine aminotransferase (ALT) levels are usually normal.

Reported rates of spontaneous clearance in acute infections have ranged from 14 to 46%. Both viral and host factors have been linked to viral persistence. The natural history of chronic HCV infection has been estimated both from prospective studies beginning with acute infection following blood transfusion, and from prospective observation of patients diagnosed with chronic HCV infection. Once chronic HCV infection has been established, there appears to be an overall risk of cirrhosis as high as 20% over the first 10 to 20 years of infection. Indeed, in the United States, the incidence of hepatocellular carcinoma (HCC) is increasing and deaths from cirrhosis secondary to chronic HCV infection are estimated to be 8,000 to 12,000 per year and are rising steadily.

Host factors that are strongly implicated in progression of chronic HC infection include older age at infection, male gender, and concomitant alcohol use. Additional factors that have been suggested include hepatic steatosis, iron loading, and human immunodeficiency virus (HIV) coinfection. In one study, cirrhosis was present in 43% of patients older than 50 years of age at the time of infection compared with 6% of those infected when younger than 20 years of age. Similarly, a prospective study from Ireland of young women infected with HCV from contaminated blood products demonstrated only a 1 to 2% rate of cirrhosis after nearly 20 years.

Clinical Implications

The health care impact of chronic HCV infection appears to be increasing due to the increased prevalence of patients with infection for more than 20 years. Chronic HC infection is now estimated to be the leading cause of end-stage liver disease necessitating liver transplants in the United States.

However, in addition to progressive liver disease the potential health care impacts include HCC—it is estimated that chronic HC infection is associated with approximately 80% of HCC in the United States—and extrahepatic manifestations (eg, hematologic [*cryoglobulinemia, aplastic anemia, thrombocytopenia, B-cell lymphoma*], renal [*glomerulonephritis, nephrotic syndrome*], dermatologic [*porphyria cutanea tarda, lichen planus, cutaneous necrotizing vasculitis*], endocrine [*diabetes mellitus, antithyroid antibodies*], salivary [*sialadenitis*], and ocular [*uveitis, corneal ulcer*].)

Diagnosis

HC may be suspected on the basis of elevated liver function tests or because of risk factors (blood transfusions before 1990, history of injection drug use, etc). A second or third generation enzyme-linked immunosorbent assay (ELISA) is the usual screening test, unless an acute infection is suspected. In acute exposure, HCV RNA will be positive early on in the vast majority of patients who have not seroconverted to HCV antibodies. However, a small proportion of patients with acute HC may be missed on the basis of serologic and RNA testing, and therefore should be observed with repeated testing for at least 6 months. Recombinant immunoblot assay testing may be done to confirm an ELISA result, if one suspects false positive antibodies to HCV.

HCV RNA quantitation is a key assay for managing treatment, and may be influenced by sample preparation and different assay methods. The dynamic ranges of these tests vary significantly and one assay cannot be reliably compared with another. Several commercial assays are now available, and the extremely sensitive transcription mediated amplification assay for HCV RNA appears to reliably detect patients who have achieved sustained virologic response versus patients with low level viremia who may later relapse (eg, *Heptimax* [Quest Diagnostics], *Quantasure* [Labcorp]). Staging underlying fibrosis by liver biopsy provides useful prognostic information that may influence the urgency of initiating treatment.

Treatment

In my practice, I often individualize decisions for treatment of chronic HC infection based on a clear understanding of (1) the natural history of chronic HC, (2) factors that influence treatment response and disease progression, (3) the required commitment for monitoring treatment adherence, tolerability, and response, and (4) the overall potential for side effects and poor outcomes. In general, my primary goal of treatment is to provide a safe and effective means to eradicate HCV infection. In addition, there are several secondary goals of treatment, including slowing disease progression, improving histology, reducing risk of HCC, and improving health-related quality of life.

The recent National Institutes of Health (NIH) Consensus Statement on the management of chronic HC emphasized that consideration of treatment should not be confined only to those patients who would have met the entry criteria of pivotal studies, but should be individualized for the goals of prevention of cirrhosis or its complications.

Interferons were among the first agents studied in the mid-1980s for treatment of viral hepatitis. The effects of interferons are multifactorial, and include induction of 2′ 5′ oligoadenylate synthetase; induction of RNA-dependent protein kinases; phosphorylation of EIF-2, a protein synthesis initiation factor; blocking viral replication; and cell membrane changes (ie, induction of HLA class I, and other immunomodulatory and antiproliferative effects). Pegylation of interferon involves a covalent attachment of polyethylene glycol (PEG), an inert, water-soluble, non-toxic substance, to the parent compound. The PEG chain size and configuration can differ (eg, straight or branched), and the various binding sites available result in mixtures of positional isomers. There are now two commercially approved peginterferons that have been approved by the US Food and Drug Administration (FDA). *Peginterferon* α-2b is a 12 kDa pegylated protein with a half-life of 22 to 60 hours and a specific activity approximately 28% of that of *interferon* α-2b. *Peginterferon* α-2a is a 40 kDa pegylated protein with a half-life of 60 to 80 hours and specific activity approximately 7% of that of *interferon* α-2a.

In 2002, the NIH Consensus Panel concluded that the combination of peginterferon and ribavirin is the most effective regimen for the treatment of chronic HC infection leading to sustained virologic responses in over 50% of treated patients. Currently FDA-approved dose regimens for peginterferons and ribavirin are as follows:

1. *Peginterferon* α-2a or *Pegasys* (monotherapy) 180 mcg (fixed dose) subcutaneously once a week
2. *Peginterferon* α-2a or *Pegasys* (combination therapy) 180 mcg (fixed dose) subcutaneously once a week along with
   i. Ribavirin (Weight < 75 kg): 1000 mg/d orally in 2 divided doses
   ii. Ribavirin (Weight > 75 kg): 1200 mg/d orally in 2 divided doses
3. *Peginterferon* α-2b or *PegIntron* (monotherapy): 1.0 mcg/kg (weight-based dose) subcutaneously once a week
4. *Peginterferon* α-2b or *PegIntron* (combination therapy): 1.5 mcg/kg (weight-based dose) subcutaneously once a week along with
   i. Ribavirin 800 mg/d orally in 2 divided doses
   ii. Ribavirin at higher doses (weight-based, 10.6 mg/kg) is currently being evaluated in prospective trials.

The recommended duration of treatment in genotype 1 patients is 48 weeks; in genotype 2 or 3 patients it is 24 weeks.

Baseline Evaluation

Interferon monotherapy and *combination therapy with ribavirin* are associated with several adverse effects, and may be contraindicated or should be used with extreme caution in patients with certain preexisting conditions. These include significant cytopenia, pregnancy, severe depression or other psychiatric conditions, cardiac diseases, poorly controlled diabetes, seizure disorders, and autoimmune or potentially immune-mediated diseases. Before initiating treatment, it is important to obtain a baseline assessment of liver tests, complete blood counts, HCV RNA levels, and genotype, and to individualize the need for cardiac stress testing and eye examinations (to exclude retinopathy, especially in patients with history of diabetes or hypertension).

Virologic Assessment of Response

This is determined using the following key tests:

1. *Baseline reference HCV RNA* (viral titer and genotype) is best measured just before starting treatment to determine optimal treatment duration and regimen, and to establish a baseline to determine later treatment end-points.
2. *Early virologic response* can be assessed after 12 weeks of therapy. Failure to achieve a decline in HCV RNA levels of at least 2 logs by week 12 predicts an extremely low likelihood of a sustained virologic response with further treatment (negative predictive value = 98%).
3. *End-of-treatment* is performed at the end of the recommended course to determine whether viral response occurred during treatment.
4. *Sustained virologic responses* is performed at the end of 6 months of observation following completion of treatment, and appears to be the gold standard for long term loss of serum HCV RNA.

Predictors of Response

Factors predictive of a sustained response include genotype (non-1), low HCV RNA levels, absence of advanced cirrhosis or fibrosis, early disappearance of HCV RNA (at 12 to 24 weeks), short duration of disease (< 5 years), younger age (< 45 years), and low hepatic iron stores. In addition, minimizing side effects, avoiding discontinuation or reduction in therapy, and maximizing adherence are important goals to achieve the highest response rates.

Management of Adverse Events

Hematologic abnormalities are frequently observed and led to dose reduction of *peginterferon* and *ribavirin* in a number of subjects in the pivotal randomized controlled trials. Ribavirin is associated with a dose-dependent, extravascular hemolytic anemia in more than 90% of treated patients. Anemia is associated with fatigue, exercise intolerance, and depression. My practice has been to assess symptoms carefully and consider ribavirin dose modifications and/or *recombinant human erythropoetin* (40,000 subcutaneously weekly). On the other hand, interferons, especially peginterferons, cause a significant decrease in peripheral white blood cell count and platelet count due to bone marrow suppression. Most clinicians often tolerate absolute neutrophil counts (ANC) as low as 500 to 750/mm^3. However, once the ANC drops below 500/mm^3, I will often consider interferon dose reduction and/or initiation of *filgrastim* (300 mcg subcutaneously once or twice weekly). Finally, the role of *oprelvekin* (IL-11) for thrombocytopenia is not well defined and currently not the standard of care because of concerns about adverse effects (papilledema [2%], cardiovascular events, including arrythmias [15%] and pulmonary edema, anasarca, and dilutional electrolyte abnormalities [15%]).

HCV/HIV Co-infection

Special consideration for HCV/HIV co-infection is warranted, because up to 30% of HIV infected individuals are co-infected with HCV, and nearly all studies indicate that HIV accelerates progression of HCV to cirrhosis and liver failure. Preliminary studies indicate the safety of peginterferon and ribavirin to be comparable to HCV mono-infected patients, despite some early concerns about fatigue, anemia, and depression. *Ribavirin* should not be co-administered with *didanosine* because of increased toxicity. Often, initiation of high active antiretroviral therapy in HCV/HIV co-infected patients will lead to a HCV disease flare from immune reconstitution injury or drug toxicity.

Mild Liver Disease

Patients who have persistent elevation in serum ALT but do not have fibrosis and have minimal necroinflammatory changes are likely to have only slow disease progression. Such patients can be monitored periodically. However, the decision to treat should be individualized.

Cirrhosis

In a patient with decompensated cirrhosis, treatment can be extremely challenging with the risk of major adverse events (eg, severe thrombocytopenia, variceal hemorrhage, etc) and further decompensation (eg, worsening hepatic encephalopathy), and should therefore, be handled in liver transplant centers with the requisite experience and infrastructure, and preferably referred for clinical trials until the safety and efficacy data of treatment are established. However, patients with advanced bridging fibrosis or early cirrhosis (Child's class A) can often be treated in the community without major complications. The efficacy of treatment in patients with advanced fibrosis or compensated cirrhosis has been derived mostly from subgroup analysis of larger clinical trials, and suggests that the response is lower than in patients without cirrhosis. The main treatment option for such patients is liver transplant.

Recurrence after Transplant

Disease progression following transplant is accelerated compared to immunocompetent patients with HCV infection. In addition, the risk of complications is higher in posttransplant HCV patients with cirrhosis compared to immunocompetent patients with cirrhosis. Recurrence correlates with HCV RNA levels at the time of the transplant, the age of the organ donor, and the degree of immunosuppression in the posttransplant period.

Acute Infection

The consensus panel recognized that studies on interferon for acute HCV have been small, heterogeneous, and lacking in randomization. The panel recommended that treatment of persons with acute HC is warranted, but the timing of therapy and the type of regimen to use remains to be determined from future trials.

Conclusions

Response to therapy is associated with clinical benefits, including reduction in hepatic inflammation and, in many cases, reduction in hepatic fibrosis and regression of septal fibrosis. New insights into the virology of HCV will likely lead to more innovative models for the discovery and evaluation of anti-HCV drugs. Second-generation recombinant interferons and albumin-stabilized interferon-α are being evaluated along with novel ribavirin-related compounds (*Levovirin, L-isomer of ribavirin,* and *Viramidine,* a ribavirin prodrug). In addition, novel immunomodulators (*Thymosin a-1*), immune-based therapies (*HCV immunoglobulin G*), therapeutic HCV vaccines (*HCV glycoprotein E1 construct*) and targeted HCV inhibitors (*NS3 protease inhibitors, helicase inhibitors*) are all contributing to make the next decade possibly the most exciting in the development of more effective treatments for chronic HCV infection.

Supplemental Reading

Alter MJ, et al. The prevalence of hepatitis C virus infection in the United States, 1988 through 1994. N Engl J Med 1999;341: 556–62.

El-Serag HB, et al. Rising incidence of hepatocellular carcinoma in the United States. N Engl J Med 1999;340:745–50.

Fried MW, et al. Peginterferon alfa-2a plus ribavirin for chronic hepatitis C virus infection. N Engl J Med 2002;347:975–82.

Jaeckel E. Treatment of acute hepatitis C with interferon alfa-2b. N Engl J Med 2001;345:1452–7.

Kenny-Walsh, et al. Clinical outcomes after hepatitis C infection from contaminated anti-D immune globulin. Irish Hepatology Research Group. N Engl J Med 1999;340:1228–33.

Manns MP, et al. Peginterferon alfa-2b plus ribavirin compared with interferon alfa-2b plus ribavirin for initial treatment of chronic hepatitis C: a randomised trial. Lancet 2001;358: 958–65.

Rodriguez-Rosado R, et al. Management of hepatitis C in HIV-infected persons [review]. Antiviral Res 2001;52:189–98.

Roudot-Thoraval F, et al. Epidemiological factors affecting the severity of hepatitis C virus-related liver disease: a French survey of 6,664 patients. The Study Group for the Prevalence and the Epidemiology of Hepatitis C Virus. Hepatology 1997;26:485–90.

Seeff LB, et al. Long-term mortality after transfusion-associated non-A, non-B hepatitis. The National Heart, Lung, and Blood Institute Study Group. N Engl J Med 1992;327:1906–11.

Seeff LB, et al. National Institutes of Health Consensus Development Conference: management of hepatitis C: 2002. Hepatology 2002;36(5 Suppl 1):S1–2.

CHAPTER 108

Viral Hepatitis in Children

Kathleen B. Schwarz, MD

Hepatitis B virus (HBV) infection is a major pediatric health problem globally; 25 to 30% of the 350 million people with this infection in the world population have acquired the virus via perinatal transmission or in early adulthood. The US Food and Drug Administration (FDA) has approved the following two antiviral therapies: (1) *interferon (IFN)-α* and (2) *lamivudine*, an HBV polymerase inhibitor. This chapter will review the indications for therapy, advantages and disadvantages of each drug, and what little data there is about combination therapy and the role of liver biopsy in both the decision about treatment and as a means of follow-up. Attention will be given to special management issues including monitoring for hepatocellular carcinoma (HCC), treatment of HBV nephropathy, and management of children with HBV infection undergoing liver transplants.

Hepatitis C virus (HCV) infection has been estimated to occur in approximately 150,000 children in the United States; global pediatric prevalence rates are unknown. In July 2003, the combination of IFN and ribavirin was approved by the FDA for treatment of chronic HCV in children ages 3 to 16 years. Given the efficacy of combination therapy and the emergence of *pegylated IFN*, *IFN* monotherapy is no longer indicated for treatment of HCV. However it is interesting to note that *IFN* monotherapy in children with chronic HCV appears to be more effective than it is in adults (sustained virologic response of 36% versus 8 to 10% for adults). This is biologically plausible because children exhibit the following three characteristics which predict a favorable response to *IFN* in adults: (1) shorter duration of infection, (2) precirrhotic liver disease, and (3) lower viral loads. A small pilot trial of *pegylated IFN* suggested that children respond well to this therapy. Because there is a suggestion that children may respond better to *IFN-based* therapies than adults, and because ribavirin is a known teratogen, there is a need for large scale prospective controlled trials to determine if addition of *ribavirin* to *pegylated IFN* will improve response rates. This chapter will review the advantages and disadvantages of IFN-α in combination with *ribavirin* as well as *pegylated IFN*. The role of liver biopsy in decisions about management and for assessing response to therapy will be discussed, as will monitoring for HCC.

HBV

Goals of Therapy

Similar to the situation in adults, the primary goals of therapy are (1) induction of disease remission, (2) prevention of progression to cirrhosis, and (3) prevention of the development of liver failure and/or HCC. Decreasing infectivity and the unpleasant social stigma accompanying chronic HBV in childhood are also important aims.

Indications for Therapy

Children with chronic HBV should be examined for possible antiviral therapy with the laboratory tests listed below under α-*IFN*. Serum α-feto protein, a relatively insensitive marker for HCC should be performed. HCV and human immunodeficiency virus (HIV) should be assessed as well because they are bloodborne pathogens which sometimes coinfect children with HBV. Baseline ultrasound for cirrhosis, HCC, and to mark a site for percutaneous liver biopsy should be performed before initiation of therapy; liver biopsy should be performed prior to initiation of therapy. Indications for antiviral treatment in children are similar to those in adults and include the following: (1) presence of hepatitis B "e" antigen (HbeAg) and HBV deoxyribonucleic acid (DNA) in serum, (2) elevated alanine aminotransferase (ALT), and (3) evidence of inflammatory activity in the liver biopsy.

α-Interferon

The IFNs exhibit antiviral and antiproliferative effects; in addition, α-*IFN* is an immunostimulant. The drug does suppress HBV replication in a small proportion of selected children. Twenty-four percent of children 1 year of age and older treated with 3 MU/m^2 subcutaneously t.i.w. times 1 week with escalation up to 6 MU/m^2 IFN subcutaneously t.i.w for 16 to 24 weeks achieved loss of HBV DNA and HBeAg at 24 weeks of follow-up as opposed to 10% of untreated control patients. The maximum weekly dosage was 10 MU t.i.w. Forty-one percent of the responders lost HBsAg compared with none of the untreated controls. Thirty-five percent of children with a low baseline HBV DNA (< 100 pg/mL) responded compared with 9% with higher levels of HBV DNA. Only 5% of children who had contracted HBV via maternal–fetal transmission achieved a response compared with 31% of those who acquired HBV via other routes. A meta-analysis of 240 children treated with *IFN* for chronic HBV infection versus untreated controls demonstrated the following odds ratios: (1) increased HBV clearance (2.2), (2) HBeAg clearance (2.2), and (3) ALT normalization (2.3).

IFN is indicated for the treatment of chronic HBV in children 1 year of age or older who have compensated liver disease. Patients should be without a history of hepatic encephalopathy, variceal bleeding, and ascites; should have a normal serum bilirubin and albumin; ≤ 2 seconds prolongation of prothrombin time; white blood cells ≥ 4000/mm^3; and platelets ≥ 150,000/mm^3.

At baseline prior to therapy, as well as at weeks 1, 2, 4, 8, 12, and 16 of therapy, the following tests should be performed:
1. Complete blood count with platelets
2. Aspartate aminotranferase
3. ALT
4. Alkaline phosphatase
5. Total and direct bilirubin
6. Albumin

HBeAg, hepatitis B surface antigen (HbsAg), and HBV DNA should be monitored at the beginning of therapy, at the end of 16 weeks of therapy, as well as at 3 and 6 months after cessation of therapy, because some patients may become virologic responders after discontinuation of therapy. Patients who respond to therapy often develop a flare (transient increase in ALT ≤ 2 times baseline value) 8 to 12 weeks after initiation of therapy (59% of responders versus 35% of nonresponders). *IFN* can be continued during the flare unless signs of liver failure ensue; patients should be monitored clinically and biochemically every 2 weeks during a flare. Adverse effects include flu-like symptoms, anxiety, depression, anorexia, weight loss, hair loss, bone marrow suppression, thyroid disorders, and autoantibody induction.

The following dose reduction/stopping rules should be used:

	White blood cells	Granulocytes	Platelet count
Reduce dose 50%	< 1.5 × 10^9/L	< 0.75 × 10^9/L	< 50 × 10^9/L
Permanently discontinue	< 1.0 × 10^9/L	< 0.5 × 10^9/L	< 25 × 10^9/L

Lamivudine

Lamivudine is a nucleoside analogue that blocks viral replication by termination of the proviral DNA chain during elongation and inhibition of the HBV polymerase. In the largest randomized controlled pediatric study of this drug to date, 191 children were treated with 3 mg/kg/d up to a maximum of 100 mg/d or placebo for one year. Twenty-three percent of treated children exhibited a virologic response (absence of HBeAg and HBV DNA in serum) at 52 weeks compared with 13% of placebo-treated patients. The higher the baseline ALT, the higher the response. Low baseline HBV DNA (< 800 mEq/mL) and a histologic activity index score > 4 were predictors of response. Nineteen percent of the lamivudine-treated patients developed drug-resistant mutations in the YMDD motif of the HBV polymerase gene. Despite development of the mutation, children exhibited median HBV DNA and ALT levels that were substantially lower at week 52 compared with baseline.

Lamivudine is indicated for children 2 years of age and older with HBeAg positivity, HBV DNA in serum, and elevated ALT. Dose reduction should be done in patients with impaired renal function, as follows (modified from recommendations for adults).

Creatinine clearance (mL/min)	Recommended dosage of *lamivudine*
≥ 50	3 mg/kg/d up to 100 mg/d
30–49	3 mg/kg/d first dose then 1.5 mg/kg/d
15–29	3 mg/kg/d first dose then 0.75 mg/kg/d
5–14	1 mg/kg/d first dose then 0.45 mg/kg/d
< 5	1 mg/kg/d first dose than 0.3 mg/kg/d

Monitoring should be as is recommended for IFN. Rare but serious side effects observed in adults include lactic acidosis and severe hepatomegaly with steatosis, most frequently observed in obese women taking antiretroviral therapy, and posttreatment exacerbation of hepatitis that usually resolves but has rarely been fatal. The major deleterious side effect with *lamivudine* usage has been the emergence of drug-resistant mutants. In one early open-label study of children with HIV and HBV, *lamivudine* therapy was associated with peripheral neuropathy and neutropenia; 14 to 15% of the children developed pancreatitis.

Drug Combinations

Dikici and colleagues (2002) found that 12 months of combined *lamivudine* and *IFN* therapy was associated with higher rates of ALT normalization and clearance of HBV DNA compared with IFN alone; however 6 months after cessation of therapy the complete response rate (as defined by HBeAg/anti-HBe seroconversion plus clearance of HBV DNA plus normalization of ALT) did not differ between groups.

Controversies

Because children with chronic HBV are usually asymptomatic, *IFN* therapy is unpleasant, and lamivudine is associated with a high rate of drug resistance, some investigators (usually adult hepatologists!) argue that therapy should be deferred until more effective agents are found. Others (usually pediatric hepatologists!) argue that an aggressive approach is warranted because eradication of the virus in a few of those treated or, more likely, at least inhibition of the progression of liver disease, could yield long lasting benefits.

Recommendations

IFN should be considered the first line of therapy for children with chronic HBV because it is the only therapy to date that has been associated with clearance of HBsAg. *Acetaminophen* and *diphenhydramine* could be given 30 minutes before bedtime to minimize unpleasant side effects; the *IFN* is then administered at bedtime. For children who fail to respond to *IFN* and/or who cannot tolerate the drug, *lamivudine* can be initiated. *IFN* can be used to treat children with HBV nephropathy. Because *IFN* is an immunostimulant and may promote liver rejection in pediatric transplant patients with chronic HBV, *lamivudine* is the drug of choice. Children with chronic HBV are at risk for HCC and should be monitored periodically with liver ultrasound and serum α-fetoprotein; the optimal frequency of monitoring has not been established. The response of children with HBeAg negativity HBV DNA in serum and elevated ALT has not been systematically studied; extrapolation from adults would suggest that 12 months of treatment as opposed to 6 months would double sustained response rates 6 months after the discontinuation of therapy.

Future Therapies

Another nucleoside analogue, *adefovir dipivoxil*, recently received FDA approval for treatment of adults with chronic HBV; a pediatric trial is being planned. A current comprehensive review discusses nine additional molecular therapies under development which aim to inhibit various aspects of the HBV life cycle.

HCV

Goals of Therapy

The aims of antiviral therapy are much the same as they are for HBV, with a much greater chance of viral eradication in children with chronic HCV as opposed to HBV.

Indications for Therapy

Children to be considered for treatment include those with viremia who are more than 2 years of age (because viral clearance may occur before this and IFN treatment in young infants may result in spastic diplegia) who have inflammation on liver biopsy consistent with chronic HCV. Because it is not yet clear whether ALT values predict response to therapy, children with normal ALT values should not be excluded from therapy. The usual inclusion and exclusion criteria for *IFN*-based trials in adults apply to children as well.

α-IFN Plus Ribavirin

There have been several uncontrolled trials using the combination of *IFN* (3 to 6 MU/m^2 3 times a week subcutaneously for 1 year) and *ribavirin* (8 to 15 mg/kg/d). HCV clearance rates 6 months or more after therapy ranged from 47 to 70%. Wirth and colleagues (2002) reported a sustained viral response (SVR) of 61% in 41 children; gender, ALT, route of transmission, and IRN pretreatment did not affect the SVR. *Ribavirin*-induced hemolysis lowered hemoglobin values at 6 and 12 months, but hemoglobin returned to baseline values after cessation of therapy.

Pegylated IFN

There has been one preliminary report of the use of *pegylated interferon* to treat children. Fourteen children ages 2 to 8 years received *pegylated IFN* α-*2a*, 180 mcg/1.73m^2 (normalized to their body surface area) subcutaneously once a week for 48 weeks. SVR was 43% 6 months after cessation of therapy. The drug was generally well tolerated but neutropenia necessitated dosage modification in 5 of the 14 children. The three major advantages of this therapy are the once weekly dosage as opposed to three injections per week with standard *IFN*, the greater antiviral efficacy of this form of *IFN* compared with standard *IFN*, and the possibility that the addition of *ribavirin*, a teratogenic drug, may not be necessary.

Controversies

Because the long term effects of the above therapies on body composition and growth as well as health-related quality of life have not been assessed, the therapies are unpleasant, the factors which predict response to therapy have not been characterized (with the exception of genotype), and because HCV in children tends to be a mild disease, there is understandable controversy as to whether or not antiviral therapy should be considered for children with this infection. In addition, it is not known whether the early viral response (a minimum of a 2 log decrease in viral load during the first 12 weeks of treatment) is predictive of SVR in children and whether children with non-I or IV genotypes could be treated for 6 months as is the case for adults. As is the case with HBV, adult hepatologists tend toward conservatism and pediatric hepatologists (who bear the burden of prevention of disease progression and are sensitive to the parental anxiety about and social stigma surrounding the child with HCV) tend to be proactive regarding antiviral therapy.

Future Therapies

A large scale multicenter trial comparing *pegylated interferon* alone or in combination with *ribavirin* is now underway and will hopefully serve to determine not only the comparative safety and efficacy of the two regimes but also long term effects on body composition, growth, and health-related quality of life.

Recommendations

Percutaneous liver biopsy should be performed on all children with chronic HCV 3 years of age or older. If there is evidence of aggressive disease (piecemeal necrosis, periportal or lobular fibrosis) then therapy should be initiated with *IFN* 3 MU/m^2 thrice weekly subcutaneously for 48 weeks in combination with *ribavirin* 15 mg/kg/d with a maximum daily dose of 1200 mg. If there is only mild disease, I suggest deferring treatment until results of the large scale multicenter trial described above are available and/or until more effective, less toxic therapies emerge.

Supplemental Reading

Barlow CF, Priebe CJ, Mulliken JB, et al. Spastic diplegia as a complication of interferon alfa-2a treatment of hemangiomas of infancy. J Pediatr 1988;132:527–30.

Bhimma R, Coovadia HM, Kramvis A, et al. Treatment of hepatitis B virus-associated nephropathy in black children. Pediatr Nephrol 2002;17:393–9.

Carithers RI, Emerson SS. Therapy of hepatitis C: meta-analysis of interferon alfa-2b trials. Hepatology 1997;26(Suppl):83–8S.

Dikici B, Bosnak M, Bosnak V, et al. Comparison of treatments of chronic hepatitis B in children with lamivudine and alpha-interferon combination and alpha-interferon alone. Pediatrics Int 2002;44:517–21.

Feld J, Lee J-y, Locarnini S. New targets and possible new therapeutic approaches in the chemotherapy of chronic hepatitis B. Hepatology 2003;38:545–53.

Jacobson KB, Murray K, Zellos A, Schwarz KB. An analysis of published trials of interferon monotherapy in children with chronic hepatitis C. J Pediatr Gastroenterol Nutr 2002;343:52–8.

Jonas MM, Kelley DA, Mizerski J, et al. Clinical trial of lamivudine in children with chronic hepatitis B. N Engl J Med 2002;346:1706–13.

Lok AS, Heathcote EJ, Hoofnagle JH. Management of hepatitis B 2000, summary of a workshop. Gastroenterol 2001;120:1828–53.

Schwarz KB. Pediatric issues in new therapies for hepatitis B and C. Curr Gastroenterol Rep 2003;5:233–9.

Schwarz KB, Mohan P, Narkewicz M, et al. The safety, efficacy and pharmacokinetics of peginterferon Alfa-2a (40KD) in children with chronic hepatitis C. DDW 2003;124(Suppl)1:A700.

Shapira R, Mor E, Bar-Nathan N, et al. Efficacy of lamivudine for the treatment of hepatitis B virus infection after live transplantation in children. Transplantation 2001;72:333–6.

Sokal EM, Conjeevaram HS, Roberts EA, et al. Interferon alfa therapy for chronic hepatitis B in children: a multicenter controlled trial. Hepatology 1996;23:700–7.

Torre D, Tambini R. Interferon-alpha treatment of chronic hepatitis B in childhood: a meta-analysis. Clin Infect Dis 1996;23:131–7.

Wirth S, Lang T, Gehring S, Gerner P. Recombinant alfa-interferon plus ribavirin therapy in children and adolescents with chronic hepatitis C. Hepatology 2002;36:585–6.

CHAPTER 109

FULMINANT HEPATIC FAILURE

TIMOTHY J. DAVERN, MD

The clinical syndrome of fulminant hepatic (FHF) was originally defined by Trey and Davidson (1970)as the development of hepatic failure with encephalopathy within 8 weeks of the onset of symptoms and in the absence of preexisting liver disease. Although there have been subsequent refinements of this definition, with varying times from symptom onset to the development of hepatic encephalopathy, all have in common the presence of severe liver injury, hepatic encephalopathy, and the absence of preexisting clinically overt liver disease. FHF results from the abrupt loss of liver function secondary to severe injury from a variety of causes and is associated with a high mortality, predominantly from cerebral edema and infection. However, some causes of FHF are associated with a better prognosis than other forms. In general, the more rapid onset forms of FHF, for example, associated with *acetaminophen* hepatotoxicity, are associated with a higher incidence of cerebral edema but an overall better prognosis, probably reflecting the lack of liver architectural derangement and thus more favorable conditions for hepatic regeneration in these cases. In contrast, FHF due to idiosyncratic drug reactions, Wilson's disease, and of indeterminate etiology, which tend to follow a subacute course, carry a particularly poor prognosis.

Incidence and Etiology

The incidence of FHF is not well defined but has been estimated at approximately 2,000 cases per year in the United States. The various causes of FHF may be grouped into five general categories (Table 109-1). Of note, there is significant geographical variation in the prevalence of various causes of FHF, for example, with drugs and toxins causing most acute liver failure (ALF) in the United States and the United Kingdom, and hepatitis B virus (HBV)causing most cases in some developing countries.

Drugs and Toxins

Drug-induced liver disease is currently the major cause of FHF in the United States and in most other Western countries, with *acetaminophen* being by far the most common single injurious agent and the leading cause of FHF overall. Hepatotoxic drugs and chemicals fall into two general classes, those that are predictable or dose-dependent hepatotoxins (eg, *acetaminophen*, *Amanita phalloides* mushroom poisoning), and those that are idiosyncratic (eg, *isoniazid* [INH], *phenytoin*, *halothane*, *troglitazone*, some *nonsteroidal anti-iflammatory drugs*, etc). The idiosyncratic group includes a far larger number of agents and, indeed, almost any drug can potentially be hepatotoxic in any given individual depending on largely undefined genetic and environmental factors. In general, women appear to be more susceptible to drug hepatotoxicity. Drug-induced liver injury appears to be increasingly common, as more drugs are marketed. Currently over 800 drugs have been associated with liver injury, and drug-induced liver injury is the major cause of drug withdrawal from the market, with *troglitazone* and *bromfenac* as two recent examples. Non-acetaminophen drug toxicity, which is idiosyncratic

TABLE 109-1. Etiology of Fulminant Hepatic Failure

Etiology	Examples	See Chapter
Drugs/Toxins	Acetaminophen	132
	amanita Phalloides	
	Isoniazid	
	Troglitazone	
	Valproic acid	
	Halothane	
	Complementary alternative medications (CAMs)	
Viruses	HBV +/-	117
	HDV	
	HAV	
	HEV	
	HSV	
Vascular	Shock	-
	BCS	
	Lymphoma	
Metabolic/Miscellaneous	Wilson's disease	137
	Autoimmune hepatitis	133
	Pregnancy-related liver disease	
	Reye's syndrome	
Indeterminate	Non-HA, non-HB, non-HC virus	–

BCS = Budd-Chiari syndrome, CAM = complementary alternative medications, HAV = hepatitis A virus, HBV = hepatitis B virus, HDV = hepatitis D virus, HEV = hepatitis E virus, HSV = herpes simplex virus.

and (at least currently) unpredictable, is responsible for approximately 10 to 15% of FHF cases in the United States and caries a relatively poor prognosis.

In addition to the heat stable toxins of *Amanita* and other mushrooms, other environmental agents such as the *Bacillus cereus emetic toxin*, which inhibits hepatic mitochondrial fatty acid oxidation, have also been associated with FHF. Likewise, recreational agents (eg, *3,4-methylenedioxy methamphetamine*, "Ecstasy") and a variety of complementary alternative herbal agents have been reported to cause FHF.

Acetaminophen hepatotoxicity, a result of both intentional and accidental overdose, is the most common single cause of FHF in the United States and in the United Kingdom, causing approximately 40% and 70% of FHF in the United States and the United Kingdom, respectively. Chronic alcohol use, a variety of medications (eg, several antituberculosis medications and anticonvulsants), as well as fasting appear to increase the risk of hepatotoxicity from acetaminophen, and individuals with one or more of these risk factors may develop hepatotoxicity with normally therapeutic doses of acetaminophen. Recognition of acetaminophen hepatotoxicity is critical, as early treatment with *N*-acetyl cysteine (NAC) is highly effective. Importantly, because of its short serum half-life, acetaminophen will often not be detectable in the blood of a patient presenting with hepatotoxcity and the lack of detectable serum acetaminophen should not prevent treatment with NAC. Clinical clues to the diagnosis of acetaminophen-induced FHF include serum aminotransferases that are often strikingly elevated (ie, approaching or even exceeding 10,000 U/L), a disproportionately low serum bilirubin, and an elevated creatinine, the latter in part reflecting the direct nephrotoxic effect of the acetaminophen. FHF associated with acetaminophen typically follows a rapid course, with encephalopathy often developing within 48 hours of an intentional overdose and death occurring within a week.

Viruses

HBV has long been thought to be the most common cause of FHF worldwide, but the incidence appears to be decreasing likely in part due to mass vaccination. Currently, HBV accounts for less than 10% of FHF in the United States, although HBV infection causing FHF is apparently still common in Asia and parts of Europe. Diagnosis of HBV-associated FHF may occasionally be challenging; hepatitis B surface antigen may not be detected by standard assays of serum and serum HBV virus deoxyribonucleic acid may also be undetectable. Hepatitis B "e" antigen negative viral mutants may also be overrepresented in cases of FHF. The delta virus can cause FHF either by coinfection or superinfection with HBV. Patients who are unrecognized "silent carriers" of HBV may present with FHF following chemotherapy or other immunosuppression.

Hepatitis A virus (HAV) infection is currently found in approximately 5% of patients with FHF in the United States. The risk of FHF developing during the course of symptomatic acute hepatitis A is low, ranging between 0.1 and 0.01%, and the survival rate of fulminant hepatitis A is relatively high. The role of hepatitis A infection superimposed on clinically silent chronic hepatitis C or B in causing severe acute liver injury including FHF is currently controversial. In the same family as HAV, hepatitis E virus (HEV) infection is endemic in subtropical and tropical regions, such as Asia, India, and Central and South America, and pregnant women appear to have a predilection for developing HEV-associated FHF. Isolated HCV infection is a very rare cause of FHF, but has been reported in Asia. In immunocompromised patients "exotic" viruses including cytomegalovirus (CMV), Ebstein-Barr virus (EBV), herpes simplex virus (HSV), varicella-zoster virus (VZV), and adenoviruses, have been associated with FHF. FHF secondary to infection with these viruses appears to extremely uncommon, but several fatal cases of disseminated infection with hepatitis due to HSVs and VZV have been reported.

Vascular Problems

Hepatic ischemia usually only produces relatively mild liver injury, but when ischemia is profound and the liver injury is massive, FHF can occur. Cardiac collapse secondary to myocardial infarction, cardiomyopathy, cardiac tamponade, pulmonary embolism, severe arrhythmia, severe bleeding, or heat stroke can result in FHF characterized by predominantly centrolobular liver cell necrosis. Typically, serum aminotransferases are markedly increased, but in those who recover, they return to normal rapidly. Obstruction of the portal or hepatic veins, as in Budd-Chiari syndrome or veno-occlusive disease, can cause FHF associated with a poor prognosis. Likewise, FHF in the setting of massive malignant infiltration of the hepatic sinusoids (see Chapter 141, "Pancreatic and Periamulla Neoplasm"), typically from leukemia, lymphoma, melanoma, metastatic breast or lung cancer, has been attributed to hepatic ischemia and is associated with a dismal prognosis.

Metabolic/Miscellaneous Etiologies

Included in this group are FHF secondary to Wilson's disease (see Chapter 124, "Management of Wilson's Disease"), autoimmune hepatitis, Reye's syndrome, and pregnancy-related ALF from acute fatty liver of pregnancy, hemolysis, abnormal liver enzymes and low platelets(HELLP) syndrome, or hepatic rupture (see Chapter 133, "Biliary Strictures and Neoplasms"). FHF may be the first clinical manifestation of Wilson's disease. Indeed, Wilson's disease should be considered in any young patient with unexplained FHF, particularly when there is evidence of hemolysis, relatively low aminotransferases (usually less than 500), and, characteristically, a normal or even low serum alkaline phosphatase. Other findings with less diagnostic specificity include an aspartate aminotransferase/alanine aminotransferase > 4 and a low serum uric acid, the former reflecting hemolysis and the latter a Fanconi syndrome from renal tubular copper deposition. Kayser-Fleischer rings may not be present, and the serum ceruloplasmin level is often nondiagnostic in this setting as it is an acute-phase reactant. Diagnosis relies on a high index of suspicion and measurement of copper concentration in a 24-hour urine collection. Fulminant Wilson's disease usually does not respond to chelation therapy, and the prognosis without transplant is poor. Screening of family members is critically important once the diagnosis of Wilson's disease is made.

Indeterminate

This heterogenous group which, by definition, defies diagnosis, is currently responsible for approximately 15 to 20% of FHF in the United States, and probably includes unrecognized viral, toxic, vascular, autoimmune, and metabolic etiologies. There has been significant interest in novel viruses and many indeterminate cases were previously attributed to "non-A, non-B, non-C, non-D, non-E" hepatitis. Certainly some cases of indeterminate FHF have viral features, including the well-described syndrome of post-FHF aplastic anemia which occasionally complicates indeterminate FHF, particularly in children and young adults.

Diagnosis

The presentation of FHF may be nonspecific. Jaundice may not be present, particularly in the hyperacute forms of FHF (eg, from *acetaminophen*), and the symptoms of hepatic encephalopathy, a cardinal feature of FHF, may be subtle. The patient may need to be carefully queried (eg, to recall his phone number, zip code, and social security number), or asked to perform simple calculations before it is apparent that his cognitive function is impaired. Subtle changes in personality and behavior may progress, often rapidly, to delirium, mania, violent behavior, somnolence, and coma. Unlike with chronic hepatic encephalopathy, fetor hepaticus is usually not present, and asterixis is not a uniform feature, especially with early encephalopathy. Because the presentation may be nonspecific, particularly in the nonjaundiced patient, these features may be misinterpreted as reflecting a primary neurological or psychological problem, or even drug intoxication, and a delay in diagnosis may result.

The history should be focused on rapidly determining the cause of FHF, as etiology influences prognosis, and on assessing whether the patient is a suitable candidate for liver transplantation (see Chapter 102, "Adult Liver Transplantation: Selection and Pre-transplant Evaluation"). The patient or his family should be queried regarding risk factors for viral hepatitis, such as exposure to blood products or needle sticks, recent travel or surgery, exposure to other ill individuals, drugs and toxins, particularly acetaminophen. Indeed, given its prevalence, acetaminophen hepatotoxicity should always be considered in the differential diagnosis, and particular attention should be focused on the patient's access to the drug, which is often combined with opiates for chronic pain relief. Requesting family members to retrieve all of the patient's medications, both prescription and nonprescription, and contacting the patient's physician and pharmacy may provide useful insights into drug exposure.

The physical examination of the patient with FHF should survey for stigmata of chronic liver disease and evidence of recreational drug use. Particular attention should be focused on the neurological examination. As mentioned above, early stages of encephalopathy may be somewhat difficult to detect, and patients who are seemingly alert and oriented should be queried extensively. The grade of hepatic encephalopathy should be quantified (Table 109 2) and the neurological examination should be frequently reassessed.

A toxicology screen should be obtained on all patients, although even patients with severe acetaminophen hepatotoxicity may have undetectable serum levels of acetaminophen by the time they present. Labs should be sent for viral and autoimmune serologies, arterial blood gas, serum lactate, serum phosphate, and glucose. Frequent assessment of serum glucose is essential. All woman of childbearing age should have a pregnancy test to exclude pregnancy-related FHF. An abdominal ultrasound should be obtained to confirm patency of hepatic vessels and assess the hepatic echotexture. Liver biopsy may be of diagnostic utility in unusual situations, including lymphomatous infiltration of the liver, which may otherwise be difficult to diagnose. The histopathology in most cases of FHF shows massive hepatic necrosis, although microvesicular steatosis is seen in certain forms of liver failure, such as those associated with pregnancy, mitochondrial toxins, valproic acid, and tetracyclines.

TABLE 109-2. Encephalopathy Grading Scheme

Encephalopathy Grade	Characteristics
0	Normal mental status/no encephalopathy
1	Subtle changes in mental status, day-night reversal, hyperreflexia
2	Drowsiness, confusion, asterixis
3	Stupor, intermittent agitation, clonus
4	Coma, decerebrate posturing

Predicting Prognosis

The prognosis for FHF has improved since the syndrome was originally described, probably reflecting a shift in the major etiologies causing FHF from HBV to acetaminophen, as well as improved medical care and, importantly, the introduction of liver transplantion. Prognosis varies by etiology; patients with acetaminophen hepatotoxicity or hepatitis A generally have a relatively good prognosis, whereas those with idiopathic drug hepatotoxicity, Wilson's disease, and FHF of indeterminate etiology have a poor prognosis, and patients with FHF from hepatitis B have a prognosis intermediate between these extremes.

The rapid and accurate prediction of prognosis is essential with FHF in order to distinguish between patients who will recover with medical therapy alone ("spontaneous survivors") and those who will not and, instead, require liver transplantation in order to survive. Ideally, this prediction should take place within a few hours of hospital admission, so decisions regarding evaluation and listing for transplant can be made in an expeditious fashion. Encephalopathy grade correlates with prognosis with more advanced encephalopathy being associated with poor prognosis. However, encephalopathy stage is not particularly useful as a means of determining prognosis, as advanced encephalopathy tends to occur relatively late in the course of the illness, often just prior to the development of irreversible neurological injury, multiorgan failure, and other complications which may preclude transplantation.

A variety of clinical parameters and biochemical tests have been used to predict prognosis, including factor V levels, unbound Gc protein (an actin scavenger), serum phosphate levels, serum lactate levels, liver histology, and serial abdominal computed tomography (CT) scans to assess liver volume changes. The most commonly used prognostic scheme in the United States is the one developed by the King's College group, which has been validated by other centers (Table 109-3). The major strength of the King's College criteria is that most of the variables used to predict prognosis can be determined rapidly after presentation, and time is of the essence, as discussed below. The King's criteria have relatively good positive predictive values, but the negative predictive value is relatively low so that patients who do not meet the criteria are still at risk for death without transplant.

Management

General Supportive Care (Table 109-4)

Patients with FHF are by definition critically ill and with few exceptions should be managed in the intensive care unit (ICU) of a liver transplant center. Whether FHF patients with FHF are best transported to such a center by land or air largely depends on distance and other logistics. Intensive medical care with meticulous attention to detail offers the best chance for patient spontaneous survival. Supportive care in this context includes maintaining blood pressure, supporting renal and respiratory function, preventing bleeding, correcting metabolic and electrolyte abnormalities, providing nutrition, and preventing and treating infection. At University of California San Francisco (UCSF), we use a multidisciplinary approach to the care of patients with FHF, and transplant hepatologists and surgeons, ICU physicians and nurses, nephrologists, neurologists, neurosurgeons, and social workers are all involved in the assessment and care of these very ill patients.

Most patients with FHF will require placement of central venous access (eg, triple lumen catheter in the femoral or internal jugular vein), a urinary catheter, and an arterial line for hemodynamic monitoring and phlebotomy. Many patients will also require dialysis access. Patients with advanced stage III or IV encephalopathy should be intubated for airway protection. Of note, high levels of positive end-expiratory pressure should be avoided as they may have deleterious effects on hepatic blood flow and intracranial hypertension by increasing intrathoracic pressure and decreasing venous return.

Coagulopathy in the setting of FHF is primarily the result of decreased hepatic production of clotting factors, although intravascular consumption and vitamin K deficiency may also contribute in particular patients. Thrombocytopenia is also quite common and probably of multifactorial etiology. Vitamin K administration (10 mg subcutaneously every day for 3 days) is safe but rarely effective in correcting coagulopathy from FHF. Because the prothrombin time is a very useful marker of prognosis in FHF, fresh frozen plasma (FFP) administration is generally reserved for clinically overt bleeding and invasive procedures. However, occasionally we administer FFP for profound coagulopathy (ie, international normalized ratio > 6) alone, particularly when a decision to proceed with liver transplantation has been made. Typically patients are given

TABLE 109-3. Predicting Prognosis with Fulminant Hepatic Failure: the King's College Criteria

Acetaminophen	Non-Acetominophen FHF	
Arterial pH < 7.3 Following fluid resuscitation and regardless of encephalopathy stage	INR > 6.5 or	
or	Any three of the following:	
In patients with grade III to IV encephalopathy:	Etiology:	indeterminate or drug/toxin
	Age:	< 10 years or > 40 years
	Jaundice duration:	> 1 week prior to encephalopathy
INR > 6.5 and	Bilirubin:	> 17 mg/dL
Creatinine > 3.4 mg/dL	INR:	> 3.5

FHF = fulminant hepatic failure; INR = international normalized ratio.

TABLE 109-4. Management of Fulminant Hepatic Failure Complications

Complication	Diagnosis	Treatment	Comment
Neurological Encephalopathy	Clinical exam	Consider lactulose	Lactulose is of unproven efficacy in the setting of FHF
Cerebral edema	Clinical exam CT ICP monitor	Intubate Elevate head of bed 20 to 30 degrees Hyperventilation Place ICP monitor Mannitol Barbituates Hypothermia	Consider lidocaine before intubation Approximately 5% risk of bleeding with ICP monitor
Infectious	Fever, leukocytosis Microbial cultures	Antibiotics Antifungal agents	*Staphylococcus* sp and gram-negative rods most common early pathogens isolated
Renal Failure	Decreased urine output Elevated creatinine	Continuous dialysis	Intermitten dialysis associated with hypotension and increased ICP
Bleeding	Exam Decreased hematocrit	FFP Factor VIIa Platelets Cryoprecipitate	Loose PT as a useful prognostic marker Large volume FFP associated with volume overload
Metabolic hypoglycemia electrolyte	Laboratory studies	Replacement	Hypokalemia and hypophasphatemia are particularly common
Hypotension	Vital signs	IV colloid Vasopressors	Norepinephrine

CT = computed tomography; FFP = fresh frozen plasma; FHF = fulminant hepatic failure; ICP = intracranial pressure; IV = intravenous; PT = prothrombin time.

a bolus of several units and then started on an FFP drip (50 to 250 mL/hour) depending on the severity of the coagulopathy. Overexuberant administration of FFP may result in volume overload and contribute to pulmonary edema. Support with continuous dialysis should be initiated early in this situation to avoid fluid overload. Recombinant activated factor VII (40 to 80 µg/kg), either alone or, more often, in combination with FFP, may also be used to correct coagulopathy in this setting.

Hypoglycemia secondary to impaired gluconeogenesis, depleted glycogen stores, and elevated circulating insulin levels, is common in FHF and must be treated vigorously. Blood glucose testing should be frequent (eg, every 4 hours) and hypoglycemia treated rapidly, usually with 10% or greater dextrose solution. Electrolyte problems, especially hyokalemia, hypomagnesiumia, and hypophosphatemia, are common and should be corrected. FHF is a catabolic state and enteral feeding should be commenced early to prevent malnutrition. This may also reduce the likelihood of gastric stress ulceration, but acid inhibition, typically with a proton pump inhibitor, is also used for this purpose. Patients with advanced FHF often require circulatory support with colloid and vasopressors (eg, *norepinephrine*). Refractory hypotension is usually caused by preterminal liver failure, sepsis or pancreatitis, the latter which may complicate FHF particularly secondary to *acetaminophen* toxicity.

Specific Medical Therapy (Table 109-5)

Early administration of NAC is a highly effective antidote for *acetaminophen* poisoning and should be promptly administered as a 140 mg/kg initially, followed by 17 doses of 70 mg/kg at 4 hour intervals when this diagnosis is suspected. If the patient is unable to tolerate oral NAC, even when given by nasogastic tube, then it should administered intravenously (IV). The usual IV dose is 150 mg/kg over 1 hour in 5% dextrose, followed by 70 mg/kg over 1 hour at 4 hour intervals for 12 doses total. Nausea and vomiting is common with both oral and IV forms of NAC. Anaphylactic reactions have been reported with the IV form of NAC, but these are relatively uncommon, and usually respond to antihistamines.

Treatment of *Amanita* intoxication includes vigorous volume replacement and forced diuresis, gastric lavage, administration of activated charcoal (50 to 100 g by mouth every 4 hours), and high dose *penicillin* (300,000 to 1,000,000 unit/kg/day IV in divided doses). Although rarely available in the United States, *silibinin* (20 to 50 mg/kg/d

TABLE 109-5. Etiology Specific Therapies for Fulminant Hepatic Failure

FHF Etiology	Specific Treatment
Acetaminophen	NAC
Pregnancy-related FHF	Delivery of fetus
	Steroids to mature fetal lungs
Hepatitis B	Lamivudine 100 to 300 mg qd
	Adefovir 10 mg qd
Autoimmune hepatitis	Corticosteroids
Amanita intoxication	Activated charcoal
	High-dose penicillin (1 million units/kg/d)
	Silymarin (50 mg/kg/d)
	NAC
Budd-Chiari syndrome	TIPS
Wilson's disease	Chelation therapy
HSV hepatitis	Acyclovir
CMV hepatitis	Ganciclovir
Lymphomatous infiltration of liver	Chemotherapy
Ischemic hepatitis	Improved hemodynamics

CMV = cytomegalovirus; FHF = fulminant hepatic failure; HSV = herpes simplex virus; NAC = N acetyl cysteine; TIPS = transjugular intrahepatic portosystemic shunt.

IV), a water-soluble form of *silimarin* (the active component of *milk thistle*), has been reported to be therapeutic with mushroom poisoning, as has NAC, given in doses similar to those for acetaminophen overdose.

Pregnancy-related FHF should be treated with early delivery along with administration of corticosteroids to foster maturation of the fetal lungs. Copper chelation is very effective for chronic Wilson's disease, but rarely effective in fulminant Wilson's in which liver transplantation is usually the only option. Other potentially beneficial but unproven therapies include high dose *corticosteroids* for fulminant autoimmune hepatitis, and *lamivudine* (and/or *adefovir*), *acyclovir*, or *ganciclovir* for FHF secondary to HBV, HSV, or CMV infection, respectively. In all of these situations, specific therapy should not delay evaluation and listing for transplant in suitable candidates.

Liver Transplantation

Liver transplantation can be lifesaving for patients with FHF. However, the scarcity of donor organs and the rapidity of clinical deterioration with FHF limit transplant as an option for many patients. The one-year survival for orthotopic liver transplant for FHF at UCSF has been approximately 90%, although this is higher than other studies suggesting a 50 to 75% one-year survival.

Early contact with a transplant center hepatologist is essential. It is better not to wait until the patient is intubated and in deep coma to contemplate transfer to a transplant center. Timing is critical once a diagnosis of FHF is established. Indeed, at UCSF we have listed particularly ill patients for transplant while arranging for transfer to our facility. The current system for organ allocation allows high-priority ("status 1") listing for patients with FHF. Early referral is important so that the patient may be listed early for transplant, and also examined while still lucid. Many patients die or develop contraindications to transplant, such as brain herniation or refractory sepsis, while awaiting a donor organ. Although patients with FHF are listed as soon as possible after presentation, the decision to actually proceed with transplant at our center is made when an acceptable organ is identified, typically within 48 to 72 hours after listing. The decision to proceed with transplant can be a very difficult one because there is the possibility, particularly with FHF of rapid onset, of complete recovery, and liver transplantation requires that the patient remain on lifelong immunosuppression. Counterbalanced against this, the patient with FHF can rapidly deteriorate, so that if transplantation is initially deferred, there may not be another opportunity because the availability of donor organs is unpredictable. The rationale for extracorporeal liver assist devices (see Chapter 121, "Primary Biliary Cirrhosis") is to support the patient and prevent complications of FHF (eg, cerebral edema), thus allowing time for liver regeneration and recovery of liver function. If successful, this would potentially obviate the need for transplant, or at least preventing progressive deterioration while awaiting transplant, thereby acting as a "bridge" to transplant. Hepatocyte transplant has a similar rationale. Living donor transplant, which has become commonplace for treatment of chronic end-stage liver disease, has also been used in the setting of FHF, although there are significant ethical concerns with the very rapid evaluation of potential donors that is required. Auxiliary or heterotopic liver transplant has also been used as a means of supporting the patient, allowing for regeneration of the patient's liver and ultimately withdrawal of immunosuppression. Total hepatectomy has also been performed while waiting for a donor organ. The rationale behind this procedure is that removal of the severely diseased liver and its byproducts may have a salutary effect on hemodynamics and intracranial pressure (ICP).

Encephalopathy

Search for and correct factors which may mimic (eg, hypoglycemia) or exacerbate (eg, hypokalemia, infection, and gastrointestinal bleeding) encephalopathy. Light restraints are preferable to sedatives for patients with mild intermittent agitation. If necessary, a short-acting sedative such as *propofol* (5 to 10 µg/kg/min) should be used for severe agitation when the violent patient puts himself or the nursing staff at risk of injury. *Lactulose* has traditionally not been used in the treatment of FHF and can result in significant fluid losses and colonic gaseous distention, and the latter may complicate subsequent transplant. However, there has been recent renewed interest in use of lactulose, in part because high serum ammonia levels correlate with a risk of neurological complications including herniation. Patients with advanced hepatic encephalopathy (stage III or IV) are sedated (eg, with *propofol*), paralyzed (eg, with *cisatricurium*) and intubated for airway protection. Because the neurological assessment of such patients limited, an ICP monitor is often placed to determine whether intracranial hypertension, a manifestation of cerebral edema, is present, as discussed below.

Cerebral Edema

Approximately 80% of patients with FHF and advanced (stage IV) encephalopathy will develop cerebral edema and this is the most common cause of death. Young patients and those with rapid onset ("hyperacute") FHF are at higher risk for developing cerebral edema. The pathogenesis of brain swelling remains incompletely defined. The adult skull is in essence a rigid box with an internal volume occupied by brain parenchyma (80%), cerebrospinal fluid (CSF) (10%), and blood (10%). The ICP, normally less than or equal to 15 mm Hg, is a function of the volume and compliance of these 3 components. Intracranial compliance is nonlinear; initially, intracranial volume may increase from brain swelling with little increase in ICP due to displacement of CSF and a decrease in the volume of the cerebral blood. Once these compensatory mechanisms are exhausted, however, ICP will increase with even small increases in volume. ICP is dictated both by the rate and the magnitude of intracranial volume change, with slow changes producing less dramatic ICP elevations than rapid changes presumably as the former allows intracranial compliance to be fully realized.

Elevated ICP damages the brain both by brain stem compression (ie, herniation) and by reduction in cerebral blood flow (ie, cerebral ischemia), the latter is measured clinically as the cerebral perfusion pressure (CPP):

$$CPP = MAP - ICP$$

where MAP is the mean arterial pressure. Pathological intracranial hypertension exists when ICP is greater than 20 mm Hg. A CPP < 40 mm Hg for greater than 2 hours has been associated with poor neurological outcome and thus is generally considered to be a contraindication to liver transplantation.

The diagnosis of increased intracranial pressure, which develops in patient with late (stage III or IV) encephalopathy and not in patients who are awake and able to follow commands, is based on clinical examination, head CT and direct pressure monitoring with an ICP monitor. Examination of the FHF patient with raised ICP may reveal systemic hypertension, pupillary abnormalities, decerebrate posturing (ie, extension and pronation of extremities), disconjugate eye movements, and loss of pupillary reflexes. Unfortunately, these clinical signs are neither sensitive nor specific in the setting of FHF. For example, both decorticate and decerebrate posturing can be due to hepatic encephalopathy in the setting of FHF without increased ICP. Furthermore, CT does not appear to be sensitive for detection of cerebral edema, and ICP can be elevated even in a patient with a normal head CT.

Empiric therapy of presumed intracranial hypertension is difficult because CPP can not be monitored without measurements of ICP. For accurate assessment of ICP direct measurement is required, and this is associated with a small but definite risk of serious complications. Although there are several types of ICP monitors, euphemistically called "bolts", for practical purposes only the epidural and subdural types are used in patients with FHF because of the higher risk of bleeding with the more invasive (ie, intraventricular and intraparenchymal) types of monitoring systems. The risk of major complications, especially bleeding, from placement of the less invasive, but inherently less accurate ICP monitors is still significant (about 5%). The Camino (Integra Life Sciences, Plainsboro, New Jersey) fiberoptic monitor, which is placed under sterile conditions at the bedside, is the most common device used at our institution. A noncontrast head CT scan is routinely obtained prior to monitor placement in order to rule out preexisting intracerebral hemorrhage. If clear-cut edema is seen on the preprocedure CT scan, we usually begin treatment (see below) of presumed intracranial hypertensison while awaiting correction of coagulopathy and ICP monitor placement, which may take several hours to accomplish. As mentioned previously, a large volume of FFP is often required to correct the coagulopathy and early consideration of renal support with continuous dialysis is appropriate to prevent fluid overload because this may exacerbate intracranial hypertension.

The use of ICP monitoring has been associated with decreased mortality in patients with traumatic brain injury, but has not been shown yet to improve the outcome of patients with FHF and brain edema. Thus the use of ICP monitoring in this setting remains controversial. Because of the lack of clear impact on patient outcome, as well as the risk of bleeding and infection with ICP monitor placement, there has been significant interest in development of less invasive systems for monitoring ICP, including jugular venous bulb saturation measurements and transcranial doppler ultrasound. However, to date, these systems have not been widely adopted.

The goals of treatment are to keep ICP < 20 mm Hg and CPP > 60 mm Hg. Interventions should generally be made for sustained ICP > 20 mm Hg. Treatment usually proceeds in a stepwise fashion and includes head elevation, sedation, head positioning to facilitate venous outflow from the brain, hyperventilation to a carbon dioxide partial pressure of approximately 30 mm Hg, IV mannitol, IV barbituates, and possibly hypothermia.

The patient's environment should be as quiet as possible and the head of the bed should be raised approximately

20 degrees above the horizontal. The patient's head should be placed in the midline to facilitate venous drainage, and agitation, gagging, excessive head turning, fever, seizures, and hypertension should be avoided or, if present, aggressively treated as they can increase ICP. The patient should be sedated and paralyzed before intubation. Care should be taken to minimize potential increases in ICP during intubation and pretreatment with intravenous *lidocaine* (1 mg/kg) has been suggested but not proven to help prevent the potential rise of ICP associated with intubation. Hypotension, hypoxemia and hypercapnia should be avoided as they can increase ICP. Cerebral blood flow, which determines the volume of intracranial blood, increases with hypercapnia and hypoxemia, thus the rationale for mild hyperventilation and maintaining normal oxygen partial pressure. Hyperventilation resulting in a moderate reduction of carbon dioxide partial pressure (to ~30 mm Hg) may decrease ICP at least transiently but excessive hyperventilation may lead to severe cerebral vasoconstriction and brain ischemia and should be avoided.

Mannitol, an osmotic diuretic, reduces brain volume by drawing free water out of brain tissue. A 20% solution of mannitol, which should be kept at the patient's bedside for rapid use, can be administered as a rapid bolus infusion (0.5 to 1.0 mg/kg over 5 minutes) for sustained rises in ICP > 30 mm Hg, or for signs of neurological deterioration. Repeat boluses can be given every 6 to 8 hours as needed, but serum osmolality should be monitored and mannitol should only be administered if the serum osmolality remains less than 320 mOsm/L. The effect on ICP is rapid, peaks at about 1 hour, and may last for up to 24 hours. However, there may be a rebound increase in ICP following mannitol administration, presumably reflecting entry of mannitol into the brain through a damaged blood-brain barrier. Other complications of mannitol therapy include volume depletion or expansion, electrolyte problems and metabolic acidosis.

If intracranial hypertension is refractory to the above measures, use of barbituates, such as *thiopental* or *pentobarbital*, may be administered in an effort to lower ICP by reducing brain metabolism and cerebral blood flow. Pentobarbital boluses (100 to 150 mg every 15 minutes for 1 hour) followed by a continuous infusion (1 to 3 mg/kg/hour) may be quite effective in controlling intracranial hypertension, but often cause hypotension necessitating pressor (eg, *neosynephrine*) administration to maintain CPP. Alternatively, thiopental may be given as an IV bolus to a maxium of 500 mg over approximately 15 minutes with a subsequent infusion of 50 to 250 mg/hour, but causes similar hemodynamic changes. Continuous electroencephalogram (EEG) monitoring is commonly performed with barbiturate coma to confirm a burst suppression pattern and an indication of maximal dosing, and is also useful to exclude subclinical seizure activity which should be treated aggressively if present. Seizures can both result from and exacerbate elevated ICP, and subclinical seizure activity was reported in one study to be common in patients with FHF and advanced coma. In this study, prophylactic *phenytoin* decreased seizure activity, pupillary changes, and cerebral edema but did not improve overall outcome. Because the neurological exam is lost and the EEG "flat lines" during barbituate coma, a cerebral perfusion scan is often used to determine brain death in this setting.

Induction of moderate hypothermia (ie, 32°C to –33°C) has recently been advocated as a method of controlling refractory intracranial hypertension in the setting of FHF based both on preclinical and early clinical studies. Hypothermia decreases cerebral metabolism, thus decreasing CBF and ICP, and may also decrease hepatic ammonia production. Hypothermia is achieved via cooling blankets or gastric lavage to a core temperature of 32°C to –34°C. However, the utility of hypothermia for improving outcome from cerebral edema, even from closed head trauma, remains controversial, and an area of continued investigation. Decompressive craniectomy may result in a prompt and dramatic reduction of ICP, and has been shown to improve outcome with brain trama and stroke, but has not been reported in FHF presumably secondary to the risk of bleeding.

Infection

Infections with both bacteria and fungi are frequent with FHF, occurring in as many as 80% of patients in some studies. Defects in immunological defenses, including complement deficiency and leukocyte dysfunction, and the presence of venous, arterial, and bladder catheters, as well as an ICP monitor, probably all contribute to the high incidence of infection. Bacterial infections, typically of the lungs, urinary tract, or blood, usually occur with in the first 3 days of admission and are most often due to *Staphylococcus aureus*, *Staphylococcus epidermidis*, or enteric gram-negative rods (eg, *Escherichia coli*). Diagnosis requires frequent surveillance cultures because the usual signs of infection, such as fever and leukocytosis, may be absent. Controversy surrounds the issue of empiric antibiotics. At UCSF we typically begin enteric antibacterial and antifungal prophylaxis, perform surveillance cultures of blood, urine and sputum on a daily basis, and initiate parenteral antibiotics for positive cultures, any signs of infection, or other clinical deterioration. In the absence of positive cultures, empiric antibiotic coverage at our center consists of an extended spectrum penicillin (eg, *piperacillin-tazobactam*) and *vancomycin*. Fungal infection, most often with *Candida* or *Aspergillus* species, usually occurs in patients with renal failure on broad spectrum antibiotics for a week or more.

Renal Failure

Approximately 70% of patients with FHF secondary to acetaminophen toxicity have renal failure compared with 30% of patient with FHF of other causes. Renal insufficiency may result from prerenal azotemia, acute tubular necrosis (ATN), or functional renal failure (hepatorenal syndrome). Determination of urine sodium concentration may be useful in distinguishing ATN from these other possibilities and measurement of central venous pressure or pulmonary capillary wedge pressure can be used to exclude prerenal azotemia. Continuous venovenous hemodialysis is the preferred means of renal support in the setting of FHF. Intermittent dialysis should be avoided as it may result in hypotension and exacerbate intracranial hypertension.

Supplemental Reading

Anand AC, Nightingale P, Neuberger JM. Early indicators of prognosis in fulminant hepatic failure: an assessment of the King's criteria. J Hepatol 1997;26:62–8.

Ascher NL, Lake JR, Emond JC, Roberts JP. Liver transplantation for fulminant hepatic failure. Arch Surg 1993;128:677–82.

Clemmesen JO, Larsen FS, Kondrup J, et al. Cerebral herniation in patients with acute liver failure is correlated with arterial ammonia concentration. Hepatology 1999;29:648–53.

Davenport A, Will EJ, Davidson AM. Improved cardiovascular stability during continuous modes of renal replacement therapy in critically ill patients with acute hepatic and renal failure. Crit Care Med 1993;21:328–38.

Davern TJ. Molecular therapeutics of liver disease. Clin Liver Dis 2001;5:381–414.

Ellis AJ, Wendon JA, Williams R. Subclinical seizure activity and prophylactic phenytoin infusion in acute liver failure: a controlled clinical trial. Hepatology 2000;32:536–41.

Hoofnagle JH, Carithers RL Jr, Shapiro C, Ascher N. Fulminant hepatic failure: summary of a workshop. Hepatology 1995;21:240–52.

Jalan R, Damink SW, Deutz NE, et al. Moderate hypothermia for uncontrolled intracranial hypertension in acute liver failure. Lancet 1999;354:1164–8.

Jones AL, Simpson KJ. Review article: mechanisms and management of hepatotoxicity in ecstasy (MDMA) and amphetamine intoxications. Aliment Pharmacol Ther 1999;13:129–33.

Lake JR, Sussman NL. Determining prognosis in patients with fulminant hepatic failure: when you absolutely, positively have to know the answer. Hepatology 1995;21:879–82.

Lee WM. Drug-induced hepatotoxicity. N Engl J Med 2003; 349:474–85.

Marcos A, Ham JM, Fisher RA, et al. Emergency adult to adult living donor liver transplantation for fulminant hepatic failure. Transplantation 2000;69:2202–5.

Munoz SJ. Difficult management problems in fulminant hepatic failure. Semin Liver Dis 1993;13:395–413.

Ostapowicz G, Fontana RJ, Schiodt FV, et al. Results of a prospective study of acute liver failure at 17 tertiary care centers in the United States. Ann Intern Med 2002;137:947–54.

Riordan SM, Williams R. Blood lactate and outcome of paracetamol-induced acute liver failure. Lancet 2002;360:573.

Rolando N, Philpott-Howard J, Williams R. Bacterial and fungal infection in acute liver failure. Semin Liver Dis 1996; 16:389–402.

Rozga J, Podesta L, LePage E, et al. Control of cerebral oedema by total hepatectomy and extracorporeal liver support in fulminant hepatic failure. Lancet 1993;342:898–9.

Schiano TD. Hepatotoxicity and complementary and alternative medicines. Clin Liver Dis 2003;7:453–73.

Schiodt FV, Balko J, Schilsky M, et al. Thrombopoietin in acute liver failure. Hepatology 2003;37:558–61.

Schiodt FV, Bondesen S, Petersen I, et al. Admission levels of serum Gc-globulin: predictive value in fulminant hepatic failure. Hepatology 1996;23:713–8.

Schiodt FV, Davern TJ, Shakil AO, et al. Viral hepatitis-related acute liver failure. Am J Gastroenterol 2003;98:448–53.

Schmidt LE, Dalhoff K. Serum phosphate is an early predictor of outcome in severe acetaminophen-induced hepatotoxicity. Hepatology 2002;36:659–65.

Shakil AO, Jones BC, Lee RG, et al. Prognostic value of abdominal CT scanning and hepatic histopathology in patients with acute liver failure. Dig Dis Sci 2000;45:334–9.

Trey C, Davidson CS. The management of fulminant hepatic failure. Prog Liver Dis 1970;3:282–98.

CHAPTER 110

Adult Liver Transplantation: Selection and Pretransplant Evaluation

Paul J. Thuluvath, MD FRCP, and Cary H. Patt, MD

Over the past 20 years, liver transplantation (LT) has evolved from an experimental procedure into a successful therapeutic option for patients with end-stage cirrhosis and those with hepatocellular cancer. The recent data from the United Network for Organ Sharing (UNOS) suggest that the 1-year and 5-year patient survival rate has reached close to 95% and 85%, respectively, in many transplantation centers. This remarkable survival rate is due to many factors, including improvements in surgical techniques, better immunosuppression, and, more importantly, better patient selection.

The improvement in outcome and better awareness has resulted in an increasing demand for LT in the United States over the past 10 years. However, the increase in organ demand has exceeded the supply resulting in longer waiting periods and higher death rates on the waiting lists. Approximately 10 to 20% of patients on the LT list die each year without receiving an organ in a timely fashion. Transplantation physicians have responded to this increased demand by developing several strategies, including the use of older donors, grafts from hepatitis C (HCV) positive donors or those with previous hepatitis B infection (positive HBV core immunoglobulin G antibody), grafts from nonheart-beating donors, domino transplantation (livers from patients with familial amyloid polyneuropathy transplanted into older recipients), split liver grafts, and, more recently, live donor liver transplantation (LDLT). There is also ongoing research in the field of xenotransplantation, artificial liver support systems, and hepatocyte transplantation. Advances in stem cell research may lead to further developments in this exciting field. However, currently there is an enormous disparity in supply and demand for liver grafts in this country. It has therefore become incumbent on the transplantation community to ration the available organs in a way that serves the best interest of the population as a whole.

When examining a potential candidate for LT, it is imperative to determine whether the recipient is going to benefit from the procedure immediately and in the long term. For instance a patient with Child A (Table 110-1) alcoholic cirrhosis without any major complication may have a comparable 5-year survival with or without transplantation. When the long term complications from immunosuppressive drugs, costs, and the immediate surgical mortality are considered, this patient may be better off with conservative treatment. Similarly, a noncirrhotic patient with primary sclerosing cholangitis (PSC) may request preemptive transplantation because of the fear of developing a cholangiocarcinoma. This patient's lifetime risk of developing cancer is around 15%, and the mortality associated with LT in the first 5-years is around 20%. This patient should be educated about the expected outcome and discouraged from early transplantation until the patient develops serious complications or when prediction models (eg, Mayo Model) suggest that the patient's life expectancy is < 2 years without transplantation. Although mortality is an important consideration, the quality of life is equally important. Patients who may not fulfill all criteria for LT may be transplanted for intractable pruritis, fatigue, repeated bouts of cholangitis, and hepatic encephalopathy. In this review, we will discuss the process of selection and examination of potential transplantation recipients, and the issues surrounding transplantation waiting lists.

Selection Process

When examining patients for LT, the transplantation team tries to answer the following questions:
1. Does the patient suffer from a disease that will benefit from LT? If so how soon does that patient require a LT?
2. Is the disease sufficiently advanced to meet the minimal listing criteria for LT?
3. Are there any comorbid conditions that would prohibit an acceptable outcome of LT?

TABLE 110-1. Childs-Turcotte-Pugh Score

Points	1	2	3
Encephalopathy	None	Grade 1 to 2	Grade 3 to 4
Ascites	None	Slight (or diuretic controlled)	At least moderate (despite diuretics)
Bilirubin (mg/dL)	< 2	2 to 3	> 3
Albumin (g/dL)	> 3.5	2.8 to 3.5	< 2.8
INR	< 1.7	1.7 to 2.3	> 2.3

Child's A = 5 to 6 points; Child's B = 7 to 9 points; Child's C = 10 to 15 points. INR = international normalized ratio.

4. Is there a past or current history of alcohol or drug use? If there is, what are the chances of recidivism? Is there a social system that allows for adequate follow-up after transplantation and a support mechanism that will take care of the patient if the patient develops serious complications?
5. Finally, will the patient benefit from an expedited LDLT?

Although many of these questions could be answered easily in some recipients, there are no rigid criteria or guidelines for the transplantation team to answer all these important questions. Published studies, experience and a multidisciplinary team approach are important resources that help the transplantation centers make these decisions. Transparent discussions in a multidisciplinary team that comprises a hepatologist, surgeon, social worker, psychologist and transplantation coordinator are essential to reduce bias and to make the right decision. The rationale for making these decisions should be clearly documented and conveyed to the referring physician or patient in a timely fashion. The process of answering the above questions is discussed in more detail below.

Does the patient suffer from a disease that will benefit from LT? If so, how soon does that patient require a LT? Is the disease sufficiently advanced to meet the minimal listing criteria for LT?

Liver disease from any cause is a potential indication for LT. Many of these conditions are common (HCV, alcohol, primary biliary cirrhosis [PBC], PSC), whereas others, such as Budd-Chiari syndrome, Wilson's disease, α-1 antitrypsin deficiency, polycystic liver, glycogen storage disease, familial amyloid polyneuropathy, and hereditary oxalosis, are extremely rare. The presence of these diseases alone does not warrant immediate evaluation or transplantation. Based on history, clinical, biochemical or radiologic examination, there should be sufficient evidence to indicate that the life expectancy of the patient is < 2 years without transplantation. The exceptions to this rule are the presence of a small, unresectable hepatocellular carcinoma (HCC) or extremely poor quality of life in an otherwise stable patient due to extreme fatigue, pruritis, or encephalopathy. There are reliable models to predict survival without transplantation in cholestatic liver diseases, such as PBC and PSC. However, for noncholestatic liver diseases, it is more difficult to predict survival. In general, patients with spontaneous bacterial peritonitis, refractory ascites, recurrent bleeding despite shunt surgery or transjugular intrahepatic portosystemic shunt, and Child C cirrhosis (which is unlikely to improve with treatment or abstinence from alcohol or medications) are good indications for immediate LT. Model for End-Stage Liver Disease (MELD) is an objective measurement that predicts short term mortality (Table 110-2). In February 2002, UNOS accepted modified MELD score to prioritize organ allocation for patients on the transplantation list. MELD score was chosen to minimize the impact of waiting time and to use objective measurements to prioritize organ allocation. Unlike Childs-Turcotte-Pugh score (see Table 110-1), serum creatinine is an important variable in the calculation of MELD score (see Table 110-2).

The decision to list a patient for transplantation does not indicate that the patient is in need of immediate transplantation. At our institution, we consider progression of liver disease to Child's class B to be a minimum requirement to consider evaluation or listing for transplantation (see Table 110-1). Patients with less advanced disease (Child's A) may also be listed if they fulfill some of the criteria discussed earlier in this section. However, patients should be listed only if they are likely to require a LT in the next 2 to 3 years. Once listed, these patients should be followed at regular intervals to assess the progression of the disease and decide timing for transplantation. Patients who are on the list and have a stable course should not be offered deceased or LDLT just because of graft availability. This is especially true for conditions such as HCV with very high recurrence rates and low 5-year survival rates.

In patients with PBC and PSC it is possible to employ mathematical models to help predict survival. The Mayo risk scores for PSC use age, bilirubin, aspartate aminotransferase, history of variceal bleed, and albumin to predict survival in years. Similarly, for patients with PBC, albumin, bilirubin, age, prothrombin time, and edema were found to be useful to predict survival without transplantation. The criteria developed by Kings College in London is widely used to predict survival in patients who present with fulminant hepatic failure. These models should be used only in conjunction with other clinical determinants to determine timing of transplantation. The selection criteria for LT in patients who have evidence of HCC are discussed below as a separate section.

TABLE 110-2 Model for End-Stage Liver Disease

MELD score = $3.8*\log_e(\text{bilirubin [mg/dL]}) + 11.2*\log_e(\text{INR}) + 9.6*\log_e(\text{creatinine[mg/dL]}) + 6.4$
Patients on dialysis arbitrarily get a creatinine of 4 mg/dL.
HCC patients with a single lesion ≤ 2 cm receive 20 points, and a single lesion 2 to 5 cm or ≤ 3 lesions which are no greater than 3 cm receive 24 points. Patients are given additional (10%) every 3 months until they are transplanted or removed from the list.

Intervals for recalculation of MELD score while on the transplant list

Points	Intervals for recalculation
> 25	7 days
19 to 24	30 days
11 to 18	3 months
< 10	1 year

Note that points for patients with hepatocellular carcinoma (HCC) are recalculated every 3 months.
MELD = Model for End-Stage Liver Disease.

Are there any comorbid conditions that would prohibit an acceptable outcome of LT?

One of the important functions of the selection process is to determine whether the recipient can withstand a transplantation operation and emerge with an acceptable quality of life. If the mortality associated with transplantation outweighs that of the liver disease, then clearly transplantion is not in the best interest of the patient. Secondly, given the limited number of organs, it is in the best interest of the transplantation community to allocate them to patients who will benefit to the greatest extent. In order to ascertain the chances for a successful outcome, it is important to obtain a detailed history of diabetes and its complications, cardiovascular and pulmonary risk factors, renal disease, and extrahepatic malignancy. Although most centers do not have an absolute age cut off, in our center, patients over 65 years are considered case by case based on their general condition, and other comorbid conditions.

Our group has determined the impact of recipient risk factors on the outcome of LT using large cohorts of patients. We found that the immediate and late outcome of orthotopic LT is dependent on many factors including age, race, body mass index (BMI), presence of diabetes, pretransplantation serum creatinine, cause and severity of liver disease, and UNOS status at the time of transplantation.

Using some of the above variables, we have developed a model that predicted mortality at 30 days, 1 year and 5 years in a reliable way and have validated this model in a large cohort of patients. In our model, the following seven pretransplantation variables had a significant influence on the posttransplantation outcome:

1. Age
2. Race
3. BMI
4. UNOS status (predictably patients who were in an intensive care unit had a worse outcome)
5. Diagnosis
6. Serum bilirubin
7. Serum creatinine

The important variables that determined 30-day mortality were serum creatinine, severity of liver disease (serum bilirubin), etiology of liver disease, and UNOS status of the patient. Although UNOS status became less important at 1 year, the influence of diagnosis, as a negative predictive factor, increased at 1 year. At 5 years, race replaced serum bilirubin as an important variable. Diagnosis and serum creatinine had a major effect on the immediate, as well as the late, outcome. Unexpectedly, age had less effect on the immediate outcome and had more negative impact with long term survival. This may well be related to the confounding influence of other comorbid conditions. In addition to the above factors, we have also identified diabetes and coronary artery disease (CAD) as important risk factors. We have shown that patients with diabetes or CAD were approximately 40% more likely to die within 5 years from transplantation compared with nondiabetics or those without CAD. Presence of both diseases had a far more negative impact than either disease alone. Although our model appeared to be very robust in validation analysis, our model has not been tested prospectively. In general, prediction models need to be treated with caution because the predicted mortality is only an approximation and may not apply to an *individual* patient. The decision not to perform a transplantation a patient should be based on sound clinical judgement and the expected outcome used only for guidance. However, our model may help transplantation physicians to give a reasonably objective probability of outcome to potential transplantation recipients and relatives who seek such information.

Is there a social system that allows for adequate follow-up after transplantation and a support mechanism that will take care of the patient if the patient develops serious complications? Is there a past or current history of alcohol or drug use? If there is, what are chances of recidivism?

Often the most difficult and challenging issue that the transplantation committee has to deal with is whether appropriate *social support* exists for a potential recipient. Many of our patients have had troubled pasts and thus will lack a nurturing environment after transplantation. Failure to follow-up with laboratory examinations and appointments, as well as missed medications, can have extremely deleterious effects on posttransplantation patients leading to rejection and late diagnosis of associated complications. Therefore, all patients undergo an examination by a social worker and psychologist dedicated to the transplantation program. The entire transplantation team discusses each case before making a decision.

Abstinence from drugs and alcohol is a prerequisite for being listed for LT. At our institution we require alcoholics and drug addicts to have completed a preapproved outpatient alcohol or drug rehabilitation program with documented abstinence for at least 6 months prior to being considered for examination. Patients who are found to be using drugs or alcohol while they are on the transplantation list are automatically removed. We believe that transplantation programs should maintain objectivity by stipulating rigid, written criteria agreed to by the members of the team regarding alcohol and other substance abuse. This is one area where bias, culture and preconceived beliefs may cause *discrimination* and unfair decisions.

Will the patient benefit from an expedited LDLT?

This is becoming an important area that deserves special attention. Selective and expedited transplantation is the major advantage of LDLT for patients with advanced cirrhosis. The other advantages of LDLT are the ability to optimize the recipient's health status, elective surgery, decrease in cold-ischemia time, and an increase of organ pool. The major disadvantage of LDLT is the potential morbidity and, in cases, mortality of the donor. The concept of performing a major operation with a potential mortality on a healthy person without any direct benefits, other than psychological, is somewhat unique. Unlike live donor renal transplantation, donation of liver to another adult (usually right lobe or 60 to 65% of liver) is associated with significant donor morbidity and a donor mortality of around 0.5%.

Expedited transplantation is of particular benefit in patients whose need for transplantation may not be accurately reflected by their MELD score. This would include patients suffering from symptoms such as fatigue or pruritis, as well as those with complications of portal hypertension (refractory ascites, spontaneous bacterial peritonitis, and encephalopathy) with a relatively low MELD score. These are the ideal candidates for LDLT, and they should be allowed to pursue this option if there are suitable donors. Although highly controversial, patients with unresectable HCC who do not fulfill the current criteria for higher MELD score (> 5 cm in diameter or > 3 lesions), and those with PSC with early cholangiocarcinoma may also be considered for potential LDLT.

The American Society of Transplant Surgeons position paper on adult-to-adult living donor transplantation suggested that recipients should be medically suitable for transplantation by the standard criteria of the institution, and understand and accept that the donor will be put at significant risk. It was also recommended that the risk to the donor should be weighed against the realistic estimate of a successful outcome, and this is an important consideration when LDLT is offered to recipients who are expected to have a poor outcome with cadaver LT. Patients, especially those with HCV, should be offered LDLT on the basis of medical necessity and not on the basis of donor *availability*. Clearly, the benefits should outweigh the immediate risks of surgery to the recipient and more importantly, to the donor.

In order to be eligible to receive an organ from a live donor, the patient should meet all the criteria necessary to be listed for a cadaver organ which allows for retransplantation with a cadaver liver should the LDLT fail. This process will confirm the medical necessity for LT. In addition, the need for LDLT should be openly discussed in the multidisciplinary, transplantation committee meeting. When patients become critically ill, LDLT may have a poor outcome, and these patients may have a more successful outcome with cadaver transplantation. It has been shown that recipients with very advanced cirrhosis may require larger donor volume compared to those with more stable patients. However, this should not be used as a justification for early LDLT because many of them may be able to wait to receive cadaver transplantation in a timely fashion. Donor safety is of paramount importance in LDLT. Therefore, LDLT should not be recommended to recipients whose predicted postoperative survival is very poor based on their pretransplantation health status (assessed by severity of liver disease, advanced liver cancer and other etiologies, comorbid conditions such as presence of diabetes, renal failure or CAD, and UNOS status).

Many studies have shown that the short term patient survival after LDLT is comparable to that of cadaver transplantation. However, the concern for donor safety and lower graft survival remains the critical issue. It is clear that the majority of donors are satisfied with the process of LDLT, but the attitude of the lay public reflects an unrealistic tolerance for adverse donor outcomes more than we as a medical community deem reasonable. Although this is a clear signal that we should continue to strive to improve outcomes and availability of LDLT, it also reinforces the importance of having a multidisciplinary team approach with objective criteria for the selection of donors and recipients for adult LDLT.

Pretransplantation Examination

If no obvious contraindications are identified on the initial clinical visit, recipients undergo comprehensive examination by the transplantation team. The diagnostic workup includes pulmonary function tests, an electrocardiogram, chest radiograph, echocardiogram, and routine blood tests, as well as serology for human immunodeficiency virus, HBV, HCV, cytomegalovirus, and syphilis. Patients over 50 years of age, those with a history of diabetes, hypertension, or family history of cardiac disease, undergo a dobutamine stress echocardiogram or thallium scan. If there is a clinical suspicion of CAD, we recommend coronary arteriogram and carotid duplex. In order to evaluate the hepatic vascular anatomy, three-dimensional computed tomography scan or magnetic resonance imaging is done. Angiogram is performed only in the presence of portal vein thrombosis to determine the extent of thrombosis. Candidates for LDLT undergo similar tests and examination as the cadaver transplantation recipients.

Recipients are interviewed by the members of the transplantation team including hepatologist, transplantation surgeon, social worker, psychologist, and the transplantation coordinator. Further consultation (cardiology, pulmonary, oncology, etc) is requested depending on the initial evaluation. The multidisciplinary transplantation team members discuss the results in a weekly meeting and make a decision regarding the suitability of the recipient for LT. If necessary, the team may request further evaluation or test before making a final decision of the candidacy.

Acute Liver Failure

Patients with acute liver failure (ALF) present a variety of unique issues with regard to LT. Because of the acuity of their illness, the luxury of detailed medical and psychosocial testing is not always feasible. When examining these patients, we attempt to make as educated a decision as possible with regards to medical comorbidity. Because the highest priority is supportive care while awaiting LT, we perform only minimal testing in these patients. Moreover, many patients who present with ALF are young with few comorbid conditions.

Although we do not perform a transplantation on a *known alcoholic* who has developed liver failure from acute alcoholic hepatitis, a history of alcohol intake would not necessarily lead to exclusion from transplantation if liver failure was secondary to another cause (acetaminophen, viral, etc). Similarly, use of illegal drugs may have different implications in these patients than someone with chronic liver diseases. At our institution these issues are decided on a case-by-case basis.

The indications and timing of LT for fulminant hepatic failure is made on the basis of published criteria (eg, King's College criteria) and will be discussed in Chapter 109, "Fulminant Hepatic Failure".

HCC

HCC has a dismal prognosis with a median life expectancy of 6 to 9 months. More than 80% of patients with hepatoma have underlying cirrhosis, and of these only 10 to 15% are potentially resectable. The remaining patients are unresectable because of the size, location, or severity of the underlying liver disease. In cirrhotic patients without local or distant metastasis, LT probably offers the best chance of long term survival because it treats the cancer as well as the underlying liver disease. Recent reports have shown an excellent outcome in carefully selected patients with hepatoma. The size (< 5cm if single, < 3 cm if > 1 and < 3), number of nodules (< 3), absence of vascular invasion and a better histology (well-differentiated) are associated with a better posttransplantation survival (Milan criteria) (see Table 110-2). Although these criteria are not mandatory, most centers have adopted these criteria for patient selection during the past decade. In addition to routine tests, patients with HCC undergo chest CT and bone scans to exclude metastases.

Shortage of donor organs and the long waiting period, allowing progression of both the tumor as well as the underlying liver disease, are two major limiting factors for transplanting HCC. The transplantation community has recognized that LT, if done expeditiously, is the optimal treatment for HCC and advanced cirrhosis. Therefore, in February, 2002, when UNOS adopted the MELD score to prioritize organ allocation, they decided to give arbitrarily chosen high MELD scores to patients who fulfill certain criteria (similar to *Milan criteria*) to expedite their transplantation. Another option that is available to these patients is LDLT that was discussed earlier in this chapter.

Follow-up of Transplantation Recipients

According to the current allocation system, patients on the transplantation list in each organ procurement area (country divided into regions and further subdivided into organ procurement areas) receive priority according to their blood type and MELD score. Waiting period is used only if there is a tie with MELD score. Patients who present with ALF are given the highest priority (UNOS status 1) and MELD score is not calculated for those patients. Waiting time is the only factor that is considered to prioritize patients on status 1. For other patients on the list, MELD scores are recalculated at fixed intervals depending on the level as depicted in Table 110-2. Whenever there is a major change in a patient's medical condition, the committee may opt to reevaluate their candidacy. If they are deemed unsuitable due to a new medical (eg, major cardiovascular event) or social condition (eg, drug or alcohol abuse), then they may be taken off the list. Patients with active infection are often temporarily deactivated until the issue is resolved.

Conclusion

LT is a lifesaving procedure and a valuable tool in the fight against liver disease. Organ constraints have demanded politicization of the process and novel approaches to increasing the organ pool. The examination and selection of patients for LT is complex and requires a team of dedicated professionals. Medical, psychological and social factors must all be taken into account in order to achieve the maximal outcome. The field of transplantation is dynamic and as new technologies become available this everchanging process will continue to evolve.

Supplemental Reading

Carithers RL. Liver transplantation. American association for the study of liver diseases. Liver Transplant 2000;6:122–35.

Hwan HY, Thuluvath PJ. Effect of insulin dependent diabetes mellitus on outcome of liver transplantation. Transplantation 2002;74:1007–12.

John PR, Thuluvath PJ. Outcome of liver transplantation in patients with diabetes mellitus: a case control study. Hepatology 2001;34:889–95.

Kamath PS, Weisner RH, Malinchoc M, et al. A model to predict survival in patients with end-stage liver disease. Hepatol 2001;33:464–70.

Lucey MR, Brown KA, Everson GT, et al. Minimal criteria for placement of adults on the liver transplant waiting list: a report of a national conference organized by the American Society of Transplant Physicians and the American Association for the Study of Liver Diseases. Transplantation 1998;66:956–62.

Markmann JF, Markmann JW, Markmann DA, et al. Preoperative factors associated with outcome and their impact on resource use in 1148 consecutive primary liver transplants. Transplantation 2001;72:1113–22.

Nair S, Eustace J, Thuluvath PJ. Effect of race on outcome of orthotopic liver transplantation. Lancet 2002;359:287–93.

Nair S, Verma S, Thuluvath PJ. Obesity and its effect on survival in patients undergoing orthotopic liver transplantation. Hepatology 2002;35:105–9.

Nair S, Verma S, Thuluvath PJ. Pretransplant renal function predicts survival in patients undergoing orthotopic liver transplantation. Hepatology 2002;35:1179–85.

Neuberger J. Liver transplantation. J Hepatol 2000;(32 Suppl 1): 198–207.

Neuberger J, Gunson B, Komolmit P, et al. Pretransplant prediction of prognosis after liver transplantation in primary sclerosing cholangitis using Cox regression model. Hepatology 1999;29: 1375–9.

Patt CH, Thuluvath PJ. Adult living donor transplantation. Med Gen Med 2003;5:26.

Ricci P, Therneau TM, Malinchoc M, et al. A prognostic model for the outcome of liver transplantation in patients with cholestatic liver disease. Hepatology 1997;25:672–7.

Thuluvath PJ, Yoo HY. Graft and patient survival after adult live donor liver transplantation compared to a matched cohort who received cadaver transplantation. Liver Transpl 2004; 10:1263–8.

Thuluvath PJ, Yoo HY, Thomson RE. A model to predict survival at one month, one year, and five years after liver transplantation based on pretransplant characterisitcs. Liver Transplant 2003;9:527–32.

CHAPTER 111

Liver Transplantation: Surgical Techniques, Including Living Donor

Luis Arrazola, MD, Ernesto Molmenti, MD, and Andrew Klein, MD

The experimental work of Welsh and Cannon in the mid-1950s, followed by its initial clinical application to liver transplantation in humans by Dr. Starzl in the 1960s, set the foundation for the development of liver transplantation. Refinements in surgical and anesthetic techniques, the application of venovenous bypass, the ability to correct coagulopathies, better understanding of the natural history of liver diseases, a significant improvement in intensive care medicine, effective viral, fungal, and bacterial prophylaxis, and the development of different immunosuppressive therapies led to significant advances in the field of liver transplantation. In 1983 the National Institutes of Health (NIH) Consensus Development Conference determined that liver transplantation was no longer an experimental modality, but a valid therapy for selected acute and chronic liver diseases. The better outcomes of liver transplantation coupled with the NIH Consensus Development Conference Statement, led to the proliferation of liver transplantation programs throughout the United States.

For the past 2 years the number of deceased liver transplantations performed in the United States has been relatively static at around 4,500. On the other hand, the number of patients on the liver transplantation waiting list has increased 15-fold, and the number of waiting list deaths has increased 5-fold over the period from 1988 to 1997. As of January 2004, there are > 17,581 patients listed on the *United Network of Organ Sharing (UNOS)* liver waiting list in the United States. In 2003, 1,501 patients died while waiting for a liver transplantation. This significant discrepancy between organ availability and need for transplantation has led liver transplantation surgeons to adopt surgical alternatives with the goal of expanding the donor pool. *These alternatives include (1) split liver transplantation from deceased donors, (2) liver transplantation from nonheart-beating donors and (3) living donor liver transplantation (LDLT).* In the following section, the surgical aspects of these transplantation modalities are discussed.

Deceased Donor Liver Procurement

A midline incision is made, and the abdominal contents explored to determine the presence of any previously undetected pathologies. A median sternotomy is also performed in order to improve exposure and maximize venous drainage into the chest at the time of cold perfusion.

The first goal in a procurement procedure is to ensure quick vascular access in case of sudden hemodynamic instability. The aorta is dissected above the bifurcation, and encircled with two umbilical tapes. Subsequently the superior mesenteric artery (SMA) is identified at the level of the left renal vein and encircled with a vessel loop. The supraceliac aorta is exposed by mobilizing the left lateral segment of the liver and dividing the diaphragmatic crura.

The hilum of the liver is addressed. The bile duct is identified, tied near to the pancreas, and transected. The gallbladder is incised and flushed with preservation solution. The hilum is also inspected for anatomical variations, such as replaced or accessory left, right, or proper hepatic arteries. In hemodynamically stable patients, the hepatic artery and celiac axis are dissected proximally to the aorta. In addition, the SMA and splenic artery are partially dissected and encircled with vessel loops.

In cases where the pancreas is being procured, the duodenum is flushed via nasogastric tube with approximately 300 mL of iodine solution, mixed with antifungal and antibiotic agents. The gastrointestinal stapler is used to divide the first and fourth portions of the duodenum from the stomach and proximal jejunum respectively.

Once the dissection is completed, *heparin* (300 Units/kg) is administered intravenously. The distal umbilical tape at the bifurcation of the aorta is then tied. A cannula is placed in the proximal end that will allow for retrograde perfusion of preservation fluid through the aorta into the abdominal organs. A smaller cannula is placed into the inferior mesenteric vein (IMV) or superior mesenteric vein (SMV) toward the portal vein for antegrade cold perfusion.

The aorta is clamped at the supraceliac level and the inferior vena cava (IVC) is incised above the diaphragm in order to allow for drainage of blood and perfusate into the chest. Simultaneously, chilled preservation fluid is instilled through the aortic and IMV/SMV cannulas in order to perfuse the organs that will be extracted. The abdominal cavity is also filled with ice to cool the organs.

The liver is removed by transecting the aorta above and below the celiac trunk and SMA respectively. The diaphragm is transected and removed with the liver. The pancreas is separated from the liver *in situ* by transecting the splenic artery, proximal vena cava, and tissues in between them. The liver can also be procured together with the pancreas and separated *ex situ* in the back table. The iliac vessels of the donor are removed for potential later use as arterial and venous conduits. If the surgeon prefers, the liver can be perfused again *ex situ* with preservation solution through the hepatic artery and portal vein. The bile duct is also flushed.

Nonheart-beating Donor Procurement

In instances in which the donor has irreversible neurologic injury but does not fulfill the criteria of brain death, the organs can be procured after pronouncement of cardiac death. Procurement from nonheart-beating donors entails withdrawing life support from the potential donor in a controlled setting. Such setting is usually the operating room or a nearby adjacent site. At the time of withdrawal of life support, *heparin* (30,000 Units, or 3,000 Units/kg) is administered. After the donor has been pronounced dead according to accepted medical criteria, a period of time following asystole (5 to 10 minutes) is allowed as a safeguard prior to performing the procurement.

The aorta is rapidly clamped at its bifurcation into iliac arteries, and preservation fluid instilled in order to perfuse the abdominal organs. The chest is opened, and the descending aorta clamped to prevent unnecessary perfusion of the supradiaphragmatic region of the body. Ice is placed within the abdominal cavity. The organs are then procured following the routine steps of cadaver donors.

Posttransplantation function of a hepatic allograft procured from a nonheart-beating donor is dependent upon factors associated with both donor and recipient. Potential donor variables include hemodynamic status prior to withdrawal of life support, time from withdrawal of life support until pronouncement, timely access to the aorta and initiation of cold perfusion, donor comorbidities, and condition of the donor liver, among others.

Implantation of the Liver Graft

The procured liver allograft is prepared in the back table just prior to its implantation by removing unnecessary tissues, including diaphragm, adrenal gland, and pericardial remnants. The vena cava, portal vein, and arterial inflow vessels are inspected and prepared for anastomosis to the recipient.

The recipient undergoes a bilateral subcostal incision with a midline upward extension. The abdomen is inspected for evidence of tumors or other unexpected findings. In the case of potential recipients with known hepatocellular tumors, the hilum should be thoroughly inspected and biopsies performed on tissue from any suspicious lesions or lymph nodes. The presence of extrahepatic malignancy is a contraindication to liver transplantation.

Once this is achieved, the hilum is addressed. The hepatic artery is identified and dissected. Its right and left branches are tied and transected as close to the liver as possible. Subsequently, the bile duct is tied and transected as close to the liver as possible. These maneuvers are intended to provide as much length as possible for the subsequent implantation of the allograft. The portal vein is identified and dissected free of surrounding structures. Small collaterals are tied and transected. Bleeding from portal vein branches may be very difficult to control in the presence of severe portal hypertension, especially during the anhepatic phase. The portal vein is then tied and transected.

At this point, the operating surgeon must determine the approach he/she will take. *There are two main approaches, including (1) standard and (2) piggyback. The standard approach entails resection of the native retrohepatic IVC.* Clamps are applied at the supra- and infrahepatic IVC and the liver is resected. Prior to removing the diseased liver, the previously prepared graft is flushed with 500 to 1000 mL of cold normal saline to remove the preservation solution, which contains high amounts of potassium. When implanting the allograft, anastomoses are constructed at the supra- and infrahepatic IVC sites. The suprahepatic IVC anastomosis is constructed first. The retrohepatic IVC is thus replaced. In some instances when the recipient becomes unstable with clamping of the IVC, venovenous bypass, which returns systemic venous blood from the distal IVC to a cervical or subclavian vein, may be necessary. *In the piggyback technique, the native retrohepatic IVC is preserved, thus preserving the return of the venous circulation from the lower extremities without the need of external venovenous bypass.* In order to proceed with the piggyback technique, thorough dissection of direct venous branches from the recipient's liver to the retrohepatic IVC is necessary. The hepatic veins are preserved, and their ostia joined. The suprahepatic vena cava of the allograft is sewn onto the common opening of the recipient's hepatic veins. The infrahepatic IVC of the allograft is left open (see below).

Once the liver has been implanted onto the vena cava (by either technique), the portal vein is addressed. An end-to-end anastomosis of donor and recipient portal veins is constructed. When doing this, it should be verified that the portal vein is stretched, preventing any kinks. As in the case of the IVC anastomoses, we routinely use running sutures. A *growth factor* is left in place in order to allow for expansion of the vein after reperfusion. The *growth factor* entails a distance equivalent to one to two diameters of the portal vein from the edge of the vein to the actual site of the tie in the suture.

At this point, reperfusion is undertaken. In livers implanted by means of the standard technique, the IVC clamps are released first. Subsequently, the portal vein clamp is released slowly. In livers with piggyback implantation, the portal vein clamp is released first, with the suprahepatic IVC clamp still in place. This allows for blood to flow through the liver, removing preservation fluid. The initial blood circulating is vented through the untied infrahepatic IVC. Once approximately 200 to 300 mL of blood have been drained, the infrahepatic IVC is tied and the suprahepatic IVC clamp released. Hemostasis is achieved.

The arterial anastomosis is addressed next. Adequate blood flow in the native artery should be verified first. The allograft artery is then inspected. We prefer to perform the arterial anastomosis using a branch patch of donor celiac artery. The recipient site usually chosen is the site of confluence of the common hepatic artery, gastroduodenal artery, and proper hepatic artery. The anastomosis is constructed either with running or interrupted sutures depending on the size of the arteries.

After the arterial inflow is reestablished, the gallbladder is removed from the allograft. Whenever possible, we construct a biliary duct-to-duct anastomosis between donor and recipient. If this is not possible, biliary drainage is reestablished by connecting the donor bile duct to the recipient jejunum (Roux-en-Y choledochojejunostomy).

After having ensured adequate hemostasis, a liver biopsy can be obtained to document the status of the allograft and to have a baseline for future comparisons.

LDLT

Introduction

The feasibility of LDLT is based on the liver's ability to regenerate after surgical resection, and the more detailed knowledge of the segmental anatomy of the liver.

LDLT was first applied in the late 1980s to the pediatric population. Because of a significant size mismatch between pediatric recipients and the (largely adult) deceased donor pool, the mortality of pediatric patients on the waiting list varied from 10 to 50%. The availability of an elective liver transplantation from a living donor source has allowed many programs to decrease their waiting list mortality rate to almost 0%. Adult to adult LDLT (ALDLT) was initially developed in Asia, in countries with no access to a deceased donor source. The initial attempts using the left hepatic lobe in the United States were disappointing. The liver volume obtained with the left lobe was not sufficient for larger size recipients in the Western world. The technique evolved towards the right hepatic lobe, which provided larger liver volumes (60% of total liver volume). The first ALDLT using the right hepatic lobe in the United States was performed in 1997. Currently, LDLT represents approximately 10% of the total liver transplantations performed in adults in the United States. As of January 31, 2003, 1,158 ALDLT had been performed in the United States. Most of these transplantations in adults involved right hepatic lobe donation.

Donor Selection and Examination

LDLT poses many questions regarding the ethical justification to place a healthy donor at risk. The complexity of these operations in the donor can lead to potential complications, such as bile leaks, bleeding, need for reexploration, pulmonary embolus, and death. The risk of death is estimated to be approximately 0.4 to 0.6%. In the United States, there have been 3 reported donor deaths (0.26%). Of these, 2 were early in the postoperative period and one at 2 years postdonation secondary to suicide. In addition, two donors were placed on the liver transplantation waiting list after undergoing a donor hepatectomy. Of these, one underwent a liver transplantation and the other improved while waiting for a liver and did not require a liver transplantation.

The true incidence of complications after undergoing a living donor hepatectomy is unclear because, until recently, there was no uniform and compulsory submission of complications to a registry. In November 2003, *UNOS*, which holds the contract from the federal government to administer the Organ Procurement and Transplant Network, established a live donor registry, which will be operational by March 2004. It is estimated that donor complications can range between 10 to 20%. A right hepatectomy for living donation has a higher rate of complications compared to a left lateral segmentectomy. The potential donors are thoroughly examined by a multidisciplinary team consisting of liver transplantation surgeons, hepatologists, social workers, psychologists, and hepatobiliary radiologists. In our institution, the living donor liver evaluation is carried out in the following three stages:
1. Preliminary screening
2. Medical and psychosocial evaluation
3. Graft evaluation

In the evaluation of the graft, before entering into the anatomical details of the liver, it is of paramount importance to determine the adequacy of the hepatic volume to be transplanted. This volume is estimated by computed tomography scan or magnetic resonance imaging using the following two formulae:
1. The graft-to-recipient body weight ratio (GRBW)
2. Graft weight as a percentage of the standard liver volume. It is considered acceptable for transplantation GRBW > 0.8% and > 40% of standard liver volume. However, in recipients with significant medical decompensation, the minimal calculated donor volume may not be sufficient.

The hepatic vasculature (hepatic artery, portal vein, and hepatic veins) and the biliary system should be evaluated in detail. The need for a liver biopsy on donor tissue is controversial.

Donor Hepatectomy

The living donor right hepatectomy should be a meticulous and careful operation. Following routine exploration of the abdomen, the hilum of the liver is addressed. The components of the portal triad are identified. Because of synthetic requirements associated with graft volume, the right lobe of the donor liver is routinely removed for LDLT.

The right branch of the hepatic artery, the right branch of the portal vein, and the right hepatic duct, are dissected but not divided. Care should be taken not to extend the plane of dissection to the left of the right portal hepatic structures. This way, injury and devascularization of the extrahepatic biliary tree is avoided. Once the right lobe is mobilized from the retroperitoneal attachments, the right hepatic vein is carefully dissected. Attempts should be made to avoid entering or injuring the IVC. The anterior surface of the IVC is dissected off the liver. The caudate lobe hepatic veins draining directly into the IVC are suture ligated and divided. The liver parenchyma is then divided. Multiple methods of transection are available, ranging from dissection and suture ligation to use of ultrasonic dissectors, harmonic scalpels, or other high energy devices. During the surgery, intraoperative ultrasound imaging can be used to guide the surgeon through the plane of transection, usually lateral to the middle hepatic vein. The vessels are clamped, the allograft removed, immediately flushed with preservation fluid, and placed in a preservation fluid bath on ice.

Certain controversies exist in regard to the technical aspects of this operation. In our institution, the donor hepatectomy of choice for an average size adult is the right hepatectomy. The intraoperative cholangiogram, in addition to determining the number and orientation of the bile ducts, allows us to better identify the bile duct bifurcation and therefore minimize dissection and devascularization. The use of the Pringle maneuver in hepatectomies for other indications is common. However, the potential ischemic injury to the graft makes most transplantation surgeons very reluctant to adopt this technique in living liver donation. Recent reports have demonstrated the safety of this technique in the donor with no adverse effects in the recipient. Most likely more transplantation centers will be adopting this technique in the near future.

Different techniques and surgical equipment can be used at the time of parenchymal transection. In our institution, we have modified our approach as we face the significant learning curve of the operation. Currently, we use no Pringle maneuver; the floating ball device (radio frequency with saline) is used for the most anterior and superficial part of the transection and the CUSA dissector for the deepest and perivascular dissection. To minimize bleeding at the time of parenchymal transection, a low central venous pressure (4 to 5 mm Hg) is maintained.

Poor hepatic venous outflow in the recipient can lead to hepatic graft swelling and graft failure. All efforts should be made to maximize hepatic venous outflow. The middle hepatic vein is routinely preserved with the donor. However, some Asian centers feel strongly about incorporating the middle hepatic vein with the graft. Accessory hepatic veins > 5 mm in diameter draining directly to the vena cava should be preserved and reimplanted in the recipient IVC. Controversy exists in the need to preserve and reimplant the anterior sector (segment V, VIII) hepatic veins draining to the middle hepatic vein.

Recipient Liver Graft Implantation

Implantation of the live donor liver is conducted in a piggyback fashion. As previously mentioned, the diseased liver is removed preserving the entire recipient IVC. Usually the middle and left hepatic veins are oversewn, preserving the right hepatic vein for implantation of the allograft. The hilum of the liver in the recipient is carefully dissected, preserving as much length of left and right hepatic arteries, portal veins, and bile ducts as possible. This will ensure optimal conditions for the implantation of the donor graft.

Ice is placed in the right upper quadrant of the donor, which is already anhepatic. The allograft lobe is placed over the ice, wrapped in an ice soaked sponge. The donor right hepatic vein is anastomosed onto the remnant of the recipient right hepatic vein. In cases of size disparities, the donor right hepatic vein opening can be enlarged by incising the adjacent IVC. The right portal vein of the donor is anastomosed onto the recipient's right branch of the portal vein (or to the portal vein itself if length and topographic dimensions permit it). The hepatic artery is subsequently anastomosed. Biliary drainage is generally established by means of a Roux-en-Y hepaticojejunostomy.

The recipient operation can be difficult and challenging. Controversies regarding the surgical aspects are numerous. The reconstruction and reimplantation of the anterior sector (segment V, VIII) hepatic veins is not routinely required. An attempt to reimplant the anterior sector hepatic vein is warranted in the presence of severe portal hypertension, prominent anterior sector hepatic veins, and a smaller than usual right posterior hepatic vein. Hepatic congestion due to inadequate hepatic venous outflow can lead to severe graft dysfunction and failure. Therefore, all efforts should be made to maximize hepatic venous outflow. This can be accomplished by maximizing the diameter of the cavotomy, reimplanting accessory posterior sector (segment VI, VII) hepatic veins > 5 mm in diameter and selectively reimplanting anterior sector hepatic veins.

The use of venovenous bypasss carries some theoretical advantages in LDLT. Venous decompression at the time of the anhepatic phase may decrease bowel edema and, therefore, facilitate the biliary reconstruction (hepaticojejunostomy). Recent reports confirm the feasibility of performing LDLT without venovenous bypass. In our center, we no longer use venovenous bypass and have not encountered any disadvantages. Biliary complications are the Achilles' heel of LDLT. The incidence of biliary complications (bile leaks and strictures) varies from 15 to 60%. The biliary reconstruction can be performed via a duct-to-duct anastomosis or hepaticojejunostomy (Roux-en-Y). The outcomes of these two techniques are comparable. In order to perform a duct-to-duct anastomosis, the arterial blood supply of the donor bile duct should be preserved and the anastomosis should be tension free. The use of biliary stents has significantly decreased the rate of biliary complications.

The rate of vascular complications (hepatic artery and portal vein thrombosis) is 3 to 10%. The techniques of microvascular surgery have been shown to minimize the rate of hepatic artery thrombosis.

Split Liver Transplantation

Split liver transplantation consists of dividing the deceased liver either *in situ* (at the time of procurement) or *ex situ* (after procurement) into two different grafts. The surgical principles followed in split liver transplantation are the same as the ones outlined above for LDLT. There are significant donor related challenges. Donor selection is of paramount importance. Donors should fulfill minimal criteria, including age (10 to 40 years), unremarkable medical history, minimal pressors, short hospital stay, normal liver function tests, and absence of hypernatremia. In addition, several logistical issues have to be sorted out prior to the procurement. The availability of appropriate surgical equipment for splitting is required. Mutual understanding among the different surgical teams regarding surgical steps and time needed to perform the operation without compromising the other organs is also necessary.

The most common splitting approach is to obtain a left lateral segment for a pediatric recipient and an extended right lobe for an adult recipient. This splitting modality in children has achieved a significant decrease in pretransplantation mortality and waiting time.

Two adult recipients can potentially be transplanted from a split liver graft. These operations are technically very challenging and should be performed by the most experienced liver transplantation or hepatobiliary surgeon. The outcomes of *in situ* split liver transplantation are comparable to regular cadaver liver transplantations. However, *ex situ* split liver transplantations are associated with a slightly higher rate of postoperative complications, such as biliary and vascular complications.

Potential Surgical Challenges Encountered During Implantation of the Liver Graft

Inadequate Arterial Inflow

In cases of inadequate arterial flow from the native hepatic or celiac artery, a direct connection to the recipient's aorta may be necessary. This is usually achieved with the aid of an iliac artery graft obtained from the donor. The infrarenal aorta of the recipient is dissected. The common iliac end of the donor iliac arterial graft is implanted in an end to side fashion onto the aorta. The graft is tunneled dorsal to the transverse colon and stomach, and ventral to the pancreas. The end of the graft is then anastomosed to the donor hepatic artery. In cases of unavailability of arterial allografts, synthetic grafts (eg, PTFE) can be used.

Inadequate Portal Venous Inflow

In some instances, recipients can exhibit partial or complete thrombosis of the portal vein. Prior to performing the transplant, the recipient must have proven patency of the splanchnic venous system at least at the level of the SMV. Angiography or other acceptable imaging modalities should be used to verify such patency.

Partial and complete thrombosis of the portal vein can be addressed by performing a thrombectomy. This technique entails removing the clot together with the intimal layer of the vein, reestablishing its entire patency. Alternatively, a venous graft can be constructed using the iliac vein from the organ donor. In order to achieve this, the root of the small bowel mesentery is dissected to identify the origin (or confluence of major veins at the origin) of the SMV. The iliac vein allograft from the donor is anastomosed onto the origin of the SMV of the recipient. The vein graft is then tunneled through the mesentery of the transverse colon and subsequently anastomosed to the donor portal vein.

In the setting of diffuse thrombosis of the portal vein and SMV, the portomesenteric venous circulation cannot provide the transplantation liver sufficient portal inflow. The systemic circulation (IVC and renal vein) can potentially be used as a source of portal inflow to the graft. This surgical modality has been described as cavoportal hemitransposition. Cavoportal transposition provides the graft with systemic portal flow but does not resolve the patient's portal hypertension. It is not uncommon for these patients to have persistent ascites and variceal bleeding postoperatively. The experience of this technique is limited to a few centers and the reported graft survival is 55%.

Conclusion

In summary, organ shortage continues to threaten the lives of thousands of patients with end-stage liver disease. Split liver and LDLT are emerging as effective alternatives to standard deceased liver transplantation. Donor examinations (psychosocial, medical, and anatomical) should be detailed and mandatory. In selected patients, living donor and split liver transplantations can be performed safely; however, appropriate surgical expertise is required.

Supplemental Reading

Broering DC. Is there still a need for living-related liver transplantation in children? Ann Surg 2001;234:713–21;discussion 721–2.

Deshpande RR. Results of split liver transplantation in children. Ann Surg 2002;236:248–53.

Deshpande RR. Surgical anatomy of segmental liver transplantation. Br J Surg 2002;89:1078–88.

Diaz GC. Donor health assessment after living-donor liver transplantation. Ann Surg 2002;236:120–6.

Emre S. Living-donor liver transplantation in children. [review]. Pediatr Transplant 2002;6:43–6.

Humar A. Split liver transplantation for two adult recipients: an initial experience. Am J Transplant 2002;1:366–72.

Keeffe E. Liver transplantation: current status and novel approaches to liver replacement. Gastroenterol 2001;120:749–62.

Malago M. Split-liver transplantation future use of scarce donor organs. World J Surg 2002;26:275–82.

Nakamura T. Anatomical variations and surgical strategies in right lobe living donor liver transplantation: lessons from 120 cases. Transplantation 2002;73:1896–903.

Neuberger J. Liver transplantation. Journal of Hepatology 2000;(Suppl 1):198–207.

Pascher A. Donor evaluation, donor risks, donor outcome, and donor quality of life in adult-to-adult living donor liver transplantation. Liver Transpl 2002;8:829–37.

Tanaka K. Living-donor liver transplantation in the new decade: perspective from the twentieth to the twenty-first century. J Hepatobiliary Pancreat Surg 2002;9:218–22.

CHAPTER 112

Pediatric Liver Transplantation

Ruba Azzam, MD, Estella M. Alonso, MD, Karan M. Emerick, MD, and Peter F. Whitington, MD

Liver transplantation is an effective and widely accepted treatment for children with liver disease. In just two decades, pediatric liver transplantation has matured from a clinical therapy performed in only a few centers in the United States and western Europe to one that is practiced worldwide in innumerable medical institutions. This transformation can be traced to a few critical developments. Improvements in immunosuppressive agents suitable for use in children have clearly been of key importance in improving survival after transplantation. The application of technical variant allografts overcame the shortage of suitable donors for children and permitted many more children to receive transplants. Finally, there has been improved understanding of where, when, and how to use transplant therapy in children. Survival rates in children at the beginning of the 1980s approximated 30%, whereas now several centers report survival rates as high as 85 to 90%.

In this chapter, we review liver transplantation, including a general overview of indications and contraindications, a discussion of some specific indications in children, a highlight of surgical approaches that have had their greatest impact in pediatrics, and some postoperative considerations peculiar to the pediatric recipient.

General Indications for Liver Transplantation in Children

Primary Liver Diseases that Lead to Hepatic Insufficiency

End-stage liver disease is the major indication for liver transplantation in pediatrics. Progressive biliary cirrhosis, particularly that due to biliary atresia, is the most common cause of end-stage liver disease in the pediatric population. Parenchymal liver diseases, including chronic active hepatitis with cirrhosis and certain metabolic diseases, are also common (Table 112-1).

Cirrhosis is neither a specific disease entity nor a general indication for transplantation. It is an anatomic diagnosis with functional implications. Developing cirrhosis in the course of disease has grave prognostic implications with regard to the prospect of requiring transplantation. However, determining when transplantation should be performed involves estimating the functional reserve of the cirrhotic liver and its potential for supporting life of reasonable quality. Cirrhosis is an indication for immediate liver transplantation when there is evidence of functional hepatic decompensation, such as coagulopathy, ascites, frequent or massive gastrointestinal (GI) hemorrhage, malnutrition and growth failure, and frequent severe bacterial infections.

The majority of children needing orthotopic liver transplantation (OLT) reach end-stage liver disease in the first 2 years of life. Predicting the time for OLT is easier when the liver disease has a characteristic progression. *Biliary atresia*, for example, has a clearly defined natural history. Even though more than 80% of children with biliary atresia will ultimately require liver transplantation, its timing

TABLE 112-1. Classification of Diseases for which Orthotopic Liver Transplantation Has Been Performed in Infants and Children for the Indication of Hepatic Insufficiency

I Metabolic diseases
  a. α_1-Antitrypsin deficiency
  b. Tyrosinemia
  c. Glycogen storage diseases types IV, III, and possibly I
  d. Wilson's disease
  e. Neonatal hemochromatosis

II Acute and chronic hepatitis
  a. Fulminant hepatic failure: viral, toxin/drug induced
  b. Chronic hepatitis: HBV, HCV, autoimmune, idiopathic

III Intrahepatic cholestasis
  a. Idiopathic neonatal hepatitis
  b. Alagille syndrome (syndromic bile duct paucity)
  c. Nonsyndromic bile duct paucity
  d. Progressive familial intrahepatic cholestasis

IV Obstructive biliary tract disease
  a. Extrahepatic biliary atresia
  b. Sclerosing cholangitis
  c. Traumatic/postsurgical biliary tract diseases

V Miscellaneous
  a. Cryptogenic cirrhosis
  b. Congenital hepatic fibrosis
  c. Caroli's disease
  d. Cystic fibrosis
  e. Cirrhosis secondary to prolonged TPN

HBV = hepatitis B virus; HCV = hepatitis C virus; TPN = total parenteral nutrition.

is determined by the success of the Kasai portoenterostomy. Patients without effective drainage will typically reach end stage and need a transplant somewhere between 9 and 18 months of age, whereas those with effective drainage have a 50% probability of living beyond 10 years without a transplant. Unfortunately, few other liver diseases in children have such a predictable course.

α_1-Antitrypsin deficiency is one of the most common liver diseases causing progressive parenchymal failure in children and the most common metabolic disease eventuating in pediatric liver transplantation. However, at the time of diagnosis, usually in infancy, the prognosis cannot be determined in most cases. Fewer than 20% of individuals with the genetic defect will have significant liver disease, and only about 15% will develop macronodular cirrhosis before the age of 20 years. There is a 2 to 3% incidence of hepatocellular carcinoma (HCC) in children and adults, and other organs may be involved, causing conditions such as early-onset emphysema and membranoproliferative nephritis. Liver transplantation should be considered for patients with cirrhosis and hepatic insufficiency or early HCC, whereas patients with neonatal cholestasis that resolves simply should be followed closely.

The decision to perform liver transplantation in a child with *acute hepatic failure* is complex. These patients have a high risk of dying without transplantation, but some may recover with medical support alone. It is not possible to predict with certainty which individual will recover without transplantation, so probabilities of recovery based on etiology and other factors are employed in the decision-making process. However, young age is one of the worst indicators of poor outcome, and all young children with fulminant liver failure should be listed for transplantation.

Growth is a sensitive measure of liver function in childhood. The integrated metabolic functions of the liver permit growth to proceed, and failure of metabolic function is often first manifested as growth failure. The infant with biliary atresia and cirrhosis may continue to grow reasonably normally, perhaps with some nutritional support, until the liver begins to decompensate. At that time, growth will cease, and no effort at nutritional support will cause it to resume. The infant cannot improve as a candidate for transplantation beyond that time even though growth arrest may precede other evidence of decompensation by several months. The point of growth arrest is, therefore, the ideal time to perform transplantation on an infant with biliary atresia and cirrhosis. Caution is required when making this assessment. If growth failure is observed in an infant with biliary atresia and otherwise normal liver function (eg, a normal bilirubin), the patient may have a correctable cause of growth failure, such as postsurgical bowel disease or bile diversion leading to malabsorption.

SYMPTOMS OF NONPROGRESSIVE PRIMARY LIVER DISEASE

Several disorders cause chronic intrahepatic cholestasis but infrequently lead to end-stage liver disease. In these diseases, the morbidity of the liver disease must be weighed carefully against the mortality associated with OLT.

Alagille syndrome is the most common example of such disease in children. This genetic disease produces severe symptoms, but few affected children progress to end-stage liver disease. Pruritus, growth failure, bone disease, hypercholesterolemia and xanthomatosis, neuropathy, and malnutrition can all be indications for transplantation. However, symptoms must be severe and have a major effect on the patient, and they must be refractory to all other treatments before considering transplant therapy.

Liver Transplantation as Primary Therapy for Inborn Errors of Metabolism

Liver transplantation is required for many metabolic diseases because they produce end-stage liver disease or carry the potential for developing malignancy. Replacement of the liver also results in correction of the metabolic defect. Liver transplantation can also benefit children with inborn errors of metabolism that do not injure the liver. The principal goal of treatment is to correct the metabolic error. Examples of disorders that have been treated in this way include the *urea cycle defects*, *Crigler-Najjar syndrome*, *homozygous familial hypercholesterolemia*, and *primary hyperoxaluria*. The decision to apply liver transplantation is determined by the knowledge that it would correct the defect and that the patient has not experienced irreversible complications.

Secondary Liver Disease

Many children and young adults with *cystic fibrosis* and *biliary cirrhosis* have undergone liver transplantation. Initially, there was concern that the use of immunosuppressants might lead to more severe infectious complications in these patients. However, survival appears to be equivalent to that of transplantation performed for primary liver disease. Many patients experience improved pulmonary function, probably as the result of improved strength, but pulmonary infections with *Pseudomonas* sp and *Aspergillus* continue to threaten the postoperative course. Successful liver transplantation has also been performed in children with destructive cholangitis secondary to *Langerhans cell histiocytosis*.

Primary Hepatic Malignancy

Malignancies involving the liver represent a difficult and controversial indication for transplantation. Liver transplantation plays an important role in the management of *primary HCC* and *hepatoblastoma*. However, that role is limited by the potential for recurrence. For transplantation to be considered, there should be little or no potential for effective nontransplant therapy and little potential for recurrence after transplantation. Meeting these criteria narrows the field of candidates and excludes patients with *cholangiocarcinoma* or *hepatic sarcoma*. Transplant therapy should not be considered in the treatment of metastatic disease to the liver.

General Contraindications to Liver Transplantations

Some patients referred for liver transplantation can benefit more from a different therapy. There is also risk involved with pursuing another therapy that turns out to be ineffective and thus delays the referral for liver transplantation. In many cases, it makes sense to place the patient on the active transplant waiting list while closely observing the effects of other therapeutic interventions.

Special consideration should be given to the young infant who presents with liver failure. Some of the causes of liver failure in this age group can be treated with medical therapy. For instance, chelation and antioxidant therapy are now used to treat neonatal hemochromatosis. Albeit the rate of survival with medical therapy is only 30 to 40%, but that may be similar to survival after OLT in neonates.

Transplantation should be withheld if the candidate has a preexisting condition that will lead to a poor quality of life following transplantation. This applies particularly to the central nervous system (CNS). Congenital malformations or secondary injury to the brain (eg, intracranial hemorrhage or hyperammonemia) often lead to severely impaired children after transplantation. Furthermore, some systemic disorders cause hepatic injury and progressive CNS disease. *Alpers' disease* is characterized by primary degeneration of cerebral gray matter in association with liver disease and can present as fulminant hepatic failure in young children. Careful review of the patient's history reveals signs of progressive neurologic impairment, such as loss of developmental milestones and new-onset seizures in the weeks to months preceding their presentation with liver failure. Liver transplantation does not halt the cerebral degeneration, and transplanted patients subsequently die of neurologic complications despite good graft function. Every effort should be made to identify and specifically diagnose these types of disorders before liver transplantation to avoid futile therapy. It may not be possible to make reasonable predictions about neurologic outcome in some cases, such as the previously healthy child with fulminant hepatic failure and deep hepatic coma. Liver transplantation almost always reverses encephalopathy, but recovery from cerebral edema is often incomplete, and sometimes brain death follows successful transplantation.

Secondary organ failure has a negative effect on outcome after liver transplantation. For example, the development of intrapulmonary shunts, with or without pulmonary hypertension, can result in respiratory failure that may not recover. *Severe pulmonary hypertension* is associated with a high risk of operative death and is considered by most to be an absolute contraindication to transplantation. In less severely affected patients, there is no way to predict which patients will recover after liver transplantation. Rather, the presence of significant intrapulmonary shunting may be an indication for transplantation, but full recovery can be expected to require prolonged ventilatory support. The patient with functional renal insufficiency (hepatorenal syndrome) is managed by establishing access for renal dialysis before or during the liver transplant procedure. Renal function recovers after liver replacement, so oliguric renal failure need not be considered an indication for combined liver and kidney transplantation. Any systemic infection is a relative contraindication to liver transplantation. In some cases, however, there is no reasonable chance that the infectious complication can be adequately treated without transplantation, as in patients with biliary atresia and unremitting cholangitis and liver transplant recipients who have developed intrahepatic infection secondary to loss of arterial flow to their graft.

Acute viral hepatitis is not a contraindication to transplantation. Survival in this group is generally good, and recurrence of the infection in the graft is uncommon. However, liver transplantation should usually be deferred in patients with *systemic viral infections*. Simple upper respiratory infections can result in viral pneumonia with respiratory failure when patients are placed on immunosuppression. Our experience with a few children with respiratory syncytial virus and parainfluenza virus who died from overwhelming infection after liver transplantation serves to underline this caution. Transplantation should be delayed if possible until any acute viral infection, no matter how trivial, is resolved. The only exception to this is when there is an effective antiviral treatment available, such as varicella and cytomegalovirus.

A final contraindication to liver transplantation is *disease that is expected to recur after therapy*. Although the recurrence rate of chronic viral hepatitis is high, cirrhosis secondary to viral hepatitis is a common indication for liver transplantation. Studies in adults have shown that recurrence of hepatitis B and hepatitis C can be delayed or prevented by medical treatment after transplantation. There is much controversy regarding offering liver transplantation to human immunodeficiency virus (HIV)-positive patients. Some centers routinely perform transplantation in such patients, whereas others deny therapy on the assumption that the reduced length and quality of life post-transplantation cannot justify the therapy.

Surgical Innovations Impacting Pediatric Liver Transplantation

Organ size is of the utmost importance in pediatric transplantation. The shortage of size-matched organs for pediatric candidates is a continuing difficult problem. When a whole liver is transplanted, the donor should be within 15 to 20% of the recipient's size. The shortage of donors for small children led to the development of "*technical variant*" *transplantation*.

Reduced-size liver transplantation is the technique in which a donor liver is divided along anatomic segments to provide a hepatic allograft for a smaller recipient. Grafts can routinely be obtained from a donor many times larger than the recipient. Left-lateral lobe grafts are generally used in the situation in which the donor-to-recipient weight ratio exceeds 4, the left lobe graft is used when the ratio is 2:4, and the right lobe is used when the ratio is 1:2.5. Not only has this technique expanded the donor pool for small recipients, it has also provided excellent long-term liver replacements, with survival results equivalent to transplantation using whole livers for grafts.

The techniques of reduced-size liver transplantation have been applied to other technical variant procedures, including orthotopic auxiliary liver transplantation for the treatment of inborn errors of metabolism, "*split-liver*" *transplantation*, and transplantation using living related donors. In auxiliary OLT, a reduced-size graft replaces the resected left lobe of the recipient's liver. The most reasonable use of the procedure is in the treatment of inborn errors of metabolism such as Crigler-Najjar syndrome, in which the recipient's liver maintains its basic capacity for life support. Split-liver transplantation is a technique whereby a donor liver is divided to provide grafts for two recipients. Despite its complexity, it is increasingly being used in pediatric centers because of the obvious advantage of doubling the supply of cadaveric hepatic allografts.

Living donor liver transplantation for infants and children has been established and has proved to have several obvious advantages. First, the earlier and more elective transplantation of small infants provides a major advantage, mitigating malnutrition and pretransplantation complications, resulting in improved survival rates, shorter hospitalization, and markedly reduced overall cost of transplantation. The quality of the graft is uniformly outstanding. Patients with living-related donor grafts are less likely to develop steroid-resistant rejection, fewer lose their grafts to chronic rejection, and, overall, in long-term follow-up, these patients appear to need less immunosuppression than recipients of cadaveric grafts. When applied to pediatric transplantation, the donor usually undergoes only a left-lateral segmentectomy, which has proven to be very safe. The donor mortality worldwide is about 0.1%.

Immunosuppression

The challenge when choosing an immunosuppressive regimen for a child is to balance the need to prevent rejection against the infectious complications of these therapeutic agents.

Cyclosporine, a calcineurin inhibitor introduced in the mid-1980s, is a potent lymphocyte-specific immunosuppressive. *Neoral*, a new oral formulation, has better intestinal absorption than the previous compounds even in the setting of poor bile flow. Monitoring of cyclosporine levels helps to avoid toxicity and ensures a therapeutic range. Most agree that a cyclosporine whole blood trough level of 200 to 300 ng/mL measured by high-performance liquid chromatography or its equivalent represents the therapeutic range. Monitoring peak cyclosporine levels at 2 hours after the dose (C2 levels) may be a more effective way to ensure adequate immunosuppression and limit toxicity. Acute nephrotoxicity correlates with high cyclosporine levels, especially in the early posttransplantation period. Gingival hyperplasia and hirsutism are common side effects.

Tacrolimus is a more potent calcineurin inhibitor than cyclosporine, which allows children treated with it to be less steroid dependent. Like cyclosporine, tacrolimus is primarily metabolized in the liver and appears to use similar degradative pathways mediated by the cytochrome P-450 system. Blood levels should be monitored with a goal range of 10 to 12 ng/mL in the immediate posttransplantation period. Some of the side effects are anorexia, chronic GI symptoms, hypertension, tremors, hyperglycemia, chronic renal tubular damage, and the predisposition to posttransplantation lymphoproliferative disease (PTLD).

Most regimens also include *corticosteroids*, *azathioprine*, or *mycophenolic acid* and sometimes *OKT3* (muromonab-CD3). *Methylprednisone* is started at a dose of 2 mg/kg/d, with a taper to 0.3 mg/kg/d at 1 month after transplantation. By 18 months, steroids are weaned to an alternate-day schedule to permit normal growth.

OKT3 is a murine monoclonal antibody directed against the CD3 complex receptor common to all T cells that is given for short courses of 10 to 14 days before initiation of the immunosuppressive regimen at some transplant centers. It is also used to treat steroid-resistant acute rejection.

Allograft Rejection

Acute rejection is common following transplantation in children, with as many as 60 to 80% of children developing at least one episode. Rejection occurs most commonly within 2 to 6 weeks after transplantation. The common signs and symptoms of rejection include fever, tachypnea, abdominal pain, pleural effusion, and jaundice. Frequent monitoring of biochemical indicators of cholestasis allows the clinician to suspect rejection before physical signs become evident. Rejection must always be confirmed by histologic diagnosis. Rejection is treated in a stepwise fashion, with the first step being an intensified corticosteroid regimen. Most centers use boluses of 10 to 20 mg/kg/d of *methylprednisone* followed by tapering doses of *corticosteroids* during the following week. If the intensified corticosteroid regimen does not result in improvement in the biochemical parameters and in the liver histology, the next step might be administration of *OKT3* or conversion from *cyclosporine* to *tacrolimus*.

Chronic rejection can occur either following an episode of refractory acute rejection or de novo, weeks to months after transplantation. It is characterized by slow progression of the clinical signs of cholestasis without many constitutional symptoms. Liver biopsies show damage to interlobular bile ducts with little inflammation. Treatment of chronic rejection is controversial. Whereas *tacrolimus* has been shown to be effective in reversing chronic rejection in children, many children with chronic rejection will improve without alteration in immunotherapy or will progress despite intense therapy. It is the most common cause of late graft loss in children.

Postoperative Considerations

Some considerations of postoperative care with particular relevance to pediatric transplantation are hepatic artery thrombosis, feeding difficulties and problems with restoring nutrition, and the development of lymphoproliferative disease.

Hepatic Arterial Thrombosis

Several factors have been related to arterial thrombosis, with probably the most important being the age of the patient. Arterial thrombosis is two- to threefold more frequent in pediatric liver recipients than in adults. This may relate to two factors: the size of the hepatic artery and the perfusion pressure. Hepatic arteries with diameters < 3 mm present a twofold higher risk of thrombosis than those with diameters > 3 mm. Obviously, smaller children have relatively smaller vessels and greater risk for thrombosis. Hepatic arterial thrombosis has variable presentations, including fulminant hepatic failure, major changes in the aminotransferase levels, enteric sepsis, and bile duct complications. If arterial thrombosis is found, retransplantation will almost certainly be required because the secondary biliary problems will not resolve. Finally, if arterial loss is discovered serendipitously at the time of Doppler ultrasonography, but there is no apparent hepatic dysfunction, the patient will probably do well.

Problems with Feeding and Restoring Nutrition

Infants are also most affected by these problems. Malnutrition is a major preoperative complication and a focus for medical postoperative care. Parenteral nutrition is usually initiated 2 to 3 days after surgery, and enteral nutrition is begun as soon as tolerated. Feeding intolerance and vomiting usually indicate delayed gastric emptying, which may be functional (unknown etiology) or mechanical (reduced-size left lobe grafts impinge on the stomach). Problems with gastric emptying may respond to prokinetic medications or may require nasojejunal feeding. Diarrhea and failure to gain weight despite adequate caloric intake indicate malabsorption owing to a secondary digestive insufficiency, such as exocrine pancreatic insufficiency and hypoplastic villous atrophy. Some infants require immense amounts of formula (> 160 kcal/kg/d) to initiate weight gain. Finally, watery diarrhea, often with perianal irritation, can indicate carbohydrate malabsorption, which can be corrected by reducing the amount in the formula. More often, it indicates bile acid malabsorption. For posttransplantation diarrhea, we empirically administer a bile acid binding substance (aluminum hydroxide antacid is usually adequate) in amounts necessary to eliminate diarrhea.

Posttransplantation Lymphoproliferative Disease

PTLD is an uncommon but serious event in children following liver transplantation. Its incidence is 4 to 9% in most series, and mortality rates reach 50%. Most cases are related to infection with Epstein-Barr virus (EBV). The spectrum of PTLD varies, ranging from polyclonal lymphoid proliferation to true lymphoma. One of the more common presentation sites is in the head and neck region in the form of tonsillar hypertrophy, cervical lymphadenopathy, or sinusitis. PTLD often presents with fever, malaise, and loss of weight and can be associated with hepatic allograft dysfunction and intestinal perforation from small bowel involvement.

Serologic investigation usually reveals high titers of immunoglobulin G antibodies against the Epstein-Barr viral capsid antigen. Confirmation of infection relies on polymerase chain reaction. Some of these cases, especially when polyclonal, respond to cessation or reduction of immunosuppression, whereas others require therapy with standard chemotherapy. More recently, immunotherapy with *anti-CD20 monoclonal antibody* (*rituximab*) has been used as first-line therapy for EBV-associated PTLD occurring early after liver transplantation. It does not prevent cerebral localization but allows a rapid decrease in the tumor size and control of PTLD and, thus, resumption of immunosuppression to prevent chronic liver graft rejection.

Quality of Life after Transplantation

It has been documented that patients with growth failure secondary to liver disease will show a dramatic increase in general energy and activity occurring within the first few months and resume normal growth during the second year after liver transplantation. Children attend school regularly and participate in physical education classes and age-related activities without difficulty. Long-term follow-up studies have shown good neurocognitive function and excellent quality of life in school-aged children transplanted as infants.

Conclusions

There have been many significant advances in the care of children with liver disease, but none have been as great as liver transplantation. The improved results reflect many improvements in surgical techniques and pre- and posttransplantation evaluation, management, and care. The quality of life for successful transplant recipients renders this expensive modality of therapy rewarding and worthwhile.

Supplemental Reading

Broelsch CE, Stevens LH, Whitington PF. The use of reduced-size liver transplants in children, including split livers and living related liver transplants. Eur J Pediatr Surg 1991;1:166–71.

Chardot C, Carton M, Spire-Bendelac N, et al. Prognosis of biliary atresia in the era of liver transplantation: French national study from 1986 to 1996. Hepatology 1999;30:606–11.

Emond JC, Aran PP, Whitington PF, et al. Liver transplantation in the management of fulminant hepatic failure. Gastroenterology 1989;96:1583–8.

Krull K, Fuchs C, Yurk H, et al. Neurocognitive outcome in pediatric liver transplant recipients. Pediatr Transplant 2003;7:111–8.

McDiarmid SV, Busuttil RW, Ascher NL, et al. FK506 (tacrolimus) compared with cyclosporine for primary immunosuppression after pediatric liver transplantation. Transplantation 1995;59:530–6.

Midgley DE, Bradlee TA, Donohoe C, et al. Health-related quality of life in long-term survivors of pediatric liver transplantation. Liver Transpl 2000;6:333–9.

Noble-Jamieson G, Valente J, Barnes ND, et al. Liver transplantation for hepatic cirrhosis in cystic fibrosis. Arch Dis Child 1994;71:349–52.

Smets F, Sokal EM. Epstein-Barr virus-related lymphoproliferation in children after liver transplant: role of immunity, diagnosis, and management. Pediatr Transplant 2002;6:280–7.

Whitington PF, Alonso EM, Boyle JT, et al. Liver transplantation for the treatment of urea cycle disorders. J Inherit Metab Dis 1998;21 Suppl 1:112–8.

Whitington PF, Soriano HE, Alonso EM. Fulminant hepatic failure in children. In: Suchy FJ, Sokol RJ, Balistreri WF, editors. Liver disease in children. Philadelphia: Lippincott, Williams and Wilkins; 2001. p. 63–88.

Woodle ES, Thistlethwaite JR, Emond JC, et al. OKT3 therapy for hepatic allograft rejection. Transplantation 1991;51:1207–12.

CHAPTER 113

Ascites and Its Complications

KE-QIN HU, MD, AND BRUCE A. RUNYON, MD

Ascites is the pathogenic accumulation of fluid in the peritoneal cavity. In the United States, 85% of ascites occurs in the setting of cirrhosis. Ascites is the most common clinical manifestation of hepatic decompensation. Approximately 50% of patients with cirrhosis will develop ascites within 10 years. The 2-year survival rate is 50% once ascites occurs. This chapter will overview the practical approach to ascites and its complications in patients with cirrhosis.

Ascites

Pathogenesis of Ascites in Patients with Liver Diseases

Portal hypertension (PHT) leads to ascites formation in patients with liver disease. Three theories of ascites formation have been proposed. The underfill theory postulates a contraction of the intravascular fluid compartment with an increase in the plasma oncotic pressure and a decrease in portal venous pressure, which results in a secondary increase in renal sodium retention in an attempt to compensate. The overflow theory proposes that primary renal sodium retention is the cause of intravascular hypervolemia, thus causing overflow of fluid into the peritoneal cavity. The peripheral arterial vasodilation theory incorporates the above two postulates. According to this theory, PHT leads to peripheral vasodilation. The reduced effective arterial blood volume triggers neurohumoral excitation, thus causing compensatory renal sodium and fluid retention. This leads to overflow of fluid into the peritoneal space.

Evaluation of Ascites

History and Physical Examination

The presence of ascites can usually be determined with a high degree of accuracy by history and physical examination. The most common symptom of ascites is an increase in abdominal girth accompanied by weight gain, frequently with lower extremity edema. Patients should be questioned about the risk factors for, symptoms associated with, and family history of liver disease.

A full bulging abdomen should prompt percussion of the flanks. If the degree of flank dullness is more than usual, then one should check for shifting. Flank dullness implies the presence of at least 1,500 mL of ascitic fluid. A fluid wave may be present with tense ascites, but this is not a very useful physical finding. Abdominal ultrasound, with a detection limit of 100 mL, may be required to confirm the presence of a small amount of ascites.

Physical findings are helpful in determining the etiology of ascites. Vascular spiders, splenomegaly, and engorged abdominal collateral veins suggest cirrhosis. Peripheral edema due to liver disease is usually confined to the lower extremities and may occasionally involve the abdominal wall.

Diagnostic Paracentesis and Ascitic Fluid Analysis

Paracentesis should be performed on all patients with new onset, clinically apparent ascites. Diagnostic paracentesis should be repeated if a patient develops fever, abdominal pain or tenderness, hypotension, encephalopathy, renal failure, peripheral leukocytosis, or acidosis. The prevalence of ascitic fluid infection was 10 to 27% at the time of hospital admission in the past. With effective prevention (see below), this is less common now. Hence, surveillance paracentesis on admission is warranted to exclude a subclinical infection.

Ascitic fluid analysis often establishes a definitive diagnosis. The initial routine screening tests consist of albumin, total protein, cell count, and culture. Serum ascites albumin gradient (SAAG) is calculated by serum albumin–ascitic fluid albumin. This is widely used to categorize ascites. Patients with significant PHT have a SAAG $\geq$ 1.1 g/dL, whereas those without PHT have a SAAG < 1.1 g/dL. SAAG predicts the presence or absence of PHT with 97% accuracy. Table 113-1 summarizes the use of SAAG, ascitic fluid total protein (AFTP), and other assays in differentiating the causes of ascites.

The cell count is the most important test for ascitic fluid infection. Ascitic fluid polymorphonuclear leukocyte (PMN) count is a much more reliable indicator of infection than the ascitic fluid white blood cell (WBC) count. Leakage of blood into the peritoneal cavity from a traumatic tap can falsely elevate the ascitic fluid PMN count. To correct for this, one PMN is subtracted from the absolute ascitic fluid PMN count for every 250 red blood cells. Patients with a corrected ascitic fluid PMN count $\geq$ 250 cells/mm^3 should be treated for ascitic fluid infection. In the setting of spontaneous bacterial peritonitis (SBP),

TABLE 113-1. Differentiation of Ascites Using Ascitic Fluid Tests

Causes of Ascites	SAAG (g/dL)	AFTP (g/dL)	Other Abnormalities
Cirrhotic ascites	≥ 1.1	Usually < 2.5	AFTP can be > 2.5 during diuresis
Cardiac ascites	≥ 1.1	> 2.5	
Peritoneal carcinomatosis	< 1.1	> 2.5	Malignant cells in AF
Tuberculosis peritonitis	< 1.1	> 2.5	WBC > 500/mm^3, lymphocyte predominance
Chylous ascites	< 1.1	> 2.5	Milky, AF triglycerides > 200 mg/dL
Nephrotic syndrome	< 1.1	< 2.5	Proteinuria
Pancreatic ascites	< 1.1	> 2.5	AF amylase (usually > 1,000 U/L) > serum amylase

AF = ascitic fluid; AFTP = ascitic fluid total protein; SAAG = serum-ascites albumin gradient; WBC = white blood cells.

the PMN count usually constitutes over 70% of the ascitic fluid WBC count and falls dramatically after antibiotic treatment is initiated.

Culturing ascitic fluid as if it were blood gives the highest yield. Bedside inoculation of 10 to 20 mL of ascitic fluid into each of 2 culture bottles has become the standard technique, with a detection rate of over 90%. Additional testing on the ascitic fluid includes glucose, lactate dehydrogenase, amylase, triglycerides, bilirubin, and cytology. Ascitic fluid and serum levels of cancer antigen 125 are almost invariably elevated in patients with cirrhosis and ascites and should not be used as surveillance markers for peritoneal carcinomatosis.

Management of Patients with Cirrhosis and Ascites

Management of the Underlying Liver Disease

The most important initial step in treating patients with cirrhosis and ascites is to permit healing of the reversible component of the underlying liver disease. Abstinence from alcohol allows healing of the reversible component of alcoholic liver disease, so that ascites becomes more responsive to medical therapy or may even completely resolve.

Sodium Balance and Diet Therapy

Positive sodium balance causes ascites formation. To achieve negative sodium balance, sodium output must exceed intake. In the absence of diuretics, many patients with cirrhosis and ascites have almost no urinary sodium excretion. Reducing dietary sodium intake below total output leads to a reduction in fluid volume and weight in these patients. Instituting a low-sodium diet maximizes urinary excretion and fluid loss. Thus, sodium restriction to 2 g (ie, 88 mmol)/d is warranted in all patients with cirrhosis and ascites (Bernardi et al, 1993). Ascites may improve with discontinuation of the precipitating agent, such as saline infusions given perioperatively or as resuscitative measures during gastrointestinal (GI) bleeding.

Diuretic Therapy

Almost all patients with clinically detectable ascites will require diuretic therapy, especially those with moderate to tense ascites and positive sodium balance while on a sodium-restricted diet. Oral diuretics are best used synergistically with the combination of *spironolactone* and *furosemide* administered as a single morning dose in the ratio of 100:40 mg. This ratio usually maintains normokalemia. The dose of *spironolactone* and *furosemide* can be initiated at 100 mg and 40 mg, respectively, and titrated up until successful diuresis is achieved or the maximum doses of 400 mg and 160 mg, respectively, are reached. Single morning dosing enhances compliance (Runyon, 2002).

Spironolactone may cause gynecomastia and a prolonged holdover effect that could be problematic if hyperkalemia develops in the setting of renal insufficiency. These adverse effects can be avoided by substituting the short acting amiloride for *spironolactone* at a dose of 10 to 40 mg.

Contraindications to diuretic use include hepatic encephalopathy, serum sodium < 120 mmol/L, and renal insufficiency with serum creatinine > 2 mg/dL. Fluid restriction is not necessary for most patients with cirrhotic ascites and should be reserved for those with serum sodium < 120 mmol/L.

Tense Ascites and Large-Volume Paracentesis

Tense ascites requires urgent management. Large-volume paracentesis (LVP) rapidly relieves tense ascites. A single 5-L paracentesis can be performed safely without colloid infusion. For patients with tense, diuretic-sensitive ascites, diuretic therapy should be initiated with LVP. Colloid replacement should be considered optional after LVP of over 5 L. Albumin infusion (8 g/L of fluid removed) may help prevent asymptomatic laboratory abnormalities, but does not prolong survival after LVP (Antillon and Runyon, 1991).

Follow-up and Assessment of Treatment Response

Regular follow-up of these patients is essential for maximal therapeutic effect and minimal adverse effects. Body weight, orthostatic symptoms and signs, serum electrolytes, urea, and creatinine should be assessed regularly during follow-up. If the fluid overload is easily controlled, the frequency of clinical visit can be reduced.

The combination of a 2-g (ie, 88 mmol) diet sodium intake with proper doses of diuretics should achieve weight loss and a negative sodium balance in approximately 90% of patients. In contrast, patients who are gaining fluid weight during treatment may either be noncompliant with the diet or diuretic-resistant. Monitoring urinary sodium excretion allows assessment of dietary compliance. Total nonurinary sodium loss is less than 10 mmol/d in afebrile cirrhotic patients without diarrhea. Patients who are eating 88 mmol/d of sodium and excreting > 78 mmol/d of sodium in a 24-hour urine specimen (or having a random urine sodium/potassium ratio > 1) should lose weight. If the patient's weight increases despite urinary sodium loss in excess of prescribed sodium intake, then dietary indiscretion is the culprit. On the other hand, diuretics should be increased if suboptimal diuresis is accompanied by 24-hour urinary sodium of less than 78 mmol or random urine sodium less than urine potassium.

Management of Refractory Ascites

Definition

Refractory ascites is defined as ascites that cannot be mobilized by dietary sodium restriction and intensive diuretic treatment. The term refractory ascites includes two different subtypes (1) diuretic-resistant ascites and (2) diuretic-intractable ascites. Diuretic-resistant ascites cannot be mobilized because of a lack of response to dietary sodium restriction and intensive diuretic treatment. Diuretic-intractable ascites cannot be mobilized because of diuretic-induced complications precluding the use of an effective diuretic dosage. Diuretic-induced complications include hepatic encephalopathy, renal insufficiency, hyponatremia, and potassium disturbances (Arroyo et al, 1996).

Serial LVPs

As discussed above, LVP results in rapid resolution of tense ascites. Serial LVP sessions remain the first line therapy for patients with refractory ascites. Albumin infusion is optional for LVP of over 5 L, but is not needed for paracentesis of lesser volume. Assuming serum and ascitic fluid sodium concentration of 130 mEq/L, a daily dietary sodium restriction of 2 g (88 mmol), zero urinary sodium excretion and 10 mmol of nonurinary sodium loss, a LVP of 10 L removes 17 days worth of accumulated sodium and water. Thus, LVPs are usually scheduled every 2 weeks.

Transjugular Intrahepatic Portosystemic Shunt

Transjugular intrahepatic portosystemic shunt (TIPS) is a side-to-side portocaval shunt created via catheterization of a hepatic vein by the transjugular approach. Overall, TIPS decreases the requirement of diuretics, and reduces or eliminates the need for paracentesis in 50 to 90% of patients with refractory ascites. However it does not improve survival and is associated with an increased frequency of hepatic encephalopathy. Patients with Child-Pugh class C or a score of Model for End-stage Liver Disease > 18 may have increased mortality after the TIPS procedure. Thus, TIPS should be considered in patients who have relatively preserved hepatic and renal function and minimal hepatic encephalopathy.

Peritoneovenous Shunt

Peritoneovenous (PV)shunt is a subcutaneously tunneled plastic tubing that returns ascitic fluid via a unidirectional valve system into the jugular vein, with flow propagated by the negative intrathoracic pressure during inspiration. Although PV shunt may decrease the diuretic requirement and frequency of rehospitalization, it is now rarely used because of its excessive complications and poor long term patency requiring prosthesis replacement.

Orthotopic Liver Transplantation

As discussed above, ascites is associated with increased morbidity and mortality. Liver transplantation should be considered in the treatment options if the patient is an acceptable candidate. Due to a supply-and-demand liver graft disparity, there has been increase in median waiting time and waiting list deaths. Referral for orthotopic liver transplantation (OLT) evaluation should not be delayed until patients present with refractory ascites or SBP, but should be initiated at the first sign of hepatic decompensation.

Complications of Ascites

Ascitic Fluid Infection

Categories and Diagnosis of Ascitic Fluid Infection

Ascitic fluid infection can be classified into three categories based on ascitic fluid PMN count, culture, and the presence or absence of a surgical source. These include spontaneous ascitic fluid infection, secondary bacterial peritonitis, and polymicrobial bacterascites. The spontaneous ascitic fluid infection is further divided into three subcategories, including (1) SBP, (2) monomicrobial non-neutrocytic bacterascites (MNB), and (3) culture-negative neutrocytic ascites (CNNA).

Table 113-2 summarizes the ascitic fluid analysis for different types of ascetic fluid infection. SBP constitutes two-thirds of all culture-positive spontaneous ascitic fluid infections. SBP is always monomicrobial. MNB contributes to the remaining one-third of all culture-positive spontaneous ascitic fluid infection. It can be regarded as an early-stage or even a common variant of ascitic fluid infection that progresses to SBP in 40% of cases and resolves without antibiotic coverage in the remaining 60%. Most episodes of CNNA are diagnosed because suboptimal cul-

TABLE 113-2. Categories of Ascitic Fluid Infection

Category	PMN	AF Culture	Other Characteristics
SBP	$\geq 250/mm^3$	Single organism	A low ascitic fluid total protein increases risk for SBP
CNNA	$\geq 250/mm^3$	Negative culture	Should rule out other causes of elevated PMN
MNB	$< 250/mm^3$	Single organism	An early stage of SBP, 40% will progress to SBP
Polymicrobial bacterascites	$< 250/mm^3$	Multiple organisms	Indicative of needle perforation by paracentesis
Secondary bacterial peritonitis	$\geq 250/mm^3$	Multiple organisms	Presence of intra-abdominal infection

Adapted with modification from Anadon and Arroyo, 2003.
AF = ascitic fluid; CNNA = culture-negative neutrocytic ascites; MNB = monomicrobial non-neutrocytic bacterascites; PMN = polymorphonuclear leukocyte; SBP = spontaneous bacterial peritonitis.

ture techniques are used. In the setting of optimal culture methodology, CNNA may represent spontaneously recovering SBP and resolving ascitic fluid PMN count.

The source of secondary bacterial peritonitis can be divided into the following two subsets: (1) free perforation of a viscus (eg, duodenal ulcer) and (2) loculated abscess without perforation. Polymicrobial bacterascites is indicative of gut perforation due to the paracentesis needle. It occurs in less than 1 of 150 paracenteses, and peritonitis affects less than 1 of 1,500 paracenteses.

TREATMENT OF ASCITIC FLUID INFECTION

Patients with a clinical presentation suggestive of ascitic fluid infection should receive empirical antibiotics. Indications for treatment include ascitic fluid PMN ≥ 250 cells/mm^3, and/or convincing signs and symptoms of infection. For symptomatic patients without an elevated ascitic fluid PMN count, empirical antibiotics should be initiated but can be then discontinued after 2 days if cultures demonstrate no growth.

Escherichia coli, streptococci (mostly pneumococci), and *Klebsiella pneumoniae* cause most episodes of spontaneous ascitic fluid infection, with only 1% contribution from anaerobes. *Cefotaxime* or a similar third-generation *cephalosporin* is the antibiotic of choice, and is superior to *ampicillin* plus *tobramycin*. Aminoglycosides should be avoided because of their nephrotoxicity. *Cefotaxime* covers 98% of the flora and does not lead to superinfection or nephrotoxicity. Intravenous (IV) dosing of 2 g every 8 hours achieves excellent levels in ascitic fluid. Five days of treatment is as efficacious as 10 days and is significantly less expensive. A follow-up paracentesis is indicated if secondary bacterial peritonitis is suspected or the typical response to cefotaxime does not occur.

The decision to treat patients with MNB depends on the presence or absence of convincing signs and symptoms of infection, regardless of the ascitic fluid PMN count. *Cefotaxime* 2 g every 8 hours should be empirically initiated for symptomatic patients, with follow-up paracentesis performed at 48 hours. On the other hand, asymptomatic patients do not need treatment immediately but require repeat paracentesis promptly for cell count and culture.

For secondary bacterial peritonitis, IV *cefotaxime* and *metronidazole* should be initiated immediately to cover both aerobic and anaerobic flora. Imaging is needed to confirm and localize the site of perforation. Emergent surgical laparotomy is mandatory for both perforation and nonperforation peritonitis. Without surgical intervention, mortality is 100%. Despite a low mortality associated with the polymicrobial bacterascites, most physicians would initiate antibiotics. A combination of *cefotaxime* and *metronidazole* should be used if decision is made to treat the patient. Repeat paracentesis is helpful to follow the ascitic fluid PMN count and culture, whether the patient has been placed on empiric antibiotic coverage.

IV VOLUME EXPANDERS IN PATIENTS WITH SBP

SBP is associated with a reduction in effective arterial blood volume and impaired renal function. The latter is the most important predictor of in-hospital mortality in these patients. IV albumin 1.5 g/kg at the time of diagnosing SBP and 1.0 g/kg on day 3 of antibiotic treatment significantly decreased the risk for renal insufficiency and SBP-related mortality in a randomized trial. It is reasonable to administer intravenous albumin in this setting.

PROPHYLAXIS AGAINST SBP

SBP occurs most often in cirrhotic patients with (1) a prior episode of SBP, (2) AFTP < 1.0 g/dL, and (3) acute episode of GI hemorrhage. Oral *norfloxacin* 400 mg daily prevents SBP in inpatients with prior SBP or a low AFTP. When given twice daily for 7 days after emergent gastroscopy in patients with GI hemorrhage, *norfloxacin* reduces the incidence of inpatient SBP by over 80%. *Trimethoprim-sulfamethoxazole* one double-strength tablet daily orally has also been shown effective in prophylaxis of SBP.

Antibiotic prophylaxis does not improve survival, but may select resistant gut flora. Prolonged antibiotic use before OLT places patients at risk for fungal infection posttransplant. Thus, prophylaxis is recommend for short term inpatient use in patients with AFTP < 1 g/dL or variceal hemorrhage, and long term outpatient use for patients who survive an SBP episode.

Hepatic Hydrothorax

Hepatic hydrothorax is a large symptomatic pleural effusion that occurs in a cirrhotic patient in the absence of primary cardiopulmonary disease. It is present in approximately 5% of patients with cirrhotic ascites. It is right-sided in 85% of the cases, with the remaining 13% left-sided and 2% bilateral. The most common clinical symptom of hepatic hydrothorax is dyspnea without chest pain.

Hepatic hydrothorax is formed by ascitic fluid transferred through diaphragmatic defects that began as tiny herniated blebs but subsequently ruptured. This can be confirmed by injecting $Tc^{99}m$-labeled sulfur colloid into the peritoneal cavity and demonstrating isotope in the chest area. The biochemical analysis of uncomplicated hepatic hydrothorax fluid resembles but is not identical to that of ascitic fluid, because pleural fluid is subject to different hydrostatic pressures. The total protein of pleural fluid is usually < 2.5 g/dL, but approximately 1 g/dL higher than that of ascitic fluid. The serum-pleural fluid albumin gradient is greater than 1.1 g/dL, similar to the high SAAG for cirrhotic ascites. The pleural fluid PMN count is less than 250 cells/mm^3 in the absence of infection.

Management of hepatic hydrothorax is similar to that for ascites. Symptomatic relief is achievable in most patients by dietary sodium restriction and diuretics. If conservative treatment fails, therapeutic thoracentesis can promptly relieve dyspnea. In patients with both symptomatic hydrothorax and massive ascites, LVP should precede therapeutic thoracentesis.

TIPS is a therapeutic option when attempts at mobilizing fluid by repeated thoracentesis and/or medical therapy have failed. However, TIPS has been associated with a variable rate in controlling hepatic hydrothorax (Rosado and Kamath, 2003). Chemical pleurodesis or chest tube insertion combined with chemical pleurodesis is generally unsuccessful and should not be attempted. OLT remains a definitive treatment for refractory hepatic hydrothorax.

Abdominal Wall Hernias

Abdominal wall hernias are common in patients with ascites and may cause serious complications (Belghiti and Durand, 1997). The hernias are usually umbilical or incisional, but occasionally are inguinal. Approximately 20% of cirrhotic patients with ascites were found to have umbilical hernias on admission. Among the affected patients, 14% developed incarcerations of hernias, 35% developed skin ulcerations, and 7% experienced hernia ruptures. Manual reduction of incarcerated hernias should be attempted. Emergent surgery should be considered for incarceration or rupture if conservative therapy fails. If the hernia of a OLT candidate is not thin-walled or incarcerated, the repair could be postponed until transplant surgery

Supplemental Reading

Anadon MN, Arroyo V. Ascites and spontaneous bacterial peritonitis. In: Schiff ER, Sorrell MF, Maddrey WC, editors. Schiff's diseases of the liver. 9th ed. Philadelphia: Lippincott Williams & Wilkins; 2003. p .559–94.

Antillon MR, Runyon BA. Postparacentesis plasma expansion prevents asymptomatic laboratory abnormalities, but does it have any impact on morbidity or mortality? Gastroenterology 1991;101:1455–7.

Arroyo V, Ginès P, Gerbes AL, et al. Definition and diagnostic criteria of refractory ascites and hepatorenal syndrome in cirrhosis. Hepatology 1996;23:164–76.

Bass NM. Intravenous albumin for spontaneous bacterial peritonitis in patients with cirrhosis. N Engl J Med 1999;341:443–4.

Belghiti J, Durand F. Abdominal wall hernias in the setting of cirrhosis. Semin Liv Dis 1997;17:219 –26.

Bernardi M, Laffi G, Salvagnini M, et al. Efficacy and safety of the stepped care medical treatment of ascites in liver cirrhosis: a randomized controlled clinical trial comparing two diets with different sodium content. Liver 1993;13:156–62.

Guarner C, Garcia-Tsao G, Navasa M, et al. Diagnosis, treatment and prophylaxis of spontaneous bacterial peritonitis: a consensus document. J Hepatol 2000;32:142–53.

Hu K-Q, Runyon BA. Ascites and spontaneous bacterial peritonitis. In: Friedman LS, Keeffe EB, editors. Handbook of liver disease. 2nd ed. [In press]

Malinchoc M, Kamath PS, Gordon FD, et al. A model to predict poor survival in patients undergoing transjugular intrahepatic portosystemic shunts. Hepatology 2000;31:864–71.

Rosado B, Kamath PS. Transjugular intrahepatic portosystemic shunts: an update. Liver Transplantation 2003;9:207–17.

Rössle M, Ochs A, Gülberg V, et al. A comparison of paracentesis and transjugular intrahepatic portosystemic shunting in patients with ascites. N Engl J Med 2000;342:1701–7.

Runyon BA. Ascites and spontaneous bacterial peritonitis. In: Feldman M, Friedman LS, Sleisenger MH, editors. Sleisenger & Fordtran's gastrointestinal and liver disease pathophysiology/ diagnosis/management. 7th ed. Philadelphia: Saunders; 2002. p. 1517–42.

Sort P, Navasa M, Arroyo V, et al. Effect of intravenous albumin on renal impairment and mortality in patients with cirrhosis and spontaneous bacterial peritonitis. N Engl J Med 1999;341:403–9.

Strauss RM, Boyer TD. Hepatic hydrothorax. Semin Liv Dis 1997;17:227–32.

Yu SA, Hu K-Q. Management of ascites. Clin Liv Dis 2001;5:541–68.

CHAPTER 114

Hepatic Encephalopathy

Challa Ajit, MD, and Santiago Munoz, MD

Hepatic encephalopathy is a neuropsychiatric syndrome consisting of altered neurological function associated with acute or chronic liver disease and portal systemic shunting. Exclusion of other disorders of the central nervous system (CNS) is important to establish the diagnosis. The development of hepatic encephalopathy in a cirrhotic patient indicates decompensation of a previously stable liver disease, or more frequently, it represents the effect of a transient precipitating factor. Hepatic encephalopathy generally implies a poor prognosis; its severity is a key component of the Child-Pugh score, an important prognostic system in chronic liver disease. In contrast, onset of hepatic encephalopathy in patients with acute liver failure (ALF), defines a fulminant course and is associated with risk of life threatening complications, including cerebral edema and intracranial hypertension.

In spite of the common occurrence of hepatic encephalopathy in patients with cirrhosis, there is no reliable laboratory method to recognize and objectively assess its severity. Recently, the final report of a working party in 1998 (Ferenci et al, 2002) proposed a new classification for hepatic encephalopathy. From a clinical presentation and course standpoints, hepatic encephalopathy can be episodic, persistent, or minimal. Most episodes of encephalopathy can be traced to precipitating factors, but some can be spontaneous and recurrent as observed in patients with decompensated cirrhosis. Minimal encephalopathy has substituted the previous term of subclinical hepatic encephalopathy. These patients appear clinically nonencephalopathic yet exhibit subtle cognitive deficits on neuropsychological testing. The clinical relevance and therapy of minimal encephalopathy is under investigation.

In the context of this revised conceptual framework, we review here the current approaches to diagnosis and management of hepatic encephalopathy.

Diagnosis

A detailed history and a thorough physical and neurological examination are essential to formulate the diagnosis. The presence of stigmata of chronic liver disease (*telangiectasis, palmar erythema, gynecomastia, ascites, jaundice, variceal bleeding*) are good reasons to include *hepatic encephalopathy* as a likely explanation for mental changes in a patient with cirrhosis. In general, alteration of mental status in a patient with cirrhosis should be considered hepatic encephalopathy until proven otherwise. Table 114-1 summarizes the frequently used New Haven bedside grading of severity of hepatic encephalopathy. *Asterixis* or flapping tremor is characteristic of early stages of hepatic encephalopathy, but is not pathognomonic, as is also observed in uremia, carbon dioxide narcosis, hypomagnesemia, and diphenylhydantoin intoxication. *Fetor hepaticus* and *hyperventilation* can often be detected in encephalopathic patients.

Laboratory investigations in patients with hepatic encephalopathy frequently reveal evidence of severe hepatic biochemical abnormalities and synthetic dysfunction. Electrolyte disturbances such as *hyponatremia* and

TABLE 114-1. Hepatic Encephalopathy: Clinical Assessment of Severity

Grade	Consciousness	Intellectual Capacity	Neurological Signs
1	Lack of awareness Change in personality Day/night reversal	Short attention span Easy forgetfulness	Slight tremor Asterixis
2	Lethargy Inappropriate behaviour	Disorientation	Slurred speech Ataxia
3	Somnolence Arousable with noxious stimulus Confused when awake	Loss of interpersonal communication	Abnormal reflexes
4	Coma	Absent	Babinski, clonus, decerebrate posturing

hypokalemia related to diuretic usage are also common. The blood ammonia level is a useful test employed to aid in the diagnosis and confirm hepatic encephalopathy. A recent report found a high correlation between blood ammonia level and the severity of hepatic encephalopathy. Furthermore, arterial blood ammonia was not better than venous blood ammonia levels in regards to correlation with encephalopathy. This information is important because in cirrhotic patients with coagulopathy and thrombocytopenia, arterial punctures are avoided whenever possible. However, for ammonia levels to be useful, blood must be drawn in heparinized Vacutainer tubes, immediately placed on ice and analyzed for ammonia content within 30 minutes. Leaving tubes at room temperatures for prolonged times yields erroneous ammonia determinations. Although ammonia levels have a high degree of correlation with severity of hepatic encephalopathy, the overlap of values between patients with and without encephalopathy is such that a single ammonia level is of limited value in the diagnosis of encephalopathy. Nevertheless, patients in hepatic coma (stage IV encephalopathy) almost always have ammonia levels greater than 130 umol/L, whereas nonencephalopathic patients (stage 0) almost always have ammonia levels lower than this value.

Other investigations including electroencephalogram, evoked potentials, and psychometric testing are generally used in clinical trial settings, but in an occasional individual patient, these tests may be useful to distinguish hepatic encephalopathy from dementia syndromes.

Arterial blood gases and biochemistries, urine analysis, blood, sputum and urine cultures, urine and blood toxic screens, and blood alcohol levels, along with neuroimaging studies, are frequently performed to exclude neurological dysfunction from causes other than hepatic encephalopathy, and to search for factors precipitating hepatic encephalopathy. Fever and leukocytosis are not features of hepatic encephalopathy and their presence makes necessary a lumbar puncture to investigate possible meningitis.

Management

Whether episodic or persistent, a critical element in the management of hepatic encephalopathy is a systematic search, identification, and correction of precipitating factors. Table 114-2 lists the most common precipitating factors of encephalopathy. Frequently, multiple precipitating factors may be operative in a given encephalopathic patient. Hepatic encephalopathy developing after installation of a transjugular intrahepatic portal systemic shunt (TIPS) can be a significant side effect of the procedure, but it may also be related to standard precipitating factors (see Table 114-2). Thus, these factors should still be considered in the evaluation and management of post-TIPS hepatic encephalopathy.

Intentional or inadvertent excess of dietary protein intake can be elicited by the intake history taken from the patient (if able) or more commonly, from a relative or household member close to the patient. This type of encephalopathy often promptly responds to protein restriction and lactulose therapy. An important corollary is that before discharge, an effort should be made to educate the patient and relatives about the dietary details of the desired level of protein intake. Constipation is another precipitating factor easily remediable by dietary measures and a preventive bowel regime. Acute gastrointestinal (GI) hemorrhage from esophagogastric varices or peptic ulcer are readily apparent causes of deteriorating mental status in a cirrhotic patient. Management should focus on control of bleeding, temporary protein restriction, and removal of blood from the GI by gastric lavage and lactulose. In patients with persistent or recurrent encephalopathy, chronic or subacute bleeding from portal hypertensive gastropathy may be less obvious as a precipitating factor for encephalopathy.

Infections of types can lead to hepatic encephalopathy. Common examples include spontaneous bacterial peritonitis, bacteremia, urinary sepsis, respiratory infections, and cellulitis. Blood and body fluids cultures should be obtained at the initial examination of a patient presenting with hepatic encephalopathy. The development of significant renal dysfunction may be sufficient to further impair the capability for ammonia excretion and lead to encephalopathy. Efforts should be made to identify diuretic-induced or cirrhosis-driven electrolyte imbalances such as hypokalemia, severe hyponatremia, hypomagnesemia, hypophosphatemia, dehydration, or disordered acid-base state. Use of sedatives, hypnotic agents, and other CNS-acting drugs are recognized causes for mental changes in cirrhosis and should be specifically investigated. Hypoxia from a variety of origens, or hypoglycemia, may be the underlying factor triggering encephalopathy.

TABLE 114-2. Common Precipitation Factors of Hepatic Encephalopathy

Excess of dietary protein
Gastrointestinal bleeding
Infections (especially, SBP, UTI, skin, respiratory, bacteremia)
Electrolyte imbalance, acidosis, dehydration
Post-TIPS stenting
Renal dysfunction
Hypoglycemia
Hypoxia
HCC
Exacerbation of chronic active hepatitis on a background of cirrhosis
Central nervous system-acting drugs (sedatives, hypnotics, etc).
Cerebral edema (in ALF)
End-stage cirrhosis

ALF = acute liver failure; HCC = hepatocellular carcinoma; SBP = spontaneous bacterial peritonitis; TIPS = transjugular intrahepatic portosystemic shunt; UTI = urinary tract infection.

Certain liver diseases such as chronic viral hepatitis, autoimmune hepatitis, or acute alcoholic hepatitis may periodically flare up and cause encephalopathy in a patient with little hepatic reserve. At the first episode of encephalopathy, a screen for hepatocellular carcinoma is warranted. Encephalopathy developing after insertion of a TIPS stent may require of institution of dietary protein restriction and lactulose. If no precipitating factors can be identified after a diligent search, it is possible that encephalopathy may be one manifestation of true end-stage liver disease. Given the erratic fluctuations of encephalopathy and impairment of cognitive and motor functions, revocation of automobile driving privileges may be reasonable for encephalopathic patients. Finally, successful liver transplantation can clearly resolve hepatic encephalopathy along with other manifestations of a failing liver.

Dietary Recommendations

Dietary protein restriction has been advocated for years for patients with hepatic encephalopathy. However, protein intakes of less than 40 g/d generally result in negative nitrogen balance and gradual malnutrition. This chain of events worsen as many of these patients undergo periodically large-volume paracentesis with considerable protein losses. We recommend protein restriction during the actual episode of encephalopathy, in a manner proportional to the severity of the mental impairment (see Table 114-1). Thus, for patients with mild to moderate, stage I or II encephalopathy, 30 to 40 g protein per day are temporarily adequate. Severe encephalopathy, stages III or IV, requires further restriction, down to 0 to 20 g daily during the stay in intensive care unit. However, once recovered from the episode of encephalopathy, the daily amount of dietary protein should be gradually titrated upwards according to the patient's neurological tolerance. The underlying concept is to maintain a balance between control of encephalopathy and avoidance of malnutrition. Vegetable proteins should constitute the bulk of proteins because of high fiber content and lower amounts of aromatic amino acids. However, it is not always realistic to expect substantial patient compliance with a vegetarian diet for the long term. We find it useful to set up a consultation for the patient and cooking relatives with a trained dietitian to review in detail the prescribed diet, preferred food types, and the range of permissible amounts.

Lactulose

As a nonabsorbable dissacharide, *lactulose* is metabolized by enteric bacteria to acetate leading to luminal acidification, catharsis, and entrapment of ammonia. In general, lactulose doses range from 30 mL orally 2 to 4 times per day. However, individual responsiveness to lactulose varies considerably and we prefer to instruct patients to self-titrate their dose gradually, aiming to achieve a target effect of three to five soft or semiliquid bowel movements per day. Unfortunately, a common error in management of encephalopathy is the omission of education of patients on the correct use of lactulose. Frequent side effects of lactulose therapy include glucose elevation in diabetics, excessive sweet taste, abdominal distention, cramping, and flatulence. Oral lactulose is appropriate for patients with stage I or II encephalopathy, but for those who have severe encephalopathy or hepatic coma (stages III or IV), a nasogastric tube should be used to instil lactulose. We prefer the use of lactulose colonic retention enemas in this setting because it allows greater dosing (enemas of 300 mL of lactulose plus 700 mL of tap water) and avoid the risks of pulmonary aspiration in these patients who have severe compromise of the mental status. Although quite effective, this route of administration clearly requires more intensive nursing care and resources. *Lactitol* (β-*galactosidesorbitol*), another dissacharide, is at least as effective as lactulose and possibly has fewer side effects.

Antibiotics

Neomycin and *metronidazole* can be useful in the management of encephalopathy that is poorly responsive to dietary protein restriction and lactulose. In spite of its poor GI absorption, prolonged usage of neomycin carries a risk of otovestibular injury and nephrotoxicity. Its efficacy in encephalopathy is similar to lactulose. We suggest starting doses of 1 to 2 g/d and gradually reduce to a minimum necessary to control encephalopathic symptoms. *Metronidazole* (750 mg/d), *vancomycin,* and *rifaximin* are other antibiotics which could be used instead of *neomycin*. *Rifaximin*, in particular, was found to be as effective as lactitol in a recent double blind controlled clinical trial. Bacterial resistance and long term toxicity are the main limitations of prolonged use of antibiotics for hepatic encephalopathy.

Combination Therapies

The combination of *neomycin* and *lactulose* is synergistic and results in greater fecal nitrogen excretion and lower stool pH. Combination triple therapy (low protein diet, lactulose, neomycin) may be required in patients with otherwise intractable hepatic encephalopathy. These patients typically have advanced liver disease and are often waiting for liver transplantation. Combinations of lactulose with *metronidazole, norfloxacin,* or *vancomycin* have not been adequately studied in clinical trials. Nevertheless, in patients with severe invalidating hepatic encephalopathy, it may be necessary to discontinue neomycin due to intervening renal dysfunction (prerenal azotemia or impending hepatorenal syndrome), and resort to trials with other agents, such as *metronidazole* or *quinolones*.

Less common treatment modalities, such as *benzodiazepine-receptor antagonists* (*flumazenil*), modification of gut bacteria with *Enterococcus faecium*, metabolic fixation of ammonia via zinc therapy, or by use of *ornithine-aspartate* or *sodium benzoate*, continue to undergo evaluation to ascertain their role, if any, in the treatment of hepatic encephalopathy.

Administration of branched chain amino acids (*leucine, isoleucine* and *valine*) to interdict entry of false neurotransmitters into the CNS has been studied for many years as a potential therapy for hepatic encephalopathy. Clinical trials have not shown consistent benefit and the available concentrates are expensive. This modality might eventually prove useful in a subset of encephalopathic patients. There are a number of attractive potential benefits of branched chain amino acids supplementation, including improved protein tolerance, stimulation of protein synthesis, inhibition of protein degradation, and energy.

Hepatic Encephalopathy of ALF

In acute (fulminant) liver failure, hepatic encephalopathy is always present to same extent, and develops due to a precipitous decrease in hepatic function. It is important to determine whether the abnormal mental status in ALF is due to cerebral edema or if it develops in the absence of increased brain water. Clinical examination and radiological methods are limited tools for making this determination, and in hepatic coma, it is frequently necessary to directly measure the intracranial pressure. The importance of confirming or excluding the presence of cerebral edema or intracranial hypertension lies in the different management strategies. In encephalopathic patients without cerebral swelling, management is not significantly different from that described above for chronic cirrhotic hepatic encephalopathy. In contrast, the presence of cerebral edema requires the use of mannitol therapy, infusion of barbiturates, and preparation for urgent liver transplantation. Dietary protein is often withheld while energy substrates are administered intravenously. Bowel cleansing with oral lactulose is reasonable in patients with ALF and mild encephalopathy (stages I and II). Lactulose enemas are better suited for patients with more severe encephalopathy who are less able to cooperate with oral medications and have a risk of aspiration. Correction of metabolic factors and precipitating factors is not different in the ALF patient. Elective endotracheal intubation is recommended at the transition of stage 3 to 4 hepatic encephalopathy in ALF, to minimize risk of pulmonary aspiration and respiratory arrest.

Supplemental Reading

Bianchi GP, Marchesini G, Fabbri A, et al. Vegetable versus animal protein diet in cirrhotic patients with chronic encephalopathy. A randomized cross-over comparison. J Intern Med 1993; 233:385–92.

Blei AT. Hepatic encephalopathy. In: Bircher J, Benhamou JP, McIntyre N, et al, editors. Oxford textbook of clinical hepatology. 2nd ed. Oxford: Oxford University Press; 1999. p. 765–83.

Conn HO, Leevy CM, Vlahcevic ZR, et al. Comparison of lactulose and neomycin in the treatment of chronic portal-systemic encephalopathy. A double blind controlled trial. Gastroenterol 1977;72(part 1):573–83.

Ferenci P, Lockwood A, Mullen K et al. Hepatic encephalopathy: definition, nomenclature, diagnosis, and quantification: final report of the working party at the 11th World Congresses of Gastroenterology, Vienna, 1998. Hepatology 2002;35:716–21.

Larsen FS, Hansen BA, Blei AT. Intensive care management of patients with acute liver failure with emphasis on systemic hemodynamic instability and cerebral edema: a critical appraisal of pathophysiology. Can J Gastroenterol 2000;14(Suppl D): 105–11D.

Marchesini G, Bianchi G, Merli M, et al. Nutritional supplementation with branched-chain amino acids in advanced cirrhosis: a double-blind, randomized trial. Gastroenterol 2003;124: 1792–801.

Mas A, Rodes J. Sunyer L, et al. Comparison of rifaximin and lactitol in the treatment of acute hepatic encephalopathy: results of a randomized, double-blind, double-dummy, controlled clinical trial. J Hepatol 2003;38:51–8.

Mullen KD, Dasarathy S. Hepatic encephalopathy. In: Schiff ER, Sorrell MF, Maddrey WC, editors. Schiff's diseases of the liver. 2nd ed. Philadelphia: Lippincott-Raven Pubs; 1999, p. 545–74.

Munoz S. Difficult management problems in fulminant hepatic failure. Sem Liv Dis 1993;13:395–413.

Munoz S. Nutritional therapies in liver disease. Sem Liv Dis 1991;11:278–91.

Ong JP, Aggarwal A, Krieger D, et al. Correlation between ammonia levels and the severity of hepatic encephalopathy. Am J Med 2003;114:188–93.

CHAPTER 115

ALCOHOLIC LIVER DISEASE

CHRISTIAN MENDEZ, MD, LUIS MARSANO, MD, DANIELL B. HILL, MD, AND
CRAIG J. MCCLAIN, MD

Alcoholic liver disease (ALD) remains a major cause of morbidity and mortality worldwide. In the western world, alcohol is the single most significant cause of liver disease, responsible for between 40 and 80% of cases of cirrhosis. In the United States, alcohol was responsible for 44% of deaths from cirrhosis between 1978 and 1988, with end-stage liver disease being the sixth leading cause of death in the age group of 45 to 64 years. The mortality rate of this form of liver disease is higher than in many forms of cancer, such as breast, colon, and prostate. In some studies, the mortality from alcoholic cirrhosis is higher than that of nonalcoholic cirrhosis. Although the per capita alcohol consumption has declined in the United States and northern Europe in the last decade, in Latin America and Asia alcohol use has increased. In the United States, almost 14 million people still meet criteria for alcoholism. Among this group, more than 2 million are suspected of having liver disease, and 14,000 people die of cirrhosis each year. The number of deaths that are alcohol-related is difficult to determine, because of inaccurate reporting of ethanol use.

Diagnosis of ALD

There appears to be a threshold in the daily amount and duration of alcohol intake for the development of ALD. Daily intake of alcohol for 10 to 12 years with doses in excess of 40 to 80 g/d for males and of 20 to 40 g/d for females is generally needed to cause alcoholic hepatitis/cirrhosis. Because alcoholic beverages have different alcohol contents, it is important to convert "usual serving" sizes to g of alcohol (Table 115-1).

Despite the need for a threshold with respect to dose and length of time for the development of ALD, there is not a particular amount of alcohol that will predictably cause ALD. The safe limits of alcohol intake are controversial but

TABLE 115-1. Alcohol Content in Common Alcoholic Beverages

- Twelve ounces of beer (5% v/v alcohol) provides 13.85 g of alcohol
- 4 ounces of wine (12% v/v alcohol) provides 10.7 g of alcohol
- 2 ounces fortified wine (20% v/v alcohol) provides 8.9 g of alcohol
- 1 ounce of "spirits" (40% v/v alcohol) provides 8.9 g of alcohol

the risk of liver disease begins at relatively low levels of alcohol consumption. A daily limit of 30 g/day in males and 20 g/day in females have been recommended.

Among heavy, long term alcohol drinkers, 90 to 100% develop fatty liver but only 10 to 35% develop alcoholic hepatitis, and 8 to 20% alcoholic cirrhosis. Alcohol acts as a "potential hepatotoxin," with development of liver disease depending on the balance of host attributes and coexisting external factors, such a gender, polymorphisms of alcohol-metabolizing enzymes, immunologic factors, exposures to other substances/drugs, hepatic viral infections, nutritional deficiencies, and obesity, etc.

The diagnosis of ALD is established with a history of alcohol intake of sufficient length and intensity together with physical signs and/or laboratory evidence of liver disease. Findings on physical examination and laboratory abnormalities may be nonspecific or even absent. The major clinical assessment necessary for diagnosing ALD is determining whether the patient is abusing alcohol. Various questionnaires such as the CAGE test are useful in screening for alcohol abuse.

The spectrum of ALD includes the three following separate pathologic diagnoses: (1) alcoholic fatty liver (steatosis), (2) alcoholic hepatitis, and (3) alcoholic cirrhosis. They may coexist in any combination.

Patients with alcoholic fatty liver are usually asymptomatic but they can have vague complaints including fatigue, nausea, or right upper quadrant discomfort. Up to 70% of hospitalized patients with steatosis have hepatomegaly and one-third have laboratory abnormalities. The clinical syndrome associated with alcoholic hepatitis includes tender hepatomegaly, jaundice, fever, ascites, hepatic encephalopathy, anorexia, and malaise. This syndrome occurs only in a minority of patients. Leukemoid reactions and hepatorenal syndrome may also occur. Portal hypertension may be present, even in the absence of cirrhosis. Once a patient has alcoholic hepatitis, the probability of developing cirrhosis is 10 to 20% per year, and up to 70% will eventually develop cirrhosis. The patients at higher risk for development of cirrhosis are those who continue drinking, have severe alcoholic hepatitis, and are female. Alcoholic cirrhosis may be present in patients with very few symptoms or signs of liver disease, but over time most patients will develop evidence of portal hypertension and hepatocellular dysfunction.

Biochemical tests may raise the suspicion of underlying ALD but if used alone, they do not correlate with the severity or exclude the presence of liver disease. Serum aspartate aminotransferase (AST) and alanine aminotransferase (ALT) levels rarely exceed 300 IU/mL. The AST:ALT ratio often exceeds 2 in patients with ALD. Aminotransferase levels greater than 300 IU/mL in an alcoholic should lead to consideration of a nonalcoholic form of hepatic injury.

Levels of alkaline phosphatase are often normal or mildly elevated in ALD. γ-Glutamyltransferase levels are commonly elevated in heavy drinkers irrespective of the presence of liver disease. The specificity of γ-glutamyltransferase is limited because many drugs induce this enzyme. In addition, γ-glutamyltransferase is increased in most forms of liver injury.

Leukocytosis and thrombocytopenia are common in alcoholic hepatitis. Chronic alcohol consumption is also often associated with hypertriglyceridemia, hyperuricemia, hypokalemia, hypomagnesemia, and elevated mean corpuscular erythrocyte volume. Carbohydrate-deficient transferrin may be specific for alcohol use but it lacks sensitivity, limiting its routine use alone in the diagnosis of active alcoholism.

Elevation of bilirubin, prolonged prothrombin time (PT) and hypoalbuminemia are markers of severe alcoholic hepatitis and/or cirrhosis. The "Maddrey's Discriminant Function" is used as a prognostic tool; it is calculated by the following equation:

$$4.6 \times [PT\ patient - PT\ control] + total\ bilirubin\ (mg/dL)$$

If this value exceeds 32, the 1-month mortality may be close to 50%. There is also evidence that serum concentrations of tumor necrosis factor (TNF)-α, interleukin (IL)-6, and IL-8 correlate with mortality in patients with alcoholic hepatitis, but levels of these cytokines are not yet used in routine clinical practice.

Liver biopsy is the most sensitive and specific test for evaluation of the degree of liver cell injury and fibrosis. It remains the only way to reliably detect steatohepatitis and cirrhosis in asymptomatic individuals. Histologic evaluation is also useful in distinguishing the cause of liver injury in patients who have more than one potential cause of liver disease.

Therapy for ALD

Major advances have been made in our understanding of mechanisms of alcohol-induced liver injury, and these concepts are being translated into clinical trials. Moreover, we are now in a position to better understand some of the mechanisms of actions of some traditionally used therapies for ALD, ranging from steroids to antioxidant therapy.

This section on therapy will focus on the importance of the following:
1. Lifestyle change, including abstinence
2. Nutrition
3. Drug therapy (conventional and alternative therapies)
4. The role of liver transplantation (Table 115-2)

Lifestyle Changes

Establishing and maintaining abstinence from alcohol is vital in order to prevent further ongoing liver injury, fibrosis, and, possibly, hepatocellular carcinoma. Abstinence allows total resolution of alcoholic steatosis. There are limited studies evaluating the effects of abstinence from alcohol on the progression of ALD, but virtually all of them show beneficial effects on survival. Moreover, data from recent Veterans Health Administration (VA) cooperative studies suggest that reducing, but not stopping, ethanol consumption also improves projected survival in ALD. The so-called "brief interventions" are the simplest form of psychological therapy for alcohol abuse and can be implemented by nonpsychiatric staff. These interventions involve educating and informing patients regarding the nature of their problem and providing them with advice as to how to change their behavior. Thus, abstinence, or a major reduction in drinking, should be encouraged in all patients with ALD. Newer agents to improve abstinence, such as Naltrexone and Acamprosate, have been shown to be effective in some chronic alcoholics; however, there are no large multicenter studies evaluating these drugs in patients with ALD. There is a separate chapter on alcoholism (Chapter 37).

Many subjects who drink alcohol also smoke cigarettes. Smoking cigarettes has been shown in European studies to increase the rate of progression of fibrosis in ALD. Moreover, hepatitis C (HC) patients who drink also have accelerated disease progression if they smoke cigarettes. Cigarette smoking causes oxidative stress, which may be the underlying mechanism for the observed accelerated liver disease in smokers.

Obesity is associated with the development of fatty liver and nonalcoholic steatohepatitis. Body mass index has been shown to be an independent risk factor for the development of ALD. Thus, the initial approach to ALD is lifestyle

TABLE 115-2. Therapy for Alcoholic Liver Disease

- Lifestyle modification (alcohol cessation, smoking, obesity)
- Proper nutrition/nutrition support
- Consider pentoxifylline or prednisone for alcoholic hepatitis
- Consider silymarin or SAMe for cirrhosis
- Correct metabolic disturbances/complications
- Transplantation in selected abstinent patients with end-stage liver disease

SAMe = S-adenosylmethionine.

modification related to issues of alcohol consumption, cigarette smoking, and obesity.

Nutrition Therapy

Malnutrition is prevalent in liver disease, especially in the more severe forms of chronic liver disease. Probably the most extensive studies of nutritional status in patients with liver disease are large studies in the Veterans Health Administration Cooperative Studies Program dealing with patients having alcoholic hepatitis. The first of these studies demonstrated that virtually every patient with alcoholic hepatitis had some degree of malnutrition. Patients had a mean alcohol consumption of 228 g/d (with almost 50% of energy intake coming from alcohol, which has little nutritional value). The severity of liver disease generally correlated with the severity of malnutrition. Similar data were generated in a follow-up VA study on alcoholic hepatitis. In both of these studies, patients were given a balanced 2500-kcal hospital diet, monitored carefully by a dietitian, and were encouraged to consume the diet. In the second study, patients in the therapy arm of the protocol also received an enteral nutritional support product high in branched-chain amino acids (BCAAs), as well as the anabolic steroid *oxandrolone* (80 mg/d). Patients were not fed by tube if voluntary oral intake was inadequate in either study (probably a study design flaw, in retrospect). Voluntary oral food intake correlated in a stepwise fashion with 6-month mortality data. Thus, patients who voluntarily consumed > 3000 kcal/d had virtually no mortality, whereas those consuming < 1000 kcal/d had > 80% six-month mortality (Figure 115-1). Moreover, the degree of malnutrition correlated with the development of serious complications, such as encephalopathy, ascites, and hepatorenal syndrome.

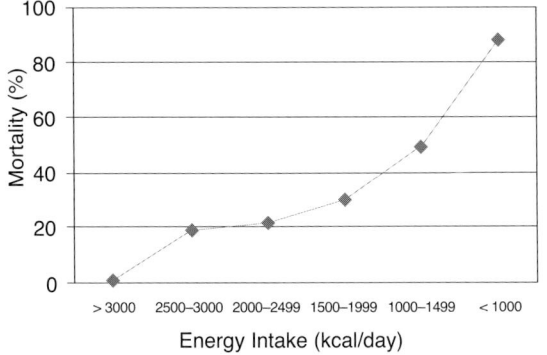

FIGURE 115-1. A direct relationship was noted between voluntary caloric intake in Veterans Health Administration studies in patients with moderate and severe alcoholic hepatitis. It is not known whether providing enteral feeding to patients with inadequate caloric intake would have improved mortality.

Interest in nutrition therapy for cirrhosis was stimulated when Patek and colleagues demonstrated that a nutritious diet improved the 5-year outcome of patients with alcoholic cirrhosis compared with patients consuming an inadequate diet. Several recent studies have further supported the concept of improved outcome with nutritional support in patients with cirrhosis. Hirsch and colleagues, demonstrated that outpatients taking an *enteral nutritional support product* (1000 kcal, 34 g protein) had significantly improved protein intake and significantly fewer hospitalizations. These same investigators subsequently gave an enteral supplement to outpatients with alcoholic cirrhosis and observed an improvement in nutritional status and immune function. Nighttime snacks and nighttime enteral BCAA supplements have been shown to improve nutritional status in cirrhotics. In the VA Cooperative Study #275 on nutritional support in ALD using both an anabolic steroid and an enteral nutritional supplement, improved mortality was seen with the combination of oxandrolone plus supplement in patients who had moderate protein-energy malnutrition. Those with severe malnutrition did not significantly benefit from therapy, possibly because their malnutrition was so advanced that no intervention, including nutrition, could help. Studies by Kearns and colleagues showed that patients with ALD hospitalized for treatment and given an enteral nutritional supplement via tube feeding had significantly improved serum bilirubin levels and liver function as assessed by antipyrine clearance. Moreover, a major randomized study of enteral nutrition versus steroids in patients with alcoholic hepatitis showed similar overall initial outcomes, and less long term infections in the nutrition group. Thus, traditional nutritional supplementation clearly improves nutritional status and, in some instances, hepatic function and other outcome indicators in alcoholic hepatitis/cirrhosis. We have no hesitation in placing a nasogastric tube (Dobhoff), if necessary for enteral nutrition, as soon as our patients with ALD are admitted to the hospital.

Drug Therapy (Conventional and Alternative Therapies)

Although ALD remains a major cause of morbidity and mortality in the United States, there is no FDA-approved therapy for either alcoholic cirrhosis or alcoholic hepatitis. However, there are several drugs that have been widely used. We will discuss only therapies available in the United States for which there generally are large randomized human studies. Our first line of therapy in ALD includes corticosteroids and pentoxifylline.

CORTICOSTEROIDS

Corticosteroids have been the most extensively studied form of therapy for alcoholic hepatitis, but their role remains limited. The rationale for steroid use is to decrease the immune response and proinflammatory cytokine response. Most meta-analyses support the use of steroids for severe acute alcoholic hepatitis, including the most recent study by Mathurin and colleagues. This study reported significantly improved survival at 28 days (85% versus 65%) in severely ill alcoholic hepatitis patients having a discriminant function (DF) of > 32. Independent prognostic factors associated with survival at 28 days in this meta-analysis were steroid treatment, age, and creatinine. It is important to note that patients studied were highly selected, and infections (eg, spontaneous bacterial peritonitis [SBP]), gastrointestinal bleeding, and many other common complications were exclusions for entry into these studies. Most investigators agree that if corticosteroids are to be used, they should be reserved for those with relatively severe liver disease (DF > 32), and possibly those with hepatic encephalopathy. Steroids have well-documented side effects, including enhancing the risk of infection, which is already substantial in patients with AH (AH). Thus, a major disadvantage to corticosteroids is their lack of applicability in many patients with AH.

Pentoxifylline

Pentoxifylline (PTX) is a nonselective phosphodiesterase inhibitor which increases intracellular concentrations of adenosine 3´,5´-cyclic monophosphate and guanosine 3´,5´-cyclic monophosphate, and decreases production of proinflammatory chemokines/cytokines, including TNF. Akriviadis and colleagues performed a prospective, randomized, double blind clinical trial of PTX in severe alcoholic hepatitis (DF > 32). Forty-nine patients received 400 mg of PTX orally 3 times daily and 52 received placebo (vitamin B_{12}) for 4 weeks. PTX treatment improved survival. Twelve patients on PTX died (24.5%) compared with 24 (46%) patients on placebo. PTX also decreased hepatorenal syndrome as a cause of death. Six of the 12 (50%) PTX-treated patients who died did so of renal failure compared with 22 of the 24 (92%) control patients who died of renal failure. Multivariate analysis revealed age, serum creatinine at randomization, and treatment with PTX as independent factors associated with survival. Our group currently uses PTX (400 mg orally 3 times daily) in patients with AH and with alcoholic cirrhosis because of its anti-inflammatory properties, its protective effects against hepatorenal syndrome, and its excellent safety profile.

Propylthiouracil

Chronic alcohol feeding in animals models produces a hypermetabolic state with increased oxygen consumption similar to the hypermetabolic state associated with hyperthyroidism. This may lead to relative hypoxia, especially in the central lobular area, or zone 3 of the liver. Propylthiouracil (PTU) has been postulated to attenuate this hypermetabolic state, to function as an antioxidant, and to improve portal blood flow. However, a recent Cochran review evaluated PTU therapy for ALD, including alcoholic steatosis, alcoholic fibrosis, alcoholic hepatitis, and/or cirrhosis, and no beneficial effect was noted. We do not recommend use of PTU in ALD.

Colchicine

Colchicine has been suggested as a treatment for ALD because of its antifibrotic effects. It has many potential therapeutic mechanisms of action including inhibition of collagen production, enhancement of collagenase activity, and anti-inflammatory functions. Initial positive studies led to a large VA cooperative study evaluating colchicine therapy in alcoholic cirrhosis and no significant benefit was observed.

TNF-α Inhibitors

Cytokine induced acute inflammatory response is one underlying basic mechanism responsible for cellular injury in alcoholic hepatitis. Serum TNF-α has been shown to be elevated in patients with acute alcoholic hepatitis, particularly in the more severe cases. TNF-α antibodies *(infliximab)* and receptor antagonists *(Entanercept)* have shown promising results in some chronic inflammatory diseases like Crohn's disease and rheumatoid arthritis. Small studies using infliximab or Entanercept in acute alcoholic hepatitis showed improvement in the Maddrey's DF, as well a reduction in TNF-inducible cytokines such as IL-6 and IL-8, and larger randomized studies are underway.

Silymarin (Milk Thistle)

Silymarin is probably the most widely used form of complementary and alternative medicine (CAM) in the treatment of liver disease in the United States. It has antioxidant activities, it protects against lipid peroxidation, and it has anti-inflammatory and antifibrotic effects. Large controlled trials of silymarin have been performed in Europe, with varying results using doses between 140 to 150 mg orally 3 times daily. In all studies performed thus far, the drug appears quite safe.

S-Adenosylmethionine

S-Adenosylmethionine (SAMe), or AdoMet, is an obligatory intermediate in the conversion of methionine to cysteine in the hepatic transsulfuration pathway. SAMe is a precursor for the synthesis of polyamines, choline, and reduced glutathione (GSH), and it is the major methylating agent for a vast number of molecules via specific methyltransferases. Patients with ALD have elevated plasma methionine levels, markedly delayed clearance of an oral methionine load, and decreased hepatic methionine adenosyltransferase (MAT) activity (the enzyme responsible for conversion of methionine to SAMe). Hepatic-specific MAT is highly sensitive to oxidative stress, and it is likely that subnormal hepatic MAT activity reported in ALD is due to oxidation of the active site. Studies from our laboratories have shown that SAMe downregulates production of the proinflammatory cytokine, TNF, in animal models of liver injury and in peripheral blood monocytes or macrophage cell lines in vitro. Mato and colleagues recently reported that patients with alcoholic liver cirrhosis who were randomized to receive SAMe (400 mg 3 times daily) for 2 years had decreased liver mortality/liver transplantation (16% versus 30%) compared to the placebo treated group.

OTHER ANTIOXIDANTS

Vitamin E *Vitamin E* deficiency has been well documented in ALD. Vitamin E has been used extensively with hepatoprotective effects in experimental models of liver injury, such as that induced by carbon tetrachloride or ischemia. Vitamin E has multiple potential beneficial effects including membrane stabilization, reduced NFκB activation and TNF production, and inhibition of hepatic stellate cell activation and collagen production. Unfortunately, the major randomized study of vitamin E in ALD did not show significant benefit and likely used an inadequate dose (500 mg).

GSH Prodrugs *GSH* is a tripeptide, which is synthesized from glutamate, cysteine, and glycine. GSH prodrugs have been used extensively in virtually every known experimental model of hepatotoxicity with beneficial results. The glutathione prodrug, *N-acetylcysteine* (given as *Mucomyst*) is the standard therapy for acetaminophen toxicity in humans. Maintaining adequate hepatocyte GSH levels has been documented to prevent acetaminophen liver injury. GSH prodrugs can directly affect the hepatocyte, and they can also positively modulate proinflammatory cytokine production with inhibition of cytokines such as TNF and IL-8. However, large, randomized studies of GSH prodrugs using mortality as an outcome indicator are lacking in ALD.

Dilinoleoylphosphatidylcholine *Dilinoleoylphosphatidylcholine* (a form of lecithin/soybean extract) has antioxidant, antifibrotic, and anticytokine activity in experimental rat models of ALD. However, a recently completed VA cooperative study failed to show significant benefit in human ALD.

Liver Transplantation

There have been multiple recent studies and reviews concerning liver transplantation in patients with severe alcoholic cirrhosis. There is a well-documented organ shortage for liver transplantation, and there are serious ethical issues concerning this controversial area that have precipitated these studies. HC and ALD are the two major reasons for liver transplantation in the United States. Data clearly demonstrate that patients transplanted for ALD do (short and long term) as well as patients transplanted for HC or other types of liver disease. However, alcoholic hepatitis clearly is not an indication for liver transplantation at the current time. Virtually all centers require that alcoholic patients undergo formal psychiatric examination and treatment before transplantation. Many centers impose a "six month rule" of abstinence before being considered for orthotopic liver transplantation; however, most centers also show some flexibility with this rule. It is unusual for ALD alone to be the cause of graft failure. The majority of patients with ALD are not listed for liver transplantation for multiple reasons including continued alcohol consumption, improvement of liver function with abstinence, lack of interest, etc. Patients with ALD appear to have a higher incidence of certain malignancies of the upper airway and upper digestive tract. Therefore, these patients should be screened for these processes prior to transplantation and monitored carefully posttransplantation.

Conclusions

In summary, all patients should stop or markedly decrease alcohol intake and employ other lifestyle modifications where appropriate (see Table 115-1). Proper nutrition and nutrition support have consistently been shown to be important. Certain drugs (eg, *corticosteroids* or *pentoxifylline*) may be effective in selected patients. Some CAM agents such as *milk thistle* and *SAMe* may be effective. Although no FDA-approved therapies are available, many new agents, such as *anti-TNF antibody*, are under investigation. Transplantation is lifesaving in certain abstinent patients with end-stage liver disease.

Complications of ALD are important events in more advanced liver disease. Diagnosing and appropriately treating these complications is vital for maintaining quality of life and decreasing morbidity and mortality. Some major complications include the following:

1. Ascites
2. SBP
3. Hepatorenal syndrome
4. Hepatic encephalopathy
5. Esophageal varices

Various therapies can attenuate or reverse these complications, but are often only palliative. Treatment of these complications is covered elsewhere in this book.

Supplemental Reading

Arteel G, Mendez C, McClain C, et al. Advances in alcoholic liver disease. Best practice and research clinical gastroenterology 2003;17:625–47.

Bellamy C, DiMartini A, Ruppert K, et al. Liver transplantation for alcoholic cirrhosis: long term follow-up and impact of disease recurrence. Transplantation 2001;72:619–26.

Diehl A. Liver disease in alcohol abusers: clinical perspective. Alcohol 2002;27:7–11.

Lieber C. Alcoholic liver disease: new insights in pathogenesis lead to new treatments. J Hepatol 2000;32:113–28.

Madhotra R, Gilmore I. Recent developments in the treatment of alcoholic hepatitis. QJM 2003;96:391–400.

Maher J. Alcoholic liver disease. In: Feldman M, Friedman L, editors. Sleisenger and Fordtran's gastrointestinal and liver disease: Pathophysiology, diagnosis and management. 7th ed. WB Saunders; 2002. p. 1375–91.

Marsano L, Martin A, Randall H. Current nutrition in liver disease. Curr Opin Gastroenterol 2002;18:246–53.

Menon N, Gores G, Shah V. Pathogenesis, diagnosis and treatment of alcoholic liver disease. Mayo Clin Proc 2001;76:1021–9.

Stewart F, Day C. The management of alcoholic liver disease. J Hepatol 2003;38:S2–13.

Stickel B, Hoehn D, Schuppan H, et al. Review article: nutritional therapy in alcoholic liver disease. Aliment Pharmacol Ther 2003;18:357–73.

CHAPTER 116

Nonalcoholic Fatty Liver Disease

Brent A. Neuschwander-Tetri, MD

Disorders of the liver characterized by fat accumulation in the absence of excessive alcohol consumption are collectively known as nonalcoholic fatty liver disease (NAFLD). Although the presence of excess amounts of fat as triglyceride in hepatocytes may not always be directly harmful, it is typically associated with progressive liver disease. In fact, in some people, NAFLD is capable of causing cirrhosis and leading to death or liver transplantation. The necroinflammatory changes associated with progressive liver disease are generally identified pathologically as steatohepatitis, and the pattern of injury and constellation of findings most commonly associated with more severe liver disease is called nonalcoholic steatohepatitis (NASH).

Insulin resistance (IR) is commonly found in patients with NAFLD and has been implicated as a causative factor in the development of NASH and the associated necroinflammatory changes (Marchesini et al, 2003). This recent finding has bolstered the emphasis on exercise and weight reduction as optimal treatment strategies, although the effectiveness of these treatments requires further verification in clinical trials.

Treatment Options

The optimal treatment of NASH remains uncertain. Treatments are generally aimed at either improving peripheral insulin sensitivity or reducing the liver's necroinflammatory response to chronic injury.

Insulin Resistance

IR is the underlying cause of type 2 diabetes. IR is an abnormal physiologic state that may exist for decades before diabetes becomes clinically evident because of increased glucose levels. Improving insulin sensitivity, ideally before the development of glucose intolerance, is a newer approach to the prevention and treatment of type 2 diabetes.

One large trial in patients with diabetes comparing a pharmacological approach (*metformin*) with aggressive changes in lifestyle found that increasing physical activity may improve insulin sensitivity more than the drug would (Knowler et al, 2002). Because IR may be the most common predisposing factor for the development of NAFLD, these findings in the diabetic and prediabetic populations may be equally relevant to people with fatty liver.

Weight Loss

Weight loss, with or without exercise, has been investigated as a therapy for fatty liver disease in several studies (Angulo and Lindor, 2001). Although weight loss is encouraged in overweight patients to prevent its many known complications, the data justifying its recommendation for liver disease remains unconvincing. Several difficulties with the interpretation of earlier studies have been suggested. The duration of weight loss in previous clinical trials was often relatively short and effective means of sustaining weight loss have been elusive. Adjuncts to weight reduction, such as the luminal lipase inhibitor orlistat, are now being investigated in clinical trials of NASH. One provocative observation is that early studies of weight loss as a treatment of NAFLD were associated with improved steatosis but possibly worsened fibrosis and inflammation. Because the histological characteristics of NAFLD as it improves during effective intervention are unknown, biopsy scoring systems developed for viral hepatitis may not properly identify resolving steatohepatitis.

For this reason, the previously used scoring systems that do not account for shifts in inflammation and key differences between the fibrosis of NAFLD and hepatitis C virus (HCV) may miss important changes that indicate resolution of NAFLD (Brunt EM, personal communication, 2003). Past studies may not have focused on specific histological abnormalities with adequate detail and their findings must be held with some circumspection. Specifically, if resolving NASH in the early weight loss trials was characterized by important shifts the inflammation and changes in the fibrosis that were missed by HCV scoring systems, such improvements would have been unnoticed. The alternate hypothesis, that weight reduction and lifestyle interventions actually worsen the underlying liver disease, especially the fibrosis, then alternative strategies must be employed to prevent progressive liver disease. Moreover, we cannot underestimate the difficulty in maintaining an altered lifestyle because of physical disabilities or societal influences, a point that further emphasizes the pragmatic need to identify effective treatment strategies besides lifestyle interventions.

Bariatric Surgery

An alternative approach to weight reduction is obesity surgery. Bariatric surgery can be offered to carefully selected patients if it is to be performed at centers with significant experience that offer a multidisciplinary approach to patient selection and postoperative management. There is a separate chapter on surgery for obesity (see Chapter 35, "Obesity"). Results of bariatric surgery suggest improvement in NASH is associated with the intended weight loss. Significant variability in the operative techniques from center to center can make generalizations difficult. Most commonly used is a reduction of gastric volume coupled with a Roux-en-Y small bowel bypass. Jejunal-ileal bypasses were abandoned several decades ago because the presence of a blind loop seems to have precipitated significant liver disease. Exacerbation of liver disease has not been the experience with currently employed surgical techniques such as gastric banding with Roux-en-Y small bowel bypass (Luyckx et al, 1999). Liver biopsies obtained at the time of surgery should be considered in all patients undergoing bariatric surgery because of the significant prevalence of unsuspected liver disease related to prior NASH in this population.

Medications for IR

One approach to IR is to improve insulin sensitivity pharmacologically. A class of drugs called *thiazolidinediones* (TZDs), has been developed as a novel treatment of type 2 diabetes and these drugs act by improving peripheral insulin sensitivity. Two such agents, *rosiglitazone* and *pioglitazone*, are indicated and available for diabetes treatment. Both drugs are being studied in clinical trials for NAFLD, and the early results are now becoming available. Improvements in NASH and NAFLD are seen with both drugs, but perhaps at the cost of important side effects. Drugs in this class cause adipocyte differentiation which may have been the cause of weight gain observed in the study subjects. Interestingly, studies in subjects with diabetes suggest that the weight gained is peripheral rather than central, and central adiposity is most associated with NAFLD and cardiovascular risk factors. Weight gain is nonetheless disheartening in these patients who are often battling obesity anyway.

The risk of idiosyncratic hepatotoxicity of TZDs may not be any greater than with any other new agent. The early experience with troglitazone, a TZD withdrawn because of its significant hepatotoxicity, appears to have been unique to this particular drug as the postmarketing experience with *rosiglitazone* and *pioglitazone* has not led to similar findings.

Another pharmacologic approach to improving insulin sensitivity is the use of *metformin*. Metformin acts by decreasing hepatic IR in the liver compared to the TZDs which primarily act by decreasing IR in muscle and adipose tissue. Early animal studies suggested that *metformin* could prevent NASH in a mouse model of obesity caused by the lack of an endogenous satiety mediator, leptin. Subsequent trials of *metformin* in humans with NASH have been less encouraging, although further studies are needed before this approach is abandoned.

In summary, pharmacologic treatment of IR may be one approach to the patients with NAFLD, although a more conservative, but possibly effective, approach is significant *lifestyle changes that increase muscle mass coupled with weight reduction*. This may prove to be the *best initial intervention for NAFLD*.

Hypolipidemic Agents

NASH has been associated with circulating hyperlipidemia, specifically hypercholesterolemia and hypertriglyceridemia. One *relatively unsuccessful treatment* approach has been to correct this circulatory abnormality with the hope that decreased circulating lipids would decrease the uptake of lipids by the liver and decrease the amount of fat in the liver. In reality, little circulating triglyceride is destined for the liver and most of the triglyceride in very low density lipoprotein is used as fuel by muscle or stored in adipose tissues. The majority of circulating triglyceride in the fasting state originates in the liver so that attempts to diminish the amount that circulates could have the theoretical disadvantage of impairing hepatic secretion of fat. Despite this concern, drugs that effectively treat hypertriglyceridemia have not been identified as significant causes of NASH; therefore, their use in NASH is typically not contraindicated. Nonetheless, the theoretical basis of correcting circulatory abnormalities as a therapy for liver disease must be questioned.

The relationship between hypercholesterolemia and NASH is *uncertain*. Most circulating cholesterol is made by the liver and secreted in lipoproteins. Drugs that specifically impair hepatic cholesterol synthesis, the 3-hydroxy-3-methyl-glutaryl-coenzyme A (HMG-CoA) reductase inhibitors, or *statins*, can increase liver enzymes independent of known preexisting liver disease. A commonly encountered clinical problem is whether to use this class of drugs in patients with known NASH or NAFLD. Because there is no evidence that statins increase the damage to the liver caused by NASH, most experts in liver disease *allow the use of statins* in patients with elevated aminotransferase due to NAFLD when these drugs are clinically indicated, as long as the liver enzymes are monitored regularly and the drug is changed if its use clearly causes a further increase above the pretreatment baseline.

Rationalizing the use of statins as therapeutic agents for NAFLD is *problematic* based on the known property of these drugs in lowering circulating cholesterol levels. However, the statins have multiple effects on inflammation in general, because of the role of cholesterol metabolites in regulating intracellular signaling. Signaling molecules such as *ras* require membrane anchoring for activation, a process that requires cholesterol metabolites such as farnesyl moieties.

Interfering with cholesterol synthesis could thus have multiple effects on proinflammatory signaling, which in turn could interfere with the steps necessary for a necroinflammatory response to excess fat in hepatocytes. How much of this theoretical framework is true will require extensive basic science investigation and confirmation in clinical studies.

Cytoprotective Strategies

Treatments aimed at improving insulin sensitivity are one way of reducing the amount of fat in the liver. Another approach is to offer patients interventions that have the potential of reducing the necroinflammatory process resulting from excessive hepatic steatosis.

Vitamin E

Oxidant stress is commonly invoked as a mechanism that ties together the accumulation of fat in the liver with the hepatocellular injury of NASH. *Vitamin E* is readily available and a biologically effective antioxidant. For these reasons, *vitamin E* is commonly used as a potentially beneficial therapy for NASH. Unfortunately, the data linking oxidant stress as a cause of the necroinflammation in humans has been scant, and data supporting the use of *vitamin E* has not been impressive. In children, *vitamin E* usually causes enzyme normalization and perhaps histological improvement (Lavine, 2000). In adults, an antioxidant approach to therapy has been more disappointing, either due to a true lack of effectiveness or failure of specific antioxidants to effectively block oxidant stress where it can cause damage. Nonetheless, *vitamin E* is commonly recommended to patients with NAFLD because in typically recommended doses (400 to 800 IU daily), little if any harm is thought to occur and the potential for benefit remains.

Betaine

Pilot studies of *betaine* have shown some promise for this agent. Perhaps one of the most controversial aspects of its use in clinical medicine is the proper pronunciation of its name. In clinical practice, *bee-tane* is commonly used, whereas chemists tend to use its original pronunciation of *beta-een*. Common use of the former may dictate its pronunciation by clinicians by affirmation. *Betaine*, or dimethyl glycine, is an alternative source for methyl groups, and as such can replace essential functions of methionine and choline in the synthesis of lecithin, an essential fatty acid for elimination of fat from the liver. It could also serve as an antioxidant by increasing the synthetic capacity for intracellular glutathione. Although the mechanisms of its actions in NAFLD remain to be fully worked out, *betaine* could be promising for the patients with NASH. Unfortunately, the doses used in the successful clinical trial were quite large and compliance was a problem for some patients.

Ursodeoxycholic Acid

Early enthusiasm for *ursodeoxycholic acid (UDCA)* was based on a report of some improvement observed in a small group of patients taking this relatively benign but expensive drug. A follow-up blinded clinical trial revealed no benefit of *UDCA* in a larger group of NASH patients (Lindor, 2003). Thus *UDCA* cannot be recommended as effective therapy for NASH.

This trial and trials by other investigators have recently shown that *spontaneous improvement in NASH can occur without specific therapy* once a diagnosis has been established. This observation is important in two respects. First is that it confirms the importance of conducting randomized placebo controlled trials to determine the efficacy of new agents in NASH. Second, it raises the important question of whether establishing the diagnosis of NASH (eg, performing a liver biopsy) provides enough impetus for lifestyle change such that patients commonly improve once a diagnosis is established. If true, this observation could provide an additional benefit of performing a liver biopsy when the diagnosis is suspected.

Liver Disease and Total Parenteral Nutrition

NAFLD and cholestasis are common complications of total parenteral nutrition (TPN) use in adults (Buchman, 2002). Since the advent of TPN four decades ago, it has been difficult to establish the etiology of these disorders with certainty. Patients receiving TPN often have multiple coexisting medical problems, potential hepatotoxic medication use, or altered bowel anatomy. Nonetheless, both choline and essential fatty acids are necessary for lecithin synthesis, a step that must occur in the liver to allow fat transport out of the liver. This essential metabolic step provides one rationale for ensuring that patients receiving

TABLE 116-1. Therapeutic Options for Nonalcoholic Steatohepatitis (NASH)

Insulin Resistance
Exercise
Weight Loss
  Diet
  Bariatric surgery
  Block absorption of calories
Drugs
  Thiazolidinediones
  Metformin
Lipid Lowering Agents
  3-hydroxy-3-methylglutaryl-coenzyme A (HMG-CoA) inhibitors (statins)
  Fibrates
Cytoprotective Agents
  Vitamin E
  Betaine

TPN also receive regular fatty acids and choline supplements. There is a concern that too much fat provided with TPN may contribute to the cholestasis that can occur in subjects receiving long-term TPN, especially children. The causes of TPN-induced cholestasis are less certain.

The approaches to NAFLD and cholestasis during TPN administration include ensuring that patients are not receiving too many calories, reducing small bowel overgrowth with antibiotics, or reducing the toxicity of bile with *ursodeoxycholic acid*. There is a separate chapter on enteral and parenteral nutrition (Chapter 54).

Supplemental Reading

Abdelmalek MF, Angulo P, Jorgensen RA, et al. Betaine, a promising new agent for patients with nonalcoholic steatohepatitis: results of a pilot study. Am J Gastroenterol 2001;96:2711–7.

Angulo P, Lindor KD. Treatment of nonalcoholic fatty liver: present and emerging therapies. Semin Liver Dis 2001;21:81–8.

Buchman A. Total parenteral nutrition-associated liver disease. JPEN J Parenter Enteral Nutr 2002;26(5 Suppl):S43–8.

Knowler WC, Barrett-Connor E, Fowler SE, et al. Diabetes Prevention Program Research Group. Reduction in the incidence of type 2 diabetes with lifestyle intervention or metformin. N Engl J Med 2002;346:393–403.

Lavine JE. Vitamin E treatment of nonalcoholic steatohepatitis in children: a pilot study. J Pediatr 2000;136:734–8.

Lindor KD, on behalf of the UDCA/NASH Study Group. Ursodeoxycholic acid for treatment of nonalcoholic steatohepatitis: results of a randomized, placebo-controlled trial. Gastroenterology 2003;124(Suppl):A–708.

Luyckx FH, Scheen AJ, Desaive C, et al. Parallel reversibility of biological markers of the metabolic syndrome and liver steatosis after gastroplasty-induced weight loss in severe obesity. J Clin Endo Metab 1999;84:4293.

Marchesini G, Bugianesi E, Forlani G, et al. Nonalcoholic fatty liver, steatohepatitis, and the metabolic syndrome. Hepatology 2003;37:917–23.

Neuschwander-Tetri BA. Betaine: an old therapy for a new scourge. Am J Gastroenterol 2001;96:2534–6.

CHAPTER 117

Portal Hypertension

Anne T. Wolf, MD, and Norman D. Grace, MD

The complications of portal hypertension—gastrointestinal hemorrhage, varices, ascites, spontaneous bacterial peritonitis, hepatorenal syndrome, portal systemic encephalopathy—present significant challenges with regard to the management of, and remain significant causes of morbidity and mortality in, patients with end-stage liver disease. These complications are manifestations of hepatic decompensation and their presence warrants consideration of liver transplantation. This chapter will discuss the management of the most morbid complication of portal hypertension, variceal hemorrhage.

Etiology and Pathophysiology

Portal hypertension develops due to a combination of increased vascular resistance coupled with a hyperdynamic circulatory state. Portal hypertension, by definition, is present when the hepatic venous pressure gradient (wedged hepatic venous pressure minus free hepatic venous pressure [HVPG]) exceeds 6 mm Hg. Resistance to outflow from the portal venous bed is the first step in the development of portal hypertension. The observed increase in resistance can be characterized anatomically as presinusoidal (eg, portal vein thrombosis, schistosomiasis), sinusoidal (eg, cirrhosis, primary sclerosing cholangitis, alcoholic hepatitis) or postsinusoidal (eg, Budd-Chiari, veno-occlusive disease) (Table 117-1). Of note, in those patients with presinusoidal and postsinusoidal portal hypertension, the increased resistance can be either intrahepatic or extrahepatic. Although some of the increased resistance is due to anatomic alterations, such as fibrosis and regenerative nodules, which are irreversible, there are also dynamic elements involving vascular tone. The alterations in vascular tone are mediated by an increase in the endogenous production of endothelin, a potent vasoconstrictor, and a decrease in the intrahepatic production of nitric oxide (NO), a potent vasodilator, leading to alterations in the level of vascular resistance. An additional site of increased vascular resistance is found in portosystemic collaterals. Although portosystemic collaterals form in response to portal hypertension, they also represent sites of increased resistance compared to normal intrahepatic resistance.

TABLE 117-1. Causes of Portal Hypertension

	Presinusoidal	Sinusoidal or Mixed	Postsinusoidal
Infectious (other than hepatitis)	Schistosomiasis	–	–
Toxin-mediated	Azathioprine	Methotrexate	–
	Chronic arsenic ingestion	Alcoholic hepatitis	–
	Vinyl chloride	Hypervitaminosis A	–
Cirrhotic	Early primary biliary cirrhosis	Chronic hepatitis	–
	–	Alcoholic cirrhosis	–
	–	Cryptogenic cirrhosis	–
	–	Primary biliary cirrhosis	–
Autoimmune/Oncologic/Primary Fibrotic	Sarcoidosis	Incomplete septal fibrosis	–
	Myeloproliferative diseases	Nodular regenerative hyperplasia	–
	Congenital hepatic fibrosis	Primary sclerosing cholangitis	–
	Early primary sclerosing cholangitis	–	–
Vascular	Splenic vein thrombosis	–	Veno-occlusive disease
	Portal vein thrombosis	–	Hepatic vein thrombosis
	Cavernous transformation of the portal vein	–	Budd-Chiari
	Extrinsic compression of the portal vein	–	Constrictive pericarditis
	–	–	Tricuspid valve disease
	–	–	Severe congestive cardiomyopathy
Other	Idiopathic portal hypertension		

In addition to increased vascular resistance, there are also significant hemodynamic alterations seen in portal hypertension which act by increasing splanchnic blood flow. In the presence of systemic and local vasodilators, such as NO and prostaglandins, peripheral vascular resistance is reduced. This leads to sodium retention and a subsequent increase in plasma volume. The net effect is increases in splanchnic blood flow and cardiac index. Thus, it is a combination of increased intrahepatic vascular resistance and systemic hemodynamic alterations that result in the observed elevations in portal pressure.

Natural History

Varices are common in patients with cirrhosis. At the time of diagnosis, approximately 40% of those with compensated cirrhosis and 60% of those with decompensated cirrhosis will have varices. Varices do not develop, however, until an HVPG of 10 to 12 mm Hg has been reached. Overall, varices will develop in 50 to 60% of cirrhotics. In those without varices at the time of diagnosis, the incidence of variceal development is 5% per year, with the severity of liver disease having the greatest influence on variceal growth and development.

The risk of hemorrhage is highest in the first year following the diagnosis of varices. Of those who bleed, 60 to 80% will bleed from esophageal varices, 7% from gastric varices, and 5 to 20% from portal hypertensive gastropathy. Patients usually present with hematemesis and melena, but occasionally melena or hematochezia is the only presenting sign. Factors influencing the risk for first variceal hemorrhage include (1) variceal size, (2) presence of endoscopic red color signs, (3) Child's classification, and (4) active alcohol use in those with alcoholic liver disease (ALD). A threshold HVPG of at least 10 to 12 mm Hg must be exceeded for variceal bleeding to occur (though there is little correlation between the risk of bleeding and HVPG once this threshold has been crossed). In patients with small varices (less than 5 mm) the risk of bleeding is on the order of 7% at 2 years, with that risk increasing to 30% in those with large varices (greater than 5 mm). The importance of variceal size is related to the increased wall tension present in larger varices, as quantified by the law of Laplace, in which wall tension is shown to be proportional to the radius of the varix. Five to 8% of patients will succumb immediately to their bleed, with an overall mortality of 20 to 50% by 6 weeks. Overall, the high mortality of variceal hemorrhage accounts for 34% of the deaths in patients with cirrhosis and esophageal varices. Risk factors for failure to control bleeding include active bleeding seen at the time of diagnostic endoscopy, bacterial infection, and HVPG > 20 mm Hg shortly after admission. However, in 40 to 50% of patients, bleeding will cease spontaneously.

Of those fortunate enough to survive their first episode of variceal hemorrhage, 70% will go on to experience recurrent hemorrhage within the first year, with 30% to 40% bleeding within the first 6 weeks. Of those who rebleed, 40% will do so in the first 5 days following their initial bleed. Risk factors for early rebleeding include bleeding gastric varices, active bleeding at emergency endoscopy, low serum albumin levels, renal failure, and an HVPG > 20 mm Hg. Mortality is high among those who survive their first bleed, especially in those who develop early rebleeding or renal failure. If patients are untreated, their median risk of rebleeding within 1 to 2 years is 63%, with an associated mortality of 33%. Given the high prevalence of varices and the high associated mortality from variceal hemorrhage, rational treatment of patients with portal hypertension is imperative.

Prevention of a First Variceal Hemorrhage

Patients with cirrhosis should be endoscopically screened for varices so that appropriate therapy can be initiated if varices are present. Because the prevalence of varices increases with the severity of liver disease, screening is based on Child's classification at the time of the diagnosis of cirrhosis. Patients with Child's Class A cirrhosis should be screened when there is evidence of portal hypertension, such as thrombocytopenia (platelets less than 140,000 per mm^3), an enlarged portal vein (diameter > 13 mm), or evidence of collateral circulation on ultrasound. Screening should occur in anyone with Child's Class B or C cirrhosis at the time of the diagnosis of cirrhosis. If the patient is free from varices at initial screening, follow up endoscopy should be carried out. The timing of follow up will vary with the etiology of the patient's liver disease. Patients with ALD require more frequent screening (every 1 to 2 years), whereas those with cirrhosis due to hepatitis C only need to be screened every 3 to 5 years. If small (< 5 mm) varices are present initially, endoscopy should be repeated every 1 to 2 years to monitor for variceal enlargement. There is currently no evidence to recommend treatment in patients who lack varices or who present with small varices. All patients with medium or large varices, however, should receive treatment aimed at preventing variceal bleeding, either pharmacologic (Table 117-2) or endoscopic.

β-Blockers

Nonselective β-blockers, such as *propranolol* or *nadalol*, are the recommended first line agents for the prevention of a first variceal bleed in compliant patients without contraindications to their use. Nonselective β-blockers act by decreasing splanchnic arterial blood flow, which results in a decrease in portal venous blood flow, and their use is associated with a 40% reduction in the risk of bleeding. Typically patients are started on a nonselective β-blocker and the dose

TABLE 117-2. Drugs Used in the Prevention of First Variceal Bleed

Drug	Starting Dose	Maximum Dose
Propranolol	40 mg bid	640 mg/d
Nadolol	40 mg qd	320 mg/d
Timolol	10 mg qd	40 mg/d
Isosorbide mononitrate	20 mg qd	240 mg/d
Spironolactone	25 mg qd	400 mg/d

bid = twice daily; qd = every day.

is titrated to either a 25% decrease in resting heart rate, a resting heart rate of 55 to 60 bpm, or until symptoms develop, in which case the highest dose that does not result in symptoms is used. Up to 27% of patients treated with *propranolol* will discontinue the drug due to side effects, which include fatigue, weakness, depression, dizziness, bronchospasm, and congestive heart failure. The rate of discontinuation appears to be less with *nadolol*, possibly because it is less lipophilic, is not metabolized by the liver, and does not cross the blood-brain barrier. *Nadolol*, therefore, may be a reasonable alternative to *propranolol*. Another alternative being studied is *timolol*, which has low liposolubility along with greater β-2 receptor antagonism, which may increase its portal hypotensive activity. Finally, *carvedilol* has also been studied and found to increase the response to β-blockade. *Carvedilol* acts both as a nonselective β-blocker and as an α-1 receptor antagonist, which results in a pronounced decrease in portal pressure, more so than that seen with *propranolol*. This may be due to a decrease in hepatic and/or portocollateral resistance from α-1 blockade. However, carvedilol is associated with excessive hypotension, especially when patients were started at a dose of 25 mg/d. When lower doses were used, tolerance was improved without a loss of the portal hypotensive response. Before *carvedilol* can be recommended, however, further prospective randomized controlled trials need to be conducted.

If available, HVPG measurement at baseline and again at 3 months is extremely useful in titrating pharmacologic treatment. Decreases in resting heart rate, which reflect the degree of β-1 blockade, fail to correlate with the decrease in portal pressure. Thus, the titration of β-blocker therapy using heart rate does not reflect the true endpoint of interest, that is, a decrease in portal pressure. Measurement of HVPG, however, does allow for the use of portal pressure to guide treatment. The target reduction in HVPG should be to < 12 mm Hg, or a reduction of at least 20% from the baseline measurement, as these are the values at which there is a significant reduction in the rate of variceal bleeding. HVPG measurement is carried out under local anesthesia by interventional radiology and is a very safe procedure. A balloon catheter is introduced into the hepatic vein via either the femoral or internal jugular vein. Pressures are then measured in the free and occluded positions to determine the HVPG. When HVPG is used to assess treatment response, 30 to 40% of patients taking β-blockers are found to have a suboptimal response to therapy (failure to achieve a 20% reduction in HVPG or to attain an HVPG < 12 mm Hg) and are thus at significant risk of variceal bleeding. There are no proven pharmacologic treatment alternatives available for patients who fail to respond adequately to βa-blocker therapy.

Diuretics

It is known that plasma volume expansion is a factor contributing to portal hypertension through its promotion of an increased cardiac output and a hyperdynamic circulatory state. In patients with compensated cirrhosis, it has been shown that the combination of a low sodium diet and administration of *spironolactone* reduces portal pressure as well as azygous blood flow and cardiac output. Based on these findings, a low sodium diet combined *spironolactone* may be a useful addition to the treatment regimen for portal hypertension.

Isosorbide Mononitrate

Long acting nitrates act as vasodilators, decreasing intrahepatic and portocollateral resistance. Despite the ability of *isosorbide mononitrate (ISMN)* to lower portal pressure, it is not effective as a lone agent for the prevention of variceal bleeding.

Endoscopic Therapy

In practice, 15 to 20% of patients will have either a relative or an absolute contraindication to therapy with a β-blocker, such as severe bradycardia, second or third degree atriovenous block, asthma, or congestive heart failure. In these patients, and in those who do not tolerate therapy with β-blockers, an alternative first line therapy for the prevention of variceal bleeding is endoscopic variceal band ligation (EVL). Studies have failed to show a consistent difference when comparing treatment with a β-blocker to EVL with regard to the prevention of variceal bleeding or mortality. Complications of EVL include superficial ulcers, transient retrosternal chest discomfort, dysphagia, and, rarely, distal esophageal stricture. In the past, endoscopic sclerotherapy was also used, as it too reduces both rebleeding and death, but due to the significant morbidity and mortality associated with endoscopic sclerotherapy, as well as a higher efficacy rate for EVL, endoscopic sclerotherapy is now reserved for the treatment of acute hemorrhage and has no role in the primary prophylaxis of variceal bleeding. There is data to suggest that combination treatment with EVL and β-blockade is superior to either therapy alone, but the data is limited and this approach is currently only recommended in patients who bleed while on standard therapy with a nonselective β-blocker or after undergoing EVL.

Transjugular Intrahepatic Portosystemic Shunts and Surgical Shunts

Surgical shunts are effective in the primary prevention of variceal bleeding, and they were historically used to this end. However, due to the high rate of postprocedure hepatic encephalopathy, and because patients undergoing portacaval shunts have decreased survival rates compared with controls, surgical shunts are no longer used for primary prophylaxis. There is no data supporting the use of transjugular intrahepatic portosystemic shunts (TIPS) for the primary prevention of variceal bleeding. TIPS is reserved for salvage therapy for variceal hemorrhage, recurrent variceal hemorrhage despite adequate first line therapy, refractory ascites, and bleeding isolated gastric fundal varices.

Future Directions

In addition to the accepted treatments of portal hypertension discussed above, there are also novel treatments being investigated. One approach involves drugs targeted at decreasing hepatic resistance. α-1 Adrenergic blockers, such as *prazosin*, markedly reduce HVPG in patients with portal hypertension, with a resultant increase in portal blood flow. However, as a result of a significant reduction in systemic vascular resistance and arterial blood pressure, there is expansion of the plasma volume and sodium retention, which in some patients results in the accumulation of ascites. Additionally, renal function can also be negatively affected by *prazosin* use. When *propranolol* is used in conjunction with prazosin, however, these adverse affects are attenuated, though this combination has not been evaluated in randomized controlled trials.

The renin-angiotensin system is often activated in patients with cirrhosis, and *angiotensin II* may increase hepatic resistance by acting on the hepatic circulation. When *losartan* was tested it was found to induce a dramatic reduction in HVPG with minimal arterial hypotension. This finding was not confirmed in subsequent randomized controlled trials, with the additional finding in follow-up studies that *irbesartan* or *losartan* were associated with a decrease in arterial pressure and glomerular filtration rate, making these agents dangerous in patients with advanced cirrhosis. They may still have a role, however, in patients with early cirrhosis, by preventing the progression of hepatic fibrosis.

Given the role of endothelin in regulating hepatic vascular resistance, there may be a place for endothelin blockers in the treatment of portal hypertension. The results of studies using endothelin blockers, however, have been conflicting and more research is required before a role for these agents can be assessed.

Finally, because it is known that NO is involved in the regulation of hepatic vascular resistance, agents acting on this system are under investigation. The goal would be to find an agent that selectively increases hepatic NO levels. Drugs, such as *ISMN*, which are not liver selective, have the problem of inducing peripheral vasodilatation. Promising agents are currently being investigated that are liver-specific NO donors. An alternative approach is to increase hepatic NO-synthase (NOS) expression, though this approach is technically complex, because it requires gene therapy with all of its inherent complexities. The final option being investigated for the regulation of NO relates to the use of inhibitors of NO and NOS systemically, with the goal being to reduce splanchnic blood flow. The problem with NO inhibition is one of selectivity, and it has been observed that many of the positive effects of systemic NO inhibition (correction of systemic hemodynamics, improved renal function, and increased sodium excretion) are offset by increased hepatic vascular resistance due to hepatic NO inhibition.

Regardless of the form of therapy chosen, patients should be treated lifelong to minimize the risk of variceal hemorrhage.

Treatment of Acute Variceal Hemorrhage
Initial Management

Regardless of subsequent intervention, the first step in the management of any patient presenting with an acute variceal hemorrhage is adequate resuscitation. This is accomplished using a combination of blood volume replacement, with a goal hematocrit of 25 to 30%, along with fresh frozen plasma to correct any coagulopathy. It is important to avoid over-transfusion, however, which can lead to an increase in portal pressure that may potentiate further bleeding or rebleeding. In actively bleeding patients, intubation should also be considered for airway protection. Finally, patients should receive prophylactic antibiotics, because they have been shown to improve survival. A reasonable choice is *norfloxacin* 400 mg every 12 hours. Once these initial steps have been taken (and in the case of pharmacologic therapy, concurrently), diagnostic endoscopy should be performed and appropriate endoscopic therapy initiated as indicated.

Pharmacologic Therapy

Pharmacologic therapy should be initiated simultaneously with resuscitation. In approximately 75% of patients, bleeding control will be achieved through a combination of pharmacologic therapy and endoscopic therapy. Initial management is with a vasoactive drug such as *terlipressin*, *somatostatin* and its analogs, or *vasopressin* combined with *nitroglycerin*. Which agent is chosen will depend on availability. A good choice is *terlipressin*, a long acting analogue of *vasopressin*, given as a bolus. It is released slowly via cleavage of it N-terminal glycyl residue and is associated with fewer side effects than *vasopressin*. It acts as a vasoconstrictor, reducing splanchnic blood flow. It is superior to *vasopressin* and is comparable to *somatostatin* and balloon tamponade for the control of acute variceal hemorrhage. It is widely used in Europe, but has not been approved by the Food and Drug Administration in the United States. *Somatostatin* and its *analogues, octreotide, lanreotide*, and *vapreotide*, also act as vasoconstrictors to decrease splanchnic blood flow (only octreotide is available in the United States). Whereas *somatostatin* is equivalent to *terlipressin* in controlling acute variceal hemorrhage, *octreotide* may be less effective, possibly due to tachyphylaxis. Both *somatostatin* and *octreotide* are well tolerated with few side effects. The final option is *vasopressin* plus *nitroglycerin*. Like its analogue *terlipressin, vasopressin* is a splanchnic vasoconstrictor. It is effective in controlling acute variceal hemorrhage, but its use is associated with significant side effects, including myocardial and peripheral ischemia, hypertension, bradycardia, hyponatremia, and fluid retention, and is thus no longer used as a single agent. When *nitroglycerin* is used in conjunction with vasopressin, many of the side effects are ameliorated. *Nitroglycerin* can be given by intravenous (IV), transdermal, and sublingual routes, though the IV route is preferred for dose titration. Pharmacologic therapy is usually maintained for up to 5 days to prevent early rebleeding.

Endoscopic Therapy

After resuscitation is complete and pharmacologic therapy has been initiated, the focus shifts to endoscopic therapy. Before endoscopic therapy, gastric lavage may be required so that blood and clots can be removed from the stomach for improved visualization. The two endoscopic options for controlling variceal hemorrhage are (1) endoscopic sclerotherapy (ES) and (2) EVL. ES is successful in controlling acute variceal hemorrhage in 75 to 90% of cases and is also effective in reducing the incidence of rebleeding. During ES, a sclerosing agent (eg, alcohol or sodium tetradecyl) is injected into the distal portion of a varix, with the goal of inducing thrombosis and scarring. The procedure is carried out in the distal 5 cm of the esophagus, as this is where varices are most superficial and where they are the most likely to bleed. In those in whom ES is successful, it is repeated every 1 to 3 weeks with the goal of achieving circumferential obliteration of the varices. The complications of endoscopic sclerotherapy are superficial ulcers, retrosternal discomfort, dysphagia, ulceration, bleeding, stricture, perforation, fever, bacteremia, sepsis, and pleural effusion. Because of its relatively high rate of complications, ES is no longer the preferred endoscopic approach for the control of variceal hemorrhage, and EVL is now the favored approach. During EVL, an endoscope equipped with a small cylinder that holds preloaded elastic bands is introduced into the esophagus and advanced to the distal esophagus. The distal portion of the varix is suctioned into the cylinder and the band is deployed. Banding leads to eventual scarring and obliteration of the varix. Five to 10 ligations may be performed during a single session. EVL is then repeated on a weekly or biweekly basis and further banding is carried out until any remaining varices are obliterated.

TIPS and Surgical Shunts

TIPS and surgical shunts are considered as salvage therapies to control acute variceal hemorrhage. Ten to 20% of patients will continue to bleed despite endoscopic treatment. TIPS and shunts are extremely effective procedures with control rates approaching 95%. TIPS involves the placement of an expandable metal stent from the hepatic vein, through the liver parenchyma, into the portal vein. Stents are the preferred form of salvage therapy as they can be successfully implanted in almost all patients and decrease the HVPG by half. An alternative to TIPS in Child's A cirrhotics is surgical shunting, which decompresses the portal system by creating a portasystemic anastomosis. Unfortunately, despite their high rate of success in controlling variceal hemorrhage, TIPS and surgical shunts are associated with many significant side effects, including hepatic encephalopathy and worsening liver failure, resulting in higher overall mortality rates.

Prevention of Recurrent Variceal Hemorrhage

Pharmacologic and Endoscopic Therapy

Once the acute bleed has been managed, the focus of treatment shifts to preventing rebleeding. As previously mentioned, rebleeding occurs in 70% of patients surviving their initial bleed, so all patients need to receive treatment aimed at preventing rebleeding. The approach to and goals of treatment are similar to the treatment aimed at preventing a first variceal bleed. First line treatment is either initiation of a nonselective β-blocker or endoscopic variceal ligation. Nonselective β-blockers decrease rebleeding by 33% and mortality by 26%. In patients who have not achieved an adequate response to a β-blocker alone, the addition of *ISMN* may result in a significant lowering of the HVPG. If *ISMN* is to be used in combination therapy to prevent rebleeding, HVPG measurement should be performed to guide therapy. Endoscopic sclerotherapy and endoscopic variceal ligation are also both effective in preventing rebleeding, but as discussed above, endoscopic variceal ligation is the preferred approach. Despite therapy, however, rebleeding still occurs in 30 to 50% of patients at 2 years. In patients who fail treatment with one modality, combination therapy with a nonselective β-blocker and endoscopic variceal ligation may result in lower rates of rebleeding.

TIPS and Surgical Shunts

TIPS and surgical shunts are more effective than pharmacologic or endoscopic therapy at preventing rebleeding, but are not recommended as first line therapy due to their side effects (see above). Additionally, there is no improvement in survival from TIPS or surgical shunts when compared with endoscopic therapy, and studies have found significantly higher mortality in patients undergoing TIPS on univariate, but not multivariate, analysis. However, in patients who fail treatment with β-blockers and endoscopic variceal ligation, TIPS and surgical shunting (for Child's A cirrhotics) may be lifesaving.

Liver Transplantation

When appropriate, liver transplantation should be considered, because it provides the definitive treatment for end-stage liver disease and portal hypertension by addressing the underling liver pathology (see Chapters 112, "Pediatric Liver Transplantation" to 125, "Hereditary Hemochromatosis" for more extensive discussions of liver transplantation). Patients are candidates for transplantation if they have complications of their liver disease that are life threatening or that significantly affect their quality of life (eg, encephalopathy, incapacitating fatigue, variceal hemorrhage, intractable ascites, and severe malnutrition). Additionally, patients must be abstinent from alcohol for at least 6 months and must not possess any absolute contraindications to liver transplantation (eg, severe cardiac or pulmonary disease, acquired immunodeficiency syndrome [AIDS], sepsis, severe pulmonary hypertension, extrahepatic cancer, portal and mesenteric vein thrombosis, inability to understand the procedure and the lifelong implications of having undergone a transplant, and severe psychologic disorders). Relative contraindications to liver transplantation include the following:

1. A history of alcohol abuse
2. Human immunodeficiency virus positivity (but not AIDS)
3. Portal vein thrombosis
4. Moderate pulmonary hypertension
5. Poor social support
6. Noncompliance

If a patient is deemed a transplantation candidate, liver transplantation is considered once hepatic decompensation has been established as assessed by the Model for End-Stage Liver Disease score (a scoring system which quantifies the degree of hepatic decompensation using measurements of the serum creatinine, bilirubin, and international normalized ratio but is not influenced by factors such as variceal hemorrhage).

Summary

All patients with cirrhosis should be monitored for the development of portal hypertension and its complications. Once large varices have developed, measures must be instituted to prevent variceal hemorrhage using either pharmacologic therapy with nonselective β-blockers or endoscopic therapy with endoscopic variceal ligation. Patients who go on to develop acute variceal hemorrhage should be managed aggressively with prompt resuscitation and the initiation of vasoactive medications, followed by endoscopic therapy. In those in whom initial efforts fail to control bleeding, more definitive portal decompression strategies, namely TIPS and surgical shunting, should be considered. In those surviving their initial bleed, it is imperative that therapy is initiated to prevent future bleeds, starting with either a nonselective β-blocker or endoscopic variceal ligation. A combination approach can then be applied for patients who continue to have episodes of hemorrhage. However, in those who continue to bleed despite maximal medical therapy, portal decompression should be carried out with TIPS or surgical shunting. Finally, liver transplantation should be considered in appropriate patients as a definitive treatment for end-stage liver disease and, thus, portal hypertension.

Supplemental Reading

Abraczinskas DR, Ookubo R, Grace ND, et al. Propranolol for the prevention of first esophageal variceal hemorrhage: a lifetime commitment? Hepatology 2001;34:1096–102.

Bass NM, Somberg KA. Portal hypertension and gastrointestinal bleeding. In: Feldman M, Scharschmidt BF, Sleisenger MH, editors. Sleisenger & Fordtran's gastrointestinal and liver disease: pathophysiology/diagnosis/management. Vol 2. 6th ed. Philadelphia: W.B. Saunders Company; 1998. p. 1284–309.

Bosch J, Abraldes JG, Groszmann R. Current management of portal hypertension. J Hepatol 2003;38:S54–68.

Conn HO. Portal hypertension, varices, and transjugular intrahepatic portosystemic shunts. Clin Liver Dis 2000;4:133–50.

Feu F, Garcia-Pagan JC, Bosch J, et al. Relation between portal pressure and response to pharmacotherapy and risk of recurrent variceal haemorrhage in patients with cirrhosis. Lancet 1995; 346:1056.

Garcia-Pagan JC, Salmeron JM, Feu F, et al. Effects of low-sodium diet and spironolactone on portal pressure in patients with compensated cirrhosis. Hepatology 1994;19:1095–9.

Garcia-Tsao G, Grace ND, Groszmann RJ, et al. Short-term effects of propranolol on portal venous pressure. Hepatology 1986; 6:101–6.

Grace ND, Bhatacharya K. Pharmacologic therapy of portal hypertension and variceal hemorrhage. Clin Liver Dis 1997; 1:59–75.

Grace ND, Groszmann RJ, Garcia-Tsao G, et al. Portal hypertension and variceal bleeding: an AASLD single topic symposium. Hepatology 1998;28:868–80.

Grace ND, Muench H, Chalmers TC. The present status of shunts for portal hypertension in cirrhosis. Gastroenterology 1966;50:684–91.

Graham D, Smith JL. The course of patients after variceal hemorrhage. Gastroenterology 1981;80:800–9.

Groszmann RJ, Bosch J, Grace ND, et al. Hemodynamic events in a prospective randomized trial of propranolol versus placebo in the prevention of a first variceal hemorrhage. Gastroenterology 1990;99:1401–7.

Gupta TK, Chen L, Groszman RJ. Pathophysiology of portal hypertension. Clin Liver Dis 1997;1:1–12.

Kamath PS, Wiesner RH, Malinchoc M, et al. A model to predict survival in patients with end-stage liver disease. Hepatology 2001;33:464–70.

Luketic VA, Sanyal AJ. Esophageal varices. II. TIPS. Gastroenterol Clin North Am 2000;29:387–421.

Slosberg EA, Keeffe EB. Sclerotherapy versus banding in the treatment of variceal bleeding. Clin Liver Dis 1997;1:77–84.

Steiber AC, Gordon RD, Galloway JR. Orthotopic liver transplantation. In: Zakim D, Boyer TD, editors. Hepatology: a textbook of liver disease. Vol 2. 3rd ed. Philadelphia: W.B. Saunders Company; 1996. p. 1759–80.

Sudan DL, Shaw BW. The role of liver transplantation in the management of portal hypertension. Clin Liver Dis 1997;1:115–20.

CHAPTER 118

NONCIRRHOTIC PORTAL HYPERTENSION

Christos S. Georgiades, MD, PhD, and Jean-Francois Geschwind, MD

Vascular Anatomy of the Liver

Understanding of the gross and microscopic anatomy of the liver is essential if one is to understand the causes, consequences, and potential treatment options of portal hypertension. The portal venous system channels the blood drainage of nearly the entire gastrointestinal (GI) system into the liver. Its main branches, the splenic and superior mesenteric veins, join to form the main portal vein, which travels for about 5 cm before it bifurcates into the right and left portal veins as it enters the substance of the liver. The portal veins branch successively until they form the terminal venules, which travel along with the hepatic arteriole and bile ductules to form the portal triad. The blood from these terminal portal venules then merges with the hepatic arteriolar blood, and the mixed blood is siphoned into the liver sinusoids (Figure 118-1). The essential functions of the liver, as well as the diffusion of oxygen and nutrients into the liver, take place during the transit of the blood through the sinusoids. The epithelium of the sinusoids is specialized and highly effective for these functions. Ultimately, the sinusoidal blood, a mixture of hepatic arterial and portal venous blood, drains into the hepatic venules, which successively join and eventually form the main hepatic veins. The three main hepatic veins then join the intrahepatic portion of the inferior vena cava just before it enters the base of the right atrium.

Definition of (Noncirrhotic) Portal Hypertension

Functional or mechanical obstruction of the above-described circulation (anywhere from the portal venous system to the right atrium) can lead to portal hypertension. Portal hypertension not caused by liver cirrhosis is termed noncirrhotic portal hypertension, though the two can coexist. Noncirrhotic portal hypertension is categorized according to the level of obstruction of the portal blood flow and its drainage, into pre-, peri- and postsinusoidal and has a large number of causes. The causes of noncirrhotic portal hypertension are listed in Table 118-1. Normally, the pressure within the portal venous system ranges between 5 and 10 mm Hg. Portal hypertension is defined as an absolute portal pressure of more than 10 mm Hg or as a > 6 mm Hg difference between hepatic and portal venous pressures (PVPs).

Measurement of Portal Pressure

Two methods are routinely used to measure PVP. The direct method, which is more technically challenging and rarely used, involves direct percutaneous, transhepatic puncture of the portal or splenic vein proximal (away from the liver and with reference to direction of normal blood flow) to the suspected site of obstruction. The indirect

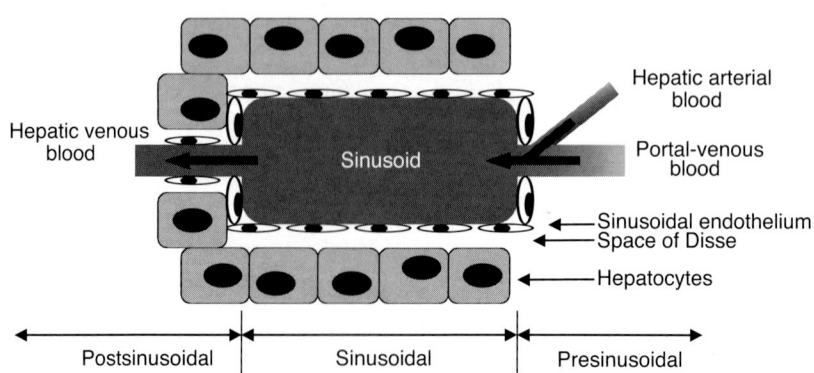

FIGURE 118-1 Schematic representation of the microvascular anatomy of the hepatic sinusoid. Hepatic arterial blood mixes with portal venous blood, crosses the sinusoid, and drains into the hepatic veins. Obstruction along this pathway can lead to portal hypertension. The sinusoid is lined with specialized, porous endothelium, and is separated from the hepatocytes by the spaces of Disse.

TABLE 118-1. Causes of Noncirrhotic Portal Hypertension

Presinusoidal	Perisinusoidal	Postsinusoidal
Portal, splenic, or superior mesenteric vein thrombosis	Congenital hepatic fibrosis	Budd-Chiari syndrome
IPH	Sarcoidosis	Veno-occlusive disease (SOS)
Mass effect (ie, tumor)	-	Chronic passive congestion (Nutmeg liver)
Schistosomiasis	-	Mass effect (ie, tumor)
Precirrhotic stage, primary biliary cirrhosis	-	-
Alcoholic central sclerosis	-	-
Endothelitis (liver rejection, radiation injury)	-	-
Arterioportovenous fistula (traumatic or Olser-Weber-Rendu)	-	-
Hyperdynamic splenomegaly (infectious or myelodysplastic)	-	-
Nodular regenerative hyperplasia	-	-

IPH = idiopathic portal hypertension; SOS = sinusoidal obstruction syndrome.

TABLE 118-2. Causes of Budd-Chiari Syndrome

Primary (60 to 70% of Cases)	Secondary (5 to 15%)	Idiopathic (25%)
Primary thrombosis (75%)	Extrinsic compression	-
Oral contraceptive pill	Benign or malignant neoplasm	-
Pregnancy	Bacterial, fungal, or parasitic collections	-
Polycythemia rubra vera	Benign cysts	-
Paroxysmal nocturnal hemoglobinuria	-	-
Factor V Leiden	-	-
Antiphospholipid antibody	-	-
Lupus anticoagulant	-	-
Idiopathic thrombocytopenic puprura	-	-
Nephrotic syndrome	-	-
Protein losing enteropathy	-	-
Myeloproliferative disorders	-	-
Protein C, S or antithrombin deficiency	-	-
Factor II, VIII, X and XI deficiency	-	-
Homocysteinuria	-	-
Hepatitis	-	-
Trauma	-	-
Membraneous web (25%) (usually suprahepatic inferior vena cava)	-	-

method is technically simpler and has significantly less complications. It involves accessing the jugular vein and selecting one of the main hepatic veins with a wedge balloon catheter. Two pressure measurements are obtained, one with the balloon deflated and the catheter nonwedged (free hepatic vein pressure [FHP]), and one with the balloon inflated and the catheter wedged as distally as possible within the hepatic vein (hepatic wedged venous pressure [HWP]). The PVP can be obtained by the following equation:

$$PVP = HWP - FHP$$

The indirect method has been shown to be accurate except in cases of perisinusoidal noncirrhotic portal hypertension and portal vein thrombosis (PVT), where the above equation underestimates the true PVP.

Causes of Noncirrhotic Portal Hypertension

Budd-Chiari Syndrome

Definition

Budd-Chiari syndrome is a constellation of signs and symptoms resulting from hepatic venous outflow obstruction. It encompasses all causes of obstruction between the hepatic venules and right atrium, but excludes the sinusoidal obstruction syndrome (SOS, formerly known as hepatic veno-occlusive disease) and all cardiac causes. Primary Budd-Chiari results from a venous endoluminal web or thrombosis of the outflow veins. In secondary Budd-Chiari the cause of obstruction does not originate in the affected vein. The most common cause of Budd-Chiari is an underlying hypercoagulable state. However, in 25% of the cases in the United States, no underlying cause is found (idiopathic).

Presentation

The clinical presentation of acute Budd-Chiari syndrome includes any combination of ascites, abdominal pain, edema, hepatomegaly and less commonly GI bleeding. Subclinical Budd-Chiari can also be found incidentally during workup of patients with hypercoagulable states. Thus the reported natural history of the disease is skewed towards the most severe forms. In a minority of patients venous outflow obstruction may lead to liver failure and be complicated by encephalopathy, elevated liver function tests, jaundice, and even death. There is also evidence that a small fraction of patients with cryptogenic cirrhosis may have an insidious chronic form of the disease.

Evaluation

The diagnosis of Budd-Chiari can easily be established once the entity is suspected and the proper diagnostic test performed. All three cross-sectional imaging modalities (computed tomography [CT], magnetic resonance imaging [MRI], and ultrasound) can be used to diagnose the disease but the standard diagnostic technique is the hepatic venogram. In the case of Budd-Chiari, contrast injection into any hepatic vein reveals many small branching vessels ("spider's-web") instead of the main hepatic veins. MRI and CT generally show a filling defect in the intra- or suprahepatic inferior vena cava, hepatomegaly with an enlarged caudate lobe, and signal/density changes in a geographic manner. Ultrasound shows no flow in the affected veins. If the diagnosis remains in doubt, liver biopsy should be performed to confirm the diagnosis. A transjugular approach is typically favored over a percutaneous one if ascites or abnormal coagulation profile are present.

Management

In the absence of conclusive studies most experts agree on a stepwise approach to the treatment of Budd-Chiari that depends on disease severity. In asymptomatic patients, and when there is no significant liver dysfunction, initial treatment should be limited with emphasis on treating the underlying cause. In the absence of contraindications, anticoagulation should be the first line of therapy. This however has met with limited success because the underlying hypercoagulable state usually results in recurrent thrombosis. In the case of hematologic disorders such as *paroxysmal nocturnal hemoglobinuria*, thrombolysis of hepatic vein clot should be closely timed with bone marrow transplant to prevent rethrombosis. Without definitive treatment most patients will progress to liver failure and will likely die within 1 to 2 years. Intensive supportive care is generally required then with diuretics, abdominal paracentesis, and endoscopic treatment of variceal bleeding as the severity of the disease increases. In the absence of a satisfactory response, more invasive intervention may be required. In selected cases, such as short-segment recent thromboses or hepatic venous web, percutaneous transluminal angioplasty with or without stenting combined with thrombolysis can be attempted. Such interventions may be ineffective either because of failure of thrombolysis or because of recurrence due to the underlying hypercoagulable state. In such cases a more definitive approach is necessary. If the disease is rapidly progressive, liver transplantation should be given priority, which provides a 5-year survival of approximately 75%. If on the other hand, liver function is adequate and stable, portocaval shunting is a viable alternative. The surgical option, mesocaval shunt, may not be technically feasible in case of inferior vena cava obstruction. The radiological option, placement of a transjugular intrahepatic portosystemic shunt (TIPS), offers a simpler and safer alternative. It is however technically challenging if there is complete thrombosis of the hepatic vein. Although, long term benefits are at best limited with either shunting technique, the greatest benefit of shunting may be delaying the need for liver transplantation.

SOS (Hepatic Veno-Occlusive Disease)

Definition

SOS results from occlusion of the sinusoids by necrotic cells (hepatocytes, red blood cells, sinusoidal epithelial cells, and lymphocytes). The initial toxic injury to the sinusoidal epithelial cells extends to involve the adjacent hepatocytes. These necrotic cells initially fill the spaces of Disse, but they then spill into the sinusoids and eventually block the sinusoidal outflow channel. Occasionally, sinusoidal obstruction may be complicated by thrombosis extending into the hepatic venules. This observation was at the origin of the old name "hepatic veno-occlusive disease." However, venule thrombosis is not a constant finding in this disease, thus SOS is a more accurate designation. *Pyrrolizidine alkaloids*, found in certain types of plants including certain bush teas, contributed the major cause of SOS until chemotherapeutic and immunosuppressive agents started being used. A list of the major causes is shown in Table 118-3. Liver irradiation, chronic hepatitis C, and concomitant administration of *norethisterone* can potentiate the toxic effect of these agents.

Presentation

The presentation of SOS can be identical to that of acute Budd-Chiari, sepsis-related cholestatic liver disease, right-sided heart failure, and graft-versus-host disease (GVHD), and includes tender hepatomegaly, ascites, weight gain, and signs of portal hypertension. Though biopsy is the only effective method that allows discrimination of these entities, the appearance of the above symptoms 10 to 30 days after cytoreductive or myeloablative treatment with the drugs listed in Table 118-3 should raise the suspicion of SOS.

Evaluation

Laboratory tests, though sensitive, are nonspecific and do not distinguish between SOS, Budd-Chiari, cholestatic disease, and GVHD. In addition, predisposing factors (such as liver transplantation, cancer chemotherapy, immunosuppression)

TABLE 118-3. Medications Implicated as Causative Agents for Sinusoidal Obstructive Syndrome

Cyclophosphamide*
Dacarbazine*
Ozogamicin*
Actinomycin D*
Dactinomycin*
Gemtuzumab*
Cytosine arabiniside*
Urethane*
Mithramycin*
Azathioprine†

* Chemotherapeutic agents.
† Immunosuppressive.

predispose patients to more than one of the above to a certain extent. Imaging studies including ultrasound, MRI and CT, are nonspecific and include early changes, such as hepatomegaly, ascites and attenuated liver venous flow, or late changes, such as reversal of portal venous flow, PVT, gastroesophageal varices, splenomegaly, and formation of spontaneous portosystemic shunts. Hepatic venograms may be normal or show hepatic venule thrombosis as a consequence of sinusoidal obstruction, which may erroneously point to Budd-Chiari. As mentioned earlier transjugular or percutaneous liver biopsy is the only definitive diagnostic test. In addition, the transjugular approach allows pressure measurements. Early biopsy specimens (1 to 2 weeks postinjury) reveal edematous changes in the subendothelial layers of the central veins, sinusoidal engorgement, adjacent hepatocellular injury, and necrotic red cells lodging in the spaces of Disse. Later changes (> 2 weeks postinjury) include perisunsinusoidal collagenization that may lead to fibrosis, and necrotic debris filling the sinusoids that eventually become obstructed.

Management

SOS is classified as mild (clinical symptoms, no treatment, complete resolution), moderate (clinical symptoms, requires treatment, complete resolution), and severe (death or clinical symptoms that persist for more than 100 days despite optimum treatment). With appropriate treatment, most patients (60 to 75%) eventually recover. Paradoxically, those who die, die not from liver failure, but rather from cardiac or renal failure. Both unimodal and bimodal forms of the disease have been identified. In unimodal disease, the symptoms appear and progress or resolve as described above. In bimodal disease, initial symptoms abate only to reappear at a later time. Prognosis is worse in bimodal disease. Prevention should be optimized by (1) avoiding SOS causing chemotherapeutic agents if possible and (2) eliminating modulating factors (liver shielding during total body irradiation and adequate treatment of sepsis). Empiric anticoagulation, usually with *heparin* or *low molecular weight heparin*, has met with limited success, attenuating the frequency of nonsevere SOS only. Once SOS has been diagnosed, treatment depends on severity. In cases with limited symptoms and no evidence of liver malfunction or significant portal hypertension/thrombosis, treatment should be supportive. Electrolyte correction (a frequent abnormality in SOS), diuretics and paracentesis for ascites may be adequate.

Idiopathic Portal Hypertension

Definition

Portal hypertension is classified as idiopathic (IPH) when all other causes have been excluded, and it is also known as noncirrhotic portal fibrosis. The most specific finding is tapering of the third and higher order portal vein branches due to periportal fibrosis, a picture that has been termed obliterative port-venopathy.

Presentation

IPH presents with all the signs and symptoms of portal hypertension of any other cause. However, presentation is heavily skewed towards variceal bleeding and splenomegaly at the expense of ascites, hepatic encephalopathy, or other complications, which are distinctly rare. There is a reported female preponderance of 2:1 to 3:1 with an average age at presentation of 45 to 50 years. The vast majority of patients will suffer at least one episode of variceal bleeding from gastroesophageal varices (90%). Splenomegaly is also a very common initial complaint (> 70%).

Evaluation

As mentioned above, IPH is a diagnosis of exclusion. In the presence of clear signs of portal hypertension and when clinical history, physical examination, imaging and laboratory studies, and biopsy rule out other causes, only then one can diagnose IPH. Biopsy invariably shows concentric fibrosis around the small portal vein branches without cirrhosis. Some authors report preferential involvement of the left lobe with associated right lobe atrophy. Liver-associated laboratory tests are normal or near normal and serve only to exclude other causes of portal hypertension. Anemia and thrombocytopenia are also common findings in IPH, the latter likely due to the significant splenomegaly that characterizes the disease.

Management

It is crucial to properly diagnose IPH from a prognostic and management point of view. With proper management of variceal bleeding and splenomegaly and its associated thrombocytopenia, life expectancy is no different from healthy individuals. Its course is stable over many years and not associated with cirrhosis or hepatic neoplasms. There is a high initial success rate for the management of bleeding varices whether banding or sclerotherapy is used, which approaches 90 to 95%. Rebleeds are uncommon (3%) but are managed equally successfully. Emergent portosystemic shunts are rarely required (< 10% of acute bleeds), with TIPS having proven to be an effective approach. Splenomegaly can be also treated effectively with percutaneous intra-arterial embolization of a portion of the spleen (initially 25 to 50% with reevaluation).

Portal (and/or Splenic) Vein Thrombosis

Definition

The presence of thrombus in the portal vein causes obstruction of the venous drainage of much of the GI system. Risk factors include cirrhosis, abdominal sepsis, pan-

TABLE 118-4. Causes of Portal Vein Thrombosis

Cirrhosis
Tumor invasion of portal vein
    Hepatocellular carcinoma
    Cholangiocarcinoma
Abdominal sepsis
Oral contraceptive pill
Pancreatitis
Prothromotic disorders
Trauma
Neonatal omphalitis

---

creatitis, hepatic malignancies, trauma/surgery, decreased portal venous flow, and hypercoagulable states, although idiopathic portal vein thrombosis (PVT) is a rare cause of presinusoidal portal hypertension in the Western world. Occasionally, thrombosis is localized to the splenic or superior mesenteric vein (SMV), which causes findings specific to the affected portion of the GI system.

Presentation

PVT can be an incidental finding on ultrasound or contrast enhanced MRI and CT studies. Cavernous transformation of the thrombosed vein (the appearance of many string-like veins that provide partial venous flow into the liver) can also be seen. Other imaging findings include enlarged SMV and splenic vein, spontaneous portosystemic shunts, splenomegaly, and edematous bowel wall with associated ascites. New symptoms and signs, such as abdominal pain, splenomegaly, and increased abdominal girth, in a patient with known hepatic disease should prompt a search for PVT. In adults, hemoptysis from esophageal varices is not an uncommon initial presentation of PVT. Causes of PVT are shown in Table 118-4.

Evaluation

The diagnosis of PVT is relatively straightforward once it is suspected. MRI and CT, as well as ultrasound, are usually diagnostic and can provide information regarding the extent of disease as well as its cause. All of these modalities can confirm the presence of varices, splenomegaly, and ascites, as well as cirrhosis. A celiac or mesenteric arteriogram can be extended to show the venous drainage into the portal vein and diagnose PVT. If required, direct transhepatic portal vein percutaneous access can be obtained and a porto-venogram performed. It is important to note that in the absence of liver disease, wedged hepatic pressures are normal, whereas preobstructive pressures (intrasplenic, SMV) are elevated. Laboratory values are usually normal with nonspecific findings, such as hypoalbuminemia and hepatocellular dysfunction, occurring late in the disease and more frequently in children.

Management

Idiopathic (no predisposing risk factors identified) PVT has a much more favorable prognosis than PVT which is caused by an underlying disease. Ten-year survival of idiopathic PVT is > 75%. In addition, variceal bleeding is more rare and easily controlled than when associated with cirrhosis because there is no underlying coagulation defect. Bleeding can be treated endoscopically with sclerotherapy or banding with excellent results (> 90% success). Because of the relatively favorable prognosis, thrombolysis of portal vein is rarely required if the disease is idiopathic. In the presence of underlying risk factors, portal vein thrombolysis should be undertaken only if the risk factor is addressed at the same time, otherwise rethrombosis is expected. Therefore, portal vein thrombolysis is rarely indicated. Exceptions include recurrent variceal bleeding despite treatment in case of idiopathic disease or when recanalization is needed for liver transplantation. Percutaneous thrombolysis performed by *interventional radiologists* is usually the easiest and safest method. First, access is achieved into the right, left, or both main portal veins using a transhepatic approach under ultrasound guidance. Multi-sideholed infusion catheters are placed along the length of the clot, which is then laced with thrombolytics. The duration of thrombolysis and amount of drugs used are specified and limited to reduce the rate of complications. Porto-venograms can be performed every 12 to 18 hours to monitor for progress.

In isolated SVT, symptoms are limited to splenomegaly and associated abdominal pain and possible gastroesophageal varices. Children may also show anemia and thrombocytopenia. If refractory to conservative treatment, such cases may require spleenectomy or preferably transarterial partial splenic embolization. This alleviates thrombocytopenia and anemia and decreases splenic blood flow, thus diminishing splenic vein pressure and possibly diminishing varices as well. Partial splenic embolization has the added advantage of preserving splenic immune function.

Other

Several other causes of noncirrhotic portal hypertension exist as shown in Table 118-1. Schistosomiasis, the most common cause worldwide, is very rare in the Western world. Of special note are the so-called hyperdynamic causes of portal hypertension, which include an arteriovenous fistula or hyperdynamic spleen. In the former, an arteriovenous fistula (most often iatrogenic rarely associated with Osler-Weber-Rendu involvement) shunts blood from an artery into the portal venous system. This can lead to rapid emergence of symptoms associated with portal hypertension in addition to left heart strain and possible failure if prolonged. Treatment is surgical ligation. If the feeding artery is accessible percutaneously, the communication channel can be embolized by *interventional radiology* (Coils, glue or detachable balloon depending on anatomic appearance and flow characteristics) in a safer and speedier manner with shorter hospital stay. In the latter, the spleen is enlarged either due to a myeloproliferative disorder or infectious disease. This is associated with thrombocytopenia due to sequestration and anemia and mass symptoms due to splenomegaly. Rarely and usually in children, transudative ascites and bleeding varices may complicate the picture. Though splenectomy is effective, partial splenic arterial embolization may relieve the above symptoms while preserving the immune function of the spleen.

In general surgical or interventional therapeutic interventions should be tailored to each patient, his/her symptomatology, and always keep the prognosis and possible complications of the intervention in mind.

TIPS

Objective

The anatomic objective of TIPS is to create a channel through the liver parenchyma connecting one of the main portal veins and one of the main hepatic veins. This artificial channel that diverts blood from the portal to the systemic venous circulation is kept open by a stent. The physiologic objective of TIPS is to help abate life threatening complications of portal hypertension without causing or worsening encephalopathy. By forming a portosystemic shunt, the portal circulation is partially decompressed, thus alleviating symptoms associated with portal hypertension. This however, is achieved at the expense of the physiologic functions of the liver, which is bypassed by the shunted blood. Thus patients should be selected carefully prior to shunt placement. Indications and contraindications are summarized in Table 118-5.

Technique

Before performing a TIPS, the patient must be stabilized because emergent TIPS have a poor outcome, and the patency of the portal vein must be confirmed with MRI, CT or ultrasound. Additionally, if there is significant ascites a large volume paracentesis before or during the procedure is indicated. Large ascites affect the patient's breathing negatively and make the procedure technically more difficult. Access is achieved in the right internal jugular vein and maintained with a long vascular sheath with its tip in the suprahepatic IVC. An angled catheter/wire combination is used to select the right hepatic vein. Free and wedged pressure measurements are taken to confirm the presence of portal hypertension and calculate in the reduction of portal vein pressure after the TIPS is performed. A wedged hepatic venogram with contrast or carbon dioxide is performed to identify the target portal vein branch. A long angled sheath is then used to select the right hepatic vein and an angled needle (Colapinto) is used to puncture the hepatic vein wall directed anteriorly towards the target portal vein. Multiple passes are usually needed until the portal vein is entered. Then a wire is advanced through the needle and into the portal vein. The needle is exchanged for a catheter over the wire. Direct portal vein pressures can be taken through the catheter. A stiff wire is placed through the catheter, which is then removed. The parenchymal tract is dilated with an over-the-wire balloon (8 or 10 mm) and then buttressed with wall stent(s). The wall stent(s) should extend from the origin of the accessed portal vein near the bifurcation to the hepatic vein/SVC junction. The portal vein pressure is measured again, and, if necessary, the stent can be ballooned to further decrease portal vein pressure. Ideally, the portal vein pressure should be brought within 10 mm Hg of the hepatic vein pressure while still maintaining hepatopedal flow in the other portal veins. A left hepatic-left portal vein shunt can be performed if the right approach is not feasible. In either case, the tract should not be too peripheral to avoid inadvertent perforation of the liver capsule.

If necessary, after placement of the TIPS, bleeding portosystemic collaterals can be embolized as the radiologist now has access to them via the newly formed shunt.

Follow-Up

The TIPS effectiveness can be monitored either indirectly by monitoring liver function and/or directly by measuring pressures via a jugular or femoral vein approach. Doppler ultrasound has become a useful tool to noninvasively document the flow and velocities through the shunt.

Recognized TIPS complications include (1) restenosis or occlusion of the shunt (20%), which, however, can be corrected with repeated balloon/stenting, and (2) new/worsening hepatic encephalopathy (18%), with 3% being refractory to medical management and liver decompensation, especially if liver reserve is severely diminished. Given the above, we feel TIPS should reserved for patients with refractory variceal bleeding or refractory ascites. In the appropriate clinical setting, patients with Budd-Chiari or hepatorenal syndrome may also benefit from a TIPS.

Table 118-5. Transjugular Intrahepatic Portosystemic Shunt

Indications	Contraindications
Recurrent variceal bleeding despite optimum therapy	Significant hepatic encephalopathy
Recurrent symptomatic ascites (or sympathetic pleural effusions) after therapeutic paracentesis	Inadequate hepatic reserve
Hepatorenal syndrome	Thrombosed hepatic or portal vein (relative, can be recanalized)
Presurgical portal vein decompression	
Budd-Chiari syndrome	-

Supplemental Reading

DeLeve LD, Shulman HM, McDonald DB. Toxic injury to hepatic sinusoids: Sinusoidal obstruction syndrome (Veno-occlusive disease). Semin Liver Dis 2002;27–42.

Janssen HLA, Garcia-Pagan JC, Elias E, et al. Budd-Chiari syndrome: a review by an expert panel. J Hepatol 2003;38:364–71.

Okudaira M, Ohbu O, Okuda K. Idiopathic portal hypertension and its pathology. Semin Liver Dis 2002;59–72.

Sobhonslidsuk A, Reddy KR. Portal vein thrombosis: a concise review. Am J Gastroenterol 2002;97:535–41.

CHAPTER 119

Drug-Induced Liver Disease

BASUKI GUNAWAN, MD, AND NEIL KAPLOWITZ, MD

Drug-induced liver disease is of great importance because it is the leading cause of acute liver failure (ALF) in the United States. It is also a major reason for withdrawal of drugs during drug development and clinical use. The latter has major medical and economic consequences, as reflected in the recent experiences when *bromfenac* and *troglitazone* were withdrawn from the market. Because drug-induced liver disease can mimic the entire spectrum of clinicopathologic features of other acute and chronic liver diseases, it is often challenging to diagnose. Establishing causality is important because the treatment of drug-induced liver disease includes discontinuation of the offending drug.

Clinical Presentations

Some drugs cause predictable liver disease, which is normally dose dependent, reproducible in animal models, and present after a short latency (hours to a few days). Hepatocellular necrosis caused by *acetaminophen* overdose is a typical example. However, the majority of drugs cause unpredictable liver disease, which is not usually dose dependent or reproducible in animal models. This type of liver injury occurs in only a small percentage of individuals (ranging from 0.01 to 1%) who use the drug but represents more than 10% of the cases of ALF. The two possible mechanisms for this unpredictable type of liver disease are as follows: (1) hypersensitivity reactions, which typically present with fever, rash, eosinophilia, an intermediate latency (1 to 6 weeks), and rapidly evolving liver injury upon rechallenge, and (2) metabolic idiosyncratic reactions, which present without hypersensitivity features and with variable latency (1 to 12 months). Drugs that can cause this type of liver disease are listed in Tables 119-1 and 119-2.

Acute Reactions

Drug-induced liver disease can also be classified as acute or chronic depending on clinical presentation. The majority of adverse reactions are acute and manifest features of acute hepatitis, cholestasis, or a mixed pattern of liver injury. The mixed reaction has biochemical features of both acute hepatitis and cholestasis. Drug-induced acute hepatitis resembles other causes of acute hepatitis, such as viral hepatitis or ischemia. Its clinical presentation ranges widely. Patients may be asymptomatic but are usually jaundiced and have elevated serum transaminases. Patients with fulminant liver failure may be brought to medical attention because of encephalopathy. At times, the histologic features of the liver injury are helpful in suggesting a particular drug toxicity. For example, *acetaminophen* and *halothane* cause centrilobular necrosis, similar to ischemic hepatitis. α-*Methyldopa* and *isoniazid* cause diffuse parenchymal necrosis and inflammation, which is indistinguishable from viral hepatitis. Hypersensitivity-type drug reactions often are associated with eosinophilic infiltration or granuloma. The mortality of drug-induced

TABLE 119-1. Hypersensitivity Drug-Induced Liver Disease

ACE inhibitors
Allopurinol
Amoxicillin–clavulanic acid
Carbamazepine
Chlorpromazine
Dihydralazine
Fluoxetine
Halogenated anesthetics
Minocycline
Phenobarbital
Phenytoin
Sulfonamides
Sulfonylureas
Tienilic acid
Tricylic antidepressants

ACE = angiotensin-converting enzyme.

TABLE 119-2. Metabolic Idiosyncratic Drug-Induced Liver Disease

Acarbose	Isotretinoin	Pyrazinamide
Amiodarone	Ketoconazole	Terbinafine
Bromfenac	Labetalol	Troglitazone
Clozapine	Nefazodone	Valproic acid
Dantrolene	Niacin	Zafirlukast
Disulfiram	Olanzapine	Zileuton
Isoniazid		

acute hepatitis approximates 10%, irrespective of the offending drug. Table 119-3 lists drugs that cause acute hepatitis.

Drug-induced acute cholestasis resembles cholestatic liver diseases caused by intra- or extrahepatic bile duct obstruction. Patients present with elevated serum alkaline phosphatase (ALP) and, often, jaundice. This type of liver disease is not normally life threatening but may lead to vanishing bile duct disease and biliary cirrhosis. Moreover, acute cholestasis may take months to resolve after discontinuation of the offending drug. Table 119-4 lists some drugs that cause acute cholestasis. In drug-induced mixed pattern disease, patients present with moderate abnormalities of serum transaminases and ALP. Phenytoin and sulfonamides exemplify this type of liver injury.

Chronic Disease

Drug-induced liver disease may also present as chronic disease, such as chronic hepatitis, granulomatous hepatitis, steatohepatitis, chronic cholestasis, and cirrhosis. There are also drugs that cause vascular disorders and hepatic tumors (Table 119-5). Again, the clinical features of these drug-induced chronic liver diseases cannot be distinguished from similar types of chronic liver disease from other etiologies.

Pathogenesis

The liver is the major organ for metabolism of many drugs. This explains its susceptibility to drug-induced injury. Drug elimination involves three phases. In phase I, drugs are metabolized by cytochrome P-450 enzymes. This process may generate toxic electrophilic chemicals or free radicals. In phase II, these metabolites or the parent drug are conjugated with glutathione or glucuronide to improve water solubility. This permits excretion of the agents from the body in bile or urine. The route of elimination is mainly determined by excretory transporters in the hepatocyte canalicular and sinusoidal membrane (phase III). Electrophilic chemicals and free radicals are potentially toxic because they can covalently bind to proteins, lipids, and deoxyribonucleic acid (DNA); cause lipid peroxidation; and deplete glutathione. Consequently, these effects may lead to hepatotoxicity in several ways, including (1) by directly causing loss of vital cell function (eg, mitochondria) and subsequent cell death; (2) by sensitizing hepatocytes to the toxic effects of the innate immune system (eg, tumor necrosis factor, Fas ligand, interferon-γ);

TABLE 119-3. Drug-Induced Acute Hepatitis

Allopurinol
Dihydralazine
Dantrolene
Fluoxetine
Herbal remedies (germander, valerian)
Isoniazid
Ketoconazole
Minocycline
Nefazodone
Paroxetine
Pyrazinamide
Sertraline
Terbinafine
Tienilic acid

TABLE 119-4. Drug-Induced Acute Cholestasis

ACE inhibitors
Amoxicillin–clavulanic acid
Androgens
Azathioprine
Chlorpromazine
Cyclosporin A
Didanosine
Erythromycin
Estrogens
Sulindac
Tamoxifen
Tricyclic antidepressants

ACE = angiotensin-converting enzyme.

TABLE 119-5. Drug-Induced Chronic Liver Disease

Chronic hepatitis
  α-Methyldopa
  Diclofenac
  Minocycline
  Nitrofurantoin
Granulomatous hepatitis
  Allopurinol
  Diltiazem
  Quinidine
  Penicillamine
  Procainamide
Steatohepatitis
  Amiodarone
  Nifedipine
  Tamoxifen
Chronic cholestasis
  Flucloxacillin
  Tetracycline
  Trimethoprim-sulfamethoxazole
Cirrhosis
  Methotrexate
  Vitamin A
Vascular disorders
  Azathioprine
  Busulfan
  Cyclophosphamide
Hepatic tumors
  Androgens
  Estrogens

or (3) by eliciting immune hypersensitivity via haptenization. The mechanisms of delayed metabolic idiosyncratic reactions are very poorly understood and may be the result of genetic or acquired differences in drug metabolism, canalicular secretion, mitochondrial defects, cell death receptor signaling, or the response of the innate immune system. Thus, it is speculated that host-dependent mechanisms render selected individuals highly susceptible to the toxicity of normally safe drugs.

The mechanisms of hepatotoxicity explained above can result in combined hepatic or cholestatic liver disease. For example, the canalicular secretion of toxic metabolites causes bile duct injury and inflammation and induces immune responses to haptenized duct cells. Because the same toxic metabolites can also injure hepatocytes, mixed patterns of liver injury may occur (cholestatic hepatitis). Some drugs (eg, *rifampicin* and *cyclosporin A*) may also cause cholestasis without producing appreciable liver damage by inhibiting bile salt excretory proteins. Reduced function of the bile salt transporters causes bile acids and other factors that are normally excreted in the bile to accumulate in liver and serum and can lead to pruritus.

Diagnosis

Because the clinical features of drug-induced liver disease are indistinguishable from other types of liver disease, diagnosis can be challenging. Success requires a thorough history (which includes a complete inquiry regarding drug and herbal remedies) and a high index of suspicion that a drug may cause the liver disease. It is important to ask about medications that were used in the previous few months because reactions to certain antibiotics (eg, *amoxicillin–clavulinic acid* and *erythromycin*) can be delayed up to 6 weeks after cessation of the medication. Serologic tests for viral hepatitis, antinuclear antibody, anti–smooth muscle antibody, and antimitochondrial antibody should be done to search for other etiologies of liver disease. In selected cases, other tests, such as iron studies, ceruloplasmin, and α_1-antitrypsin phenotype, may need to be performed. Ultrasound and biliary studies are often needed to exclude biliary tract disease. Hypotension, sepsis, congestive heart failure, and alcoholism need to be identified and related to the clinical picture. After ruling out other causes of liver disease, a temporal relationship between ingestion of a drug and the onset of clinical presentation or abnormality in liver enzymes and bilirubin should be assessed.

The signature pattern of liver disease, that is, whether it is acute or chronic or hepatitis, cholestasis, or mixed, can be helpful in pinpointing the offending drug. *Hepatitis* is defined as alanine transaminase (ALT) > 2 times the upper limit of normal or an ALT-to-ALP ratio ≥ 5. *Cholestasis* is defined as ALP > 2 times the upper limit of normal or an ALT-to-ALP ratio ≤ 2. *Mixed disease* is defined as ALT and ALP > 2 times the upper limit of normal and an ALT-to-ALP ratio between 2 and 5.

A review of the medical literature, as well as the *Physicians' Desk Reference*, should be performed when the drug is not commonly known to cause liver disease or the physician is unfamiliar with the adverse effects of the drug. Liver biopsy is often nondiagnostic and unnecessary but occasionally may be useful if diagnosis or the severity of the liver disease remains uncertain despite less invasive tests. A rechallenge with the offending drug that results in recurrent abnormality in liver tests may give the definitive diagnosis. However, the risks should be weighed against the benefits, and, usually, this approach is not justified.

Several standardized scoring systems for assessing the probability of a drug as the cause of liver disease have been developed. The most reliable system is the Roussel Uclaf causality assessment method. It was developed by an international panel of experts and uses various factors, such as temporal relationship, use of concomitant drugs, search for other etiologies, previous information on the hepatotoxicity of the drug, and response to rechallenge, to assess the probability of a drug as the cause. The system has been validated using drug-induced liver disease cases with positive rechallenge.

Autoantibodies against particular neoantigens that are formed by cytochrome P-450 proteins and drug metabolites have been identified and have been associated with hypersensitivity reactions to certain drugs. Although their significance is still unclear, their determination may help in diagnosis (Table 119-6).

Risk Factors

Certain individuals are far more susceptible than others to develop drug-induced liver disease. This susceptibility may be due to inherited or acquired risk factors. Chronic liver disease, such as hepatitis B and C, and human immunodeficiency virus (HIV) have been suggested to increase the risk for toxicity from certain drugs, such as *isoniazid*. The exact mechanism is still unclear, but it is speculated that an activated or altered innate immune system caused by the viral infection is important. Chronic alcohol use has also been reported to be a risk factor for *methotrexate*-, *isoniazid*-, and

TABLE 119-6. Autoantibody Targets in Drug-Induced Liver Disease

Autoantibody Target	Drug
CYP2C9	Tienilic acid
CYP1A2	Dihydralazine
CYP3A1 (CYP8, CYP5A1, CYP52A)	Anticonvulsants (eg, phenytoin)
CYP2E1	Halothane
Microsomal epoxide hydrase	Germander

acetaminophen-induced hepatotoxicity. Concomitant drug use, such as *rifampicin* and *pyrazinamide* with *isoniazid* or *phenobarbital* with *valproic acid*, can increase the risk for developing hepatotoxicity.

Managment

The treatment of drug-induced liver disease is focused mainly on discontinuation of the offending drug. If the offending drug cannot be pinpointed with certainty, discontinuation of drugs that have a strong temporal relationship with the clinical presentation of the patient should not be delayed. At the same time, workup to rule out other etiologies of liver disease should be initiated. Liver enzymes and measures for liver synthetic function, including bilirubin and prothrombin time, should be monitored closely until they show improvement. Most hepatitis-type reactions improve within 1 to 2 weeks of discontinuation of the offending drug. In contrast, drug-induced cholestatic liver disease resolves much more slowly. For many individuals, discontinuation of the offending drug may be all the therapy that is needed, and the patient may not need to be hospitalized. However, for others with more severe presentations, such as ALF, supportive management in hospital is required. Symptomatic treatment may also be required, such as opioid receptor blockers for intractable pruritus or antiemetics for nausea. If the clinical condition deteriorates, transfer to a hospital that performs liver transplantation should be arranged so that liver transplantation evaluation is expedited. In general, suspected drug-induced hepatitis with overt jaundice and any degree of coagulopathy should be viewed as potentially life threatening. Transplantation evaluation is prudent so that further deterioration can be dealt with expeditiously.

Acetaminophen

For *acetaminophen* overdose, the treatment includes N-*acetylcysteine*. The mechanism for *acetaminophen* hepatotoxicity is related to its toxic metabolite, N-*acetyl-p-benzoquinoneimine* (NAPQI). *Acetaminophen* is primarily metabolized by sulfation and glucuronidation to derivatives that are excreted in urine. However, a small amount of acetaminophen is metabolized by cytochrome P-4502E1 (CYP2E1) to NAPQI. NAPQI is preferentially conjugated with glutathione and excreted as a nontoxic mercapturic acid. When glutathione is depleted, NAPQI covalently binds to cell proteins and ultimately causes hepatic necrosis. Oxidative stress owing to depletion of mitochondrial glutathione and covalent binding to mitochondrial proteins may both contribute. *Acetaminophen* causes toxicity after single or daily doses of 7.5 g or above because the metabolism pathway using sulfation and glucuronidation is saturated by high doses of *acetaminophen*, and the surplus is then available to be metabolized by the CYP2E1 pathway. As a result, large amounts of NAPQI are produced, and once glutathione is depleted, hepatic necrosis occurs. N-*Acetylcysteine* is a cysteine precursor for glutathione synthesis that replenishes glutathione in hepatocytes. It is noteworthy that therapeutic doses of *acetaminophen* (< 4 g/24 hours) have been reported to cause liver toxicity. This rare toxicity owing to low-dose *acetaminophen* probably represents a variant of idiosyncratic drug-induced liver disease in which individual susceptibility is heightened by altered metabolism (eg, induction of CYP2E1 by ethanol, isoniazid, or fasting; by depletion of glucuronic acid or glutathione by fasting; or by altered response of the innate immune system).

Once patients admit to taking *acetaminophen* at a supratherapeutic dose, a detailed history of the time of consumption and the amount of acetaminophen should be performed. Patients may be asymptomatic or present with minor gastrointestinal symptoms, especially early after *acetaminophen* ingestion. Liver tests and serum *acetaminophen* level should be drawn. If the patient presents within 4 hours after drug consumption, gastric lavage should be performed. The use of activated charcoal may also decrease *acetaminophen* absorption. However, the institution of N-acetylcysteine should not be delayed in patients who admit to recent consumption of more than 7.5 g or 150 mg/kg body weight. However, because estimation of *acetaminophen* consumed by patients is not always reliable, the serum *acetaminophen* level is very important. If the patient's *acetaminophen* level falls above a line between a serum *acetaminophen* of 200 mg/L at 4 hours after ingestion and 30 mg/L at 15 hours, there is a significant chance of developing severe liver disease (ALT > 1,000). All patients with *acetaminophen* levels above this line should receive N-*acetylcysteine*. For high-risk patients, such as chronic alcohol users, malnourished individuals, or those on epileptic medicine, the threshold line is lower, between 100 mg/L at 4 hours and 15 mg/L at 15 hours. Ideally, N-*acetylcysteine* treatment is given within 8 hours after the *acetaminophen* overdose. In the past, N-*acetylcysteine* was not administered beyond 24 hours after *acetaminophen* ingestion. However, recent data suggest that N-*acetylcysteine* treatment improves mortality even when it is initiated more than 24 hours after the overdose. For cases of inadvertent overdose who present with overt liver injury, the blood levels and nomogram are not useful. Although there is no proof of efficacy, we recommend using N-*acetylcysteine* in this setting. In the United States, N-*acetylcysteine* is given orally because the intravenous (IV) preparation is not available. The standard dose for N-*acetylcysteine* is 140 mg/kg body weight as a loading dose, followed by 70 mg/kg every 4 hours for 17 doses. In Europe and Canada, the standard dose is 150 mg/kg IV bolus over 15 minutes followed by 50 mg/kg over 4 hours and then 100 mg/kg over 16 hours. The oral preparation has an unpleasant taste and smell and may need to be given with carbonated soda or antiemetic medication. A feeding tube may be needed in patients who cannot tolerate the medication orally. Oral N-*acetylcysteine* has no serious side effects, but the IV preparation may rarely cause an anaphylactic reaction.

Other Therapies

Apart from N-*acetylcysteine* treatment for *acetaminophen* poisoning, therapy for drug-induced liver injury is scant. A short course of high-dose corticosteroid may be used for severe drug-induced liver disease, especially in patients with systemic features of a hypersensitivity reaction. However, corticosteroids have not been proven to be of value in controlled trials. Nevertheless, we recommend a short course of corticosteroids when systemic features of immune hypersensitivity accompany acute hepatitis (eg, phenytoin skin rash and liver injury). In patients with prolonged drug-induced cholestatic liver disease, ursodeoxycholic acid treatment may be of use, although the efficacy is unproved.

Prevention

Because there is little specific therapy for drug-induced liver disease, prevention is of great importance. This process starts during drug development. It is important to monitor for ALT abnormality, as well as signs and symptoms of liver disease, during clinical studies with new drugs. Even after a drug receives approval from the US Food and Drug Administration, surveillance and report of suspected cases should continue to identify hepatotoxicity that may not have been apparent during the initial clinical studies.

For patients who take drugs that are known to have hepatotoxic potential, monitoring liver enzymes should be considered. Careful follow-up may identify emerging hepatotoxicity and, thus, prevent severe drug-induced liver disease. However, this approach is most rational for delayed-onset, idiosyncratic, drug-induced liver disease. When starting any drug, all patients should be educated about the signs and symptoms of liver disease and urged to report such symptoms to health care professionals immediately. This practice is particularly important for patients who take multiple medications because immune cross-sensitization has been known to occur among drugs in the same class, such as anticonvulsants, macrolides, or phenothiazines. If patients have a history of an immune hypersensitivity reaction to one drug, they may need to avoid other drugs from the same class.

Supplemental Reading

Ballet F. Hepatotoxicity in drug development: detection, significance and solutions. J Hepatol 1997;26 Suppl 2:26–36.

Danan G, Benichou C. Causality assessment of adverse reactions to drugs—I. A novel method based on the conclusions of international consensus meetings: application to drug-induced liver injuries. J Clin Epidemiol 1993;46:1323–30.

Degott C, Feldmann G, Larrey D, et al. Drug-induced prolonged cholestasis in adults: a histological semiquantitative study demonstrating progressive ductopenia. Hepatology 1992;17:244–51.

Farrell G. Liver disease caused by drugs, anesthetics, and toxins. In: Feldman M, Friedman LS, Sleisenger MH, editors. Sleisenger & Fordtran's gastrointestinal and liver disease: pathophysiology, diagnosis, and management. 7th ed. Philadelphia: Saunders; 2002.

Kaplowitz N. Drug-induced liver disorders: implications for drug development and regulation. Drug Saf 2001;24:483–90.

Kaplowitz N, Aw TY, Simon FR, Stolz A. Drug-induced hepatotoxicity. Ann Intern Med 1986;104:826–39.

Keays R, Harrison PM, Wendon JA, et al. Intravenous acetylcysteine in paracetamol induced fulminant hepatic failure: a prospective controlled trial. BMJ 1991;303:1026–9.

Liu ZX, Kaplowitz N. Immune-mediated drug-induced liver disease. Clin Liver Dis 2002;6:755–74.

Makin AJ, Wendon J, Williams R. A seven year experience of severe acetaminophen-induced hepatotoxicity (1987–1993). Gastroenterology 1995;109:1907–16.

O'Grady J. Paracetamol-induced acute liver failure: prevention and management. J Hepatol 1997;26 Suppl 1:41–6.

Ostapowicz G, Fontana RJ, Schiodt FV, et al. Results of a prospective study of acute liver failure at 17 tertiary care centers in the United States. Ann Intern Med 2002;137:947–54.

Schiødt FV, Rohling FA, Casey DL, Lee WM. Acetaminophen toxicity in an urban county hospital. N Engl J Med 1997;337:1112–7.

Seeff LB, Cuccherini BA, Zimmerman HJ, et al. Acetaminophen hepatotoxicity in alcoholics: a therapeutic misadventure. Ann Intern Med 1986;104:399–404.

Smilkstein MJ, Knapp GL, Kulig KW, Rumack BH. Efficacy of oral N-acetylcysteine in the treatment of acetaminophen overdose. N Engl J Med 1988;319:1557–62.

Stieger B, Fattinger K, Madon J, et al. Drug- and estrogen-induced cholestasis through inhibition of the hepatocellular bile salt export pump (BSEP) of rat liver. Gastroenterology 2000;118:422–30.

CHAPTER 120

LIVER DISEASE AND PREGNANCY

ANNE M. LARSON, MD

Normal pregnancy induces physiologic, hormonal, and biochemical changes which are adaptive and do not represent significant pathology. These changes may cause confusion about the true status of the liver and the presence or absence of disease. Liver test abnormalities are seen in about 10% of all pregnancies and represent disorders commonly seen in the nongravid state (ie, viral hepatitis), disorders related to pregnancy, or disorders unique to pregnancy.

Normal Changes during Pregnancy

Anatomic Changes

The enlarging uterus rotates the liver superiorly and posteriorly, however, the liver's size and gross appearance do not change. Nonspecific histologic changes include hepatocyte variability, cytoplasmic granularity, centrilobular fat vacuoles, and a minimal increase in Kupffer cells. Despite increases in global maternal blood volume of 20 to 70%, and a 30 to 50% increase in maternal cardiac output, liver blood flow remains unchanged.

Laboratory Studies

The major liver test changes during pregnancy are outlined in Table 120-1. Increases in alkaline phosphatase levels represent an influx of the placental isoenzyme. Decreases in serum γ-glutamyl transpeptidase (GGT) are secondary to impaired hepatic release. Maternal hemodilution and decreased hepatic synthesis lead to a relative decrease in serum albumin. Decreased hepatic synthesis of antithrombin III and increased synthesis of fibrinogen lead to the prothrombotic state seen in pregnancy. There is a marked increased hepatic synthesis of lipoproteins, cholesterol, and triglycerides. Increased concentrations of cholesterol found in the bile.

Physical Examination

Spider angiomata occur in 60 to 70% of women, with palmar erythema in as many as 63% of white women and 39% of black women. These changes are likely due to the hyperestrogenemia seen during pregnancy and disappear in the majority of women by about 7 weeks postpartum. The liver is normally not palpable.

Liver Disease During Pregnancy

Cholelithiasis and gallstone disease are seen in 3 to 12% of pregnant women, with higher incidence in the second and third trimesters. Most women are asymptomatic, however, up to 50% will have recurrent pain and worsening symptoms as pregnancy advances. Asymptomatic cholelithiasis requires no treatment. Symptomatic disease should initially be managed conservatively, but up to 35% will fail medication management and require surgical intervention. If possible surgery should be delayed until the second trimester. Likewise, medical management during the third trimester is preferable with surgical intervention following delivery.

Variable outcomes are seen in pregnant women with cirrhosis and portal hypertension. Significant hepatic decompensation (jaundice, ascites, and encephalopathy) can occur. Preexisting portal hypertension may be worsened by increased total blood volume, possibly increasing the risk of bleeding from esophageal varices. Pregnancy is generally uneventful in patients with chronic hepatitis B or C virus infections. Women with autoimmune hepatitis have had successful pregnancies and should continue to be treated with *corticosteroids* and/or *azathioprine*. Women with untreated Wilson's disease are generally anovulatory, but can undergo successful pregnancy with following copper chelation treatment. *Penicillamine* or *trientine* therapy

TABLE 120-1. Normal Changes During Pregnancy

Serum Test	Usual Change
Albumin	Decreased (mean value 3 g/dL)
AST	Normal
ALT	Normal
Alkaline phosphatase	Two- to fourfold increase
GGT	Normal or slight decrease
Bilirubin	Slight decrease
5′-nucleotidase	Slight increase
Prothrombin time	Normal
Ferritin	Decreased
Ceruloplasmin	Decreased
Cholesterol/Triglycerides	Marked increase
Bile acids	No change

ALT = alanine aminotransferase; AST = aspartate aminotransferase; GGT = γ-glutamyl transpeptidase.

should be continued in this setting because discontinuation can lead to fulminant liver failure (the potential effects of these medications on the fetus should be discussed with the patient). Alcoholic women with significant liver disease may be anovulatory and thus infertile.

Pregnancy-Associated Liver Disorders

Hyperemesis Gravidarum

Nausea and vomiting occur in up to 90% of all pregnancies. Hyperemesis gravidarum (HG) has a prevalence of 0.35 to 1%, and is characterized by severe, persistent nausea and vomiting during the first trimester. Intractable vomiting requires aggressive support, including, at times, parenteral nutrition. Risk associations include increased body weight, multiple gestations, hyperemesis in a prior pregnancy, and nulliparity.

Up to half of women hospitalized for HG have liver enzyme abnormalities, generally occurring within the first 1 to 3 weeks following onset of vomiting. Aminotransferase levels may be as high as 2 to 3 times normal, but rarely above 1000 IU/L. The more severe the vomiting, the higher the elevation. Mild elevations in bilirubin (rarely above 4 mg/dL) and jaundice, occasionally with pruritus, occur. Alkaline phosphatase levels are usually elevated beyond those seen with normal pregnancy.

The etiology of the hepatic abnormalities is unknown, but it is a relatively benign process. Liver abnormalities resolve rapidly with resolution of emesis. HG was at one time a lethal disease, however, with early diagnosis and aggressive support, both maternal and fetal mortality is now negligible.

Intrahepatic Cholestasis of Pregnancy

Intrahepatic cholestasis of pregnancy (IHCP) is heralded by the development of pruritus, liver enzyme abnormalities, and occasionally jaundice. Most cases occur within the third trimester of pregnancy (Table 120-2). The worldwide incidence varies; ICHP occurs in less than 1 to 2% of all pregnancies in the United States, Asia, Australia, and Europe, but in Bolivia, Chile, and Scandinavia, the incidence is as high as 14%, with rates of 24% in the Araucanian Indians of Chile. There is a greater prevalence among woman from the Indian subcontinent and the disease is rare in black patients. IHCP recurs in 60 to 70% of subsequent pregnancies and is 5 times more frequent in women with multiple gestation.

The etiology of ICHP is uncertain and is probably multifactorial. Seasonal variations suggest environmental influ-

TABLE 120-2. Features of Liver Disease of Pregnancy

	IHCP	AFLP	HELLP
Maternal age of onset (years)	Any	26 (range, 16 to 39)	25 (range 14 to 40)
Gestational age of onset (weeks)	29 (range, 7 to 40) 70%: 3rd trimester 30%: before 3rd trimester	36 (range, 26 to 40) 100%: 3rd trimester	33 (range, 22 to 40) 60%: 3rd trimester 30%: postpartum 13: 5% 1st/2nd trimester
Parity	Any Fivefold increase with twin pregnancy	42 to 70% Primagravida 60 to 76% male fetus 10 to 15% twin pregnancy	52-81% Primagravida -
Incidence (in all pregnancies)	1 to 24 %	1 in 7,000 to 15,000	0.17 to 0.85%
Recurrence	60 to 70%	Rare	2 to 3%
Malaise	-	100%	100%
Nausea/Vomiting	5 to 75%	> 70%	up to 90%
Abdominal Pain	9 to 24 %	~ 60%	≥ 80%
Headache	–	40%	25%
Increased alkaline phosphatase	~67%	100%	–
Increased bilirubin	25%	≥ 95%	47 to 62%
Increased AST/ALT	20 to 60%	≥95%	≥95%
Increased PT	≤ 20%	≥ 90%	≤ 15%
Hypertension	Rare	30 to 40%	> 90%
Preeclampsia	Rare	≥ 50%	≥ 80%
Maternal mortality	Low	15 to 50%	up to 8%
Fetal mortality	1 to 2%	40 to 50%	8 to 37%

Adapted from Larson AM. Liver disease in pregnancy. Clin Perspectives Gastroenterol 2001; 4:351(17).
AFLP = acute fatty liver of pregnancy; ALT = alanine aminotransferase; AST = aspartate aminotransferase; HELLP = hemolysis, elevated liver enzymes, and low platelets syndrome; ICPH = intrahepatic cholestasis of pregnancy; PT = prothrombin time.

ences. Genetic components are suggested given that female relatives of patients with IHCP often develop IHCP and it is seen in successive generations (30 to 50% report a positive family history). Further support for this is the high recurrence rate in subsequent pregnancies. Nearly half of the women who develop IHCP will also develop jaundice when using oral contraceptives, suggesting that the genetic defect is in estrogen processing.

Estrogen concentrations peak in the third trimester of pregnancy, perhaps explaining the onset of illness during this time. Serum bile acids are also markedly increased (10 to 100 times normal), suggesting decreased hepatic capacity to either process or transport them. Both estrogens and monohydroxy bile acids are conjugated within the liver. It has been postulated that a genetic defect in sulfotransferase activity leads to the accumulation of toxic metabolites via glucuronidation. Mutations have been described in the *MDR3* gene, which encodes for a biliary canalicular phospholipid translocater. *MDR3* has been associated with familial forms of intrahepatic cholestasis and in women with IHCP associated with an elevated GGT. Exogenous progesterone administration or impaired secretion of progesterone metabolites has also been implicated as a trigger for IHCP in predisposed women.

Nearly all affected women report intense pruritus, which typically involves the palms and soles, but may be diffuse. Pruritus is often worse at night and becomes progressively severe as the pregnancy progresses. It may precede abnormalities in liver tests. There appears to be no correlation between serum levels of bile acids and the severity of pruritus.

Pruritus gravidarum, clinical jaundice within 1 to 4 weeks after onset of pruritus, develops in 10 to 60% of patients. The skin appears normal but patients may have excoriations secondary to scratching. Systemic symptoms are generally mild (see Table 120-2). Elevation in bilirubin correlates with jaundice and is rarely greater than 5 to 6 mg/dL. GGT levels are normal to minimally elevated. Prolonged prothrombin time (PT) generally reflects the vitamin K deficiency resulting from impaired bile salt formation. Serum bile acids are often as high as 100 times normal (bile acid concentrations change little during normal pregnancy) and are the most sensitive marker for IHCP. They may be the only abnormality, however, absolute levels do not correlate with maternal symptoms, other liver tests, or with prognosis.

Diagnosis is made clinically, based upon history, symptoms, and laboratory studies. Other causes of liver disease, such as viral hepatitis or gallstone disease, must be ruled out. Liver biopsy is rarely needed and histopathology reveals normal portal tracts, and bland cholestasis, with bile plugs predominating in zone 3.

Maternal management of IHCP is symptomatic and the most common approach is early delivery (generally 37 to 38 weeks). *Oral vitamin K* should be started at the time of diagnosis and, when given before delivery, can minimize postpartum hemorrhage. Treating pruritus is more problematic. *Antihistamines* and *benzodiazepines* have been used with little success. Studies using *phenobarbitol* have been contradictory and it may cause neonatal respiratory depression. *Dexamethasone* (12 mg/d for 7 days with 3 day taper) has been shown to improve pruritus. Controlled trials have not been done, however, and there is a report of worsened liver function with *dexamethasone* use. Studies with *S-adenosyl-methionine* have shown conflicting results. In two randomized controlled trials, it significantly decreased pruritus (800 mg/d intravenously or 1,600 mg/d orally). In a third double blind randomized controlled trial, no improvement was seen. Pruritus has been successfully treated with *cholestyramine* at 8 to 16 g per day, although it is usually poorly tolerated. It must be used with caution as it may worsen maternal absorption of *Vitamin K* and maternal steatorrhea.

Therapy with *ursodeoxycholic acid (UDCA)* at dosages of 15 mg/kg/d leads to a reduction in pruritus, a reduction in maternal serum bile acids and maternal aminotransferases, and a reduction in delivery of bile acids to the fetus. *UDCA* also appears to decrease negative maternal and fetal sequelae. *UDCA* can cross the placenta, but there have been no reports of fetal toxicity. Because *UDCA* appears safe to mother and fetus, it is reasonable to consider its use, keeping in mind that it is not approved for this indication in the United States. Larger randomized controlled trials are needed.

Maternal prognosis is excellent with IHCP and there are usually no hepatic sequelae. Symptoms progress until delivery and then promptly disappear. Jaundice resolves rapidly and serum laboratory tests resolve over weeks to months. Acute liver failure does not occur. IHCP is associated with an increased incidence of primary postpartum hemorrhage (20 to 22%), likely due to vitamin K deficiency. The incidence of cholelithiasis is also increased.

Fetal prognosis is less benign. Fetal morbidity and mortality are significantly increased. Premature labor (6 to 60%), meconium-stained amniotic fluid (26 to 58%), fetal distress (17 to 22%), and stillbirth (1 to 3%) are all seen. Early reports of fetal mortality were as high as 10 to 15%; however, with more aggressive management, this is improving (1.7 to 3.5%). Unfortunately, there are no antepartum tests, which predict fetal compromise.

Acute Fatty Liver of Pregnancy

Acute fatty liver of pregnancy (AFLP) was first described in 1934 and is a rare, idiopathic, potentially fatal disease presenting in the third trimester of pregnancy. Incidence ranges from 1 of 7,000 to 1 of 16,000 deliveries and it constitutions 16 to 43% of severe liver disease seen during pregnancy. In its most severe form, it is manifest by fulminant hepatic failure. Seen worldwide, there appears to be no ethnic or geographic variation.

The average maternal age at onset is 26 years (range, 16 to 39 years) with gestational age of onset at about 36 weeks (range, 22 to 40 weeks). AFLP can rarely occur earlier in pregnancy or shortly postpartum. Primagravidas with male gestations comprise most cases (see Table 120-2). Recurrence with subsequent pregnancies, once thought to be uncommon, is increasingly being reported.

AFLP has little or no association with the hormonal changes of pregnancy. Its etiology is unknown, but may stem from decreases in fetal mitochondrial fatty acid β-oxidation by the enzyme long-chain 3-hydroxyacyl-CoA dehydrogenase (LCHAD). Cholestatic liver disease with microvesicular steatosis is often seen in patients with LCHAD deficiency and an association between LCHAD and AFLP has been described. In many cases, the defect appears to reside in the α-subunit of a trifunctional protein gene, which includes LCHAD activity. This may lead to poor fetal processing of triglycerides and free fatty acids, which are toxic to the maternal hepatocytes. Testing for the genetic variants of the LCHAD enzyme is available. When the deficiency is present, recurrent disease can be seen in subsequent pregnancies. Not all investigations have confirmed this specific association and other genetic variants, such as a defect in short-chain acyl-coenzyme A dehydrogenase, have been associated with AFLP.

Asymptomatic elevations in liver tests may be the only abnormality, but the majority of severe cases present with malaise, fatigue, anorexia, headache, nausea, and vomiting (see Table 120-2). Right upper quadrant or epigastric pain may mimic acute cholecystitis or reflux esophagitis. Within 1 to 2 weeks of onset of symptoms, and within days following clinical jaundice, the disease may rapidly worsen, leading to acute liver failure, with hepatic encephalopathy, ascites, edema, and renal insufficiency. Hallmarks of preeclampsia (hypertension, proteinuria) are seen in over 50% of cases.

Serum aminotransferases are generally less than 1,000 IU/L and do not reflect severity of liver dysfunction. Hyperbilirubinemia averages 10 to 15 mg/dL, but levels up to 30 to 40 mg/dL have been reported. In the setting of eclampsia and preeclampsia, hyperbilirubinemia is predominantly unconjugated and hemolysis is present. Increases in alkaline phosphatase are difficult to interpret because they overlap the normal values seen late in pregnancy. A left-shifted leukocytosis and some degree of thrombocytopenia are nearly universal.

Clinical and laboratory findings suggest the diagnosis of AFLP. The differential diagnosis includes acute viral hepatitis, acute toxic or drug-induced hepatitis, preeclampsia-related liver disease (including hemolysis, elevated liver enzymes, and low platelets syndrome [HELLP]), and biliary tract disorders. Imaging studies are useful in assessing the biliary tree. Virologic markers and history can help to rule out viral and toxic hepatitis.

Liver biopsy provides the diagnostic gold standard, but it is problematic if coagulopathy is present, and is rarely needed (Figure 120-1). Fatty changes in pancreatic acinar cells and renal tubular epithelia have also been described and likely account for the findings of renal failure and pancreatitis in these patients.

Upper gastrointestinal hemorrhage (in 30 to 40% of cases) occurs from a variety of causes. Renal dysfunction is generally mild to moderate, but 25% of patients develop severe renal failure and may require dialysis. Coagulopathy (elevated PT), decreased antithrombin III levels, and thrombocytopenia) probably represents both hepatic synthetic dysfunction and peripheral consumption. Frank disseminated intravascular coagulation (DIC) is common (up to 70%). Pancreatitis develops in up to 30% of patients. Severe hypoglycemia may be seen in 25 to 50% of patients and can occur at any stage in the disease.

AFLP is a medical and obstetrical emergency. It is often difficult to distinguish from toxic or viral hepatitis. Patients may progress to fulminant liver failure and death or require liver transplantation. No specific therapy is available. Patients should promptly be admitted to an experienced liver failure unit, since it is impossible to predict which patients will progress to liver failure. The patient should be medically stabilized and delivery attempted as soon as reasonably possible; ALFP never resolves before delivery. Aggressive maternal supportive care is required and fresh frozen plasma or cryoprecipitate may be necessary prior to delivery. Blood glucose levels should be followed frequently. Likewise, PT must frequently be checked as this helps to assess the severity of disease. With early diagnosis and management, severity of disease and need for liver transplantation can be minimized.

Maternal mortality has been reported as high as 70%, but can be improved to 10 to 20% with early delivery and intensive clinical support. Fetal death occurs in 42 to 90%

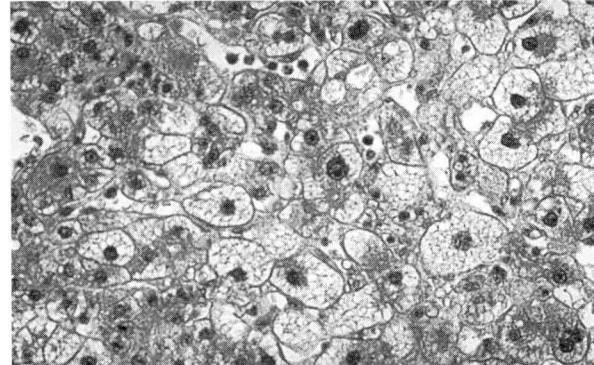

FIGURE 120-1. Acute fatty liver of pregnancy. The zone 3 centrilobular hepatocytes are swollen with microvesicular fat globules. Sinusoidal compression can be seen but signs of hepatic necrosis and inflammation are often subtle. Hepatic necrosis is a minor feature. Courtesy of Carolyn A Riely, MD.

of cases with only minimal improvement with early delivery (36%). After delivery, affected women improve slowly; full recovery often takes up to a month. There are no hepatic sequelae. Infants who survive should be tested for LCHAD deficiency and other fatty acid transport and mitochondrial oxidation disorders.

Toxemia and Preeclampsia/Eclampsia

Pregnancy-induced hypertension (toxemia) is seen late in pregnancy and remains a major medical challenge. Five to 10% of pregnant women with toxemia may develop preeclampsia (hypertension plus proteinuria and nondependent edema). Preeclampsia generally occurs during the second and third trimesters, and is most frequent in young primagravidas. Risk factors associated with preeclampsia include nulliparity, a positive family history, preeclampsia in a prior pregnancy, obesity, chronic hypertension or renal disease, diabetes mellitus, a multiple gestation pregnancy, low socioeconomic status, and cigarette smoking.

The cause of preeclampsia is unknown. Laboratory abnormalities are nonspecific. Hepatic involvement is seen in 10 to 30% of women with preeclampsia. Mild elevations of serum transaminases and, rarely, an increase in indirect bilirubin can be seen in the absence of HELLP syndrome. Histologically, periportal fibrin deposition and hemorrhage with hepatocellular necrosis are seen (Figure 120-2). Preeclampsia can also have a similar histological pattern to AFLP (both may develop microvesicular steatosis).

The clinical course may be mild or rapidly progressive. Onset of seizures signals development of true eclampsia (usually young primagravidas), accounting for approximately 8% of all maternal deaths. Control of the hypertension is associated with reduced morbidity and mortality in both the mother and the fetus. Definitive therapy requires delivery.

HELLP Syndrome

The HELLP syndrome is a severe, life-threatening form of preeclampsia reported as early as 1922. The acronym HELLP was coined by Weinstein in 1982 to describe preeclampsia associated with microthrombi, thrombocytopenia, and coagulopathy. HELLP syndrome has an incidence of 0.11 to 0.85% of all live births and occurs in 20 to 25% of women with preeclampsia. Ethnic variations exist; risk is higher in white and Chinese populations (relative risk of 2.2) when compared to East Indian populations and is higher in black Americans when compared to white Americans. Patients are usually young primagravidas (see Table 120-2).

The pathophysiology of preeclampsia and HELLP syndrome are unknown. They may represent a single disease spectrum, with the HELLP syndrome the most severe form of preeclampsia. An imbalance between endothelial vasodilatative (ie, nitric oxide) and vasoconstrictive (ie, endothelin) substances probably occurs and increased vascular tone leads to increased platelet adhesion and aggregation. Thrombin-induced activation of intravascular coagulation subsequently occurs and can rapidly progress to disseminated intravascular coagulation (DIC ~20%). The resultant severe coagulopathy leads to fatal hemorrhagic complications and multiorgan failure. These changes may be more common in preeclampsia than in HELLP syndrome.

Clinically, onset may be without warning. Nonspecific symptoms of nausea, vomiting, and malaise are seen in up to 90% of women (see Table 120-2). Abdominal pain precedes biochemical abnormalities in as many as 20 to 40% and visual changes (15 to 30%) have been reported. Hypertension may be absent in as many as 20% of cases and 5 to 15% of patients have little to no proteinuria. Thus, about 15 to 20% of women presenting with HELLP syndrome have no signs of preeclampsia. HELLP syndrome also appears to be associated with eclampsia, although reports of incidence are conflicting. Generalized edema (50 to 77% of cases) and development of ascites (8 to 10% of cases) carries an increased risk of congestive heart failure and adult respiratory distress syndrome. Pulmonary edema (6%) and acute renal failure may develop and, in association with ascites, often coexist with DIC. Transient nephrogenic diabetes insipidus has been reported.

Gestational thrombocytopenia is seen in 4 to 8% of uncomplicated pregnancies, whereas thrombocytopenia in preeclampsia ranges from 15 to 50%. Those who develop gestational thrombocytopenia are sevenfold more likely to develop HELLP. Platelet levels in HELLP syndrome are frequently less than 100,000/μL, and there is a positive correlation between the extent of platelet decline and the severity of liver abnormalities. Elevations of serum aminotransferases

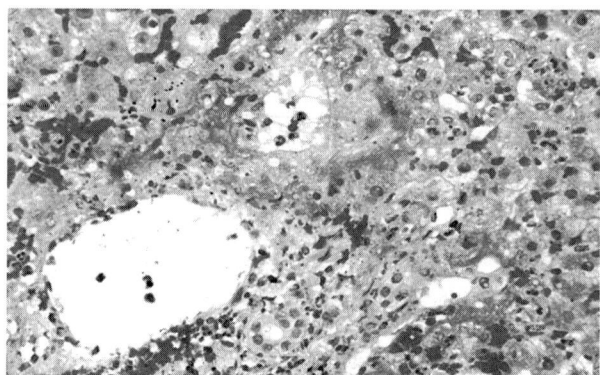

FIGURE 120-2. Eclampsia/ hemolysis, elevated liver enzymes, and low platelets syndrome (HELLP). Periportal fibrin deposition, hemorrhage, and hepatocellular necrosis seen in severe eclampsia. The classic histologic picture of HELLP is one of periportal or focal parenchymal necrosis, hyaline deposits, and vascular microthrombi. In some cases, fibrin exudate has been reported similar to that seen in eclampsia. Courtesy of Carolyn A Riely, MD.

precede platelet drop off in HELLP syndrome. Leukocytosis also correlates with the severity of disease.

Measurement of serum haptoglobin is the most sensitive measure of hemolysis and it will be significantly reduced in 95 to 97% of cases. Elevations in serum bilirubin do not occur in all patients and are therefore a less reliable measure of hemolysis (see Table 120-2). Other less specific measures include schistocytes and burr cells on peripheral blood smear (54 to 86%) and elevated serum lactate dehydrogenase levels.

The definitive diagnosis of HELLP syndrome requires clinical suspicion as well as timely and appropriate laboratory screening. The differential diagnosis includes other causes of hematologic and/or liver abnormalities, such as AFLP, appendicitis, viral hepatitis, gallbladder disease, gastroenteritis, ulcer disease, idiopathic thrombocytopenia purpura, hemolytic-uremic syndrome, or thrombotic thrombocytopenic purpura. Microangiopathic hemolytic anemia, thrombocytopenia, and elevated serum aminotransferase activity are essentially always seen in the HELLP syndrome. Liver biopsy is rarely needed to establish the diagnosis, and women with the HELLP syndrome may not have evidence of hepatic synthetic dysfunction (see Figure 120-2).

The clinical course of HELLP syndrome is unpredictable. Maternal complications occur in up to 65% of cases, including DIC (4 to 38%), placental abruption (10 to 16%), acute renal failure (1 to 8%), severe ascites (5 to 8%), pulmonary edema (2 to 10%), cerebral edema (1%), adult respiratory distress syndrome (ARDS, 1%), and hepatic infarction or rupture (1%). Eclampsia with maternal seizures can be seen. Events associated with maternal death include cerebral hemorrhage, cardiopulmonary arrest, DIC, ARDS, hepatic hemorrhage, and hypoxic ischemic encephalopathy.

Several authors have attempted to define and classify HELLP syndrome based upon laboratory parameters (Table 120-3). These classifications have been used to predict the rapidity of recovery, risk of recurrence, perinatal outcome, and need for plasmapheresis.

Intensive care in a tertiary care setting if appropriate remains critical to the management of HELLP syndrome. Medical stabilization and careful maternal monitoring are crucial. Ultimately, prolongation of the pregnancy would improve fetal outcome. Complete bed rest is indicated and complete reversal of symptoms with conservative treatment has been reported in individual cases. The development of DIC requires immediate delivery following correction of coagulopathy. Aggressive treatment of severe hypertension and antiseizure prophylaxis with magnesium sulfate are indicated. It may not be possible to prolong the pregnancy, and immediate delivery may be necessary. The baby should be delivered in an obstetric intensive care unit (fetal management is beyond the scope of this chapter and will not be discussed).

Corticosteroids have shown significant benefit in stabilizing maternal status, inducing fetal lung maturation, and prolonging the gestation. Optimal dosages for maternal therapy have yet to be determined. In one trial, intravenous *dexamethasone* (10 mg twice daily) was superior to intramuscular *betamethasone* (12 mg once daily) in the stabilization of maternal blood pressure, urinary output, and liver studies. This group recommended initiation of treatment in all patients with Class 1 and 2 HELLP (see Table 120-3), with discontinuation upon resolution of symptoms. *Corticosteroids* given postpartum have also been shown to accelerate maternal recovery and lower maternal morbidity.

Laboratory studies may actually worsen after delivery. Haptoglobin and LDH levels generally normalize within 24 to 48 hours postpartum. Liver enzymes return to normal within 3 to 5 days. Platelets begin to recover within 23 to 29 hours postpartum, with normalization within 6 to 11 days. Failure of the platelets to recover within the first 96 hours postpartum is an indication of a severe declining postpartum course. Plasamapheresis may be needed in this setting, however, it's use remains controversial.

Hepatic infarction is usually associated severe right upper quadrant pain, fever, and significantly elevated serum aminotransferases (1,000 IU/L or higher). Hepatic infarction and unruptured hepatic hematoma can be managed expectantly and generally resolve without sequelae. Hepatic rupture may develop in a small percentage of women (~1%) leading to massive hemoperitoneum and shock requiring early intervention by a skilled surgeon and may be an indication for liver transplantation. HELLP syndrome may lead to fulminant hepatic failure, requiring intensive care management at a specialized liver failure unit. Those patients who survive generally have no hepatic sequelae.

Overall, maternal mortality may be as high as 8%. Maternal outcome following hepatic infarction is generally favorable. When hepatic hematoma with rupture occurs, it is responsible for maternal mortality of up to 50% and fetal mortality of 60 to 70%. The risk of recurrent HELLP is about 2 to 37%, but has been reported to be as high as 61% if the prior pregnancy ended before 32 weeks.

Fetal mortality is high (8 to 37%) and is associated with placental insufficiency, fetal hypoxia, and intrauterine

Table 120-3 Hemolysis, Elevated Liver Enzymes, and Low Platelets Syndrome Classification Systems

Mississippi System	Tennessee System
Class 1—platelets < 50,000/mm^3	Complete Syndrome
Class 2—platelets 50,000 to 100,000/mm^3	AST and/or ALT > 40 IU/L
Class 3—platelets 100,000 to 150,000/mm^3	Platelets < 100,000/mm^3
hemolysis plus elevated liver enzymes	LDH > 600 IU/L
LDH > 600 IU/L	AST > 70 IU/L
	Incomplete Syndrome
	any one or two of the above

ALT = alanine aminotransferase; AST = aspartate aminotransferase; LDH = lactate dehydrogenase.

growth restriction. Prematurity at delivery also complicates fetal survival. In babies who survive, outcome is similar to children of similar gestational age.

Summary

Pregnancy-induced liver diseases carry a significant morbidity and mortality for both mother and fetus. Fortunately, with early recognition and aggressive management, survival rates have improved. A multidisciplinary approach and high level intensive care are crucial to enhanced patient outcome.

Supplemental Reading

Abell TL, Riely CA. Hyperemesis gravidarum. Gastroenterol Clin North Am 1992;21:835–9.

Audibert F, Friedman SA, Frangieh AY, Sibai BM. Clinical utility of strict diagnostic criteria for the HELLP (hemolysis, elevated liver enzymes, and low platelets) syndrome. Am J Obstet Gynecol 1996;175:460–4.

Bacq Y. Acute fatty liver of pregnancy. Semin Perinatol 1998; 22:134–40.

Bacq Y, Zarka O, Brechot JF, et al. Liver function tests in normal pregnancy: a prospective study of 103 pregnant women and 103 matched controls. Hepatology 1996;23:1030–4.

Goodwin TM. Nausea and vomiting of pregnancy: an obstetric syndrome. Am J Obstet Gynecol 2002;185(5 Suppl Understanding): S184-9.

Ibdah JA, Yang Z, Bennett MJ. Liver disease in pregnancy and fetal fatty acid oxidation defects. Mol Genet Metab 2000;71:182–9.

Kenyon AP, Piercy CN, Girling J, et al. Obstetric cholestasis, outcome with active management: a series of 70 cases. BJOG 2002;109:282–8.

Lammert F, Marschall HU, Matern S. Intrahepatic cholestasis of pregnancy. Curr Treat Options Gastroenterol 2003;6:123–32.

Magann EF, Martin JN Jr. Twelve steps to optimal management of HELLP syndrome. Clin Obstet Gynecol 1999;42:532–50.

Mattar F, Sibai BM. Preeclampsia: clinical characteristics and pathogenesis. Clin Liver Dis 1999;3:15–29.

Palmer DG, Eads J. Intrahepatic cholestasis of pregnancy: a critical review. J Perinat Neonatal Nurs 2000;14:39–51.

Rahman TM, Wendon J. Severe hepatic dysfunction in pregnancy. QJM 2002;95:343–57.

Rath W, Faridi A, Dudenhausen JW. HELLP syndrome. J Perinat Med 2000; 28:249–60.

Reyes H. Acute fatty liver of pregnancy: a cryptic disease threatening mother and child. Clinics in Liver Disease 1999;3:69–81.

Tsang IS, Katz VL, Wells SD. Maternal and fetal outcomes in hyperemesis gravidarum. Int J Gynaecol Obstet 1996;55:231–5.

Yates MR, Baron TH. Biliary tract disease in pregnancy. Clin Liver Dis 1999;3:131–46.

CHAPTER 121

Primary Biliary Cirrhosis

Jordan J. Feld, MD, and E. Jenny Heathcote, MD

Primary biliary cirrhosis (PBC) is a chronic inflammatory disease of the interlobular and septal intrahepatic bile ducts. Destruction of these small ducts leads to ductopenia and retention of bile in hepatocytes. Cholestasis causes hepatocyte damage, which promotes progressive fibrosis and eventual cirrhosis. Ultimately, liver failure and death ensue unless liver transplantation is available.

Diagnosis

Antimitochondrial Antibodies

The identification of antimitochondrial antibodies (AMAs) as the serologic hallmark of PBC greatly improved the diagnostic sensitivity and specificity of this disease. These nonorgan-, nonspecies-specific antibodies are directed at the 2-oxoacid dehydrogenase enzymes located on the inner mitochondrial membrane. Using sensitive enzyme-linked immunosorbent assay or immunoblotting, AMAs can be detected in 95% of patients with histologic and clinical features of PBC, and they are rarely associated with any other clinical condition. They may occasionally be found in otherwise clear-cut autoimmune hepatitis but, fortunately, are not seen with any other chronic cholestatic liver diseases. Along with AMAs, other laboratory features of PBC include elevation of serum alkaline phosphatase and γ-glutamyl transpeptidase, a pattern typical of anicteric cholestasis, an elevated immunoglobulin (Ig)M, and high total cholesterol.

Liver Biopsy

Because of the high degree of specificity of AMAs, some authors have questioned the need for liver biopsy in all patients with PBC. In middle-aged women with fatigue, pruritus, cholestatic enzyme pattern, high IgM, and positive AMAs, a liver biopsy is certainly not necessary to make a diagnosis of PBC. However, it does potentially provide some utility in terms of prognostication. The staging system initially introduced by Scheuer in 1967 and further developed by Ludwig and colleagues in 1978 is still in common use. The histologic pattern is graded from I to IV, with stage I disease showing only portal inflammation with duct injury (+/− granulomata) and stage IV disease representing established cirrhosis. Although it has been suggested that the disease progresses steadily from early stage to cirrhosis (about one stage per 2 years), this is not the case for all patients. In fact, there is evidence that sampling error is common in PBC. Early-stage lesions may be seen in one part of a biopsy, whereas fibrosis and/or cirrhosis are noted in other areas of the same specimen. That being said, in patients with preserved liver synthetic function (normal albumin, normal international normalized ratio, no ascites), aside from liver biopsy, there is no other means to prognosticate. Early-stage disease on biopsy, with adequate core size, is still predictive of a better outcome than the finding of significant fibrosis or cirrhosis. In addition, recent data suggest that the presence of a lymphoplasmacytic interface hepatitis portends rapidly progressive disease, and more rapidly progressive bile duct loss has been reported to precipitate liver failure even in the absence of cirrhosis. Therefore, we tend to biopsy patients at diagnosis largely for prognostic reasons unless they are over the age of 70 years or have significant other comorbid illnesses, making it unlikely that PBC will alter their life expectancy. Naturally, in cases in which the diagnosis is not crystal clear, a biopsy is imperative to confirm features typical of PBC.

Some Caveats

Along with AMAs, patients will typically have evidence of anicteric cholestasis with mild elevation of the serum aminotransferases on routine liver biochemistry. Aspartate aminotransferase and alanine aminotransferase greater than four- to five-fold normal should prompt consideration of an alternative or concomitant diagnosis. Similarly, patients who present with jaundice that subsequently resolves spontaneously are unlikely to have PBC. In such patients, investigations to exclude biliary obstruction, drug or alcohol toxicity, and viral hepatitis must be carried out. A small proportion of patients with PBC will also have evidence of autoimmune hepatitis (AIH)—so-called PBC-AIH overlap syndrome. Identification of such individuals is important because it may affect clinical management. Although no specific diagnostic criteria have been established for overlap syndrome, other suggestive features include IgG elevation (> 2 × upper limit of normal), positive smooth muscle and/or antinuclear antibodies, and, most importantly, interface hepatitis on liver biopsy.

Although corticosteroid therapy has been advocated for this group of patients, they appear to respond as well to ursodeoxycholic acid (UDCA) therapy as patients with PBC alone.

In a small number of patients, the clinical, biochemical, and histologic features of PBC will be present in the absence of AMA (even on repeated testing using highly sensitive methods). These patients tend to have circulating antinuclear antibody or smooth muscle antibodies, often in high titer. Before making a diagnosis of AMA-negative PBC, biliary tract imaging with magnetic resonance cholangiopancreatography or endoscopic retrograde cholangiopancreatography is imperative to exclude primary sclerosing cholangitis and/or biliary obstruction.

Natural History

As PBC is diagnosed at earlier and earlier stages of the disease, the natural history is becoming more clearly defined. It seems that there is likely a preclinical stage in which patients test AMA positive in serum but have normal liver biochemistry. Some of these patients will already have the histologic features of PBC on liver biopsy, and at 10-year follow-up, the majority develop cholestasis, many with symptomatic disease. Once biochemical cholestasis occurs, patients may be symptomatic or asymptomatic, and this appears to affect prognosis. The initial report on asymptomatic PBC suggested that over 10 years, 50% become symptomatic. Data from the controlled treatment trials of PBC suggest that about one-third of asymptomatic patients will develop symptoms within 5 years. The longest studies of natural history suggest that asymptomatic PBC tends to progress considerably more slowly than symptomatic PBC, with a mean survival of 8 years for symptomatic disease and 16 years for asymptomatic disease. Because many patients do not present until later life and PBC is a slowly progressive disease, it is important to consider that PBC may not affect a given individual's life expectancy. In fact, in a study from northern England, 54% of asymptomatic patients with PBC died of causes other than their liver disease.

Risk Scores

A number of risk scores have been developed to predict prognosis in PBC. None have found the severity of symptoms, titer or presence of AMA, or height of serum alkaline phosphatase or aminotransferases to be of prognostic value. In contrast, serum bilirubin has proven useful in all of the various risk scores. The most widely used risk score comes from the Mayo Clinic and, conveniently, does not require a liver biopsy to be performed for calculation. It takes into account age, serum albumin, prothrombin time, and the presence of fluid retention with or without diuretic use. The Mayo risk score has been shown to be valid in patients on UDCA therapy and those undergoing liver transplantation.

Therapy

Management of PBC can be divided into the following major components: (1) *symptomatic/preventive therapy* and (2) *disease-modifying therapy* (Table 121-1). Although much attention is focused on disease-modifying therapy, often preventive strategies and alleviation of symptoms are more important to patients.

Symptomatic Therapy

The most prevalent symptoms affecting patients with PBC are *fatigue* and *pruritus*. Both can be extremely debilitating and significantly impact on patients' quality of life.

Fatigue

Unfortunately, to date, no good therapy exists to manage fatigue in patients with PBC. There are many anecdotal reports that *UDCA* improves fatigue, and pilot studies of *methotrexate (MTX)* suggested that it may be effective for this purpose as well. Although targeted therapy may not markedly affect fatigue in PBC, it is important to ensure that there are no other contributing factors. *Hypothyroidism* is commonly associated with PBC and should be excluded. Fatigue is extremely common in the general population and is often multifactorial. It is important to take a good *sleep history* and to identify and correct any bad habits that may be worsening fatigue. Some common problems include

TABLE 121-1. Strategies for Prevention and Management of Primary Biliary Cirrhosis Symptoms and Complications

Problem	Management Strategy
Fatigue	Ensure no contributing factors, exclude hypothyroidism
Pruritis	Cholestyramine 1 pkt before and after breakfast
	Rifampicin 150 mg bid
	Naltrexone 50 mg od (use cautiously)
	Ultraviolet light exposure
Sialoadenitis/Sjögren's syndrome	Artificial teardrops
	Water, sugarless gum, pills with ++ water
	Regular dental follow-up
	Pilocarpine
Osteoporosis	All—calcium 1,500 mg/d + vitamin D 800 IU/d
	If osteoporosis—bisphosphonates
	Hormone replacement therapy (use cautiously)
	Calcitonin
Hepatocellular carcinoma	Ultrasound screening every 6 mo for cirrhotics
Esophageal varices	Screen once platelets < 200,000/μL
	β-Blocker/band ligation therapy as needed
Hypercholesterolemia	Not assisted with heart disease
	Cholestyramine (first line)
	"Statins" safe (if needed)

bid = twice daily; od = once daily.

excessive caffeine and/or nicotine use, obesity with or without sleep apnea, use of sedatives that may impair sleep quality, and lack of exercise. Often improvement of one or more of these factors may make the difference between manageable and unmanageable fatigue.

Pruritus

Although the specific cause of pruritus is unknown, there is a range of therapeutic options for this troublesome symptom. Although bile acids per se are not likely the cause of pruritus, there is clearly a pruritogen in bile. Consequently, the use of *cholestyramine* as a binding agent is generally very successful for cholestasis-induced pruritus. It is given before and after breakfast to coincide with maximal gallbladder emptying. Although effective, it is important to warn patients that it may cause constipation and that it will bind all medications taken within 4 hours of ingestion, including UDCA. If patients take *cholestyramine* in the morning, it is best that they take UDCA, calcium, and vitamin D in the evening. If cholestyramine is not well tolerated or is ineffective, the antituberculous medication rifampicin can be used. Although *rifampicin* can occasionally cause a hepatitis, this is generally seen only when used in combination with isoniazid. At the dose of 150 mg twice daily, adverse effects (aside from orange urine) are not generally seen. However, a recent report of three cases of rifampicin-induced hepatitis in patients with PBC stresses the importance of clinical follow-up in all patients on this medication. *Opiate antagonists* can be used if the above two medications are ineffective. It is believed that endogenous opioids may be overproduced in the liver in PBC and other chronic cholestatic conditions. Although reportedly effective, these agents should be used with caution because severe opiate withdrawal-type reactions have been reported. Generally, *naltrexone* is used at a dose of 50 mg daily. Some patients have also reported improved fatigue with opiate antagonists. Antihistamines should not be used to treat PBC-induced pruritus because they will not be effective and may contribute to fatigue. Exposure to ultraviolet light in the absence of sunblock is often helpful for pruritus as well. If pruritus is intractable and unresponsive to all agents, consideration of liver transplantation on this basis alone should be given. It is noteworthy that pruritus often improves as the disease progresses.

Sjögren's Syndrome

A symptom that is often underappreciated by physicians is sialoadenitis or full-blown Sjögren's syndrome. This is present in up to 93% of patients with PBC and can be quite troublesome. Patients may not report symptoms of dry eyes or dry mouth unless directly asked. Dry eyes can usually be managed with artificial teardrops. It is important that patients with complaints of dry mouth regularly see a periodontist to ensure that they do not develop gingival disease. If drinking water and chewing sugarless gum are inadequate, use of pilocarpine and other standard therapies for Sjögren's syndrome has been reported with good success. All affected individuals should be advised to swallow pills with plenty of water while standing up. Finally, women should be asked directly if they have problems with vaginal dryness because they rarely report this spontaneously. Management with lubricants is usually adequate.

In addition to the specific symptoms of PBC, it is also worthwhile to consider associated diseases. Rheumatoid arthritis; Raynaud's phenomenon with or without scleroderma; calcinosis, Raynaud's phenomenon, esophageal dysfunction, sclerodactyly, and telangiectasia (CREST syndrome); thyroiditis; and celiac disease are all associated with PBC and should be investigated as necessary.

Preventive Therapy

Because PBC is a progressive disease that often eventually results in the need for liver transplantation, it is particularly important that patients remain as healthy as possible to improve their long-term outcome. The major preventable complications of PBC include *osteoporosis* and *variceal hemorrhage*. However, it is important to counsel patients on other modifiable *lifestyle* choices as well. Particular attention should be paid to *smoking* and *obesity* because both have the potential to modify transplantation outcome.

Osteoporosis

It remains somewhat controversial whether osteoporosis is truly a complication of PBC. Although it is common among patients with PBC, this disease affects predominantly middle-aged women who are at risk for osteoporosis for other reasons. In any case, patients should be screened for osteopenia or osteoporosis using bone densitometry. All patients with PBC should take *calcium* and *vitamin D*, either as a supplement or as part of their regular diet. The bisphosphonate *etidronate* has been shown to be safe in PBC, stabilizing bone loss in corticosteroid-treated patients. Caution should be used with these agents if patients have significant esophageal varices because of the risk of esophageal ulceration. Newer-generation bisphosphonates such as *risedronate* (*Actonel*) are likely safer, although no data specifically addressing this question are currently available. Other options include *hormone replacement therapy*, which has been shown not to worsen cholestasis in PBC but must be used with caution given the recent Women's Health Initiative trial, and *calcitonin*. UDCA therapy has not been shown to improve osteoporosis in PBC.

Esophageal Varices

Unlike with most forms of chronic liver disease, the presence of esophageal varices in PBC does not necessarily indicate the presence of cirrhosis. The granulomatous destruction of the bile ducts can also obliterate small portal vein branches, resulting in presinusoidal noncirrhotic portal hypertension, similar to that seen in hepatic sarcoidosis. As a consequence, patients with PBC may have significant portal hypertension even with fairly early, noncirrhotic-stage PBC; therefore, *upper endoscopy to screen for varices* should be performed at diagnosis. If present, varices should be managed with *β-blockade* and *band ligation* as appropriate. No validated interval for variceal screening has been identified. We have shown that it is very unlikely for patients to have varices with a platelet count of ≥ 200,000/μL as a surrogate marker for hypersplenism secondary to portal hypertension. Consequently, endoscopy is performed every 1 to 2 years in those with platelets < 200,000/μL. Because variceal hemorrhage may not be a consequence of end-stage liver disease in PBC, a single bleed is generally not considered an indication for liver transplantation.

HEPATOCELLULAR CARCINOMA

Although not preventable, hepatocellular carcinoma (HCC) is another important complication of PBC that requires mention. Although the prevalence of HCC in patients with PBC ranges widely in different studies, recent data suggest that the incidence of HCC among cirrhotic patients with PBC is similar to that found in patients with hepatitis C–induced cirrhosis. Consequently, as for patients with cirrhosis from chronic hepatitis C virus infection, patients with PBC should have *screening sonograms* once they have radiographic or histologic evidence of cirrhosis.

HYPERCHOLESTEROLEMIA

One final point regarding preventive therapy is the issue of hypercholesterolemia. Increased total cholesterol is common in PBC and is believed to result from chronic cholestasis. This has naturally raised concerns about cardiovascular effects. A recent study confirmed earlier findings that there was no increased cardiac death among patients with PBC. In general, cholesterol levels will fall with cholestyramine therapy for pruritus and tend to come down as the disease progresses. If patients have other cardiac risk factors, there is no concern with using 3-hydroxy-3-methylglutaryl coenzyme A (HMG CoA) reductase inhibitors (statins), although they may not be necessary.

Disease-Modifying Therapy

Many randomized controlled trials (RCTs) of a number of different agents have been performed in patients with PBC. Because PBC is such a slowly progressive disease, it takes many years with large numbers of patients to perform an adequately powered trial of a new therapy. Unfortunately, most of the studies in PBC have been significantly underpowered and of short duration and have lacked valid end points, making the results very difficult to interpret. As a compromise, meta-analyses have been performed combining the raw data from numerous small trials. Although generally a reasonable strategy, it is important to ensure that all trials included are of similar quality; this has not always been the case.

A variety of different types of agents have been used to treat PBC. Because it is thought to be an autoimmune disease, many different *immunosuppressive agents* have been tried. In addition, *antifibrotic* and *anticholestatic agents* have been studied to see if they may slow down disease progression. Because of the likely need for very prolonged therapy to combat this slowly progressive disease, long-term complications of therapy are critical to consider. It is imperative to ensure that such complications are not worse than the disease itself.

Immunosuppressive agents that have been studied in PBC include *azathioprine, cyclosporine, MTX, prednisolone, chlorambucil, thalidomide,* and *budesonide* (Table 121-2). None of these agents have been shown to be useful in a properly conducted RCT. *MTX* has probably received the most attention because of early promising pilot studies. In the only RCT, no benefit was seen, and, in fact, the patients taking MTX had higher serum bilirubin values and Mayo risk scores with a trend to worsened survival at the end of 5 years, suggesting that MTX may, in fact, be toxic in PBC.

D-Penicillamine and *colchicine* have been studied to see if they may reduce fibrogenesis in PBC. There have been eight RCTs of *D-penicillamine*, but the results have been uniformly disappointing, with significant adverse effects and no survival benefit. *Colchicine* has been studied in three small RCTs. Although two of the three studies showed an improvement in liver synthetic function (ie, albumin and bilirubin), the benefit on histology or survival is doubtful.

URSODEOXYCHOLIC ACID

UDCA is a hydrophilic bile acid that appears to have its effect by reducing exposure of hepatocyte membranes to the toxic effects of retained endogenous hydrophobic bile acids. It also reduces bile acid absorption in the terminal ileum and up-regulates the canalicular transporter Mrp2, which may explain its pronounced effect on serum bilirubin levels. UDCA was first studied in the early 1980s, and now a total of 16 RCTs have been performed and analyzed in multiple meta-analyses. The most recent meta-analysis comes from the Cochrane Library in which Gluud and Christensen combined the data from all of these rather heterogeneous studies; treatment periods ranged from 6 months to 4 years, with a daily dose of UDCA from 7.7 to 15 mg/kg, and there was a range of disease severity. In addition, the majority of the trials (11 of 16) were of poor methodologic quality. Attempting to take all of this into consideration, the authors concluded that there was no survival benefit at 2 years, *but patients who received UDCA for 4 years or longer had a significant delay to time for liver transplantation.* Examining liver

TABLE 121-2. Disease-Modifying Agents in Primary Biliary Cirrhosis

Agent	Trials	Benefits	Adverse Effects	Comment
Azathioprine	1 uncontrolled, 1 RCT	Only seen after adjustment for baseline factors	—	Underpowered, high dropout rates, survival benefit of months after adjust for baseline factors only—questionable
Cyclosporine	2 pilot, 1 RCT	Only seen after adjust for baseline factors	Renal 9%, HTN 11%	Unequal groups at baseline, survival benefit seen after adjust baseline factors only—significant adverse events
Methotrexate	1 pilot, 1 RCT	Decreased ALP, no history or survival benefit	—	Higher Mayo risk score and bilirubin in treated patients, questionable toxicity in PBC
Prednisolone	2 RCTs	Reduced bilirubin	Significant osteoporosis	Decreased bilirubin at 3 yr, addition of bisphosphonate stabilized bone loss
Chlorambucil	1 pilot	Decreased ALP	30% dropout, BM suppression	High toxicity and very small study (13 patients)
Thalidomide	1 RCT	No	—	Only 6-mo study in 18 patients; no benefit seen
Budesonide	2 RCTs	Improved histology in early disease	Osteoporosis	Initial trial showed histology benefit; second study worse Mayo score and osteoporosis? 2° to shunting past liver
D-Penicillamine	8 RCTs	No	+++	High withdrawal rates; no benefit
Colchicine	3 RCTs	Two-thirds improved albumin/bilirubin	32% dropout in 1 study	All underpowered, high dropout; may be promising; needs further study
UDCA	16 RCTs	Survival improved at 4 yr and maybe at 2 yr	Minimal	Most recent meta-analysis less encouraging results, but questionable study inclusion

ALP = alkaline phosphatase; BM = bone marrow; HTN = hypertension; PBC = primary biliary cirrhosis; RCT = randomized controlled trial; UDCA = ursodeoxycholic acid.

histology, UDCA does not reduce existing fibrosis but does appear to slow its progression.

Based on the data to date, *UDCA is the only treatment that has any effect on long-term outcome in PBC*. Currently, a study is ongoing looking at the combination of UDCA with *MTX*, and small studies looking at other combinations have been performed in the past. *Until these data are available, UDCA remains the mainstay of treatment for this disease.* The major advantage to UDCA is that, in addition to being moderately effective, it is harmless. Rarely, patients report gastrointestinal intolerance with diarrhea or constipation, and, curiously, UDCA occasionally makes pruritus worse. Some important considerations about UDCA therapy are that the dosing is (15 mg/kg, which can be taken once daily), AMAs may disappear on therapy, and enzymes will remain elevated (albeit less elevated) in up to 50% of patients. Although patients may progress on UDCA (even if liver tests return to and remain normal) and it is tempting to try additional therapies, it is important to consider that none have been shown effective and most are associated with at least moderate adverse effects. Although this is rather conservative advice, until better data are available supporting other treatments, we would not advocate their use.

In patients who progress to liver failure despite treatment, *liver transplantation* remains the only alternative. Fortunately, patients with PBC tend to do extremely well, with > 70% with 5-year survival and > 60% with 10-year survival. Although PBC can recur in the new liver, this is uncommon and usually inconsequential. To date, no transplantations have been done for recurrent PBC, although this may be misleading because it can be difficult to differentiate between chronic ductopenic rejection and recurrent PBC.

Supplemental Reading

Caballeria L, Pares A, Castells A, et al. Hepatocellular carcinoma in primary biliary cirrhosis: similar incidence to that in hepatitis C virus-related cirrhosis. Am J Gastroenterol 2001;96:1160–3.

Corpechot C, Carrat F, Bonnard AM, et al. The effect of ursodeoxycholic acid therapy on liver fibrosis progression in primary biliary cirrhosis. Hepatology 2000;32:1196–9.

Corpochet C, Carrat F, Poupon R, Poupon RE. Primary biliary cirrhosis: incidence and predictive features of cirrhosis development in ursodiol-treated patients. Gastroenterology 2002;122:652–8.

Dickson ER, Grambsch PM, Fleming TR, et al. Prognosis in primary biliary cirrhosis: model for decision making. Hepatology 1989;10:1–7.

Gluud C, Christensen E. Ursodeoxycholic acid for primary biliary cirrhosis (Cochrane Review). Cochrane Database Syst Rev 2002;1:CD000551.

Guanabens N, Pares A, Monegal A, et al. Etidronate versus fluoride for treatment of osteopenia in primary biliary cirrhosis: preliminary results after 2 years. Gastroenterology 1997;113:219–24.

Locke GR III, Therneau TM, Ludwig J, et al. Time course of histological progression in primary biliary cirrhosis. Hepatology 1996;23:52–6.

Longo M, Crosignani A, Battezzati PM, et al. Hyperlipidaemic state and cardiovascular risk in primary biliary cirrhosis. Gut 2002;51:265–9.

Metcalf JV, Mitchison HC, Palmer JM, et al. Natural history of early primary biliary cirrhosis. Lancet 1996;348:1399–402.

Prince M, Chetwynd A, Newman W, et al. Survival and symptom progression in a geographically based cohort of patients with primary biliary cirrhosis: follow-up for up to 28 years. Gastroenterology 2002;123:1044–51.

Prince MI, Burt AD, Jones DE. Hepatitis and liver dysfunction with rifampicin therapy for pruritus in primary biliary cirrhosis. Gut 2002;50:436–9.

Tinmouth J, Tomlinson G, Heathcote EJ, Lilly L. Benefit of transplantation in primary biliary cirrhosis between 1985–1997. Transplantation 2002;73:224–7.

Wolfhagen HF, Sternieri E, Hop WC, et al. Oral naltrexone treatment for cholestatic pruritus: a double-blind, placebo-controlled study. Gastroenterology 1997;113:1264–9.

CHAPTER 122

Chronic Cholestasis and Its Sequelae

Nora V. Bergasa, MD

Cholestasis is defined as impaired secretion of bile. It is a complication of liver disease characterized by the accumulation in plasma of substances that are excreted in bile under physiological conditions, including bile acids, cholesterol, and bilirubin. In this chapter the sequelae of cholestasis with emphasis on management will be discussed.

The Pruritis of Cholestasis

Pruritus is one of the most common complications of cholestasis, but its etiology is unknown. It is a well-recognized manifestation of primary biliary cirrhosis (PBC) and primary sclerosing cholangitis (PSC), but conditions not usually associated with a serum liver profile classic for cholestasis (eg, predominantly increased activity of alkaline phosphatase and γ-glutamyl transpeptidase), including liver disease secondary to chronic hepatitis C (HC), can also be associated with pruritus. The pruritus of cholestasis can be severe; it is an indication for liver transplantation in cases of intractability.

It is inferred that the pruritus of cholestasis results from the accumulation of pruritogens that are excreted in bile under normal conditions and that accumulate in tissues, including plasma, as a result of cholestasis. In support of a hepatic origin of the pruritogen(s) is the disappearance of the pruritus after liver transplantation; in support of the biliary excretion of pruritogen(s) is the relief of the symptom after resolution of biliary tract obstruction.

Bile acids, which accumulate in tissues as a result of cholestasis, have been implicated in the pathogenesis of the pruritus. Thus far, there are no scientific data that convincingly support a role of bile acids in this type of pruritus. Histamine, which was reported to accumulate in plasma in patients with cholestasis, has also been implicated in the pathogenesis of the pruritus. The characteristics of histamine-mediated pruritus (ie, cutaneous edema and erythema), however, are absent from the skin of patients with the pruritus of cholestasis, although skin lesions secondary to chronic scratching are common.

The opiate withdrawal-like reaction that patients with cholestasis can experience after the administration of *opiate antagonists* suggests that in cholestasis central neurotransmission by the opioid system is increased. Increased opioidergic neurotransmission by pharmacologic means (eg, central administration of *morphine*) is associated with pruritus, which can be effectively treated with *opiate antagonists*. *Opiate antagonists* have been shown to decrease the pruritus of cholestasis and the behavioral manifestation of pruritus, scratching, in controlled clinical trials that applied objective methodology. These results support the idea that the pruritus of cholestasis results from increased opioidergic tone, at least in part. A central mechanism for the pruritus is hypothesized. The nature of the pruritogenic compound(s) with affinity for opioid receptors, however, is not known.

In examining patients with pruritus associated with cholestasis it is necessary to rule out contributing causes to the pruritus, including dermatological conditions, which, in contrast to the pruritus of cholestasis, manifest with pruritic skin lesions, in general. Pruritus can result from nondermatologic conditions different from cholestasis including medications, altered thyroid function, and malignancy. It is prudent, therefore, to rule out possible contributing factors to the pruritus, even in patients with cholestasis, by performing a well-planned investigation (eg, thyroid function tests, dermatologic examination).

Therapy for the Pruritis of Cholestasis

A list of some of the therapies for the pruritus of cholestasis is provided in Table 122-1.

Interventions Aimed at the Removal of the Pruritugen(s)

The interventions that aim at the removal of the pruritogen(s) in cholestasis have not been submitted to properly controlled clinical trials. *Cholestyramine*, *colestipol*, and, more recently *colesevalam*, are nonabsorbable anion exchange resins used to lower serum cholesterol. The resins are not absorbable, bind anions in the small intestine, and aim to enhance the fecal excretion of pruritogen(s). *Cholestyramine* is the most widely used medication prescribed to treat the pruritus of cholestasis. Many patients respond to *cholestyramine* with a decrease in their pruri-

TABLE 122-1. Selected Publications on the Treatment of Pruritis on Cholestasis

Medication	Aim	Dose/Mode of Administration/ Frequency	Type of Study/Duration	N	Endpoints	Results
Cholestyramine	Removal of pruritogen(s)	3.3 to 12 g/po/d	Single blind/open label/placebo controlled crossover 1 of 6 to 32 months	27	Not reported	23 patients experienced relief of symptoms*
Rifampicin	Unknown	150 mg PO bid if serum > 3 mg/dL; 150 mg PO tid if serum bilirubin < 3	Double-blind, randomized placebo-controlled crossover for 4 weeks†	9	Change in VAS*	Highly significant decrease in the 7-day summed VAS†
Nalozone	To decrease opioidergic tone	0.2 µg/kg/min IV continuous infusions preceded by 0.4 mg IV bolus	Double-blind placebo-controlled, randomized crossover for 4 consecutive days	29	Change in HAS	Geometric mean HAS 34% lower on naloxone than on placebo
Naltrexome	To decrease opiodergic tone	25 mg PO bid on day 1 followed by 50 mg PO daily	Randomized placebo-controlled for 4 weeks‡	16	Change in VAS	Daytime VAS down by 54% and nighttime VAS down by 44%
Ondansetron	To decrease in serotoniergic tone	8 mg IV (followed by 4 mg in 3 patients) on day of study	Placebo-controlled single-blind/single dose	10	Change in VAS	Decrease in mean VAS by 50% at 6 hours posttreatment
		8 mg IV followed by 8 mg PO bid	Randomized double-blind placebo-controlled for 5 days	19	Change in VAS and scratching activity index during first 24 hours	No significant difference between the effect of drug and placebo

bid = twice daily; HAS = hourly scratching activity; IV = intravenous; N = total number of patients; PO = by mouth; tid = 3 times daily; VAS = mean visual analogue scale.
*Compared with an observational control group that did not receive cholestyramine but that received norethandrolone or no treatment.
†Patients were allowed to continue taking cholestyramine; during the study, the number of cholestyramine packs per day was counted. Mean change in VAS not reported; VAS graphed per patient.
‡ Concomitant use of antipruritic medications were allowed.

tus, but some do not respond at all and some respond transiently. The use of *colesevalam* for pruritus has been published in abstract form.

Based on the assumption that the pruritogen(s) is excreted in bile, *cholestyramine* powder (4 g/dose) mixed with some fluid can be prescribed right before and after breakfast to take advantage of the pouring of the gall bladder contents into the small bowel after breaking the overnight fast. When the first 2 doses are not associated with relief of pruritus, the dosage can be increased by adding 4 g at lunch and at dinnertime. It is recommended that 16 g per day not be exceeded. The most common side effects of resin treatment are bloating and constipation. Malabsorption of fat-soluble vitamins, a complication of cholestasis (see below), may arise or may be worsened by resin treatment; accordingly, follow up of the prothrombin time (PT) and serum concentration of fat-soluble vitamins is prudent while these resins are prescribed for chronic use. Patients who take medications need to space out their intake at least 2 hours from the dose of the resin to assure drug absorption. Well-informed patients can work out the times at which they can take their drugs.

Plasmapheresis and, more recently, the technique of extracorporeal albumin dialysis (the MARS procedure) have been implemented to remove hypothetical pruritus-inducing compound(s) from the circulation. The experience with MARS is anecdotal and limited. As it relates to plasmapheresis, the effect of this procedure on the pruritus appears to be inconsistent. In general, these procedures are used in patients in whom pruritus is considered severe and/or intractable. None of these modalities have been submitted to clinical trials, which, due to the nature of the interventions, require special considerations. The idea of removing pruritogens has also led to surgical interventions such as partial external diversion of bile and ileal diversion in children with chronic cholestasis and pruritus, which was reported to be associated with a decrease in pruritus and improved quality of life. The nature of any relevant substance(s) removed by these interventions is not known.

Antihistamines

Antihistamines are frequently administered to patients with cholestasis and pruritus, although there is no evidence to support a role of histamine in this type of pruritus. Antihistamines (eg, *hydroxyzine*) do not consistently induce amelioration of the pruritus of cholestasis. Prescribing antihistamines in a patient in whom there is no relief associated with that class of drugs serves little purpose unless the sedative effect of antihistamines helps patients to sleep. A limiting factor to the use of antihistamines is the dryness of mucous membranes with which they are associated and which in patients with PBC and Sjögrens's syndrome is problematic.

Hepatic Enzyme Inducers

Hepatic enzyme inducers including *phenobarbital* and *rifampicin* are used to manage patients with the pruritus of cholestasis. The reported ameliorating effect of the pruritus of cholestasis by *phenobarbital* is not sustained for a prolonged period of time. The risk and benefits of sedation have to be taken into account when prescribing this drug. *Rifampicin* has been used to treat the pruritus since the late 1980s. At doses between 300 to 450 mg/d or 10 mg/kg, *rifampicin* has been reported to improve the pruritus of cholestasis secondary to PBC as assessed subjectively. In one of the controlled studies, this drug appeared to be more effective than *phenobarbital* in inducing ameliorations of pruritus. The mechanism of the reported antipruritic effect of *rifampicin* is unknown. There are reservations to the use of *rifampicin* to treat patients with cholestasis and pruritus because of its potential for liver toxicity. Follow-up of liver tests is necessary if this drug is to be prescribed.

Opiate Antagonists

Opiate antagonists to treat patients with the pruritus of cholestasis have been studied in controlled studies in which quantitative methodology was applied to generate an objective efficacy endpoint (change in scratching activity). Continuous infusions of the opiate antagonists *naloxone* (0.2 µg/kg/hr) preceded by 0.4 mg administered as an intravenous (IV) bolus and the oral administration of the drug *nalmefene* were associated with significant reductions in scratching activity, the behavioral manifestation of pruritus, and in its perception. These results support the hypothesis that the pruritus of cholestasis is mediated, at least in part, by a mechanism that involves the endogenous opioid system and provide a rationale for the use of opiate antagonists in the treatment of this form of pruritus. Thus, the treatment is specific. *Naltrexone*, an orally bioavailable opiate antagonist, has also been studied in clinical trials that applied subjective methodology including two placebo controlled studies. Doses of 25 mg twice a day increased to a single 50 mg dose per day were associated with decreased pruritus at short term.

A concern regarding the use of opiate antagonists in patients with cholestasis and pruritus is the opiate withdrawal-like reaction that this class of drugs may precipitate in these patients. The only opiate antagonist available in the United States for oral administration is *naltrexone*, in 50 mg capsules, which could be high at initiation of treatment in some patients. To prevent or minimize the potential opiate withdrawal-like reaction, patients can be admitted to the hospital for initiation of treatment with ultra low doses of IV *naloxone* (0.002 µg/kg/min) by continuous infusion, gradually increasing the dosage of 0.2 to 0.8 µg/kg/min for 48 hours, for example, depending on the patients' response, and to start oral *naltrexone* at the lowest possible dose. This option requires that the tablet be divided, ideally, in the hospital pharmacy (eg, 4 pieces, 12.5 mg/quarter pill). The final oral dose depends on the response of the patient. As oral *naltrexone* is introduced, the *naloxone* infusion is gradually decreased and discontinued. A recent publication on *naltrexone* in patients with alcoholism did not report hepatotoxicity; however, the potential hepatotoxicity of *naltrexone* exists, especially in patients with liver disease. Pharmacokinetic studies revealed that in decompensated liver disease, there is accumulation of *naltrexone* metabolites, but it is unusual for patients whose hepatic function has deteriorated to experience pruritus because pruritus tends to cease as synthetic function decreases. Nevertheless, monitoring of serum activity of liver-associated enzymes is recommended when patients with liver disease are treated with *naltrexone*.

Patients who are very distressed by their pruritus warrant admission to the hospital for management and for psychiatric examination for general support or treatment if suicidal actions are a concern. In these patients naloxone infusions can be tried as described above.

Serotonin Antagonists

Pruritus is a nociceptive stimulus. The serotonin system is involved in the mediation of nociception. Like the opioid system, the serotonin system may also mediate pruritus. There are no data in support of altered neurotransmission via the serotonin system in cholestasis, but increased central opioidergic tone can result in increased serotoninergic tone. *Ondansetron* is an antagonist at the type-3 serotonin receptor ($5-HT_3$), which is found both in the central nervous system and in peripheral nerves. IV bolus administrations of *ondansetron* (4 or 8 mg) were reported to be associated with a decrease in pruritus lasting for several hours in a placebo controlled study. In a short term placebo controlled study that included 18 patients, oral *ondansetron* was associated with a small, but significant decrease in pruritus, as measured by a visual analogue scale. In contrast to these studies that applied subjective methodology, in a study in which scratching activity was measured, IV *ondansetron* followed by its oral preparation was not associated with a decrease in scratching activity or in the perception of pruritus over placebo. The different results obtained in these studies may be attributable to the differences in their design, but they also emphasize the importance of behavioral methodology in studies of pruritus.

Along the lines of serotonin neurotransmission, a retrospective review published in abstract form stated that patients with PBC had reported improvements in their pruritus associated with *sertraline*, a selective serotonin reuptake inhibitor (SSRI). How a SSRI (ie, *sertraline*) as well as an antagonist at the serotonin type-3 receptor (ie, *ondansetron*) may relief the pruritus of cholestasis is not known. If these reports are confirmed in properly controlled clinical trials, studies of the serotonin system in cholestasis may be warranted.

Three patients with cholestasis were reported to experience relief of their pruritus after the administration of *dronabinol*, an agonist at the cannabinoid receptor. Experimental data suggest that the endocannabinoid system participates in the mediation of nociception, but how this relates, if at all, to pruritus is unknown.

Modalities That Escape Classification As Antipruritic Interventions

Propofol is an anesthetic with some anti-opiate activity. At subhypnotic doses, *propofol* was reported to ameliorate the pruritus of cholestasis in an open label study and in a double-blind cross-over placebo-controlled trial that included 10 patients. *S-adenosylmethionine (SAMe)* was reported to ameliorate the pruritus of cholestasis in a group of patients. It has antidepressant properties. If the antipruritic effect of *SAMe* is real, a central mood-enhancing effect of the drug, which may have an impact on how pruritus is experienced or may change the central component of pruritus, may play a role in the reported antipruritic actions. Phototherapy to the skin with ultraviolet (UV) light B is used by some clinicians. UV B treatment in erythemogenic doses is one of the treatments of psoriasis. There is no apparent rationale to use this intervention in the treatment of the pruritus of cholestasis. The effect of UV B treatment on this type of pruritus is highly questionable.
It is not possible to make general recommendations regarding the use of the treatments described in this last section because of the limited available data.

Other therapeutic modalities that have been used to treat the pruritus of cholestasis include *flumecinol, lignocaine, antioxidants,* and *androgens,* and are stated here for completion. *Ursodeoxycholic acid (UDCA)* is a drug approved to treat PBC. *UDCA* treatment may be associated with some improvement in pruritus by virtue of the impact it has on the liver disease per se. The effect of *UDCA* as a specific antipruritogen has not been studied and based on clinical trials of *UDCA* in PBC, it is uncertain; however, the choleretic effect of *UDCA* may have a beneficial impact on the pruritus by the presumed enhanced biliary excretion of pruritogen(s). Exacerbation of pruritus upon starting a regimen with *UDCA* is reported by some patients (NV Bergasa, unpublished observations).

The Fatigue of Cholestasis

Patients with cholestasis can experience fatigue, which can be profound. It is one of the most common symptoms associated with PBC. Patients with HC commonly report fatigue. It is uncertain whether the fatigue experienced by patients with HC is specific for that condition and different from the fatigue of liver disease in general.

The etiology of the fatigue of cholestasis is unknown. Central and peripheral components for the fatigue of cholestasis have been suggested. In one of the first studies that addressed fatigue in PBC, the presence of this symptom, as measured by questionnaires, was associated with poor sleep quality and with depression; this finding suggested that fatigue may be, in part, centrally mediated as it had been editorialized previously.

Increasing serotoninergic tone by the administration of *paroxetine* was associated with worse performance in male athletes on a bicycle ergometer. These results could not be explained by variations in exercise intensity or by metabolic or respiratory factors. Supporting the idea that enhanced serotonin neurotransmission may be associated with fatigue is a case report of a patient with HC and fatigue who reported increased energy level (ie, "decreased fatigue") associated with the administration of *ondansetron*, a serotonin antagonist at the type-3 receptor. Increased opioidergic tone in cholestasis (for review) may also contribute to the fatigue. In a study of patients with cholestasis, most of who had PBC, a decrease in fatigue, as assessed by a visual analogue scale, was reported after the administration of the opiate antagonist *nalmefene*. Recently, a beneficial effect of *naloxone* infusions (0.2 μg/kg/min) on the degree of fatigue, assessed by a visual analogue scale, was reported. A severe opiate withdrawal-like reaction was also reported in this patient. This side effect supports the idea of increased opioidergic tone in cholestasis.

Serotonin Antagonists

There is no specific treatment for the fatigue of cholestasis at present. The methodology to study fatigue is subjective; thus, there is substantial uncertainty in interpreting any data on fatigue. Some patients with PBC report that taking naps during the day facilitates the performance of their daily activities (NV Bergasa, unpublished). The examination of patients with fatigue and liver disease includes the exclusion of conditions that have a negative impact on energy level, including anemia, thyroid dysfunction, adrenal and renal insufficiencies, and depression, in order for specific treatments to be prescribed if those conditions are present.

The use of *ondansetron* at doses of 4 mg orally 3 times a day in patients with PBC was associated with a decrease in fatigue scores as assessed by the Fisk Fatigue Impact Score (FFIS), as published in abstract form. Headache and constipation were the most common side effects associated with ondansetron. These preliminary results may support the idea that altered serotoninergic neurotransmission contributes to the pathogenesis of fatigue in liver disease. Table 122-2 summarizes the experience with ondansetron in the treatment of fatigue to date.

Aerobic Exercise

Aerobic training increases maximal work capacity, which leads to a reduction in the percentage of total capacity required for activities of daily living. This reduction is associated with decreased fatigue. Aerobic training achieved during an 8-week structured exercise program was associated with a decrease in fatigue as assessed with questionnaires in 3 patients with chronic HC. These preliminary results support the conduct of studies of aerobic training for the treatment of fatigue secondary to liver disease.

Hypercholesterolemia

Hypercholesterolemia is a complication of cholestasis. Hypercholesterolemia has been classically reported in patients with PBC. Xanthomas and xanthelasmas can be identified in the skin of patients with PBC and hypercholesterolemia. Data available tend to suggest that high density lipoprotein is the dominant lipid fraction present in the serum of patients with PBC and hypercholesterolemia. Higher concentration of Apo(a) in the plasma of patients with PBC than in that of the control groups that have been included in the studies has been interpreted as being protective against complications secondary to atherosclerosis. The limited epidemiologic data available from retrospective studies indeed do not suggest that patients with PBC have a high risk for complications due to atherosclerosis. This observation, in conjunction with the characteristic lipid profile of PBC, has not supported the specific treatment of hypercholesterolemia in these patients. One study reported that patients with PBC and marked hypercholesterolemia were not at an increased risk for cardiovascular complications, whereas patients with moderate hypercholesterolemia were; this finding suggested the existence of protective factors in the former group. It may be that patients with PBC and hypercholesterolemia who have risk factors for adverse cardiovascular events in addition to high cholesterol benefit from treatment with lipid lowering drugs. Indeed, myocardial infarction was reported in patients with PBC in one published series. At present, there are no recommendations on the treatment of hypercholesterolemia in patients with PBC but it seems prudent to refer patients with hypercholesterolemia at risk for cardiovascular events, as determined by calculated lipid ratios, to lipid experts for an evaluation and recommendation.

PSC can also be associated with hypercholesterolemia. There is less information in PSC than in PBC from which to build recommendations regarding treatment; thus, referral to lipid experts is the best approach. It is emphasized that in contrast to PBC, there are no data suggesting a low risk for adverse cardiovascular events in patients with PSC.

Malabsorption

Cholestasis results in decreased concentrations of bile acids in the intestine. Malabsorption of fat and fat-soluble vitamins ensue when the concentration of bile acids fall below a critical micellar concentration. Deficiency of fat-soluble vitamins, A, D, E, and K, tend to correlate with duration and degree of cholestasis. Some degree of maldigestion may also exist in liver disease.

Fat Malabsorption

Fat malabsorption can accompany chronic liver disease but the degree of steatorrhea is modest, with over 70% of the ingested fat being absorbed. In patients with PBC, an association with celiac disease has been reported. Thus, in patients with PBC and suggestion of malabsorption of fat or other specific deficiencies (eg, magnesium, iron) celiac disease should be excluded because the treatment for this condition is specific (ie, gluten-free diet). Screening for

TABLE 122-2. Selected Reports on the Treatment of Fatigue of Liver Disease

Intervention	Aim	Dose/Mode of Administration/ Frequency	Type of Study/ Duration	N	Endpoints	Results
Ondansetron	To decrease serotoninergic tone	4 mg PO bid	Case report/NA	1*	NA	Increased energy level
Ondansetron	To decrease serotoninergic tone	4 mg PO tid	Double-blind randomized placebo-controlled crossover design for 4 weeks	56	Change in fatigue scores[†]	Decrease in FISS

bid = twice daily; FFIS = Fisk Fatigue Impact Score; NA = not applicable; PO = by mouth; tid = 3 times daily.
*Patients had fatigue associated with liver disease secondary to chronic hepatitis C infection.
[†]Fatigue assessed with a questionnaire from which the FFIS is derived.

celiac disease in patients with PBC and vice versa is a topic of current discussion that will not be addressed in this chapter.

Important fat malabsorption in patients with cholestasis can be treated with the administration of medium chain triglycerides. It is noted that pancreatic insufficiency can be associated with PBC, considered to result from decreased pancreatic secretion, resulting from the "dry gland syndrome" as PBC has been suggested to be. Pancreatic insufficiency requires specific treatment with supplemental pancreatic enzymes as described in another section of this book.

Vitamin Deficiencies

Vitamin A is available from animal dietary sources as retinol and from plant sources as β-Carotene. The uptake of retinol by intestinal cells is regulated by retinol binding protein. β-Carotene depends on bile acid availability in the small intestine for absorption. In addition to poor absorption secondary to bile acid deficiency, decreased availability of retinol binding protein, which results from chronic hepatobiliary disease, contributes to vitamin A deficiency because of impaired released of the vitamin from liver stores. Enhanced urinary clearance of retinol due to deficiency in transhyretin, a thyroxine binding globulin to which retinol binding globulin is bound in the circulation, may also occur. Deficiency in vitamin A usually manifests itself as impaired dark adaptation, of which patients may not be aware; accordingly, opthalmological referral is necessary for a complete examination in patients at risk for deficiency. The activation of retinol to a photochemical compound and the hepatic secretion of retinol binding protein depends on zinc; thus, it is necessary to check zinc levels and correct a deficiency if present. Oral doses of 25,000 IU/d to 30, 000 IU 3 times a week have been recommended for vitamin A supplementation. Vitamin A can be toxic to the liver and to other organs; accordingly, it has to be administered under supervision not to exceed what are considered normal levels.

The most important source of *vitamin D* in human beings is endogenous production. The metabolism of vitamin D has been reported to be normal at least in patients with PBC. These facts have suggested that in cholestasis poor exposure to sunlight by debilitated chronically ill patient is the main cause of vitamin D deficiency, in addition to its decreased absorption and renal losses of its metabolites, which can be enhanced, at least, in PBC. Vitamin D, parathyroid hormone and calcitonin regulate plasma calcium and phosphorus homeostasis, thus, these compounds may be abnormal in cases of vitamin D deficiency. Doses that have been recommended for vitamin D supplementation include 400 to 4,000 IU orally per day or 50, 000 IU orally 3 times a week. Prolonged supplementation of vitamin D can lead to hypocalcemia and soft tissue calcifications.

Naturally occurring tocopherols, which require micellar solubilization for absorption, is the most abundant source of *vitamin E* activity. Vitamin E inhibits the oxidation of unsaturated fatty acids, prevents lipid peroxidation and it is a scavenger of free radicals. Vitamin E deficiency manifests itself with a neurological syndrome characterized by peripheral neuropathy, cerebellar degeneration, and abnormal eye movements. Retinal degeneration has been ascribed to vitamins E and A deficiencies alone or combined. In children the complications of vitamin E deficiency are more severe than in adults with cholestasis. Recommendations to treat deficiency of vitamin E include 2 to 20 IU of α-tocopherol by mouth daily, 100 mg twice a day or 10 to 25 IU/kg/d.

Two forms of *vitamin K* contribute to vitamin K activity; K_1, or *phytonadione*, is found in most vegetables and K_2, a series of menaquinones, is formed by gram-positive bacteria in the intestine. Other compounds that have vitamin K activity are structurally related to *menadione*. Vitamins K_1 and K_2 require micellar solubilization for absorption in the small intestine. Vitamin K deficiency may present with coagulopathy, as measured by prolonged PT secondary to deficiency of vitamin K dependent clotting factors, or it may subclinical. Coagulopathy from vitamin K deficiency secondary to cholestasis resolves upon administration of the vitamin, which can be administered subcutaneously. Vitamin K deficiency can be corrected with doses of 1 to 10 mg of vitamin K_1 by the subcutaneous route daily for 3 consecutive days. In patients with chronic cholestasis, vitamin K deficiency may be prevented by monthly administration of 10 mg of vitamin K. The intramuscular administration of vitamin K, or of any medication, should be avoided in patients with coagulopathy because of the risk of intramuscular hemorrhage. If the coagulopathy results from hepatocellular failure, it will not resolve with treatment with vitamin K.

Prolonged treatment with *cholestyramine* for pruritus in patients with cholestasis can worsen vitamin deficiencies and can even contribute to bleeding complications secondary to coagulopathy due to deficiency of vitamin K dependent clotting factors. Vitamin supplementation is necessary is cases of deficiencies as documented by blood levels. Periodic check up of serum vitamin levels to provide sufficient but not excessive amounts can guide the process of vitamin supplementation, in general. Some of the recommended regimens to supplement vitamins when deficient are listed in Table 122-3.

Cutaneous Sequelae of Cholestasis

Hyperpigmentation

The skin of patients with cholestasis may darken. Hyperpigmentation is a classic finding in patients with PBC. The pigment is melanin. The etiology of the hyper-

TABLE 122-3. Selected Regimens for Vitamin Supplementation in Patients with Cholestasis and Vitamin Deficiencies

Deficient Vitamin	Preparation	Dose/Mode of Administration/Frequency
A	Vitamin A	30,000 IU/orally/3 times per week (105)
D	Cholecalciferol	50,000 IU/orally/3 times per week (105)
E	α-tocopherol	100 mg bid (105)
K	K$_1$	10 to 10 mg SC daily for 3 consecutive days or monthly* (112)

bid = twice daily; SC = subcutaneously.
*For patients who have chronic cholestasis.

pigmentation of cholestasis is not known. Increased availability of β-melanocyte stimulating hormone has been proposed as an etiologic factor in PBC. There are no treatments recommended for this complication.

Complications Secondary to Chronic Scratching

Excoriations and prurigo nodularis are apparent in the skin of patients who suffer from pruritus due to chronic scratching. Any of the lesions that result from chronic scratching can get secondarily infected in which case specific antibiotic treatment is indicated.

Cholelithiasis

The prevalence of cholelithiasis in patients with cirrhosis is higher than in the general population. In a series that included 23 patients with PBC, 39% were found to have gallstones. There are specific recommendations on the management of gallstones associated with symptoms, which will not be reviewed in this section; however, it is important to state that in patients with cirrhosis gallbladder surgery carries an important risk for complications. The effect of UDCA, the treatment approved for PBC, on the incidence of gallstones in this disease has not been published.

In summary, cholestasis leads to systemic complications. Metabolic complications of cholestasis tend to correlate with its degree. In contrast, pruritus and fatigue do not appear to correlate with degree of cholestasis; furthermore, they can precede the diagnosis of liver disease (eg, PBC) for years because, in part, these two symptoms may not be recognized as symptoms of liver disease Awareness of complications of cholestasis leads to their early recognition and prevention of their sequelae in many cases.

Supplemental Reading

Bachs L, Parés A, Elena M, et al. Comparison of rifampicin with phenobarbitone for treatment of pruritus in biliary cirrhosis. Lancet 1989;1:574–6.

Berg C. Use of colesevelam hydrochloride (Welchol) as a novel therapeutic agent for the management of refractory pruritus in chronic liver disease. Hepatology 2001;34:541.

Bergasa NV, Alling DW, Talbot TL, et al. Naloxone ameliorates the pruritus of cholestasis: results of a double-blind randomized placebo-controlled trial. Ann Intern Med 1995;123:161–7.

Bergasa NV, Alling DW, Talbot TL, et al. Oral nalmefene therapy reduces scratching activity due to the pruritus of cholestasis: a controlled study. Journal of the American Academy of Dermatology 1999;41:431–4.

Borgeat A, Wilder-Smith OHG, Mentha G. Subhypnotic doses of propofol relieve pruritus associated with liver disese. Gastroenterol 1993;104:244–7.

Datta DV, Sherlock S. Cholestyramine for long term relief of the pruritus complicating intrahepatic cholestasis. Gastroenterol 1966;50:323–32.

Frezza M, Surrenti C, Manzillo G, et al. Oral S-adenosylmethionine in the symptomatic treatment of intrahepatic cholestasis. A double-blind, placebo-controlled study. Gastroenterol 1990;99:211–5.

Ghent CN, Carruthers SG. Treatment of pruritus in primary biliary cirrhosis with rifampin. Results of a double-blind, crossover, randomized trial. Gastroenterol 1988;94:488–93.

Jeffrey GP, Muller DP, Burroughs AK, et al. Vitamin E deficiency and its clinical significance in adults with primary biliary cirrhosis and other forms of chronic liver disease. J Hepatol 1987;4:307–17.

Joannidis M, Bellmann R, Graziadei I, et al. In: Current indications for the albumin dialysis: intractable pruritus. 4th International Symposium on Albumin Dialysis in Liver Disease; 2002; Rostock-Warnemünde: 2002. p. 27.

Jones EA. Relief from profound fatigue associated with chronic liver disease by long-term ondansetron therapy. Lancet 1999;354:397.

Jones EA, Neuberger J, Bergasa NV. Opiate antagonist therapy for the pruritus of cholestasis: the avoidance of opioid withdrawal-like reactions. QJM 2002;95:547–52.

Lauterburg BH, Pineda AA, Dickson ER, et al. Plasmaperfusion for the treatment of intractable pruritus of cholestasis. Mayo Clin Proc 1978;53:403–7.

Longo M, Crosignani A, Battezzati PM, et al. Hyperlipidaemic state and cardiovascular risk in primary biliary cirrhosis. Gut 2002;51:265–9.

Muller C, Pongratz S, Pidlich J, et al. Treatment of pruritus of chronic liver disease with the 5-hydroxytryptamine receptor type 3 antagonist ondnsetron: a randomized, placebo-controlled, double-blind cross-over trial. European Journal of Gastroenterology and Hepatology 1998;10:865–70.

Neff GW, O'Brien CB, Reddy KR, et al. Preliminary observation with dronabinol in patients with intractable pruritus secondary to cholestatic liver disease. Am J Gastroenterol 2002;97:2117–9.

Ng VL, Ryckman FC, Porta G, et al. Long-term outcome after partial external biliary diversion for intractable pruritus in patients with intrahepatic cholestasis. J Pediatr Gastroenterol Nutri 2000;30:152–6.

O'Donohue JW, Haigh C, Williams R. Ondansetron in the treatment of the pruritus of cholestasis: a randomised controlled trial. Gastroenterol 1997;112:A1349.

Sokol RJ. Fat-soluble vitamins and their importance in patients with cholestatic liver diseases. Gastroenterol Clin North Am 1994;23:673–705.

Theal J, Toosi MN, Girlan LM, et al. Ondansetron ameliorated fatigue in patients with primary biliary cirrhosis (PBC). Hepatology 2002;36(Part 2):296A.

Turner IB, Rawlins MD, Wood P, James OF. Flumecinol for the treatment of pruritus associated with primary biliary cirrhosis. Aliment Pharmacol Ther 1994;8:337–42.

Walt R, Daneshmend T, Fellows I. Effect of stanozolol on itching in primary biliary cirrhosis. BMJ 1988;296:607.

Walt RP, Kemp CM, Lyness L, et al. Vitamin A treatment for night blindness in primary biliary cirrhosis. Br Med J (Clin Res Ed) 1984;288:1030–1.

CHAPTER 123

Primary Sclerosing Cholangitis and Cholangiocarcinoma

Paul Angulo, MD, and Gregory J. Gores, MD

Primary Sclerosing Cholangitis

Primary sclerosing cholangitis (PSC) is a chronic cholestatic disorder of unknown causation that is frequently associated with inflammatory bowel disease (IBD). PSC is characterized by diffuse inflammation and fibrosis of the biliary tree and usually leads to biliary cirrhosis, which can be complicated by portal hypertension and liver failure.

Before the widespread availability of endoscopic retrograde cholangiopancreatography (ERCP) in the late 1970s, PSC was considered a rare disease. It is now seen as an important cause of chronic cholestasis in adults and is increasingly diagnosed in the pediatric population. It is unclear whether the prevalence of the disease has increased, but emerging data suggest that it has. The recognized association of PSC and IBD and the common screening of IBD patients with liver enzymes have also probably increased the frequency with which the diagnosis of PSC is made. This greater recognition of the disease and increased experience have led to greater understanding of the course of the disease, although the cause and identification of specific beneficial therapies have eluded investigators so far.

The etiology of PSC has remained poorly understood since the earliest description of the disease. The current thinking is that PSC occurs as a consequence of a genetically determined dysregulated immune system, resulting in an uncontrolled inflammatory response in the bile ducts with destruction and fibrosis and, ultimately, biliary cirrhosis. The allo- and/or autoantigen(s) that trigger this restricted inflammatory response in the bile ducts are unknown. Putative agents include bacterial antigens absorbed through a diseased bowel mucosa, particularly in patients with underlying IBD, as well as cytotoxic bile acids, viral infections, and ischemic injury.

Clinical Manifestations, Imaging, and Histologic Features

PSC can affect any age group, and it has been described in most racial groups. It usually occurs among men twice as commonly as it does among women. The average age at diagnosis is the early forties, but the disease has been described in children as young as 1 year and adults as old as 90 years. When PSC occurs in children, however, the liver disease seems to share features with autoimmune hepatitis. The overlap of PSC and autoimmune hepatitis in adults occurs in 5% of patients. PSC can be identified in patients without symptoms who come into medical attention solely because of abnormal results of function tests. Symptoms such as jaundice, pruritus, abdominal pain, fever, and weight loss or manifestations of portal hypertension in advanced stages of liver disease are uncommon initial manifestations. Physical examination may be unrevealing. Hepatomegaly, splenomegaly, hyperpigmentation, and excoriation can be found, but patients are now coming to medical attention earlier with a diagnosis established before some of the physical findings of more advanced liver disease have developed. Health-related quality of life is significantly impaired among patients with PSC compared with individuals from the healthy population, although it is similar to other liver disease, such as primary biliary cirrhosis (PBC), and chronic infection with hepatitis B or C virus.

Chronic cholestasis of at least 6 months duration is the biochemical hallmark of PSC. Alkaline phosphatase is the most commonly elevated liver enzyme, usually to a higher level than aminotransferases, which are seldom more than 5 times normal. In children, however, aminotransferase levels may be markedly elevated. Serum bilirubin levels usually are normal, but they may be slightly elevated, and in patients with advanced PSC, they can reach very high levels. Hypergammaglobulinemia occurs in approximately 25% of patients, immunoglobulin M levels being the most commonly elevated component. About 80% of patients test positive for perinuclear antineutrophil cytoplasmic antibodies, but these antibodies can also be found in patients with PBC and autoimmune hepatitis, rendering this test nonspecific.

Typical cholangiographic findings of PSC include multifocal structuring and beading, usually involving the intrahepatic and extrahepatic biliary systems. Often the strictures are diffusely distributed and are short and annular. Cystic duct and gallbladder are affected in 15% of patients. The presence of gallbladder polypoid masses should raise the suspicion of gallbladder cancer.

Liver biopsy findings usually are not enough to establish a diagnosis of PSC. The classic onion-skin fibrosis may be seen in less than 15% of biopsy specimens but, when seen, is highly suspicious of PSC. The most commonly used histologic grading system, proposed by Ludwig and colleagues (1986), has the four following stages: stage 1, portal; stage 2, periportal; stage 3, septal; and stage 4, cirrhosis. Unfortunately, the histologic changes in patients with PSC seem to be quite varied from segment to segment of the same liver at any given point in time.

Course of Disease and Prognostic Survival Models

PSC is usually a progressive disease. An earlier study reported a median survival rate from the time of diagnosis of 12 years, which was significantly shorter than the expected survival for the age- and gender-matched general population. Patients with PSC who presented with symptoms, however, had a median shorter survival rate of about 8 years, whereas in asymptomatic patients, a median survival rate of up to 17 years has been reported in more recent studies, but survival of these asymptomatic patients is still less than expected for the general age- and gender-matched population.

Diagnosis

DIAGNOSTIC CRITERIA AND DIFFERENTIAL DIAGNOSIS

Visualization of the biliary tree is essential for establishing the diagnosis of PSC. ERCP is the diagnostic test of choice, although magnetic resonance cholangiography (MRC) is reasonably sensitive and specific for the detection of PSC and may be a more cost-effective alternative for establishing the diagnosis in patients with suspected PSC. Percutaneous approaches also can be used, but because of the frequently sclerotic intrahepatic bile ducts, gaining access to the intrahepatic biliary system by the percutaneous route can be challenging. The availability of MRC as a screening test for patients with suspected PSC made non-invasive diagnosis possible. The diagnosis criteria for PSC include typical cholangiographic abnormalities involving any part of the biliary tree, compatible clinical and biochemical findings (typically prolonged cholestasis), and exclusion of other causes of secondary sclerosing cholangitis, such as *previous biliary tract surgery, bile duct neoplasm, acquired immunodeficiency syndrome cholangiopathy, choledocholithiasis, congenital abnormalities*, history of *caustic sclerosis* of the bile ducts, *ischemic strictures* after transplantation, or *caustic* or *chemical injury* to the bile ducts caused by infusion. Liver biopsy has been used in the past to help confirm the diagnosis, although the diagnostic specificity and sensitivity of the biopsy have come under question, particularly in those patients with typical cholangiographic features of PSC. A liver biopsy with features compatible with PSC in patients with IBD and chronic cholestasis, but a normal cholangiogram, is called *small-duct PSC* and represents about 5 to 10% of histologically confirmed cases of PSC. Small-duct PSC can progress to classic PSC with typical cholangiographic features in some patients whose cases are followed for several years.

Given the uncertainty of natural history studies, prognostic models based on actual data obtained from patients at a given point in time have been developed to help more accurately predict an individual patient's prognosis. A variety of models have been created; among them, the Mayo risk score is the most widely used. The Mayo PSC risk score is calculated by the following formula:

$$R = 0.03 \text{ (age in years)} + 0.54 \times \log \text{ (bilirubin in mg/dL)} + 0.54 \times \log \text{ (aspartate aminotransferase [AST] in U/L)} + 1.24 \text{ (history of variceal bleeding)} - 0.84 \times \text{ (albumin in g/dL)}$$

Thus, a 50-year-old man with a serum bilirubin of 5 mg/dL, an AST of 140 U/L, one prior gastrointestinal bleed, and an albumin of 2.8 g/dL would have a Mayo PSC risk score of 1.92. If this patient had another episode of variceal bleeding, his Mayo risk score would increase significantly, even if all other parameters remained unchanged.

Treatment

MANAGEMENT OF COMPLICATIONS OF PSC

Pruritis Although not common, pruritus can be disabling and associated with a diminished quality of life, but its severity does not parallel the severity of the liver disease. *Cholestyramine* (4 g 3 to 4 times daily), several antihistamines, and *rifampicin* (150 to 900 mg by mouth daily), as well as opioid receptor antagonists (*naltrexone* 50 mg by mouth daily), have been used with varying results to treat patients with cholestatic pruritus. First-line therapy is usually *cholestyramine*; however, *rifampicin* is effective and is frequently needed for patients not responding to the bile acid binding resins. There is a separate chapter on chronic cholestasis (see Chapter 122, "Chronic Cholestasis and Its Sequelae").

Vitamin Deficiency As many as 40% of patients are deficient in vitamin A, whereas 14% are deficient in vitamin D and 2% are deficient in vitamin E. These vitamin-deficient patients should receive vitamin replacement therapy (vitamin A, 100,000 IU PO per day for 3 days, then 50,000 IU/day PO for 14 days; vitamin D, 25,000 to 50,000 U 2 to 3 times a week; vitamin E, 400 U daily). Vitamin K deficiency is uncommon, but if suspected, a short trial of water-soluble vitamin K (*Mephyton* [phytonadione], 5 mg/dL) can be considered. If the prothrombin time responds after a few doses, long-term therapy should be recommended.

Osteoporosis Metabolic bone disease, usually caused by osteoporosis instead of osteomalacia, is relatively common in patients with PSC. Glucocorticoids used to treat accom-

patients, but there are exceptions where these may be present earlier on, even under the age of 10 years, or are present in conjunction with symptoms of liver disease.

The diagnosis of Wilson's disease is established by the presence of KF rings and a decreased level of serum ceruloplasmin, KF rings and neurologic or psychiatric symptoms, and in those with liver disease and appropriate histology, an elevated hepatic copper (typically > 250 µg/g dry weight). Urinary copper excretion is elevated above 100 µg/24 h in most symptomatic patients, and in those with fulminant hepatic failure (FHF) due to Wilson's disease. Genetic studies, haplotype or polymorphism analysis can identify affected siblings with the caveat that the diagnosis must be first firmly established in the proband. Direct identification of *ATP7B* mutations is possible, but limited by the size of the gene and the greater than 250 disease causing mutations and the limited availability of this testing (http://www.uofa-medical-genetics.org/wilson/index.php). In populations with a high frequency of specific mutations, molecular diagnostic testing for these mutations is useful.

The management of Wilson's disease depends upon the firm establishment of the diagnosis because treatment is lifelong. Therapy is directed at the removal of copper or the prevention of its further accumulation in the liver and in other body sites where it may be injurious.

Treatment options for Wilson's disease include medical therapy with oral chelating agents or zinc, and liver transplantation. Dietary restrictions in copper intake are recommended along with medical therapy, especially during the initial phase of treatment. The chelating agents *penicillamine* and *trientine* promote renal copper excretion and are recommended as first line therapy for symptomatic patients with hepatic or neurological disease. These chelating agents may be used at lower dosages for maintenance therapy. *Tetrathiomolybdate* is an effective copper chelator that is under investigation for initial treatment of patients with neurologic disease. *Zinc* functions by blocking copper absorption from the gut by induction of the endogenous chelator *metallothionein* in enterocytes. Zinc is mainly used for maintenance therapy or initial therapy for asymptomatic patients, but may also have a role as an adjunct to initial chelation therapy. Liver transplantation restores a normal phenotype with respect to copper metabolism, and therapy specific for Wilson's disease is no longer required.

Management of Wilson's Disease

Hepatic Disease

Patients with liver disease may be asymptomatic or they may experience symptoms of chronic liver disease, such as fatigue or jaundice, or manifest signs or symptoms of portal hypertension, such as ascites and varices without or with bleeding. Some may have chronic hepatitis with features indistinguishable from autoimmune hepatitis. In about 5%, the sudden onset of jaundice or ascites with associated hemolysis heralds the onset of acute FHF.

Patients that are asymptomatic with compensated liver disease may be treated with *zinc monotherapy* or with a *chelating agent*, typically *trientine* or *penicillamine* (see Table 124-2). *Tetrathiomolybdate* is a very potent chelator that may be useful for initial therapy for patients with Wilson's disease, however it is still undergoing further testing and is not commercially available in the United States. Patients with active disease should be treated initially with a chelator or a chelator with zinc supplementation. Chelation therapy must be begun slowly and with careful monitoring for side effects. Specific concerns for penicillamine are hypersensitivity reactions and marrow suppression. For patients with complications of the chronic liver disease due to Wilson's disease additional therapy is the same as that for other chronic liver diseases. The most common problems are that associated with portal hypertension or with portosystemic shunting. Patients with ascites are treated with *diuretics*; those with variceal bleeding are treated with β-*blockers, somatostatin infusion, endoscopic band ligation,* and *portosystemic shunting,* or *liver transplantation.* Encephalopathy is present in the acute fulminant setting, or in patients with end-stage liver disease. In this latter group, encephalopathy may exacerbate neuropsychological symptoms due to the Wilson's disease, and should be considered and treated separately.

For Wilson's disease patients with liver disease, the initial period of treatment with a chelator should range from 2 to 12 months, with close monitoring maintained during this initial period of treatment. For most patients, there is a general trend towards stabilization of hepatic function over the first 8 weeks of therapy. Biochemical parameters of hepatic inflammation and insufficiency should show a trend towards gradual improvement over the next 6 to 12 months, though may improve further for up to about 4 years after the initiation of treatment in some individuals. For those with ascites and edema that respond to the primary treatment of the Wilson's disease, requirements for diuretics decrease with time. Similarly, the need for treatment of encephalopathy, if necessary, may also improve with primary treatment for Wilson's disease. Once stabilization is achieved, then either the chelator can be continued at a reduced dosage, or patients can be maintained on zinc therapy. For those individuals with severe hepatic insufficiency but not fulminant liver failure due to Wilson's disease, a trial of medical therapy is warranted. However these individuals should also be followed by a liver transplantation center because some may fail to respond to therapy or suffer serious complications of their liver disease before stabilization.

Patients presenting with FHF due to Wilson's disease typically have a nonimmune hemolytic anemia, relatively low

TABLE 124-2. Therapies for Wilson's Disease

Medication	Mode of Action	Dosages (total/24 h)	Adverse Effects
d-Penicillamine (Cuprimine)	Chelating agent, induces cupriuresis	750 to 2000 mg in 2 to 3 divided doses apart from meals; maintenance 750 to 1000 mg; requires supplemental pyridoxine	Worsening of neurologic symptoms in 10 to 50% after initiation of treatment; initial hypersensitivity reactions; marrow suppression; lupus-like syndrome; nephrosis; dermatologic toxicity; rare Goodpastures syndrome
Trientine (Syprine)	Chelating agent, induces cupriuresis	750 to 1500 mg in 2 to 3 divided doses apart from meals; maintenance 750 to 1000 mg	Lupus-like syndrome; nephrosis; marrow suppression
Zinc (Galzin)	Blocks intestinal copper uptake by enterocytes	75 to 150 mg in 2 to 3 divided doses apart from meals	Gastric irritation

alkaline phosphatase level compared to total bilirubin (ratio < 4), aminotransferases less than 500 IU/L and significant hypoalbuminemia and coagulopathy. In this setting, urine and hepatic copper concentrations are markedly elevated. Liver transplantation is lifesaving for these individuals, and most have good long term survival. While awaiting a donor liver, the use of albumin dialysis, plasma exchange or plasmapheresis, or other devices equipped for these functions will acutely lower serum copper that was released into the serum by the severe hepatocellular injury. Although these treatments may help decrease hemolysis and the continued insult to the liver and other organs, specifically the kidneys, they have not been shown to eliminate the need for transplantation. Wilson's disease accounts for approximately 5% of all patients presenting with acute liver failure (ALF) worldwide.

Special consideration must be made for patients who become pregnant or are contemplating pregnancy while being treated for their Wilson's disease, and for those Wilson's disease patients who are undergoing elective surgical procedures. Treatment of Wilson's disease must continue through pregnancy. Successful pregnancies have been reported with patients using penicillamine, trientine, and zinc. FHF has occurred following discontinuation of therapy during pregnancy. No dosage reduction is needed for zinc therapy, whereas the smallest effective dosage of penicillamine or trientine should be administered during pregnancy and afterward in those who undergo cesarean section to promote wound healing. A separate issue is the potential problem of portal hypertension and varices and the risk of variceal bleeding in pregnancy, a state where vascular volume typically increases. If varices are detected, patients should be treated with a β-blocker with the consent of the obstetrician. In Wilson's disease patients undergoing elective surgical procedures, dosages of chelating agents should be minimized until wound healing is achieved. Zinc dosages should remain unaltered for those undergoing elective surgery.

Neurologic Disease

Neurologic manifestations of Wilson's disease are due to copper induced injury of the brain. The main sites for copper-induced injury are the basal ganglia, but many different parts of the brain may be affected. Neurologic symptoms may include *impaired motor coordination, tremor, drooling, dysarthria, dystonia,* and *spasticity.* Autonomic dysfunction has recently been recognized in some patients with other neurological manifestations of Wilson's disease. KF rings are present in approximately 98% of patients with neurologic and psychiatric Wilson's disease, and are often accompanied by abnormalities detectable on magnetic resonance imaging or computed tomography imaging of the brain.

Treatment of the patient with neurologic manifestations of Wilson's disease, although focused on treatment of the underlying Wilson's disease, should also include potential therapies aimed at symptomatic relief or prevention of complications that may result from the neurologic disease. Treatment of the Wilson's disease with *penicillamine* has resulted in worsening disease and irreversible neurologic damage in some patients. However worsening can occur even with *trientine* or with *tetrathiomolybdate,* though it is thought to occur at a reduced rate compared to penicillamine. Stabilization and then improvement in signs and symptoms of the disease occurs with time. Most improvement occurs in the first 24 to 48 months, though continued slow improvement may occur up to 4 years following start of therapy for Wilson's disease.

Several problems are more frequently encountered in patients with significant neurologic disease. The presence of *dysphagia* necessitates precautions against aspiration, and measures to enhance swallowing, or the use of enteral feedings sometimes must be considered. *Dystonia* can lead to great discomfort or contractures, and use of muscle relaxants or direct injection of muscle groups with *botulinum toxin* can give relief. *Dysarthria* can inhibit communication, and assistance from a speech therapist may be helpful in improving certain aspects of speech. The use of a signboard or electronic communication devices has helped for some individuals. Physical and occupational therapy may help maintain strength and assist with problems with coordination. Tremor can at times be disabling, and muscle relaxants or other therapies may be sought. Some patients may have the severe *bradykinesia* and gait disturbance of *parkinsonism.* In these individuals, consultation with a neurologist with an interest in movement disorders can be helpful in characterizing the degree of disability and its course during treatment, and in assisting the patient with therapies directed at the neurological symptoms.

Psychiatric Disease

Psychiatric symptoms due to Wilson's disease range from *behavioral changes* and *anxiety disorders* to *depression* and *psychosis*. In very young patients, the initial manifestations of psychiatric symptoms may be behavioral problems, withdrawal, and difficulty concentrating or performing higher cognitive tasks. In some patients, the psychiatric symptoms may precede any other symptoms of the disease. In adults, depression is the most commonly recognized symptom, occurring even in treated patients. There may be components of reactive depression in some newly diagnosed individuals to the realization that they are afflicted with a chronic illness or disability, or there may be no apparent trigger for the depression. The failure to recognize psychiatric symptoms in patients can lead at times to serious consequences. Depression can deepen and patients can become suicidal. In some, psychosis may be severe and require inpatient psychiatric attention.

Treatment of psychiatric signs and symptoms in patients with Wilson's disease requires the treatment of the underlying disease, but may also necessitate the use of specific therapies aimed at the treatment of the psychiatric disorder. Counseling, including family counseling, may be very helpful for some individuals. The use of pharmacotherapy for depression, anxiety or psychosis associated with Wilson's disease should be guided by psychiatrists, though initiation of therapy with antidepressants and anxiolytics by internists or other medical specialists while formal consultation is awaited may be warranted.

Prognosis

Medical treatment of asymptomatic patients prevents the development of liver or neurologic disease. The long term survival of patients with Wilson's disease with medical therapy is excellent, even when chronic liver disease and cirrhosis are present at the outset. Patients with cirrhosis still may manifest signs or symptoms due to portal hypertension, including esophageal or gastric varices or ascites. In some patients, neurologic symptoms may improve with therapy, whereas in others they may worsen during the initial phase of treatment or patients may develop neurologic disease no longer responsive to therapy aimed at Wilson's disease.

Liver transplantation also offers excellent survival approaching 90% for patients with ALF due to Wilson's disease, well above the survival of approximately 60% for all others transplanted for fulminant liver failure. Patients with Wilson's disease surviving beyond 1-year post-liver transplant typically have excellent long term survival.

Supplemental Reading

Brewer GJ, Dick RD, Johnson VD, et al. Treatment of Wilson's disease with zinc: XV Long-term follow-up studies. J Lab Clin Med 1998;132:264–78.

Brewer GJ, Dick RD, Johnson VD, et al. Treatment of Wilson's disease with zinc XVI: treatment during the pediatric years. J Lab Clin Med 2001;137:191–8.

Brewer GJ, Hedera P, Kluin KJ. Treatment of Wilson's disease with ammonium tetrathiomolybdate: III. Initial therapy in a total of 55 neurologically affected patients and follow-up with zinc therapy. Arch Neurol 2003;60:379–85.

Brewer GJ, Johnson VD, Dick RD, et al. Treatment of Wilson's disease with zinc. XVII: treatment during pregnancy. Hepatology 2000;31:364–70.

Emre S, Atillasoy EO, Ozdemir S, et al. Orthotopic liver transplantation for Wilson's disease: a single center experience. Liver Transpl 2001;72:1232–6.

Roberts EA, Schilsky ML. A practice guideline on Wilson disease. Hepatology 2003;37:1475–92.

Schilsky ML. Wilson's disease—genetic basis of copper toxicity and natural history. In: Tavill AS, Bacon BR, editors. Seminars in liver disease. Vol. 16. New York: Thieme Medical Publishers Inc; 1995. p. 83–95.

Shah AB, Chernov I, Zhang HT, et al. Identification and analysis of mutations in the Wilson disease gene (*ATP7B*): population frequencies, genotype-phenotype correlation, and functional analyses. Am J Hum Genet 1997;61:317–28.

Sternlieb I. Wilson's disease and pregnancy. Hepatology 2000;31: 531–2.

CHAPTER 125

HEREDITARY HEMOCHROMATOSIS

STEPHEN A HARRISON, MD, AND BRUCE R BACON, MD

Iron overload is commonly seen in clinical practice and can be divided into two distinct categories based on specific etiology and distribution of iron loading within the liver (Table 125-1). Primary iron overload is due to inherited metabolic defects that result in inappropriate iron absorption relative to total body iron stores, and is termed hereditary hemochromatosis (HH). Iron overload not associated with known genetic defects is called secondary iron overload and typically results from ineffective erythropoiesis, hepatic diseases that predispose to associated iron loading, and parenteral iron loading (Harrison and Bacon, 2003). The diagnosis and management of HH will be discussed in this summary of iron overload.

The most common form of HH has an autosomal recessive inheritance pattern and is found in approximately 1 in 250 persons of northern European descent. The inheritance pattern of HH was originally described by Joseph Sheldon in 1935, but the specific genetic defect went unrecognized until 1996, when the *HFE* gene was cloned. The *HFE* gene encodes for a major histocompatibility complex class 1-like protein, and mutations in this gene result in excessive iron absorption and subsequent deposition in organs such as the liver, pancreas, other endocrine organs, heart, joints, and skin (Feder et al, 1996). It is now known that the HFE protein binds with β_2-microglobulin (β_2M), which together interact with transferrin receptor-1, thereby affecting cellular iron transport. Mutations in the *HFE* gene alter the cellular trafficking of HFE protein and the interaction with β_2M, resulting in inappropriate iron absorption. The exact cellular mechanism(s) by which this occurs are currently being investigated (Parkkila et al, 2001).

Two major missense mutations of *HFE* have been identified. The first mutation results in the change of the amino acid cysteine to tyrosine at position 282 (*C282Y*). The second mutation results in the change of the amino acid histidine to aspartate at position 63 (*H63D*). Studies have demonstrated that approximately 85% of patients with typical HH phenotype are homozygous for the *C282Y* mutation. Additionally, 3 to 5% of these patients are compound heterozygotes (*C282Y/H63D*). In addition to *HFE*-associated HH, it is now recognized that non–*HFE*-associated HH can result from mutations in other iron-related genes such as the following: (1) ferroportin-1, which is involved in export of iron across the basolateral membrane of the duodenal enterocyte, (2) transferrin receptor-2, which is primarily expressed in hepatocytes, and (3) hepcidin, which is a peptide synthesized in the liver that down-regulates iron absorption.

Historically, HH was diagnosed if patients had abnormal iron studies with stainable iron in hepatocytes on liver biopsy and/or if patients had symptomatic disease with development of end-organ damage, including cirrhosis, heart failure, diabetes, arthritis, or skin pigmentation. The availability of commercial tests for the *C282Y* and *H63D* mutations of *HFE* provides an important diagnostic tool in patients with iron overload (Tavill, 2001). However, recent large population studies indicate that a substantial proportion of *C282Y* homozygotes do not have clinically

TABLE 125-1. Iron Overload Conditions

Hereditary Hemochromatosis
  HFE-associated
    C282Y/C282Y
    C282Y/H63D
    Other *HFE* mutations
  Non-*HFE*-associated
    Juvenile hemochromatosis (*HFE* 2)
    Transferrin receptor-2 mutations (*HFE* 3)
    Ferroportin 1 mutations (*HFE* 4)
Secondary Iron Overload
  Acquired iron overload
    Iron-loading anemias
      Thalassemia major
      Sideroblastic anemia
      Chronic hemolytic anemia
      Aplastic anemia
      Pyruvate kinase deficiency
  Pyridoxine-responsive anemia
    Parenteral iron overload
      Red blood cell transfusions
      Iron-dextran injections
      Long term hemodialysis
  Chronic liver disease
    Porphyria cutanea tarda
    Hepatitis C
    Hepatitis B
    Alcoholic liver disease
    Nonalcoholic steatohepatitis

significant iron overload (Beutler et al, 2002). Thus, the *C282Y* mutation has incomplete penetrance and additional genetic modifiers may influence the impact of *C282Y*.

Clinical Features of HH

Before the advent of genetic testing, the diagnosis of HH was based on the recognition of symptoms and physical examination findings of iron overload. Currently, most patients with HH are detected at a much earlier stage, prior to the development of end-organ damage, as a result of (1) routine health maintenance examinations, which include testing for serum iron, ferritin and liver enzymes, (2) genetic testing of relatives of a HH patient as part of family screening, and (3) population studies of either serum iron studies or of *HFE* mutations. When individuals are identified in these ways, the vast majority are asymptomatic.

In normal individuals, approximately 1 mg/d of dietary iron is absorbed to maintain a total body iron storage pool of 2 to 3 g. This absorption rate maintains homeostasis, as daily iron loss is approximately 1 mg/d. In *HFE*-associated HH, iron absorption is increased, with about 1.5 to 2.5 mg/d of iron being absorbed through the duodenum. Although the rate of accumulation of iron is variable in *HFE*-associated HH, total iron stores of > 20 g are usually required to develop symptomatic disease.

Those patients who are *symptomatic* at the time of diagnosis tend to be *older* than 40 years of age and are predominantly *male*. Weakness, lethargy, abdominal pain, arthralgias, and loss of libido are common. The *arthropathy* seen in *HFE*-associated HH tends to be symmetric and involves multiple joints. Specifically, the proximal interphalangeal, metacarpophalangeal, wrist, knee and vertebral joints are most commonly involved. *Hepatomegaly* and *cirrhosis* may be present, along with skin *pigmentation* and *clinical diabetes*.

However, patients identified through routine screening physicals and familial screening typically are much less symptomatic (Bacon and Sadiq, 1997). The most common symptom in one study evaluating HH patients discovered by familial screening was *arthralgias* and *loss of libido*. The most common clinical finding was *diabetes*.

Diagnosis of HH

Three groups of patients will present clinically for evaluation of HH. The first group includes symptomatic patients presenting with stigmata of chronic liver disease and elevated iron indices. This group also includes diabetic patients with hepatomegaly, patients with evidence of cardiac dysfunction, skin pigmentation or sexual dysfunction, and patients presenting with de novo sexual dysfunction or symmetric polyarthropathy. The second group comprises asymptomatic patients who present with abnormal iron indices, incidentally discovered hepatomegaly, or imaging studies of the liver suggesting iron deposition. The third group consists of first degree relatives of patients with known HH.

Blood Iron Studies

Once there is some degree of clinical suspicion or in a patient for whom screening studies are proposed, initial examination should include a fasting transferrin saturation and a ferritin level. A fasting serum sample is preferred as serum iron may be elevated following meals and has a diurnal variation. Transferrin saturation (TS) is calculated by dividing the serum iron level by the total iron binding capacity or transferrin. A TS > 45% is commonly used as a trigger for *HFE* mutation analysis. Serum ferritin is also helpful, but lacks specificity as it is often elevated in systemic inflammatory processes. The TS and ferritin are best used in combination.

Genetic Testing

Genetic testing for *HFE* mutations should be performed in all patients with elevated TS and ferritin as well as in first degree relatives of patients with *HFE*-associated HH. Those relatives determined to be homozygous for the *C282Y* mutation should be carefully assessed for evidence of iron overload. Individuals who are compound heterozygotes (*C282Y/H63D*) should also be examined for iron overload and for clinical evidence of concomitant liver disease, and a liver biopsy may be useful in these patients.

Liver Biopsy

Liver biopsies are no longer required to make a definitive diagnosis of HH and are much less commonly performed in suspected HH. However, a liver biopsy can be helpful in several different ways, including the following: (1) it gives the clinician an assessment of the amount of iron and its cellular and lobular distribution, (2) it provides an important assessment of hepatic fibrosis, and (3) it allows for the investigation of other concomitant liver diseases that may not be readily detectable using noninvasive analysis.

The hepatic iron concentration (HIC) can be measured in fresh or paraffin-embedded biopsy material, and the normal level is less than 1,500 μg/g dry weight. Evidence suggests that most patients with *HFE*-associated HH do not develop hepatic fibrosis until the HIC exceeds 14,000 μg/g dry weight; concomitant ethanol consumption is a potentiating factor in the development of cirrhosis in patients with iron overload (Fletcher et al, 2002).

Although liver biopsy can provide useful information, it remains an invasive test with well-documented risks. Consequently, recent studies have evaluated several clinical and biochemical factors in an attempt to predict the absence of cirrhosis in patients with *HFE*-associated HH to obviate the need for liver biopsy. It has been reported that *C282Y* homozygotes with serum ferritin levels < 1000 ng/mL, with normal liver enzymes, and who are < 40 years of age are unlikely to have cirrhosis, so that liver biopsy may be unnecessary in such patients (Bacon et al, 1999).

Treatment of Hemochromatosis

Therapy for HH is relatively simple and quite effective. Phlebotomy has been shown to effectively remove excess iron stores without significant side effects. If therapeutic phlebotomy is started before the development of cirrhosis, morbidity and mortality are significantly reduced. Some clinical features of iron overload respond better to phlebotomy than others. Malaise, fatigue, abdominal pain, skin pigmentation, and insulin requirements in diabetic patients tend to improve, whereas arthropathy and hypogonadism are less responsive. Given these findings, early identification and initiation of therapeutic phlebotomy should be the goal.

Therapeutic phlebotomy (500 mL of blood) should be initiated weekly with approximately 250 mg of iron removed with each unit of blood. Some patients can tolerate biweekly phlebotomy; in contrast, some petite older women can only tolerate half a unit every other week. The goal should be to continue weekly phlebotomy until the patient's serum ferritin level is < 50 ng/mL and the transferrin saturation is < 50%. Before each phlebotomy, the hematocrit should be checked. According to the American Association for the Study of Liver Diseases practice guidelines, the hematocrit should not fall > 20% with each phlebotomy. In the uncomplicated patient, each unit of blood removed will result in a decrease in the serum ferritin level by about 30 ng/mL. This can be used as a rough guideline to predict phlebotomy requirements to deplete excess iron stores. It is important to remember that some patients with symptomatic HH may have in excess of 30 g of stored iron, and thus may require several years of weekly to biweekly phlebotomy to remove the excess stored iron. The goal of treatment is not to make patients iron deficient and/or anemic, but rather to deplete excess iron stores and to achieve serum iron values in the low normal range.

Once initial therapeutic phlebotomy has been accomplished, maintenance phlebotomy should be performed. In most patients, one unit of blood should be removed every 2 to 4 months with subsequent assessment of iron status by measuring serum ferritin and transferrin saturation. Some patients will require more frequent maintenance phlebotomies, whereas others will be on a less frequent maintenance schedule.

Occasionally, patients with significant iron loading will present with anemia that precludes frequent phlebotomy. This rarely occurs in HH, and is more often seen in patients with anemia due to ineffective erythropoiesis with secondary and/or parenteral iron overload when it can be used. In these patients, chelation therapy may be warranted. Chelation therapy with deferoxamine using continuous subcutaneous infusion results in urinary excretion of 50 to 100 mg iron per day. However, it should be noted that phlebotomy remains the easier, quicker, and less expensive therapy for iron reduction.

Cirrhosis does not improve with iron reduction therapy. Despite therapeutic phlebotomy, hepatocellular carcinoma (HCC) continues to be a threat in patients who have cirrhosis. In fact, HCC accounts for about 30% of all deaths in HH patients. Orthotopic liver transplantation is a viable alternative for patients who develop decompensated liver disease due to HH. However, it is important to note that in undetected and thus untreated HH patients, the post-transplant survival rate is lower than for other types of chronic liver disease, largely in part to increased perioperative cardiac and infection-related complications.

Family Members Screening for Hemochromatosis

All first degree relatives of patients with *HFE*-associated HH should be offered screening for HH. Screening of adults should include both a genetic test for *HFE* mutations and serum iron studies to measure fasting transferrin saturation and ferritin. The tested relative is unlikely to have HH if the fasting iron studies are normal and the patient is neither homozygous for the *C282Y* mutation or a compound heterozygote (*C282Y/H63D*). Alternatively, if the tested relative is either homozygous for the *C282Y* mutation or is a compound heterozygote with an elevated ferritin or transferrin saturation, then the patient has HH and a therapeutic phlebotomy program should be initiated. Screening of minors raises the potential for genetic discrimination in regards to future insurance and/or job candidacy. Therefore, it is appropriate to first perform *HFE* analysis in the other parent. This may obviate the need to test the children if the other parent has no *HFE* mutations. Family screening for *HFE* mutations has been shown to be beneficial. Recent studies have shown grade 3 or 4 iron stores on liver biopsies in > 25% of siblings; 10 to 15% had some degree of hepatic fibrosis with 3% having cirrhosis.

Population

It has been suggested that population screening using genetic testing might be ideally suited for *HFE*-related HH. This is because the disorder is common, there is a long latent phase before the development of disease manifestations, treatment is simple, safe, and effective and tests of phenotypic markers are available. However, it has quickly become apparent that not all *C282Y* homozygotes have phenotypic expression and this raises questions about the advisability of large scale population screening. A recent study by Beutler and colleagues (2002) of 41,038 subjects from the San Diego area showed that about 25% of males and about 50% of females who are *C282Y* homozygotes do not have an elevated ferritin level. This suggests that there are large numbers of *C282Y* homozygotes that do not have evidence of phenotypic expression. As a result of these and other studies, it has been suggested that population screening using genetic testing may not be appropriate.

Liver Disease Patients

Studies evaluating the frequency of *HFE* mutations and abnormalities in iron metabolism have been done in groups of patients with porphyria cutanea tarda (PCT), nonalcoholic steatohepatitis (NASH), chronic hepatitis C (HC), and alcoholic liver disease (ALD). In PCT, about half the patients have mutations in *HFE* and it is well known that this disorder responds favorably to iron reduction therapy by phlebotomy. Accordingly, all patients with PCT should have *HFE* mutation analysis and serum iron studies performed. In ALD, it appears that *HFE* mutations are not responsible for the mild degrees of secondary iron overload that are occasionally seen in this disorder. Also, there is no clear benefit by phlebotomy therapy in patients who have ALD with our without abnormalities in iron metabolism. In patients with chronic HC, about a dozen studies have been performed looking at *HFE* mutations and parameters of iron metabolism. Almost all studies have shown the same prevalence of *HFE* mutations in patients with HC as in control populations; some studies have shown a relationship between increased iron and *HFE* mutations, as well as in worse liver disease with increased fibrosis. At the present time, it is recommended that if iron studies are performed in patients with HC and they are abnormal, then *HFE* mutation analysis should be considered. Finally, in NASH the data are mixed showing that some groups of patients have an increased frequency of *HFE* mutations and there are some data suggesting benefit of phlebotomy therapy. More formal and complete studies still need to be performed.

Summary and Conclusions

HH is a common disorder that is increasingly being recognized in clinical practice. The quality of diagnosis has been improved with the use of genetic testing that has come about since the gene for hemochromatosis was discovered in 1996. Over the last few years, we have learned that approximately 50% of patients who are *C282Y* homozygotes may not have evidence of phenotypic expression. Also, many other patients will have mild degrees of iron overload. Because iron overload is so easy to treat, it makes sense to use phlebotomy as definitive therapy for patients even if they have mild degrees of iron loading. The use of genetic testing (*HFE* mutation analysis) has superseded the use of *HLA*-typing in the performance of family studies once a proband was identified, and its use in population surveys is still being debated. Finally, the reasons for the differences in phenotypic expression in patients who are genotypically identical (*C282Y* homozygotes) probably relates to other genetic abnormalities identified in genes involved in cellular iron transport.

Supplemental Reading

Bacon BR, Britton RS. Hereditary hemochromatosis. In: Feldman M, Friedman LS, Sleisenger MH, and Scharschmidt BF, editors. Sleisenger and Fordtran's gastrointestinal and liver disease. Vol. 2. 7th ed. Philadelphia: Harcourt Health Sciences; 2002. p. 1261–8.

Bacon BR, Olynyk JK, Brunt EM, et al. *HFE* genotype in patients with hemochromatosis and other liver diseases. Ann Intern Med 1999;130:953–62.

Bacon BR, Sadiq SA. Hereditary hemochromatosis: presentation and diagnosis in the 1990s. Am J Gastroenterol 1997;92:784–9.

Beutler E, Felitti VJ, Koziol JA, et al. Penetrance of 845G-A (C282Y) *HFE* hereditary haemochromatosis mutation in the USA. Lancet 2002;359:211–8.

Feder JN, Gnirke A, Thomas W, et al. A novel MHC class I-like gene is mutated in patients with hereditary haemochromatosis. Nature Genetics 1996;13:399–408.

Fletcher LM, Dixon JL, Purdie DM, et al. Excess alcohol greatly increases the prevalence of cirrhosis in hereditary hemochromatosis. Gastroenterol 2002;122:281–9.

Harrison SA, Bacon BR. Herditary hemochromatosis: update for 2003. J Hepatol 2003;38:S14–23.

Parkkila S, Niemela O, Britton RS, et al. Molecular aspects of iron absorption and HFE expression. Gastroenterol 2001;121:1489–96.

Powell LW, Subramaniam N, Yapp TR. Haemochromatosis in the new millennium. J Hepatol 1999;32(Suppl 1):48–62.

Tavill AS. Diagnosis and management of hemochromatosis. Hepatology 2001;33:1321–8.

CHAPTER 126

THE PORPHYRIAS

JOSEPH R. BLOOMER, MD

The porphyrias are metabolic disorders which are characterized biochemically by the increased production, accumulation and excretion of porphyrins and/or porphyrin precursors, compounds which are intermediates of the heme biosynthetic pathway. The liver and bone marrow are the major sites of expression of the biochemical abnormality. The clinical manifestations are varied and include complications for which the gastroenterologist or hepatologist may be consulted for evaluation and management. Principally these occur in patients with porphyria cutanea tarda, erythropoietic protoporphyria, and the acute (inducible) types of porphyria. Because there is a relationship between the clinical manifestations and biochemical abnormalities, the cornerstone of therapy is to use measures which will decrease the excess production and accumulation of the porphyrins and porphyrin precursors.

The Acute Porphyrias

Diagnosis

Acute intermittent porphyria is the most common type of inducible porphyria. Variegate porphyria and hereditary coproporphyria also cause acute porphyric attacks. A fourth disorder, delta-aminolevulinic acid (ALA) dehydrase deficiency, is very rare and is unlikely to be encountered by most physicians.

Several signs and symptoms may occur during an acute porphyric attack, reflecting widespread involvement of the nervous system. The most frequent is abdominal pain which is caused by an autonomic neuropathy. Other features of autonomic neuropathy are tachycardia, hypertension, constipation, and urinary retention. Peripheral neuropathy may develop as the attack progresses and can lead to paralysis in its most severe form. Central nervous system manifestations include organic brain syndrome, depression, and seizures.

The diagnosis of an acute porphyric attack is made by demonstrating increased urinary excretion of the porphyrin precursors ALA and porphobilinogen (PBG). The measurement of urinary porphyrin excretion is not used to establish the diagnosis and may be misleading if the excretion of the porphyrin precursors is not measured. Between attacks the diagnosis is more difficult, but in acute intermittent porphyria the urinary excretion of porphyrin precursors usually remains elevated. The measurement of erythrocyte PBG deaminase activity can also be used to establish the diagnosis of acute intermittent porphyria. In variegate porphyria there is a plasma porphyrin fluorescence marker which is specific for the disorder. Increased fecal excretion of coproporphyrin is found in hereditary coproporphyria.

Management

Therapy for the acute porphyric attack involves several steps. First, the precipitating factors of the attack should be defined and corrected. If the patient is taking a drug which may have precipitated the attack, it should be stopped. Infections should be promptly treated. Adequate caloric intake should be given, because diminished oral intake is recognized as a precipitant of attacks. Glucose should be given orally and intravenously to provide at least 400 grams daily. Intravenous (IV) fluids should be administered to maintain a fluid intake > 2 L/d. Normal saline is preferable to guard against the development of hyponatremia, which may be caused by inappropriate secretion of antidiuretic hormone during the acute attack.

If the patient does not show improvement within 24 hours of therapy, *hematin* should be administered (Mustajoki et al, 1989). Some experts in the field start hematin initially if the patient has previously had severe acute attacks. *Hematin* is obtained commercially as *Panhematin* through Ovation Pharmaceuticals in Deerfield, Illinois. *Hematin* is administered over 15 to 30 minutes in a dose of 3 to 4 mg/kg body weight IV once daily for 4 days. This usually produces a significant decline in serum and urinary levels of ALA and PBG, along with clinical improvement. The course of therapy can be repeated if there is not satisfactory improvement. *Hematin* should be given as soon as possible after dissolving in sterile water because it is unstable in aqueous solution. The most common side effect is thrombophlebitis, which can be prevented by administering the solution in a large arm vein. If peripheral venous access is poor, administration should be through a central venous catheter. A mild coagulopathy may occur during *hematin* therapy, but this has not caused bleeding unless the patient is also taking on anticoagulant.

These problems can be avoided by reconstituting *hematin* in 25% human serum albumin (Bonkovsky et al, 1991), but this will increase the cost of therapy.

Management of the signs and symptoms of the acute porphyric attack should be done while *hematin* is being given. Pain should be controlled with *acetaminophen* if pain is mild, whereas *meperidine* or *morphine* is used for more severe pain. Hypertension and tachycardia can be treated with a β-blocker such as *propranolol*. *Ondansetron* is used to control nausea and vomiting, and anxiety is managed with *chlorpromazine* or *haloperidol*. Seizure management may be difficult because anticonvulsants such as barbiturates and phenytoin are major causes of porphyric attacks. *Clonazepam* in low doses may be used, and *gabapentin* also appears to be safe. Status epilepticus can be controlled with *diazepam* (up to 10 mg IV) or *paraldehyde* (8 to 10 mL rectally).

Many patients with acute porphyria have only a limited number of porphyric attacks and do well if they avoid precipitating factors such as certain drugs (Moore and Hift, 1997), diminished food intake, excessive alcohol intake, and prolonged infections. Information regarding drugs and nutrition can be obtained through the American Porphyria Foundation. However, some patients have frequent attacks, which pose a particularly challenging problem. If recurrent attacks in women are regularly related to the menstrual cycle, the cautious use of oral contraceptive therapy with ethiny estradiol is justified. Alternatively, use of an analog of luteinizing hormone releasing hormone to inhibit gonadotropin secretion may be done. The prophylactic use of IV hematin infusions to prevent attacks should also be considered, although available studies have shown uncertain benefit. If this is done, it should be noted that 100 mg of hematin will provide 8.2 mg of iron, thus potentially causing iron overload over an extended period of time. There are no good data regarding the effect of liver transplantation in severe acute porphyria, but this may also be a consideration. Siblings and children of an individual with acute porphyria should be screened for the disorder by biochemical testing after they have reached puberty.

Porphyria Cutanea Tarda

Diagnosis

The major clinical feature in porphyria cutanea tarda (PCT) is fragility of sun-exposed skin which causes the formation of blisters and erosions after minor trauma, particularly on the backs of the hands. Chronic skin damage may lead to scarring and thickening of the skin which resembles scleroderma. Skin lesions are accompanied by liver abnormalities which vary from mild portal inflammation to cirrhosis. In patients with long standing untreated PCT there is an increased incidence of hepatocellular carcinoma. Neurological symptoms do not occur in PCT. Alcoholism and use of estrogens are precipitating factors of PCT. Patients also have an increased prevalence of chronic hepatitis C (HC) and mutations in the HFE gene which occur in hereditary hemochromatosis (Bloomer, 2000).

The diagnosis is established by demonstrating a marked increase in the excretion of *octacarboxyl porphyrin* (*uroporphyrin*) and *hepatcarboxyl porphyrin* in the urine. In patients in whom the history indicates there is the familial form of PCT (10 to 20% of patients) the measurement of *uroporphyrinogen decarboxylase activity in erythrocytes* may also be used to establish the diagnosis.

Management

Patients with active PCT should *stop the ingestion of alcohol, estrogens, and iron containing compounds*. Sun exposure should be limited. *Phlebotomy* is the preferred therapy based on the observation that hepatic iron overload is common in PCT and probably plays an important role in the pathogenesis of active disease. The liver usually has an excess of 2 to 4 g of iron, and the amount of phlebotomy needed is on the order of 3 to 8 L of blood. The schedule for phlebotomy is to remove 500 mL of blood every 1 to 3 weeks until the ferritin level is at the lower limit of normal and transferrin saturation is normal. The urinary excretion of uroporphyrin usually decreases below 500 μg daily. This will be accompanied by an improvement in skin fragility, and patients will no longer develop blisters and erosions in sun exposed areas. Chronic skin changes such as scarring, hyperpigmentation, and hirtusism take much longer to resolve, however. Approximately 10% of patients will relapse within 1 year but usually respond to a second course of phlebotomy. Resumption of heavy alcohol intake and ingestion of iron containing compounds may lead to a recurrence of active disease and should be avoided. In women who had been previously treated with estrogens, there is usually not a recurrence of active disease when estrogens are restarted. Following successful therapy patients may resume normal sun exposure.

For patients who do not tolerate phlebotomy, or in whom cutaneous symptoms continue despite an adequate course of phlebotomy, *chloroquine* or related compounds is an alternative treatment. These compounds appear to mobilize excess porphyrin from the liver and enhance its excretion in urine. They should be administered in a low dose, starting with 100 mg of hydroxychloroquine 3 times a week and increasing to 200 mg 3 times weekly. The small doses seldom cause eye problems. Larger doses are not used because they may cause significant liver damage related to the massive removal of uroporphyrin from the liver.

PCT may be particularly severe in the patient with *end-stage renal disease*. In this situation *deferoxamine* infusion (2 to 4 g IV during hemodialysis) or small volume *phlebotomy* (100 to 200 mL removed at time of hemodialysis) along with erythropoietin therapy may be used successfully. Chloroquine is not used when there is renal failure.

For the patient who also has chronic HC it does not appear that treatment of the HC is needed to manage PCT successfully. Indeed, ribavirin may potentially worsen PCT because of increased iron absorption due to hemolysis. Thus, treatment of the HC should be delayed until the PCT has been adequately managed, and the patient should be monitored for recurrence of PCT if HC is subsequently treated.

Erythropoietic Protoporphyria

Diagnosis

The major clinical feature in erythropoietic protoporphyria (EPP) is photosensitivity which usually begins in childhood. Patients report burning, itching, swelling and redness of the skin following sun exposure that varies in length from a few minutes to several hours. Some patients also develop hepatobiliary disease because of the toxic effects of protoporphyrin on liver structure and function. In a small number of patients, probably no more than 5%, this may cause progressive hepatic fibrosis that leads to liver failure and necessitates liver transplantation.

The diagnosis of EPP is established in the patient with typical photosensitivity by demonstrating an increased level of free erythrocyte protoporphyrin. Fecal protoporphyrin excretion may also be increased. Urine porphyrin levels are normal except in the patient with liver disease, where coproporphyrin excretion may be secondarily increased.

Management

Most sunscreens do not prevent photosensitivity in EPP because they do not block transmission of the wavelength of light (400 to 410 nm) which activates protoporphyrin, and patients thus require *opaque sunblocks* and/or *protective clothing*. Ordinary window glass also does not prevent transmission of this wavelength of light, but a *clear film* is available which can be installed on windows (including car windows), providing protection (CLS-200-X film, Madico, Woburn, MA). The oral intake of pharmaceutical grade β-carotene also may ameliorate photosensitivity in EPP. Most patients increase their duration of sun exposure at least threefold by taking 60 to 180 mg of *Lumitene* daily (Tishcon Corporation, Westbury, NY). The only side effects reported have been loose stools and the development of carotinemia. Vitamin A toxicity does not occur.

For the patient with EPP in whom liver disease develops, therapeutic approaches are used to diminish the production of excess protoporphyrin, and interrupt its enterohepatic circulation. *Correction of iron deficiency* may dramatically reduce the erythrocyte protoporphyrin level, although iron therapy has caused worsening of EPP in some patients. *Transfusion* with red cells and the IV administration of *hematin* have also diminished erythrocyte protoporphyrin levels, presumably through an effect on the bone marrow. Oral administration of *cholestyramine* (8 to 12 g daily) may be used to interrupt the enterohepatic circulation of protoporphyrin and thereby reduce the amount of protoporphyrin which the liver is required to excrete. Drugs which have a potentially cholestatic effect should be stopped. *Ursodiol* may be administered to enhance the secretion of protoporphyrin into bile, but this must be done cautiously because ursodiol does not solubilize protoporphyrin in bile.

Patients with advanced liver disease should be considered for *liver transplantation*. They are also susceptible to a crisis which is characterized by abrupt worsening of liver chemistries and the erythrocyte protoporphyrin level, severe abdominal pain that often radiates into the back, mild hypertension, and tachycardia. These symptoms are felt to be caused by the neurotoxic effect of protoporphyrin when high blood levels are reached. The crisis may be stabilized and reversed by the combination of *plasmaphoresis* and *hematin administration*. A 1.5 to 2.0 volume plasmaphoresis should be done 3 times weekly, following each plasmaphoresis with the intravenous administration of hematin in a dose of 3 to 4 mg/kg body weight. During the peri-operative transplant period the patient is susceptible to a number of unique problems because of the high blood and tissue levels of protoporphyrin. Photodamage to the skin and abdominal tissue may occur during exposure to fluorescent lights in the operating rooms, which should be covered with CLS-200-X film. Skin and abdominal organs should also be protected from light as much as possible during the operation. Transfusion with red cells should be minimized because transfused red cells are sensitive to photohemolysis caused by circulating protoporphyrin. Axonal neuropathy has also occured in the immediate postoperative period and causes severe motor weakness that necessitates prolonged mechanical ventilation. Nevertheless, liver transplantation has been successful in the majority of patients with EPP, and the 5-year survival of patients has been good (Bloomer et al, 2000). Unfortunately, liver transplantation does not significantly alter the bone marrow production of protoporphyrin, and patients may develop protoporphyrin induced damage in the graft as time progresses. Bone marrow transplantation in such patients should be considered as this will change the EPP phenotype (Poh-Fitzpatrick et al, 2002).

Supplemental Reading

Anderson KE. The porphyrias. In: Zakim D, Boyer T, editors. Hepatology. A textbook of liver disease. 4th ed. Philadelphia: WB Saunders Company; 2003. p. 291–346.

Bloomer JR. Chronic hepatitis C and porphyria cutanea tarda. In: Liang TJ, Hoofnagel JH, editors. Hepatitis C. Biomedical Research Reports. San Diego: Academic Press; 2000. p 3551–61.

Bloomer J, Brenner D. The porphyrias. In: Schiff E, Sorrell M, Maddrey W, editors. Schiff's diseases of the liver. 9th ed.

Philadelphia: Lippincott Wiliams and Wilkins; 2003. p. 1231–60.

Bloomer JR, Rank JM, Payne WD, et al. Follow-up after liver transplantation for protoporphyric liver disease. Liver Transpl Surg 1996;2:269–75.

Bonkovsky HL, Healey JF, Lourie AN, et al. Intravenous heme-albumin in acute intermittent porphyria: evidence for repletion of hepatic hemoproteins and regulatory heme pools. Am J Gastro 1991;86:1050–6.

Moore MR, Hift RJ. Drugs in the acute porphyrias—toxicogenetic diseases. Cell Mol Biol 1997;43:89–94.

Mustajoki P, Tenhunen R, Pierach C, et al. Heme in the treatment of porphyrias and hematological disorders. Sem Hematol 1989;26:1–9.

Poh-Fitzpatrick MB, Wang X, Anderson KE, et al. Recessive erythropoietic protoporphyria: altered phenotype after bone marrow transplantation. J Am Acad Dermatol 2002;46:861–6.

Rocchi E, Gibertini P, Cassanelli M, et al. Serum ferritin in the assessment of liver iron overload and iron removal therapy in porphyria cutanea tarda. J Lab Clinc Med 1986;107:36–42.

The porphyrias. Sem Liver Dis 1998; 18:1–101.

CHAPTER 127

PRIMARY HEPATIC NEOPLASMS

JORGE A. MARRERO, MD, MS, AND ANNA S. LOK, MD

Hepatic tumors may originate from liver tissue, including from the hepatocytes, bile duct epithelium, or mesenchymal tissue, or spread to the liver from primary lesions in other organs. In this chapter we will concentrate on hepatocellular carcinoma (HCC) and cholangiocarcinoma, the most common primary hepatic neoplasms.

HCC

HCC is currently the fourth most common tumor worldwide. Once thought to be rare in the United States, the incidence of HCC has risen from 2.2 per 100,000 persons in 1990 to 3 per 100,000 persons in 1996 to 1998, an increase of 25% during the last 10 years (Davila et al, 2003). Chronic hepatitis C infection has been shown to be the most important factor for the increase in incidence of HCC in the United States, Europe and Japan, whereas chronic hepatitis B infection is the most important etiologic agent worldwide. Cirrhosis remains the most important risk factor for the development of HCC regardless of the etiology, with 5-year probability of developing HCC among cirrhotics around 20%. Thus, cirrhotic patients, particularly those with Child-Pugh class A and B, are the target population for surveillance for HCC. Patients with Child class C cirrhosis should be considered for liver transplantation so the impact of HCC surveillance on survival is less clear, except in the context of ranking on the transplantation waiting list.

The current recommendation for HCC surveillance is to perform α-fetoprotein (AFP) measurement and hepatic ultrasonography every 6 months. The best recall policy determined at a recent consensus conference is depicted in Figure 127-1 (Bruix et al, 2001). The level of AFP that should trigger a workup to detect HCC is controversial, but most investigators will initiate radiologic investigations when the AFP value exceeds 20 ng/mL. Because of the difficulty in detecting small tumor nodules in a cirrhotic liver, dynamic magnetic resonance imaging (MRI) or computed tomography (CT) is preferred to ultrasound (US) in evaluating elevated AFP values. MRI is in general slightly more sensitive and specific than CT scan for the evaluation of HCC (Semelka et al, 2001). One important technique to improve the sensitivity of CTs and MRIs in the detection of HCC is dynamic triple-phase scanning (arterial, portovenous, and venous delayed phases). The gold standard for the diagnosis of HCC remains the pathologic confirmation by histology or cytology. However, because of risks of needle track-seeding and improvements in hepatic imaging, noninvasive criteria have been developed for the diagnosis of HCC in patients with cirrhosis (Table 127-1). The United Network of Organ Sharing (UNOS) accepts listing of patients with HCC based on the following criteria: a vascular lesion on spiral CT or dynamic MRI plus one of (1) pathological confirmation, (2) AFP > 200 ng/mL, or (3) confirmation of vascular mass

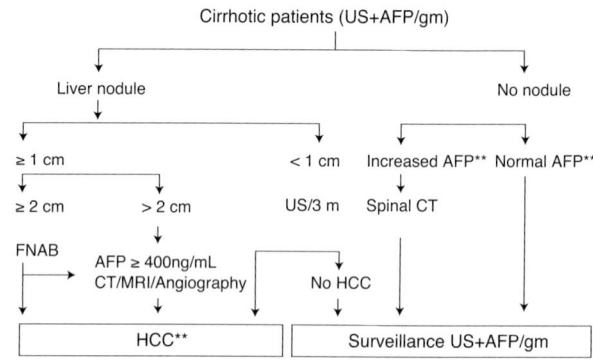

FIGURE 127-1. Surveillance and recall strategy for hepatocellular carcinoma. Reproduced with permission from Bruix J et al, 2001. AFP = α-fetoprotein; CT = computed tomography; HCC = hepatocellular cancer; US = ultrasound.

TABLE 127-1. Definition of Hepatocellular Carcinoma Based on the 2001 EASL Consensus Conference

A. Histology
B. Noninvasive Criteria
  Two imaging* techniques showing a lesion of > 2 cm with arterial hypervascularization
  One imaging technique showing a lesion of > 2cm with arterial hypervascularization *plus* AFP > 400 ng/mL

AFP = α-fetoprotein.
*Four techniques, including ultrasound angiography, spiral computed tomography, dynamic magnetic resonance imaging, and angiography.

by angiogram, chemoembolization or ablation of the lesion. Currently none of the staging systems for HCC is able to stratify patients according to their predicted survival or help determine the best treatment option. In the United States, most liver centers follow UNOS TNM staging as liver transplantation is the best treatment of HCC.

Treatment

Great advances have been made with regards to the treatment of HCC. Treatment can be divided into effective (potentially curative) or palliative interventions. Effective therapies include tumor resection, orthotopic liver transplantation (OLT), and ablative techniques, all of which offer the hope of achieving a long term response and, thereby, improving survival. However, only about 30% of patients with HCC will be diagnosed at a stage when effective treatment can be applied; the remaining 70% will only be eligible for palliative interventions. Palliative therapies are those that aim to prolong survival but evidence supporting improvement in survival is lacking for most of these therapies. Palliative therapies for HCC include intra-arterial chemoembolization, radiation, and systemic chemotherapy. What follows is a review of the efficacy of the available treatment options.

LIVER TRANSPLANTATION

OLT is theoretically the best treatment option for HCC because it removes the tumor together with the entire diseased liver, thereby eliminating the risk for development of de novo HCC. In the early 1990s the results of OLT for HCC were dismal with 1-year survival of 10 to 70% and 3-year recurrence rates up to 69%. In 1996, Mazzaferro and colleagues published a seminal paper on OLT for HCC. By restricting OLT to patients with a *single tumor 5 cm or less, and no more than 3 tumors each less than 3 cm in diameter*, the 4-year actuarial survival rate was 75% and recurrence-free survival was 83%. At transplantation, some patients were found to have tumors that exceeded the restrictive criteria. Of the 35 (73%) patients that met the predefined criteria, the overall and recurrence-free survivals were 85% and 92%, respectively, whereas in the 13 patients (27%) that had tumors exceeding the criteria the overall survival was 50% and recurrence-free survival was 59%. These criteria have been adopted by UNOS. Table 127-2 summarizes the findings of major studies assessing OLT for HCC. With 5-year survival around 60 to 75%, the results of OLT for HCC are close to that of OLT for non-HCC patients.

However, OLT has several drawbacks. Not all patients with HCC can afford or have access to liver transplantation. In addition, waiting time for liver transplantation is increasing worldwide from 6 months to more than 1 year. Therefore, some patients will not be able to proceed to OLT because of tumor progression or deterioration in medical condition. A recent study from Barcelona (Llovet et al, 2002) showed a decrease in survival from 84 to 54% as the waiting time to OLT increased from 62 to 162 days. In the United States, patients with HCC receive higher ranking scores to shorten their waiting time and to prioritize them. The impact of the adjusted score on the posttransplant survival of HCC patients and the wait-list mortality of patients with end-stage liver disease and no HCC remains to be determined.

The size limitations described by Mazzaferro and colleagues (1996) have been challenged. The group in San Francisco (Yao et al, 2001) reported 1- and 5-year survival of 90% and 75%, respectively, among 70 patients undergoing OLT for HCC including 25% with solitary tumors 5 to 6.5 cm in diameter or < 3 tumor nodules each < 4.5 cm

TABLE 127-2. A Summary of Studies Comparing the Outcome of Patients Undergoing Liver Transplantation or Surgical Resection for Hepatocellular Carcinoma

		Actuarial Survival (%)							
	Number of Patients	Overall				Recurrence-free			
		1-year	3-year	5-year	10-year	1-year	3-year	5-year	10-year
Transplant									
Mazzaferro	48	92	—	75	—	90	—	83	—
Bismuth	60	—	50	—	—	—	46	—	—
Figueras	85	84	74	60	—	83	72	60	—
Llovet	87	84	69	69	—	86	80	80	—
De Carlis	121	—	—	62	60	—	—	86	86
Hemming	112	78	63	57	—	—	—	68	—
Resection									
Bismuth	60	—	47	—	—	—	27	—	—
Figueras	35	83	57	51	—	70	44	31	—
Llovet	77	85	62	51	—	73	39	25	—
De Carlis	154	—	—	47	28	—	—	43	30
Michel	102	—	—	31	—	—	—	14	—

with a total diameter < 8 cm. The authors suggested loosening the criteria of OLT for HCC, but these results should be confirmed by other centers before changing the current criteria.

Live donor transplantation can potentially eliminate the significant waiting time and allow the surgery to be performed electively. A recent case series from Japan described 56 patients who underwent live donor transplantation for HCC. The 1- and 3-year survival rates were 73% and 55%, respectively, and 6 tumor recurrences were noted. The authors stated that the 3-year survival rate was lower than that in patients who underwent live donor transplantation for nonmalignant liver disease (73%). However, in this study 35% of the patients had tumors that exceeded the Mazzaferro criteria, which likely led to the poor results. A national study is needed to determine the safety and efficacy of live donor transplantation for HCC in the United States.

Surgical Resection

Resection is second to OLT in effectiveness as a treatment of HCC. Its main disadvantages are the high recurrence rates because it does not remove the diseased liver that lead to the development of HCC, and it does not improve the overall liver function. In addition, surgical resection is feasible only in patients with preserved hepatic function. Table 127-2 summarizes the long term results of resection compared with OLT. Patient selection is of outmost importance in order to achieve a long term response. In selected individuals with Child's class A cirrhosis, who have normal bilirubin level and no portal hypertension by hepatic venous pressure measurements, the 5-year survival reaches 50%. A recent study showed that Child's class A patients with single tumor nodule and a preoperative aspartate aminotransferase < 2 times the upper limit of normal were independent predictors of no recurrence after resection. In these excellent candidates, the decision to perform liver transplantation or resection depends on the local resources, expertise, and organ availability. In most series of surgical resection for HCC recurrence rates of 50% at 3 years and 70% at 5 years were reported making resection an unattractive option to many patients. However, in patients with HCC and no cirrhosis liver resection is the best option. A series of 68 noncirrhotic patients from France who underwent resection for HCC with a mean tumor diameter of 8.8 cm showed a survival of 40% and 26% at 5 and 10 years, respectively (Bismuth et al, 1995). In Western countries where the overwhelming majority of HCC patients have cirrhosis, resection will remain the second option after transplantation. The availability of live donor transplantation may shift some HCC patients towards transplantation that otherwise would undergo surgical resection.

Local Ablation

Local ablation of HCC is usually performed while patients await liver transplantation or as a curative treatment in patients with one or a few small tumor nodules but who are not candidates for surgical intervention because of other medical comorbidities. Ablation may be accomplished by chemical (eg, *100% ethanol or 50% acetic acid*) or physical (eg, *radiofrequency, cryoablation,* or *microwave*) techniques. Table 127-3 summarizes the studies involving the more common methods for percutaneous ablation. Ethanol ablation has been the most widely used technique. The procedure is safe and is performed under US guidance and conscious sedation. The long term outcome after ethanol injection was compared with surgical resection in a European study. A cohort of 30 patients underwent percutaneous ethanol injection and another cohort of 33 contemporary patients underwent surgical resection. The survival rates were similar among the 2 groups, with 81% and 44% at 1 and 4 years for resection, and 83% and 34%, respectively, for ethanol injection. However, a mean of 4.8 sessions were required for complete ethanol ablation. Even

TABLE 127-3. A Comparison of the Outcome of Local Ablative Techniques for Hepatocellular Carcinoma

Ablation	Number of Patients	Tumor Size (cm)*	Survival		Recurrence	
			3-year	5-year	3-year	5-year
PEI						
Livraghi	746	< 5	78	37	51	67
Lencioni	184	< 3	78	54	51	67
	-	3.1 to 5	61	32	-	-
Ebara	95	< 3	65	28	66	-
Castells	84	< 5	68	37	53	71
RFA	-	-	-	-	-	-
Buscarini	88	< 3.5	62	33	24	4
Fontana	33	3.6	58	-	44	-
Microwave	-	-	-	-	-	-
Dong	234	4.1	72	56	20	-

*Maximal tumor diameter.
Microwave = percutaneous microwave coagulation; PEI = percutaneous ethanol injection; RFA = radiofrequency ablation.

though the groups were not comparable (resection patients were all Child's class A), this study showed for the first time that percutaneous ablation achieved similar survival to hepatic resection (Castells et al, 1993).

Radiofrequency ablation (RFA) is a relatively new technique compared to ethanol injection. Its ability to destroy HCC tissue at one session, its tolerability and the paucity of side effects make it the preferred local ablative therapy in many liver centers. The principle of RFA involves inserting an insulated cannula into the tumor where alternating current is passed, resulting in heating of the area around the tumor to about 100°C. The cannula contains about 8 to 10 individual electrodes that when deployed within the tumor allow a sphere of up to 5 cm diameter to be destroyed. As seen in Table 127-3, RFA for HCC has achieved comparable survival and recurrence rates to surgical resection and ethanol injection. Table 127-4 shows the 3 studies that have directly compared radiofrequency ablation versus ethanol injection in patients with tumors < 5 cm. RFA was more efficient at achieving complete ablation, 90 to 100% compared with 80 to 94% for ethanol, with fewer sessions. The largest study by Lencioni and colleagues (2003) also showed a better 2-year overall survival for RFA of 98% versus 88%, and a better recurrence-free survival of 96% versus 62%. Thus, RFA outperforms ethanol injection for the treatment of HCC less than 5 cm in maximal diameter.

Microwave, acetic acid injection and cryoablation have also been performed to ablate HCC. As seen in Table 127-3, microwave ablation can achieve complete coagulative necrosis in up to 90% of patients with 3-year survival rates of 73%. One study compared microwave coagulation with RFA of lesions less than 3 cm; complete necrosis was achieved in 96% of those who underwent RFA versus 89% in those with microwave coagulation ($p = .26$); RFA required less sessions for tumor ablation (1.1 versus 2.5 [$p < .001$]).

The risks involved with ablation techniques include puncture site bleeding, fever, abdominal pain, and transient elevations of the aminotransferases. Both RFA and ethanol injection have been associated with needle track seeding of tumors, especially when the lesions are > 2cm. A recent report from Italy examined the safety of RFA in 2,320 HCC patients with 3,554 lesions of 3.1±1.1 cm in maximal tumor diameter. A total of 6 (0.3%) patients died from complications related to the procedure including intestinal perforation (2), peritonitis (1), massive tumor hemorrhage (1), biliary strictures (1), and one unknown. An additional 50 patients (2.2%) had major complications, such as peritoneal hemorrhage, neoplastic seeding, intrahepatic abscess, and intestinal perforation. The authors concluded that RFA is a well tolerated and safe procedure for the treatment of HCC.

Ablative therapies are safe and effective at achieving tumor necrosis. However, the high recurrence rates at 3 and 5 years and the development of de novo tumors indicate that this is not a cure for most patients. Local ablative therapy is most effective for lesions < 3 cm diameter, although some studies found that complete ablation can be achieved with tumors up to 5 cm diameter. Local ablation is best suited for patients with no more than 2 to 3 tumor nodules. Among the various techniques, RFA and ethanol injection have been more extensively studied. Both techniques are similar in efficacy and safety. RFA has the advantage that tumor ablation can be achieved in fewer sessions and has been shown to improve survival in randomized clinical trials compared with ethanol injection. The main advantages of ethanol injection are low cost and ease of the technique. However, the disadvantages include the requirement of multiple sessions, and changes in echo features of the tumor after the initial injection make subsequent visualization of the tumor more difficult. The choice of ablative technique to be used for HCC will depend on the local expertise.

Intra-Arterial Chemoembolization

HCC is a vascular tumor that derives its blood supply from the hepatic artery, whereas the rest of the liver is perfused by both hepatic artery and portal vein. Therefore, selective intra-arterial administration of chemotherapeutic agents followed by embolization of the major tumor artery has been

TABLE 127-4. Randomized Controlled Trials Comparing Percutaneous Ethanol Injection and Radiofrequency Ablation

Author	Number of Patients	Complete Necrosis (%)		Number of Sessions		Survival		Recurrence	
	RFA/PEI	RFA	PEI	RFA	PEI	RFA	PEI	RFA	PEI
Livraghi	42/44	90	80	1.2	4.8	NA		NA	
Ikeda	23/96	100	94	1.5	4.0	NA		15*	14
Lencioni	52/50	91	82	1.1	5.4	98†	88	‡96	62

All studies included patients with a maximal tumor diameter < 5 cm.
*1-year recurrence rate;
†2-year recurrence-free survival;
‡2-year survival.
PEI = percutaneous ethanol injection; RFA = radiofrequency ablation.

performed to treat HCC. This procedure may be complicated by liver failure possibly due to ischemic infarct of adjacent nontumorous liver. A metanalysis evaluating the impact of arterial embolization and arterial chemoembolization was performed (Llovet and Bruix, 2003). There was a survival benefit with chemoembolization versus control, but no survival benefit with embolization alone versus control. A recent randomized study compared chemoembolization versus embolization alone with supportive care in 112 patients with unresectable HCC (Llovet et al, 2002). The groups were equally matched and two-thirds of the patients had multinodular tumors with a maximal tumor diameter of about 5 cm. Only chemoembolization showed a survival benefit compared to conservative treatment (hazard ratio 0.47; 95% CI 0.25 to 0.91). The tumor-free survival at 2 years was 63% for chemoembolization, 50% for embolization, and 27% for conservative management. These studies showed that in carefully selected patients with compensated or mildly decompensated liver function (78% Child's A and 22% Child's B), absence of tumor-related symptoms, renal failure or portal vein invasion and a maximal tumor diameter of about 5 cm, intra-arterial chemoembolization can lead to a survival benefit. However, patients with lesions of about 5 cm are also eligible for local ablation. Therefore, local expertise and underlying liver function will dictate whether patients with small HCC (< 5 cm) will undergo chemoembolization or ablative techniques.

Systemic Chemotherapy/Radiation/Hormonal Therapy

A variety of chemotherapeutic regimens have been used for patients with HCC not amenable to any of the treatments discussed previously. The results have been dismal and may in part be elated to the limitations in choice of chemotherapeutic agents and the dose that can be used in patients have underlying cirrhosis. Focal liver radiation targeted to the tumor has been shown to result in complete responses in 17 to 92% of unresectable HCC but is most effective in smaller (< 7 cm) lesions. However, about one-third of patients develop radiation induced liver damage, which may lead to hepatic decompensation. There have been no randomized control trials comparing radiation against local ablation or chemotherapy. A new form of radiation therapy is direct intratumoral injection of ^{90}Y spheres, has been reported to result in complete destruction of nonresectable HCC. This technique needs to be further evaluated in randomized clinical trials. Three large double-blind randomized clinical trials have shown no benefit for tamoxifen in HCC (Bruix et al, 2001). Antiangiogenic agents have also shown promise in pilot trials, but studies in larger number of patients in comparison to other established therapies are needed to determine the role of antiangiogenic agents in the treatment of HCC.

Summary

The incidence of HCC is rising in the United States likely due to the hepatitis C epidemic. Surveillance should be performed in patients with cirrhosis given that there are effective therapies, such as liver transplantation, resection and ablation that may achieve longterm survival. Figure 127 2 shows an algorithm for the treatment of patients with HCC. The choice of therapy is dependent on the extent of the tumor, the underlying liver function, general medical condition of the patient, and local expertise.

Cholangiocarcinoma

Three epidemiologic studies have shown an increase in the incidence of cholangiocarcinoma in the United States. The incidence is about 8 per million (1973 to 1997) with one-third being intrahepatic cholangiocellular cancers and two-thirds ductal cholangiocarcinomas (Gores, 2003). The lifetime risk for developing cholangiocarcinoma in patients with primary sclerosing cholangitis (PSC) is approximately 1.5% per year of disease. A TNM pathologic staging has been developed but is of little clinical value. Figure 127-3 shows the algorithm for examining a patient suspected of having a malignant stricture or cholangiocarcinoma. Surgery is the best treatment option for patients with intrahepatic cholangiocarcinoma, with 3-year survival rates close to 60%. However, only about 10% of these patients will be eligible for surgical interventions. For patients with ductal cholangiocarcinoma, surgical extirpation should be performed with a curative intent and partial hepatic resection is often necessary. In patients with tumor-free margins, the 5-year survival rates are only 20 to 40%, and the operative mortality is approximately 10%. There is no proven adjuvant therapy. Surgical resection of cholangio-

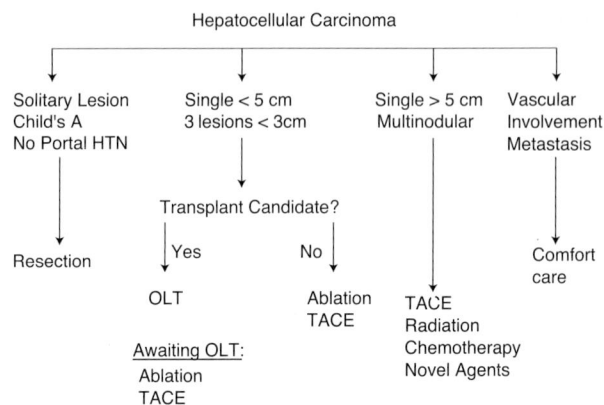

FIGURE 127-2. Algorithm for the treatment of hepatocellular carcinoma. OLT = orthotopic liver transplantation; TACE = transarterial chemoembolization.

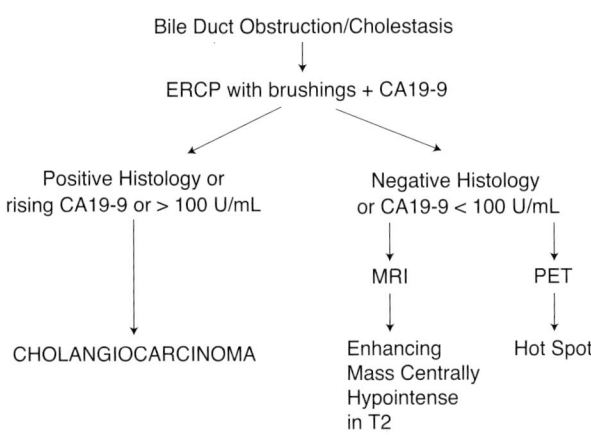

FIGURE 127-3. Algorithm for the evaluation of malignant strictures. ERCP = endoscopic retrograde cholangiopancreatography; MRI = magnetic resonance imaging; PET = positron emission tomography.

carcinoma in patients with PSC is controversial due to their often advanced fibrotic stage, and the 5-year survival rates are dismal (< 10%). Results with OLT are poor with recurrence rates of 60%; most transplantation centers will not transplant patients with cholangiocarcinoma because of the poor results. Recently, a few centers have reported long term survival following OLT for intraductal cholangiocarcinoma (De Veede et al, 2000). The recent update from the Mayo Clinic reports a 5-year survival of more than 80% among patients who had chemoirradiation followed by exploratory laparotomy showing no more than TNM stage I and II disease before transplant. However, only a small percentage of patients with cholangiocarcinoma fulfill the criteria for transplantation. Palliative interventions include pain relief and biliary drainage. No survival benefit has been shown with chemotherapy.

Supplemental Reading

Bismuth H, Chiche L, Castaing D. Surgical treatment of hepatocellular carcinoma in noncirrhotic liver: experience with 68 liver resections. World J Surg 1995;19:35–41.

Bruix J, Sherman M, Llovet JM, et al. Clinical Management of Hepatocellular Carcinoma. Conclusions of the Barcelona 2000 EASL Conference. J Hepatology 2001;35:421–30.

Buscarini L, Buscarini E, Di Stasi M, et al. Percutaneous radiofrequency ablation of small hepatocellular carcinoma: long-term results. Eur Radiol 2001;11:914–21.

Castells A, Bruix J, Bru C, et al. Treatment of small hepatocellular carcinoma in cirrhotic patients: a cohort study comparing surgical resection and percutaneous ethanol injection. Hepatology 1993;18:1121–6.

Davila JA, Petersena NJ, Nelson HA, El-Serag HB. Geographic variation within the United States in the incidenceof hepatocellular cancer. J Clin Epidemiol 2003;56:487–93.

De Carlis L, Giacomoni A, Pirotta V, et al. Surgical treatment of hepatocellular cancer in the era of hepatic transplantation. J Am Coll Surg 2003;196:887–97.

De Veede I, Steers JL, Burch PA, et al. Prolonged disease-free survival after orthotopic liver transplantation plus adjuvant chemoirradiation for cholangiocarcinoma. Liver Transpl 2000;6:309–16.

Dong B, Liang P, Yu X, et al. Percutaneous sonographically guided microwave coagulation therapy for hepatocellular carcinoma: results in 234 patients. Am J Roentgenol 2003;180:1547–55.

Ebara M, Ohto M, Sugiura N, et al. Percutaneous ethanol injection for the treatment of small hepatocellular carcinoma. Study of 95 patients. J Gastroenterol Hepatol 1990;5:616–26.

Figueras J, Jaurrieta E, Valls C, et al. Resection or liver transplantation for hepatocellular carcinoma in cirrhotic patients: outcomes based on indicated treatment strategy. J Am Coll Surg 2000;190:580–7.

Fontana RJ, Hamidullah H, Nghiem H, et al. Percutaneous radiofrequency ablation of hepatocellular carcinoma: a safe and effective bridge to liver transplantation. Liver Transpl 2002;12:1165–74.

Gores GJ. Cholangiocarcinoma: current concepts and insights. Hepatology 2003;37:961–9.

Hemming AW, Cattral MS, Reed AI, et al. Liver transplantation for hepatocellular carcinoma. Ann Surg. 2001;233:652–9.

Ikeda M, Okada S, Ueno H, et al. Radiofrequency ablation and percutaneous ethanol injection in patients with small hepatocellular carcinoma: a comparative study. Jpn J Clin Oncol 2001;31:322–6.

Kaihara S, Kiuchi T, Ueda M, et al. Living-donor liver transplantation for hepatocellular carcinoma Transplantation. 2003;75:S37–40.

Lencioni RA, Allgaier HP, Cioni D, et al. Small hepatocellular carcinoma in cirrhosis: randomized comparison of radiofrequency ablation versus percutaneous ethanol injection. Radiology 2003;228:235–40.

Lencioni R, Pinto F, Armillota N, et al. Long-term results of percutaneous ethanol injection therapy for hepatocellular carcinoma in cirrhosis: a European experience. Eur Radiol 1997;7:514–9.

Livraghi T, Giorgio A, Marin G, et al. Hepatocellular carcinoma and cirrhosis in 746 patients: long-term results of percutaneous ethanol injection. Radiology 1995;197:101–8.

Livraghi T, Goldberg SN, Lazzaroni S, et al. Small hepatocellular carcinoma: treatment with radiofrequency ablation versus ethanol injection. Radiology 1999;210:655–61.

Livraghi T, Solbiati L, Meloni MF, et al. Treatment of focal liver tumors with percutaneous radiofrequency ablation: complications encountered in a multicenter study. Radiology 2003;226:441–51.

Llovet JM, Bruix J. Systematic review of randomized controlled trials for unresectable hepatocellular carcinoma: chemoembolization improves survival. Hepatology 2003;37:429–42.

Llovet JM, Real MI, Montana X, et al. Arterial embolisation or chemoembolisation versus symptomatic treatment in patients with unresectable hepatocellular carcinoma: a randomised controlled trial. Lancet 2002;359:1734–9.

Mazzaferro V, Regalia E, Doci R, et al. Liver transplantation for the treatment of small hepatocellular carcinomas in patients with cirrhosis. N Engl J Med 1996;334:693–9.

Michel J, Suc B, Montpeyroux F, et al. Liver resection or transplantation for hepatocellular carcinoma? Retrospective analysis of 215 patients with cirrhosis. J Hepatol 1997;26:1274–80.

Semelka RC, Martin DR, Balci C, Lance T. Focal liver lesions: comparison of dual-phase CT and multisequence multiplanar MRI including dynamic gadolinium enhancement. J Magn Reson Imaging 2001;13:397–401.

Yao FY, Ferrell L, Bass NM, et al. Liver transplantation for hepatocellular carcinoma: expansion of the tumor size limits does not adversely impact survival. Hepatology 2001;33:1394–403.

MANAGEMENT OF HEPATOCELLULAR CARCINOMA

Timothy M. Pawlik, MD, MPH, Melanie B. Thomas, MD, and
Jean-Nicolas Vauthey, MD

Prevalence and Natural History

Hepatocellular carcinoma (HCC) is the fifth most common malignancy in men and the ninth most common malignancy in women, accounting for 500,000 to 1 million cancer cases annually worldwide. Although the incidence in the United States is considerably less, it is estimated that 17,300 patients were diagnosed with HCC and 14,400 patients died of liver cancer in 2003. Unlike the incidence and death rate of most cancers that have stabilized or decreased during the past two decades, the incidence of HCC has been steadily increasing. Surgical resection remains the therapy of choice for HCC because primary treatment with traditional medical therapy yields a median survival of only 6 to 9 months. Although hepatectomy for HCC can be associated with a significant risk of morbidity and mortality, over the past two to three decades, the mortality rate has fallen from 20% in patients operated on before 1980 to usually less than 5% in patients undergoing liver resection thereafter. This improvement in morbidity and mortality is multifactorial and is undoubtedly related to better patient selection, improved anesthetic monitoring, greater understanding of hepatic anatomy, advances in surgical technique, and improved perioperative critical care.

Etiologies and Prognostic Factors

Worldwide, most cases of HCC occur in areas where viral hepatitis is endemic and develop in a background of cirrhosis. In contrast, in the United States, it is estimated that only 25% of patients with HCC have evidence of hepatitis C virus (HCV) infection, and hepatitis B virus and HCV together account for no more than 40% of HCC cases (El-Serag, 2001). HCC also frequently presents in the setting of severe parenchymal liver disease. Both cirrhosis and fibrosis represent a state of chronic liver injury, which may act as a stimulus for ongoing hepatic regeneration, leading to eventual malignant transformation. The presence of hepatitis, cirrhosis, and fibrosis is also important for postresection prognosis because several studies have documented an association between cirrhosis, hepatitis status, and tumor recurrence that is presumably due to continued carcinogenesis in the affected liver remnant. In fact, we have previously reported that 5-year survival rates were significantly higher for patients without fibrosis or cirrhosis compared with those with fibrosis or cirrhosis, regardless of tumor stage. Other risk factors implicated in HCC include several metabolic disorders, such as type I glycogen storage disease, α_1-antitrypsin deficiency, Wilson's disease, and hemochromatosis.

Diagnosis and Staging

HCC is usually diagnosed at a late stage, with many patients presenting with upper abdominal pain, weight loss, ascites, and other sequelae of portal hypertension. An elevated α-fetoprotein (AFP), especially greater than 400 ng/mL, should raise one's suspicions for HCC, although patients with small tumors may have normal levels. In addition to its diagnostic use, AFP measurements are also used to monitor for tumor recurrence because levels should fall to normal after curative resection. Radiologic confirmation of a liver mass is usually initially made with either ultrasonography (US) or computed tomography (CT). Although US is used as a screening tool, all patients presenting to the University of Texas M. D. Anderson Cancer Center for examination of HCC undergo a three-phase helical CT scan. The early arterial phase is especially useful in imaging hypervascular tumors such as HCC. Although histologic diagnosis can be obtained by CT or US-guided percutaneous needle biopsy, we do not recommend that this be performed routinely. Most often the diagnosis of HCC can be obtained based on the patient's history, physical presentation, laboratory findings, and radiologic examinations. If the lesion is deemed to be unresectable and an alternative therapy is being planned, a liver biopsy to document the diagnosis may be warranted.

Several clinical staging systems that rely on liver function parameters are often used to guide initial therapy in patients with HCC. The Okuda staging system, which accounts for both liver function and tumor extension, has traditionally been used for predicting the prognosis of patients with cirrhosis and HCC. A new prognostic score proposed by the Cancer of the Liver Italian Program (CLIP) group (2000) includes Child-Pugh stage, tumor morphology and extension, the presence of portal vein thrombosis, and the serum level of AFP. Compared with the Okuda score, the CLIP score has been shown to give more accurate prognostic information, to be statistically more efficient, and to have a greater survival predictive power.

Whereas clinical staging systems are used for patients with advanced-stage HCC, the American Joint Committee on Cancer/International Union Against Cancer (AJCC/UICC) staging system has been used for accurate prognostic assessment after resection. The AJCC/UICC staging system uses a tumor-node-metastasis (TNM) classification scheme to stratify patients with respect to predicted survival after resection (Table 128-1). In the latest edition of the AJCC staging manual, the tumor categories have been redefined and simplified. All solitary tumors without vascular invasion, regardless of size, are classified as T1 because of similar prognosis. One of the most important changes from the previous AJCC/UICC TNM staging is that the cutoff value for tumor size in the prognostic classification was shifted from 2 to 5 cm, and the influence of tumor size was limited only to patients with multiple tumors. All solitary tumors with vascular invasion, regardless of size, are combined with multiple tumors ≤ 5 cm and are classified as T2 because of similar prognosis. Multiple tumors > 5 cm and tumors with evidence of major vascular invasion are combined and classified as T3 because of a similar poor prognosis. T4 tumors are classified as those with direct invasion of adjacent organs other than the gallbladder or with perforation of visceral peritoneum. Another important feature of the new AJCC/UICC TNM staging is the provision of a separate reporting of fibrosis in every resected case of HCC. The fibrosis scoring system proposed by Ishak and colleagues (1995) has been incorporated into the most recent AJCC/UICC staging system (Ishak 0 to 2, no or minimal fibrosis; Ishak 3 to 4, incomplete bridging fibrosis; Ishak 5 to 6, complete fibrosis and nodules). Patients with severe fibrosis or cirrhosis (Ishak score of 5 to 6) are staged as F1, whereas those patients with no or moderate fibrosis (Ishak score 0 to 4) are staged as F0. The new scoring of severity of fibrosis provides a more precise method to evaluate the impact of fibrosis and cirrhosis on prognosis and should enhance the prognostic value of the new TNM staging system.

Therapy

Selection of Candidates for Surgical Resection

The extent of underlying liver disease is a variable known to have a significant effect on operative morbidity and mortality. The presence of steatosis, fibrosis, and cirrhosis is associated with an increased perioperative risk. Studies have shown that only patients with severe fibrosis are at a higher risk for complications and death from liver failure after resection. In one study, 32% of patients with severe fibrosis (cirrhosis) who underwent a right hepatectomy died from liver failure compared with none of the patients with grade 0 to 3 fibrosis (Farges et al, 1999). As a rule, we do not operate on patients who are Child-Pugh class B or C. Similarly, we do not recommend resection for those patients who manifest clinical or radiologic signs of portal hypertension, including splenomegaly, abdominal collaterals, or thrombocytopenia. In fact, the preoperative portal pressure has been found to be an important factor in determining the risk of postoperative liver decompensation in cirrhotic patients (Bruix et al, 1996). Portal hypertension can lead to increased hemorrhage and decreased capacity to tolerate bleeding, as well as an early coagulopathy in the course of treatment. For this reason, we measure portal pressure preoperatively in patients who are suspected of having occult portal hypertension. By advancing a venous introducer into the main right hepatic vein, measurements of the preoperative wedged (occluded) and free hepatic venous pres-

TABLE 128-1. New AJCC/UICC Tumor-Node-Metastasis, Histologic Grade, and Fibrosis Score Classification Scheme for Hepatocellular Cancer

Primary tumor (T)
TX	Primary tumor cannot be assessed
T0	No evidence of primary tumor
T1	Solitary tumor without vascular invasion
T2	Solitary tumor with vascular invasion or multiple tumors, none more than 5 cm
T3	Multiple tumors more than 5 cm or tumor involving a major branch of the portal or hepatic vein(s)
T4	Tumor(s) with direct invasion of adjacent organs other than the gallbladder or with perforation of visceral peritoneum

Regional lymph nodes (N)
NX	Regional lymph nodes cannot be assessed
N0	No regional lymph node metastasis
N1	Regional lymph node metastasis

Distant metastasis (M)
MX	Distant metastasis cannot be assessed
M0	No distant metastasis
M1	Distant metastasis

Stage grouping
I	T1	N0	M0
II	T2	N0	M0
IIIA	T3	N0	M0
IIIB	T4	N0	M0
IIIC	Any T	N1	M0
IV	Any T	Any N	M1

Histologic grade (G)
GX	Grade cannot be assessed
G1	Well differentiated
G2	Moderately differentiated
G3	Poorly differentiated
G4	Undifferentiated

Fibrosis score (F)
F0	Fibrosis score 0 to 4 (no fibrosis to moderate fibrosis)
F1	Fibrosis score 5 to 6 (severe fibrosis to cirrhosis)

AJCC/UICC = American Joint Committee on Cancer/International Union Against Cancer.

sures and the hepatic venous pressure gradient (HVPG) can be obtained. Patients with elevated HVPG (greater than 12 to 13 mm Hg) are at a significantly higher risk of postoperative hepatic decompensation and are therefore not appropriate for surgical resection.

Although there is a general consensus that the extent of safe resection is limited mainly by the size and function of the residual liver after resection, there are emerging data regarding what minimal volume of residual liver is sufficient to avoid postoperative liver failure. Based on volumetric studies, we feel that a liver remnant volume of > 20% is the minimal safe volume that can be left following extended resection in patients with a normal underlying liver. In a diseased liver (cirrhosis or hepatitis), we use > 40% of the total liver volume as the cutoff for the minimally safe liver remnant. CT can now provide an accurate, reproducible method for preoperatively measuring the volume of the future liver remnant (FLR). We routinely measure the FLR directly by three-dimensional CT volumetry. The ratio of the measured FLR volume to the total estimated liver volume is determined using a formula that is derived from the association between total liver volume and body surface area (BSA), as follows:

$$\text{Total liver volume (cm}^3\text{)} = -794.41 + 1{,}267.28 \times \text{BSA (m}^2\text{)} \text{ (Vauthey et al, 2002)}$$

Based on this method of FLR volume calculation, we have established a correlation between FLR volume and operative outcome, with the postoperative complication rate being significantly increased in patients with FLR volume ≤ 20% of the total estimated liver volume. Based on our experience, a small FLR is associated with an increased length of stay and morbidity after extended hepatic resection. We do not use other measures to evaluate hepatic metabolic function, such as the indocyanine green retention rate, galactose elimination, and animopyrine clearance. These tests are impractical for surgical planning because they provide an overall measurement of function and do not differentiate between the liver to be resected and the anticipated liver remnant.

Strategies to Optimize Surgical Success

Given that a small FLR is correlated with an increase in morbidity, we have been interested in developing methods to initiate hypertrophy of the FLR before resection. Portal vein embolization (PVE) has been proposed to induce hypertrophy of the anticipated liver remnant. This concept emerged from the recognition that portal invasion by tumor leads to ipsilateral hepatic lobar atrophy and contralateral lobar hypertrophy. At our institution, PVE involves the percutaneous cannulation of the ipsilateral portal vein under direct fluoroscopic control followed by portography and selected PVE using polyvinyl alcohol and microcoils. PVE is safe, with a < 5% complication rate, causes little periportal reaction, and generates durable portal vein occlusion, especially when used in combination with coils. Others have shown that PVE increases both the size of the FLR and the function of the remnant liver, as demonstrated by an increase in biliary excretion (Uesaka et al, 1996). In addition, in patients with chronic liver disease, PVE has also been reported to decrease the incidence of postoperative complications, intensive care unit stay, and total hospital stay after major hepatic resection. Thus, we use PVE selectively in those patients in whom a remnant volume of ≤ 20% (normal underlying liver) or ≤ 40% (diseased underlying liver) is anticipated. After PVE, repeat CT scans are obtained at 3 to 4 weeks to assess for the extent of compensatory hepatic hypertrophy. Surgical decision making is then appropriately based on post-PVE CT volumetric analysis.

After the selection of appropriate candidates for operative resection, the next most significant determinant of morbidity and mortality in patients undergoing liver resection is the intraoperative course. Expert anesthetic support is critical in obtaining a good surgical outcome. In most cases, general anesthesia is accompanied by a thoracic epidural regional anesthetic. This allows for decreased intraoperative anesthetic use and decreased postoperative narcotic use, which facilitates early mobilization and postoperative pulmonary mechanics. All patients have large-bore intravenous (IV) access established and have a central venous catheter placed to allow for continual intraoperative assessment of central venous pressure. Although there are no data to support their routine use, most patients routinely receive perioperative IV antibiotics. One group of patients who clearly should receive antibiotics are those patients with biliary stents because there are data to suggest that patients with biliary stents are at a significantly higher risk of infectious complications (52% versus 28%) (Hochwald et al, 1999). Blood loss and transfusion requirements are well-established independent intraoperative predictors of patient morbidity. Multiple studies have shown that as the blood loss and transfusion requirement increase, there is a significant corresponding linear increase in the risk of serious morbidity and death from surgery. Massive blood transfusions can add to the risk of coagulopathy and exert immunosuppressive effects. Given this, a familiarity with the techniques to minimize intraoperative blood loss becomes critical. Arguably, the most important factor relating to intraoperative blood loss is the pressure within the inferior vena cava (IVC). In a prospective study examining blood loss and IVC pressure, there was a direct linear correlation between mean caval pressure and blood loss (Johnson et al, 1998).

Surgical Techniques for HCC Resection

The operative approach to the tumor mass is dictated, to some degree, by the results of the intraoperative ultrasonography (IOUS). After completely mobilizing the liver, we routinely use IOUS to determine the size of the tumor and its relation to adjacent vascular and biliary structures. The tumor's proximity to vascular and biliary structures, the size of the mass, and the degree of underlying liver disease dictate, to some degree, the amount of liver to be resected. In performing the actual resection, several different parenchymal dissection techniques are available, none of which have been shown in randomized trials to be superior with regard to blood loss. Currently, we use the ultrasonic aspirator in association with the argon beam. Major resections are usually performed following one or several anatomic fissures of the liver, sparing intraparenchymal division of large vessels and intrahepatic bile ducts, thereby minimizing the risk of incurring the two most common operative complications: blood loss and bile leaks.

Techniques of vascular control are also critical in minimizing blood loss. Vascular control can range from total vascular exclusion (TVE) with control of the hepatic pedicle and vena cava above and below the liver to the Pringle maneuver, in which only hepatic inflow is occluded. We use the Pringle maneuver as the vascular control technique of choice for most major hepatic resections. When performing the maneuver, one must be cognizant of the total time that hepatic inflow is occluded. Although the upper limit to inflow occlusion has been reported to be up to 200 minutes, we apply the Pringle maneuver by intermittently occluding the hepatic artery and portal vein for 15-minute periods separated by 5 minutes of restored flow. Although TVE can be useful in cavohepatic junctional tumors, we believe it is, in general, unnecessary. In addition, roughly 14% of patients will be unable to hemodynamically tolerate TVE, and it may lead to an actual increase in blood loss and complications when used by surgeons inexperienced in the technique. For this reason, we favor the selective use of venovenous bypass instead of TVE when cavohepatic resection is anticipated.

Abdominal drainage, which once was considered mandatory, is now used selectively. Several studies have shown that the routine use of drains is unnecessary and may lead to an overall increase in the rate of infection. For these reasons, routine abdominal drainage is unnecessary and should be employed only on an individual basis. We currently use drains after thoracoabdominal incisions, biliary reconstructions, and extended resections.

Orthotopic Liver Transplantation

For those patients whose poor underlying liver function and tumor number or location preclude hepatic resection, we advocate total hepatectomy with orthotopic liver transplantation (OLT). Although the initial series of OLT for HCC reported poor results, the selection criteria for OLT have subsequently undergone major revision, and more recent results have been favorable. Currently, patients with HCC and cirrhosis with three or less tumor nodules up to 3 cm in maximum diameter or a single tumor not exceeding 5 cm and no signs of vascular invasion should be considered for transplantation. Recent survival data obtained from Milan revealed 4-year survival rates of 75% in patients with solitary tumors that were less than 5 cm who had no vascular invasion (Mazzaferro et al, 1996). Many of the risk factors that predict cancer recurrence following OLT are similar to those that predict a high risk of recurrence after partial hepatectomy, with the major factor being the presence of vascular invasion.

Radiologic Intervention

Because of the shortage of donors and the risks of tumor progression while patients who are not candidates for traditional surgical resection are waiting for OLT, several strategies have been developed in an attempt to achieve local control. These methods include percutaneous ethanol injection, transcatheter arterial chemoembolization (TACE), and radiofrequency ablation (RFA). Although the majority of studies have not shown an improved survival with the use of TACE as primary therapy for HCC, most studies do report significant response rates. At M. D. Anderson Cancer Center, TACE is used selectively. Exclusion criteria include advanced liver disease (Child-Pugh class C), active gastrointestinal bleeding, encephalopathy, refractory ascites, main portal vein thrombosis, extrahepatic spread, hepatofugal flow, renal failure, and severe thrombocytopenia. In well-selected patients, chemoembolization has been shown to improve survival in two recent randomized controlled studies (Llovet et al, 2002; Lo et al, 2002).

Another treatment aimed at local control in patients who are not candidates for traditional resection has been RFA. RFA is a localized thermal treatment technique that produces tumor destruction by heating tumor tissue to temperatures over 50°C, which causes cytodestruction by denaturation of intracellular proteins, as well as dissolution and melting of the phospholipid membranes. Experience from our institution has shown that RFA can produce effective local control of disease while being performed safely with minimal complications. In our experience, although local tumor recurrence at the RFA site was only 3.6%, new liver tumors or extrahepatic metastasis developed in 45.5% of patients. Thus, although local tumor control may be achieved to some measure with RFA, the high recurrence rate emphasizes the need for novel effective therapies.

Systemic Chemotherapy

Systemic chemotherapy for HCC has historically resulted in very low response rates and no improvement in the 5-year survival rate of approximately 5%. Response rates of only 0 to 20% have been reported with treatment of unresectable HCC with cytotoxic agents such as *5-fluorouracil*, *paclitaxel, doxorubicin, cisplatin, vinblastine, etoposide,* and *mitoxantrone,* as single agents or in combinations. Given the modest response rates to traditional chemotherapy, new innovative regimens that "target" molecular abnormalities are warranted. At M. D. Anderson Cancer Center, we have been interested in strategies aimed at inhibiting the epidermal growth factor (EGF) receptor, which has been shown to induce mitogenic activity in vivo in numerous cell types, including hepatocytes. OSI-774 (*Tarceva*) is an orally active, potent, selective inhibitor of the EGF receptor tyrosine kinase that blocks cell-cycle progression in the G_1 phase. OSI-774 is currently being studied in both a phase II clinical trial in HCC and a phase I trial in hepatoma patients with some degree of hepatic dysfunction.

Supplemental Reading

Barbara L, Benzi G, Gaiani S, et al. Natural history of small untreated hepatocellular carcinoma in cirrhosis: a multivariate analysis of prognostic factors of tumor growth rate and patient survival. Hepatology 1992;16:132–7.

Bilimoria M, Lauwers G, Doherty D. Underlying liver disease but not tumor factors predict long-term survival after hepatic resection of hepatocellular carcinoma. Arch Surg 2001;136:528–35.

Bruix J, Castells A, Bosch J, et al. Surgical resection of hepatocellular carcinoma in cirrhotic patients: prognostic value of preoperative portal pressure. Gastroenterology 1996;111:1018–22.

Cancer of the Liver Italian Program (CLIP) Investigators. Prospective validation of the CLIP score: a new prognostic system for patients with cirrhosis and hepatocellular carcinoma. Hepatology 2000;31:840–5.

El-Serag HB. Epidemiology of hepatocellular carcinoma. Clin Liver Dis 2001;5:87–107, vi.

Farges O, Malassagne B, Flejou JF, et al. Risk of major liver resection in patients with underlying chronic liver disease: a reappraisal. Ann Surg 1999;229:210–5.

Hochwald SN, Burke EC, Jarnagin WR, et al. Association of preoperative biliary stenting with increased postoperative infectious complications in proximal cholangiocarcinoma. Arch Surg 1999;134:261–6.

Ishak K, Baptista A, Bianchi L, et al. Histological grading and staging of chronic hepatitis. J Hepatol 1995;22:696–9.

Johnson M, Mannar R, Wu AV. Correlation between blood loss and inferior vena caval pressure during liver resection. Br J Surg 1998;85:188–90.

Llovet JM, Real MI, Montana X, et al. Arterial embolisation or chemoembolisation versus symptomatic treatment in patients with unresectable hepatocellular carcinoma: a randomised controlled trial. Lancet 2002;359:1734–9.

Lo CM, Ngan H, Tso WK, et al. Randomized controlled trial of transarterial lipiodol chemoembolization for unresectable hepatocellular carcinoma. Hepatology 2002;35:1164–71.

Mazzaferro V, Regalia E, Doci R, et al. Liver transplantation for the treatment of small hepatocellular carcinomas in patients with cirrhosis. N Engl J Med 1996;334:693–9.

Okuda K, Ohtsuki T, Obata H, et al. Natural history of hepatocellular carcinoma and prognosis in relation to treatment. Study of 850 patients. Cancer 1985;56:918–28.

Uesaka K, Nimura Y, Nagino M. Changes in hepatic lobar function after right portal vein embolization. An appraisal by biliary indocyanine green excretion. Ann Surg 1996;223:77–83.

Vauthey JN, Abdalla EK, Doherty DA, et al. Body surface area and body weight predict total liver volume in Western adults. Liver Transpl 2002;8:233–40.

Vauthey JN, Lauwers GY, Esnaola NF, et al. Simplified staging for hepatocellular carcinoma. J Clin Oncol 2002;20:1527–36.

CHAPTER 129

Metastatic Cancer of the Liver

Michael A. Choti, MD

Metastatic disease is the most common malignancy of the liver in the United States. The liver is the most common site for developing metastases, accounting for more than half of the cases of advanced cancer. Although primary tumors that drain principally into the portal circulation are more likely than others to develop hepatic metastases, many tumors arising in other sites, including those of the breast and lung, also commonly develop hepatic metastases. Colorectal and neuroendocrine tumors account for the majority of primary tumors with isolated liver metastases.

Cancer of the colon and rectum is the third most commonly diagnosed cancer in the United States. Approximately 20% of patients have clinically recognizable liver metastases at the time of their primary diagnosis. After resection of a primary colorectal cancer in the absence of apparent metastatic disease, approximately 50% of patients will subsequently manifest metastatic liver disease. Given these figures, one can expect that at least 30,000 patients per year in the United States will develop metastatic colorectal cancer confined to the liver.

The potential for developing liver metastases from neuroendocrine tumors depends upon the tumor type. Appendiceal carcinoid tumors and insulinomas rarely develop liver metastases, whereas small bowel carcinoid tumors and other islet cell tumors, including gastrinoma and glucagonoma, develop hepatic metastatic disease in up to 40% of cases. Liver metastases from carcinoid and islet cell tumors are often slow growing, and prolonged survival is often possible even with untreated bilobar and multicentric disease. Other less common malignancies can also demonstrate a pattern of liver-predominant metastases. These include gastrointestinal (GI) stromal tumors, retroperitoneal sarcoma, and ocular melanomas. Other tumor types, including renal cell carcinoma, Wilm's tumor, and breast cancer, although they do not metastasize principally to the liver, can occasionally develop isolated liver metastases.

Assessment of Patients with Hepatic Metastases

The diagnostic approach in patients with hepatic metastases is based on the available treatment options. In patients for whom further treatment is not being considered due to comorbid factors or patient choice, an exhaustive examination for the extent of disease may be unwarranted. In patients for whom systemic chemotherapy is being considered, an examination should facilitate monitoring of the response to treatment at all sites.

Before considering local treatment of liver metastases, particularly colorectal cancer, a thorough preoperative assessment is essential. The goal of the evaluation is to identify the best candidates for resection and discriminate these from those with limited survival benefit or those who will be found at operation to have unresectable disease. The performance status of the patient must also be considered. Although age alone is not a contraindication to resection, comorbid diseases, including especially significant cardiac, pulmonary, and/or renal conditions, increase postoperative morbidity and mortality and may preclude major surgical resection.

Computed tomography (CT) is the imaging modality used most frequently to assess the extent of disease both within and outside the liver. Within the liver, the sensitivity and specificity can vary widely, depending upon equipment and contrast enhancement methods. Although CT detects the presence or absence of liver metastases in approximately 85% of cases, the accuracy of detecting any individual lesion is < 70%, particularly when < 1 cm in diameter. Abdominal CT can detect other intra-abdominal disease, whereas chest CT is most sensitive for identifying pulmonary metastases, detecting 95% of lesions > 1 cm in diameter. Although controversial, chest CT should be considered prior to resection of liver metastases, even in patients with a normal chest radiograph.

Magnetic resonance imaging (MRI) is becoming more commonly used for preoperative evaluation, particularly when assessing the liver. In addition to the ability to accurately detect metastases within the liver and characterize indeterminate lesions, MRI can provide information about the vascular anatomy of the liver, which may be important in planning hepatic surgery. *MRI angiography* can also demonstrate hepatic or portal venous patency, as well as characterize hepatic arterial anatomy. *MRI cholangiography*, though rarely necessary to resection of liver metastases, can be used in selected cases to assess both the intrahepatic and extrahepatic biliary tree. Diagnostic hepatic angiography has a limited role in the management of hepatic colorectal metastases. *CT arterioportography (CTAP)* is a variation of hepatic CT imaging performed after the selective injection of contrast material into the celiac and/or superior mesenteric arteries. Although reported in some series to be more sensitive at detecting small hepatic lesions, false positive findings can occur. Because of the associated morbidity, expense, and lower specificity, CTAP is rarely used for preoperative evaluation in most centers.

Perhaps the most promising imaging modality for the assessment of metastatic sites is *whole body position emission tomography (PET)*. Unlike CT and MRI, which provide anatomic information, PET provides functional information related to metabolic activity. Although a number of radiopharmaceuticals have been labeled with positron emitters, *18F fluorodeoxyglucose (FDG)* is presently the most widely used PET radiopharmaceutical in oncology. A wide spectrum of malignancies can be successfully staged by FDG-PET, including colorectal, lung, and breast cancer. PET has been reported to have a sensitivity as high as 92 to 100%, with a specificity of 85 to 100%. In patients with colorectal liver metastases in whom resection is planned, preoperative FDG-PET appears to be especially useful to exclude extrahepatic disease. Recent studies report identifying additional disease by PET alone, which alters the patient management in up to 20% of the patients undergoing planned liver resection for colorectal metastases. Newer technology that combines PET and CT offers advantages over PET alone, which is limited by poor anatomic localization. This ability to precisely localize the areas of increased PET activity can both increase the overall specificity and improve identification of the site of disease.

Treatment Options

After the patient has been examined for the location and extent of disease, a number of therapeutic options are available. These include *systemic chemotherapy, surgical resection, intratumoral ablation, chemoembolization,* and *regional chemotherapy*.

Systemic Chemotherapy

The choice of systemic chemotherapeutic agents and their efficacy varies with respect to the tumor type. For advanced colorectal cancer, a variety of cytotoxic agents have been tested in patients with advanced disease in the liver and elsewhere. The most useful chemotherapeutic regimens are typically drug combinations including *5-fluorouracil, leucovorin,* and either *irinotecan* or *oxaliplatin*. Newer biologic agents, such as *cetuximab* and *bevacizumab*, are showing early promising results in advanced colorectal cancer as well. Recent studies with these newer regimens demonstrate response rates exceeding 50% with significant improvement in survival. Systemic therapy for metastatic neuroendocrine cancer is of limited benefit.

Liver Resection for Colorectal Metastases

In 1963 Woodington and Waugh first reported a 20% 5-year survival in 20 patients undergoing liver resection for a variety of malignancies, including colon, stomach, gallbladder, pancreas, and melanoma. Since that time there has been an increasing acceptance of this approach to treat liver metastases, particularly in light of the poor outcome obtained with other treatment modalities. A more accurate understanding of liver structure, based on functional segmental anatomy, as well as advances in operative technique and postoperative care, have resulted in the capability to perform this operation with very low morbidity and mortality.

Before considering liver resection, a thorough preoperative examination is essential. As discussed, careful preoperative examination with CT or MRI, and perhaps FDG-PET, is needed to determine the extent and resectability of disease within the liver, and to exclude extrahepatic disease. Intraoperative exploration and evaluation of the extent of disease within the abdominal cavity and liver is critical prior to proceeding with surgical resection. If the site of the primary tumor was intra-abdominal, this area should be inspected and palpated if accessible to rule out local or regional recurrence. Bimanual palpation of the liver is carried out, after inspection and palpation of the peritoneal surfaces and periportal nodal region. Nodal involvement in the periportal area is associated with a significantly poorer long term outcome, and should preclude curative resection in most cases.

Intraoperative ultrasonography (IOUS) is the most sensitive modality currently available for detecting otherwise occult liver metastases. Its overall sensitivity is reported to be up to 98%. By improving the capability of detecting clinically occult metastases, patients with multiple unresectable metastases may be spared unnecessary hepatic resection. IOUS may also contribute to improved survival by helping to detect and excise or ablate otherwise occult residual disease. Moreover, IOUS facilitates the careful examination of intrahepatic vascular structures and their relationship to the hepatic tumors, often allowing for safer resections with more adequate resection margins.

In some centers, laparoscopic examination of the liver and abdominal cavity just prior to laparotomy has been used to identify additional patients who have unresectable disease, reducing the number of patients unnecessarily undergoing full surgical exploration. With recent refinements in laparoscopic ultrasonographic devices, intraoperative hepatic ultrasonography can now complement visual laparoscopic assessment. Despite such enthusiastic initial reports, the role of laparoscopy prior to surgical exploration for patients with isolated hepatic metastases remains to be defined.

The main goal of the liver resection is to precisely remove the involved portion of liver with an adequate surgical margin and preserve sufficient hepatic reserve.

Although most patients with metastases do not have cirrhosis and can tolerate extended resections, increased morbidity can be associated with larger resections, particularly in patients heavily pretreated with chemotherapy. Therefore, an attempt should be made in most cases to preserve as much liver as possible.

Overall, the perioperative mortality of liver resection for colorectal metastases is < 3% in most reported series. In experienced hands, even major hepatic resections (*hemihepatectomy* or *extended hemihepatectomy*) result in perioperative mortalities of < 5%. The potential for adverse outcome and the complexity of these operations, however, justifies the recommendation that major liver resection be performed at centers and by surgeons with more than occasional experience with such procedures.

Outcomes of Liver Resection for Colorectal Metastases

The overall 5-year survival reported following hepatic resection with curative intent for metastatic colorectal cancer in most series ranges from 28 to 50%. In these reports, the median survival was as high as 46 months. More recent studies demonstrate a favorable trend in improved long term outcome in recent years. Although the reasons for this trend are not definitive, multiple factors, including improved preoperative and intraoperative imaging and use of adjuvant chemotherapy, are likely contributors.

Although surgical resection results in prolonged survival and perhaps cure in some patients, the majority will eventually develop recurrent disease. For this reason, many investigators have attempted to identify factors that might improve patient selection, thereby improving the long term outcome of those resected. Clearly, some features of the metastatic disease, including the number, size, and location of the metastases, correlate with prognosis. Although prognosis appears worse in patients with an increased number of metastases, long-term survival can be achieved, at least in selected patients, with resection of even four or more metastatic lesions. Similarly, the size of the metastasis or direct invasion into adjacent structures should not preclude resection if the disease can be completely removed. Concomitant extrahepatic metastatic disease, although associated with poorer prognosis in many series, should not be an absolute contraindication to hepatectomy provided the extrahepatic disease is also resected.

The stage of the primary colorectal tumor does appear to correlate with long term outcome. Both positive nodal status and high histologic grade of the primary tumor are associated with poor prognosis following liver resection in several reported series. However, these differences are small and do not appear to weigh heavily on the decision for liver resection. Technical factors at the time of surgery can also impact on the prognosis. These are of particular significance as they may be avoidable. A positive histologic surgical resection margin has been shown to be clearly associated with poor long term survival. The optimal width of the negative surgical margin, however, remains controversial. Some investigators have reported an improved survival when clearance margins were ≥ 1 cm, whereas others have shown no differences, provided the margin is grossly negative. The type of resection performed and the technique of parenchymal dissection does not appear to affect long term recurrence rates, independent of margin status.

Although a variety of factors appear to be associated with differences in prognosis, including the stage of the primary tumor, the number of hepatic metastases, the disease-free interval, and the resection margin, patients should not be excluded from an attempt at curative resection solely on the basis of one or more of these poor prognostic factors. However, the presence of unresectable extrahepatic disease, probably including periportal nodal disease, or lack of control of the locoregional primary disease, is generally considered a contraindication to resection.

Liver Resection for Noncolorectal Metastases

The role of liver resection for hepatic metastases from noncolorectal tumors has not been studied as well as that for metastases from colorectal primaries. Selected patients with neuroendocrine metastases may benefit from aggressive complete surgical resection and even (incomplete) cytoreductive surgery because of the slow tumor growth and often significant symptoms related to hormone production and tumor bulk. Even when all disease cannot be resected, uncontrolled reports suggest that when symptomatic or when > 90% of disease can be resected, palliative or cytoreductive surgery may also be of benefit in patients with hepatic metastases from neuroendocrine primaries.

Local Ablative Therapies

Although surgical resection may afford the only potential for cure in patients with hepatic metastases, many patients may not be candidates for surgical resection for a variety of reasons. Novel methods for local ablation have been developed with a goal of increasing the number of patients eligible for surgical resection. The early experiences with metastasis ablation have been primarily with *hepatic cryosurgery*. More recently, *radiofrequency ablation (RFA)* has been applied for the treatment of liver tumors in much the same manner. With this technique, a needle is inserted within the selected tumor and electric current is employed to generate heat, resulting in thermal ablation. RFA can be performed laparoscopically or even percutaneously, as well as via open laparotomy. For these reasons, RFA has largely replaced other ablative techniques as the preferred method of interstitial ablation in most centers.

Summary

Metastatic disease is the most common malignant process affecting the liver. Although metastatic disease can develop in the liver via systemic spread from most solid malignancies, certain tumor types have the propensity to develop liver-dominant disease and, often, isolated liver metastases. These include primarily colorectal cancer and, less commonly, neuroendocrine tumors, GI sarcomas, ocular melanoma, and others. There is a preponderance of uncontrolled studies strongly suggesting that surgical resection offers the best potential cure for colorectal cancer metastatic to the liver. Careful preoperative evaluation of the liver, primary tumor, and extrahepatic sites, is important to exclude unresectable disease and select those patients who may benefit most from resection. Potential strategies currently under investigation for improving outcomes include combining resection with adjuvant regional or systemic chemotherapy. For unresectable disease, other local ablative approaches, including RFA or regional chemotherapy may offer some benefit.

Supplemental Reading

Altendorf-Hofmann A, Scheele J. A critical review of the major indicators of prognosis after resection of hepatic metastases from colorectal carcinoma. Surg Oncol Clin N Am 2003;12:165–92.

Bleicher RJ, Allegra DP, Nora DT, et al. Radiofrequency ablation in 447 complex unresectable liver tumors: lessons learned. Ann Surg Oncol 2003;10:52–8.

Chen H, Hardacre JM, Uzar A, et al. Isolated liver metastases from neuroendocrine tumors: does resection prolong survival? J Am Coll Surg 1998;187:88–92.

Choti MA, Sitzmann JV, Tiburi MF, et al. Trends in long-term survival following liver resection for hepatic colorectal metastases. Ann Surg 2002;235:759–66.

Conlon R, Jacobs M, Dasgupta D, Lodge JP. The value of intraoperative ultrasound during hepatic resection compared with improved preoperative magnetic resonance imaging. Eur J Ultrasound 2003;16:211–6.

Figueras J, Valls C. The use of laparoscopic ultrasonography in the preoperative study of patients with colorectal liver metastases. Ann Surg 2000;232:721–3.

Fong Y, Fortner J, Sun RL, et al. Clinical score for predicting recurrence after hepatic resection for metastatic colorectal cancer: analysis of 1,001 consecutive cases. Ann Surg 1999;230:309–18.

Gill S, Thomas RR, Goldberg RM. New targeted therapies in gastrointestinal cancers. Curr Treat Options Oncol 2003; 4:393–403.

Harrison LE, Brennan MF, Newman E, et al. Hepatic resection for noncolorectal, nonneuroendocrine metastases: a fifteen-year experience with ninety-six patients. Surgery 1997;121:625–32.

Kamel IR, Bluemke DA. MR imaging of liver tumors. Radiol Clin North Am 2003;41:51–65.

Louvet C, de Gramont A. Colorectal cancer: integrating oxaliplatin. Curr Treat Options Oncol 2003;4:405–11.

Rohren EM, Paulson EK, Hagge R, et al. The role of F-18 FDG positron emission tomography in preoperative assessment of the liver in patients being considered for curative resection of hepatic metastases from colorectal cancer. Clin Nucl Med 2002;27:550–5.

CHAPTER 130

LAPAROSCOPIC CHOLECYSTECTOMY

DON J. SELZER, MD, AND KEITH D. LILLEMOE, MD

Laparoscopic cholecystectomy, reported by Reddick in 1989, began a revolution in surgical practice. Improvements in video imaging and instrumentation, in addition to changing patient expectations, have fueled an explosion in the breadth, availability, and number of laparoscopic procedures. A videoscopic minimally invasive approach is available for treatment of diseases ranging from parathyroid adenoma to morbid obesity to varicose veins. Benefits of a laparoscopic approach over a traditional open technique include less pain, shorter hospital stay, faster return to activities of daily living, and improved cosmesis.

Since the National Institutes of Health Consensus Statement in 1992, the laparoscopic approach has become the preferred technique for cholecystectomy. Laparoscopic cholecystectomy is now the most commonly performed elective abdominal procedure in the United States. During the last decade, significant experience gained in preoperative selection, surgical technique, and intraoperative decision making has dramatically improved results. However, complications continue to occur and controversies remain. Indications, surgical technique, and outcomes for laparoscopic cholecystectomy are reviewed.

Indications and Evaluation

Currently, the Centers for Disease Control and Prevention estimates 600,000 to 750,000 cholecystectomies are performed annually in the United States. Cholecystectomy is classically indicated to treat signs, symptoms, and complications of gallstones. Despite the relatively low risks associated with laparoscopic cholecystectomy, the procedure should be limited to symptomatic patients. These patients are at increased risk of developing complications including acute cholecystitis, common bile duct obstruction, cholangitis, and pancreatitis. Evidence exists that these complications seldom develop at initial presentation, so asymptomatic patients are generally treated with watchful waiting. Laparoscopic cholecystectomy is also indicated for patients without gallstones but typical biliary colic. These patients may have acalculous cholecystitis or biliary dyskinesia diagnoses made by quantitative gallbladder emptying or radio-nucleotide study.

The quick recovery and excellent outcomes of laparoscopic cholecystectomy have reduced the reluctance of patients to undergo gallbladder surgery, leading to an increase in the number of cholecystectomies performed annually. During the 1990s, there was a 29% increase in the number of cholecystectomies performed, with over a 100% increase in cholecystectomy for acute acalculous cholecystitis and 300% increase for biliary dyskinesia. Although nonsurgical methods of gallstone removal, including pharmacologic dissolution, shock wave lithotripsy, and endoscopic laser ablation, were once considered alternatives to the traditional open surgical approach, widespread use of laparoscopic cholecystectomy with its increased patient acceptance, has generally lead to the elimination of these treatments as alternatives.

Despite advances in radiologic methods, ultrasonography remains the mainstay of gallbladder imaging. Information obtained from a right upper quadrant sonogram (ie, including the presence of gallstones, gallbladder wall thickening, pericholecystic fluid, and common bile duct dilatation) surpasses other diagnostic studies at a fraction of the cost. Radioscintigraphy of the biliary tree has two indications. First, it confirms gallbladder uptake or cystic duct obstruction in the diagnosis of acute cholecystitis in patients with confounding symptoms, signs, and medical conditions. Second, a calculated gallbladder ejection fraction below 35% following administration of intravenous cholecystikinin during scintigraphy is used to diagnose biliary dyskinesia. In addition to radiologic tests, laboratory evaluations, including complete blood count, liver function tests, and serum amylase and lipase, help confirm disease processes and determine treatment plans.

The choice of surgical treatment may be affected by a patient's medical comorbidities and presentation. Severely limiting cardiac and pulmonary disease processes may prevent a patient from withstanding the rigors of even laparoscopic surgical intervention. Creation of a pneumoperitoneum leads to multiple cardiovascular effects including decreased stroke volume, cardiac output, and venous return. Patients also develop increased systemic and pulmonary vascular resistance, mean arterial pressure, central venous pressure, and pulmonary artery wedge pressure. Most of these effects are directly related to the mechanical effects of increased intra-abdominal pressure, but sympathetic stimulation and biochemical effects of the gas used to create the pneumoperitoneum add to the insult.

Early in its development, some surgeons limited the use of laparoscopic approach, avoiding patients with acute cholecystitis, gallstone pancreatitis, choledocholithiasis, hepatitis or cirrhosis with portal hypertension, previous abdominal surgery, severe obesity, sepsis, and pregnancy. As surgeons have surpassed the "learning curve," the relative contraindications to the laparoscopic approach have been reduced or eliminated. In fact, preoperative concern for gallbladder carcinoma remains the only absolute contraindication to laparoscopic cholecystectomy because of the risk of dissemination of cancer cells by the turbulent flow of gas in the pneumoperitoneum.

Perioperative Care and Surgical Technique

Patient preparation for laparoscopic cholecystectomy does not typically include a bowel cleansing regimen, but no oral intake is restricted a minimum of 6 hours prior to induction of general anesthesia. Preoperative prophylactic antibiotics are typically administered intravenously, ideally one half hour before surgical incision. Choice of antibacterial agent is commensurate with the spectrum of biliary infectious agents.

Following induction of general anesthesia and preparation of the patient's abdomen with antibacterial agents, the procedure begins with insertion of a 10 mm diameter laparoscopic port at the umbilicus. Gas is delivered, or insufflated, through the port into the abdomen and a laparoscope with attached fiber optic video camera is introduced. Carbon dioxide is almost exclusively used to create the pneumoperitoneum, but other gases including air, helium, and nitrous oxide have been used. Intra-abdominal pressures are limited to approximately 15 mm Hg because of the previously mentioned secondary hemodynamic and pulmonary effects created by the pneumoperitoneum. A brief laparoscopic examination of the abdomen is performed and 3 more laparoscopic ports, typically 5 mm in diameter, are introduced through small incisions in the epigastrium and right subcostal regions.

Laparoscopic graspers allow manipulation of intra-abdominal contents including the gallbladder. The dome of the gallbladder is elevated in a cephalad fashion to reveal Calot's triangle. Inflammation secondary to acute or chronic cholecystitis may lead to regional adhesions, limit exposure of Calot's triangle, and render the laparoscopic approach precarious.

Dissection begins with stripping of the peritoneal lining from the gallbladder infundibulum and cystic duct. Absolute, positive identification of the cystic duct and cystic artery are essential to performing a safe and successful laparoscopic cholecystectomy. Strong evidence exists that misidentification of the common bile duct as the cystic duct leads to most major bile duct injuries, the so-called "classic bile duct injury." Difficult identification of important anatomical landmarks requires the surgeon to maintain a low threshold to convert from the laparoscopic approach to an open cholecystectomy. Conversion to an open procedure for prevention of inadvertent injury is not considered a complication; it is considered good clinical judgment. Selective use of laparoscopic intraoperative cholangiography (IOC) can help to determine anatomical variants, diagnose choledocholithiasis, and identify inadvertent injuries. A normal cholangiogram is followed by ligation of the cystic duct and cystic artery with clips or sutures and separation of the gallbladder from its liver attachments. The gallbladder is removed from the peritoneal cavity through one of the laparoscopic port incisions, commonly the umbilical site. Hemostasis is confirmed and the gas is removed, or desufflated, from the abdomen.

Duration of the procedure is dependent on regional inflammatory changes and patient anatomy. However, an elective laparoscopic cholecystectomy may be performed in < 1 hour on a routine basis. Although patients are routinely admitted for overnight observation following the procedure, outpatient laparoscopic cholecystectomies are becoming more common. A liquid diet is instituted immediately following surgery and the patients is instructed to advance to regular food as tolerated. Patients generally recover and return to normal activities in < 2 weeks after surgery.

Although the surgical technique of laparoscopic cholecystectomy remains essentially unchanged since the early days of its development, technological refinements continue to provide improvements. Improved digital imaging provides better visualization and allows the use of smaller diameter equipment, smaller incisions, and fewer laparoscopic ports.

Laparoscopic Cholecystectomy for Expanded Indications

With growing experience, surgeons are now successful in performing laparoscopic cholecystectomy on the majority of patients regardless of presentation. However, several clinical scenarios continue to provide challenging settings for the laparoscopic technique and controversies with regard to methods of treatment. Acute cholecystitis, gallstone pancreatitis, choledocholithiasis, hepatitis or cirrhosis with portal hypertension, previous abdominal surgery, severe obesity, sepsis, and pregnancy are areas where dramatic improvements have occurred.

Acute cholecystitis is no longer considered an absolute contraindication to laparoscopic cholecystectomy. Recent experience shows cholecystectomy should be performed within 24 to 48 hours of admission or 72 to 96 hours after development of symptoms. During this brief window, pericholecystic fluid and edema aid surgical dissection. After this period has passed, this edema leads to dense fibrosis and impedes or even prevents safe completion of the cholecystectomy. Laparoscopic cholecystectomy performed during the initial 72 hours after presentation has a conversion rate of approximately 25%; whereas procedures performed > 3 days after initial presentation lead to conversion in 30 to 60% of cases. The method of "cooling down" acute cholecystitis with interval cholecystectomy 6 weeks later has fallen out of favor, because the residual chronic inflammation often makes dissection difficult.

Complication rates in patients with acute cholecystitis are similar for the laparoscopic and open approach. However, conversion from the laparoscopic approach to an open technique occurs in < 5% of patients undergoing elective laparoscopic cholecystectomy compared with the higher conversion rates noted previously for patients with acute cholecystitis. Judicious conversion to an open approach has limited inadvertent biliary injuries in patients with acute cholecystitis and prevented other major complications. Patients that undergo successful laparoscopic cholecystectomy for acute cholecystitis frequently experience the same rapid recovery as elective procedures. However, with the addition of the preoperative hospital stay and a brief postoperative observation period, total length of the hospital stay is generally longer for patients with acute cholecystitis.

Gallstone pancreatitis, once considered a contraindication for the minimally invasive approach, is now successfully treated with laparoscopic cholecystectomy on a regular basis. Timing of cholecystectomy remains controversial and is determined by severity of the pancreatitis. Recovery from an attack of mild acute pancreatitis is signaled by normalization of white blood cell count, serum amylase and lipase, and resolution of pain. Long delay in removing the gallbladder leads to recurrent attacks and raises risk of severe necrotizing pancreatitis. Therefore, laparoscopic cholecystectomy and IOC performed during the same hospital admission and immediately following resolution of signs and symptoms is the recommended course of treatment.

In the presence of pancreatitis, persistent signs of biliary obstruction and choledocholithiasis typically lead to endoscopic intervention with endoscopic retrograde pancreatography (ERCP), endoscopic sphincterotomy (ES), and stone removal prior to considering laparoscopic cholecystectomy. Successful preoperative ERCP with ES has not shown to significantly increase morbidity. In fact, early ERCP with duct clearance appears to benefit patients. Despite this evidence, most surgeons do not routinely employ preoperative ERCP in mild, self-limited gallstone pancreatitis, because stones have frequently passed and patients are exposed to the risk of the ERCP with ES and needlessly experience a longer hospital stay. Following resolution of pancreatitis, laparoscopic cholecystectomy exhibits the same low rates of morbidity and mortality and rapid surgical recovery as seen in other patients.

Minimally invasive methods of treating choledocholithiasis have advanced dramatically. IOC during open cholecystectomy with common bile duct exploration and stone removal as indicated was considered the standard of care. Increasing use of ERCP with ES and stone removal has experienced great success. However, ERCP is associated with recognized morbidity. Postprocedure pancreatitis occurs in 0.5 to 2% of elective ERCPs, but therapeutic ERCP may cause pancreatitis in as many as 26% of cases. Duodenal perforation following sphincterotomy occurs in approximately 1% percent of patients. Therefore, use of preoperative ERCP should be limited to clinical scenarios with high likelihood for common bile duct stones, including jaundice and cholangitis. Unfortunately, attempts to identify statistically significant predictive signs for choledocholithiasis have been unsuccessful, including abnormal liver function tests and ultrasound findings. Therefore, a more common approach now includes laparoscopic cholecystectomy with IOC and laparoscopic common bile duct exploration with a transcystic duct or transcholedochal approach. Attempts to clear the common bile duct laparoscopically include administration of glucagon, infusion of saline, fluoroscopic guided insertion of stone retrieval wire baskets, or placement of a flexible choledochoscope for common bile duct exploration via the cystic or common bile duct.

Laparoscopic common bile duct exploration is a complicated and technically demanding procedure practiced by few surgeons on a regular basis. Failure to clear the common bile duct of stones during the laparoscopic procedure leads to either postoperative ERCP or conversion to an open common bile duct exploration. Success of ERCP in this setting is excellent and preserves the benefits of minimally invasive procedures. The availability of skilled ERCP technicians or radiologic interventionalists has lead many surgeons to complete the cholecystectomy laparoscopically and allow duct clearance to be performed by one of these alternative minimally invasive approaches. Unsuccessful ERCP or percutaneous transhepatic stone removal leading to another surgical procedure with open common bile duct exploration is an infrequent occurrence.

Patients with cirrhosis and portal hypertension remain a challenge for the surgeon to perform any surgical procedure. However, laparoscopic cholecystectomy can be performed safely and effectively in patients with Child's A or B cirrhosis. In addition, increased experience with laparoscopic lysis of adhesions allows surgeons to successfully complete laparoscopic cholecystectomy in patients who have had previous surgical procedures. Obesity is no longer considered a contraindication to the laparoscopic approach. Successful completion of the laparoscopic cholecystectomy in the morbidly obese patient may require insertion of additional ports for retraction of adipose tissue or use of longer laparoscopic trochars, and is clearly associated with an increased risk for conversion to open approach.

Although bedside diagnostic laparoscopy is performed in septic patients at some centers, percutaneous cholecystostomy or traditional open cholecystectomy are preferred forms of therapy in hemodynamically unstable patients with acute calculous or acalculous cholecystitis. Gasless laparoscopy or pneumoperitoneum laparoscopy performed with an alternative gas, like helium, that does not cause acidosis or other hemodynamic effects of carbon dioxide, are also options in this patient group.

Finally, pregnancy remains a controversial setting to treat symptomatic gallstones. Conservative nonsurgical therapy is frequently considered in mild cases of biliary colic or acute cholecystitis to reduce risk to the patient and fetus. Although, laparoscopic cholecystectomy is a safe procedure in all three trimesters, the second trimester remains the preferred timing for any elective surgical intervention. A lower risk of spontaneous abortion during the first trimester and lower risk of preterm labor during the third trimester favor the laparoscopic approach over the open technique, if surgery is indicated during those time periods.

Complications and Outcomes

During the early development of laparoscopic cholecystectomy, controversy raged over the dramatically increased risks of complications associated with the new procedure and credentialing of practicing surgeons in this technique. Many at academic institutions initially dismissed this apparently radical and potentially dangerous approach.

The result was that many surgeons gained their initial experience with the procedure through short animal courses with limited clinical proctoring. Therefore, an understandably steep learning curve was associated with frequent complications. Fortunately, with the passage of time and wide acceptance of the procedure, laparoscopic cholecystectomy is now performed safely and acquisition of surgical skills is no longer a problem. Although controlled trials, necessary to demonstrate the procedure's worth to academia, lagged behind the overwhelming public support, large retrospective reviews have eventually confirmed the safety and efficacy of laparoscopic cholecystectomy.

Elective laparoscopic cholecystectomy for calculous disease is a safe and successful procedure with a morbidity of < 5% and a mortality of < 0.25%. Greater than 90% of patients with a classic presentation of right upper quadrant pain and ultrasonographic diagnosis of gallstones experience relief of symptoms following laparoscopic cholecystectomy. Although elective laparoscopic cholecystectomy for uncomplicated symptomatic cholelithiasis may have a conversion rate of < 2 or 3% in skilled hands, the majority of reported series have demonstrated a consistent conversion ratio of 5 to 6% over the last decade. The most common predictive factors for conversion to an open approach include surgeon's experience, morbid obesity, acute cholecystitis, chronic cholecystitis with thickened gallbladder wall on preoperative ultrasound, previous surgical procedures, and patients with multiple medical comorbidities. As previously mentioned, patients with acute cholecystitis may experience a conversion rate as high as 25%. Patients with acalculous disease and atypical symptoms have not experienced the same results following laparoscopic cholecystectomy. As previously mentioned, acute acalculous cholecystitis frequently occurs in clinical scenarios limiting the role of surgical intervention. Hemodynamically unstable patients who are unable to tolerate general anesthesia are frequently treated with percutaneous ultrasound guided placement of a cholecystostomy tube or urgent open cholecystectomy. Patients with biliary dyskinesia, experience only an 80% relief of symptoms following laparoscopic cholecystectomy.

Common complications following laparoscopic cholecystectomy include those seen with operations of any type including bleeding, infection, and risks of general anesthesia, and those complications specific for the laparoscopic cholecystectomy, including conversion to an open procedure, bile duct injury, injury to surrounding organs, and bile or gallstone spillage into the peritoneal cavity. Although considered a complication by patients and many physicians, conversion to an open procedure more often demonstrates good clinical and technical judgment rather than surgical misadventure. Persistence with a laparoscopic approach despite difficulty with visualization and identification of anatomical landmarks may lead to other more severe complications like bile duct injury.

Inadvertent bile duct injury is an uncommon but devastating complication that fortunately occurs less frequently with growing surgical experience. Common bile duct injury occurs in 0.5% of laparoscopic cholecystectomies. Suspicion of a biliary injury based on unclear anatomy, bile leak, or demonstration on IOC, requires immediate conversion to an open procedure to delineate the injury and repair it or reconstruct with a bilioenteric drainage procedure. Unfortunately, most bile duct injuries are missed at the initial laparoscopic cholecystectomy and remain undiagnosed until several days after surgery. This leads to the need for additional radiologic, endoscopic, or surgical drainage procedures, and a reoperation for eventual bilioenteric anastomosis. Although specific clinical scenarios, errors in skill, or lapses in judgment may lead to increased risk of injury, misperception appears to be the most common culprit. Recent surgical literature promotes regular use of IOC to help identify and perhaps reduce inadvertent biliary tree injuries. Although considered devastating and clearly associated with significant pain, suffering, and short term disability, long term results following reconstruction are good. Repair of a bile duct injury is associated with an overall success rate of 90% and an excellent quality of life.

Bleeding during laparoscopic cholecystectomy may occur from avulsion of the cystic artery or a tear in the liver. These are typically controlled successfully with ligation and cautery respectively. An inexperienced surgeon, when faced with persistent bleeding from the cystic artery stump, may rashly place superfluous metallic clips and cause inadvertent injury to other vascular structures or the remaining extrahepatic biliary tree. Errant introduction of the initial laparoscopic trochar has lead to injury of the mesenteric vessels, or more seriously, the iliac vessels. Injury to a major vascular structure including the portal vein, inferior vena cava, or hepatic artery is an extremely uncommon occurrence in only 0.11% of procedures, but it requires conversion to a laparotomy for immediate repair.

Injury can occur to internal structures, including the intestine or mesentery, during insertion of laparoscopic ports, retraction of the liver or duodenum, or application of cautery to bleeding foci. Immediately identified injuries are repaired with laparoscopic or open surgical techniques. The most troublesome intestinal injury occurs from errant transmission of electrical cautery arcing to other inserted instruments or breakdown in the insulation of the electrical current applicator. These injuries may go unnoticed until 2 to 3 days have passed and peritonitis is present. Injuries are avoided by judicious use of electrical cautery under direct visualization.

Bile spillage happens frequently during cholecystectomy. Inflammation alters surgical dissection planes and creates a friable and easily torn gallbladder wall. Bile is easily irrigated and aspirated with little residual effects. On the other hand, gallstones spilled into the peritoneal cavity should be located and removed to reduce infectious foci and possible complications. Wound infection, an infrequent occurrence, is limited by extraction of the gallbladder from the peritoneal cavity with a plastic pouch.

Conclusion

Time has provided surgeons with experience to surpass the "learning curve" associated with laparoscopic cholecystectomy. The surgical technique has changed little during the last several years. However, improved technology and growing experience have allowed surgeons to offer the laparoscopic approach to patients who were once considered to have relative contraindications with similar low rates of morbidity and mortality. Routine use of IOC and preoperative ERCP remain controversial issues. The greatest changes have occurred with increasing push to perform laparoscopic cholecystectomy early in the chronology of the disease process and in acalculous disease. Over 15 years ago, laparoscopic cholecystectomy started the dramatic shift toward the minimally invasive approach, a process that continues to change the practice of general surgery.

Supplemental Reading

Byrne MF, Suhocki P, Mitchell RM, et al. Percutaneous cholecystostomy in patients with acute cholecystitis: experience of 45 patients at a US referral center. J Am Coll Surg 2003; 197:206–11.

Canal DF, Broadie TA. Results of laparoscopic cholecystectomy for the treatment of gallstone pancreatitis. Am Surg 1994;60:495–9.

Carroll BA. Preferred imaging techniques for the diagnosis of cholecystitis and cholelithiasis. Ann Surg 1989;210:1–12.

Fan ST, Lai ECS, Mok FPT, et al. Early treatment of acute biliary pancreatitis by endoscopic papillotomy. New Engl J Med 1993;328:228–32.

Fiore NF, Ledniczky G, Wiebke EA, et al. An analysis of perioperative cholangiography in one thousand laparoscopic cholecystectomies. Surgery 1997;122:817–23.

Flum DR, Dellinger EP, Cheadle A, et al. Intraoperative cholangiography and risk of common bile duct injury during cholecystectomy. JAMA 2003;289:1639–44.

Graham G, Baxi L, Tharakan T. Laparoscopic cholecystectomy during pregnancy: a case series and review of the literature. Obstet Gynecol Surv 1998;53:566–74.

Johanning JM, Gruenberg JC. The changing face of cholecystectomy. Am Surg 1998;64:643–8.

Lillemoe KD, Melton GB, Cameron JL, et al. Postoperative bile duct strictures: management and outcome in the 1990's. Ann Surg 2000;232:430–41.

MacFadyen BV, Vecchio R, Ricardo AE, Mathis CR. Bile duct injury after laparoscopic cholecystectomy: the United States experience. Surg Endosc 1998;12:315–21.

National Institutes of Health. Gallstones and laparoscopic cholecystectomy. NIH Consensus Statement 1992;10:1–26.

Pessaux P, Tuesch JJ, Rouge C, et al. Laparoscopic cholecystectomy in acute cholecystitis: a prospective comparative study in patients with acute vs chronic cholecystitis. Surg Endosc 2000;14:358–61.

Reddick EA, Olsen DO. Laparoscopic laser cholecystectomy: a comparison with mini-lap cholecystectomy. Surg Endosc 1989;3:131–3.

Romano F, Franciosi CM, Caprotti R, et al. Pre operative selective endoscopic retrograde cholangiopancreatography and laparoscopic cholecystectomy without cholangiography. Surg Laparosc Endosc & Perc Tech 2002;12:408–11.

Rosen M, Brody F, Ponsky J. Predictive factors for conversion of laparoscopic cholecystectomy. Am J Surg 2002;184:254–8.

Rutledge D, Jones D, Rege R. Consequences of delay in surgical treatment of biliary disease. Am J Surg 2000;80:466–9.

Uhl W, Warshaw A, Imrie C, et al. IAP guidelines for the surgical management of acute pancreatitis. Pancreatology 2002;2: 565–73.

Usal H, Sayad P, Hayek N, et al. Major vascular injuries during laparoscopic cholecystectomy: an institutional review of experience with 2589 procedures and literature review. Surg Endosc 1998;12:960–2.

Way LW, Stewart L, Gantert W, et al. Causes and prevention of laparoscopic bile duct injuries: analysis of 252 cases from a human factors and cognitive psychology perspective. Ann Surg 2003;237:460–9.

Acute and Chronic Cholecystitis

Alexandra L. B. Webb, MD, and Aaron S. Fink, MD FACS

Acute cholecystitis is usually caused by obstruction of the cystic duct or Hartmann's pouch with gallstones, leading to painful gallbladder distention. Edema of the gallbladder and lymphatic and venous congestion then occur. Superinfection of the bile may then supervene.

This illness is more frequent in females; the female to male ratio is 3:1 for patients under the age of 50 years and decreases to 1.5:1 after the age of 50 years. Acute cholecystitis is most common in the fourth to eighth decades of life and occurs with increased frequency in overweight patients as well as in those who are multiparous. Most patients who develop acute cholecystitis have a prior history of symptomatic cholelithiasis.

Presentation

The most common symptom is right upper quadrant pain and is often associated with anorexia, nausea, or vomiting. Fever is frequently present, but is not required for the diagnosis. On physical examination, right upper quadrant tenderness is common and may be severe with localized guarding or rebound. The gallbladder may be palpable in some patients, but a Murphy's sign (inspiratory arrest during palpation of the gallbladder) is almost always present. Mild jaundice is not uncommon, although bilirubin rarely exceeds 6 mg/dL. Laboratory examination frequently reveals leukocytosis of 12,000 to 15,000 cells/mm^3, but a normal white blood cell count does not exclude the diagnosis of acute cholecystitis. Liver function tests (bilirubin, transaminases, and alkaline phosphatase) may be elevated or normal.

Diagnosis

Ultrasonography (US) is the most helpful study in diagnosing acute cholecystitis. US findings suggestive of acute cholecystitis include the presence of gallstones, gallbladder wall thickness > 4 mm, pericholecystic fluid, or a sonographic Murphy's sign. Gallbladder distention with dimensions > 8 × 5 cm may also suggest acute cholecystitis.

Computed tomographic (CT) scan is frequently obtained in patients with right upper quadrant pain and may also demonstrate evidence of acute cholecystitis. Gallbladder wall thickening and pericholecystic fluid are typically well visualized on CT scan (Figure 131-1). Gallstones may also be seen, although CT is much less sensitive than US in detecting gallstones. CT scan may also

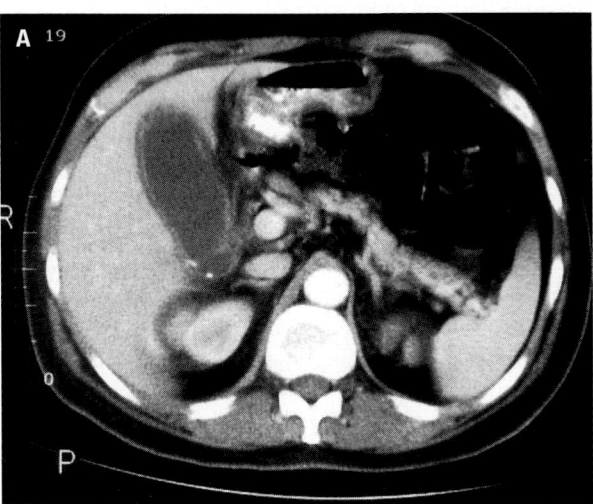 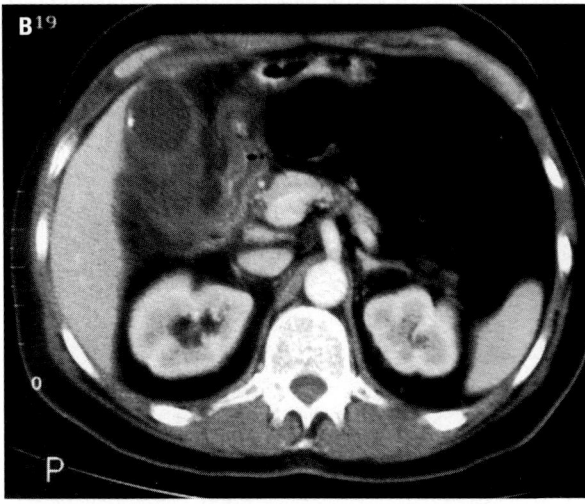

FIGURE 131-1. A computed tomographic scan image demonstrating findings of acute cholecystitis. Thickened gallbladder wall, calcified gallstones, pericholecystic fluid (A). Pericholecystic inflammation, calcified gallstones (B). Images courtesy of Dr. Todd Fibus.

demonstrate air in the gallbladder or gallbladder wall, indicative of advanced disease with progression to emphysematous cholecystitis. Emphysematous cholecystitis requires immediate surgical intervention, most frequently via laparotomy.

Patients who have a classic clinical picture of acute cholecystitis in conjunction with confirmatory US or CT scan do not require further diagnostic examination. In patients in whom the diagnosis remains unclear, cholescintigraphy is the diagnostic procedure of choice for establishing the diagnosis of acute cholecystitis. Technetium-99m labeled iminodiacetic acid derivatives are injected intravenously. These acids are cleared by the liver and excreted in bile, allowing imaging of the biliary tree. Normal time for gallbladder filling with radiotracer is 30 minutes. Nonfilling of the gallbladder in 4 hours confirms the diagnosis of acute cholecystitis. This test has a sensitivity of 97% and a specificity of 90% for acute calculous cholecystitis.

Therapy

Initial management for all patients with acute cholecystitis consists of hospital admission, intravenous (IV) hydration, cessation of oral intake, and treatment with IV antibiotics. Only 50 to 75% of patients with acute cholecystitis have positive bile cultures, giving weight to the theory that bacterial infection is a consequence rather than a cause of cholecystitis. Although bacterial contamination of the bile is uncommon in uncomplicated acute cholecystitis, antibiotics are given to all patients, as it is difficult to determine when superinfection occurs. The antibiotic chosen should cover both gram-negative organisms and anaerobes and cover the three most commonly isolated organisms: *Escherichia coli, Klebsiella, and Enterococcus.*

Laparoscopic cholecystectomy was rapidly adopted for treatment of patients with chronic cholecystitis, but was not initially recommended for patients with acute cholecystitis because of concern over increased conversion and complication rates. This concern is based on technical issues often encountered in patients with acute cholecystitis (ie, the distended, thickened gallbladder wall may be difficult to grasp, making retraction difficult) (Figure 131-2). Additionally, inflammatory changes may make exposure of Calot's triangle and clear identification of the cystic duct and artery more difficult. However, the benefits of laparoscopic over open cholecystectomy are clear in terms of decreased pain, shorter hospital stay, and lower cost. As experience has increased, laparoscopic cholecystectomy is being used more frequently in patients with acute cholecystitis.

Nonetheless, there is an increased incidence of conversion from laparoscopic to open access when attempting cholecystectomy for acute versus chronic cholecystitis. Although the frequency of conversion to open cholecystectomy was initially reported to be as high as 60% in early series, most recent studies describe a conversion rate of 5 to 20%. This conversion rate compares favorably with that usually reported (< 5%) for elective laparoscopic cholecystectomy.

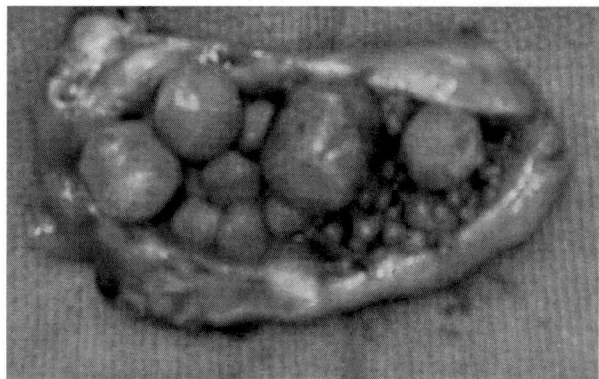

FIGURE 131-2. Surgically removed gallbladder, demonstrating a thickened wall and multiple gallstones.

Although the incidence of bile duct injury is difficult to determine, some have suggested that this dreaded complication is increased following laparoscopic cholecystectomy for acute cholecystitis. Early studies revealed an incidence as high as 5.5%. However, the data from prospective studies of laparoscopic cholecystectomy for acute cholecystitis do not demonstrate a marked increase in bile duct injury. Indeed, many recent series have not identified any bile duct injuries following laparoscopic cholecystectomy for acute cholecystitis. However, because the overall incidence is low, most of the studies contain insufficient numbers of patients to adequately address this issue. Current data suggests a very slight or no increased chance of sustaining bile duct injury, justifying the use of laparoscopic cholecystectomy in acute cholecystitis. Maintaining a low threshold for conversion from laparoscopic to open cholecystectomy is important in this situation and will minimize bile duct injuries.

Immediate laparoscopic cholecystectomy is recommended in those patients who present within 48 to 72 hours of the onset of symptoms. During this time period, edema is present, but fibrosis usually has not yet developed, allowing safe dissection. Many studies indicate that in the majority of patients, the procedure can be completed safely in this time period. In this setting, early aspiration of the gallbladder may facilitate cholecystectomy by improving one's ability to retract the tense, thickened gallbladder wall.

Patients who present after 48 to 72 hours of symptoms may require a different approach. By this time, the inflammatory process may be so advanced that laparoscopic cholecystectomy becomes much more difficult or impossible. The risk of conversion to open cholecystectomy is 23% at this point, compared with a conversion rate of 9% when laparoscopic cholecystectomy is performed within the first 72 hours. Often, these patients are admitted to the hospital, maintained in a fasting state, and given IV antibiotics until abdominal pain resolves, leukocytosis reverses, and fever ceases. Patients usually improve within 48 hours, allowing resumption of enteral feeding; interval laparoscopic cholecystectomy is performed in 6 to 8 weeks.

Patients who fail to respond to the above conservative measures should undergo cholecystectomy. An attempt at laparoscopy is warranted, but many patients in this group require conversion to open cholecystectomy. Cholecystostomy is an appropriate surgical (or radiologic) option if the patient is too ill for surgery or if the gallbladder cannot be removed. This can be followed by laparoscopic cholecystectomy once the patient is more stable. A treatment algorithm for acute cholecystitis is presented in Figure 131-3.

The role of cholangiography is controversial. Some authors routinely perform intraoperative cholangiogram, whereas others only perform cholangiogram when alkaline phosphatase or bilirubin is abnormal or when common bile duct dilation is present. Several retrospective series show a benefit of cholangiography in the prevention of bile duct injuries. However, Lorimer and Fairfull-Smith described their experience of 500 successive laparoscopic cholecystectomies without cholangiography with no biliary injuries. As suggested by these authors, we concur that any patient with dilated common bile duct on US or persistently elevated bilirubin or alkaline phosphatase should undergo cholangiography, regardless of the indication for cholecystectomy. Additionally, cholangiography should be performed any time the biliary ductal anatomy is unclear at operation.

Acute Acalculous Cholecystitis

Between 2 and 15% of patients with acute cholecystitis have no gallstones identified on US. Such patients appear to have a different clinical entity, acute acalculous cholecystitis.

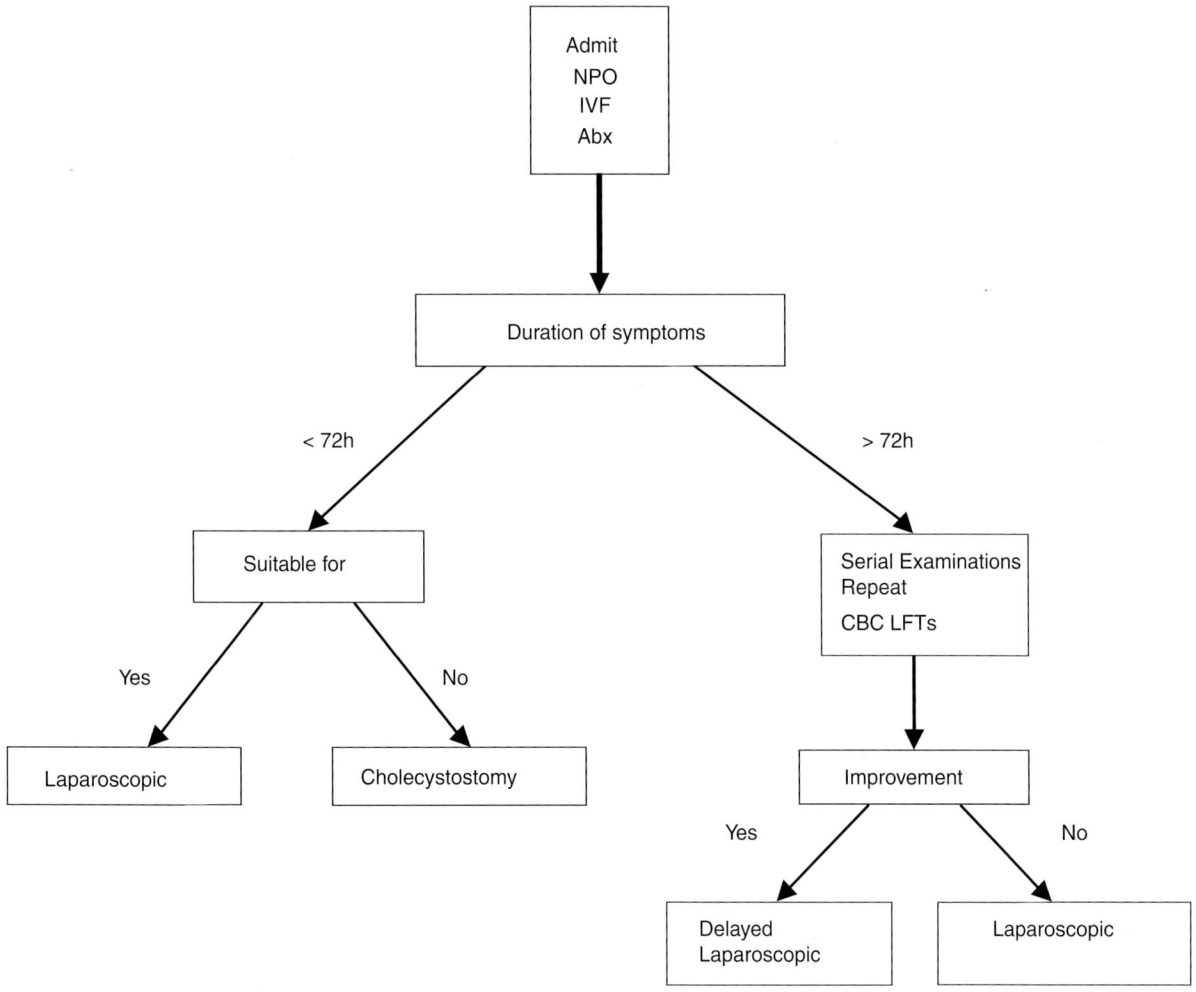

FIGURE 131-3. Treatment algorithm for acute cholecystitis. Abx = antibiotics; CBC = complete blood count; IVF = intravenous fluids; LFT = liver function tests; NPO = nil per os.

Presentation

This syndrome is traditionally described in the critically ill patient population. It is often associated with severe trauma or burn injury, nonbiliary tract surgery, and prolonged fasting. It usually has a more fulminant course with an increased incidence of gangrene, empyema, and perforation. Affected patients present with fever, increasing abdominal pain, elevated liver function tests, and leukocytosis. These patients are often deemed too ill for cholecystectomy due to their underlying disease processes. Therefore, cholecystostomy tube placement is frequently undertaken. The latter may be performed under either general anesthesia or with conscious sedation.

Etiology

Bile stasis is considered a primary etiologic factor which results in increased mucosal susceptibility to injury. Systemic bacterial or fungal infection then colonizes the static bile in the biliary tree, providing a medium for bacterial growth. Ischemic mucosal injury is also thought to play an etiologic role. Thus, a history of hypotensive episodes and atherosclerotic disease is frequently present in patients who develop acute acalculous cholecystitis. Increased intraluminal pressure due to increased bile viscosity may also produce gallbladder wall ischemia.

In a retrospective chart review, Kalliafas and colleagues (1998) found 14% of cholecystectomies performed for acute cholecystitis did not reveal gallstones. Fifty-two percent of patients with acute acalculous cholecystitis were critically ill, and 63% were in patients recovering from nonbiliary tract surgery. Of the patients with acute acalculous cholecystitis, 19% presented as outpatients. There were no mortalities in this group, in contrast to the inpatient group, which suffered a 50% mortality rate.

A recent series describes 22 patients with acute acalculous cholecystitis. Surprisingly, 20 of these patients were outpatients at the time of diagnosis. There were no deaths in this series. There was an increased need for open cholecystectomy (54%) in this group, compared with 20% for acute calculous cholecystitis. This is likely reflective of the fact that advanced gallbladder disease was more prevalent in patients with acute acalculous cholecystitis. Fifty-nine percent had gangrenous gallbladders upon exploration.

Diagnosis

US may demonstrate gallbladder distention, gallbladder wall thickening, or pericholecystic fluid, but stones are absent. Hepatobiliary iminodiacetic acid (HIDA) scans are less useful in acalculous cholecystitis because false positives are frequent, as most of these patients are in the fasting state and may be receiving hyperalimentation. However, the addition of morphine to cholescintigraphy in fasted patients improves the specificity to 88%. CT scan is often of diagnostic benefit because of its increased sensitivity for pericholecystic inflammatory changes.

Therapy

Because of the rapid progression of the disease and the increased incidence of complications, prompt recognition of acute acalculous cholecystitis is essential. As with acute calculous cholecystitis, antibiotic therapy should be initiated using agents which cover the common biliary pathogens. Tube decompression or cholecystectomy is then performed. It is important to continue to reassess patients treated with cholecystostomy tube placement. Progression of pain, persistent leukocytosis, or worsening of symptoms may signal the presence of gangrene or perforation, necessitating emergent cholecystectomy.

Chronic Cholecystitis

Laparoscopic cholecystectomy is one of the most frequently performed operations performed in the United States. The most frequent indication for surgery is symptomatic cholelithiasis or chronic cholecystitis.

Presentation

Patients with chronic cholecystitis typically present with right upper quadrant pain, nausea, vomiting, and occasionally right shoulder pain; symptoms are often worse after fatty meals. Duration of episodes ranges from a few hours to 2 to 4 days. Fever is usually absent. Patients frequently have right upper quadrant tenderness on examination, but abdominal examination may be normal. Attacks are often recurrent over a period of several months or years.

Diagnosis

Examination of patients is similar to the examination of patients for acute cholecystitis, except that it is more frequently undertaken on an outpatient basis. Diagnosis is most frequently confirmed by the presence of gallstones on ultrasonography. Pericholecystic fluid and gallbladder wall thickening may or may not be present. Ultrasonographic demonstration of gallstones combined with a history compatible with biliary colic is sufficient for the diagnosis of chronic cholecystitis.

Treatment

Laparoscopic cholecystectomy should be recommended to all patients who are appropriate operative candidates deemed to manifest symptoms attributable to their gallstones. Given the low morbidity of laparoscopic cholecystectomy, there are very few contraindications to this minimally invasive procedure. The main contraindications are a contraindication to general anesthesia and extensive prior open upper abdominal surgery. Patients with a long-standing history of severe symptoms face an increased risk of requiring conversion to open cholecystectomy, as they are more likely to have significant fibrosis surrounding the gallbladder and ducts.

Chronic Acalculous Cholecystitis

Presentation

This diagnosis is synonymous with gallbladder dyskinesia. Patients present with similar complaints as those with chronic cholecystitis; however, gallstones are absent on US. Typical presenting symptoms include nausea, bloating, fatty food intolerance, vomiting, weight loss, irregular bowel habits, and fever. There is a strong female predominance; approximately 80% of patients with this disease entity are female. Gallbladder dyskinesia is frequently associated with other gastrointestinal (GI) motility disorders, such as irritable bowel syndrome.

Diagnosis

Ultrasonography is normal in these patients, but if a biliary etiology of pain is suspected, cholescintigraphy should be obtained. Cholecystokinin infusion allows quantitative assessment of gallbladder emptying (ejection fraction). A gallbladder ejection fraction of < 35% and/or reproduction of symptoms with cholecystokinin infusion are considered positive results.

ERCP with bile aspiration may also be performed. The bile is then examined for cholesterol crystals. When present, these crystals predict a favorable response to cholecystectomy. This "microlithiasis" may represent a form of calculus disease, albeit with a low stone burden; outcomes more likely parallel those for patients with calculous cholecystitis rather than those with acalculous disease.

Treatment

Laparoscopic cholecystectomy is the treatment of choice for gallbladder dyskinesia. The success rate is lower than for acute or chronic calculous cholecystitis. Tabet and Anvari (1999) studied 123 patients with gallbladder dyskinesia. Laparoscopic cholecystectomy decreased pain in 93% of patients with low gallbladder ejection fraction, 75% of patients with normal gallbladder ejection fraction and symptoms suggestive of biliary colic, and 93% of patients who had reproduction of pain with cholecystokinin infusion. Symptoms of pain, nausea, vomiting, and fever were most likely to improve postoperatively, whereas symptoms of flatulence, loose stools, belching, and indigestion were the least likely to resolve. More than 90% of patients were pain free at follow up. The lower success rate may be due in part to the presence of other GI motility disorders in this patient population.

Summary

Acute cholecystitis is a common disease that can usually be treated laparoscopically. If a patient presents within the 48 to 72 hours of the onset of symptoms, immediate laparoscopic cholecystectomy is recommended. If the presentation is delayed, a "cooling off" period of hydration and IV antibiotics are instituted, followed by delayed laparoscopic cholecystectomy in 6 weeks. There is a slight increase in the risk of conversion to open cholecystectomy when compared with elective laparoscopic cholecystectomy. Cholecystostomy tube placement is reserved for patients who are too ill to withstand general anesthesia, often encountered when treating acute acalculous cholecystitis.

Chronic cholecystitis is likewise treated with laparoscopic cholecystectomy. Chronic acalculous cholecystitis, also referred to as gallbladder dyskinesia, frequently afflicts patients with associated gastrointestinal motor disorders. These patients frequently have relief of their symptoms following cholecystectomy, particularly in those who have a low preoperative gallbladder ejection fraction.

Supplemental Reading

Bender JS, Zenilman ME. Immediate laparoscopic cholecystectomy as definitive therapy for acute cholecystitis. Surg Endosc 1995;9:1081–4.

Flancbaum L, Choban PS. Use of morphine cholescintigraphy in the diagnosis of acute cholecystitis in critically ill patients. Intensive Care Med 1995;21:120–4.

Fletcher DR, Hobbs MS, Tan P, et al. Complications of cholecystectomy: risks of the laparoscopic approach and protective effects of operative cholangiography: a population-based study. Ann Surg 199:229:449–57.

Jones DB, Soper NJ, Brewer JD, et al. Chronic acalculous cholecystitis laparoscopic treatment. Surg Laparosc Endosc 1996;6:114–22.

Kalliafas S, Ziegler DW, Flancbaum L, et al. Acute acalculous cholecystits: incidence, risk factors, diagnosis, and outcome. Am Surg 1998;64:471–5.

Kum C-K, Eypasch F, Lefering R, et al. Laparoscopic cholecystectomy for acute cholecystitis: is it really safe? World J Surg 1996;20:43–9.

Lillemoe KD. Surgical treatment of biliary tract infections. Am Surg 2000;66:138–44.

Lorimer JW, Fairfull-Smith RJ. Intraoperative cholangiography is not essential to avoid duct injuries during laparoscopic cholecystectomy. Am J Surg 1995;169:344–7.

Ryu JK, Ryu KH, Kim KH. Clinical features of acute acalculous cholecystitis. J Clin Gastroenterol 2003;36:166–9.

Schwesinger WH, Sirinek KR, Strodel WE. Laparoscopic cholecystectomy for biliary tract emergencies: state of the art. World J Surg 1999;23:334–42.

Shea J, Berlin JA, Escarce JJ, et al. Revised estimates of diagnostic test sensitivity and specificity in suspected biliary tract disease. Arch Intern Med 1994;154:2573.

Soper NJ, Stockman PT, Dunnegan DL, Ashley SW. Laparoscopic cholecystectomy: the new gold standard? Arch Surg 1992;127:917–23.

Tabet J, Anvari M. Laparoscopic cholecystectomy for gallbladder dyskinesia: clinical outcome and patient satisfaction. Surg Laparosc Endosc Percutan Tech 1999;9:27–42.

Willsher PC, Sanabria JR, Gallinger S, et al. Early laparoscopic cholecystectomy foracute cholecystitis: a safe procedure. J Gastrointest Surg 1999;3:50–3.

Woods MS, Traverso LW, Kozarek RA, et al. Biliary tract complications of laparoscopic cholecystectomy are detected more frequently with routine intraoperative cholangiography. Surg Endosc 1995;9:1076–80.

CHAPTER 132

CHOLELITHIASIS

CYNTHIA W. KO, MD, MS, AND SUM P. LEE, MD, PHD

Gallstones are commonly found but are often asymptomatic. In general, the risk of developing biliary colic in asymptomatic patients is low, but once a person develops symptoms, the risk of ongoing biliary colic or more serious complications of cholelithiasis is substantial (Gracie and Ransohoff, 1982). However, serious complications of cholelithiasis, such as cholecystitis, cholangitis, or acute pancreatitis, are frequently preceded by attacks of biliary colic. Therefore, in patients with gallstones who are otherwise asymptomatic, treatment is not recommended. However, once symptoms or complications develop, treatment of cholelithiasis, either surgical or medical, should be strongly considered (Table 132-1). In general, cholecystectomy is the treatment of choice for symptomatic or complicated gallstones. However, in selected patients, dissolution with ursodeoxycholic acid (UDCA) or fragmentation of stones with extracorporeal shock wave lithotripsy can be useful.

Surgical Therapy

Open Cholecystectomy

Cholecystectomy is one of the most commonly performed operations, with over 700,000 performed annually in the United States. Cholecystectomy is the only definitive therapy for symptomatic gallstones. Elective cholecystectomy is usually safe, with mortality rates of less than 0.1 to 0.2%. The

TABLE 132-1. Management Options for Symptomatic Gallstones

-	Indications and Inclusion Criteria	Stone Clearance (%)	Comments
Open cholecystectomy	Symptomatic gallstones Able to tolerate general anesthesia	100	Invasive Requires general anesthesia Definitive treatment for gallstones Possible bile duct injury Prolonged recovered compared to laparoscopic approach Overall mortality < 1%
Laparoscopic cholecystectomy	Symptomatic gallstones Able to tolerate general anesthesia	100	Invasive Requires general anesthesia Definitive treatment for gallstones Possible bile duct injury May require additional procedures to remove common bile duct stones
ERCP	Retained common bile duct stones Severe acute pancreatitis Bile leak after cholecystectomy Acute cholangitis	> 90% of common bile duct stones	Risk of hemorrhage, pancreatitis, perforation Not definitive therapy for gallstones Symptoms may recur in up to 47% if cholecystectomy not also done
Oral bile acid dissolution	Symptomatic gallstones Unwilling or unable to undergo patent cystic duct–cholecystectomy Functioning gallbladder Floating radiolucent stones, < 10 mm in diameter	20 to 70%	Useful only for cholesterol stones Recurrent stones in 50% at 5 years follow-up Few side effects
Extracorporeal shock wave lithotripsy, with or without oral bile acid supplementation	Symptomatic gallstones Unwilling or unable to undergo cholecystectomy Patent cystic duct functioning gallbladder Fewer than 3 radiolucent stones < 20 mm in diameter	40 to 70%	Procedure occasionally requires intravenous analgesia Contraindicated in patients with bleeding diatheses and pregnancy Biliary colic in 30 to 40% as stones fragment and pass Stones recur in up to 44% at 5 years follow-up

ERCP = endoscopic retrograde cholangiopancreatography.

majority of these operations are performed using a laparoscopic approach. However, open cholecystectomy remains an important and necessary option for many patients.

Laparoscopic Cholecystectomy

Laparoscopic cholecystectomy was first performed in France in 1987, and was rapidly adopted by patients and physicians. The procedure is now the standard of care for the treatment of symptomatic cholelithiasis and its complications. There have been few randomized, controlled trials comparing laparoscopic with open cholecystectomy, but prospective case series examining results in several thousand patients have shown that laparoscopic cholecystectomy is safe and effective. Compared with open cholecystectomy, the laparoscopic approach produces shorter hospital stays with more rapid return to normal activities and fewer complications. Overall mortality appears to be similar to or even less than with open cholecystectomy.

Cholecystectomy can be performed laparoscopically in most patients. The only absolute contraindications to a laparoscopic approach are an inability to tolerate general anesthesia and uncontrollable coagulopathy. Even in patients with prior abdominal surgery or peritonitis, the laparoscopic approach can still be attempted, although conversion to an open procedure may be required. Experienced surgeons can often perform the procedure in obese or anticoagulated patients, those with recent cholecystitis, or pregnant women.

The mortality rate with laparoscopic cholecystectomy is low and is < 0.5%, with morbidity rates around 5% in most series (MacFayden et al, 1998). This is comparable to the mortality and morbidity rates seen with open cholecystectomy. Most complications are relatively minor, such as urinary retention or infections, wound infections or seromas. Complications related directly to cholecystectomy include bile duct injury, bile leak, and acute pancreatitis. Of these, bile duct injury is the most serious, but relatively uncommon (< 1% of cases). Nevertheless, bile duct injuries can be difficult to repair and lead to biliary strictures. Bile duct injuries are commonly the result of unrecognized variations in bile duct anatomy or problems in identifying normal anatomy. Other factors influencing the risk of bile duct injury include use of intraoperative cholangiogram and surgeon experience. The risk of common bile duct injury may be decreased by the use of intraoperative cholangiography, both with laparoscopic and open procedures. However, routine use of cholangiogram remains controversial. In laparoscopic procedures, the risk of common bile duct injury is highest in a surgeon's initial experience. The risk of bile duct injury eventually plateaus as surgeons gain experience, and becomes similar to that with open cholecystectomy. Bile leaks can be recognized using ultrasonography and hepatobiliary scintigraphy, and are usually managed with endoscopic retrograde cholangiography and stent placement.

Conversion to open cholecystectomy is required in 2 to 8% of procedures. It is more commonly required if there is difficulty in identifying the anatomy of the porta hepatis or with underlying inflammation, such as in patients with acute cholecystitis. Conversion should not be considered as a complication of a procedure, but rather as a necessary alternative in some patients.

Intraoperative cholangiogram is not standardized, and is often not performed in community practice. Use of intraoperative cholangiogram is often advocated to decrease the risk of common bile duct injuries (Flum et al, 2003). It is also useful to identify patients with unsuspected common bile duct stones, in whom further intervention may be necessary. Further options for extraction of discovered common bile duct stones include conversion to an open procedure with stone extraction, laparoscopic common bile duct exploration, or endoscopic retrograde cholangiography. Expertise with laparoscopic stone extraction is relatively uncommon in general practice. Techniques for laparoscopic stone removal include flushing of the duct (for small stones), retrograde balloon or basket extraction through the cystic duct, or extraction under direct visualization with a choledochoscope. In experienced hands, stones can be successfully extracted in over 90% of patients, with overall operative morbidity rates of less than 10%.

In patients with acute cholecystitis, the timing of surgery has been controversial. Although laparoscopic cholecystectomy can be performed successfully in these patients, there may be a higher incidence of common bile duct stones. Because of the local inflammation the procedure is often technically more difficult. In this setting, intraoperative cholangiograms may be more difficult to obtain and bile duct injuries more common. Randomized trials comparing early (< 3 days) versus delayed (4 to 6 weeks) surgery for acute cholecystitis have showed no benefit to delaying surgery. Although patients in the early surgery group have longer operating times, they had similar rates of conversion to open cholecystectomy and shorter hospital stays. Thus, early operation for acute cholecystitis can be beneficial.

Endoscopic Retrograde Cholangiopancreatography with Stone Removal

Endoscopic retrograde cholangiopancreatography (ERCP) is a commonly used technique used in patients with common bile duct stones. It is now widely available, and endoscopic techniques continue to evolve. It is the modality of choice for emergent management of cholangitis unresponsive to conservative measures. ERCP may also be useful in selected patients with severe acute biliary pancreatitis or pancreatitis accompanied by bile duct obstruction. It is also the standard of care for management of common bile duct stones remaining after laparoscopic cholecystectomy (Carr-Locke, 2002).

Endoscopic sphincterotomy is the most commonly used initial technique to overcome the sphincter of Oddi and facilitate stone removal. More recently, the technique of endoscopic balloon dilation of the sphincter has been developed, and can be used in selected patients with smaller and less numerous stones. Sphincterotomy or balloon dilatation is generally followed by stone extraction using balloon catheters or baskets. In certain patients, mechanical lithotripsy must also be used to crush large stones before they can be extracted into the duodenum. Using combinations of these techniques, stones can be successfully extracted in > 95% of patients. Rarely, stones must be fragmented using extracorporeal shock-wave lithotripsy before they can move into the duodenum. Complications of ERCP and sphincterotomy include hemorrhage, acute pancreatitis, and perforation, and occur in 1 to 5% of patients (Freeman et al, 1996). Operator experience and case volume are major factors in determining the complication rate of ERCP.

Use of endoscopic sphincterotomy alone can be considered in patients who are either unable or unwilling to undergo cholecystectomy. However, endoscopic sphincterotomy alone may be associated with an unacceptably high risk of recurrent symptoms or complications (Boerma et al, 2002). Thus, in most patients, endoscopic sphincterotomy should be accompanied by cholecystectomy for definitive management of gallstones.

Extracorporeal Shock-Wave Lithotripsy

Large gallbladder stones in patients who are not surgical candidates or common bile duct stones that cannot be removed using standard endoscopic techniques may need to be fragmented using extracorporeal shock-wave lithotripsy. This is only available in selected centers within the United States. Several different types of lithotripters are available, which differ in their method of generating the shock waves and in specific operating characteristics. To be a candidate for *lithotripsy*, patients should have *few stones* (usually < 3) and a *functioning gallbladder with a patent cystic duct*. The stones should be *radiolucent*, and *generally < 20 mm in diameter*. Very small stones may be difficult to target, and some centers will *exclude* patients with stones less < 5 to 10 mm in diameter. Patients who have coagulation or platelet abnormalities, vascular anomalies of the liver, acute gallstone-related complications, or who are pregnant are not good candidates for lithotripsy.

Stones are generally localized using sonographic or fluoroscopic guidance. High frequency shock waves are focused on the stones, producing fragmentation of the stones. Some of these stone fragments are small enough to pass from the gallbladder. However, it is often useful to use oral bile acids in conjunction with lithotripsy. The fragments produced by lithotripsy can be more easily dissolved by the administered bile acids, enhancing the overall success of stone clearance. At established centers, stone clearance can be achieved in 77% of patients with single stones less than 2 cm in diameter, 60% of those with larger solitary stones, and 41% of those with multiple stones (Sackmann et al, 1991).

Pain during the procedure is not uncommon, and occurs more frequently with spark gap lithotriptors. In some patients, this may require intravenous analgesia. There can also be some local discomfort or bruising associated with the therapy. Microscopic hematuria has been found in 1 to 2% of patients. Biliary colic will develop in 30 to 40% of patients as stones fragment and pass from the gallbladder, usually within the first few weeks after therapy. However, few patients develop more severe complications such as pancreatitis. Up to 3% of patients may require cholecystectomy for persistent stones or symptoms.

As with bile acid dissolution therapy, stone recurrence is frequent. Up to 12% of patients will have recurrent stones within 1 year, and up to 44% at 5 years of follow-up (Sackmann et al, 1994). Patients who are obese and those with poor gallbladder function are at higher risk of recurrence. Patients with recurrent stones can again develop biliary symptoms, such as biliary colic or cholecystitis. Repeat treatment with oral bile acids or lithotripsy can be considered, but some patients will need cholecystectomy for recurrent stones.

Medical Therapy

Oral Bile Acid Dissolution Therapy

Dissolution of cholesterol gallstones with oral bile acid supplementation is appropriate in selected candidates. The two bile acids which have been studied are *chenodeoxycholic acid* and *UDCA*. However, *UDCA (ACTIGAL)* has very few side effects, and has become the preferred bile acid for this indication. *UDCA* works by decreasing biliary cholesterol secretion and thus inducing the secretion of undersaturated bile. This favors the dissolution of cholesterol stones. To be considered for this therapy, patients should have *small cholesterol gallstones* (preferably < 10 mm) with a *patent cystic duct*. Stones with a diameter greater than 15 mm cannot usually be treated successfully. The number of stones is not an absolute contraindication to bile acid dissolution therapy. Cystic duct patency can be documented by hepatobiliary scintigraphy or, occasionally, by oral cholecystography. Some experts recommend *evaluating stones by computed tomography* to be sure they are buoyant and isodense or hypodense to bile, which are indicators that stones are composed primarily of cholesterol. Patients with calcified stones, which are generally not composed of cholesterol, are not candidates for dissolution therapy. The usual dose of *UDCA* for dissolution is 10 to 15 mg/kg of body weight daily. It can be administered either as single bedtime dose, or divided in 2 daily doses. Patients should be treated until stones are sonographically documented to resolve. Rarely, dissolution therapy can be accompanied by attacks of biliary colic as stones fragment and pass through to the duodenum. In addition, the risk of *recurrent stones* after *UDCA* is discontinued is not insubstantial (up to 50% at 5 years) (Villanova et al, 1989). Thus, bile acid dissolution is not curative for gallstones. This therapy should only be applied in patients who are unwilling or unable to undergo a definitive cholecystectomy.

Successful treatment is defined by complete stone disappearance, as confirmed by two consecutive ultrasound exams. Complete dissolution can be achieved in 20 to 70% of patients treated with *UDCA* (May et al, 1993). The success of dissolution therapy depends on adhering to strict selection criteria. Generally, the best results are obtained in patients with *stones < 5 mm in diameter* (up to 70% dissolution rate). Complete dissolution is seen in < 30% of patients with stones larger than 10 mm. There is also wide variation in the time needed for stone dissolution. However, on average, *stone diameter will decrease* by 0.7 to 1 mm per month of treatment.

In some patients, symptoms of *biliary colic* often improve before gallstones are documented to disappear. However, in some patients, biliary colic continues as stones dissolve and the fragments pass from the gallbladder. Long term therapy with bile acids may result in a lower risk of biliary colic and acute cholecystitis, whether or not stones completely resolve. Therefore, in patients with severe comorbidities who are not surgical candidates, long-term bile acid therapy could be considered to prevent recurrence of gallstone complications. If patients do now show evidence of gallstone dissolution after 6 months of therapy, or if stones shrink but do not eventually resolve, oral bile acid therapy should be discontinued.

Summary

In evaluating treatment options for cholelithiasis, there are two important questions. The first is: are the stones causing symptoms or complications? If they are not, then management should be watchful waiting. If stones are causing symptoms or complications, then the patient's ability and willingness to undergo surgery must be assessed. For patients who are able and willing to undergo surgery, cholecystectomy is the treatment of choice and provides definitive management. In most cases, it can be completed laparoscopically with minimal risk of morbidity or mortality. In certain cases, an open approach may be necessary. For patients who are not able or willing to undergo surgery, consideration should be given to dissolution with *UDCA* or to fragmentation with lithotripsy. Only rarely should symptomatic or complicated stones be treated with endoscopic sphincterotomy alone. With any management option short of cholecystectomy, there is a substantial risk of recurrent stones and symptoms.

Supplemental Reading

Boerma D, Rauws EA, Keulemans YC, et al. Wait-and-see policy or laparoscopic cholecystectomy after endoscopic sphincterotomy for bile-duct stones: a randomised trial. Lancet 2002;360:761–5.

Carr-Locke DL. Therapeutic role of ERCP in the management of suspected common bile duct stones. Gastrointest Endosc 2002;56:S170–4.

Flum DR, Dellinger EP, Cheadle A, et al. Intraoperative cholangiography and risk of common bile duct injury during cholecystectomy. JAMA 2003;289:1639–44.

Freeman ML, Nelson DB, Sherman S, et al. Complications of endoscopic biliary sphincterotomy. N Engl J Med 1996;335:909–18.

Gracie WA, Ransohoff DF. The natural history of silent gallstones. N Engl J Med 1982;307:798.

MacFadyen BV, Vecchio R, Ricardo AE, Mathis CR. Bile duct injury after laparoscopic cholecystectomy. The United States experience. Surg Endosc 1998;12:315–21.

May GR, Sutherland LR, Shaffer EA. Efficacy of bile acid therapy for gallstone dissolution: a meta-analysis of randomized trials. Aliment Pharmacol Ther 1993;7:139–48.

Orlando R III, Russell JC, Lynch J, Mattie A. Laparoscopic cholecystectomy. A statewide experience. The Connecticut Laparoscopic Cholecystectomy Registry. Arch Surg 1993;128:494–9.

Sackmann M, Miller H, Klueppelberg U, et al. Gallstone recurrence after shock-wave therapy. Gastroenterology 1994;106:225–30.

Sackmann M, Pauletzki J, Sauerbruch T, et al. The Munich gallbladder lithotripsy study. Ann Intern Med 1991;114:290–6.

The Southern Surgeons Club. A prospective analysis of 1,518 laparoscopic cholecystectomies. N Engl J Med 1991;324:1073.

Villanova N, Bazzoli F, Taroni F, et al. Gallstone recurrence after successful oral bile acid treatment. A 12-year follow-up study and evaluation of long-term postdissolution treatment. Gastroenterology 1989;97:726–31.

Chapter 133

Biliary Strictures and Neoplasms

Sergey V. Kantsevoy, MD, PhD

Multiple congenital and acquired illnesses can lead to the development of biliary tree strictures. The most common causes of biliary strictures are intra-abdominal surgeries, especially operations on the biliary tree, such as open or laparoscopic cholecystectomy, biliary-enteric anastomosis, liver transplantation, etc. The risk factors that predispose to intraoperative bile duct injuries include poor visualization of anatomic structures, misidentification of the common bile duct for the cystic duct, inaccurate placement of sutures and clips, excessive use of cautery or laser, and development of ischemic stricture after damage of ductal vascular supply. Unrecognized congenital anomalies of the biliary tree may also lead to accidental injury with the future development of strictures.

Biliary strictures can develop after blunt or penetrating abdominal trauma, infectious, inflammatory or autoimmune conditions affecting the liver, pancreas, and biliary ducts (primary sclerosing cholangitis, acute and chronic pancreatitis, and sarcoidosis, etc). Various benign and malignant tumors located in the gallbladder, bile ducts, major duodenal papilla, liver, pancreas, and adjacent organs can also cause obstruction of the biliary tree.

Presentation

The main presenting symptoms in patients with benign and malignant biliary strictures are abdominal pain, fever, chills, cholangitis, and obstructive jaundice. Abdominal pain is usually localized in the right upper quadrant or epigastric area. Usually the pain starts gradually and has a constant (not crampy) character. Infection in the obstructed portion of the biliary tree manifests with low grade fever and chills or with overt cholangitis (high fever, pain, jaundice, and changed mental state). Often patients with biliary strictures present with painless jaundice raising suspicion of possible underlining malignancy.

Examination of patients with suspected biliary tree obstruction usually starts with clinical and laboratory evaluation. Careful history taking can lead to recollection of abdominal trauma or previous surgery, which can lead to development of the biliary stricture or reveal other illnesses potentially involving biliary ducts (ulcerative colitis, Crohn's disease, sarcoidosis, acquired immunodeficiency syndrome). Physical examination can reveal abdominal scars post previous surgery or trauma of the anterior abdominal wall, icterus, skin scratches due to pruritus, and palpable intra-abdominal masses. The degree of tenderness on right upper quadrant palpation varies from patient to patient: patients with low grade stricture usually have no tenderness on examination of the right upper quadrant, but patients with biliary leak or cholangitis may have peritoneal signs and severe tenderness on palpation. In patients with biliary tree obstruction below the level of cystic duct, enlarged, distended gallbladder can be palpable below the right rib margin (*Courvoisier's* sign). Patients with cholangitis are usually very sick, often lethargic. Patients with underlying malignancy may have dramatic weight loss and appear debilitated and malnourished.

Diagnosis

Laboratory data in patients with biliary tree obstruction usually demonstrate "obstructive pattern" in liver function tests, including elevated total and direct bilirubin and alkaline phosphatase. The degree of blood bilirubin and alkaline phosphatase elevation usually correlates with the degree and duration of obstruction of the biliary ducts. Patients with incomplete ductal occlusion may have isolated elevation of alkaline phosphatase with a normal level of bilirubin. Infection in obstructed portion of the biliary tree usually causes leukocytosis with a left shift.

We now have multiple imaging techniques for examination of patients with suspected benign or malignant biliary strictures. Transabdominal ultrasound (US) is painless, has no contraindications or side effects, does not require special preparation, and is usually used as a first step in the examination of patients with suspected biliary duct obstruction to determine the level of biliary tree obstruction; dilatation of the entire biliary tree (extra- and intrahepatic ducts) is suggestive of obstructive lesion located in the distal common bile duct, the head of the pancreas, or major duodenal papilla. In patients with dilatated intrahepatic ducts and normal diameter of the extrahepatic duct, the obstructing lesion is usually located on the level of the bifurcation of the right and left hepatic ducts. Unfortunately, to penetrate the distance from the skin to the biliary tree, transabdominal US uses low frequency US beam (3.5 MHz), which usually does not provide enough resolution to determine the nature of biliary tree obstruction (benign or malignant). Transabdominal US can define the level of obstruction in 95% of patients and the cause in up to 88% of patients. Transabdominal US is usually followed by abdominal computed tomography (CT) scan, which can not only determine the degree and level of biliary tree obstruction, but can also frequently provide additional information about the obstructing lesion itself, helping to distinguish benign biliary strictures from cholangiocarcinoma or pancreatic cancer.

Magnetic resonance cholangiopancreatography (MRCP) is another noninvasive test that can provide very useful and accurate information about intra- and extrahepatic biliary ducts comparable with the data from endoscopic retrograde cholangiopancreatography (ERCP) and transcutaneous transhepatic cholangiography (TTC). A recent prospective study of 50 patients with biliary strictures reported the sensitivity and specificity for malignancy as follows: (1) 85% and 75% for ERCP/TTC, (2) 85% and 71% for MRCP, and (3) 77% and 63% for CT.

Endoscopic ultrasound (EUS) is the latest addition to noninvasive diagnostic tests for evaluation of the biliary and pancreatic lesions. EUS delivers an US beam into direct proximity to biliary ducts and pancreas and allows use of high frequency US waves (7.5, 12.5 or even 20 to 30 MHz), providing high resolution pictures of biliary tree and pancreas. Erickson and Garza (2001) demonstrated that use of EUS as a first test in patients with obstructive jaundice eliminates use of more invasive ERCP in 47% of patients and saves an estimated $1,007 to $1,313 per patient.

ERCP is still considered the gold standard for examination of patients with suspected biliary ducts obstruction. ERCP is especially useful in patients with benign or malignant ductal *strictures*, demonstrating the precise location of the obstruction, diameter of the ducts below and above the obstruction, and length and shape of the obstructing lesion, and differentiating benign biliary strictures from malignant neoplasms. The biopsy from the lesion using endoscopic brushes or forceps can provide material from the site of obstruction for cytological or histological examination. However, if the patient has *complete obstruction* of the biliary tree, contrast injected during the ERCP through the major duodenal papilla may not be able to fill the ducts above the obstruction and will not provide any information about the biliary tree proximal to the obstruction site. In this situation the patient will need TTC for direct opacification of the proximal biliary ducts.

Management

Endoscopy is currently not only an important diagnostic tool but also provides important therapeutic options for patients with benign and malignant biliary ducts obstruction. The endoscopic guide wire should be placed into the bile ducts proximal to obstruction. The next key step is endoscopic biliary sphincterotomy to provide easier and reliable access to the common bile duct. In patients with high grade obstruction, the place of obstruction may need to be dilatated with Sohendra dilators over the wire and then a dilatating biliary balloon advanced over the wire and inflated for 30 seconds on 2 occasions. If the obstructive lesion is longer than the length of the dilation balloon, it usually requires several placements of the dilatating balloon. It is technically easier first to place the balloon to the most proximal portion of the lesion and dilatate it and then to pull the balloon down to dilatate middle and more distal portions of the lesion.

Patients with benign strictures require dilatation followed by placement of the biliary plastic stents. It is recommended to place the stent of maximal diameter (10 F) and if possible, to place 2 or even 3 stents along side of each other to keep the maximal residual diameter possible. These plastic stents should be electively exchanged every 2 to 3 months over the period of 12 months to prevent restricturing after the dilatation. The goals of endoscopic therapy are to keep the patient symptom-free with sustained normalization of liver function tests. Unfortunately, some of the biliary strictures can recur many years after treatment. Close monitoring of liver function tests and abdominal USs (to evaluate the diameter of biliary ducts) are recommended every 3 months during the first year after treatment and at 6-month intervals thereafter.

Surgery

When endoscopic management of benign biliary strictures is not successful, surgical intervention should be considered. These operations are technically quite demanding and usually consist of resection of the stricture with end-to-side, Roux-en-Y choledochojejunostomy or hepaticojejunostomy. Success of surgery depends on complete dissection of the strictured segment, and the creation of a tension-free anastomosis with accurate mucosa-to-mucosa approximation. Preservation of the ductal blood supply during surgery is extremely important to prevent development of ischemic strictures. Results of surgical and endoscopic correction of benign bile ducts strictures are comparable; Eighty-three percent have good to excellent results and the recurrence rate is 17%.

In patients with malignant biliary lesions, placement of a stent can be a temporary or final therapeutic option. If the patients are good surgical candidates, 10 F temporary plastic stents are usually placed to relieve the obstruction and to eliminate the jaundice in order to prepare the patient for the following palliative or radical surgery. If the patient is not a surgical candidate, the endoscopic stent placement will be used for palliation of the obstruction. If the patient's life expectancy is less than 6 months, temporary palliation is usually achieved with plastic biliary stents. These stents commonly last for 2 to 3 months and should be exchanged electively or if the signs of obstruction develop. If the patient is not a surgical candidate and his/her life expectancy is longer than 6 months, placement of self-expandable metal stents is recommended. These stents are larger in diameter and last longer than plastic stents, eliminating the need for repeated endoscopy for stent exchange. In patients with preserved gallbladder, covered metal stents over the confluence of common bile duct and the cystic duct should not be used to prevent blockage of the duct followed by acute cholecystitis.

If the guide wire cannot be passed proximal to the biliary tree obstruction, the patient may benefit from TTC with antegrade dilatation of the biliary tree, followed by the transcutaneous placements of 12 to 16 F polymeric catheters. If a malignant tumor occludes the bifurcation of the right and left hepatic ducts, separate percutaneous tubes are inserted into the right and left biliary system and advanced through the side of the occlusion into the distal common bile duct or duodenum. These percutaneous transhepatic biliary stents are usually exchanged at regular intervals to prevent occlusion and infectious complications. Percutaneous, self-expendable metallic stents are recommended as a definitive method of palliation in patients with cholangiocarcinoma who are not surgical candidates.

In patients with resectable neoplasms of the biliary ducts, the choice of surgical procedure will depend on the location and size of the malignant lesion; hilar cholangiocarcinomas require resection of the right and left hepatic ducts and its bifurcation followed by bilateral hepaticojejunostomy on Roux-en-Y intestinal loop above the transhepatic plastic biliary stents. For tumors of the proximal third of the extrahepatic ducts, surgical options include resection of the tumors with subsequent hepaticojejunostomy. Tumors located in the middle third of the extrahepatic duct require resection of the mass with possible primary end-to-end bile duct anastomosis (for small tumors) or hepaticojejunostomy (if a large portion of the biliary ducts is resected). Whipple procedure is recommended for tumors located in the distal common bile duct, major duodenal papilla, or head of the pancreas.

Chemotherapy and radiation have very little effect and are not usually used for patients with unresectable biliary neoplasms, although successful palliation of malignant biliary duct obstruction was recently reported with use of photodynamic therapy.

Summary

In conclusion, multiple benign and malignant lesions can cause obstruction of the biliary ducts. Numerous invasive and noninvasive diagnostic modalities are now available for examination of patients with suspected biliary tree obstruction. ERCP continues to be a key step in management of patients with benign and malignant biliary lesions, serving as a gold standard for diagnosis and providing main therapeutic options for patients with benign bile duct stricture and temporary (before surgery) or final palliation in patients with malignant tumors of the biliary tree.

Supplemental Reading

Ahmad NA, Shah JN, Kochman ML. Endoscopic ultrasonography and endoscopic retrograde cholangiopancreatography imaging for pancreaticobiliary pathology: the gastroenterologist's perspective. Radiol Clin North Am 2002;40:1377–95.

Davids PH, Tanka AK, Rauws EA, et al. Benign biliary strictures. Surgery or endoscopy? Ann Surg 1993;217:237–43.

Eisen GM, Dominitz JA, Faigel DO, et al. An annotated algorithmic approach to malignant biliary obstruction. Gastrointest Endosc 2001;53:849–52.

Erickson RA, Garza AA. EUS with EUS-guided fine-needle aspiration as the first endoscopic test for the evaluation of obstructive jaundice. Gastrointest Endosc 2001;53:475–84.

Foutch G. Disorders of the bile ducts related to surgery. In: DiMarino AJ, Benjamin SB, editors. Gastrointestinal disease: an endoscopic approach. Vol. 2. Malden (MA): Blackwell Science; 1997. p. 906–17.

Gonzalez D, Gouma DJ, Rauws EA, et al. Role of radiotherapy, in particular intraluminal brachytherapy, in the treatment of proximal bile duct carcinoma. Ann Oncol 1999;10:215–20.

Hamy A, d'Alincourt A, Paineau J, et al. Percutaneous self-expandable metallic stents and malignant biliary strictures. Eur J Surg Oncol 1997;23:403–8.

Iwatsuki S, Todo S, Marsh JW, et al. Treatment of hilar cholangiocarcinoma (Klatskin tumors) with hepatic resection or transplantation. J Am Coll Surg 1998;187:358–64.

Kalloo AN, Kantsevoy SV. Biliary diseases. In: Benjamin SB, editor. Educational review manual in gastroenterology. New York: Castle Connolly Graduate Medical Publishing, LLC; 2000. p. 1–20.

Mulvihill S. Surgical management of gallstone disease and postoperative complications. In: Feldman M, Scharschmidt BF, Sleisenger MH, editors. Sleisenger & Fordtran's gastrointestinal and liver disease: pathophysiology/diagnosis/management. Vol. 1. Philadelphia: WB Saunders Company; 1998. p. 973–84.

Osei-Boateng K, Ravendhran N, Haluszka O, Darwin PE. Endoscopic treatment of a post-traumatic biliary stricture mimicking a Klatskin tumor. Gastrointest Endosc 2002;55:274–6.

Rosch T, Meining A, Fruhmorgen S, et al. A prospective comparison of the diagnostic accuracy of ERCP, MRCP, CT, and EUS in biliary strictures. Gastrointest Endosc 2002;55:870–6.

Rumalla A, Baron TH, Wang KK, et al. Endoscopic application of photodynamic therapy for cholangiocarcinoma. Gastrointest Endosc 2001;53:500–4.

Sutton D. A textbook of radiology and imaging. New York: Churchill Livingstone; 1998.

Taylor AC, Little AF, Hennessy OF, et al. Prospective assessment of magnetic resonance cholangiopancreatography for noninvasive imaging of the biliary tree. Gastrointest Endosc 2002;55:17–22.

Vazquez-Sequeiros E, Baron TH, Clain JE, et al. Evaluation of indeterminate bile duct strictures by intraductal US. Gastrointest Endosc 2002;56:372–9.

Yeoh KG, Zimmerman MJ, Cunningham JT, Cotton PB. Comparative costs of metal versus plastic biliary stent strategies for malignant obstructive jaundice by decision analysis. Gastrointest Endosc 1999;49:466–71.

CHAPTER 134

Endoscopic Management of Bile Duct Obstruction and Sphincter of Oddi Dysfunction

David J. Novak, MD, and Firas Al-Kawas, MD

The advent of endoscopic retrograde cholangiopancreatography (ERCP) in the early 1970s revolutionized the diagnosis and management of biliary disorders. This section will focus on endoscopic management of bile duct stones, benign ampullary tumors, and sphincter of Oddi (SO) dysfunction.

Choledocholithiasis

Approximately 15% of Americans have gallstones, with roughly 20% of the patients developing symptoms over their lifetime. Bile duct stones are classified as primary if they form within the bile ducts, or secondary if associated with gallstones (cholecystolithiasis). The majority of bile duct stones in Western society are secondary, and composed of almost pure cholesterol (yellow stones). Primary bile duct stones are less common in Western countries and contain higher concentrations of bilirubin. Bacterial infection and biliary stasis have been postulated as important factors in the formation of primary bile duct stones.

Common bile duct (CBD) stones are seen in 15% of patients undergoing cholecystectomy for symptomatic gallbladder disease. Choledocholithiasis may be asymptomatic or present with acute cholangitis, pancreatitis, and, rarely, with hepatic abscesses. In most cases, the obstruction is incomplete, but in a minority of cases the obstruction may be complete and persistent, leading to jaundice. The clinical presentation of choledocholithiasis is often difficult to differentiate from cholecystolithiasis based on physical examination and history. However, the presence of jaundice or biochemical evidence of cholestasis in the setting of known cholecystolithiasis should make one suspect the presence of choledocholithiasis or *Mirizzi syndrome*. On the other hand, the finding of normal liver enzymes does not exclude the presence of CBD stones.

Imaging

Abdominal ultrasonography (US) is highly sensitive for the detection of gallstones. However, it is far less sensitive for detecting CBD stones. The finding of a dilated CBD on US in the presence of elevated alkaline phosphatase and/or serum aminotransferases is suggestive of choledocholithiasis. On the other hand, abdominal US is very specific when stones are identified in the CBD. Computed tomography (CT) scan of the abdomen provides slightly better sensitivity. Other imaging modalities such as magnetic resonance cholangiography (MRCP), computed tomography cholangiography (CTC), and endoscopic ultrasonography (EUS) have greater sensitivity than transabdominal US. MRCP is very sensitive for stones larger than 10 mm, and in experienced hands compares favorably with ERCP. MRCP has a reported sensitivity and specificity of > 90% in multiple studies, when ERCP was used as the reference standard. EUS is highly sensitive for the detection of CBD stones, but is operator dependent. There have been a total of nine studies comparing EUS and ERCP in the detection of CBD stones. The results of the studies have been split, with three studies showing EUS was superior to ERCP, and three studies showing ERCP superior to EUS; two studies were equivocal. Based on these studies one can assume that EUS and ERCP have similar sensitivity and specificities in detection of CBD stones. Both EUS and MRCP are ideal diagnostic modalities for the detection of CBD stones where there is a low pretest probability for finding CBD stones. CTC has a slightly lower sensitivity compared to ERCP, with sensitivities of 80 to 88% and specificities of 97 to 100% when ERCP was used as the standard.

ERCP is the preferred approach in patients with known CBD stones or in those patients with high pretest probability of CBD stones. As described below, endoscopic management using sphincterotomy, lithotripsy, and other therapeutic interventions are considered the initial steps in the management of most patients with CBD stones.

Management

The role of ERCP in the management of choledocholithiasis and its related complications has evolved dramatically over the last decade. The availability of new devices and technology, such as wire guided baskets and balloons, through the scope mechanical lithotripsy, and electrohydraulic lithotripsy (EHL), has enabled ERCP to play a pivotal role in the management of diseases such as cholangitis, gallstone pancreatitis, and CBD stones.

ERCP using standard procedures such as endoscopic sphincterotomy and balloon/basket stone extraction should be successful in up to 90% of all cases (Figure 134-1). Failure to remove CBD stones endoscopically may be related to the inability to access the bile duct due to anatomic alterations from prior surgery (ie, Billroth II gastrectomy or Roux-en-Y anastamosis), papillary stenosis, or inexperience. However, in experienced hands, cannulation of the bile duct can be achieved in > 90% of cases. Most CBD stones are between 8 to 10 mm, and are unable to pass freely through the CBD. Therefore, the factors that determine whether a stone can be removed by the standard techniques are diameter of the distal CBD, shape of the stone, and the size of the sphincterotomy performed. When dealing with large stones it is important to extend the sphincterotomy to the maximal safe diameter. Recent European and Japanese data suggest that endoscopic balloon sphincteroplasty may be an appropriate method to remove small stones from the CBD. However, current data from the United States demonstrates an increased risk of postprocedure pancreatitis.

Stones up to 1 cm in diameter are frequently removed easily, whereas larger stones usually require the use of lithotripsy before extraction. Mechanical lithotripsy is the most cost effective, dependable, and easily performed method of stone fragmentation. A variety of mechanical lithotriptors are commercially available. Through the scope lithotriptors are composed of a wire basket, a plastic catheter, an outer metal sheath, and a handle with a metal winding device. In the majority of cases the stones are successfully extracted, with stone fragmentation achieved in 75 to 85% of cases (Figure 134-2). Failure of stone extraction using this device is usually secondary to the inability to position the wire basket around the stone. Basket impaction may be encountered when using a standard basket or when through the scope mechanical lithotripter fails. Thus, it is imperative to have a basket retrieval device available (Soehendra lithotriptor, Wilson-Cooke, Winston Salem, NC). This problem can be minimized if a through the scope mechanical lithotripror is used when large stones are encountered.

In cases where the stone(s) are too large for mechanical lithotripsy, electrohydraulic lithotripsy or laser lithotripsy is used for stone fragmentation. Both standard laser lithotripsy and EHL systems require the use of a cholangioscope to gain access to the stone (Figure 134-3). After sphincterotomy, the cholangioscope is inserted through the therapeutic channel of the ERCP scope and into the CBD. The cholangioscope allows the proper positioning of the laser or EHL fiber in the CBD adjacent to the stone. Both systems produce energy bursts that are converted to acoustic shock waves in a water medium. Newer "smart" laser lithotripsy systems are commercially available in Europe and do not require cholangioscopy. Our preference is to use an EHL system for fragmentation of stones not amenable to mechanical lithotripsy. Following stone fragmentation, the fragments can then be removed using baskets and/or balloons. If complete stone clearance is not possible, then a stent is left in the CBD to reduce the risk of sepsis and the procedure is repeated in a few weeks for complete clearance.

There are reports of stone clearance in patients who have had stents placed for large/residual CBD stones after unsuccessful ERCP extraction using standard techniques. In most patients, the use of long term stenting is not a good option because of increased risk of cholangitis. Depending on local expertise, open or laproscopic surgical extraction of large stones continues to be an option with patients who are a low operative risk.

Complications

ACUTE CHOLANGITIS

ERCP plays a key role in the management of acute cholangitis. The most common cause of cholangitis is choledocholithiaisis, and it occurs in approximately 80% of cases of cholangitis. Other causes of acute cholangitis include congenital abnormalities of the biliary tree (choledochal cyst), and malignant obstruction of the biliary tree from ampullary tumors, cholangiocarcinoma, and pancreatic tumors. The management of malignant biliary obstruction and congenital abnormalities will be discussed in other sec-

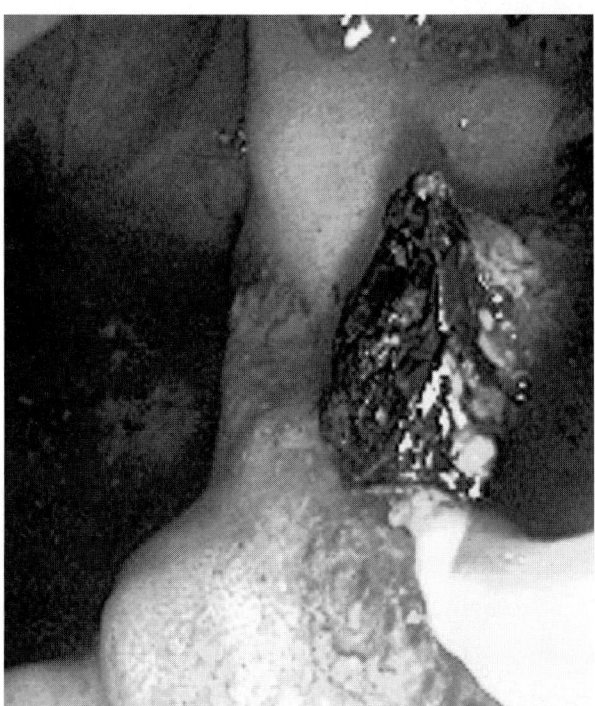

FIGURE 134-1. Stone retrieval of common bile duct stone with balloon extraction following sphincterotomy.

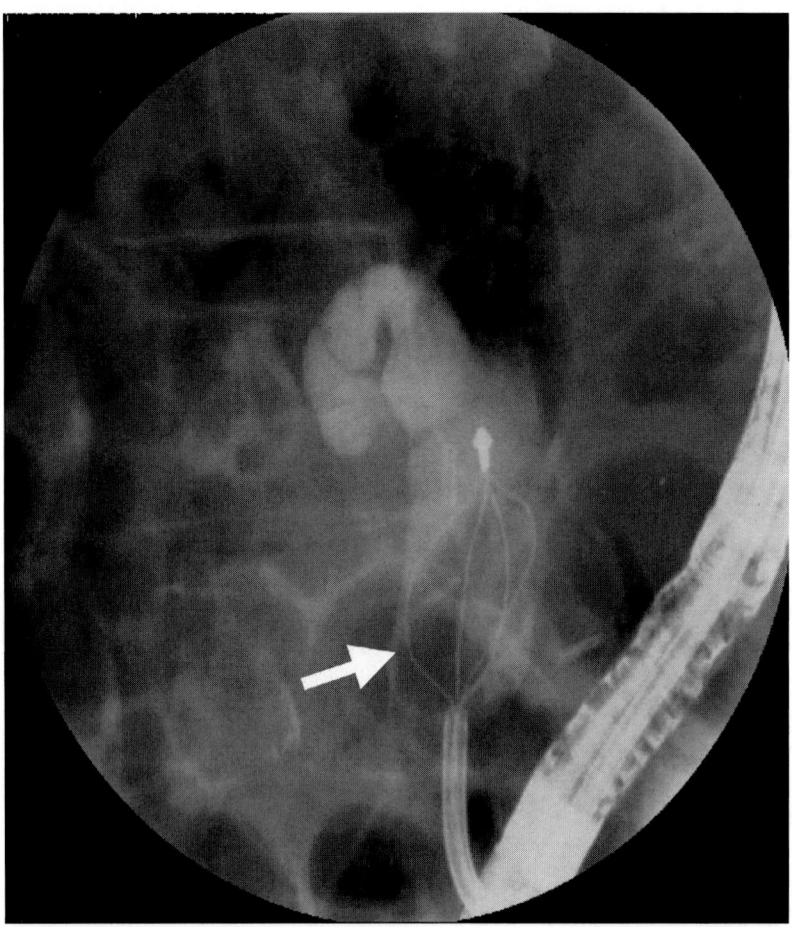

FIGURE 134-2. Fluoroscopic image of through the scope mechanical lithotriptor in the common bile duct during stone extraction. *Arrow* indicates basket around stone.

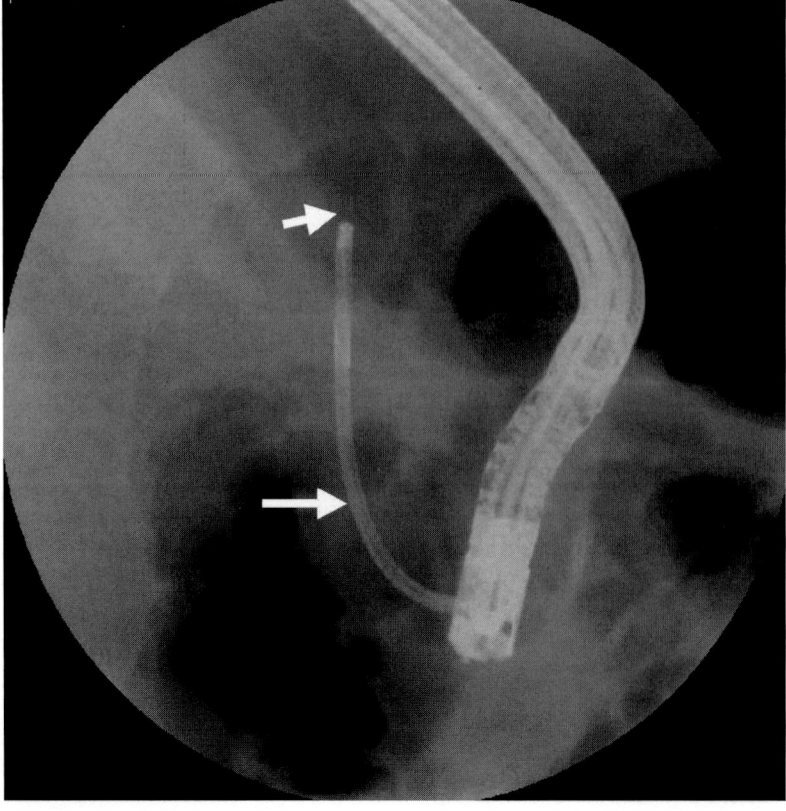

FIGURE 134-3. Fluoroscopic image of electrohydraulic lithotripsy. *Long arrow* indicates cholangioscope; *short arrow* indicates electrohydraulic lithotripsy fiber.

tions of this text. In patients with benign strictures such as primary sclerosing cholangitis and CBD stricture due to chronic pancreatitis, cholangitis can be the presenting symptom or the result of duct manipulation during ERCP or percutaneous cholangiography. The classic presentation of acute cholangitis includes Charcot's triad (right upper quadrant pain, fever, and jaundice). Most cases of cholangitis are mild, but 15 to 20% of cases are severe, and require emergent intervention. In severe cases, patients may present with Reynolds pentad of right upper quadrant pain, fever, jaundice, altered mental status, and shock. Patients with suspected cholangitis usually have elevation of the bilirubin, alkaline phosphatase, and transaminases. Initial management of patients should include blood cultures, administration of broad spectrum antibiotics, intravenous fluids, and urgent right upper quadrant US to detect presence of cholelithiasis and biliary dilatation. If the patient fails to quickly respond to conservative management, then urgent ERCP is necessary. The goal of endoscopic management with ERCP is affecting drainage of infected bile. Endoscopic sphincterotomy with complete clearance of the bile duct of stones is the goal of treatment in stable patients. However, placement of a stent or nasobiliary drain is all that is required to stabilize the patient. Cholangitis can reoccur despite endoscopic sphincterotomy due to retained stones. If complete clearance of the CBD cannot be achieved, then a plastic stent should be left in the CBD, and antibiotics should be continued for 10 to 14 days. Clogged biliary stents are another common cause of cholangitis. The clinical presentation of these patients may be mild with subtle symptoms such as malaise, low grade fever, and mild jaundice. The clogged stent should be removed/exchanged urgently to avoid the development of more severe cholangitis.

Gallstone Pancreatitis

The role of ERCP in acute pancreatitis involves the treatment of an impacted or ball-valving CBD stone. Gallstones are implicated in 50 to 80% of cases of acute pancreatitis. Supportive care is the mainstay of treatment for acute gallstone pancreatitis, but early recognition of gallstone pancreatitis is imperative. Abdominal imaging with US demonstrating the presence of cholelithiasis and elevated transaminases have a high predictive value for diagnosing acute gallstone pancreatitis. The timing of endoscopic sphincterotomy with stone extraction should be performed in specific clinical scenarios either before or after cholecystectomy. ERCP should be performed before cholecystectomy if the patient has concomitant cholangitis, obstructive jaundice, or severe pancreatitis not responding to conservative measures. However, preoperative ERCP is of low yield and is not indicated in the majority of patients with resolving or normal liver enzymes. Patients should undergo intraoperative cholangiography with ERCP reserved to those with positive findings.

Benign Ampullary Tumors

Ampullary neoplasms are rare, but they are becoming more recognized over the last decade, with the increased use of endoscopy in the examination of patients with upper gastrointestinal symptoms. Endoscopic management of benign ampullary neoplasms has supplanted the traditional surgical approach of pancreaticoduodenectomy in specific clinical settings at many referral centers, such as ours. However, the sessile nature of some of these lesions may make endoscopic resection technically challenging.

Clinical Presentation

In many patients, ampullary adenomas are asymptomatic, and are found when endoscopy is performed for evaluation of dyspepsia or reflux symptoms or for screening in patients with familial polyposis. The presenting symptom of patients with ampullary adenomas is variable and usually relates to obstruction of the biliary or pancreatic ducts, anemia, or duodenal obstruction. Jaundice is the most frequent presenting symptom, seen in up to 75% of symptomatic patients, with weight loss and nonspecific abdominal pain seen in up to 40% of patients, and anemia in up to 20% of patients. Duodenal obstruction and pancreatitis are less common.

Endoscopic Management

The clinical decision for endoscopic management of an ampullary lesion depends on accurate histologic differentiation between adenoma and carcinoma. A negative mucosal biopsy does not completely rule out the presence of carcinoma, as carcinoma may still be present in adjacent tissue or deeper layers. Ulceration of the lesion is the only endoscopic finding that predicts adenocarcinoma. Biopsy of an ulcerated lesion should be obtained from the margin of the ulcer, rather than the necrotic base of the ulcer. Ampullary neoplasms can extend into the bile duct or pancreatic duct. The presence of malignancy may be missed in up to 30% of cases if mucosal biopsies were obtained alone. Endoscopic sphincterotomy can increase the diagnostic yield of endoscopic mucosal biopsy, by facilitating intraductal or submucosal sampling. ERCP should be performed to identify intraductal extension, as this usually warrants surgical resection. EUS may be helpful in further assessing deep layer disruption suggesting malignancy. Papillary adenomas, like adenomatous polyps elsewhere in the gastrointestinal tract are premalignant. Therefore, the therapeutic goal should be complete endoscopic removal of adenomatous tissue using a combination of snare excision and thermal ablation. Saline injection with methylene blue may facilitate removal of small or sessile portions. Small lesions may be removed en bloc, whereas larger lesions may be removed piecemeal. Current data suggests that the placement of a 3 cm, 5 F pancreatic stent can reduce the risk of postprocedure pancreatitis (Figure 134-4). Residual tumor may be ablated with argon plasma coagulation (ERBE APC, ERBE USA Inc, Marietta, GA), or YAG laser. Complications of snare ampullectomy include those of ERCP, including pancreatitis, local bleeding, and rarely perforation. In a series of 26 patients undergoing endoscopic snare excision of duodenal ampullary adenomas, the incidence of pancreatitis (14%), bleeding (7%), and perforation (3.5%) was significantly higher than the complication rates seen in ERCP.

Sphincter of Oddi Dysfunction

Structurally, the SO is a segment of circular and longitudinal smooth muscle that incorporates the distal CBD and pancreatic duct. The SO is often treated as a single sphincter, but the SO is composed of a biliary sphincter (sphincter choledochus) and a pancreatic sphincter (sphincter pancreaticus). The normal function of the SO is to regulate bile and pancreatic juice flow into the duodenum, prevent reflux of duodenal contents into the bile and pancreatic ducts, and promote gallbladder filling. The SO has both sympathetic and parasympathetic innervation, with its activity increased by cholinergic stimulation. Cholecystokinin (CCK) appears to provide the major hormonal regulation of the SO. CCK release results in inhibition of the sphincter and contraction of the gallbladder.

SO dysfunction is a benign, noncalculous obstruction of the flow of bile or pancreatic juice at the level of the pancreaticobilliary junction. SO dysfunction refers to a functional motor disorder involving the biliary or pancreatic portion of the sphincter leading to intermittent abdominal pain or pancreatitis. Patients are subdivided into those with sphincter stenosis and sphincter dyskinesia. True structural stenosis occurs at the level of the sphincter and papillary orifice, and is believed to be secondary to inflammation and fibrosis. The passage of small CBD stones or recurrent episodes of pancreatitis may contribute to the inflammation and fibrosis of the papillary orifice. Please see Chapter 135, "Postcholecystectomy Syndrome."

Epidemiology

SO dysfunction occurs in both the pediatric and adult population at any age, but it is predominately seen in postcholecystectomy middle-aged women. The diagnosis of SO dysfunction should be considered in the following three groups: (1) patients with postcholecystectomy abdominal pain, (2) patients with idiopathic recurrent pancreatitis, and (3) patients with episodic right upper quadrant or epigastric pain (biliary-type pain) with intact gallbladders and negative diagnostic tests (abdominal US and gallbladder ejection fraction). Postcholecystectomy pain that resembles preoperative biliary pain is reported to occur in up to 20% of patients.

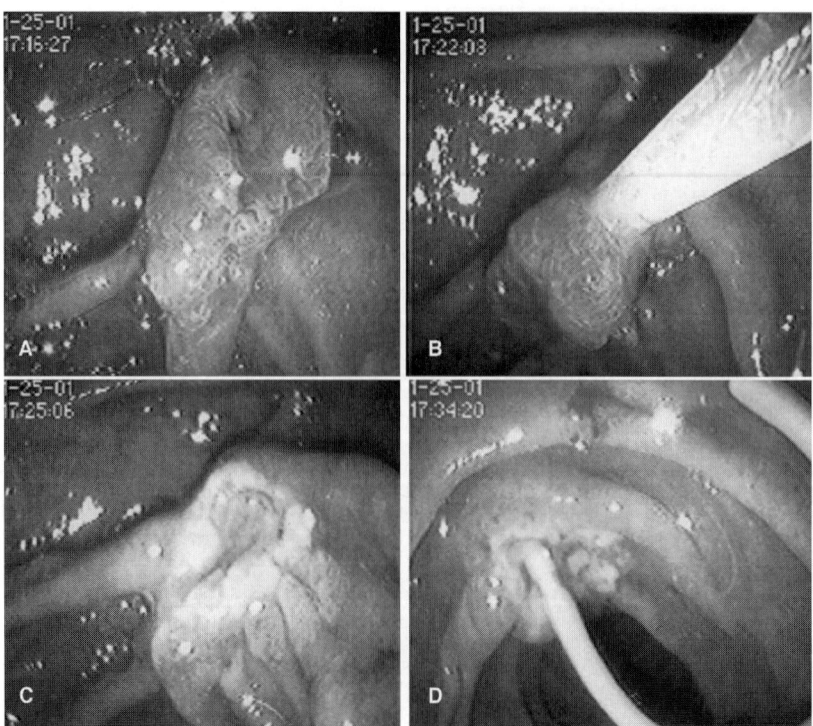

FIGURE 134-4. Ampullectomy of ampullary adenoma. *A*, ampullary adenoma, *B*, snare electrocautery, *C*, post-ampullectomy, *D*, pancreatic duct stent.

Clinical Presentation

Most patients diagnosed with SO dysfunction have undergone prior cholecystectomy, but SO dysfunction may exist with an intact gallbladder and biliary tree. It is important to remember that symptoms of SO dysfunction can mimic those of gallbladder dysfunction, and the diagnosis should not be made until after the patient has had a cholecystectomy or after proper investigations have ruled out the presence of gallbladder dysfunction. In postcholecystectomy pain, the patient often has temporary improvement of their pain following cholecystectomy, but pain similar in character and location to the pain experienced before cholecystectomy often returns. The pattern of pain is variable, with patients experiencing episodes of pain occurring infrequently, lasting several hours, to patients whose pain frequency and severity increases to a chronic baseline pain syndrome with intermittent acute attacks. The pain relationship to food intake is also variable, with some patients noting the onset of pain 1 to 3 hours postprandially. Other patients note no relationship to food ingestion. The ROME II diagnostic criteria were developed to better characterize the pain associated with SO dysfunction (Table 134-1). The physical examination between episodes of pain is often normal, but patients may have nonspecific abdominal tenderness. Elevations of liver associated enzymes or pancreatic enzymes during episodes of pain, are noted in < 50% of patients.

Clinical Evaluation

The evaluation of patients with suspected SO dysfunction based on ROME II criteria should begin with noninvasive diagnostic testing. The Milwaukee Classification (Table 134-2) provides an objective means to classify the subjective nature of pain into three distinct groups (I, II, and III). All three groups share biliary or pancreatic pain as their common thread. Liver or pancreatic enzymes should be ordered at least once during the evaluation, and preferably during or soon after the episodes of pain. Mild elevations (< 2 times the upper limit of normal) are often seen in SO dysfunction. More significant elevations (> 2 times normal) are suggestive of biliary pathology, such as stones, or tumors. Common upper gastrointestinal tract diseases, such as gastroesophageal reflux disease and irritable bowel syndrome (IBS) should be evaluated and appropriately treated before examination of patients with suspected biliary-type abdominal pain. Noninvasive imaging modalities, such as abdominal US, abdominal CT scan, or MRCP, should be performed to rule out structural abnormalities of the biliary tree and pancreas.

Hepatobiliary scintigraphy (HBS) is a noninvasive test that assesses bile flow through the biliary tract. Impairment of bile flow results in abnormal radionucleotide flow. However, HBS does not evaluate the pancreatic sphincter. The sensitivity of HBS has been reported to range from 44 to 100%, and the specificity from 80 to 100%, among 4 studies using the results of SO mannometry as the reference standard. Therefore, HBS can be helpful if SO mannometry is unsuccessful or is not available.

ERCP is an invasive test that is helpful in ruling out other pancreaticobiliary conditions that may cause similar pain, such as retained stones, strictures, papillary tumors, and chronic pancreatitis. However, in view of the availability of the less invasive modalities, such as MRCP, ERCP should be reserved for patients with a high pretest probability of SO dysfunction or those with significant or disabling abdominal pain and should be combined with SO mannometry. ERCP should not be performed unless definitive therapy (sphincter ablation) is planned in the event SO dysfunction is diagnosed.

SO mannometry is considered by most authorities to be the reference standard for examining patients with suspected sphincter dysfunction. Indications for SO mannometry include the following: (1) for examining patients with unexplained, disabling pancreaticobiliary pain, (2) for examining patients with idiopathic pancreatitis, and (3) to assess for residual sphincter hypertension in patients who had sphincterotomy for SO dysfunction. This procedure requires a high level of technical expertise and is usually only available at referral centers. SO mannometry directly measures sphincter pressure with a triple lumen, water-perfused catheter that is passed through the duodenoscope into the bile duct or pancreatic duct. The proximal end of

TABLE 134-1. ROME II Diagnostic Criteria for Biliary Pain

Patients have episodes of severe steady pain located in the RUQ or epigastrum associated with following criteria:
(1) episodes last 30 minutes or more with pain-free intervals
(2) symptoms have occurred on one or more occasions in the last 12 months
(3) pain is steady and interrupts daily activities or requires consultation with a physician
(4) no evidence of structural abnormalities in the biliary tree to explain symptom

RUQ = right upper quadrant.

TABLE 134-2. Milwaukee Classification

(a) biliary-type pain (ROME criteria)
(b) abnormal AST or alkaline phosphatase > 2 × normal, measured on two or more occasions
(c) delayed drainage of contrast from biliary tree on ERCP > 45 minutes and dilated common bile duct > 12 mm in diameter
Patient group
Type 1   all of the above (a, b, and c)
Type 2 (a) *plus* (b) or (c)
Type 3 (a) only

Adapted from Prajapati and Hogan, 2003.
AST = aspartate aminotransferase; ERCP = endoscopic retrograde cholangiopancreatography.

the catheter is attached to a transducer and a paper or computer recording device. Sphincter pressures are measured as the catheter is slowly withdrawn from the duct and stationed within a sphincter zone. Duodenal pressure is the zero reference point. The basal resting pressures of the sphincter ranges from 10 to 40 mm Hg (Figure 134-5). Elevated basal pressures may be secondary to both structural stenosis of the sphincter and dyskinesia. Therefore, most experts agree that an ERCP or MRCP should be performed to rule out structural abnormalities before proceeding with SO mannometry.

Endoscopic sphincterotomy is the current approach for the management of patients with SO dysfunction. The clinical response rate to endoscopic sphincterotomy ranges from 55 to 95%. Patients classified as Type 1 will benefit from sphincter ablation. These patients have a high prevalence of SO dysfunction diagnosed at SO mannometry (80 to 90%), making SO mannometry an unnecessary intervention. Type 2 biliary pain patients should undergo SO mannometry. Two large studies, have found that patients with Type 2 biliary pain and elevated SO dysfunction pressure benefited from biliary sphincterotomy. Abnormal SO mannometry in Type 2 biliary pain is seen in approximately 50% of patients, making SO mannometry useful in diagnosing SO dysfunction and predicting response to therapy. Data on Type 3 patients is limited. Approximately 30 to 40% of type 3 patients have SO dysfunction. Many of these patients have symptoms similar to IBS and visceral hyperalgesia. Type 3 patients have only a 50 to 60% chance of positive clinical improvement following endoscopic sphincterotomy for SO dysfunction.

Pancreatic SO dysfunction can present as recurrent acute pancreatitis, or pancreaticobiliary pain. A modification of the Milwaukee classification system is used (Table 134-3). Isolated pancreatic SO dysfunction is seen in 25% of patients undergoing manometry and in 15 to 20% of patients with pancreatitis of unknown etiology. There is a growing body of evidence suggesting that patients who fail to respond to biliary sphincterotomy may have pain secondary to elevated pancreatic sphincter pressures. A recent study suggests that 72% of patients who had continued pain despite prior biliary sphincterotomy, became symptom-free following pancreatic sphincterotomy. Therefore, pancreatic sphincter pressures should be measured during SO mannometry, if technically feasible, followed by pancreatic sphincterotomy if pressure is elevated. SO mannometry should be included in the diagnostic examination of all patients with pancreatitis of unknown etiology. Several studies have shown that endoscopic pancreatic sphincterotomy has led to a significant reduction in pancreatitis in this subset of patients.

Post-ERCP Pancreatitis

The risk of post-ERCP pancreatitis ranges from 5 to 25%. SO mannometry appears to significantly increase the risk of post-ERCP pancreatitis and, perhaps, identifies patients with untreated pancreatic sphincter hypertension or postprocedure ampullary edema. At our institution, it is general practice to place a prophylactic pancreatic stent to reduce the risk of post-ERCP pancreatitis, in those patients at high risk for post-ERCP pancreatitis (ie, SO dysfunction or difficult cannulation). A recent prospective randomized trial validated this approach by demonstrating a significant reduction in post-ERCP pancreatitis in this subset of patients.

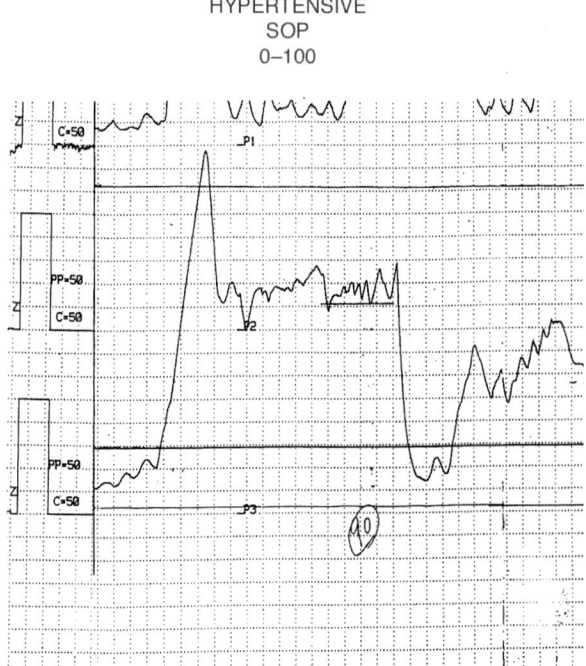

FIGURE 134-5. Sphincter of Oddi mannometry tracing from a patient with sphincter of Oddi dysfunction.

TABLE 134-3. Modified Milwaukee Classification for Pancreatic Type Sphincter of Oddi (SO) Dysfunction

(a) pancreatic-type pain
(b) amylase/lipase > 1.5 to 2.0 × normal
(c) pancreatic duct diameter > 6 mm in head or > 5 mm in body
Patient group
    Type 1 all of the above
    Type 2 (a) *plus* (b) or (c)
    Type 3 (a) only

Adapted from Prajapati and Hogan, 2003.

Supplemental Reading

Bergman JJ, van Berkel AM, Bruno MJ, et al. Is endoscopic balloon dilation for removal of bile duct stones associated with an increased risk for pancreatitis or a higher rate of hyperamylasemia. Endoscopy 2001;33:416–20.

Black NA, Thompson E, Sanderson CFB, ECHSS group. Symptom and health status before and six weeks after open cholecystectomy: a European cohort study. Gut 1994;35:1301–5.

Cahen DL, Fockens P, De Witt LT, et al. Local resection or pancreaticoduodenectomy for villous adenoma or the ampulla of Vater diagnosed before operation. Br J Surg 1997;84:948–51.

Elfant AB, Haber GB. Endoscopic management of ampullary neoplasms. In: Jacobson IM, editor. ERCP and its applications. Philadelphia: Lippincott-Raven Publishers; 1998. p. 239–47.

Fazel A, Quadri A, Catalano MF. Does a pancreatic duct stent prevent post-ERCP pancreatitis? A prospective randomized study. Gastrointest Endosc 2003;57:291–4.

Fry SW, Al-Kawas FH. Endoscopic retrograde cholangio-pancreatography. In: Evans SR, Ascher SM, editors. Hepatobiliary and pancreatic surgery. New York: Wiley-Liss Inc; 1998. p. 207–52.

Green PH, Kjandelwal M. ERCP for acute cholangitis and biliary pancreatitis. In: Jacobson IM, editor. ERCP and its applications. Philadelphia: Lippincott-Raven Publishers; 1998. p. 105–13.

Greenen JE, Hogan WJ, Dodds WJ, et al. The efficacy of endoscopic sphincterotomy after cholecystectomy in patients with suspected sphincter of Oddi dysfunction. N Engl J Med 1989;320:82–7.

Kaw M, Brodmerkel GJ. ERCP, biliary crystal analysis and sphincter of Oddi mannometry in idiopathic recurrent pancreatitis. Gastrointest Endosc 2002;55:157–62.

Ko CW, Lee SP. Epidemiology and natural history of common bile duct stones and prediction of disease. Gastrointest Endosc 2002;56:S165–73.

Kozarek P. Role of ERCP in acute pancreatitis. Gastrointest Endosc 2002;56:S231–6.

Lee JG, Leung JW. Choledocholithiasis, bacterial cholangitis, oriental intrahepatic stone disease, and parasitic disorders of the biliary tree. In: Benjamin SB, DiMarino AJ, editors. Gastointestinal disease: an endoscoic approach. 2nd ed. New Jersey: Slack Inc; 2002. p. 1133–44.

Mark DH, Flamm CR, Aronson N. Evidence-based diagnostic modalities for common bile duct stone. Gastrointest Endosc 2002;56:S190–4.

Norton ID, Gostout CJ, Baron TH, et al. Safety and outcome of endoscopic snare excision of the major duodenal papilla. Gastrointest Endosc 2002;56:239–43.

Prajapati DN, Hogan WJ. Sphincter of oddi dysfunction and other functional biliary disorders: evaluation and treatment. Gastroenterol Clin 2003;32:601–18.

Sherman S. What is the role of ERCP in the setting of abdominal pain of pancreatic or biliary origin (suspected sphincter of Oddi dysfunction)? Gastrointest Endosc 2002;56:S258–66.

Touli J, Roberts-Thompson IC, Kellow J, et al. Mannometry based randomized trial of endoscopic sphincterotomy for sphincter of Oddi dysfunction. Gut 2000;46:98–102.

CHAPTER 135

POSTCHOLECYSTECTOMY SYNDROME

AYMAN KOTEISH, MD, AND ANTHONY N. KALLOO, MD

The postcholecystectomy syndrome (PCS) refers to a recurrence or persistence of symptoms following cholecystectomy. This is not a true syndrome in that it may be a result of different disease processes as opposed to a classic syndrome that is usually attributable to a single disease. PCS has been incorrectly used synonymously with Sphincter of Oddi dysfunction (SOD). SOD is a malfunction of sphincter of Oddi (SO) contractility and is a benign noncalculous hindrance to the flow of bile and/or pancreatic juice through the SO muscle. It is, however, a relatively common cause of PCS. Furthermore, there are differences in nomenclature that are a major source of confusion when referring to SOD, and these include *papillary stenosis, biliary spasm, biliary dyskinesia,* and *sclerosing papillitis*. Knowledge of the specific cause of PCS is important to the appropriate management of these patients. Table 135-1 lists the more common causes of PCS. In this chapter we will delineate our approach to address this syndrome, with special attention to SOD diagnosis and management.

Symptoms after Cholecystectomy

Overall, it has been estimated that 5 to 40% of patients have persistent biliary-type symptoms after cholecystectomy. Diarrhea, on the other hand, is a physiologic consequence of cholecystectomy. It has been reported that about 8% of patients develop persistent diarrhea postcholecystectomy (PC). The actual number may be much higher, however, as only patients with severe diarrhea seek medical attention. Milder cases remain unrecognized unless patients are specifically asked about their bowel habits. The pathophysiology of diarrhea PC has not been established, although some investigators hypothesized that it is due to an increased intestinal transit by excess intraluminal bile acids.

The most common postoperative symptoms after cholecystectomy are dyspepsia, bloating, and flatulence, which mostly precede the surgery. A smaller subset of patients, however, will present with severe abdominal pain, nausea, vomiting, and/or jaundice. Diagnostic workup is more likely to yield a specific disorder in the latter group. In patients with more severe symptoms, especially if accompanied by fever, leukocytosis, and/or jaundice, bile peritonitis, secondary to a bile leak, has to be suspected and ruled out.

TABLE 135-1. Common Causes of Postcholecystectomy Syndrome

- Irritable bowel syndrome
- Peptic ulcer disease
- Retained bile duct stone
- Chronic pancreatitis
- GERD
- Sphincter of Oddi dysfunction

GERD = gastroesophageal reflux disease.

Management of PCS

Management of PCS has to address the specific cause. *Irritable bowel syndrome* (see Chapter 39, "Irritable Bowel Syndrome"), *peptic ulcer disease* (see Chapter 25, "Peptic Ulcer Disease"), *cholelithiasis* (see Chapter 132, "Cholelithiasis"), and *chronic pancreatitis* (see Chapter 139, "Chronic Pancreatitis") are important diagnostic considerations in the management of this syndrome. However, in this chapter we will focus on SOD. One study that systematically examined patients after cholecystectomy found that IBS was the most common cause of PCS.

SOD

SOD is an important consideration in the examination of patients with PCS, and is thought to be the cause of pain in up to 14% of these patients. It manifests as pancreatic or biliary pain, or a combination thereof, and in some patients, may present as pancreatitis or cholestasis. We recognize the following two separate entities within this disorder:

1. *SO stenosis* is an anatomic abnormality that may have resulted from prior inflammatory processes leading to fibrosis (eg, pancreatitis, passage of stones, operative trauma, etc). It is associated with elevated basal sphincter pressures and a lack of manometric response to smooth muscle relaxants.
2. *SO dyskinesia* is a functional disorder of the SO resulting in intermittent biliary and/or pancreatic obstruction also associated with elevated sphincter pressure but with a manometric response to smooth muscle relaxants. The etiology is unknown, and may be related to local hormonal or neurologic disturbance.

Abdominal pain is the major symptom. Pain is epigastric to right upper quadrant in location, may be severe, lasts from 30 minutes to several hours, and may radiate to the back or right shoulder, and it may be accompanied by nausea and vomiting. The pain may begin from weeks to several years after a cholecystectomy. Alternatively, in a subset of patients, SOD is suspected upon continued biliary pain, not relieved by prior cholecystectomy. Moreover, pain is refractory to medications for acid suppression or IBS. Fever, chills, and jaundice are rare.

Clinical Classification

In addition, diagnosis of SOD is supported by liver and/or pancreatic enzyme abnormalities. A history of unexplained acute intermittent pancreatitis may result from SOD. The best-studied classification system is the Hogan-Geenen classification (also known as the Milwaukee Biliary Group Classification [Table 135-2]), where three categories were identified (types 1, 2, and 3). Note, that a similar classification has been adopted for patients with SOD and predominant pancreatic symptoms (presenting with recurrent idiopathic pancreatitis), and an otherwise negative workup.

Diagnosis

The diagnosis of SOD requires a high index of suspicion, and the systematic exclusion of more common gastrointestinal disorders (eg, IBS, peptic ulcer, and gastroesophageal reflux diseases). Patients with suspected SOD may demonstrate abnormal elevation of serum liver biochemistry and pancreatic enzymes especially in association with pain. Abdominal ultrasound (US) or computed tomography scan usually shows normal findings, although, occasionally, a dilatated bile duct or pancreatic duct may be described (especially in type 1). Moreover, in the absence of choledocholithiasis or mass lesions, SOD should be suspected.

Hepatobiliary Scintigraphy

Hepatobiliary scintigraphy (after stimulation with cholecystokinin [CCK]) uses technetium-99 labeled dyes and provides a semi-quantitative assessment of biliary drainage in PC patients (where obstruction was ruled out). We have devised a scoring system (Hopkins' scintigraphic score), using several scintigraphic parameters (Table 135-3). A score of 5 or more is considered abnormal and highly indicative of SOD (Jaganath and Kalloo, 2001). In our hands, scores have correlated closely with manometric readings, although other groups have had weaker strong correlations. We will perform therapy for SOD based on the results of scintigraphy alone. One drawback of biliary scintigraphy is that it provides no information on the pancreatic sphincter, which may be abnormal in up to 40% of patients with biliary sphincter dysfunction.

Other noninvasive tests such as the morphine-Prostigmin test (also known as the *Nardi test*), and *CCK- or fatty meal-stimulated US* are provocative tests. A positive test is defined by reproduction of symptoms and/or biochemical abnormalities. These tests have relatively low sensitivity and specificity and have been largely abandoned. *Secretin stimulated endoscopic US (EUS)* has been promising in evaluating pancreatic-type SOD, but results are still preliminary, and EUS has not gained a role in the actual diagnostic workup of SOD.

Sphincter Manometry

Sphincter manometry (SOM) remains the gold standard for diagnosing SOD. Its invasive nature, however, in addition to its potential complications, makes it reserved as a last diagnostic step, only used when it is likely to lead to a therapeutic intervention. We reserve SOM for patients with a history suggestive of pancreatic type pain or recurrent

TABLE 135-2.

	Biliary-type Pain	Abnormal LFTs (a)	Dilatated CBD (b)	Delayed Drainage (c)
Type 1	+	+	+	+
Type 2	+	One of two of above		
Type 3	+	None of the above		

Reproduced with permission from <www.hopkins-gi.org>.
(a) Alanine aminotransferase and aspartate aminotransferase levels are > 2 times normal values on at least 2 separate occasions.
(b) Common bile duct diameter > 12 mm on ultrasonography, or > than 10 mm on cholangiography.
(c) More than 45 minutes at endoscopic retrograde cholangiopancreatography while patient is in supine position.
CBD = common bile duct.

TABLE 135-3. The Hopkins Scintigraphic Scoring System for Sphincter of Oddi Dysfunction

	Criteria	Score
Peak Time	(a) < 10 minutes	0
	(b) ≥ 10 minutes	1
Time of Biliary Visualization	(a) < 15 minutes	0
	(b) ≥ 15 minutes	1
Prominence of Biliary Tree	(a) Not prominent	0
	(b) Prominent major intrahepatic ducts	1
	(c) Prominent small intrahepatic ducts	2
Bowel Visualization	(a) < 15 minutes	0
	(b) 15 to 30 minutes	1
	(c) > 30 minutes	2
CBD Emptying	(a) > 50%	0
	(b) < 50%	1
	(c) No change	2
	(d) Shows increasing activity	3
CBD-to-Liver Ratio	CBD_{60} < $Liver_{60}$	0
	CBD_{60} > $Liver_{60}$ but < $Liver_{15}$	1
	CBD_{60} > $Liver_{60}$ and = $Liver_{15}$	2
	CBD_{60} > both $Liver_{60}$ and $Liver_{15}$	3

Reproduced by permission <www.hopkins-gi.org>.
Hepatobiliary scintigraphy has no value in evaluating the pancreatic portion of the Sphincter of Oddi.
CBD = common bile duct.

pancreatitis of unclear etiology, and for patients who have had biliary sphincterotomy for biliary sphincter dysfunction and continue to have persistent symptoms.

Therapy

The prime aim of therapy is to relieve symptoms by reducing the resistance to bile or pancreatic juice flow. Several types of therapy exist that have been studied to variable degrees.

Medical Therapy

A limited number of studies evaluated this type of therapy. Because the SO is composed of smooth muscle, drugs that relax smooth muscle were evaluated, namely calcium channel blockers (*nifedipine*) and nitrates. Both have been used and have shown a reduction in sphincter pressures in both patients and controls, although a more profound effect was noted in the former group. Short term studies have revealed up to 75% improvement among patients with SOD. Although medical therapy is an attractive concept, several drawbacks limit its widespread application; these mainly include medication side effects (in close to 30% of the patients), tolerance (eg, to nitrates), and an ineffectiveness in situations such as SO stenosis. There still may be room for medical therapy, however, in less severe forms of SOD.

Surgical Therapy

Transduodenal sphincteroplasty and *pancreatic septoplasty* were the most common form of therapy for SOD. With the advent of endoscopic therapy, however, *endoscopic sphincterotomy* (ES) has largely replaced surgery as a standard SOD therapy. There still exists some role for surgical intervention in situations where endoscopy fails, or is inaccessible. However, it is highly recommended that patients being considered for surgery be referred to specialized centers with expertise in the field.

Endoscopic Therapy

ES is the current standard of care for patients with SOD. Sixty to 95% of patients have reportedly improved with this form of therapy. Variability in outcome is due to the variability of different types of SOD treated (eg, type 1 has better response than types 2 and 3). Better responses could also be achieved in more than half of nonresponders.

Balloon dilatation of the SO is yet another approach that is attractive because it is "sphincter-sparing" but it is currently not recommended because of the increased risk of pancreatitis, including severe pancreatitis and death. Balloon dilatation may play a role in patients who have restenosed after demonstrating a good response to ES *and* if from a technical standpoint it is not possible to extend the ES.

Stent placement has been studied as a means of predicting response to ES. Although improvement following stent placement has been suggested to be a good predictor of response to ES, pancreatitis has been a major complicating factor to this approach. Moreover, this approach has a disadvantage of requiring an additional procedure. Stent placement is not recommended as a therapeutic trial.

Botulinum toxin (Botox) is a potent inhibitor of acetylcholine release. Intrasphincteric injections of Botox into the SO have decreased sphincter pressures by close to 50%, increased bile flow, and resulted in symptomatic relief. A single shot of 100 units of Botox injected with a sclerotherapy needle into the apex of the papilla has been shown to be effective. Botox effect, however, may wane in 6 months to 1 year, and repeated injections may then be needed. This procedure is safe and without significant complications. It may have usefulness as a therapeutic trial when SM and scintigraphy are not available because a good response to Botox has been shown to predict a favorable response to ES.

Conclusion

PCS encompasses a wide spectrum of diagnoses. Approach and management follow general guidelines, but should be tailored to the individual patient. SOD remains the most challenging entity of this syndrome, both diagnostically and therapeutically. In patients with Type 1 SOD, we perform ES without further testing, such as SM, because there is a general consensus that a structural disorder of the sphincter is at the basis of this disorder (ie, stenosis). In patients with PC biliary-type pain, and a hepatobiliary score ≥ 5, we perform biliary ES. In situations were the Hopkins' scintigraphic score is < 5 (and less commonly, if the score is > 5 in the setting of an atypical presentation), we perform endoscopic retrograde cholangiopancreatography with SOM. In patients requiring pancreatic sphincterotomy, we invariably place a pancreatic stent for up to 2 weeks to minimize the risk of postsphincterotomy pancreatitis.

Supplemental Reading

Corazziari E, Shaffer EA, Hogan WJ, et al. Functional disorders of the biliary tract and pancreas. Gut 1999;45(Suppl 2):II48–54.

Desautels SG, Slivka A, Hutson WR, et al. Postcholecystectomy pain syndrome: pathophysiology of abdominal pain in sphincter of Oddi type III. Gastroenterol 1999;116:900–5.

Kalloo AN. Overview of differential diagnoses of abdominal pain. Gastrointest Endosc 2002;56:S255–7.

Jagganath S, Kalloo AN. Efficacy of biliary scintigraphy in suspected sphincter of Oddi dysfunction. Curr Gastroenterol Rep 2001;3:160–5.

Shaffer EA. Review article: control of gall-bladder motor function. Aliment Pharmacol Ther 2000;14(Suppl 2):2–8.

Sherman S. What is the role of ERCP in the setting of abdominal pain of pancreatic or biliary origin (suspected sphincter of Oddi dysfunction). Gastrointes Endosc 2002;56(Suppl):S258–66.

CHAPTER 136

ACUTE PANCREATITIS

ANIL B. NAGAR, MD, AND FRED S. GORELICK, MD

Acute pancreatitis is a clinical syndrome of pancreatic inflammation with discrete episodes of abdominal pain and elevations in serum pancreas enzyme levels. Inciting factors result in a cascade of events, beginning with the intra-acinar activation of zymogens, generation of harmful cytokines and other pro-inflammatory mediators, and ischemia, which result in tissue injury. Patients usually present with severe abdominal pain and elevation of the amylase and lipase. Most attacks of acute pancreatitis are mild and resolve without therapy or complications. Severe pancreatitis is seen in 10 to 20% of cases and results in complications including necrosis, infection, abscesses and pseudocysts, a systemic inflammatory response, and organ failure. Patients with severe disease may have a mortality rate of up to 30%. After an attack of acute pancreatitis, there is usually full recovery of function, unless there is underlying chronic pancreatitis. Early in the course of acute pancreatitis the clinician should predict the severity of disease so that therapy may be directed to patients with severe disease and possibly reduce complications. There is no specific treatment for acute pancreatitis; supportive care, fluid resuscitation and treatment of complications are the foundation of management.

Etiology

Many conditions predispose to disease development (Table 136-1). Gallstones and alcohol abuse account for at least 75% of acute pancreatitis in the United States. Many patients with idiopathic pancreatitis may have unidentified hereditary pancreatitis or other gene mutations that predispose them to disease. There is a separate chapter on cystic fibrosis (see Chapter 140, "Cystic Fibrosis and Other Hereditary Diseases of the Pancreas").

Pathogenesis

Gallstone pancreatitis is caused by acute obstruction of the pancreatic duct by gallstones. Although alcohol has many potentially harmful effects, the reason it causes pancreatitis remains unclear. Because < 10% of individuals who chronically abuse alcohol (> 80 g ethanol/d for 10 years) will develop pancreatitis, additional environmental or inherited factors must affect disease development.

Definition of Terms

The Atlanta symposium helps classify mild and severe pancreatitis (Table 136-2). Pancreatic necrosis is nonviable pancreatic parenchyma. During the course of acute pancreatitis, it may remain sterile or become infected. Using contrast enhanced computed tomography (CT) scan, an area of necrosis is observed as nonenhanced parenchyma (Figure 136-1).

Prognostic Assessment

The early assessment of disease severity may be critical to optimize therapy. Clinical signs of severe pancreatitis

TABLE 136-1. Etiology of Acute Pancreatitis

Structural
  Gallstones or microlithiasis
  Sphincter of Oddi dysfunction
  Pancreas divisum
  Trauma
Toxins
  Alcohol
  Medications and toxins
Infectious
  Viral
  Parasitic
Metabolic
  Hypertriglyceridemia
  Hypercalcemia
Iatrogenic
  ERCP
  Pancreatic biopsy
Other specific etiologies
  Vasculitis (autoimmune)
  Cholesterol emboli
  Coronary bypass
  Peritoneal dialysis
  Cystic fibrosis
  Fibrocalculous (tropical)
  Hereditary (trypsinogen gene mutations)
  Inflammatory bowel disease
  Neoplasia
Idiopathic

ERCP = endoscopic retrograde cholangiopancreatography.

TABLE 136-2. Definitions of Mild and Severe Pancreatitis

Mild acute pancreatitis
    Minimal organ dysfunction and an uneventful recovery
Severe acute Pancreatitis
    End organ failure
        Shock: systolic blood pressure < 90 mm Hg
        Respiratory insufficiency: PaO_2 < 60 mm Hg
        Renal failure: serum creatinine > 2 mg/dL
        Gastrointestinal bleeding: > 500 mL/24 hr
    And/or local pancreatic complications
        Necrosis
        Abscess
        Pseudocyst
    Unfavorable early prognostic signs
        > 3 Ranson's signs
        > 8 APACHE-II points
Pancreatic necrosis
    Nonviable pancreatic parenchyma
Acute fluid collection
    Early fluid collection around pancreas lacking a wall
Pseudocyst
    Persistent fluid collection (> 4 weeks) encapsulated by granulation tissue
Pancreatic abscess
    Circumscribed purulent collection

APACHE = Acute Physiological and Chronic Health Evaluation.

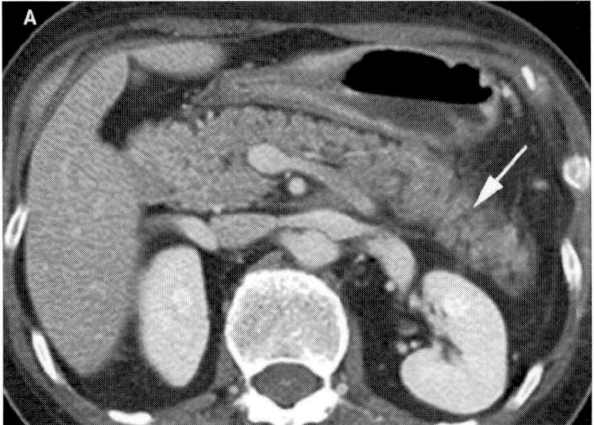
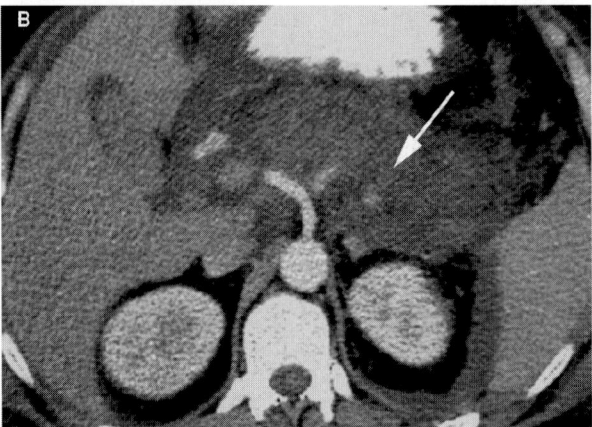

FIGURE 136-1. Contrast enhanced computed tomography (CT) scan in acute pancreatitis. *A*, Contrast enhanced CT scan in mild pancreatitis. *B*, Contrast enhanced CT scan in severe necrotizing pancreatitis. Note the unenhanced pancreatic parenchyma (*arrows*) indicative of pancreatic necrosis.

include signs of peritonitis, shock, coma, and respiratory insufficiency. An admission hematocrit of > 47% or pleural effusions may be a poor prognostic signs. Ranson's prognostic criteria are often used (Table 136-3). A score of ≥ 6 is correlated with > 60% mortality. Drawbacks include that it requires all 11 measures, takes 48 hours to evaluate and has a sensitivity and specificity for severe disease of 60 to 80%. The APACHE-II (Acute Physiological and Chronic Health Evaluation) is commonly used to score disease severity and uses 14 routinely measured parameters. It predicts severity in acute pancreatitis with a sensitivity and specificity of 70 to 80% (Wilson et al, 1990). A score > 8 predicts severe disease. A major shortcoming is its complexity. Contrast enhanced CT dynamic scan is useful to document necrosis and fluid collections. Because necrosis progresses during the first 3 days of disease, we usually wait 48 to 72 hours after disease onset to perform a contrast-enhanced study. The CT findings are the basis for a *CT severity index* (Table 136-4). This severity index correlates with mortality and is the current standard for assessment of severity in acute pancreatitis (Balthazar, 1989). Patients who are obese (body mass index > 27), have C-reactive proteins > 150 mg/dL, or have organ failure, or who develop it during their hospitalization, have a worse prognosis.

Approach to the Management

The first step in the management of acute pancreatitis is to make the correct diagnosis. This should be done while the patient is receiving resuscitation with intravenous (IV) flu-

TABLE 136-3. Ranson's Criteria for Severity of Pancreatitis*

At Admission	During Initial 48 Hours
Age > 55 years	Hematocrit decrease of > 10 mg/dL
White blood cell count > 16,000/mm³	Blood urea nitrogen increase of > 5 mg/dL
Glucose > 200 mg/dL	Calcium < 8 mg/dL
Lactate dehydrogenase > 350 IU/L	PaO_2 < 60 mm Hg
Aspartate aminotransferase > 250 U/L	Base deficit > 4 mEq/L
	Fluid sequestration > 6 L

*A score of 6 or more correlates with > 60% mortality.

ids in the emergency room. The correct diagnosis is important in patients presenting with severe disease, because conditions such as acute mesenteric ischemia and acute cholecystitis may present in a similar fashion and have a different management. Once the diagnosis of acute pancreatitis is established, an attempt should be made to define the etiology of the acute attack. This is important since the

TABLE 136-4. CT Finding in Acute Pancreatitis and CT Severity Index

Staging	Score
A. Normal	0
B. Focal or diffuse enlargement of gland	1
C. As B plus involvement of peripancreatic fat	2
D. As C plus single, ill defined fluid collection	3
E. As D plus ≥ 2 ill-defined fluid collections and/or intrapancreatic gas	4
Degree of Necrosis (%) (Nonenhancement with IV contrast)	Score
0	0
< 33 of pancreas	2
33 to < 50 of pancreas	4
≥ 50 of pancreas	6

From Balthazar et al, 1989.
CT = computed tomography; IV = intravenous.
CT score + necrosis score = CT Severity Index (CTSI).

management of acute biliary pancreatitis may include urgent endoscopic retrograde cholangiography (ERCP). We perform an ultrasound scan at admission on patients with suspected biliary pancreatitis, the severity of acute pancreatitis should be assessed clinically and by scoring systems such as the APACHE II. Patients who have severe acute pancreatitis should receive a contrast enhanced CT scan. It confirms the clinical diagnosis, establishes severity, and documents the extent of necrosis. MRI and serological markers such as CRP may prove to be useful markers of disease severity and necrosis. Patients with severe acute pancreatitis should be admitted to an intensive care unit whereas mild pancreatitis can be managed on a regular medical floor (Figure 136-2).

Treatment

The cornerstone of therapy is to provide supportive care, with adequate volume resuscitation and monitoring of hemodynamic, respiratory, and renal function. The aims of therapy are to reduce pancreatic necrosis and enhance tissue perfusion, limit complications, recognize infected necrosis early, and prevent future attacks.

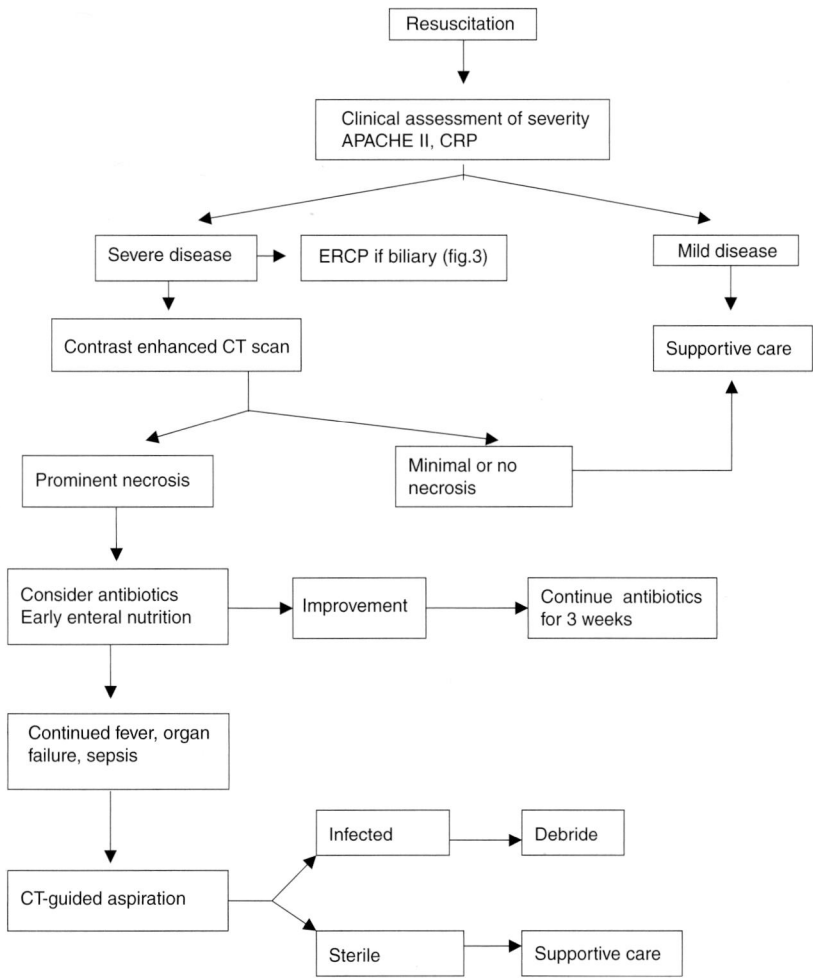

FIGURE 136-2. Management algorithm for acute pancreatitis. APACHE = Acute Physiological and Chronic Health Evaluation; CT = computed tomography; ERCP = endoscopic retrograde cholangiopancreatography.

General Measures

Severe acute pancreatitis is like a burn with patients developing intravascular volume depletion due to "third spacing" of fluid. Resuscitation begins in the emergency room with normal saline; patients with severe pancreatitis will require 4 to 10 L over the first 24 hours. Intravascular volume assessment should be made regularly using the urine output, vital signs, and mental status. Adequate electrolyte replacement should accompany fluid infusion. In severely ill patients central venous pressure monitoring is useful. A persistently elevated hematocrit may be a sign of inadequate volume replacement and a poor prognostic sign. Abdominal pain is treated with meperidine (Demerol) (50 to 100 mg) given every 4 hours; fentanyl is an alternative medication for this purpose. We avoid the use of morphine because it causes more increase in sphincter of Oddi (SO) pressure. Patients are kept NPO on admission and nasogastric (NG) tube placement is only used for patients with severe disease and an ileus. Gastric acid secretion should be suppressed to prevent stress ulceration. Nasal oxygen should be used for oxygen saturation < 90%. Mechanical ventilation may be required in patients who hypoventilate or develop adult respiratory distress syndrome (ARDS).

Mild Pancreatitis

Patients by mild pancreatitis have a good prognosis and can be managed on a regular medical floor. In addition to supportive care described above, patients are kept NPO until there is a prominent reduction in their abdominal pain. This usually takes 3 to 5 days after which they are started on a low fat diet. There is no indication for enteral feeding or prophylactic antibiotics in this group of patients. NG tube placement is not necessary. When patients are hungry and their symptoms have resolved, they should be fed even if the serum levels of pancreatic enzymes are elevated. If pain occurs with feeding it may reflect unresolved pancreatitis or a disease complication (eg, duct leak).

Severe Pancreatitis

Patients with severe acute pancreatitis are admitted to an intensive care unit for hemodynamic and respiratory monitoring and support. Following adequate resuscitation, a contrast enhanced CT scan of the abdomen is obtained on day 2 or 3, because pancreatic necrosis is best observed at 48 to 72 hours after onset and this delay may minimize the harmful effects of the CT contrast. The patient is kept NPO; NG tube decompression is used in patients with a symptomatic ileus. Hyperglycemia is sometimes observed but it is often mild and transient and requires treatment only when glucose levels are very high. Multiple factors cause a decrease in serum calcium levels during acute pancreatitis. The most common cause is hypoalbuminemia, which results in normal serum ionized calcium, is asymptomatic, and requires no treatment. Reduced ionized serum calcium with neuromuscular irritability is rare, but requires treatment with cautious administration of IV calcium. Because hypocalcemia may be accompanied by hypomagnesemia, serum magnesium levels need to be measured in the symptomatic patient. Hypertriglyceridemia observed during an episode of acute pancreatitis generally does not require any specific therapy. Only those with persistently elevated triglyceride levels need to be considered for treatment. A very rare exception may be patients with ARDS and hypertriglyceridemia who may benefit from acute plasmapharesis.

Specific Organ Involvement in Severe Pancreatitis

Pulmonary Patients may develop respiratory failure from pain and ascites, pleural effusions, and ARDS. Respiratory failure form ARDS is the most serious complication and is usually seen in the first week of severe acute pancreatitis. Pulmonary artery wedge pressure (PAWP) measurement must be performed to determine if hypoxemia is due to congestive heart failure (elevated PAWP) or ARDS (normal or low PAWP). There is no specific treatment and patients require support by mechanical ventilation with positive end-expiratory pressure.

Renal Renal dysfunction is common and initially is due to volume depletion and prerenal azotemia. Aggressive volume resuscitation is necessary early in the course of disease. If the renal dysfunction does not resolve, the patient has developed acute tubular necrosis and fluid management requires central venous pressure monitoring.

Cardiovascular Patients may develop congestive cardiac failure or myocardial ischemia. This should be considered in those who do not respond to adequate fluid resuscitation. Once again PAWP determination is helpful in management and patients may require support with pressors.

Gastrointestinal Gastrointestinal bleeding in acute pancreatitis may be due to erosive gastritis, duodenitis from acute pancreatitis, bleeding from a pseudoaneurysm of the gastroduodenal or splenic arteries, gastric variceal bleeding from splenic vein thrombosis (usually associated with chronic pancreatitis), and hemosuccus pancreaticus. Patients should receive blood transfusions to maintain a hematocrit of about 30 and upper endoscopy may be indicated. Arterial embolization is the treatment of choice for pseudoaneurysms. The inflammation of pancreatitis may extend into the transverse mesocolon and result in colonic inflammation presenting as a "colon cut off sign" on abdominal radiograph. No specific treatment is required and this usually resolves, but rarely surgery is required for perforation or bleeding.

Pancreatic Necrosis and the Role of Antibiotics

Deaths in acute pancreatitis occur in two patterns; early (first week after the onset) death is due to multisystem organ failure and late (after week two) death is due to infection of pancreatic necrosis or organ failure. If pancreatic necrosis remains sterile, the mortality is much less than if it becomes infected. Management of pancreatic infection involves the following issues. First, can infection be prevented? Second, how can infection be detected? Third, once detected how should it be treated? Fourth, in the absence of infection how should sterile necrosis be managed? Prospective studies by Bassi and colleagues (1998) demonstrate that prophylactic IV antibiotic therapy in patients with severe pancreatitis and extensive pancreatic necrosis results in some reduction of infectious complications and may improve survival. Gram-negative bacteria are most often cultured from infected necrosis. Antibiotics such as *imipenem* and *cefuroxime* have been used in an effort to prevent infection. Prophylactic decontamination of the gut with orally administered, nonabsorbable antibiotics may also have efficacy. The incidence of resistant bacteria and fungal infections has increased in patients given prophylactic antibiotics, and guidelines for antibiotic use are still evolving. It is possible that the use of antibiotics postpones the occurrence of infection to the third and fourth week of disease. We consider the use of *imipenem* or *ciprofloxacin* plus *metronidazole* in patients with extensive necrosis (> 50%), starting early (day two to three) and continued for 2 weeks. Infection of pancreatic necrosis occurs in the second to third week of presentation. Pancreatic infections usually present with increased abdominal pain, high fevers with leukocytosis, worsening renal and respiratory function, and occasionally bacteremia. The diagnosis of pancreatic infection is made using CT guided needle aspiration of the necrotic areas in the pancreas. Immediate Gram's stain of the aspirate should be performed along with cultures. This method is safe and accurate. If the suspicion for infection is high and aspirates do not demonstrate infection, the procedure should be repeated. Multiple areas of necrosis in and around the pancreas should be sampled. It should be noted that early needle aspiration (before 2 weeks) does not have a significant yield for infection, with the highest yield seen on day 17. Once infected necrosis is diagnosed the patient should be treated with prompt surgical debridement, because untreated necrosis has a mortality of 100%. Late complications of infection in a walled off area (pancreatic abscess) may be managed by percutaneous drainage catheters. Patients with sterile necrosis can be managed without surgery. Early surgical intervention was associated with a high mortality and experience has now shown that it is best to avoid surgery in patients with sterile necrosis regardless of the extent of necrosis (Bradley 1993; Buchler et al, 2000). Most patients can be treated conservatively, with a mortality of 1 to 5%. A small group of patients with sterile necrosis and persistent severe pancreatitis will fail to improve with conservative therapy. Patients with sterile necrosis may benefit from surgery even in the absence of infection, but this should be delayed past the third or fourth week of disease. This gives time for organization of necrosis and reduces the risk of bleeding and loss of viable pancreatic tissue.

Role of ERCP in Acute Gallstone Pancreatitis

The exact mechanism through which gallstones induce pancreatitis is still debated, but the most likely explanation is acute obstruction of the pancreatic duct. Most gallstones will pass spontaneously into the duodenum following an attack of acute pancreatitis. Studies of urgent (within 72 hours of admission) ERCP with biliary sphincterotomy have demonstrated an improved outcome in patients with severe acute gallstone pancreatitis (Neoptolemous et al, 1988) and evidence of persistent biliary obstruction. These are patients with hyperbilirubinemia, common bile duct dilatation, or sepsis. The improvement appears to result from treatment of cholangitis. The role of urgent ERCP in severe acute gallstone pancreatitis without clinical biliary obstruction is controversial with at least one study by Flosch and colleagues (1997) demonstrating an increased mortality. In these patients we would perform an endoscopic ultrasound (EUS) to detect common duct stones, prior to ERCP. It should be noted that ERCP with endoscopic sphincterotomy has been demonstrated to be safe in the setting of acute pancreatitis, and, when performed by experienced endoscopists, does not appear to increase morbidity or mortality. One setting in which ERCP with biliary sphincterotomy should always be considered is acute biliary pancreatitis during pregnancy, when timely cholecystectomy is precluded.

Nutrition

There are several important issues related to nutrition and acute pancreatitis. These include the approach to the patients with mild versus severe disease, the type of nutritional support, and when to begin feeding. Traditionally patients have been kept NPO for fear that that feeding would worsen acute pancreatitis by stimulating the inflamed pancreas. The standard of nutritional support has been total parenteral nutrition (TPN). However, TPN is associated with higher infection rates and has not been demonstrated to reduce mortality. Additionally the gut barrier function is compromised during acute pancreatitis; this may be a factor in bacterial translocation and bacterial seeding of pancreatic necrosis. It is tempting to consider that early enteral feeding may preserve gut barrier function. In 1997 Kalfarentzos and colleagues (1997) demonstrated that enteral feeding (via a nasojejunal tube) in severe acute pancreatitis is possible, safe, less expensive, and may reduce pancreatic infections compared to TPN.

Since then there have been several studies that have reproduced these results, although a convincing benefit in mortality has not been demonstrated (Imrie et al, 2002). Most recently there have been reports that NG feeding is well tolerated in these patients. Our practice is to begin enteral feeding in patients by an endoscopically or radiologically placed nasojejunal feeding tube after day 2 or 3 in patients with severe pancreatitis. Feeding is started at low rate of 20 cc/hr. Although this does not provide complete caloric requirements, small amounts of feeding are usually tolerated and may preserve the intestinal barrier. If nausea and vomiting are present, a NG tube can be placed and kept to drainage. A small group of patients (between 10 to 20%) will not tolerate this method of feeding and require TPN. Triglyceride levels should be checked after the onset of feeding, especially in patients with known hypertriglyceridemia.

Pharmacotherapy with Cytokines, Enzyme Inhibitors, and Anti-Inflammatory Agents

Multiple cytokines and anti-inflammatory mediators have been implicated in the pathogenesis of acute pancreatitis. Thus, blockage by a single agent (eg, interleukin-10, lexipafant) has not been effective in the treatment of pancreatitis.

Surgical Therapy and Management of Other Complications

Surgical therapy is used to treat infected necrosis or complications. The following chapter is on surgical management of pancreatitis. Surgical management includes *necrosectomy* to remove necrotic tissue with intraoperative and postoperative lavage of debris and pancreatic fluids. Percutaneous catheter-directed debridement of infected necrosis has been described, but is best directed to patients who are hemodynamically and clinical stable. Further, a number of these patients will subsequently require surgery. It is not our practice to recommend *percutaneous drainage*, except in carefully selected patients with pancreatic abscesses. Endoscopic drainage with placement of transgastric and tranduodenal catheters and nasopancreatic tubes for irrigation has been described. The experience with this method is limited and it requires specific endoscopic experience, with experienced surgical backup. *Acute fluid collections* can be observed early in the course of acute pancreatitis and will usually resolve spontaneously; treatment is required only if they become symptomatic or infected. *Pseudocysts* are localized collections of necrotic debris and fluid within a wall of granulation tissue that persist for > 4 weeks. Regardless of its size, an asymptomatic pseudocyst does not require any therapy and may be observed indefinitely. If the cyst is symptomatic (pain, obstruction), it may be drained using a variety of methods including endoscopic, percutaneous, and surgical. Cysts may be drained endoscopically either by cyst-gastrostomy or cyst duodenostomy or by transampullary stent drainage. There is a separate chapter on endoscopic management of pancreatitis (see Chapter 138, "Pancreatitis: Endoscopic Therapy"). Percutaneous drainage is attempted if the location precludes endoscopic cystgastrotomy or when multiple noncommunicating cysts are observed. If the pseudocyst does not resolve with drainage, a *proximal pancreatic duct stricture* may be present and an ERCP should be performed. ERCP prior to cyst drainage should *only be attempted if the pseudocyst can be immediately drained*, because if there is contrast entry into the pseudocyst (as in communicating cysts) it increases the chance of infection in the event that drainage is not performed. Pseudocysts may become infected, rupture, or hemorrhage.

Post-ERCP Pancreatitis

Approximately 1 to 10% of ERCPs may be complicated by acute pancreatitis. This is usually mild, but severe pancreatitis and death may occur. Table 136-5 summarizes risk factors and preventive measures. The judicious use of non-imaging procedures (magnetic resonance cholangiopancreatography and EUS) to circumvent diagnostic ERCP is important because preventative measures have limited success. Short duration (1 to 2 days) pancreatic duct stenting appears to be effective in high risk patients, including those undergoing pancreatic sphincterotomy, SO dysfunction, and pancreatic endotherapy.

Prevention of Recurrence

In patients with predicted biliary pancreatitis, if gallstones are not observed on an initial ultrasound, the procedure should be repeated after the pancreatitis has resolved. Patients with biliary pancreatitis have a significant risk of recurrence unless a cholecystectomy is performed. In patients with mild to moderate pancreatitis, this can be accomplished prior to discharge. Patients who refuse surgery or are very high operative risks benefit from endoscopic biliary sphincterotomy to prevent recurrence. Patients with alcohol use should be counseled about cessation. The treatment of patients with *pancreas divisum* is controversial, but those with recurrent pancreatitis in whom no other etiology is identified may benefit from pancreatic sphincterotomy of the minor ampulla. *Hyperlipidemic* patients should receive appropriate lipid lowering medications and patients with acute recurrent pancreatitis may benefit from further endoscopic workup including ERCP, EUS, and SO manometry. Ampullary or pancreatic cancer may present in pancreatitis. Young patients or those with a family history should be offered genetic testing in the appropriate setting.

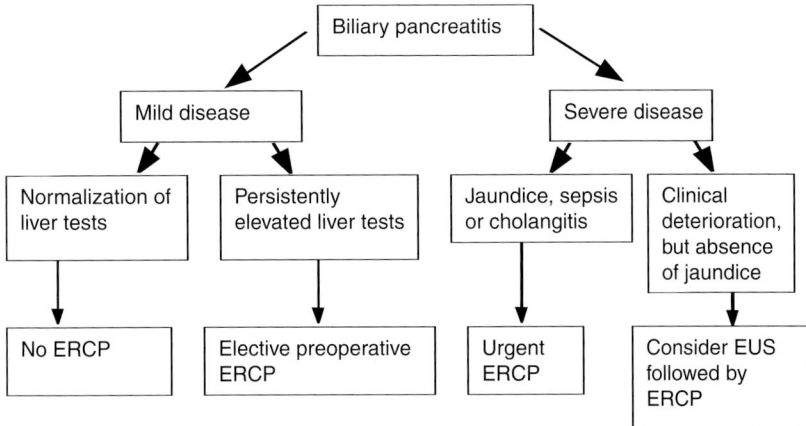

FIGURE 136-3 Role of endoscopic retrograde cholangiopancreatography in acute gallstone pancreatitis. ERCP = endoscopic retrograde cholangiopancreatography.

TABLE 136-5. Post-ERCP Pancreatitis

Increased Risk of ERCP-Pancreatitis	Measures to Prevent ERCP-Pancreatitis
Patient Factors	Most Useful
Sphincter of Oddi dysfunction	Proper technique and patient selection
Young age	Pancreatic duct stent in high risk patients
Female gender	Potentially useful: require further study
Procedure factors	Diclofenac
Sphincter of Oddi manometry	Nitroglycerine
Difficult cannulation	Probably not useful
Multiple injections of pancreatic duct	Interleukin-10
Precut sphincterotomy	Somatostatin
Pancreatic sphincterotomy	Gabexate mesilate (protease inhibitor)

ERCP = endoscopic retrograde cholangiopancreatography.

Supplemental Reading

Balthazar EJ. CT diagnosis and staging of acute pancreatitis. Radiol Clin North Am 1989;27:19–37.

Bassi C, Falconi M, Talamini G, et al. Controlled clinical trial of pefloxacin versus imipenem in severe acute pancreatitis. Gastroenterol 1998;115:1513–7.

Bradley EL III. A clinical based classification system for acute pancreatitis. Arch Surgery 1993;128:586–90.

Bradley EL III, Allen K. A prospective longitudinal study of observation versus surgical intervention in the management of necrotizing pancreatitis. Am J Surg 1991;161:19–24.

Buchler MW, Gloor B, Muller CA, et al. Acute necrotizing pancreatitis: treatment strategy according to the status of infection. Ann Surg 2000;232:619–26.

Flosch UR, Nitsche R, Ludtke R, et al. Early ERCP and papillotomy compared conservative treatment for acute acute biliary pancreatitis. N Engl J Med 1997;336:237–42.

Imrie CW, Carter CR, McKay CJ. Enteral and parnteral nutrition in acute pancreatitis. Best Pract Res Clin Gastroenterol 2002;16:391–7.

Isenmann R, Rau B, Beger HG. Bacterial infection and extent of necrosis are determinants of organ failure in patients with acute necrotizing pancreatitis. Br J Surg 1999;86:1020–4.

Kalfarentzos F, Kehagias J, Mead, et al. Enteral nutrition is superior to parenteral nutrition in severe acute pancreatitis: results of a randomized prospective trial. Br J Surg 1997;84:1665–9.

Neoptolemous JP, Carr-Locke CL, London NJ, et al. Controlled trial of urgent endoscopic retrograde cholangiopancreatography and endoscopic sphincterotomy versus conventional treatment for acute pancreatitis due to gallstones. Lancet 1988;ii: 979–83.

Ranson JHC, Rifkind RM, Roses DF. Prognostic signs and the role of operative management in acute pancreatitis. Surg Gynecol Obstet 1975;139:69–80.

Wilson C, Heath DI, Imrie CW. Prediction of outcome in acute pancreatitis: a comparative study of APACHE II, clinical assessment and multiple factor scoring systems. Br J Surg 1990;77:1260–4.

CHAPTER 137

CHRONIC PANCREATITIS: SURGICAL CONSIDERATIONS

OSCAR JOE HINES, MD, AND HOWARD A. REBER, MD

Chronic pancreatitis is characterized by chronic inflammation with fibrosis and obliteration of both the endocrine and exocrine components of the gland. These changes are irreversible, progressive, and may culminate in clinically significant pancreatic insufficiency and diabetes. Although chronic alcoholism is the usual etiology, some patients develop the disease because of chronic ductal obstruction, some because of genetic predisposition, and a substantial number for reasons as yet unknown. Regardless of the cause, the most common symptom of the disease is chronic abdominal pain, and pain relief is the most frequent reason for surgical intervention. Other reasons include various intra-abdominal complications of pancreatitis (eg, bile duct or duodenal obstruction, pseudocyst), and the concern that pancreatic cancer may be present. We will describe the surgical considerations related to each.

Chronic Abdominal Pain

The etiology of the pain is multifactorial and, in general, is not well understood. Factors include continued alcohol consumption that results in local release of oxygen-derived free radicals, diminished pancreatic blood flow and tissue acidosis, perineural sheath destruction with exposure to various nociceptive agents, and elevated pancreatic ductal and parenchymal pressures. The initial therapy for pain in all of these patients should be nonoperative and includes recommendations for the cessation of alcohol intake, and the administration of oral analgesic agents.

Referral for consideration of surgery requires (1) an assessment of the *significance of the pain* for the individual patient, which is highly subjective, (2) a determination of the *type of surgical procedure* that might be appropriate, and (3) an evaluation of the ability of the patient to deal with any long term *morbidity* that an operation might produce.

PAIN ASSESSMENT

In general, operation may be indicated in patients whose pain interferes with the quality of their lives. For example, the attacks of pain may require frequent hospitalizations that interfere with school or employment. The patient may be unable to function productively because of the depression that often accompanies the chronic pain state. Nutrition may be impaired because oral intake is limited by the pain that it produces. The patient may be addicted to narcotics.

Type of Surgical Procedure

The type of operation depends on the anatomy of the pancreatic ductal system, and whether or not the pancreas is diffusely involved with the disease or it involves one part of the gland more than the others. Thus, patients with a dilated pancreatic duct (> 7 mm in the body of the gland) are candidates for a drainage operation that decompresses the duct. Those with a duct that is of normal caliber will probably require resection of a part of the pancreas, usually the head of the gland.

Morbidity

Patients who undergo a pancreatic resection may develop *exocrine insufficiency* and/or *diabetes* if enough pancreas is removed. Whereas this may be an acceptable price to pay for pain relief in some patients, others might be unable to manage the dietary and insulin requirements that would ensue (eg, patients who are addicted to narcotics and/or alcohol). So a resection operation might be contraindicated in them. However, even in patients with narcotic and/or alcohol addiction and a dilated duct, a duct decompression operation may be appropriate, because it almost never produces exocrine or endocrine insufficiency. Preoperative psychiatric examination may help the surgeon to decide about whether or not operation should be considered.

Preoperative Imaging

All patients require preoperative imaging studies to help with decisions about the kind of operation that may be indicated. The goals of imaging are (1) to assess the diameter of the duct, (2) to determine the presence of any associated disease (eg, cysts, bile duct obstruction), and (3) to search for an unsuspected pancreatic malignancy. All patients should undergo a high resolution computed tomography (CT) scan with fine cuts through the pancreas during the arterial phase of the study. Endoscopic ultrasound (EUS) with fine needle aspiration (FNA) of any suspicious area may be indicated if the results of the CT scan raise a question about malignancy. There is a separate chapter on EUS and FNA (see Chapter 5, "Endoscopic Ultrasonography and Fine-Needle Aspiration").

Operations to relieve pain in these patients either (1) drain a dilated pancreatic ductal system or (2) resect diseased pancreatic tissue if the duct is not enlarged. The main pancreatic duct normally measures 4 to 5 mm in the head, 3 to 4 mm in the body, and 2 to 3 mm in the tail of the pancreas. The duct is considered dilated when it is at least 7 mm in diameter in the body of the gland.

Ductal Drainage Operation

In patients with a dilated pancreatic duct, a ductal drainage operation *(longitudinal pancreaticojejunostomy, Puestow procedure)* is likely to be effective. The operation involves wide exposure of the anterior surface of the pancreas, and incision of the anterior wall of the duct throughout the length of the gland. Pancreatic duct stones are removed and a Roux-en-Y jejunal limb is constructed and sewn along the length of the duct, so that pancreatic secretions empty directly into the bowel.

The operative results for longitudinal pancreaticojejunostomy are summarized in Table 137-1. The morbidity and mortality (< 2%) rates are minimal and there is almost no risk of diabetes because little if any pancreatic tissue is resected. Pain is relieved in 85% of patients for the first several years. Most patients gain weight because they no longer experience pain with eating, although the degree of malabsorption does not change. The major drawback of this operation is that within 5 years, pain recurs in as many as 40 to 50% of patients. In a small number, this may be due to stricturing of the anastomosis, but in most, it is probably associated with disease progression or the development of a complication. Recurrence of pain may also herald the appearance of pancreatic cancer.

Pancreatic Resection

Patients with a normal diameter or narrowed duct may be candidates for *pancreatic resection*. This is especially true when the pancreatic head is enlarged and contains multiple cysts and calcifications. Pancreaticoduodenectomy (Whipple resection) or pylorus-preserving pancreaticoduodenectomy are performed most commonly, and we prefer the latter. Pylorus preservation is felt by many to allow for better postoperative nutrition and weight gain, but little objective data support this. The operative mortality rate is < 3% and *permanent* pain relief is to be expected in 85 to 90%. These operations are more likely to produce endocrine (22%) and exocrine (55%) insufficiency, which is their major drawback. Of course, some patients develop these problems anyhow as the disease progresses.

In an effort to design an operation that would provide permanent pain relief and avoid the exocrine and endocrine insufficiency of a major resection, surgeons have designed several new procedures that combine *limited resection of the head of the pancreas with a pancreaticojejunostomy*. The so-called *Beger or Frey operations* remove most of the head of the pancreas except for a shell of pancreatic tissue posteriorly. The cavity thus created is drained into a Roux-en-Y limb of jejunum; gastroduodenal continuity is not disturbed. This operation can be performed whether or not the pancreatic duct is dilated. If it is, the

TABLE 137-1. Results of Longitudinal Pancreaticojejunostomy for Chronic Pancreatitis

Author	Year	Number of Patients	Mortality (%)	Mean follow-up (mo)	Pain Relief (%)
Leger	1973	45	4.5		63
Prinz	1978	42	5	108	76
Prinz	1981	43	4.5	95	65
Sarles	1982	69	4.2	60	85
Warshaw	1984	33	3	43	88
Bradley	1986	48	0	69	66
Nealon	1988	41	0	14.8	93

TABLE 137-2. Results of Resection for Chronic Pancreatitis

Study	Year	Type of Resection	Number of Patients	Operative Mortality (%)	Pain Relief (%)	New Onset DM (%)	New Endocrine Insufficiency (%)
Heise	2001	PPW	41	4.8	54	19	67
		Drainage	59	—	59	16	54
		DP	26	—	89	21	50
Jimenez	2000	PPW	39	1.4	60	10	63
		SW	33	—	70	12	77
Martin	1996	PPW	45	2.2	92	46	77
Beger	1999	DPPHR	504	0.8	91	21	—
Frey	1994	LRLPJ	50	0	87	11	11

DM = diabetes mellitus; DP = distal pancreatectomy; DPPHR = duodenum-preserving pancreatic head resection; LRLPJ = local pancreatic head resection with longitudinal pancreaticojejunostomy; PPW = pylorus-preserving Whipple; SW = standard Whipple.

pancreaticojejunostomy is extended over the body of the pancreas to incorporate the dilated duct in that area. Early results suggest that pain relief is excellent in 85 to 90% of patients, that the relief persists beyond several years, and that exocrine or endocrine insufficiency are not precipitated by the surgery. In those patients whose bile duct has also been obstructed by the fibrotic pancreas, this "coring" of pancreatic tissue from the head of the gland may decompress that duct as well. This operation is contraindicated if there is a concern about the presence of a malignant neoplasm in the head of the pancreas; a pancreaticoduodenectomy should be performed in these cases.

Uncommonly, chronic pancreatitis is localized predominantly in the body or tail of the pancreas. In these cases, a distal pancreatectomy (with or without splenectomy) may be effective. The surgeon should investigate the possibility that an occult malignancy may have produced a more proximal duct obstruction, and that a neoplastic duct stricture is the reason for such localized pancreatitis. Otherwise in patients with predominantly distal disease, distal pancreatectomy is safe and pain relief can be expected in as many as 90% of patients after 4 years. For the usual patient who has diffuse disease involving the entire pancreas, distal pancreatectomy is ineffective, however. Because it results in a brittle diabetes which is often difficult to control, and because lesser procedures are likely to be effective, total pancreatectomy for chronic pancreatitis is almost never done today.

Complications of Chronic Pancreatitis

Pseudocyst

A pancreatic pseudocyst is a collection of fluid usually in the vicinity of the pancreas, which develops in association with a leak of pancreatic juice from the inflamed parenchyma or from a disrupted duct. The wall of the pseudocyst is comprised of fibrous nonepithelialized tissue. Occasionally a pseudocyst may present at great distance from the pancreas (eg, thorax, groin), when the fluid dissects through tissue planes. The majority of acute pseudocysts that appear during an episode of acute pancreatic inflammation resolve without intervention. However, most pseudocysts that develop on a background of chronic pancreatitis are unlikely to resolve spontaneously, and they may need treatment. Asymptomatic pseudocysts up to 5 to 6 cm in diameter may be safely observed, and are usually followed with either serial ultrasound or CT examinations. Larger cysts or pseudocysts of any size that are symptomatic require intervention. Symptoms are most often from gastrointestinal (GI) obstruction when the cyst distorts or compresses the stomach, duodenum, or bile duct, or produces abdominal pain. Serious complications also can occur, although they are uncommon (< 5% of cases). These include hemorrhage into the cyst, perforation of the cyst, or cyst infection. Hemorrhage is usually caused by erosion of the splenic or gastroduodenal artery or other major vessel within the wall of the cyst, and the bleeding is often confined to the cyst lumen. The diagnosis should be suspected if there are clinical signs of hypovolemia and a falling hematocrit. There may be abdominal pain, and a mass may be palpable. An abdominal CT scan shows the cyst with the contained blood clot. Angiography confirms the diagnosis, and the radiologist should attempt to embolize the bleeding vessel. If not, emergency surgery with ligation of the vessel or excision of the cyst is required. Perforation of a pseudocyst is a surgical emergency that is characterized by the sudden onset of intense abdominal pain with peritonitis. Patients require urgent surgery with irrigation of the peritoneal cavity and usually external cyst drainage. Infection of a pseudocyst should be suspected if signs of sepsis develop. Diagnosis by CT scan and treatment by percutaneous cyst aspiration and drainage are usually effective.

In the absence of a life threatening complication, elective surgery of pseudocysts is usually delayed until the cyst has developed a mature wall that will hold sutures at the time of repair. For those cysts that develop following an episode of acute pancreatitis, this requires 4 to 6 weeks. In most cases the patient can eat and be discharged from the hospital during the interval. Pseudocysts that resolve spontaneously usually will do so during this time. If no episode of clinically significant acute pancreatitis preceded the development of the cyst, as is often the case in patients with chronic pancreatitis, usually no waiting period is necessary.

Pseudocysts may be treated *surgically*, or by *endoscopic or radiologic drainage*. Endoscopic methods require the placement of a plastic stent through the stomach or duodenal wall into the adjacent cyst. The stent is eventually removed, and in about 80% of cases, the cyst is permanently eradicated. These endoscopic techniques require expertise, which still is not widely available. They are discussed in the next chapter (see Chapter 138, "Pancreatitis: Endoscopic Therapy"). Radiologic approaches usually consist of percutaneous external drainage of the cyst with eventual removal of the drainage catheter many weeks later. Many of these pseudocysts recur. Surgical treatment usually consists of drainage of the cyst internally to either the stomach (cystgastrostomy) or to a Roux-en-Y limb of jejunum (cystjejunostomy). Both are safe and effective, with recurrence rates < 10%. If the pseudocyst is in the tail of the pancreas, a distal pancreatectomy with excision of the cyst may be best.

Pancreatic Fistula

In the setting of chronic pancreatitis, a pancreatic fistula is usually the result of a ductal disruption from an episode of acute pancreatitis. The diagnosis is made by finding a high amylase level (usually many thousands of U/L) in the fistula effluent. Some fistulas will close spontaneously, provided that ductal continuity can be re-established as healing occurs, infection is eradicated, and nutrition is adequate. However, the frequent presence of duct obstruction in chronic pancreatitis may make it less likely that the fistula will close. Parenteral nutrition is usually not required and most patients are able to eat a regular diet. There is no evidence that oral intake delays resolution of fistula. The use of somatostatin does not appear to hasten fistula closure, although if it is a high output fistula (ie, > 200 mL/d), the secretory inhibitor may simplify management of the patient. Fistulas that persist for as long as 1 year, or those whose anatomic characteristics preclude spontaneous closure (eg, duct obstruction between fistula and duodenal lumen, duct discontinuity), will require operative repair. This is best done by creating an anastamosis between the pancreatic duct at the point of the leak and a Roux-en-Y limb of jejunum. The success rate of operative repair is > 90%.

Biliary Stricture or Obstruction

Jaundice may occur in up to one-third of patients with chronic calcific pancreatitis at some point during the disease, usually when there is pancreatic swelling at the time of an episode of acute pancreatitis. This often resolves as the acute inflammation subsides, but as many as 10% of patients are left with obstruction of the common duct. This is due to fibrosis of the head of the pancreas resulting in constriction of the duct as it passes through this portion of the gland. The stricture usually appears as a long, symmetrical narrowing when it is visualized by magnetic resonance cholangiopancreatography or endoscopic retrograde cholangiography. The proximal duct and gallbladder may be distended, but obstruction of the duct is almost never complete, which differentiates it from a malignant obstruction. A simple biliary bypass using a Roux-en-Y choledochojejunostomy effectively treats such a biliary stricture. Endoscopic procedures are discussed in the next chapter.

Intestinal Compression or Obstruction

A minority of patients will present with obstruction of the second or third portion of the duodenum. Upper endoscopy and CT scan should be performed to rule out the presence of a neoplastic process. Then a loop gastrojejunostomy can be done to bypass the obstruction.

Obstruction of the colon (usually the transverse or splenic flexure) can also occur from chronic pancreatitis. If this is due to an episode of acute inflammation, the obstruction will likely resolve. If it persists, then a colonoscopy should be performed to rule out malignancy. Persistence of the obstruction requires a resection of the involved segment of colon and an end-to-end anastomosis.

Pancreatic Malignancy

Patients with long standing chronic pancreatitis are at a 10% lifetime risk for the development of pancreatic adenocarcinoma. During examination for surgery in a patient with chronic pancreatitis, imaging studies may show focal changes in the pancreas that suggest malignancy, or other aspects of the clinical presentation (eg, rising or markedly elevated CA19-9, change in character of pain, accelerated weight loss) may have raised the clinician's index of suspicion about the possibility that cancer is present.

If there is concern about malignancy, we recommend EUS examination, which is currently the most sensitive diagnostic study to identify small cancers, and also can be used to obtain tissue from the lesion that could confirm the diagnosis. EUS and FNA are discussed in Chapter 5 ("Endoscopic Ultrasonography and Fine-Needle Aspiration").

However, whether or not the diagnosis is confirmed preoperatively, patients in whom the surgeon suspects the coexistence of pancreatic cancer with underlying chronic pancreatitis require pancreatic resection. This means a pancreaticoduodenectomy for head and uncinate lesions and a distal pancreatectomy for body and tail lesions. Even if cancer is not found when the resected specimen is examined by the pathologist, this approach represents the current standard of care in such circumstances. This is because resection operations are safe, they are one of the standard operations normally done for chronic pancreatitis without coexisting cancer, and pancreatic cancer is uniformly fatal when it is not surgically resected.

Conclusion

The surgical considerations for patients with chronic pancreatitis include procedures to address chronic pain, various complications of the disease, and pancreatic cancer. The decision to operate in any single patient with pain from the disease is complex, and should be based on a variety of factors that include the psychosocial makeup of the patient as well as pancreatic anatomy. If surgery is indicated, the type of operation hinges on the appearance of the pancreatic ducts (Figure 137-1). In patients with a dilated duct, a drainage procedure is often the best option because this offers good pain relief and the least long term morbidity. If the ducts are not enlarged, failed prior ductal drainage, or there is concern about the presence of cancer, then resection should be performed. Newer operations that resect most of the head of the pancreas but still preserve GI continuity (Beger et al, 1999; Frey and Amikura, 1994) may provide the best long term pain relief with the least long term morbidity. Patients with chronic pancreatitis can develop pseudocysts, pancreatic fistulas, and biliary or intestinal obstruction. The pancreatic surgeon must be prepared to deal with all of these issues.

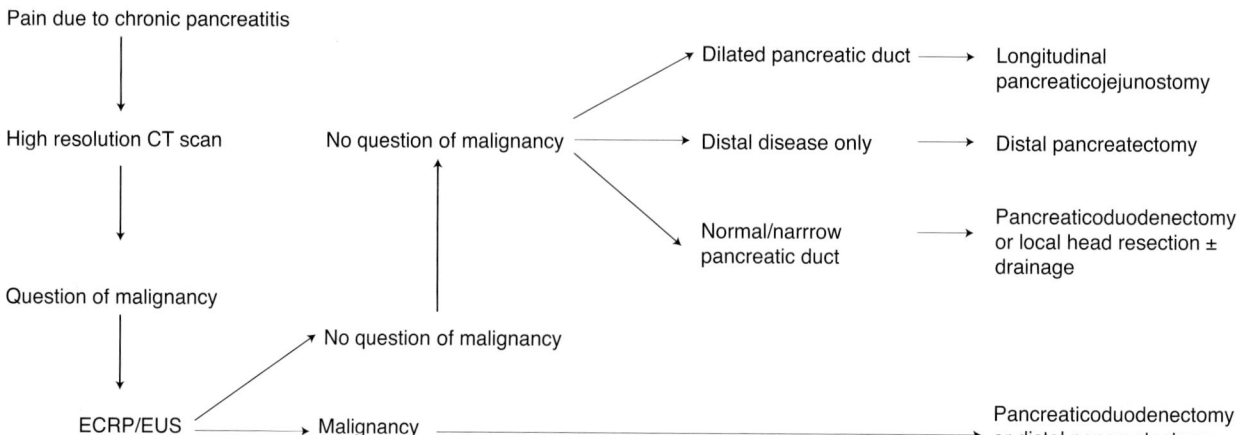

FIGURE 137-1. Surgery for chronic pancreatitis algorithm. CT = computed tomography; ERCP = endoscopic retrograde cholangiopancreatography; EUS = endoscopic ultrasound.

Supplemental Reading

Beger HG, Schlosser W, Friess HM, Buchler MW. Duodenum-preserving head resection in chronic pancreatitis changes the natural course of the disease: a single-center 26-year experience. Ann Surg 1999;230:512–23.

Bradley EL. Long-term results of pancreatojejunostomy in patients with chronic pancreatitis. Am J Surg 1987;153:207–13.

Frey CF, Amikura K. Local resection of the head of the pancreas combined with longitudinal pancreaticojejunostomy in the management of patients with chronic pancreatitis. Ann Surg 1994;220:492–507.

Heise JW, Katoh M, Luthen R, Roher H-D. Long-term results following different extent of resection in chronic pancreatitis. Hepatogastroenterology 2001;48:864–8.

Jimenez RE, Fernandez-del Castillo C, Rattner DW, et al. Outcome of pancreaticoduodenectomy with pylorus preservation or with antrectomy in the treatment of chronic pancreatitis. Ann Surg 2001;231:293–300.

Leger L, Lenriot JP, Lemaigre G. Five to twenty year follow up after surgery for chronic pancreatitis in 148 patients. Ann Surg 1974;180:185–91.

Martin RF, Rossi RL, Leslie KA. Long-term results of pylorus-preserving pancreatoduodenectomy for chronic pancreatitis. Arch Surg 1996;131:247–52.

Nealon WH, Townsend CM Jr, Thompson JC. Operative drainage of the pancreatic duct delays functional impairment in patients with chronic pancreatitis: a prospective analysis. Ann Surg 1998;208:321–9.

Prinz RA, Greenlee HB. Pancreatic duct drainage in 100 patients with chronic pancreatitis. Ann Surg 1981;194:313–20.

Prinz RA, Kaufman BH, Folk FA, Greenlee HB Pancreaticojejunostomy for chronic pancreatitis: two- to 21-year follow-up. Arch Surg 1978;113:520–5.

Sarles J-C, Nacchiero M, Garani F, Salasc B. Surgical treatment of chronic pancreatitis: report of 134 cases treated by resection or drainage. Am J Surg 1982;144:317–21.

Warshaw AL. Conservation of pancreatic tissue by combined gastric, biliary, and pancreatic duct drainage for pain from chronic pancreatitis. Am J Surg 1985;149:563–9.

Chapter 138

Pancreatitis: Endoscopic Therapy

Lee McHenry Jr, MD, and Glen A. Lehman, MD

Since the inception of diagnostic endoscopic retrograde cholangiopancreatography (ERCP) in 1968 the therapeutic approaches to a variety of biliary, ampullary and pancreatic disorders has burgeoned. Endoscopic therapy for pancreatic diseases has been used over the past several decades, particularly in treating patients with acute and chronic pancreatitis. As well, the complications of acute and chronic pancreatitis, such as pancreatic pseudocysts and pancreatic leaks, may be approached via ERCP. Similar techniques to endoscopic treatment of biliary tract diseases, including sphincterotomy, stricture dilatation, basket and balloon extraction of stones, and stent placement, have been extended to treat patients with pancreatic disorders.

Acute Pancreatitis

The endoscopic approach to a patient with acute pancreatitis most commonly is in the setting of acute gallstone-induced pancreatitis. Acute pancreatitis related to bile duct stones is suspected in patients with gallstones, elevated liver function tests, particularly those with alanine aminotransferase levels greater than three times the upper limit of normal, and a dilatated common bile duct (CBD) by ultrasonography or computed tomography (CT) scan. Biliary sphincterotomy of the major papilla affords removal of stones in the bile duct, if present, and also affords a patent biliary sphincter to allow for future stone passage in the setting of gallbladder stones or microlithiasis. The challenge to endoscopists is to determine which patients with suspected acute gallstone pancreatitis would benefit from ERCP and biliary sphincterotomy. Four prospective studies have addressed early ERCP within 72 hours of admission in patients with gallstone pancreatitis (Fogel and Sherman, 2003). ERCP, if performed early in patients with suspected gallstone pancreatitis, showed the presence of CBD stones in 63% of patients with severe pancreatitis as compared to 25% of patients with mild gallstone pancreatitis (Neoptolemos et al, 1988). Endoscopic therapy with early ERCP and biliary sphincterotomy in patients with severe gallstone pancreatitis reduced morbidity in all four studies and reduced mortality in three of the four studies published to date. The timing of ERCP in patients with acute gallstone pancreatitis does not appear to influence the rate or severity of post-ERCP pancreatitis. We adhere to the practice of early ERCP (preferably within 24 hours) for patients with severe gallstone pancreatitis. A biliary sphincterotomy is performed if bile duct stones are visualized at ERCP. For patients with mild acute gallstone pancreatitis with gallbladder in situ, ERCP may not be necessary as intraoperative cholangiography can be obtained by surgeons at most centers at the time of cholecystectomy. If bile duct stones are present at the time of cholecystectomy, postoperative ERCP can be subsequently performed with a high level of success.

When acute pancreatitis occurs and is not related to gallstones or alcohol, a search ensues to attempt to define the incriminating cause of the pancreatitis. "Idiopathic" acute pancreatitis may have a myriad of causes, including medication related (ie, azathioprine), metabolic (ie, hypertriglyceridemia), infectious (ie, cytomegalovirus), or collagen vascular disease. The role of endoscopy focuses on determining whether an obstructive etiology for the pancreatitis is present, as outlined in Table 138-1. ERCP with biliary sphincterotomy, major or minor papilla sphincterotomy, pancreatic stricture dilatation and/or pancreatic stent placement has been shown to benefit patients with recurrent bouts of unexplained pancreatitis (Tarnasky and Hawes, 1998). At the time of ERCP, our approach to patients with idiopathic pancreatitis is to proceed with pancreatography and cholangiography with manometry of both biliary and pancreatic sphincters. If pancreatic sphincter dysfunction, pancreatic ductal stricture, pancreatic duct stones or pancreatic duct disruption are visualized on the

TABLE 138-1. Obstructive Etiologies of Idiopathic Pancreatitis

Biliary microlithiasis
    Pancreas divisum
        Sphincter of Oddi dysfunction
            Neoplasms
    Pancreatic ductal stricture and/or stones
    Pseudocyst or duct disruption
    Duodenal diverticulum
    Choledochal cyst
    Annular pancreas

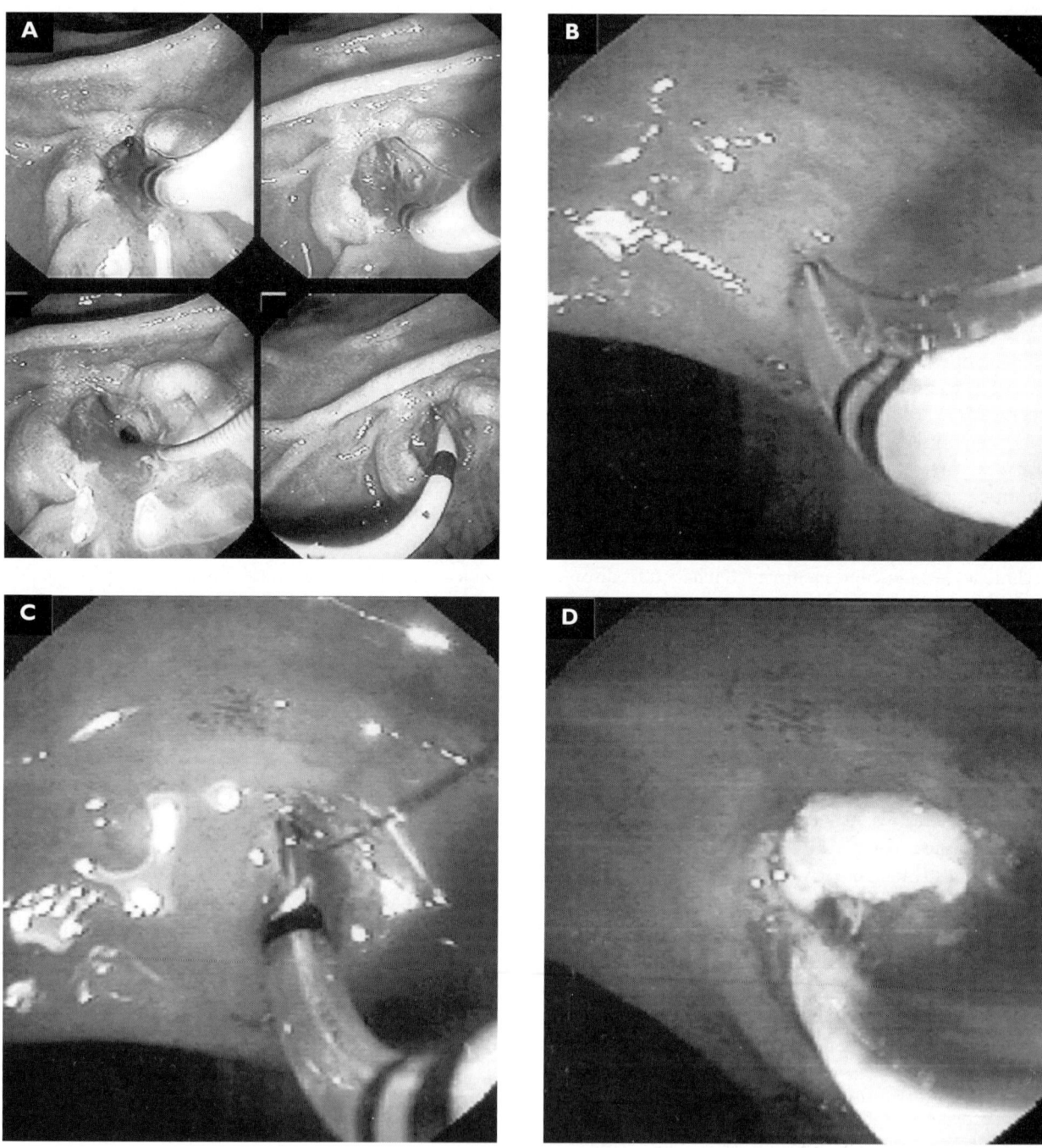

FIGURE 138-1. (A) Technique of pancreatic sphincterotomy using a pull type sphincterotome. (*Left top*) Biliary sphincterotomy is performed using a standard pull type sphincterotome. (*Right top*) Pancreatic spincterotomy performed with a pull type sphincterotome cutting in the 1 o'clock direction. (*Left bottom*) Completed biliary and pancreatic sphincterotomy. A guidewire is in the pancreatic duct. (*Right bottom*) A 6 F pancreatic stent is placed following performance of the pancreatic sphincterotomy. (B) Traction sphincterotome positioned in minor papilla. Note the extent of the minor papilla mound (*arrows*). Duodenal juice at the minor papilla orifice is aspirated away before cutting to prevent heat dissipation to juice and boiling the adjacent tissues during the sphincterotomy. (C) Wire is bowed taught and cut is performed rapidly with minimal coagulation utilizing the ERBE generator. The optimal cut length in this setting is unknown. The 5 mm length minor papilla sphincterotomy is complete without white tissue coagulum. (D) White pancreatic stone removed through patent sphincterotomy orifice with balloon catheter.

ventral pancreatogram, a major papilla pancreatic sphincterotomy is usually performed to facilitate access to the duct prior to attempts at stricture dilation and stent placement. There are two methods to cut the major pancreatic sphincter. A standard pull-type sphincterotome (with or without a guide wire) is inserted into the pancreatic duct and oriented along the axis of the pancreatic duct (usually in the 12 to 1 o'clock position). Although the landmarks to determine the length of incision are imprecise, authorities recommend a cutting length of 5 to 10 mm. The cutting wire of the sphincterotome should not extend more than 6 to 7 mm up the duct when applying electrocautery, so as to prevent deep ductal injury. Alternatively, a needle-knife can be used to perform the sphincterotomy over a previously placed pancreatic stent. Performing a biliary sphincterotomy first can expose the pancreaticobiliary septum and allow the length of the cut to be gauged more accurately.

Cannulation of the ventral pancreatic duct may be unsuccessful in patients with recurrent, idiopathic pancreatitis and should heighten the suspicion that pancreas divisum may be present. If the pancreatogram from the major papilla is successful, a fine branching of the ventral duct typical of pancreas divisum must be ascertained. In patients over the age of 40 years with pancreatic duct cut-off in the head of the pancreas, the endoscopist must be wary of underlying pancreatic malignancy causing an abrupt cut-off of the ventral pancreatic duct masquerading as pancreas divisum. If the ventral pancreatogram is typical of pancreas divisum, the minor papilla is sought.

Approaches to the minor papilla for cannulation begin with an endoscopic still photo of the minor papilla orifice to refer to during attempted minor papilla cannulation (Lehman and Sherman, 1995). The use of intravenous secretin (Secreflo, Repligen Inc.) 16 μg to induce pancreatic ductal secretion may aid in identifying the minor papilla orifice and successful cannulation. We have reported our experience with spraying the minor papilla with methylene blue prior to secretin administration to more accurately locate the minor papilla and improve success of minor papilla cannulation (Park et al, 2003). For cannulation, we commonly use the highly tapered 3-4-5 F catheter loaded with the 0.018 inch roadrunner guide wire (Wilson-Cook, Winston-Salem, NC). Once the dorsal duct is accessed and the anatomy is defined, minor papilla therapy is considered. We reserve minor papilla therapy for patients who have experienced at least two bouts of documented pancreatitis or for patients with chronic pancreatitis with strictures, duct disruptions or stones in the dorsal duct. In patients with pancreas divisum, a minor papilla sphincterotomy is usually necessary. The minor papilla sphincterotomy may be performed with a needle-knife sphincterotome over a 3 or 4 F pancreatic stent or with a standard pull-type sphincterotome. The technique is similar to that of major papilla pancreatic sphincterotomy, except that the direction of the incision is usually in the 10 to 12 o'clock position and the length of the sphincterotomy is limited to 4 to 8 mm.

Chronic Pancreatitis

Endoscopic therapy is now being applied in the setting of chronic pancreatitis for patients presenting with pain and/or clinical episodes of acute pancreatitis. One of the aims of endoscopic therapy is to alleviate the obstruction to exocrine juice flow. Outflow obstruction may be caused by ductal strictures (biliary or pancreatic), pancreatic stones, pseudocysts, and minor or major papilla stenosis. Although the endoscopic approach has never been directly compared with surgery, endoscopic drainage is appealing in that it may offer an alternative to surgical drainage procedures, with generally less morbidity and mortality. Furthermore, endoscopic procedures do not preclude subsequent surgery, should it be necessary. Moreover, the outcome from reducing the intraductal pressure by endoscopic methods may be a predictor for the success of surgical drainage.

Benign strictures of the main pancreatic duct may be a consequence of generalized or focal inflammation or necrosis around the main pancreatic duct. Given the putative role of ductal hypertension in the genesis of symptoms (at least in a subpopulation of patients), the utility of pancreatic duct stents for treatment of dominant pancreatic duct strictures is being evaluated. Underlying malignancy must be considered and excluded by tissue sampling at ERCP or by endoscopic ultrasonography with fine-needle aspiration of the strictured segment. Most pancreatic stents are simply standard polyethylene biliary stents with extra side holes at approximately 1 cm intervals to permit better side branch juice flow. Stents made of other materials have received limited evaluation. The technique for placing a stent in the pancreatic duct is similar to that used for inserting a biliary stent. In most patients, a pancreatic sphincterotomy (with or without a biliary sphincterotomy) via the major or minor papilla is performed to facilitate placement of accessories and stents. A guide wire must be maneuvered upstream to the narrowing. Hydrophilic flexible tip wires are especially helpful for bypassing strictures. Torqueable wires are occasionally necessary to achieve this goal. High-grade strictures require dilatation prior to insertion of the endoprosthesis. This may be performed with hydrostatic balloon dilating catheters or graduated dilating catheters. Extremely tight strictures may permit passage of only a small caliber guide wire. Such wires may be left in situ overnight and usually permit dilator passage the next day. Alternatively, 3 F angioplasty balloons or the Soehendra stent retriever may be helpful to effectively dilate the stricture. Although one preliminary report suggested that luminal patency of the duct persisted at a mean time

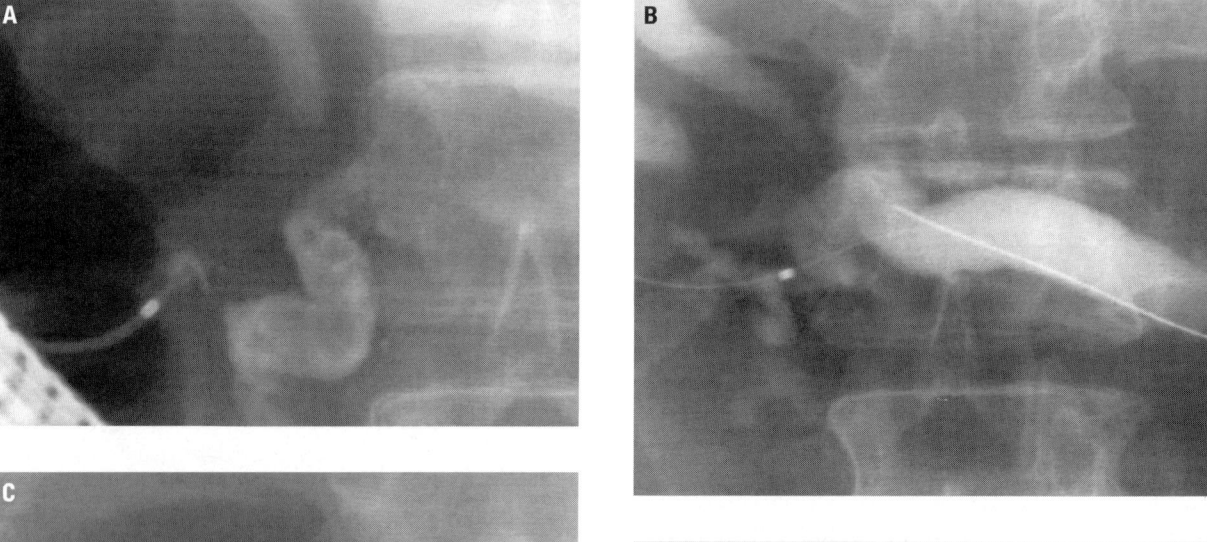
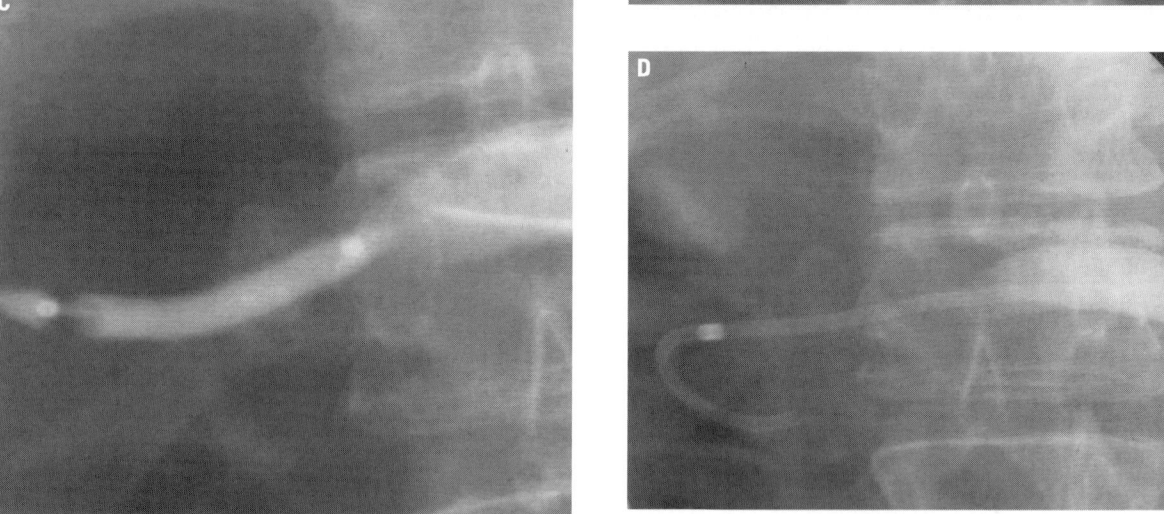

FIGURE 138-2. A 57-year-old male with history of alcohol-induced chronic pancreatitis with recurrent monthly attacks of pain requiring multiple hospitalizations. Pancreatogram via major papilla reveals tight stricture of downstream pancreatic duct with multiple filling defects in the dilated upstream pancreatic duct (A). A hydrophilic 0.025 inch guide wire is used for engagement of the stricture and access to the dilated duct (B). A 4 mm diameter hydrostatic balloon catheter is used for stricture dilatation after a 5-7-10 F dilation catheter was not successfully passed through the stricture (C). One 7 F by 8 cm long with a three-quarter external pigtail and single internal flap was placed into the pancreatic duct. This stent was removed 1 month later and the patient has been without pain 1 year later (D).

of 5 months following balloon dilation alone, most authorities have observed recurrence of strictures after onetime dilation and therefore advocate stenting. As a rule, the diameter of the stent should not exceed the size of the downstream duct. Therefore, 5, 7, or 8.5 F stents are commonly used in smaller ducts, whereas 10 to 11.5 F stents or dual side-by-side 5 to 7 F stents may be inserted in patients with severe chronic pancreatitis and a dilatated main pancreatic duct. The tip of the stent in the pancreas must extend upstream to the narrowed segment and into a straight portion of the pancreatic duct to avoid stent tip erosion through the duct wall. For diagnostic trials of pancreatic stenting in patients with nearly daily pain, most stents are left in place for 3 to 4 weeks.

The appropriate duration of pancreatic stent placement and the interval from the placement to change of the pancreatic stent is not known. The following two options are available: (1) the stent can be left in place until symptoms or complications occur and (2) the stent can be left in place for a predetermined interval (eg, 3 months). If the patient fails to improve, the stent should be removed, because ductal hypertension is unlikely to be the cause of pain. If the patient has benefited from stenting, one can remove the stent and observe the patient clinically, continue stenting for a more prolonged period, or perform a surgical drainage procedure.

The majority of patients with a stricture have associated calcified pancreatic duct stones. For optimal results, the

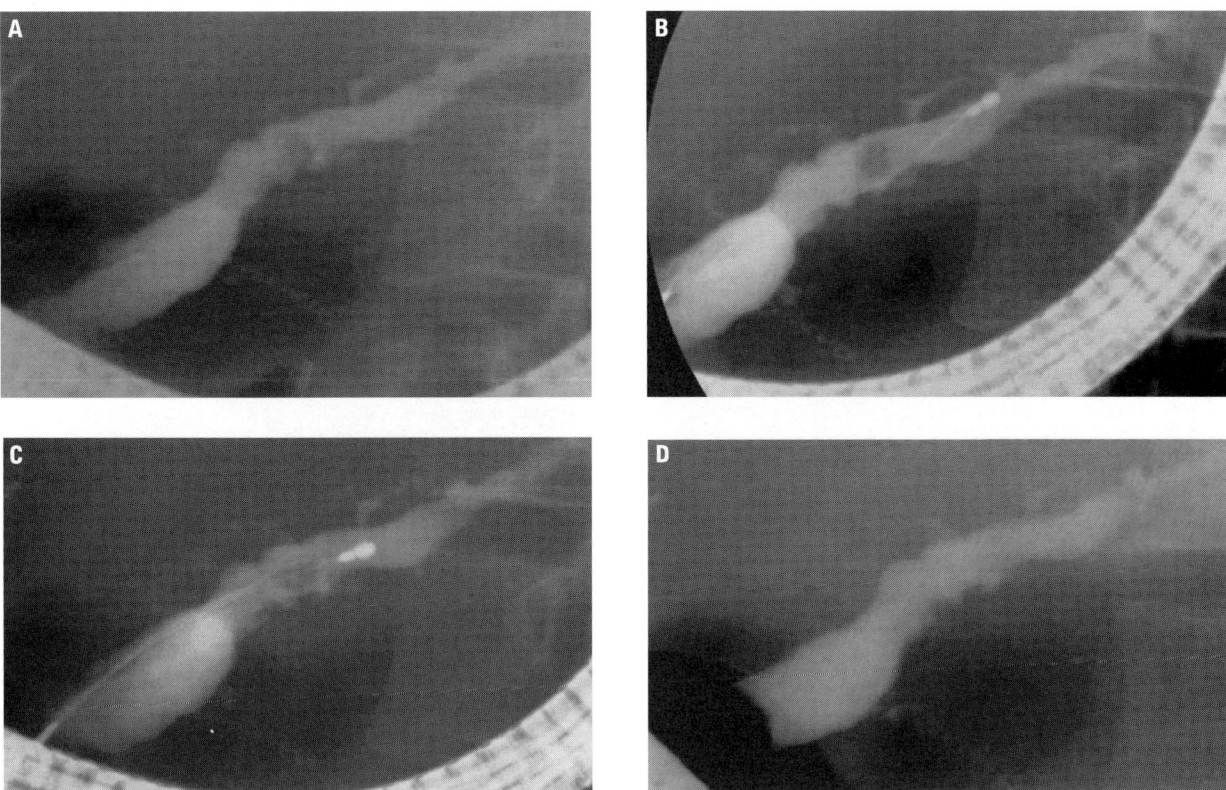

FIGURE 138-3. A 40-year-old female with alcohol-induced chronic pancreatitis complicated by pancreatic main duct stones. Pancreatogram revealing dilatated pancreatic duct with 5 mm diameter filling defect consistent with a pancreatic stone (A). After pancreatic sphincterotomy, a non-wire guided stone extraction basket was used. The basket is opened fully in the dilatated pancreatic duct and the stone is engaged (B). Basket is slowly closed on the stone (C). Stone is extracted and follow-up pancreatogram with a balloon catheter reveals no residual filling defects. No further stenting was performed (D).

therapy must address both the stones and stricture. In the largest multicenter trial, Rosch and colleagues (2002) reported on the long-term follow up of over 1000 patients with chronic pancreatitis undergoing initial endoscopic therapy during the period 1989 to 1995. One thousand two hundred and eleven patients from eight centers in Europe with pain and obstructive chronic pancreatitis underwent endoscopic therapy, including endoscopic pancreatic sphincterotomy, pancreatic stricture dilation, pancreatic stone fragmentation by extracorporeal shock wave lithotripsy and pancreatic stone removal, pancreatic stent placement, or a combination of these methods. One thousand eighteen patients (84%) were observed for symptomatic improvement and need for pancreatic surgery over a mean of 4.9 years (range 2 to 12 years). Success of endoscopic therapy was defined as a significant reduction or elimination of pain and reduction in pain medication. Partial success was defined as reduction in pain, though further interventions were necessary for pain relief. Failure of endoscopic therapy was defined as the need for pancreatic decompressive surgery or patients that were lost to follow-up. Over long-term follow-up, 69% of patients were successfully treated with endoscopic therapy and 15% experienced a partial success. Twenty percent of patients required surgery, with a 55% significant reduction in pain. Five percent of patients were lost to follow-up. The group of patients that had the highest frequency of completed treatment were patients with stones alone (76%) as compared to patients with strictures alone (57%) and patients with strictures and stones (57%) ($p < .001$). Interestingly, the percentage of patients with no or minimal residual pain at follow-up was similar in all groups (strictures alone 84%, stones alone 84%, and strictures plus stones 87%) ($p = .677$). The authors of this report concluded that endoscopic therapy for chronic pancreatitis in experienced centers is effective in the majority of patients and the beneficial response to successful endoscopic therapy in chronic pancreatitis is durable and long term.

Endoscopic methods alone will likely fail in the presence of large or impacted stones and stones proximal to a stricture. Extracorporeal shock wave lithotripsy can be used to fragment stones and facilitate their removal. Thus, this procedure is complementary to endoscopic techniques and improves the success of nonsurgical ductal decompression.

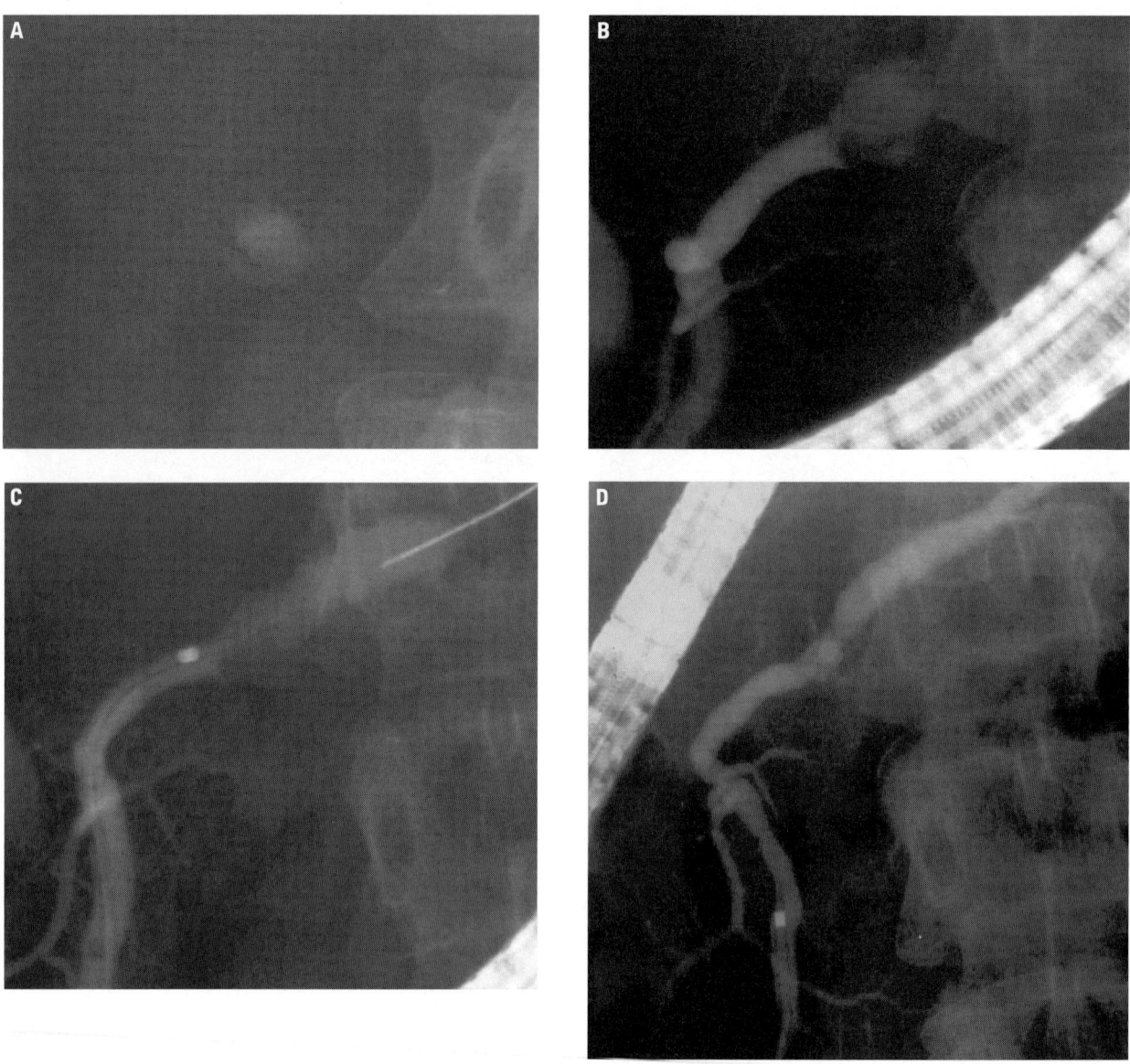

FIGURE 138-4. A 41-year-old woman with a history of abdominal pain, pancreatitis and pancreatic calcification on computed tomography scan. Abdominal radiograph reveals solitary radio-opaque stone in head/body region (A). Pancreatogram reveals an 8 mm obstructing stone in body of pancreas pancreatic duct (B). A 0.018 inch diameter guide wire was advanced beyond the stone. Further contrast filling of duct demonstrating upstream dilatation. Stone extraction with basket was unsuccessful (C). Extracorporeal shock wave lithotripsy performed with excellent fragmentation of stone. Pancreatogram 1 week post-ESWL. Mild duct irregularity in body of pancreas duct with minimal upstream dilatation. All stone fragments were removed and no pancreatic stent was placed. (Patient reported a history of abdominal injury in an auto accident over 10 years before the onset of symptoms) (D).

In a recent retrospective review of the efficacy of ESWL as an adjunct to endoscopic therapy, Kozarek and colleagues (2002) examined 40 patients who underwent a total of 46 ESWL sessions (average 1.15 sessions per patient). Eighty percent (80%) of patients did not require surgery and had significant pain relief, reduced number of hospitalizations, and reduced narcotic use as compared to the pre-ESWL period over a mean 2.4 years follow-up.

Only randomized controlled studies comparing surgical, medical, and endoscopic techniques will allow us to determine the true long-term efficacy of pancreatic duct stenting for stricture therapy. There remain many unanswered questions: Which patients are the best candidates? Is proximal pancreatic ductal dilatation a prerequisite? Does the response to stenting depend on the etiology of the chronic pancreatitis? Finally, as noted, how does endoscopic therapy compare with medical and surgical management?

Pancreatic Pseudocysts

Pancreatic pseudocysts as complications of acute and chronic pancreatitis are being tackled more frequently by experienced endoscopists (Lehman, 1999). A word of caution if you as the endoscopist consider wading into pseudocyst territory: Obtain and review a pre-ERCP high quality pancreas CT scan, become very familiar with transpapillary and transluminal drainage techniques, have experienced interventional radiology and surgical back-up, and have an understanding of potential complications. A high quality CT scan of the pancreas and surrounding structures will define the proximity of the pseudocyst to the luminal wall (< 10 mm thickness between lumen and pseudocyst is optimal), contents of pseudocyst, the presence of splenic artery aneurysm, splenic thrombosis and/or gastric varices, and the extent of pancreatic necrosis. At the initial ERCP, a pancreatogram is attempted to evaluate whether duct communication is present. Transpapillary drainage of pseudocysts may be performed by placing the stent either into the duct upstream from the communication ("bridging the disruption") or placing the stent into the pseudocyst cavity itself. Pancreatic sphincterotomy is commonly performed to ablate the sphincter pressure gradient, and downstream pancreatic strictures, if present, are dilated with balloon or passage catheter dilators. In a large series of endoscopic therapy for acute and chronic pancreatic pseudocysts by Baron and colleagues (2002), 63% of 136 patients had communication of the collection, with the main pancreatic duct affording the potential for transpapillary therapy.

Transluminal drainage via transduodenal or transgastric approach may be the preferred technique in patients with pancreatic duct cut-off, noncommunicating pseudocysts, large tail of pancreas pseudocysts. Endoscopy with the therapeutic duodenoscope is performed to assess for a bulge on the gastric wall or duodenal wall. Once localized, sampling or injection of the pseudocyst with the Howell aspiration needle (Wilson-Cook Inc, Winston-Salem, NC) may be performed prior to needle-knife puncture into the pseudocyst. The needle-knife puncture is performed perpendicular to the lumen with short bursts of cautery and a forceful entry into the pseudocyst cavity. This perpendicular approach will minimize tracking into the gut wall and reduce bleeding. A guide wire is placed into the pseudocyst and coiled in the cavity to maintain access. Balloon catheter dilation of the fistulous tract is performed and single or multiple double-pigtail stents are placed. Technical success with proper patient selection approaches 90% in most series. In Baron's series, complete endoscopic resolution was achieved in 113 of 138 patients. Patients with chronic pseudocysts obtained the best result (59 of 64 resolved, 92%) as compared to patients with acute pseudocysts (23 of 31, 74%) or necrosis (31 of 43, 72%). Complications of transluminal endoscopic drainage of pseudocysts, including bleeding, infection, and perforation, total 20% in combined series. Death has been reported in 1% of over 500 patients undergoing endoscopic drainage of pseudocysts, similar to the reported mortality of surgically treated patients.

Conclusion

Endoscopic therapy for acute pancreatitis, chronic pancreatitis and pancreatic pseudocysts has continued to evolve with improved innovative techniques and better patient selection. Results of endoscopic therapy for pancreatic diseases, in experienced hands, rivals the results obtained with surgery. Early ERCP in the setting of severe acute gallstone pancreatitis is routinely performed in academic and community practices with success. Endoscopic therapy for chronic pancreatitis with stricture dilatation, pancreatic stone extraction, and pancreatic sphincterotomy afford short- to medium-term relief in the majority of patients. Endoscopic pseudocyst drainage is the most technically demanding procedure in managing patients with pancreatic disease, but with proper patient selection, good results may be achieved by experienced endoscopists in the majority of patients

Supplemental Reading

Baron TH, Harewood GC, Morgan DE, et al. Outcome differences after endoscopic drainage of pancreatic necrosis, acute pancreatic pseudocysts, and chronic pancreatic pseudocysts. Gastrointest Endosc 2002;56:7–17.

Fogel EL, Sherman S. Acute biliary pancreatitis: When should the endoscopist intervene? Gastroenterology 2003;125:229–35.

Kozarek RA, Brandabur JJ, Ball TJ, et al. Clinical outcomes in patients who undergo extracorporeal shock wave lithotripsy for chronic calcific pancreatitis. Gastrointest Endosc 2002;56:496–500.

Lehman GA. Pseudocysts. Gastrointest Endosc 1999;49(Part 2):S81–4.

Lehman GA, Sherman S. Pancreas divisum: diagnosis, clinical significance, and management alternatives. Gastrointest Endosc Clinics N America 1995;5:145–70.

Neoptolemos JP, Carr-Locke DL, London NJ, et al. Controlled trial of urgent endoscopic retrograde cholangiopancreatography and endoscopic sphincterotomy versus conservative treatment for acute pancreatitis due to gallstones. Lancet 1988;2:979–83.

Park S-H, de Bellis M, McHenry L, et al. Use of methylene blue to identify the minor papilla or its orifice in patients with pancreas divisum. Gastrointest Endosc 2003;57:358–63.

Rosch T, Daniel S, Scholz M, et al. Endoscopic treatment of chronic pancreatitis: a multicenter study of 1000 patients with long-term follow-up. Endoscopy 2002;34:765–71.

Tarnasky PR, Hawes RH. Endoscopic diagnosis and therapy of unexplained (idiopathic) acute pancreatitis. Gastrointest Endosc Clinics N America 1998;8:13–34.

CHAPTER 139

CHRONIC PANCREATITIS

PETER DRAGANOV, MD, AND PHILLIP P. TOSKES, MD

Overview

Patients with chronic pancreatitis come to medical attention because of abdominal pain and/or maldigestion. The management of patients with maldigestion (steatorrhea) is relatively easy with the use of potent pancreatic enzymes. The management of abdominal pain continues to be a frustration for both the patient and the physician managing that patient. The pathogenesis of the pain associated with chronic pancreatitis is ill understood. Clinicians must appreciate that chronic pancreatitis is not one disease, but that there are subsets of patients labeled with chronic pancreatitis who must be approached based on the pathophysiology present. It is helpful to divide patients with chronic pancreatitis into those with *big duct disease* and those with *small duct disease*. The diagnostic and therapeutic approaches to patients with chronic pancreatitis are greatly influenced by the degree of damage to the exocrine pancreas. The cornerstone of medical management for either abdominal pain or maldigestion is the employment of *pancreatic enzyme formulations*. If severe damage to the pancreas is present, *endoscopic or surgical decompression of the main pancreatic duct or suppression of pancreatic secretion* with agents such as octreotide may afford pain relief.

Presentation

Patients with chronic pancreatitis seek medical attention because of abdominal pain or symptoms of maldigestion (chronic diarrhea, steatorrhea, weight loss, and fatigue). The abdominal pain is quite variable in location, severity, and frequency. The pain of chronic pancreatitis often does not follow a classical pattern, such as that seen in acute pancreatitis where the pain is mid-epigastric and radiates to the back. Indeed, chronic pancreatitis pain may mimic other causes of abdominal pain and may be quite nonspecific in its clinical presentation. The pain can be constant or intermittent and there may be frequent pain-free intervals. Eating may exacerbate the pain, leading to fear of eating and weight loss. The spectrum of abdominal pain ranges from mild to severe and narcotic addiction is often a frequent complication of chronic pancreatitis pain.

In those patients with abdominal pain secondary to big duct disease, often as a result of alcohol abuse, the patient's exocrine function may deteriorate even if the patient stops drinking. That progression of exocrine dysfunction does not occur in patients with small duct disease and their problem continues to be pain and not steatorrhea. Approximately 20% of patients with chronic pancreatitis may present with endocrine or exocrine dysfunction in the absence of abdominal pain (Layer et al, 1995). Progression to end-stage pancreatitis is associated with significant morbidity, mortality, and utilization of societal resources.

Pathogenesis

Alcohol abuse continues to be the most common cause of chronic pancreatitis worldwide, accounting for 60 to 70% of all patients with chronic pancreatitis. In the 30 to 40% of subjects with chronic pancreatitis where the etiology is not due to alcohol, the most common setting is that of *idiopathic pancreatitis*, which may account for 20% of the cases. Table 139-1 lists the causes of chronic pancreatitis, and it is important to point out that *cystic fibrosis (CF)* is the most common cause in children. There is a separate chapter on cystic fibrosis (see Chapter 140, "Cystic Fibrosis and Other Hereditary Diseases of the Pancreas"). As more knowledge about the pathophysiology of chronic pancreatitis is gained, it is becoming appreciated that there are several subsets of patients with chronic pancreatitis. It is likely that with the recognition that a *cholecystokinin (CCK)-releasing factor* is important in the feedback control of pancreatic exocrine secretion, an appreciation is emerging that there may be

TABLE 139-1. Causes of Chronic Pancreatitis

Alcohol-induced (60%)
Idiopathic (20%)
Other (20%)
- Cystic fibrosis
- Genetic abnormalities
- Tropical
- Tumor
- Pancreatic resection
- Congenital abnormalities
- Trauma
- Hypertriglyceridemia
- Autoimmune

forms of pancreatitis that are related to abnormalities in CCK homeostasis (Chey, 1997). This *CCK-releasing factor* has been isolated and sequenced, and it may be available as a diagnostic test in the very near future. One issue that must be faced is that clinicians have attempted to treat all patients with chronic pancreatitis in a similar fashion, which has generally not been successful. It is helpful to begin to look at chronic pancreatitis subsets by dividing the patients into those with *big duct disease* and those with *small duct disease*. The diagnostic approach, clinical course, and therapeutic management are quite different in patients with these two kinds of chronic pancreatitis. These differences will be stressed throughout the discussion.

A great deal of attention has been paid recently to the finding of whether or not genetic defects can account for the majority of patients with idiopathic chronic pancreatitis. Despite enthusiastic expectations, it is becoming quite clear that most cases of idiopathic chronic pancreatitis represent a complex interaction of genetic and environmental factors rather than resulting from a single gene mutation. Indeed at the present time, it appears that most experts would agree that *genetic abnormalities* may account for approximately *15%* of those patients in the idiopathic category. Optimistic clinicians among us had thought that this percentage would be much CF fibrosis conductance regulator (*CFTR*) gene account for the chronic pancreatitis noted in most patients with idiopathic chronic pancreatitis. Other genetic mutations that may be important in chronic pancreatitis include the secretory trypsin inhibitor gene (*SPINK1*) and polymorphisms in genes modulating inflammation such as interleukin (*IL*)-*1, IL-10,* and tumor necrosis factor (*TNF*). *CFTR* mutations are common in the general population. It is believed that the *pancreatitis risk* is increased *approximately 40-fold by having two CFTR mutations, 20-fold by having a SPINK1 mutation, and 900-fold by having both two CFTR mutations and a SPINK1 mutation* (Grendell, 2003).*

Diagnosis

The diagnosis of chronic pancreatitis is rather easy in patients with *big duct disease* and quite challenging in patients with *small duct disease*. Table 139-2 lists diagnostic tests that are carried out worldwide in the examination of patients with chronic pancreatitis. Tests of function usually precede tests of structure in regard to sensitivity. The most sensitive and most specific tests are at the top of each column with the least sensitive and specific at the bottom. In 2004, the most appropriate way of detecting whether or not chronic pancreatitis is present is a combination of a *secretin hormone stimulation test* and *endoscopic ultrasonography*

---

*Editor's Note: Interestingly, two mutations in NOD 2/CARD 16 gene increase the risk of Crohn's disease 20- to 40-fold.

(*EUS*). In big duct disease, just about any test chosen will be abnormal. In our experience, we have used a *serum trypsinogen* as a first line test in patients who appear to have severe pancreatic insufficiency (PI) and present with malabsorption/maldigestion. That test is now commercially available from general diagnostic laboratories. In our laboratory, the normal values are 29 to 58 ng/mL. Patients with chronic pancreatitis of a mild to moderate degree have values of 20 to 28 ng/mL; patients with values < 20 ng/mL have severe PI and this value usually correlates well with the presence of steatorrhea. A new test that has been introduced into the United States and is now US Food and Drug Administration (FDA)-approved is *fecal elastase*. This is a stool determination from an aliquot of stool, not a quantitative collection, and is measured by a radioimmunoassay of human fecal elastase. Normal values are > 200 µg/g of stool. A value < 200 µg/g but > 100 µg/g usually reflects mild to moderate chronic pancreatitis. A value < 100 µg/g is severe PI and correlates well with an abnormal fecal fat excretion or steatorrhea. These function tests reflect severe damage and often confirm the abnormalities found on computed tomography (CT) or magnetic resonance imaging (MRI). In patients with *small duct disease* who present largely just with pain and do not have maldigestion, those function tests just mentioned are often normal. Indeed in up to 40% of patients with small duct chronic pancreatitis, radiographic tests including CT, MRI, magnetic resonance cholangiography (MRCP) and endoscopic retrograde cholangiography (ERCP) may be normal. It is those patients with small duct disease that have radiographic negative findings that are the real challenge, particularly if the secretin hormone stimulation test is not available. Patients suspected of having small duct chronic pancreatitis should be referred to a center that is proficient in performing these tests. When compared against any radiographic test or function test as listed in Table 139-2, the *secretin hormone stimulation test* has consistently been found to be more sensitive and more specific. The secretin test has been evaluated against histology in over 100 patients from Japan. In this study, the bicarbonate concentration of pancreatic secretion was the most accurate parameter; ERCP was 60% as accurate as the bicarbonate concentration (Hayakawa et al, 1992).

TABLE 139-2. Diagnostic Tests for Chronic Pancreatitis

Tests of Function	Tests of Structure
Secretin Test	EUS
Fecal Elastase	ERCP
Serum Trypsinogen	CT
Fecal Chymotrypsin	MRI/MRCP
Fecal Fat	US
	KUB

CT = computed tomography; ERCP = endoscopic retrograde cholangiography; EUS = endoscopic ultrasound; MRCP = magnetic resonance cholangiography; MRI = magnetic resonance imaging; US = ultrasound.

Secretins

Until recently, the world supply of biologic porcine secretin had been depleted because of the unproven use of this agent to decrease the symptoms of autism. Synthetic porcine secretin and synthetic human secretin have been evaluated against the biologic porcine secretin and both synthetic preparations are equal to the biologic preparation when evaluated against each other in normal subjects and patients with proven chronic pancreatitis (Somogyi et al, 2003).

Synthetic porcine secretin is FDA-approved and the application to approve synthetic human secretin for clinical use is pending.

EUS

In recent years, EUS has emerged as a forerunner among radiographic tests evaluating pancreatic structure. The use of EUS overcomes two disadvantages that occur with transabdominal ultrasonography, including the ability to provide high resolution and not to be obscured by overlying bowel gas. At our medical center, we have had extensive experience with EUS and EUS has replaced ERCP as a diagnostic test. Whereas ERCP can image only the pancreatic ductal system, EUS can evaluate both the pancreatic ducts and the parenchyma. We are continuing to evaluate EUS and secretin against each other in patients with suspected small duct disease who present with chronic abdominal pain and negative radiographic testing. A preliminary report from our laboratory indicates that EUS was only 57% as sensitive and 64% as specific as a secretin test in patients with unexplained abdominal pain who ultimately where shown to have small duct chronic pancreatitis (Chowdhury et al, 2001). More studies have to be carried out comparing EUS to the secretin hormone stimulation test in patients suspected of having early chronic pancreatitis of the small duct variety. In those patients with a normal secretin test and EUS evidence of changes of chronic pancreatitis, it is not clear whether the EUS is more sensitive in some patients for early changes or if it is truly over-diagnosing chronic pancreatitis (Draganov and Toskes, 2002). This is particularly problematic because similar changes on EUS have been found in an appreciable number of normal control subjects and in people with nonulcerative dyspepsia. Exactly what the criteria should be for making a firm diagnosis of chronic pancreatitis is still under discussion. EUS is an important modality in the diagnosis and management of patients with chronic pancreatitis particularly if fine needle aspiration (FNA) is carried out. Cystic lesions within the pancreas, which may either be due to chronic pancreatitis or due to neoplastic causes, can be sorted out quite well with EUS. There is a separate chapter on EUS and FNA (see Chapter 5, "Endoscopic Ultrasonography and Fine-Needle Aspiration").

Management

The cornerstone in medical therapy is the use of potent pancreatic enzyme preparations whether the clinician is managing maldigestion or abdominal pain. Table 139-3 lists some of the more commonly used pancreatic enzyme formulations in the United States. They are divided into conventional or nonenteric-coated preparations and enteric-coated preparations. For the treatment of maldigestion, one to two capsules of an enteric-coated pancreatic enzyme preparation with meals is usually quite effective. With the use of these preparations, patients usually cease having diarrhea, gain weight, and have an improved quality of life. Indeed if one measures in a quantitative fashion fecal fat excretion under a controlled high fat diet, it will be shown that most patients treated with pancreatic enzymes do not completely correct their steatorrhea. Is there any danger in not correcting steatorrhea? This issue has not been very clear but recent observations from several laboratories, including our own, have indicated that patients with pancreatic steatorrhea may have bone changes of osteopenia and osteoporosis despite being on good enzyme treatment and being asymptomatic. It is also interesting that patients with small duct pancreatitis and pain but no steatorrhea have had similar bone changes. The numbers of patients in these studies is small but work is in progress to see whether or not this is of significant import to patients with chronic pancreatitis. Most experts have not recommended that patients with chronic pancreatitis and PI take supplements of calcium and vitamin D because it was thought that the normal small intestine could compensate for the loss of calcium. Indeed, our own observations are such that when one calculates how much calcium is lost per gram of fat lost, the presently allowed levels of supplementation would fall far short of correcting this problem in such patients.

Pain

In respect to managing pain in patients with chronic pancreatitis, the pathogenesis is multifactorial and, thus, one therapy is not apt to help all patients in a similar fashion.

TABLE 139-3. Pancreatic Enzyme Preparations

Enteric-Coated	Units of Lipase
Ultrase MT6, 12, 18, 20	6,000–20,000
Creon 10, 20	10,000–20,000
Pancrease MT4, 10, 16	4,000–16,000

Nonenteric-Coated	Units of Lipase
Viokase 8, 16	8,000; 16,000
Kuzyme HP	8,000
Cotazym	8,000 Protease content is usually three times lipase content

The following three pathophysiologic mechanisms may explain the pain in chronic pancreatitis: (1) acute pancreatic inflammation, (2) increased intrapancreatic pressure, and (3) alterations in pancreatic nerves. Pancreatic enzyme therapy, CCK antagonists and octreotide decrease pancreatic secretion thus decreasing intrapancreatic pressure in both large and small ducts, as well as the pancreatic gland itself. Endoscopic procedures attempt to decrease the pain by decreasing pressure through improved drainage. There is a separate chapter on endoscopic treatment (see Chapter 138). Surgery affords decompression of the major pancreatic duct and is successful in some patients. There is also a chapter on surgical treatment (see Chapter 137, "Chronic Pancreatitis: Surgical Considerations"). Celiac plexus block and thorascopic splanchnicectomy interrupt neural transmission of pain signals. There is also a chapter on chronic pain management (see Chapter 41, "Chronic Abdominal Pain").

It must be appreciated that often the diagnosis of chronic pancreatitis in a given patient is based on very little evidence. Mild elevations of pancreatic enzymes in the blood of patients with chronic abdominal pain usually do not mean chronic pancreatitis. The clinician must eliminate other causes of abdominal pain because the pain of chronic pancreatitis is often nonspecific and can mimic many other kinds of pain. In particular, it is now being appreciated that dysmotility syndromes both in the form of gastroparesis and small bowel dysmotility can present with abdominal pain indistinguishable from that of chronic pancreatitis. Patients with these dysmotility syndromes may even manifest a mild elevation in serum amylase and/or lipase. There are separate chapters on nonulcer dyspepsia (see Chapter 30, "The Management of Nonulcer Dyspepsia"), chronic abdominal pain (see Chapter 41) and intestinal pseudo-obstruction (see Chapter 63, "Chronic Intestinal Pseudo-Obstruction").

A recent study at our medical center presented preliminary data on 74 patients referred to our pancreatitis clinic who were suspected by the referring gastroenterologist and surgeons as having radiographic negative chronic pancreatitis or small duct chronic pancreatitis (Chowdhury et al, 2001; Chowdhury et al, 2003). The examination of these patients with unexplained pain of presumed pancreatic origin revealed that 40% actually had chronic pancreatitis diagnosed by the secretin stimulation test and did well with pancreatic enzyme treatments. Fifty percent had dysmotility most commonly of the stomach, and 10% had no cause that could be found. Prokinetic therapy in the form of erythromycin ethyl succinate suspension given orally in a dose of 100 mg 4 times a day, if the delayed gastric emptying was mild to moderate, and erythromycin 200 mg intravenously 4 times a day, if the gastroparesis was very severe, decreased the abdominal pain in these dysmotility patients. Even retrospectively, the pain of chronic pancreatitis could not be distinguished in any accurate manner from the pain caused by dysmotility. There is a separate chapter on gastroparesis (see Chapter 31, "Gastroparesis").

Coexistent Motility Disturbances

This interaction of *motility disturbances* with *chronic pancreatitis* takes on an even more complex connection because our laboratory has recently reported that the prevalence of gastroparesis is significantly increased in patients with chronic abdominal pain and small duct chronic pancreatitis. In 56 patients with small duct chronic pancreatitis documented by the secretin test, 25 of the 56 (44%) had gastroparesis. The etiology of this delay in gastric emptying is unclear, but it may be related to the high levels of CCK that such patients with small duct chronic pancreatitis demonstrate. In addition, many of these patients are receiving narcotics and that may lead to gastroparesis. Our laboratory has been quite successful in using *nonenteric-coated pancreatic enzymes to treat the pain in patients with small duct chronic pancreatitis*. However, if the stomach is not emptying properly, those enzymes will not be delivered into the proximal small bowel where feedback inhibition of pancreatic secretion is operative. The documentation of gastroparesis allows the administration of *prokinetics* with the *pancreatic enzymes* to allow this feedback process to be restored. Because motility disturbances are quite frequent in patients with chronic pancreatitis, it is strongly recommended that *potent narcotic analgesics be avoided* if possible and anodynes, such as nonsteroidal anti-inflammatory drugs, propoxyphene, or tramadol, be used. These latter three medications do not slow down gastric emptying. Despite all these efforts, narcotic addiction is quite common in patients with chronic pancreatitis and constant pain (see Chapter 41).

Feedback Control of Exocrine Secretion

Nonenteric Coated Pancreatic Enzyme Perspective

The basis for the use of nonenteric-coated pancreatic enzyme preparations to decrease abdominal pain in patients with chronic pancreatitis is based on the concept of feedback control of pancreatic exocrine secretion (Isaksson and Ihse, 1983; Slaff et al, 1984). *Nonentericcoated pancreatic enzyme preparations* appear to inhibit pancreatic secretion through a negative feedback mechanism involving intraduodenal serine proteases in the exocrine pancreas. These serine proteases modulate pancreatic secretion by regulating CCK release. Because patients with chronic pancreatitis often have decreased intraduodenal protease activity, they may not be capable of inactivating the CCK-releasing peptide that exists in the proximal small bowel and is largely responsible for stimulating CCK release. In these patients, it can be demonstrated that there are high levels of CCK in the blood. This is a proximal small intestine phenomenon and the pancreatic proteases must be delivered to the upper small intestine. This can be done consistently only by the administration of nonenteric-coated pancreatic enzyme preparations. Such nonenteric-coated enzyme preparations are *susceptible to acid degradation* as they pass through the stomach; therefore, it is recommended that a *proton pump inhibitor (PPI) be given along with the pancreatic enzymes.* We have found that the most consistent preparation that affords control feedback inhibition and relieves abdominal pain is the preparation of *Viokase-16*. This preparation should be given orally in a dose of *four tablets, four times a day, along with the acid suppressive agent*. These enzyme preparations are remarkably devoid of side effects. The remarkable side effect of *colonic strictures* noted in patients with CF receiving very large doses of enteric-coated pancreatic enzymes (see Chapter 140, "Cystic Fibrosis and other Hereditary Diseases of the Pancreas") does not occur in adult patients with chronic pancreatitis.

Six randomized trials have evaluated the effectiveness of pancreatic enzymes in the reduction of chronic pancreatitis pain (Warshaw et al, 1998). Of these, two trials using nonenteric-coated enzymes were effective in reducing pain, whereas the four trials using the enteric-coated preparations showed no statistical improvement in pain relief. In patients with big duct disease, there was, at best, a 25% response rate in decreasing abdominal pain, whereas the response rate was approximately 70% in those with small duct disease. A meta-analysis of these trials indicates that pancreatic enzyme therapy did not decrease abdominal pain in patients with chronic pancreatic (Brown et al, 1997). It should be pointed out that this meta-analysis has been sharply criticized for lumping together patients receiving nonenteric-coated and enteric-coated enzymes. Abundant information now exists both from randomized trials and extensive clinical experience that *nonenteric-coated enzyme preparations are preferable* for relief of the abdominal pain in such patients. Table 139-4 contrasts the nonenteric and the enteric-coated enzymes in this feedback control process.

Thus if one wants to optimize pancreatic enzyme therapy in treating the pain of chronic pancreatitis, the appropriate enzyme preparation must be employed in a suitable patient. A *nonenteric enzyme preparation should be given along with a PPI to a patient with small duct chronic pancreatitis who does not have steatorrhea*. Great success will not be achieved when a patient with large duct disease and steatorrhea is treated with an enteric-coated preparation.

Duration of Enzyme Therapy

Our extensive experience indicates that those patients who are receiving pancreatic enzyme therapy for pain and who attain appreciable pain relief should be evaluated for discontinuation of enzyme therapy if they have been pain-free for at least 6 months. In our experience, about half of the patients no longer have pain when enzymes are discontinued, whereas the other half experience a relapse and must continue enzyme therapy indefinitely. We have not yet been able to identify those markers that will allow us to predict in which group a given patient will fall.

Octreotide

In patients with big duct disease, pancreatic enzyme therapy is not very effective and may be beneficial in only 25% of patients. Following the principle feedback inhibition, it was proposed that *octreotide,* an analog of *somatostatin,* might be effective in controlling pain. Octreotide markedly inhibits pancreatic secretion and significantly lowers CCK levels. Several small short-term studies result in variable findings with regard to pain control with this agent. Results from a multicenter, double-blind, placebo-controlled, dose-ranging pilot study suggests that a dose of 200 µg administered subcutaneously 3 times a day was effective. In that study of over 100 patients, 65% of patients showed a decrease in abdominal pain with that dose of octreotide and a decrease in anodyne (pain relief medication) usage. Not all patients respond to this agent, but it appears that those that respond are those that demonstrate at least a 50% reduction in blood CCK levels. Studies are now being launched from our laboratory that will be looking at a long acting form of octreotide that can be given once every 28 days in the dose equivalent to the 200 µg 3 times a day (Draganov and Toskes, 2002). Thus in patients with small duct chronic pancreatitis, the treatment of choice should be nonenteric-coated pancreatic enzymes with a PPI. Treatment should be started and carried out for 4 to 6 weeks before an evaluation of success or failure has been made. If the patient fits all the criteria of small duct pancreatitis and is not benefiting from the enzyme approach described above, then a gastric emptying study should be done and, if there is gastroparesis, a prokinetic should be added to the plan.

CCK Receptor Antagonists

A recent multicenter, dose-response controlled trial was conducted in Japan to evaluate the efficacy of the CCK receptor antagonist, *loxiglumide*, in patients with abdom-

TABLE 139-4. Pancreatic Enzyme Preparations and Feedback Control of Pancreatic Secretion

Criteria	Nonenteric-Coated	Enteric-Coated
Release proteases into duodenum	Yes	No
Lower CCK level	Yes	No
Decrease pancreatic secretion	Yes	No
Reduce pain	Yes	No

CCK = cholecystokinin.

inal pain associated with chronic pancreatitis (Shiratori et al, 2002). Two hundred and seven patients were randomly assigned to several dosages of loxiglumide for 4 weeks or a placebo. The overall clinical improvement was 46 to 58% in the loxiglumide categories versus 34% in the placebo group. In another study, a patient with abdominal pain associated with chronic pancreatitis had elevated blood CCK levels and analgesia produced by morphine appeared to be reduced. The patient was treated with *proglumide*, a nonspecific CCK receptor antagonist, and analgesia improved markedly. The patient derived consistent analgesia from the use of proglumide alone. It was theorized that proglumide-induced analgesia would be reduced in chronic pancreatitis patients who have elevated CCK levels.

Surgical Therapy

In patients with big duct pancreatitis and significant abdominal pain, the treatment of choice is surgical ductal decompression of the main pancreatic duct. Usually in such patients, 80% receive relief immediately, but if the patients are followed for 3 years, there will be a decrease in the number of patients who have pain relief to the extent that 30 to 40% of patients will be free of pain (Howell et al, 2001). There is a chapter on surgical therapy (see Chapter 137).

Endoscopic Therapy

In regard to endoscopic treatment, pancreatic stents have been used in patients with chronic pancreatitis to reduce intraductal pressure. Such interventions are quite appropriate if there is a dominant stricture or a stone within the duct. There is no good evidence that a diffusely dilated pancreatic duct without any dominant stricture will respond to stenting. The possible benefits of pancreatic ductal stenting must be balanced against the risk of further damage induced by the stent to the pancreatic duct and the pancreatic parenchyma. There is a chapter on endoscopic therapy (see Chapter 138, "Pancreatitis: Endoscopic Therapy").

Celiac Plexus Block

Celiac plexus block has had mixed results and, in our opinion, is at best, a temporizing measure. *EUS-guided celiac plexus block* has been used in patients with both pancreatic cancer and chronic pancreatitis. When EUS-guided versus *CT-guided blocks* are looked at in a prospective, randomized fashion, the EUS-guided celiac block seems to provide more pain relief than the CT-guided block. In patients treated with ultrasonography-guided celiac plexus block, a significant improvement in pain score occurred in 55% of patients. The benefit persisted beyond 12 weeks in only 26% of patients, and it appears that was not very effective in patients under 45 years of age or those who have had previous surgery (Gress et al, 2001). It appears that this procedure is well tolerated with temporary results that are quite impressive but its role at this time should probably be limited to treating flares of chronic pain in patients with otherwise limited options. This is discussed in the chapter on chronic abdominal pain (see Chapter 41).

Conclusion

The management of the abdominal pain in patients with chronic pancreatitis continues to pose significant challenges to gastroenterologists and surgeons. The subjective nature of the pain, the heterogeneity of the patients, and the poor understanding of the pathophysiology are potential pitfalls. This situation is exacerbated by concurrent alcohol abuse in some patients and narcotic dependence in many, and it is further compounded by the lack of predictors for the response to pain. Patients with chronic abdominal pain are quite common and often present to their primary care physician for examination and management. If the cause of abdominal pain is not obvious by radiographic examination, a gastroenterologist should be consulted for further diagnostic testing. It is very important that a proper diagnosis be made and that the pathophysiology of the pain be considered rather than just treating the symptoms. What should not be done is an expedient referral to a pain clinic without proper diagnosis. A clinical diagnosis of chronic pancreatitis based on scant evidence leads to the administration of narcotics for an indefinite period by such pain clinics. With new awareness that coexisting motility problems are common in such patients and the observation that narcotics commonly used by physicians that direct pain clinics make such motility patients worse, greater efforts should be made to probe the pathogenesis of the abdominal pain.

Chronic pancreatitis should seriously be considered in all patients with unexplained abdominal pain. It is again important to stress that chronic pancreatitis is not one disease and all patients with chronic pancreatitis cannot be treated the same. The importance of small duct versus large duct disease must be emphasized. If radiographic tests do not provide a diagnosis of chronic pancreatitis but the clinical suspicion is still high, then more sophisticated testing such as a direct hormone stimulation test or EUS should be sought. A nonenteric-coated pancreatic enzyme preparation along with a PPI is the treatment of choice for that subset of patients who have chronic pain and small duct disease. Octreotide is increasingly being used for abdominal pain that is unresponsive to pancreatic enzyme therapy. If medical therapy fails, an expertise must sought to attempt possible endoscopic and surgical management. Clinical trials with very high doses of pancreatic proteases, long acting forms of octreotide, and CCK antagonists in selected patients are underway.

Supplemental Reading

Brown A, Hughes M, Tenner S, et al. Does pancreatic enzyme supplementation reduce pain in patients with chronic pancreatitis: a meta-analysis? Am J Gastroenterol 1997;92:2032–5.

Chey WY. Neurohormonal control of the exocrine pancreas. Curr Opin Gastroenterol 1997;13:375–80.

Chowdhury R, Bhutani M, Forsmark C, et al. The association of gastroparesis with chronic pancreatitis. Gastroenterology 2001; 20:A648.

Chowdhury R, Bhutani M, Mishra G, et al. Comparative analysis of pancreatic function testing versus morphologic assessment by EUS for evaluation of chronic unexplained abdominal pain. Gastroenterology 2001;120:A647.

Chowdhury RS, Forsmark CE, Davis RH, et al. Increased prevalence of gastroparesis in small duct chronic pancreatitis. Pancreas 2003;26:235–8.

Draganov P, Toskes PP. Chronic pancreatitis. Curr Opin Gastroenterol 2002;18:558–62.

Grendell JH. Genetic factors in pancreatitis. Curr Gastroenterology Reports 2003;5:105–9.

Gress F, Schmitt C, Sherman S, et al. Endoscopic ultrasound-guided celiac plexus block for managing abdominal pain associated with chronic pancreatitis: a prospective single-center experience. Am J Gastroenterol 2001;96:409–16.

Hayakawa T, Kondo T, Shibata T, et al. Relation between pancreatic exocrine function and histological changes in chronic pancreatitis. Am J Gastroenterol 1992;87:1170–4.

Howell JG, Johnson LW, Sehon IK, et al. Surgical management for chronic pancreatitis. Am Surg 2001;67:487–90.

Isaksson G, Ihse I. Pain reduction by an oral pancreatic enzyme preparation in chronic pancreatitis. Dig Dis Sci 1983;28:97–102.

Layer P, Yamamoto H, Kalthoff L, et al. The different courses of early and late onset idiopathic and alcoholic pancreatitis. Gastroenterology 1995;107:1481–6.

Shiratori K, Takeuchi T, Satake K, et al. Clinical evaluation of oral administration of a cholecystokinin-A receptor antagonist (loxiglumide) to patients with acute painful attacks of chronic pancreatitis: a multi-center, dose-response study in Japan. Pancreas 2002;25:E1–5.

Somogyi L, Ross AS, Cintron M, Toskes P. Comparison of biologic porcine secretin, synthetic porcine secretin, and synthetic human secretin in pancreatic function testing. Pancreas 2003;27:230–4.

Slaff J, Jacobson D, Tillman CR, et al. Protease-specific suppression of pancreatic enzyme secretion. Gastroenterology 1984;87:44–52.

Warshaw AL, Banks PA, Fernandez-delCastillo C. AGA technical review: treatment of pain in chronic pancreatitis. Gastroenterology 1998;115:765–76.

CHAPTER 140

CYSTIC FIBROSIS AND OTHER HEREDITARY DISEASES OF THE PANCREAS

MARGARET P. BOLAND, MD, AND DAVID R. MACK, MD

Cystic Fibrosis

Cystic fibrosis (CF) has long been known as the most common lethal inherited disease in Caucasians. For gastroenterologists it is of some interest to realize that the name of the disease comes from a pathologic description of the fibrotic and cystic changes in the pancreas of infants as described by Dorothy Andersen more than 60 years ago. Over the last 14 years, since the discovery of the CF gene on the long arm of chromosome 7, and investigations into the nature of the CFTR protein coded by that gene, CF has become much more commonly identified and diagnosed in adults. The mean age at death has also increased to about 37 years, and with over 1,000 mutations identified, the spectrum of the disease is known to be widely variable and not confined to Caucasians. All this is to say that both pediatric and adult gastroenterologists will be asked to see and treat these individuals.

Gastrointestinal (GI) disease in CF involves all segments of the gut and its embryologic derivatives, including the pancreas and liver. (This also accounts for the lung involvement, as the lungs are outgrowths of the foregut in early embryologic life). The easiest approach, then, to discussing the problems is to travel the tract mouth to anus discussing liver and pancreatic disease along the way (Table 140-1).

Gastroesophageal Reflux

This is an extremely common entity in CF patients, occurring in about 20 to 25% of young patients (< 5 years) and up to 80% of older patients. Increased numbers of transient relaxations of the lower esophageal sphincter (LES), and decreased basal pressure at the LES both play a role. Patients with chronic CF chest disease also have abnormal pressure gradients between the abdomen and thorax, exacerbated by cough and at times postural change. All this can lead to the problem of erosive esophagitis, and the complications of esophageal peptic stricture or Barrett's esophagus. Chest complications related to reflux can be significant in these patients and include aspiration pneumonia and laryngitis. Treatment needs to be aggressive and the index for investigating low. Treatment options include positional change such as elevating the head of the bed and avoiding head down tilting during chest percussions. Medications are limited to histamine-2 receptor antagonists (H_2RAs) and proton pump inhibitors (PPIs) to limit acid injury. Treatment is similar to other causes of erosive gastroesophageal reflux disease (GERD). Both medications are well tolerated and are used chronically. There is no evidence that long term use leads to susceptibility to GI infections, nor vitamin B_{12} deficiency. Some patients may have reflux exacerbated chest disease that does not respond to medication, and a fundoplication, either complete wrap (Nissen) or partial, will have a role. Laparoscopic fundoplications are widely performed, and although the surgical procedure time may not be much less than an open fundoplication, the limited size of incisions on the abdominal wall make recovery and resumption of routine airway clearance techniques significantly easier in these patients. Other newer procedures to tighten the LES with endoscopically placed sutures, or injections have not been studied sufficiently in CF to recommend their use at this time.

TABLE 140-1. Gastrointestinal Manifestations in Cystic Fibrosis

Intestinal	Relative Incidence (%)
Meconium ileus	10 to 15 (pancreatic insufficient)
Intestinal atresia	
Rectal prolapse	
GERD	10 to 20
PUD	1 to 10
Intussusception (recurrent?)	
DIOS	10 to 20 (pancreatic insufficient, increases with age)
Constipation	
Fibrosing colonopathy	< 1
Pancreatic	
Pancreatic insufficiency	60 to 85 increases with age
Pancreatitis	2 to 3 (pancreatic sufficient)
Hepatobiliary	
Neonatal cholestasis	1 to 5
Steatosis	15 to 30
Focal biliary fibrosis	10 to 60 increases with age
Multilobular cirrhosis with portal hypertension	1 to 15 increases with age
Cholelithiasis	4 to 12

DIOS = distal intestinal obstruction syndrome; GERD = gastroesophageal reflux disease; PUD = peptic ulcer disease.

Peptic Ulcer Disease

The majority of patients with CF with pancreatic insufficiency (PI) have greatly reduced pancreatic production of bicarbonate and consequent inability to raise the pH within the duodenum. This lower pH and the use of anti-inflammatory medication in some patients, such as ibuprofen and prednisone, predispose patients to acid-peptic injury in the duodenum. This is another cause of symptoms of abdominal pain, and may be difficult to diagnose without endoscopic investigation. Assessment of the chest disease by the attending respirologist or an anesthetist is warranted prior to undertaking endoscopy. Again, as with GERD, the treatment is chronic acid suppression medication.

Malabsorption and Maldigestion

The pancreatic disease, with severe fibrosis and cystic changes on pathologic examination (Figure 140-1), is present in the severe mutations, and accounts for the PI of these patients. *CFTR* in the pancreas is localized to the luminal surface of ductular cells, and malfunction of this channel, which is known to transport both chloride and bicarbonate ions, leads to acidic and viscous secretions blocking pancreatic exocrine outflow. With screening for pancreatic function in early life, about 40% of infants have pancreatic sufficiency (PS) (defined as < 7% loss of ingested fat on a 72-hour fecal fat collection), but by the age of about 5 years, this has declined to approximately 15% of cases. This screening for pancreatic function is not an easy task, as the methods of checking for PS are difficult or invasive. The standard clinical test is a 72-hour fecal fat measure (Van de Kamer et al, 1949). Loss of any stool during collection would favour a more normal report of fecal fat loss. In addition to stool collection, a diet record of weighed food ingested should be obtained for 5 days, with the stool collection occurring during the last 3 days. The average daily fat lost in the stool is then assessed as a percent of the average daily fat ingested. The normal value is fecal loss of < 7 % of ingested fat. Patients with PI will have a loss of fat usually in the range of 20 to 50%. This testing should be performed on all patients at the time of diagnosis to assess pancreatic function. It should also be repeated on patients who are initially assessed as having PS when there is a change in GI symptoms or any faltering of growth.

Other testing for pancreatic function includes the use of a monoclonal antibody based enzyme-linked immunoassay test for human pancreatic elastase 1 in the stool. An aliquot from a 24-hour stool collection is assayed. Human elastase 1 is not present in porcine pancrease supplemental enzymes, so this test is convenient to perform while the patient is receiving pancreatic enzyme supplements. This test is both sensitive (96%) and specific (100%) for CF patients with PI when compared with healthy subjects and those with nonpancreatic diseases (Gullo et al, 1997; Soldan et al, 1997). It is also somewhat more acceptable than a 72-hour fecal fat for those asked to perform the test. This test will sort patients into those that have PS and those who have PI, and can be used to judge the requirement for pancreatic enzymes. More recently it has also been used to track the decline in exocrine pancreatic function in PS CF patients (Walkowiak et al, 2003). It cannot be used to test for the efficacy of enzyme therapy, or to monitor the effect of changes or additions to therapy, such as the use of acid suppressants. A 72-hour fecal fat is needed for this.

A further test for pancreatic function, the pancreatic stimulation test, involves insertion of a nasoduodenal tube and the administration of secretagogues (secretin/cholecystokinin) to stimulate the flow of pancreatic juice. The collected secretions can then be assessed for pH and enzyme content. Technical challenges make these tests very demanding, and patients with PS have a significant chance of being misclassified as having PI (Schibli et al, 2003); therefore, this is not usually performed in the clinical setting, but is very useful for research clinical investigations. Endoscopic aspiration of pancreatic fluid following secretin stimulation is not recommended as it has even greater potential for misclassification of pancreatic functional status.

Nutrition

The majority of CF patients have PI, and consequent steatorrhea and azotorrhea, and are predisposed to gross malnutrition. We know that the growth failure of children and youth with CF is not intrinsic to the disease, but remediable with provision of sufficient energy and protein along with supplemental pancreatic enzymes as needed. There is also evidence that improved nutrition helps stabilize lung function, improves quality of life, and may prolong life. Estimates of energy requirements for patients with CF are clearly higher than normal and should be based on weight gain and body fat stores. The quality of the diet can fit with

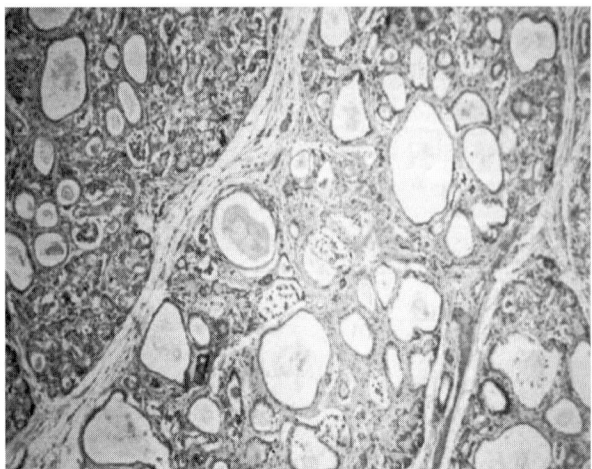

FIGURE 140-1. Pathologic examination of pancreatic disease.

normal recommendations for nutrient mix, recognizing the importance of fat as the most energy dense nutrient, and the one that makes our food most palatable. Formerly recommended *restrictions* on fat intake to improve GI discomfort and other symptoms *should be entirely abandoned*. *Pancreatic replacement enzymes* on the market at present are derived from pig pancreas (eg, trade names *Pancrease*, *Cotazym*, *Creon*, *Ultrase*), although newer crystalline synthetic enzymes are in trials. The appropriate use of enzymes has been carefully examined in the last decade since the first appearance of *fibrosing colonopathy*. The Consensus Statement (Borowitz et al, 2002,) of the Cystic Fibrosis Foundation recommends the following dosing guidelines:

Infants: 2,000 to 4,000 Units lipase per 120 mL formula or breast feed

Children < 4 years: 1,000 to 2,500 Units lipase per kg per meal

Children and adults: 500 to 2,500 Units lipase per kg per meal

Plus: half the standard meal dose with snacks

Or

Enzyme dose < 10,000 Units lipase per kg per day

Beyond these recommendations, lipase dosing based on grams of fat in the diet is a rational approach. Standards of care support a maximum dose of 4,000 U lipase per gram fat per day (Fitzsimmons et al, 1998). This cut off keeps doses of lipase *well below* those reported with *colonic strictures*. The differential diagnosis of patients with ongoing abdominal complications while taking the maximum enzyme dose is listed in Table 140-2.

As most of the enzymes in clinical use are enteric coated to protect them from stomach acid, use of an H$_2$RA or PPI to raise duodenal pH can enhance enzyme function. The best test of improved absorption is a 72-hour fecal fat measure.

Monitoring success in treating malabsorption and malnutrition is done in children by the careful assessment of *growth* throughout childhood and adolescence. For adults, maintenance of a normal and stable body mass index (BMI) should be sought. We want our young patients to achieve normal growth, not only when compared with the National Center for Health Statistics (NCHS)/Centers for Disease Control and Prevention (CDC) growth curves (CDC Web site, <http://www.cdc.gov/growthcharts>), but when assessed by growth potential as estimated by midparental height. Diligence should be taken in obtaining accurate heights with a wall-mounted stadiometer, and weights with minimal standard clothing, and plotting the values on the CDC growth charts, including values for head circumference and weight for height or BMI. As well as the standard measures, the Consensus Report on Nutrition (Borowitz et al, 2002) recommends mid-arm circumference and triceps skinfold be measured annually as a marker of body composition. Special vigilance on growth and nutritional status should be given at the time of diagnosis, during infancy, and during the pubertal growth spurt. We are much closer now to achieving normal growth of our patients when comparing height and weight to population standards, but there is room still for improvement.*

Along with the loss of macronutrients, pancreatic insufficient patients are at risk for deficiencies in fat-soluble vitamins (A, D, E, and K), and essential fatty acids, and for the consequences of these deficiencies particularly on bone mineral accretion, neurological function, and membrane integrity. Patients with PI are routinely supplemented with *fat-soluble vitamins* at between one and two times the normal. Much work on *essential fatty acid levels* (linoleic acid [18:2n-6] and alpha-linolenic acid [18:3n-3], and the longer products, arachidonic acid [20:4n-6] and eicosapentanoic acid [20:5n-3] and docosahexaenoic acid [22:6n-3]) has been done. Although recommendations for routine supplementation have not been made, assurance of intake of these fatty acids within the high fat diet is a prudent recommendation. The quality of supplemental dietary fat should be assessed by the dietitian to minimize saturated and trans fatty acids. As well, an emphasis on medium chain triglycerides as a source of energy is unnecessary. Routine *annual monitoring* of *fat-soluble vitamin levels (vitamin A, 25-OH-D, α-tocopheral* and *prothrombin time*) is currently recommended. Other micronutrients including iron, calcium and zinc, although clearly essential, have no specific recommendations, except for a yearly *hemoglobin* and *hematocrit* as surrogates for iron nutriture, and ensuring at least normal intake of the others.

Nutrition support for those starting to fall below channel (percentile line) on the growth curves can be enhanced in a step-wise fashion as required, including oral supplementation, nasogastric (NG) feeds for short term gain, and surgically-placed enteral tube feeds for long term nocturnal nutrition support (gastrostomy or jejunostomy tubes). There is some evidence that oral supplements merely replace food (Pencharz and Durie, 2000), but with some patients weight gain occurs. The energy provided by these additional supplements is often > 50% of the patients total

TABLE 140-2. Differential Diagnoses of Patients With Ongoing Abdominal Complaints While Taking the Maximum Enzyme Dose

Lactose intolerance
Giardiasis
Biliary disease
Short bowel syndrome
Bacterial overgrowth
Enteric bacterial infection
Celiac disease
Crohn's disease
Fibrosing colonopathy

---

*Editor's Note: This same attention to growth should be exercised when caring for prepubescent adolescents with Crohn's disease.

energy intake. However, with increased severity of pulmonary disease, increased inflammation and anorexia, patients are not able to ingest the required additional energy, but do tolerate enteral infusions, usually provided overnight. This care is an additional significant burden for families and requires a lot of support and encouragement from the care team.

Meconium Ileus

This is a neonatal disorder, which most often occurs in the term infant, and is the presenting sign in about 15% of children diagnosed with CF, usually those with PI. Although no specific *CFTR* mutations have been identified with meconium ileus (MI), a modifier locus on human chromosome 19 has been determined (Zielenski et al, 1999). Suspicion for MI may be raised with fetal ultrasounds (USs) demonstrating dilated loops of bowel on the second or third trimester scan. Meconium plug syndrome, attributed to a tight anus, should be ruled out. In this disorder, light-coloured gelatinous firm stool is present in the lower colon and rectum. The likelihood of MI is confirmed with a barium enema showing a microcolon. About 50% of infants have complications of the disorder with *perforation, meconium peritonitis, atresias,* or *volvulus*. A history of this should be sought when seeing these patients later in life.

For patients with uncomplicated ileus, a trial of medical management may be successful in alleviating the obstruction, but the infant should be at a center where surgical intervention is available, if and when required. As with distal intestinal obstruction syndrome (DIOS) (see later in chapter), a combination of *acetyl-cysteine, polyethylene glycol (PEG)* or *water-soluble contrast* can be used to clear the obstruction. For complications, a *resection* with primary or secondary anastomosis may be performed. For some patients this results in loss of the ileocecal valve, loss of absorptive surface in the ileum, and vitamin B_{12} or bile salt malabsorption. This will then add to the PI of the child and make malnutrition a greater risk. Some patients with atresia or volvulus may end up with a true short gut.

DIOS

Previously known as *meconium ileus equivalent*, DIOS is obstruction of the distal small bowel with inspissated stool and mucous. This occurs more frequently in the older child adolescent or adult, and may present acutely, or have a prodrome of weeks or even months of nonspecific crampy abdominal pain. The patient presents with a partial or, less commonly, complete distal small bowel obstruction with crampy abdominal pain, vomiting, abdominal distension, and decreased stooling. Although the patients who have DIOS are usually those with PI, fat per se is not likely the major culprit, and decreasing the amount of fat in the diet is never an appropriate measure. There is some evidence that it is the thick tenacious intestinal mucous that initiates the intestinal block. Some patients have problems with adherence to appropriate use of supplemental pancreatic enzymes, and encouraging better enzyme use does decrease the bulkiness of the stool. There is some evidence that motility of the bowel in CF is decreased, but there is no evidence the presently available prokinetic agents have any role. In my experience, those who are chronically undernourished, or maintain poor fluid intake, or experience acute dehydration (eg, children who participate in a soccer tournament with inadequate drinking) put themselves at risk for these events, and may have recurrent episodes, or a chronic rumbling history. On physical examination, tenderness in the right lower quadrant is usually present, and there is a fullness or palpable mass in some patients.

Diagnosis

Conventionally, plain films of the abdomen, with supine and upright or lateral decubitus views, confirm air/fluid levels, often with some dilation, in most of the small bowel. Frequently, there is a *foamy appearance* to the bowel contents in the right lower quadrant. The rectum is devoid of air or stool, differentiating DIOS from constipation. At our center, this is followed by a real-time *US* of the bowel, which is very helpful in examining intestinal contents, ruling out intussusception, and observing bowel motility. The ultrasonographer can often point out sluggish motility, or virtual absence of motility in the bowel segments clogged with "toothpaste" consistency stool. The amount of motility then guides the attending physician in the use of therapy, whether a lavage solution from above, or enemas from below, or a combination. Physicians need to be mindful of the differential diagnosis (Table 140-3) and take some care with the examination. As stated above, simple constipation should be ruled out as this involves the rectosigmoid, or whole colon, and not the distal small bowel.

Therapy includes use of products to clear the block, from above, if the obstruction is incomplete and there is some motility on the US examination, or from below, if the obstruction is fairly complete. PEG 3350—electrolyte solutions (Golytely or others) can be given by lavage through

TABLE 140-3. Differential Diagnoses for Patients Presenting with Abdominal Pain and Small Bowel Obstruction

Intussusception
Adhesions (especially if patient had surgery for MI as newborn)
Inflamed or ruptured appendix
Volvulus
Crohn's disease
Fibrosing colonopathy

MI = meconium ileus.

an NG tube or other enteral feeding tube (G-tube or J-tube) if available. Most patients will not tolerate drinking the quantity of these solutions required to clear DIOS. The volume to infuse varies from 5 to 15 mL/kg/hr to a maximum of 250 to 750 mL/hr. Start slowly (50 to 100 mL/hr), and increase every 10 to 15 minutes as tolerated until the maximum rate tolerated is reached, and continue the lavage until the effluent is clear and bile stained. If the patient becomes overly distended, or vomits, hold the lavage, and clear from below, before advancing with the lavage solution again. Although PEG solutions do not cause fluid shifts, in my practice, patients have an intravenous solution running to provide maintenance fluids, and to correct dehydration if present. We allow patients to have small quantities of clear fluids orally if desired, understanding that some of the glucose in the fluids may then be cotransported with the electrolytes and thus absorbed; however, this has not interfered with the GI clearance. For patients who are totally obstructed, who have little to no motility on US, we would avoid lavage until some obstruction is relieved. Enemas from below can also be both diagnostic and therapeutic. Isotonic contrast will loosen the stool block, and may also help rule out intussusception, strictures, and non-DIOS lesions. We also use *acetyl-cyteine* (*Mucomyst*) as enemas. This comes as a 20% solution, and we dilute to 4%, and provide repeat enemas of 50 to 150 mL. This helps to break up disulfide bonds in the mucous, and although the literature is sparse (Hodson et al, 1976), this does work.

Patients with one episode of DIOS may go on to repeat events, and chronic therapy should be instituted to prevent recurrence if possible. Discuss with patients the need to titrate enzymes appropriately and to not miss doses. This may not be the whole answer, but will decrease stool bulk. Use of a regular stool softener, such as lactulose, milk of magnesia, mineral oil, or PEG, can be given on a routine basis. Patient preference and adherence to care should guide the choice of product. Miralax may be an option where available because it is far more palatable. Usual doses for all the above are those used to treat simple constipation. In the past, chronic use of acetyl-cysteine has been advocated, but there is only anecdotal evidence for its use. It can be given as a 4% solution (4 mL acetyl-cysteine with 16 mL beverage) mixed with a stronger beverage such as cola, taken once or twice a day. Mineral oil should not be given at the same time as vitamin supplements.

Intussusception

This is a relatively common occurrence in children with CF, and may occur intermittently. It is also an important cause of intestinal obstruction in the adult with CF (Di Sant'Agnese et al, 1979). As with DIOS, inspissated mucous may play a role, in this case as the lead point for the intussuscipiens. We have noted patients who have this appearing and disappearing over a few minutes when examined by US. Clearly, it is only when the blood flow is compromised, with swelling and bowel obstruction, that treatment is required. Insufflation of the colon with air, or the use of a contrast enema, may decompress the intussusception. Failing this, surgery will be required.

Constipation

Patients with CF may have constipation, just as do other adults and children. History, physical examination including digital rectal examination, and a plain abdominal film is of help in differentiating this from DIOS. Patients with PI at times decrease their enzyme dose with the mistaken thought that this will loosen the stool and treat the constipation. Physicians need to ensure that patients are taking appropriate doses of enzymes. Usual measures of increasing dietary fluid and fiber should be taken, but attention needs to be given to ensure the energy content of the diet does not suffer with this decrease in energy density. The usual stool softeners, such as mineral oil, milk of magnesia, or PEG solutions, can be titrated to effect.

Fibrosing Colonopathy

This disease was first described in CF patients from Britain in 1994 in a report from Dr. R. Smyth. About 2 years before the report, very high dose supplemental pancreatic enzyme products became available on the market, with lipase content of 20,000 or 25,000 U/capsule. Although this was done to limit the number of capsules the patient had to take, these higher lipase capsules could more easily provide patients with exceptionally high lipase doses. This was especially true when patients made little change in the number of capsules when switching from a lower dosage to a higher dosage. This initial report described five children with CF who developed strictures, chronic obstructive symptoms, and eventually underwent colectomy. The pathologic description of the surgical specimens was *marked submucosal fibrosis* primarily affecting the proximal colon. Subsequent work indicates that before that final stage is reached, the endoscopic appearance may be that of a *few nonspecific ulcers*. Again the microscopic appearance of mucosal biopsies shows nonspecific changes with fairly marked eosinophilia, but no granulomas. The epidemiology of the disease from a good case-control study in the United States points to the dose of pancreatic enzyme as the causative factor. The fibrosis is the final outcome for colons that have been irreparably damaged by very high dose enzymes. Based on observations in the rat, one hypothesis about the nature of the injury involves the increased intestinal permeability in CF patients (Mack et al, 1992), in addition to high dose pancreatic enzymes leading to enteropathy, fibrosis, and possibly hepatic injury (Lloyd-Still et al, 1998). Current recommendations limit the dose of enzymes that patients ingest. The *maximum dose* should be *2,500 Units lipase per kg per meal* or *10,000 Units lipase per kg per day*. All the currently marketed enzymes function best at a ≥ pH 6.5. Due to the loss of bicarbonate production by the pancreas to optimize duodenal pH, a *PPI* may assist with both the activity of the enzymes in the proximal small intestine, and improving intestinal permeability (Hendriks et al, 2001) by increasing tight junction function. Although reports of this entity have declined, ongoing vigilance should be maintained.

Carcinoma

With the survival of patients with CF improving, we are beginning to see an increased risk of GI cancers in adult patients (Neglia et al, 1995). Although there are many causes of abdominal pain in this population, an awareness that carcinoma is on the list of potential causes may prevent delayed diagnosis.

Liver Disease in CF

As with the pancreas, the CFTR protein is localized to the apical membrane of bile duct cells, and the biliary fluid is more viscous and less alkaline than normal due to this defect of cholangiocyte transport. The small ducts become obstructed, and the reaction to this obstruction is proliferation of small ducts, cholangitis, and fibrosis. The liver damage, therefore, affects the hepatocyte late in the process, and patients may present with cirrhosis and portal hypertension, with relatively preserved overall hepatic function. Efforts to correlate a specific CF mutation with liver disease have been unsuccessful. Although cirrhosis seems to occur more commonly in those with the more severe mutations, these patients may have mild to moderate lung disease, and are candidates for liver transplant. Monitoring for liver disease should be part of routine care for all patients. Biochemical testing of transaminases, γ-glutamyl transpeptidase (GGT), and alkaline phosphatase on an annual basis is complemented by liver US, which can detect abnormalities in patients with or without clinical or biochemical liver disease (Lenaerts et al, 2003).

Neonatal Cholestasis

CF is one of the differential diagnoses for prolonged *conjugated hyperbilirubinemia* in the first 4 to 12 weeks of life. Infants presenting at this time should have a sweat chloride done as part of the initial workup. CF patients may have a small, shrunken gall bladder on US. In most CF infants with prolonged jaundice, the discoloration improves over weeks, and entirely resolves, although this may take up to 6 months. In my experience, infants with CF and jaundice should also have testing done for *α-1-antitrypsin (α-1-AT) deficiency*, as the severe forms of this disease may occur with CF resulting in rapidly deteriorating, aggressive cirrhosis and liver failure, and the need for early transplant referral. Testing here should include not only the α-1-AT level, which is an acute phase reactant, but also the *Pi (protease inhibitor) typing*, which is done in a few centers in North America.

Hepatic Steatosis

Some patients with CF may develop fatty infiltration of the liver, with hepatomegaly. This is not uncommon as part of refeeding of malnourished patients, and I have seen this arise over a few days in an inpatient on NG tube feeds. Most of the time, this is an entity diagnosed by US (hyperechogenicity) or computed tomography (CT), and rarely has a biopsy been performed. Ensuring normal nutrition for both macronutrients and micronutrients is important and will help to resolve the problem. It needs to be remembered that many patients with CF will have a palpable liver on examination when they have pulmonary hyperinflation. This should not be confused with hepatomegaly.

Focal Biliary Fibrosis/Cirrhosis

This is a description of the pathology in the liver of CF patients. The scarring around the biliary tree is not generalized, but patchy, and likely occurs to some degree in most patients, although clearly some patients are more affected and go on to an extensive lesion with cirrhosis and consequent portal hypertension. The fibrosis alone does not produce symptoms. Biochemical tests of liver enzymes (aspartate aminotransferase, alanine aminotransferase, GGT, alkaline phosphatase) may, however, be mildly elevated (1.5 to 4 times normal), and if this is sustained for > 3 months while the patient is otherwise well, then treatment with *ursodeoxycholic acid* (20 mg/kg/d) is started. Once initiated, this would continue as *lifelong therapy* at most centers.

Liver disease, including focal biliary fibrosis, may be entirely silent until a patient presents with cirrhosis. About 15% of patients have or will develop cirrhosis or important liver disease, and liver disease is the third most common cause of death, accounting for about 2.5% of CF deaths each year. The basic genotype likely comes under the influence of modifier genes and other environmental influences in these patients.

The presentation of cirrhosis may be that of hepatosplenomegaly and portal hypertension with GI bleeding. Usually this bleeding is from esophageal varices, although of course not all bleeding in patients with cirrhosis is from varices; therefore, endoscopy will be needed not just for therapy, but to diagnose the bleeding site and lesion. Endoscopy confirms the site of bleeding and rules out gastric varices, hypertensive gastropathy, or peptic ulcer disease. Usual treatment for varices is then applied, including banding or sclerotherapy. For those where bleeding is not controlled, or those who have gastric varices that cannot be banded, surgical decompression by transjugular intrahepatic portosystemic shunt or surgical shunt such as splenorenal shunt may be required. Some patients who continue to bleed despite these aggressive measures, may need to be listed for transplant as the ultimate means of decompressing the portal circulation.

Many gastroenterologists will also think about going on to secondary prevention of bleeding varices with nonselective β-blockers, such as propranolol, to decrease splanchnic pressure and cardiac output (Shashidhar et al, 1999). The respirologist caring for the patient needs to be consulted before starting this therapy to ensure it will not interfere with other therapy, such as the use of bronchodilators for lung disease. Some centers would avoid the use of β-blockers except in those cases where bleeding cannot be controlled by banding, such as patients with gastric varices or portal hypertensive gastropathy. Should the drug need to be stopped at some point, the risk for rebleeding appears to return to baseline risk. Primary prevention of variceal bleeding in CF has not been well studied. Gastroenterologists who consider either β-blockers or banding must take into account the severity of the pulmonary disease, other medications the patient may be on, and the risk for general anesthesia. All these may argue against treatment before the first bleed.

Patients with complications of portal hypertension, such as bleeding, ascites, and malnutrition, are candidates for *liver transplant*, and referral should be made at an early stage, taking into account the severity of the lung disease in the patient. We have shown that survival is good and quality of life is improved posttransplant (Mack et al, 1995). Some patients do well with transplant of liver and lungs.

Biliary Obstruction

The viscous biliary secretions may also lead to extrahepatic biliary obstruction, with gallbladder sludge and cholelithiasis occurring more commonly than normal. There is also some work demonstrating extrinsic compression of the common bile duct by the fibrotic pancreas. Standard imaging studies for these presentations should be performed and endoscopic retrograde cholangiopancreatography (ERCP) is also a useful tool.

Shwachman-Diamond Syndrome

Shwachman-Diamond syndrome (SDS) is an autosomal recessive genetic disorder that is caused by mutations of the *SBDS* gene (Boocock et al, 2003). Although the exact function of the SBDS protein is currently unknown, the most common clinical manifestations are characterized by exocrine pancreatic dysfunction, bone marrow dysfunction, and skeletal abnormalities (Mack et al, 1996). Other organs may be involved including the liver, kidneys, heart, central nervous system, and teeth. The difficulty in diagnosis lies in the variability of disease expression among individuals and the clinical symptoms can vary with age (Ginzberg et al, 2000).

Diagnosis

There are several mutations in the *SBDS* gene discovered to date and with the phenotypic variation among individuals, gene testing may become a tool similar to its use in CF as this form of testing becomes more available. By and large the diagnosis is made in infancy and is based on the constellation of clinical features, along with blood tests and radiologic investigations. Acinar and ductal exocrine pancreatic dysfunction may be quantified by pancreatic stimulation tests but they are demanding and no standard methodology has been established. Serum testing for pancreatic enzymes may be useful as a diagnostic tool in suspected patients because serum pancreatic isoamylase remains low in SDS patients in contrast to the serum cationic trypsinogen that may increase with advancing age. Bone marrow dysfunction is characterized in peripheral blood counts by persistent or intermittent anemia, leukopenia, and/or thrombocytopenia (Dror et al, 2002). Radiologic investigations reveal abnormal development in growth plates and metaphyses (Makitie et al, 2004) and imaging studies show a small fatty pancreas.

Management Issues

Stature and Skeletal Phenotypes

It is not unusual for the patients with SDS to have short stature throughout life. The mean height and weight of patients is below the 5th percentile but after infancy growth velocity normalizes and so longitudinal measurements show height and weight measurements paralleling but below the 5th percentile. However, as in all manifestations of SDS, there is variability and some SDS patients can have heights above the 25th percentile. Pancreatic enzyme replacement therapy to normalize digestion will not reverse the short stature. No phenotype-genotype correlations have been recognized for skeletal findings.

Skeletal changes are present in all patients but any given specific abnormality is age-dependent. Due to the effects of metaphyseal chondrodysplasia of the femur, patients can have persistent asymmetrical growth resulting in valgus deformities of the head and neck of the femur and varus deformities of the knees. In addition, some patients can have structural failure of metaphyseal bone of the femoral necks giving rise to fractures and varus deformities. Osteopenia and compression fractures have been documented in SDS patients. Patients should have their bone mineral density monitored. Serial radiographic determinations in patients with skeletal deformities or examinations of sites of bony pain (eg, spinal radiographs for vertebral compression fractures) should be performed.

Orthopedic interventions may be needed. With exocrine pancreatic involvement being a prominent feature of SDS patients, vitamin D status should be monitored and corrected by ensuring good calcium and vitamin D intake and adequate pancreatic enzyme replacement therapy for pancreatic insufficient patients.

EXOCRINE PANCREAS FUNCTION

SDS is the second most common inherited cause of exocrine PI after CF. Unlike pancreatic disease in CF, pancreatitis is not a feature of SDS and there is normal pancreatic fluid and bicarbonate secretion (Stormon and Durie, 2002). Virtually all patients have some degree of exocrine pancreatic dysfunction though the degree of dysfunction is variable. Thus, quantitative tests of exocrine pancreatic function remain abnormal but some patients may not require pancreatic enzyme replacement therapy for normal fat digestion (ie, they are pancreatic sufficient). Furthermore, about 50% of patients may show improvement in exocrine pancreatic function with advancing age such that they become pancreatic sufficient and no longer need pancreatic enzyme replacement therapy. Consequently, if a patient with this condition has not been re-evaluated for some time to verify whether there is a continued need for pancreatic enzyme replacement therapy then obtaining a serum trypsinogen would be useful. If the serum trypsinogen is in the intermediate or normal range (> 6 µg/L) then performing a 72-hour fecal fat collection to evaluate fat digestion is indicated. One must remember that even though the serum trypsinogen and fecal fat determinations may improve with age, the serum pancreatic isoamylase and possibly other pancreatic digestive enzymes do not. Consequently, there may continue to be benefit from pancreatic enzyme replacement capsules as they contain a mixture of enzymes. Fat-soluble vitamin deficiencies should be monitored and corrected with supplementation.

HEMATOLOGY DYSFUNCTION

All cellular lines of the bone marrow may be abnormal. The most common hematologic abnormality is neutropenia and it is usually intermittent. As well, anemia with low reticulocytes and thrombocytopenia may be identified. As a result of bone marrow dysfunction SDS patients are at risk of bleeding, developing severe infections, and suffering from periodontal disease. In cases of life threatening infection, granulocyte-colony stimulating factor (G-CSF) may be required. All three cell lines can be involved, and patients with this complication are at a greater risk of developing severe aplasia, advanced myelodysplastic syndrome, or acute myeloid leukemia. SDS-related leukemia carries a poor prognosis. Ongoing consultation with an hematologist would be advisable to decide how often to perform blood tests and bone marrow aspirations. One suggestion has been to recheck blood work every 4 months and perform yearly bone marrow aspirations in SDS patients without complications and, for patients with severe cytopenia, to have blood tests repeated every 1 to 3 months with bone marrow aspirations performed every 3 to 6 months.

LIVER ABNORMALITIES

Hepatomegaly and biochemical abnormalities tend to normalize with increasing age.

Chronic Pancreatitis

Mutation Analysis

The development of chronic pancreatitis is the end-result of a process whereby recurrent acute pancreatitis events occur because of increased susceptibility, triggering events and the development of a fibrotic and destructive response. Pancreatitis may develop as the result of both intra-acinar or intraductal events. Molecular techniques applied to groups of patients and families with a high prevalence of pancreatitis are yielding information as to mechanisms whereby gene mutations increase susceptibility in the development of acute pancreatitis events. In the pancreatic parenchymal cells an imbalance in the activation of proteases and their inhibition may be integral to the process. Small amounts of active trypsin are normally generated from its inactive precursor, most notably cationic trypsinogen. Trypsin molecules are kept in check by protease inhibitors, such as serine protease inhibitor Kazal type 1 (ie, SPINK1; also known as pancreatic secretory trypsin inhibitor or PST1) and autolysis. However, when 10 to 20% of cationic trypsinogen (ie, protease, serine 1; PRSS1) becomes activated, the inhibitory SPINK1 mechanism becomes overwhelmed and a cascade of events can follow with the end result of pancreatitis (Whitcomb, 2002; Witt, 2003; Naruse, 2003). Some mutations in *PRSS1* (eg, arginine-histidine substitution at residue 122 [R122H]) result in increased autoactivation and yield a trypsin resistant to autolysis, whereas other mutations, such as the asparagine-isoleucine substitution at residue 29 (N29I), appear to have increased autoactivation only. Mutations in *SPINK1* (eg, asparagines-serine substitution at residue 34-N34S) result in loss of the SPINK1 line of defense resulting in more intracellular trypsin. It is the acinar ductal cells where expression of CFTR occurs. *CFTR* mutations have been classified by the CF genetic analysis into various classes based on their predicted molecular dysfunction, and there are a number of proposed mechanisms whereby pancreatitis can develop based on the fluid and electrolyte alterations in the duct with the resultant effect of acinar inflammation (Freedman et al, 2000). Disparate clinical consequences might be predicted at different gene mutation sites but interestingly any given mutation has a spectrum of phenotypic expression. A number of mutations in the above 3 genes have been described, including over 1,000 for *CFTR* and around 10 so far for *PRSS1* and *SPINK1* (http://archive.uwcm.ac.uk/uwcm/mg/hgmd0.html). The spectrum of phenotypic expression between individuals remains unexplained but may be as a result of combinations of mutations. For instance, CF individuals homozygous for the most common *CFTR* mutation (deletion of the phenylalanine residue at position 508 [ie, ΔF508]) have evidence of pancreatitis early in life (fetal and neonatal) and generally are pancreatic insufficient. Individuals that present with chronic pancreatitis rather than typical CF manifestations may be compound heterozygotes for *CFTR* (Cohn et al, 2002). As well, there may be synergism with non-*CFTR* gene modifiers. For instance, mutational analysis of patients with chronic pancreatitis has yielded individuals trans-heterozygous for a *CFTR* mutation and a mutation in *SPINK1* (Audrezet et al, 2002; Noone et al, 2001). Thus, mutations in genes associated with pancreatic functioning can create an environment in the pancreas that modifies responses to pancreatic insults and places individuals at risk of developing pancreatitis. Then, other processes lead to the development of chronic pancreatitis and tissue destruction.

Patient Counseling and Monitoring

The clinical signs and symptoms of pancreatitis in individuals with genetic mutations such as R122H in *PRSS1* are not different from those induced by other causes, such as alcohol (Whitcomb et al, 2002). However, the presence of hereditary mutations such as *R122H* in *PRSS1*-hereditary pancreatitis and *CFTR* in CF are significant risk factors for development of pancreatic cancer (Lowenfels et al, 2000). The presence of pancreatitis-associated mutations (eg, *ΔF508*, *R122H*) themselves is not important in the development of pancreatic cancer. However, the pancreatitis-associated genes result in an environment of chronic inflammation that is postulated to increase the penetrance of other germline mutations that promote oncogenesis of the pancreas. It would seem quite reasonable to counsel patients to *avoid alcohol intake* because it is a controllable environmental risk factor in the etiology of pancreatitis. *Smoking* appears to double the high risk of pancreatic cancer and *lower* the mean age of development of pancreatic cancer by 20 years for those with hereditary pancreatitis. Thus, *avoidance of cigarette smoking* should be advocated because it is also a controllable environmental factor associated with the development of pancreatic cancer. There is a separate chapter on smoking and GI diseases (see Chapter 45, "Smoking and Gastrointestinal Disease"). Because of the significant risk in the development of pancreatic cancer, screening for it (endoscopic US, helical CT, ERCP) should be offered to those patients at the age of 40 years with known gene mutations (Ulrich, 2001). There is a separate chapter on cysts and precancerous lesions of the pancreas (see Chapter 143, "Neoplastic Cysts and Other Precancerous Lesions of the Pancreas"). Other long term concerns related to the destruction of the pancreas include the development of PI in 20% of patients and the development of diabetes mellitus in 7.5%. Assessment and appropriate therapy for both should be part of the long term follow-up of these patients (Sossenheimer et al, 1997).

Gene Screening

Phenotype penetrance is not 100% related to genotype, and genetic testing can have significant psychological and practical implications for the individual regarding lifestyle, work, and insurability. Information gained from gene analysis must be balanced with patient implications. A consensus conference recommended testing for *PRSS1* R122H and N29I for patients with unexplained recurrent acute pancreatitis, unexplained chronic pancreatitis, and a family history of chronic pancreatitis. Additionally, for children with unexplained pancreatitis the consideration of the above *PRSS1* mutations and *SPINK1* N34S mutation can be justified (Ellis et al, 2001). Screening of a greater number of mutations has been also advocated since the consensus conference report but still only half of chronic pancreatitis patients were found to have one of the currently known mutations.

Supplemental Reading

Andersen DH. Cystic fibrosis of the pancreas and its relation to celiac disease. Am J Dis Child 1938;56:344–99.

Audrezet MP, Chen JM, Le Marechal C, et al. Determination of the relative contribution of three genes—the cystic fibrosis transmembrane conductance regulator gene, the cationic trypsinogen gene, and the pancreatic secretory trypsin inhibitor gene—to the etiology of idiopathic chronic pancreatitis. Eur J Hum Genet 2002;10:100–6.

Boocock GRB, Morrison JA, Popover M, et al. Mutations in SBDS are associated with Shwachman-Diamond syndrome. Nat Genet 2003;33:97–101.

Borowitz D, Baker RD, Stallings V. Consensus report on nutrition for pediatric patients with cystic fibrosis. J Pediatr Gastroenterol Nutr 2002;35:246–59.

Borowitz D, Grand RJ, Durie PR. Use of pancreatic enzyme supplements for patients with cystic fibrosis in the context of fibrosing colonopathy. J Pediatr 1995;127:681–4.

Cohn JA, Noone PG, Jowell PS. Idiopathic pancreatitis related to *CFTR*: complex inheritance and identification of a modifier gene. J Invest Med 2002;50:247–55S.

Di Sant'Agnese PA, David PB. Cystic fibrosis in adults: 75 cases and a review of 232 cases in the literature. Am J Med 1979;66:121–32.

Dror Y, Freedman MH. Shwachman-Diamond syndrome. Br J Haematol 2002:118:701–13.

Ellis I, Lerch MM, Whitcomb DC, et al. Genetic testing for hereditary pancreatitis—guidelines for indications, counseling, consent and privacy issues. Pancreatology 2001;1:405–15.

Fitzsimmons SC, Burkhart GA, Borowitz D, et al. High-dose pancreatic-enzyme supplements and fibrosing colonopathy in children with cystic fibrosis. N Engl J Med 1998;336:1283–9.

Fomon SJ, Ziegler EE, Thomas LN, et al. Excretion of fat by normal full-term infants fed various milks and formulas. Am J Clin Nutr 1970;23:1299–313.

Freedman SD, Blanco P, Shea JC, et al. Mechanisms to explain pancreatic dysfunction in cystic fibrosis. Gastroenterol Clin North Am 2000;84:657–64.

Ginzberg H, Shin J, Ellis L, et al. Segregation analysis in Shwachman-Diamond syndrome: evidence for recessive inheritance. Am J Hum Genet 2000;66:1413–6.

Gullo L, Graziano L, Babbini S, et al. Faecal elastase 1 in children with cystic fibrosis. Eur J Pediatr 1997;156:770–2.

Hendriks HJE, van Kreel B, Forget PP. J Pediatr Gastrenterol Nutr 2001;33:260–5.

Hodson ME, Mearns MB, Batten JC. BMJ 1976;2:790–1.

Lenaerts C, Lapierre C, Patriquin H, et al. Surveillance for cystic fibrosis-associated hepatobiliary disease: early ultrasound changes and predisposing factors. J Pediatr 2003;143:343–50.

Lloyd-Still JD, Uhing MR, Arango V, et al. The effect of intestinal permeability on pancreatic enzyme-induced enteropathy in the rat. J Pediatr Gastroenterol Nutr 1998;26:489–95.

Lowenfels AB, Maisonneuve P, Whitcomb DC. Risk factors for cancer in hereditary pancreatitis. Med Clin North Am 2000;84:565–72.

Mack DR, Flick JA, Durie PR, et al. Correlation of intestinal lactulose permeability with exocrine pancreatic dysfunction. J Pediatr 1992;120:696–701.

Mack DR, Forstner GG, Wilschanski M, et al. Shwachman syndrome: exocrine pancreatic dysfunction and variable phenotypic expression. Gastroenterology 1996;111:1593–602.

Mack DR, Traystman MD, Colombo JL, et al. Clinical denouement and mutation analysis of patients with cystic fibrosis undergoing liver transplantation for biliary cirrhosis. J Pediatr 1995;127:881–7.

Makitie O, Ellis L, Durie PR, et al. Skeletal phenotype in patients with Shwachman-Diamond syndrome and mutations in *SBDS*. Clin Genet 2004;65:101–12.

Naruse S. Molecular pathophysiology of pancreatitis. Intern Med 2003;42:288–9.

Neglia JP, Fitzsimmons SC, Maisonneuve P, et al. The risk of cancer among patients with cystic fibrosis. N Engl J Med 1995;11:434–7.

Noone PG, Knowles MR. 'CFTR-opathies': disease phenotypes associated with cystic fibrosis transmembrane regulator gene mutations. Respir Res 2001;2:238–332.

Noone PG, Zhou Z, Silverman LM, et al. Cystic fibrosis gene mutations and pancreatitis risk-relation to epithelial ion transport and trypsin inhibitor gene mutations. Gastroenterology 2001;121:1310–9.

Pencharz PB, Durie PR. Pathogenesis of malnutrition in cystic fibrosis, and its treatment. Clin Nutr 2000;19:387–94.

Schibli S, Corey M, Durie P. The pancreatic stimulation test– factors that influence validity [abstract]. J Pediatr Gastroenterol Nutr 2003;37:361–2.

Shashidhar H, Langhans N, Grand RJ. Propranolol in prevention of portal hypertensive hemorrhage in children: a pilot study. J Pediatr Gastroenterol Nutr 1999;29:12–7.

Smyth RL, Van Velzen D, Smyth AR, et al. Strictures of ascending colon in cystic fibrosis and high-strength pancreatic enzymes. Lancet 1994;343:85–6.

Soldan W, Henker J, Sprossig C. Sensitivity and specificity of quantitative determination of pancreatic elastase 1 in feces of children. J Pediatr Gastroenterol Nutr 1997;24:53–5.

Sossenheimer MJ, Aston CE, Preston RA, et al. Clinical characteristics of hereditary pancreatitis in a large family, based on high-risk haplotype. Am J Gastroenterol 1997;92:1113–6.

Stormon MO, Durie PR. Pathophysiologic basis of exocrine pancreatic dysfunction in childhood. J Pediatr Gastroenterol Nutr 2002;35:8–21.

The Cystic Fibrosis Genetic Analysis Consortium. Population variation of common cystic fibrosis mutations. Hum Mutat 1994;4:167–77.

Ulrich CD II. Pancreatic cancer in hereditary pancreatitis—concensus guidelines for prevention, screening, and treatment. Pancreatology 2001;1:416–22.

Van de Kamer JH, Huinunk HTB, Weyers HA. Rapid method for the determination of fat in feces. J Biol Chem 1949;177:347–55.

Walkowiak J, Nousia-Arvanitakis S, Agguridaki C, et al. Longitudinal follow-up of exocrine pancreatic function in pancreatic sufficient cystic fibrosis patients using the fecal elastase-1 test. J Pediatr Gastroenterol Nutr 2003;36:474–8.

Whitcomb DC, Pogue-Geile K. Pancreatitis as a risk factor for pancreatic cancer. Gastroenterol Clin North Am 2002;31:663–78.

Whitcomb DC. How to think about SPINK and pancreatitis. Am J Gastroenterol 2002;97:1085–8.

Witt H. Chronic pancreatitis and cystic fibrosis. Gut 2003;52:ii31–41.

Zielenski J, Corey M, Rozmahel R, et al. Detection of a cystic fibrosis modifier locus for meconium ileus on human chromosome 19q13. Nat Genet 1999;22:128–9.

CHAPTER 141

Pancreatic and Periampullary Neoplasms

Richard D. Schulick, MD

Incidence

Pancreatic and periampullary neoplasms are a diverse group of tumors. The great majority of these lesions are pancreatic cancers, which have an annual incidence of approximately 28,000 cases per year in the United States (Lillemoe et al, 2000). Pancreatic cancer is the fifth leading cause of cancer-related deaths (following lung, colon, breast, and prostate), and is responsible for 5% of all cancer-related deaths. A more rare cause of pancreatic and periampullary neoplasms are neuroendocrine tumors with a reported incidence of 4 to 10 per million (Ahrendt and Demeure, 2001). The incidence of pancreatic cystic neoplasms is not well characterized, but with the more frequent use of cross-sectional imaging, many more patients with asymptomatic lesions are being discovered. There is a separate chapter on this topic (see Chapter 143, "Neoplastic Cysts and Other Precancerous Lesions of the Pancreas"). The causes of pancreatic and periampullary neoplasms are listed in Table 141-1 and Table 141-2. For anatomic and technical reasons, neoplasms of the pancreas can be divided into distal lesions (potentially require resection of the neck, body, and/or tail) and periampullary (potentially require pancreaticoduodenectomy). As can be seen by Table 141-1 and Table 141-2, the neoplasms that comprise this group of diseases are quite numerous and diverse. Pancreatic adenocarcinoma (AC) will be covered in detail. Secretory diarrhea and gastrinoma are discussed in separate chapters.

Presentation

Patients may present with mass-related signs or symptoms or conditions caused by excess hormones or vasoactive peptides. Any of the lesions may present with pain but typically, patients with periampullary ACs present with painless obstructive jaundice and/or gastric outlet obstruction. All tumors that secrete hormones or vasoactive peptides may present with the signs and symptoms of the specific hormonal excess. If not hormonally active, distal lesions tend to present with pain and or signs and symptoms of widespread metastases.

Work-Up

The great majority of patients presenting with pancreatic or periampullary neoplasms are studied with helical computed tomography (CT) scan, which anatomically places the lesion and gives information about morphology, such as whether it is solid or cystic. A multidetector, dual-phase CT scan of the pancreas with three-dimensional reconstructions is preferable. This technique gives exquisite detail about the possible involvement of the nearby vascular structures, such as the portal vein, superior mesenteric vein (SMV), superior mesenteric artery (SMA), celiac axis, and hepatic artery. Additionally, the liver and peritoneal cavity can be screened for possible involvement at the same time. Because the chest also represents a potential site of metastatic spread, it should also be screened. This may be accomplished by either a chest CT or chest radiograph.

Patients who present with biliary duct obstruction can be further worked up with biliary imaging. These include both invasive and noninvasive techniques. The most common

TABLE 141-1. Pancreatic Neoplasms

Pancreas adenocarcinoma
Pancreatic islet cell tumors
    Insulinomas
        Gastrinomas
        Glucagonomas
    VIPoma
    Nonfunctioning
Acinar cell carcinoma
Giant cell carcinoma
Solid pseudopapillary tumor
Lymphoma
Cystic
    Malignant potential
        Intraductal papillary mucinous neoplasm
        Mucinous cystic neoplasm
    Usually behave in benign fashion
        Serous cystic neoplasm

TABLE 141-2. Periampullary Neoplasms (Including Adenocarcinomas)

Pancreatic neoplasms (see Table 141-1)
Distal bile duct neoplasms
Ampulla of Vater neoplasms
Duodenal neoplasms

technique is magnetic resonance cholangiopancreatography. This technique has the advantage of being noninvasive and can be accomplished without bacterial seeding of the obstructed biliary system, and without the risk of bleeding or pancreatitis. This technique has the disadvantages of being without the possibility of making a tissue diagnosis or draining an obstructed biliary system. The common invasive techniques include endoscopic retrograde cholangiopancreatography and percutaneous transhepatic cholangiography with or without drainage. These techniques have the converse advantages and disadvantages just previously discussed. Obstructive jaundice does not need to be relieved prior to bringing a patient to the operating room if the patient is not suffering any septic or nutritional consequences of the obstruction. Several authors have reported on the increased rate of infectious and bleeding complications in patients who have undergone manipulation of their biliary trees prior to definitive resection.

In certain cases, endoscopic ultrasound (EUS) with or without biopsy may be of benefit. This technique can especially be helpful in smaller lesions not well characterized by CT or magnetic resonance imaging. This test should only be used in situations where the outcome will effect subsequent management. For example, it is rare that EUS and biopsy changes the decision to explore an elderly patient with painless obstructive jaundice, a good quality CT scan demonstrating a resectable solid mass in the head of the pancreas, no evidence of metastatic disease, and who is a good operative candidate. Additionally, patients with a good quality three-dimensional CT demonstrating resectability might be best served with exploration even if the EUS shows possible vessel involvement because of the low but real false-positive rate of the test. EUS and fine needle aspiration are discussed in a separate chapter (see Chapter 5, "Endoscopic Ultrasonography and Fine-Needle Aspiration").

Patients who present with signs and symptoms of hormonal excess or who are suspected of having a neuroendocrine tumor may benefit from other specialized testing. The value of performing the various specific biochemical and imaging tests are quite variable from patient to patient and often depend on the degree of suspicion and possible clinical consequences. Each of the specific neuroendocrine disorders that can affect the pancreas or the periampullary region has specific hormones or peptides that can be assayed for in the blood or urine. Additionally, the majority of pancreatic and periampullary neuroendocrine lesions will be detectable with octreotide scan. It is sometimes of benefit to place patients with functional carcinoid lesions on octreotide prior to resection to block the potential systemic consequences of a sudden release of serotonin with manipulation. There are separate chapters on secretory diarrhea (see Chapter 72, "Secretory Diarrhea") and on gastrinoma (see Chapter 31, "Gastroparesis").

Potentially Curative Treatment
Periampullary Lesions

It is beyond the scope of this chapter to describe in detail the operative steps in all of the potential resections. However, it is of benefit for all clinicians that take care of patients with periampullary and pancreatic neoplasms to understand the basic steps of pancreaticoduodenectomy and distal pancreatectomies, as these operations are commonly performed. Additionally, it is important for all clinicians involved to understand the potential limitations of the operation and why patients are deemed unresectable. Resections of periampullary neoplasms are usually accomplished with *pancreaticoduodenectomy*. Patients are sometimes explored first with the intent of trying a transduodenal ampullectomy and/or bile duct exploration for small and superficial lesions thought to have a high chance of being benign and/or to rule out stone disease. The decision to proceed with pancreaticoduodenectomy can be made at the time of the transduodenal procedure, depending on the operative findings or frozen sections.

Once the decision has been made to proceed with a *pancreaticoduodenectomy*, exposure is accomplished either through a vertical midline or a bilateral subcostal incision. The first portion of this procedure is devoted to assessing the extent of disease and resectability. There is debate as to the benefits of staging laparoscopy versus open staging in anticipation of surgical resection or palliation. At open exploration, the entire peritoneal cavity is assessed for the presence of metastases not seen by preoperative imaging in studies. Tumor-bearing nodes within the resection zone do not contraindicate resection because long-term survival is sometimes achieved with peripancreatic nodal involvement. An extensive Kocher maneuver is performed by elevating the duodenum and head of the pancreas out of the retroperitoneum and into the midline, allowing the visualization of the SMA at its origin at the aorta. The porta hepatis is assessed by mobilizing the gallbladder out of its fossa and dissecting the cystic duct down to the junction of the common hepatic and common bile duct. The hepatic artery is also assessed to determine that it is free of tumor involvement.

If the intraoperative assessment reveals localized disease without tumor encroachment upon resection margins, the resection is performed in relative standard fashion. If assessment reveals evidence of local tumor extension giving the early impression of unresectability, the normal sequence for performing the pancreaticoduodenectomy is modified so that the easiest and safest portions of the resection are performed first, and the more difficult portions are performed later. In cases with localized disease without tumor encroachment upon resection margins, the distal common hepatic duct is divided close to the level of the cystic duct entry site early during the operation. The gastroduodenal artery is next identified and divided. For a pylorus-preserving pancreaticoduodenectomy, the proximal gastrointestinal (GI) tract is divided 2 to 3 cm distal to the pylorus with a linear stapling device. A plane is then formed between the neck of the pancreas and the underlying anterior surface of the portal vein. For a classic Whipple procedure, a 30 to 40% distal gastrectomy is performed using a linear stapling device (Figure 141-1). The GI tract is divided distally at a point of mobile jejunum, typically 20 cm distal to the ligament of Treitz. The proximal jejunum is then separated from its mesentery and delivered dorsal to the superior mesenteric vessels from the left to the right side. The SMV caudal to the neck of the pancreas is identified while performing an extensive Kocher maneuver. The plane anterior to the SMV is developed under the neck of the pancreas. The neck of the pancreas is then divided. The specimen now remains connected by the head and uncinate process of the pancreas. These structures are separated from the portal vein, SMV, and SMA. With these areas dissected, the specimen is removed and the pancreatic neck margin, uncinate margin, bile duct margin, and duodenal or gastric margin are analyzed by intraoperative frozen section to confirm that they are free of tumor.

There are multiple options for *reconstruction* after pancreaticoduodenectomy. Most commonly the reconstruction first involves the pancreas, followed by the bile duct, ant then the duodenum. The issues and controversies surrounding the pancreatic and biliary reconstruction are outlined by multiple papers specifically addressing these issues. In brief, the pancreatic anastomosis can be performed to the jejunum or to the stomach. If the jejunum is used for reconstruction, some groups favor a separate Roux-en-Y reconstruction for pancreas or even a double Roux-en-Y reconstruction for the pancreas and bile duct. Controversy continues regarding the best type of pancreaticojejunostomy, the importance of duct-to-mucosa sutures, and the use of pancreatic duct stents. At the Johns Hopkins Hospital, the pancreatic reconstruction is typically performed with an end-to-end or end-to-side pancreaticojejunostomy to the proximal jejunum brought through a defect in the mesocolon to the right of the middle colic artery. The biliary anastomosis is typically performed with an-end-to-side hepaticojejunostomy approximately 10 to 15 cm distal from the pancreaticojejunostomy. If the patient has a percutaneous biliary stent, then this is left in place, traversing the anastomosis. The third anastomosis performed is the duodenojejunostomy in cases of pylorus preservation, or the gastrojejunostomy in patients who have undergone classic pancreaticoduodenectomy. This anastomosis is typically performed downstream from the hepaticojejunostomy, either proximal or distal to the segment of jejunum traversing the defect in the mesocolon. Figure 141-1 depicts the resection specimen and reconstruction after a pylorus preserving and classic pancreaticoduodenectomy. After reconstruction is completed, closed suction drains are left in place to drain the biliary and pancreatic anastomosis. Some groups prefer not to place closed suction drains, accepting that if a fluid collection becomes clinically evident postoperatively, percutaneous drainage by interventional radiology may be required.

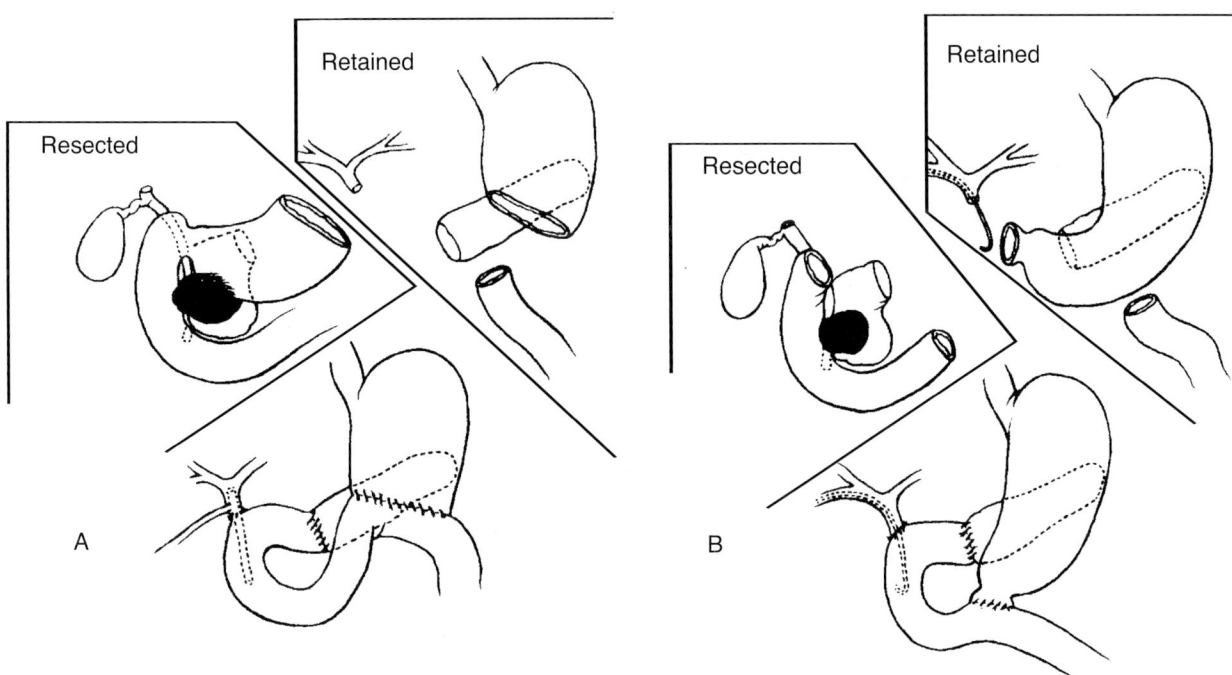

FIGURE 141-1. Classic pancreaticoduodenectomy (A) and pylorus preserving pancreaticoduodenectomy (B). From Yeo and Cameron, 1988.

Distal Lesions

Staging with laparoscopy is often of benefit with patients with distal pancreatic cancers. If metastatic disease is found, distal pancreatectomy and splenectomy are unlikely to help in the palliation of the patient. Exposure for a distal pancreatectomy and splenectomy can be obtained through a vertical midline incision, or alternatively, a bilateral subcostal incision. The spleen can technically be preserved for benign disease, however, for cancer most groups prefer to remove the spleen en bloc to gain wider margins and incorporate the lymph nodes in the splenic hilum. The spleen is mobilized towards the midline by dividing the lienorenal ligament. The short gastric vessels in the lienogastric ligament are also divided. A plane is then developed behind the pancreatic tail and body, also mobilizing the splenic artery and vein. This dissection is continued several centimeters beyond the tumor. The splenic artery and vein are isolated and suture ligated. The body or tail of the pancreas is then divided after placing a row of overlapping "U" stitches in the remnant. A frozen section is performed on the pancreatic margin to confirm clearance of the lesion and a closed suction drain is generally left in place in case of leak from the pancreatic duct. Several centers are now beginning to use laparoscopic techniques for distal lesions, especially if they have benign characteristics.

Palliative

Unfortunately, only a minority of patients with AC of the pancreas are suitable for resection and potential cure at presentation. Optimal palliation of symptoms to maximize remaining quality of life is of primary importance to most patients. Nonoperative palliation is generally readily available in most centers. The three main components of palliation of unresectable periampullary ACs include (1) drainage of the biliary tree, (2) relief of gastric outlet obstruction, and (3) pain control. The biliary tree may be drained internally or externally with *endoprostheses*, as well as *metallic wall stents* that can be inserted endoscopically or percutaneously. Some patients require percutaneous access to the biliary tree and may be best palliated via a percutaneous transhepatic drain that can be externalized when obstructed. There is a chapter on biliary tract endoscopy (see Chapter 134, "Endoscopic Management of Bile Duct Obstruction and Sphincter of Oddi Dysfunction"). New approaches for palliative endostenting of gastric outlet obstruction are now being tried with variable results. *Chemical celiac splanchnicectomy* may be performed via a transcutaneous approach and is sometimes quite effective at relieving the pain of locally invasive pancreatic cancer.

Some centers also rely on surgical palliation. Surgical palliation offers the only chance for long term palliation of the three major symptoms of periampullary AC. Biliary bypass can be performed with hepaticojejunostomy. Unlike endoscopic and percutaneous approaches, biliary bypass may be more durable. In a series reported from Johns Hopkins, recurrent jaundice developed in only 2% of patients receiving a palliative biliary bypass prior to death. (Lillemore et al, 1993) A second reason that some favor surgical palliation is that nonoperative palliation is frequently associated with late complications of gastric outlet obstruction. In a prospective randomized trial of performing a prophylactic gastrojejunostomy in patients with unresectable periampullary AC, 19% of patients not undergoing gastrojejunostomy developed late duodenal obstruction requiring intervention (Lillemore et al, 1999). The final major advantage of operative palliation is the management of pain. A prospective randomized study has demonstrated that intraoperative celiac axis injection with 50% alcohol can both successfully relieve pain in patients with pain and prevent the development of pain in patients without pain at the time of exploration (Lillemore et al, 1993).

Postoperative Results

During the 1960s and 1970s, many centers reported operative mortality rates following pancreaticoduodenectomy in the 20 to 40% range, with postoperative morbidity rates as high as 40 to 60%. During the last two decades, a dramatic decline in operative morbidity and mortality following this operation has been reported at a number of centers, with operative mortality rates in the range of 2 to 3%. Some centers have reported large series in excess of 100 patients without 1 perioperative death (Gilsdorf and Spanos, 1973). These dramatic improvements might be attributed to concentration of these patients in high volume centers with fewer but more experienced surgeons performing the operation and improved perioperative care (Sosa et al, 1997). Unfortunately, complications rates following pancreaticoduodenectomy remain high, usually in excess of 25 to 35%. Pancreatic fistula remains the most common serious complication following pancreaticoduodenectomy, with incidence raging from 5 to 15% (Lillemore et al, 1993). The overall mortality associated with pancreatic fistula has greatly diminished over the last several decades, thanks to improved management. The most frequent complication following pylorus-preserving pancreatic resection is delayed gastric emptying, with incidence ranging from 5 to 20%. In most cases, *delayed gastric emptying* is temporary and resolves spontaneously after a variable period of time, resulting in a delay in hospital discharge.

Long-Term Survival

Survival following pancreaticoduodenectomy for periampullary carcinoma is highly dependent on the tumor's site of origin. For instance, survival after resection of distal bile duct, ampullary, and duodenal AC has always been significantly greater that that for pancreatic AC, with 5-year survival rates ranging from 30 to 50% (Yeo et al, 1997) In contrast, 5-year survival rates for patients with AC in the head of the pancreas managed by pancreaticoduodenectomy have been reported to reach 21%. A number of variables have been evaluated by univariate and multivariate analyses in an attempt to identify other factors predictive of long-term survival. Tumor characteristics found by most investigators to be important predictors of survival include tumor size, lymph node status, and resection margin status.

Survival following pancreaticoduodenectomy for periampullary lesions that are not AC are strongly dependent on the histology and biologic behavior of the primary lesion resected. Benign lesions that are completely resected generally result in very high long-term survival. Neuroendocrine tumors of the pancreas that are resected may have a variable and somewhat indolent course.

Supplemental Reading

Ahrendt GM, Demeure MJ. Pancreatic islet cell tumors excluding gastrinoma. In: Cameron JL, editor. Current surgical therapy, 7th ed. St. Louis: Mosby; 2001.

Gilsdorf RB, Spanos P. Factors influencing morbidity and mortality in pancreatico-duodenectomy. Ann Surg 1973;177:332–7.

Lillemoe KD, Cameron JL, Hardacre JM, et al. Is prophylactic gastrojejunostomy indicated for unresectable perimapullary cancer? A prospective randozimed trial. Ann Surg 1999;230:322–30.

Lillemoe KD, Cameron JL, Kaufman HS, et al. Chemical splanchnicectomy in patients with unresectable pancreatic cancer. A prospective randomized trial. Ann Surg 1993;217:447–57.

Lillemoe KD, Sauter PK, Pitt HA, et al. Current status of surgical palliation of periampullary carcinoma. Surg Gynecol Obstet 1993;176:1–10.

Lillemoe KD, Yeo CJ, Cameron JL. Pancreatic cancer: state-of-the-art care. CA Cancer J Clin 2000;50:241–68.

Sosa JA, Bowman HM, Bass EB, et al. Importance of hospital volume in the surgical management of pancreatic cancer. Surg Forum 1997;48:584–6.

Yeo DJ, Cameron JL. The pancreas. In: Jardy JD, editor. Hardy's textbook of surgery, 2nd ed. Philadelphia: JB Lippincott; 1988. p. 717–8.

Yeo CJ, Cameron JL, Lillemoe KD, et al. Pancreaticoduodenectomy for cancer of the head of the pancreas. 201 patients. Ann Surg 1995;221:721–33.

Yeo DJ, Cameron JL, Sohn TA, et al. Six hundred fifty consecutive pancreaticoduodenectomies in the 1990's: Pathology, complications, outcomes. Ann Surg 1997;226:248–60.

CHAPTER 142

Pancreatic Cancer Therapy

Dan Laheru, MD

The challenges in managing patients with pancreatic cancer (PC) are underscored by the seemingly immutable survival data, including a 5-year survival of 15 to 20% with a median survival of 15 to 19 months for resectable disease and 3% survival for all stages combined. For patients with locally advanced unresectable disease, median survival is 6 to 10 months, and for patients with metastatic disease it is 3 to 6 months. This chapter will describe the current treatment recommendations as well as highlight the most recent therapy advances for resected and advanced disease.

Therapy for Adjuvant Disease

The current standard of 5-fluorouracil (5-FU) based combined modality chemoradiotherapy is originally based on data from the Gastrointestinal Tumor Study Group (GITSG). This study was the first to document that adjuvant therapy following surgical resection for pancreatic surgery prolonged survival (Kalser and Ellenberg, 1985). A number of groups have further developed this approach and have, in general, also used 5-FU based chemotherapy (Table 142-1).

Recently the Virginia Mason Medical Center published their experience of 53 patients with resected pancreatic adenocarcinoma (AC) who received combined radiotherapy (external beam at a dose of 45 to 54 Gy in standard fractions d1-35) and chemotherapy (5-FU 200 mg/m^2/d as continuous infusion, weekly cisplatin 30 mg/m^2 intravenous [IV] bolus, and interferon [IFN]-α 3 million units subcutaneously every other day) during radiation or GITSG type chemotherapy with radiation therapy. Following combined modality chemoradiotherapy, chemotherapy alone was administered (5-FU 200 mg/m^2/d as a continuous infusion) in two 6-week courses during weeks 9 to 14 and 17 to 22. There were *significant grade 3 and 4 gastrointestinal (GI) toxicities,* including vomiting, mucositis, diarrhea, and GI bleeding in the IFN-based chemotherapy, *requiring hospitalization in 43%* of patients. However, the majority of patients were still able to receive > 80% of planned therapy. The *median survival* and *2-year survival were 46 months and 53% respectively* for the IFN-based chemoradiotherapy (Picozzi et al, 2003). The American College of Surgery Oncology Group (ACOSOG) will coordinate a similar multi-institutional phase II trial in patients with pancreatic AC who are candidates for resection that has begun accrual in December 2003.

In July 2002, the Radiation Therapy Oncology Group (RTOG) closed R97-04. This phase III trial randomized 518 resected PC patients to 5-FU continuous infusion (250 mg/m^2/d for 3 weeks), followed by 5-FU continuous infusion (250 mg/m^2/d) during radiation therapy (50.4 Gy in 1.8 Gy/fractions), followed by 2 cycles 5-FU continuous

TABLE 142-1. Selected Adjuvant Studies in Pancreatic Cancer

Adjuvant Study	Number of Patients	EBRT Dose (Gy)	Chemotherapy	Median Survival (mo)	1-Year Survival	2-Year Survival	5-Year Survival
GITSG (1985)	22 surgery alone	none	none	11	49%	15%	NR
	21 to chemorad	40 split course	5-FU bolus	20 $p = .01$	63%	42%	NR
Sohn (2000)	119 surgery alone	none	none	11	48%	22 (est)	9%
(retrospective study)	333 adjuvant tx	40–50	5-FU/+/− MMC, DPM	19 $p < .001$	71%	38% (est)	20%
Picozzi (2003)	53	45–50	5-FU CI with cisplatin and IFN-α	46	88%	53%	49%
EORTC (1999)	54 surgery alone	none	none	12.6	40% (est)	23%	10%
	60 chemorad	40	5-FU bolus	17.1 $p = .099$	65% (est)	37%	20%
ESPAC1 (2001)	200 surgery alone	none	none	16.1	N/A	N/A	NR
	103 chemorad	40 split course	none	15.5	N/A	N/A	NR
	166 chemo alone	none	5-FU	19.7	60% (est)	39% (est)	16% (est)
	72 chemorad with additional chemo	40 split course	5-FU bolus	N/A	N/A	N/A	NR

CI = continuous infusion; DPM = dipyridamole; 5-FU = 5-fluorouracil; IFN = interferon-α; N/A = not applicable; NR = not reported; MMC = mitomycin; tx = treatment.

infusion, versus Gemcitabine 1000 mg/m² weekly for 3 weeks, followed by 5-FU continuous infusion during radiation therapy, followed by 3 cycles Gemcitabine alone. The experimental question being asked was whether Gemcitabine before and after 5-FU based chemoradiotherapy would be more efficacious than continuous infusion 5-FU before and after the same 5-FU based chemoradiotherapy. In 1997, when this study was designed, there was inadequate knowledge regarding how to safely administer Gemcitabine concurrently with irradiation to allow for concurrent Gemcitabine and radiotherapy. This study was the first North American Co-operative group trial since the GITSG trial. Although the survival results for this trial will not be known until 2004, a number of important observations have already been made. These include that neither arm was associated with unacceptable acute toxicity during the trial, that accrual was quite rapid (12 to 14 patients per month) reflecting both the support of the Eastern Co-operative Oncology Group (ECOG) and the Southwest Oncology Group, and the willingness of patients and their physicians to participate in adjuvant trials for PC.

Inconclusive Study Results

Despite a growing body of literature seemingly supporting the benefit of adjuvant combined modality therapy following potentially definitive resection in *patients with high risk for recurrence*, adjuvant chemoradiation *has not been universally accepted* as standard of care. A major criticism has been that none of these studies included an observation only arm.

There have now been two additional major studies that have demonstrated inconsistent or negative conclusions. A European Organization for Research and Treatment of Cancer (EORTC) trial randomized 218 patients with pancreatic and nonpancreatic periampullary AC 2 to 8 weeks following potentially curative resection to either observation or to combined radiotherapy (40 Gy using a 3 or 4 field technique in 2 Gy fractions with a 2 week break at mid-treatment) and chemotherapy (5-FU administered as a continuous infusion 25 mg/kg/d during the first week of each 2 week radiation therapy module only). No postradiation chemotherapy was administered. Median progression-free survival was 16 months in the observation arm versus 17.4 months in the treatment arm ($p = .643$). Median survival was 19 months in the observation group versus 24.5 months in the treatment group, but was not statistically significant ($p = .737$). For the subgroup of patients with pancreatic AC ($n = 114$), the median survival was 12.6 months in the observation group versus 17.1 months in the treatment arm but was not statistically significant ($p = .099$). Of note, 21 of 104 patients randomized to the treatment arm were not treated. In addition, although the original dose of 5-FU was already modest, 35 patients in the treatment arm received only 3 days of 5-FU during the second module of radiotherapy secondary to grade 1 and 2 toxicities (Klinkenbijl et al, 1999). Therefore, this study could be better described as an underpowered positive study (see Table 142-1)

Recently, the European Study Group for Pancreatic Cancer (ESPAC) randomized 541 patients with pancreatic AC in a 4 arm design based on a 2 × 2 factorial design, which included the following:

1. Observation
2. Concomitant chemoradiotherapy alone (20 Gy in 10 fractions over 2 weeks with 500 mg/m² 5-FU IV bolus during the first 3 days of radiation therapy); the module is repeated after a planned 2-week break, followed by no additional chemotherapy
3. Chemotherapy alone (leukovorin 20 mg/m² bolus followed by 5-FU 425 mg/m² administered for 5 consecutive days repeated every 28 days for 6 cycles)
4. Chemoradiotherapy followed by chemotherapy

There was *no significant difference in survival* between patients assigned to chemoradiotherapy (median survival 15.5 months) versus observation (median survival 16.1 months, $p = .24$). The survival data was similar in the subset ($n = 285$ patients) randomized through the 2 × 2 design. In contrast, there was a *survival advantage* for those patients treated with *chemotherapy alone* (median survival 19.7 months) versus the observation arm (median survival 14 months, $p = .0005$). For the same subset randomized through the original 22 design, survival demonstrated a trend towards survival for chemotherapy alone (median survival 17.4 months) versus observation alone (15.9 months) but was not statistically significant ($p = .19$). Multivariate analysis for known prognostic factors including margin status, lymph node involvement, and tumor grade and size did not alter the effect for chemoradiotherapy treatment. The study authors concluded that there was no survival benefit for adjuvant chemoradiotherapy. In addition, the authors concluded that a *potential benefit* existed for adjuvant chemotherapy alone following surgical resection (Neoptolemos et al, 2001). Although this was a randomized study consisting of over 500 patients, the *conclusions* of the *study should be carefully measured*. To encourage maximal patient recruitment, the study was modified in that 68 patients were assigned separately and randomized to either chemoradiotherapy or observation. In addition, 188 patients were subsequently assigned separately and randomized to either chemotherapy alone or observation. In a sense, three randomizations were possible for inclusion into the same study. Also, patients in the additional two randomizations could have potentially received "background chemotherapy or chemotherapy" which was not specifically defined. The background treatment was not known in 82 eligible patients. Of note, these patients were still assigned into an arm of the study despite lack of definitive knowledge of prior therapy. Finally, 25 of the eligible 541 patients refused to accept their randomization and an additional 25 patients withdrew secondary to treatment toxicities.

As the debate continues, there are several studies that have recently opened or have been proposed by either the cooperative groups or through single institutions. Table 142-2 summarizes open or planned studies in the adjuvant setting. These future studies will be characterized by the addition of multi-agent chemotherapy to irradiation at the cooperative group level, by the addition of Gemcitabine to the period of chemoradiation and by the use of conformal, three-dimensional irradiation planned to patient specific anatomic and surgical pathologic data.

CURRENT PRACTICE

Nonetheless, most practitioners in the United States employ radiation therapy (typically 54 Gy in 1.8 Gy fractions) with simultaneous chemotherapy, the standard being 5-FU. Although 5-FU can be administered in a number of different schedules, most practitioners choose either continuous infusion 200 to 250 mg/m^2/d during radiation therapy, or 500 mg/m^2 bolus given on the first 3 days and last 3 days of radiation. There is some interest in substituting an oral formulation of 5-FU known as Capecitabine for continuous infusion 5-FU. Although there is preliminary data primarily from the rectal cancer literature demonstrating that Capecitabine can be safely combined with radiation therapy, the comparison studies in PC have not been completed.

TABLE 142-2. Active or Planned Adjuvant or Neoadjuvant Studies

Study	Regimen	Study Phase
RTOG1091	Gem 1000 mg/m^2 for 2 wks, EBRT 50 Gy fx/Gem 600 mg/m^2 weekly followed by gem for 3 cycles	II
ACOSOG Z05031	EBRT (50 Gy/5-FU CI/cisplatin/IFN, 5-FU CI for 2 cycle)	
Johns Hopkins	GM-CSF allo vaccine, 5-FU CI, 5-FU CI/XRT, 5-FU CI for 2 cycles followed by GM-CSF allo vaccine for 4 cycles	II
ECOG 1200	Arm A: Gem 500 mg/m^2 over 50 min weekly for 6 wks with EBRT 50.4 Gy followed by surgery, gem 1000 mg/m^2 over 100 min for 5 cycles Arm B: Gem 175 mg/m^2 over 30 min day 1, 5, 28, 33/ cisplatin 20 mg/m^2 days 1–4, 29–33, 5-FU 500 mg/m^2 over 21 hrs days 1–4, 29–32 followed by EBRT 50.4, surgery, gemzar for 3 cycles	

allo = allogeneic; CI = continuous infusion; 5-FU = 5-fluorouracil; Gem = gemcitabine; GM-CSF = granulocyte macrophage colony stimulating factor; IFN = interferon-α; LV = leukovorion; MMC = mitocycin.

Role of Neoadjuvant Therapy

POTENTIAL ADVANTAGES

Neoadjuvant therapy is a potentially attractive alternative to current standard adjuvant chemoradiation for several reasons, including the following:

1. Radiation is more effective on well-oxygenated cells that have not been devascularized by surgery
2. Contamination and subsequent seeding of the peritoneum with tumor cells secondary to surgery could theoretically be reduced
3. Patients with metastatic disease on restaging following adjuvant therapy would not need to undergo definitive resection and might benefit from palliative intervention
4. The risk of delaying adjuvant therapy would be eliminated because it would be delivered in the neoadjuvant setting

There is significant published data primarily from MD Anderson Cancer Center and Fox Chase Cancer Center using chemoradiotherapy in a neoadjuvant approach for resectable PC. To date, the current data demonstrate that although neoadjuvant chemoradiotherapy can be administered safely, there is no clear advantage to this strategy when compared with postoperative therapy. In patients with marginally resectable disease, it remains to be seen whether there is a meaningful cohort of patients for whom this approach may represent an important therapeutic advantage based on "downstaging" and improved surgical outcomes.

Currently, the ECOG is planning to open a prospective randomized trial randomizing patients to intensified Gemcitabine based or Gemcitabine/5-FU/platinum based chemoradiotherapy. This trial makes an important distinction between clearly unresectable disease and potentially resectable disease, especially around the issues of partial versus complete encasement of the superior mesenteric artery and the length of superior mesenteric vein involved by tumor at initial presentation.

Treatment of Locally Advanced Disease

Pancreatic tumors frequently invade adjacent structures, such as superior mesenteric and celiac vascular structures, making curative resection difficult if not impossible. The Memorial Sloan Kettering group recently reviewed their experience of 163 patients with locally advanced PC. A number of chemotherapy regimens were integrated with radiation therapy and administered to 87 patients. Only three patients had sufficient radiographic response to justify surgical exploration. Of these selected patients, one of these underwent resection for curative intent (Kim et al, 2002). For the approximately 30 to 40% of PC patients who present with such locally advanced, nonmetastatic disease, optimal management is controversial. Palliative surgery, chemoradiation, chemotherapy alone, and locally directed therapies have all been employed in this setting.

Metastatic Disease

In patients with metastatic disease, the current standard of care is single agent Gemcitabine. Burris and colleagues (1997) randomized 126 patients with unresectable PC to either *Gemcitabine* (1000 mg/m^2 weekly over a 30 minute infusion 7 times followed by 1 week rest then weekly 3 times every 4 weeks) or 5-FU (600 mg/m^2 weekly). Although the primary endpoints were issues related to quality of life (performance status, weight gain, analgesic consumption, and pain), median survival was 5.7 months in the Gemcitabine arm compared with 4.4 months in the 5-FU arm. In addition, 1-year survival was 18% in the Gemcitabine arm compared with 2% in the 5-FU arm ($p = .0025$) with median time to progression also favoring Gemcitabine (9 weeks compared with 4 weeks in the 5-FU arm, $p = .0002$). Gemcitabine was well tolerated with the majority of side effects related to grade 3 or 4 neutropenia (26%) without associated infections, low grade fevers (30%), and nausea and vomiting (9.5% and 3.2%) (Burris et al, 1997). Based on this study, Gemcitabine was approved for the treatment of patients with advanced PC in the United States and many other countries and is currently considered the standard agent for the treatment of this disease as well as the accepted control with which to compare new drugs and interventions.

Recent efforts have focused on developing strategies that would enhance the efficacy of Gemcitabine and ultimately improve on median survival. These strategies include identifying alternative dosing schedules of Gemcitabine that might enhance drug delivery to tumor cells, as well as identifying synergistic combinations with other chemotherapeutic agents. Tempero and colleagues (2003) randomized 92 patients to either Gemcitabine (2200 mg/m^2) over the standard 30-minute infusion or Gemcitabine (1500 mg/m^2) at a rate of 10 mg/m^2/min. The drug was given weekly for 3 consecutive weeks every 4 weeks in both arms of the study. Patients treated with the fixed-dose-rate regimen experienced more toxicity, with a 49 and 37% occurrence of neutropenia and thrombocytopenia versus a 28 and 10% occurrence, respectively, in patients treated in the conventional schedule (Tempero et al, 2003). Patients on the fixed-dose-rate had a higher response rate (11.6 vs 4.1 %), median survival (8 vs 5 months, $p = .013$) and 1-year survival (23.8 vs 7.3 %) than patients treated on the conventional schedule. This strategy is now being tested in randomized phase III studies.

Other potentially synergistic agents that have been used with Gemcitabine include Cisplatin, Irinotecan, 5-FU, antifolates, such as raltitrexed and pemetrexed, and Taxotere and Oxaliplatin. Some of these studies are highlighted in Table 142-3. Although some of these studies appear promising, the results are preliminary.

New Drugs in PC

During the last few years, an increasing number of new drugs, many of them targeted to specific alterations in malignant cells, have been tested in PC. The rationale to develop these drugs in PC comes from the better understanding of the biological basis of the disease that has made possible the identification and validation of some of these targets in PC. In addition, the poor prognosis of patients with this disease and the evidence from clinical trials discussed above that conventional chemotherapy may have reached a plateau with regards to improving outcome has also motivated an aggressive evaluation of new drugs in PC. To date, targeted drugs such as the matrix metalloproteinase inhibitors (marimastat and Bay12-9566), inhibitors of angiogenesis (bevacizumab), agents targeted to the *ras* oncogene (R115777 and Lonafarnib), and inhibitors of the epidermal growth factor receptor (EGFR) family of membrane receptors (trastuzimab, ceuximab),

TABLE 142-3. Selected Studies in Advanced Pancreatic Cancer

Study	Patient Number	Chemotherapy	PR/CR Rate	Median Survival (mo)	1-Year Survival
Burris (1997)	63	5-FU bolus	0 (0%)	4.4	2%
	63	Gemcitabine	3 (5.4%)	5.7 $p = .0025$	18%
Tempero (2003)	49	Gem standard infusion	2 of 22 (9.1%)	5	9%
	43	Gem fixed infusion	1 of 17 (5.9%)	8 $p = .13$	28.80%
Heinemann (2003)	96	Gem	NR	6	NR
	99	Gem+cisplatin	NR	8.3 $p = .12$	NR
Rocha Lima (2003)	173	Gem	8 (4.4%)	6.6	NR
	169	Gem+irinotecan	27 (16%)	6.3 $p = ns$	22%
Louvet (2003)	156	Gem	25 (16%)	NR	NR
	152	Gem+oxaliplatin	39 (26%)	NR	NR
Fine (2002)	33	Gem/Taxol/Xeloda	20 (66%)	Not reached	NR

5-FU = 5-fluorouracil; Gem = gemcitabine; NR = no response; PR = partial response.

immunotherapy and gene therapy have been evaluated in this patient population with mixed results.

Summary

Gemcitabine is currently the only approved chemotherapeutic agent that has demonstrated significant antitumor effects in advanced PC. Although the efficacy of Gemcitabine may be augmented by innovative dosing schedules or by the use of synergistic drug combinations, the standard regimen to date remains single agent Gemcitabine. This strategy is also appropriate for patients with locally advanced disease, though these patients are commonly managed with combined modality approaches. Either a conventional 30-minute or fixed-dose-rate infusion is appropriate based on existing data. Combinations of Gemcitabine with other agents such as cisplatin, irinotecan, oxaliplatin, and fluoropyrimidines have not consistently resulted in significant improvement in survival or quality of life in studies available thus far and should not be considered the standard of care at the present time; however, this could change as the results of randomized studies are available. Given the data with conventional treatments, enrollment in a clinical trial should still be the preferred approach to these patients.

Supplemental Reading

Burris HA, Moore MJ, Anderson J, et al. Improvements in survival and clinical benefit with gemcitabine as first-line therapy for patients with advanced pancreas cancer: a randomized trial. J Clin Oncol 1997;15:2403–13.

Fine RL, Sherman W, Chabot J, et al. Biochemically synergistic chemotherapy for advanced pancreatic cancer [abstract 575]. Proc ASCO 2002;21:145a.

Heinemann V, Quietzsch D, Gieseler F, et al. A phase III trial comparing gemcitabine plus cisplatin vs gemcitabine alone in advanced pancreatic carcinoma [abstract 1003]. Proc ASCO 2003;22:250.

Kalser MH, Ellenberg SS. Pancreatic cancer: adjuvant combined radiation and chemotherapy following curative resection. Arch Surg 1985;120:899–903.

Kim HJ, Kzischke K, Brennan MF, et al. Does neoadjuvant chemoradiation downstage locally advanced pancreatic cancer? J Gastrointest Surg 2002;6:763–9.

Klinkenbijl JH, Jeekel J, Sahmoud T, et al. Adjuvant radiotherapy and 5-Fluorouracil after curative resection of cancer of the pancreas and periampullary region. Ann Surg 1999;230:776–84.

Louvet C, Labianca R, Hammel P, et al. Gemcitabine versus GEMOX (Gemcitabine + oxaliplatin) in nonresectable pancreatic adenocarcinoma: interim results of the GERCOR/GISCAD Intergroup Phase III [abstract 1004]. Proc ASCO 2003;22:250.

Neoptolemos JP, Dunn JA, Stocken DD, et al. Adjuvant chemoradiotherapy and chemotherapy in resectable pancreatic cancer: a randomized controlled trial. Lancet 2001;358:1576–85.

Picozzi VJ, Kozarek RE, Jacobs AD, et al. Adjuvant therapy for resected pancreas cancer (PC) using alpha-interferon (IFN)-based chemoradiation: completion of a phase II trial [abstract 1061]. Proc ASCO 2003;22:265.

Rocha Lima CMS, Rotche R, Jeffery M, et al. A randomized phase III study comparing efficacy and safety of gemcitabine (GEM) and Irinotecan (I), to gemcitabine (GEM) alone in patients with locally advanced or metastatic pancreatic cancer who have not received prior systemic therapy [abstract 1005]. Proc ASCO 2003;22:251.

Sohn TA, Yeo CJ, Cameron JL, et al. Resected adenocrcinoma of the pancreas-616 patients: results, outcomes, and prognostic indicators. J Gastrointest Surg 2000;4:567–79.

Tempero M, Plunkett W, van Haperan VR, et al. Randomized phase II comparison of dose-intense Gemcitabine: thirty-minute infusion and fixed dose rate infusion in patients with pancreatic adenocarcinoma. J Clin Oncol 2003;21:1–7.

CHAPTER 143

Neoplastic Cysts and Other Precancerous Lesions of the Pancreas

Ralph H. Hruban, MD, Michael Goggins, MD, and Charles J. Yeo, MD, FACS

Pancreatic cancer (PC) is an almost uniformly fatal disease and the vast majority of patients do not come to clinical attention until after the cancer has spread. One of the few opportunities to cure patients with a malignant pancreatic neoplasm is to identify and remove it prior to invasion. The three most common preinvasive neoplasms of the pancreas are intraductal papillary mucinous neoplasms (IPMNs), mucinous cystic neoplasms (MCNs), and the recently defined pancreatic intraepithelial neoplasia. This chapter will review the current state of our knowledge for each of these three entities.

IPMNs

IPMNs were first recognized by Japanese gastroenterologists in 1980 (Ohhashi et al, 1982). IPMNs are now much more widely recognized and currently account for 20% of all cystic neoplasms of the pancreas. As the name suggests, IPMNs are large, intraductal proliferations of usually papillary mucinous epithelium. These distinctive neoplasms occur with similar frequency in both men and women, and the average age at diagnosis is 65 years (range 25 to 94 years). Clinically, most patients present with abdominal pain, weight loss, anorexia, or pancreatitis. Remarkably, by the time a diagnosis can be established, most patients will report that these symptoms have been present for years. Abdominal imaging will often reveal dilatation of the main pancreatic duct, usually in the *head of the gland. Mucin oozing* from a *patulous ampulla of Vater* is an almost diagnostic finding on endoscopic retrograde pancreatography (ERCP). Clinical laboratory data are generally nonspecific.

IPMNs are pathologically distinctive neoplasms. Grossly they are characterized by dilatation of the main pancreatic duct or one of its branches by a prominent papillary mucin-producing neoplasm. As noted earlier, these neoplasms arise in the head of the gland more frequently than they arise in the tail of the gland. Microscopically, IPMNs are papillary growths of columnar mucin-producing epithelium. This epithelium can show varying degrees of atypia. IPMNs without significant cytologic or nuclear atypia are designated *IPMN-adenoma*, those with moderate cytologic and/or nuclear atypia *IPMN-boderline*, and those with significant dysplasia *IPMN-carcinoma in situ*.

IPMNs primarily involving the main pancreatic duct are designated "main duct IPMNs," whereas those involving a side branch are appropriately designated "side branch variants." *One-third of all IPMNs have an associated invasive adenocarcinoma (AC).* In half the cases this invasive carcinoma has a "*colloid*" or "*muconodular*" pattern of invasion, and in the other half a "*tubular*" or "*ductal*" pattern. The diagnosis of an invasive carcinoma is based on the presence of tissue invasion by the neoplastic cells. Metastases to lymph nodes are seen in a third of IPMNs that harbor an associated invasive carcinoma. IPMNs with an invasive colloid carcinoma may have a better prognosis than IPMNs with an invasive tubular type of AC.

Surgery and Survival

Surgical resection is the therapy of choice for both noninvasive and invasive IPMNs. Surgical strategies at present include the appropriate resection of the neoplasm with negative resection margins. In most patients this is followed by periodic *postoperative surveillance* for recurrent disease. For example, if an IPMN of the head of the gland is resected and the tail left in place, then the residual duct system can be followed with *annual magnetic resonance cholangiopancreatography. Most* patients with an IPMN are *surgically resectable* (between 80 and 98%). The *5-year survival* rate for patients with surgically resected noninvasive IPMNs is > 90%, whereas the 5-year survival rate for patients with surgically resected IPMN with an *associated invasive carcinoma is only 40%*. The surgically resected patients with noninvasive IPMNs who recur presumably had multifocal disease in the pancreas because the 5-year survival rate for patients with noninvasive IPMNs who undergo total pancreatectomy approaches 100%.

The long history of symptoms experienced by most patients, the association of noninvasive IPMNs with an invasive cancer, and molecular genetic analyses of IPMNs, *all suggest that noninvasive IPMNs can and do progress to invasive cancer over time.* Although the time course or natural history of this progression is not known at present, the fact that some IPMNs do progress suggests an enormous opportunity to save lives that would otherwise be lost to invasive PC. If noninvasive IPMNs can be detected and surgically resected before an invasive cancer develops, then lives could be saved. The large size of most noninvasive IPMNs (3 cm in some series), suggests that it should be possible to detect these neoplasms using conventional imaging techniques such as endoscopic ultrasound (EUS) or computerized tomography. Indeed, we have recently reported an asymptomatic patient who was found to have a noninvasive IPMN by EUS. He underwent EUS because of a history that suggested he was at increased risk for developing a pancreatic neoplasm (see later section on familial PC). The IPMN was resected and this patient is presumably cured before a life threatening invasive cancer developed.

MCNs

MCNs of the pancreas are distinctive cystic neoplasms that arise *primarily (90%) in women*. In contrast to IPMNs, which usually arise in the head of the gland and in the larger pancreatic ducts, MCNs usually arise in the *tail* of the gland. *MCNs almost never connect to the larger pancreatic ducts.* The mean age at diagnosis is between 40 and 50 years (range 14 to 95 years) and most patients present with nonspecific symptoms including epigastric pain or a sense of abdominal fullness. These patients can also develop gastrointestinal (GI) symptoms, including nausea and vomiting, diarrhea, anorexia, and weight loss. Remarkably, as many as 20% of MCNs are discovered incidentally during abdominal imaging for unrelated indications. This percentage can be expected to increase with the growing use of screening imaging studies in asymptomatic individuals.

Pathologically, MCNs are usually large (mean 7 to 10 cm) cystic masses filled with thick tenacious mucin. In contrast to IPMNs, these neoplasms typically do not connect with the larger pancreatic ducts, and therefore these patients do *not* have mucin oozing from the ampulla of Vater. MCNs are lined by a columnar mucin-producing epithelium, and, of note, they have a dense underlying stroma that resembles the stroma seen in the ovary ("ovarian stroma"). Just as was true for IPMNs, MCNs can show varying degrees of atypia. Noninvasive MCNs without significant cytologic or architectural atypia are designated *mucinous cystadenoma*, those with moderate architectural and/or cytologic atypia are designated *MCNs with moderate dysplasia*, and those with significant architectural and cytologic atypia are designated *MCN-in situ carcinoma*. *One-third* of all MCNs are *associated with an invasive AC*. These neoplasms are designated as *mucinous cystadenocarcinomas with an associated invasive carcinoma*. The invasive carcinomas are usually a tubular/ductal type of invasive AC. The diagnosis of an invasive carcinoma is based on the presence of tissue invasion by the neoplastic cells. *Lymph node metastases* are identified in about one-fourth of all surgically resected mucinous cystadenocarcinomas with an associated invasive carcinoma.

Surgery and Survival

Surgical resection is the treatment of choice for all MCNs. The 5-year disease-specific survival rate for patients with surgically resected noninvasive MCNs is 100%. If an invasive cancer is present, the 5-year disease specific survival rate drops to 50%. The survival rate for patients with unresectable mucinous cystadenocarcinomas with an associated invasive carcinoma is even worse (20% at 2 years). *The goal of surgical resection of MCNs is complete resection of the neoplasm with negative margins.* It may be possible to preserve the spleen in patients with left-sided tumors without an invasive component.

Just as is true for patients with IPMNs, the long history of symptoms experienced by most patients with MCNs, the association of noninvasive MCNs with an invasive cancer, and molecular genetic analyses of MCNs, all *suggest that noninvasive MCNs can and do progress to invasive cancer over time*. This has enormous clinical implications. It suggests that the lives of patients with MCNs can be saved if their neoplasms can be detected and surgically resected before an invasive cancer develops.

MCNs should be distinguished from *serous cystadenomas* of the pancreas because the latter are almost always *benign*. The presence of a central stellate scar and innumerable small cysts should suggest the diagnosis of a serous cystadenoma.

Pancreatic Intraepithelial Neoplasia

Pancreatic intraepithelial neoplasms (PanINs) are microscopic lesions in the small pancreatic ducts and ductules. Although these lesions have been recognized for decades, their clinical importance as the likely noninvasive precursors to invasive AC of the pancreas has only recently been established.

PanINs are not recognizable grossly. Instead, these are *small microscopic lesions*. PanINs can show varying degrees of atypia, and a system to classify these lesions has recently been adopted. *PanIN-1A* is the designation given to flat lesions without significant atypia and *PanIN-1B* to papillary lesions without atypia. Lesions with moderate dysplasia are designated *PanIN-2*, and those with significant architectural and cytologic atypia are designated *PanIN-3* (carcinoma in situ).

Three lines of evidence strongly suggest that PanINs are the precursors to invasive AC of the pancreas. First, PanINs are often found in the pancreatic parenchyma adjacent to an invasive AC. Second, there have been several anecdotal case reports of patients with histologically proven PanINs who later develop an invasive AC. Third, molecular genetic analyses of PanINs have shown that they harbor many of the same genetic alterations found in invasive pancreatic ACs. Therefore, just as there is a progression in the colorectum from adenoma to invasive carcinoma, so too do *we believe that there is a progression in the pancreas from PanIN-1 to PanIN-2 to PanIN-3 and eventually to invasive AC*. This has enormous clinical potential, considering the almost uniformly fatal outcome of invasive AC of the pancreas. We also know from autopsy studies of patients without known pancreatic disease that PanINs occur with increasing frequency with advancing age, but in the absence of an invasive cancer these are almost always low grade PanINs (PanIN-1).

Clearly, if techniques can be developed to prevent, detect, and treat PanINs, particularly high grade PanINs, before they develop into an invasive AC, then lives will be saved. Unfortunately, PanINs are extremely small lesions; they are significantly smaller than the resolution of most currently available imaging modalities. A great deal of effort is therefore going into the development of *molecular based screening/diagnostic tests* that have the potential to detect neoplasms as small as PanINs.

At-Risk Publications

Clearly, as exciting as the characterization of each of these noninvasive precursor lesions in the pancreas is, the challenge is to define subgroups in the population who might best benefit from screening for early pancreatic neoplasia. Individuals with a strong family history of PC and individuals with certain genetic syndromes may represent a subgroup at great enough risk to warrant screening.

Familial PC

Although the familial aggregation of other forms of cancer has been recognized for decades, the importance of family history as a risk factor for PC has become clearer in the past several years. Individuals with a strong family history of PC have an increased risk of developing PC themselves. Tersmette and colleagues (2001) studied kindreds enrolled in the National Familial Pancreas Tumor Registry at Johns Hopkins <http://pathology.jhu.edu/PANCREAS_NFPTR/> and found that healthy individuals in kindreds in which 3 or more family members had previously been diagnosed with PC had a 56-fold increased risk of developing PC themselves. The risk of developing PC in these kindreds may be particularly high among cigarette smokers. Clearly, because of their increased risk, individuals with a strong family history of PC would be one of the first groups to benefit from screening for early pancreatic neoplasia.

Although the genetic basis for the aggregation of PC in most kindreds has not yet been identified, five genetic syndromes have been identified that increase the risk of PC (Table 143-1). These include the following:

1. Second breast cancer gene (BRCA2) syndrome
2. Peutz-Jeghers syndrome
3. Familial atypical multiple mole melanoma (FAMMM) syndrome
4. Hereditary nonpolyposis colorectal cancer (HNPCC) syndrome
5. Familial pancreatitis

In addition, recent studies by van der Heijden and colleagues (2003) have identified *inherited mutations* in the *Fanconi anemia genes, FANCC* and *FANCG*, in a small percentage of patients with *young age of onset PC*.

The *BRCA2 syndrome* is caused by germline mutations in the *BRCA2* gene and these patients not only have an increased risk of developing breast, ovarian, and prostate cancer, but they also have a 3.5 to 10-fold increased risk of developing PC. To date, germline mutations in the *BRCA2* gene account for 16% of the kindreds with an aggregation of PC.

The *Peutz-Jeghers syndrome* is characterized by pigmented macules on the lips and buccal mucosa and hamartomatous polyps of the GI system. Peutz-Jeghers is caused by germline (inherited) mutations in the *STK11/LKB1* gene on chromosome 19. Giardiello and colleagues (2000) have recently shown that patients with the Peutz-Jeghers syndrome have a 132-fold increased risk of developing PC.

The *FAMMM syndrome* is characterized by nevi, atypical nevi, melanomas, and a 20 to 34-fold increased risk of PC. It is caused by germline mutations in the *p16* gene on chromosome 9p.

HNPCC is associated with an increased risk of colorectal, endometrial, gastric, ovarian, small intestinal, ureter, and PC. HNPCC is caused by germline mutations in one of the deoxyribonucleic acid (DNA) mismatch repair genes (particularly *hMLH1* and *hMSH2*), and, as a result, cancers in patients with HNPCC are characterized by microsatellite instability, the hallmark of a mismatch repair defect.

Familial (hereditary) pancreatitis is characterized by the autosomal dominant inheritance and young age of onset of pancreatitis. Familial pancreatitis has been shown to be caused by germline mutations in the cationic trypsinogen gene (*PRSS1*) and patients with familial pancreatitis have a 50 to 80-fold increased risk of developing PC.

IMPLICATIONS

The identification and characterization of well-defined genetic syndromes associated with an increased risk of PC has several important implications. First, most of these syndromes are also associated with an increased risk of other cancer types. For example, FAMMM is associated with an

TABLE 143-1. Risks of Pancreatic Cancer

Individual	Risk	Age 50	Age 70
No history	RR = 1	0.05%	0.50%
BRCA2	3.5 to 10 times	0.5%	5%
Familial PC	18 times	0.9%	9%
FAMM	20 to 34 times	1%	10 to 17%
Hereditary pancreatitis	50 to 80 times	2.5%	25 to 40%
Peutz-Jeghers	132 times	6.6%	30 to 60%

BRCA2 = second breast cancer gene syndrome; FAMM = familial atypical multiple mole melanoma.

increased risk of both melanoma and PC. The recognition of a patient with FAMMM should therefore lead to increased screening for melanoma, and this screening may save lives.

Second, in selected instances patients with one of these syndromes may elect to undergo pancreatectomy. For example, older patients with hereditary pancreatitis may have evidence of both pancreatic endocrine and exocrine insufficiency, and yet harbor a 25 to 40% lifetime risk of developing PC. In patients with chronic abdominal pain (narcotic dependent) and hereditary pancreatitis, total pancreatectomy can be offered, to alleviate pain and reduce cancer risk. Additionally, it is not unreasonable to discuss "prophylactic" total pancreatectomy for patients with markedly increased risk, noting that patient education about the consequences of pancreatectomy (endocrine and exocrine insufficiency) is mandatory.

Prophylactic total pancreatectomy is, however, a high risk procedure with a high rate of long term morbidity and mortality. A third option, effective screening for early pancreatic neoplasia, is urgently needed. Brentnall and colleagues, (1999) have suggested screening for pancreatic dysplasia with EUS. Abnormal EUS findings can be sampled using fine needle aspiration and further investigated with other imaging techniques, such as ERCP. Patients with suspicious cytology and imaging findings can then be considered for surgical resection. Such an approach has been shown to detect early noninvasive pancreatic neoplasms, including IPMNs, and it is predicted to increase patient life expectancy, hopefully in a cost effective manner.*

Future Screening Modalities

Because of the low prevalence of PC in the population, any useful screening modalities will only target individuals at high risk of developing PC, such as those with a strong family history of PC and those with germline mutations in one of the PC causing genes. The main goals of screening are to detect pancreatic neoplasia before invasive PC develops and, failing that, to detect asymptomatic PCs while they are still resectable. In this regard, using current imaging tests such as EUS, experienced investigators can detect prevalent small (1 to 2 cm) pancreatic neoplasms. More challenging is detecting microscopic high grade PanIN lesions. The detection of these microscopic lesions will probably require molecular assays.

Molecular assays will need to be able to distinguish pancreatic neoplasia from chronic pancreatitis. For a molecular assay to succeed as a screening test, it will need to be applied to the appropriate clinical sample. *Apoptotic pancreatic carcinoma* cells including *tumor DNA* and *proteins* are released through the pancreatic ducts into *pancreatic juice*, duodenal fluid, stool, and, to a lesser extent, into the blood. Although all of these secondary sources can be sampled, an ideal diagnostic marker of pancreatic neoplasia would be measurable in serum. Unfortunately, in the setting of early invasive PC, existing serum markers are often normal. This suggests that in order to detect pre-invasive lesions of the pancreas, a more direct sampling of the pancreas will be required. Pancreatic juice can be collected during routine upper GI endoscopy after secretin stimulation. Higher levels of cancer DNA and proteins make pancreatic juice a potentially optimal specimen to use when screening high risk patients for PC, analogous to sputum for lung cancer or nipple aspirates for breast cancer.

The ideal marker or marker panel of pancreatic neoplasia has not yet been identified. Potential biomarkers of PC can be divided into three biochemical targets. DNA-based techniques aim to detect cancer specific DNA alterations, such as mutations in genomic DNA, CpG island methylation, and mutations in mitochondrial DNA. Ribonucleic acid-based detection methods have been used to identify overexpressed genes in secondary fluids, and global gene expression profiles using oligonucleotide microarrays could be obtained from clinical samples, such as *fine needle aspirates* of suspicious lesions or from *pancreatic juice*. Finally, protein-based detection methods remain the mainstay of cancer markers. Tumor markers can be identified as proteins upregulated in cancer cells using mass spectrometry-based approaches, or by using antibody-based methods to the protein product of genes known to be overexpressed in cancer.

Among DNA markers, because of their prevalence and ease of detection, DNA methylation abnormalities have potential for use in early detection strategies. One limitation to DNA methylation as a marker of cancer is that the abnormal methylation changes that arise during neoplastic development in one tissue may be present in histologically normal cells of adjacent tissues.

Given the current limitations of DNA markers, an ideal PC marker may be protein based. Large-scale analyses of the proteins in biological fluids (known as "proteomics") are underway. Thus, perhaps the most promising molecular strategies for early PC detection and for detecting advanced PanINs are through proteomics profiling of the serum and pancreatic juice of individuals at high risk of developing PC.

Supplemental Reading

Adsay NV, Longnecker DS, Klimstra DS. Pancreatic tumors with cystic dilatation of the ducts: intraductal papillary mucinous neoplasms and intraductal oncocytic papillary neoplasms. Semin Diagn Pathol 2000;17:16–30.

Brentnall TA, Bronner MP, Byrd DR, et al. Early diagnosis and treatment of pancreatic dysplasia in patients with a family history of pancreatic cancer. Ann Intern Med 1999;131:247–55.

---

*Editor's Note: Investigators working with families with hereditary pancreatitis have been considering surveying protocols for that population.

Giardiello FM, Brensinger JD, Tersmette AC, et al. Very high risk of cancer in familial Peutz-Jeghers syndrome. Gastroenterol 2000;119:1447–53.

Hruban RH, Petersen GM, Ha PK, Kern SE. Genetics of pancreatic cancer: from genes to families. Surg Oncol Clin N Am 1998;7:1–23.

Hruban RH, Canto MI, Yeo CJ. Prevention of pancreatic cancer and strategies for management of familial pancreatic cancer. Dig Dis 2001;19:76–84.

Hruban RH, Adsay NV, Albores-Saavedra J, et al. Pancreatic intraepithelial neoplasia (PanIN): a new nomenclature and classification system for pancreatic duct lesions. Am J Surg Pathol 2001;25:579–86.

Jones JB, Song JJ, Hempen PM, et al. Detection of mitochondrial DNA mutations in pancreatic cancer offers a "Mass"-ive advantage over detection of nuclear DNA mutations. Cancer Res 2001;61:1299–304.

Murphy KM, Brune KA, Griffin CA, et al. Evaluation of candidate genes MAP2K4, MADH4, ACVR1B, and BRCA2 in familial pancreatic cancer: deleterious BRCA2 mutations in 17%. Cancer Res 2002;62:3789–93.

Ohhashi K, Murakami Y, Takekoshi T. Four cases of "mucin producing" cancer of the pancreas on specific findings of the papilla of Vater [abstract]. Prog Diagn Endosc 1982;20:348–51.

Rosty C, Christa L, Kuzdzal S, et al. Identification of hepatocarcinoma-intestine-pancreas/pancreatitis-associated protein I as a biomarker for pancreatic ductal adenocarcinoma by protein biochip technology. Cancer Res 2002;62:1868–75.

Rulyak SJ, Lowenfels AB, Maisonneuve P, Brentnall TA. Risk factors for the development of pancreatic cancer in familial pancreatic cancer kindreds. Gastroenterol 2003;124:1292–9.

Rulyak SJ, Kimmey MB, Veenstra DL, Brentnall TA. Cost-effectiveness of pancreatic cancer screening in familial pancreatic cancer kindreds. Gastrointestinal Endoscopy 2003;57:23–9.

Tersmette AC, Petersen GM, Offerhaus GJA, et al. Increased risk of incident pancreatic cancer among first-degree relatives of patients with familial pancreatic cancer. Clin Cancer Res 2001;7:738–44.

Ueki T, Toyota M, Sohn TA, et al. Hypermethylation of multiple genes in pancreatic carcinoma. Cancer Res 2000;60:1835–9.

van der Heijden, Yeo CJ, Hruban RH, Kern SE. Fanconi anemia gene mutations in young-onset pancreatic cancer. Cancer Res 2003;63:2585–8.

Wilentz RE, Albores-Saavedra J, Zahurak M, et al. Pathologic examination accurately predicts prognosis in mucinous cystic neoplasms of the pancreas. Am J Surg Pathol 1999;23:1320–7.

Wilentz RE, Albores-Saavedra J, Hruban RH. Mucinous cystic neoplasms of the pancreas. Semin Diagn Pathol 2000;17:31–42.

CHAPTER 144

PANCREATIC AND ISLET CELL TRANSPLANTATION

ANTONELLO PILEGGI, MD, AND CAMILLO RICORDI, MD

The field of reparative medicine is rapidly evolving and significant progress has been made during the last three decades. Transplantation of tissues or cells is intended to replace functional cell loss due to infection, trauma, toxicity, or autoimmune destruction, and to restore or complement genetically dysfunctional and/or deficient cells, as in the case of inherited metabolic diseases. Advancement in tissue harvesting and preservation methods, and safer transplantation techniques, together with the availability of powerful immunosuppressive agents, are making possible the increasing success of the recent years.

The *insulin producing β-cells* of the islets of Langerhans can be transplanted either as *vascular (whole pancreas)* or *nonvascular (isolated islets)* grafts in patients with insulin-dependent diabetes, and both treatments offer the enormous advantage of achieving a more physiologic glucose metabolic control than exogenous insulin administration. We will review the current status of insulin producing cell transplantation.

Benefits of β-Cell Replacement

Type 1 Diabetes Mellitus

Loss of islet β-cell function is consequent to a number of pathologic conditions, most of which may virtually benefit from transplantation of insulin-producing tissue. Type 1 diabetes mellitus (T1DM) is the main cause of insulin-dependent diabetes worldwide, and it is consequent to the destruction of the β-cells in the pancreatic islets by a T-cell mediated autoimmune process (Joslin, 1994). The onset of T1DM in juvenile age influences the natural history of the disease, which is associated with microvascular, neuropathic, and macrovascular complications of the long lasting instable glycemic control, dramatically affecting both quality of life and life expectancy. Proper management of diabetes obtained by combining diet, physical activity and exogenous insulin treatment can substantially improve glycemic metabolic control. The Diabetes Control and Complication Trial (DCCT, 1998) has shown that intensive insulin therapy with tight glycemic control in patients with T1DM could reduce and delay the risk of dreadful complications associated with long lasting diabetes (Herman and Eastman, 1998). Tight glucose control is also cost effective in terms of health care expenses. Although intensive insulin treatment cannot sustain euglycemia throughout the day and is associated with an increased frequency of severe hypoglycemic episodes, the DCCT data strongly supports the beneficial effect of strict metabolic control on the progression of diabetes complications (DCCT, 1998). The extreme value of endocrine tissue replacement to achieve physiologic control of glucose metabolism is supported by the evidence that transplantation of the pancreas or of isolated pancreatic islets can reverse lesions of diabetic nephropathy, retinopathy, and neuropathy (Fioretto et al, 1998, Fiorina et al, 2003).

Iatrogenic Diabetes

Diabetes following surgical removal of the pancreas for organic diseases is one other possible indication for β-cell replacement. Total pancreatectomy performed to relieve the pain associated with *chronic pancreatitis* invariably results in insulin-dependent diabetes. Approximately 50% of the patients develop diabetes within 5 to 10 years from onset of chronic pancreatitis, even in the absence of surgery. After surgery, one of the main reasons for hospital readmission is poor management of diabetes mellitus in these patients, suggesting the importance of preserving endocrine function by β-cell replacement. Additional causes of iatrogenic diabetes that could benefit of β-cell transplantation include total pancreatectomy following *trauma* or *benign neoplasm*.

METABOLIC DISORDERS

Diabetes can also be associated with *metabolic disorders*. A proportion of patients affected by *cystic fibrosis (CF)* may develop diabetes, and its development appears to have substantial impact on pulmonary function and significantly increases morbidity and mortality rates. Most patients with *cirrhosis* have insulin resistance and impaired glucose tolerance, and about 20% eventually develop type 2 diabetes (Bahtiyar et al, 2004). Patients with *type 2 diabetes* may require insulin treatment and develop diabetes-related complications, including kidney failure. Transplantation of insulin producing cells in these patients may provide the same benefits discussed for patients with T1DM, although advanced age and obesity may represent contraindications due to the increased risk of morbidity (Sutherland et al, 2001; Friedman and Friedman, 2002).

Pancreas Transplantation

Transplantation of the pancreas as a whole organ is generally performed in uremic patients receiving a kidney transplantation (Robertson et al, 2003), allowing for long term graft function with sustained euglycemia and insulin independence in the vast majority of patients, although the procedure is still associated with perioperative mortality and morbidity (Sutherland et al, 2001; International Pancreas Transplant Registry, 2003). A body of literature supports the beneficial effect of restoring endocrine function by transplanting the pancreas on the performance of the transplanted kidney as well as on the overall survival of both graft and patient (Fioretto et al, 1998; Sutherland et al, 2001; International Pancreas Transplant Registry, 2003). The transplantation can be performed as a *simultaneous kidney and pancreas* (SKP) procedure using the organs obtained from the same donor. Alternatively, pancreas transplantation can be performed in patients who had already received kidney (*pancreas after kidney*, PAK) transplantation. *Pancreas transplantation alone* (PTA) in preuremic patients has been performed in the recent years in selected patients with brittle diabetes that, despite strict compliance to the treatment, experience glycemic instability and unawareness to the life threatening hypoglycemic episodes (Robertson et al, 2003). In this category of patients the risk of associated with the surgical procedure and with lifelong immunosuppression is considered justified by the potential improvements that may follow restoration of endocrine function, including the effects on glycemic metabolic control and on its complications.

The main indication for pancreas transplantation (SPK, PAK, or PTA) is T1DM. A series of patients with T2DM have been transplanted worldwide (SPK and PAK), following strict candidate selection criteria (ie, obesity and age > 55 years are considered contraindications), and graft outcome rates are comparable to those of T1DM patients (Sutherland et al, 2001; Friedman and Friedman, 2002). The overall outcome of allogeneic pancreas grafts is generally analyzed by eras, based on the progress in immunosuppressive management introduced over the years. Since the late 1970s up to mid-2003 over 19,600 (> 14,300 from United States centers, > 5,300 from outside the United States) pancreas transplantations have been reported to the International Pancreas Transplant Registry, most of which were SPK (~ 79% of all transplantation in the United States, and 92% abroad); less, but increasing, were both PAK (~ 14% in United States, ~ 5% abroad) and PTA (~ 6% in United States, 3% abroad). Graft survival for cadaveric pancreas transplantations performed in the United States since 1999 ($N = 5129$) at 1 year was close to 80% for all categories, with a slight advantage for SPK when compared with PAK and PTA (84.7% versus 78.5% and 78.2%, respectively), that was more pronounced at 3 years (SPK 80%; PAK and PTA ~ 60%). Patient survival at 1 and 3 years was respectively 95.5% and approximately 90% for SPK, 94.9% and approximately 89% for PAK, and 98.4% and approximately 94% for PTA.

Pancreas transplantation for iatrogenic diabetes (total pancreatectomy for chronic pancreatitis, trauma, or benign neoplasm) is performed in a relative small proportion of patients (Sutherland et al, 2001; Watkins et al, 2003). *Segmental pancreas autotransplantation* (generally body and tail of the gland) in patients undergoing pancreatectomy to relieve the pain associated with chronic pancreatitis has been proposed as a means to preserve endocrine function, but is often associated with high morbidity (Sutherland et al, 2001; Watkins et al, 2003). Transplantation of allogeneic pancreas is performed in selected patients undergoing multivisceral cluster transplantation, generally including the intestine and the liver. For allogeneic pancreas transplantation, the whole gland or a pancreatic segment is generally obtained from *cadaveric multiorgan donors*. Transplantation of pancreas segment obtained from *living donors* undergoing hemipancreatectomy (50% of the pancreas) to provide the graft to a relative with T1DM has been performed in selected cases in a number of centers in the recent years (Sutherland et al, 2001; Sammartino et al, 2004). The procedure may be associated with an increased morbidity risk in both donor and recipient, whereas graft survival rates are comparable to those of cadaveric pancreas. It is noteworthy that this approach may have serious repercussions on the health of the living-related donors with appreciable increased incidence of diabetes after surgery; many of the donors experience a decrease in oral glucose tolerance and onset of diabetes by 1 year from surgery (Kendall et al, 1990).

Several surgical transplantation techniques are used worldwide (Sutherland et al, 2001; International Pancreas Transplant Registry, 2003). In the case of whole pancreas transplantation, the *exocrine secretion* of the pancreas graft can be drained into the recipient's jejunum (*enteric drainage*) or into the bladder (*bladder drainage*). The technique of choice may vary between centers. The bladder drainage offers the practical advantage of performing immunologic monitoring of the pancreatic graft by measuring urine amylase concentration, but may be associated with side effects of secreting pancreatic enzymes in the urinary tract (digestion of urethra, uncorrectable metabolic acidosis subsequent to the loss of bicarbonate). The *venous drainage* of the pancreatic graft (and therefore of insulin release) can be performed with the systemic venous system (*systemic drainage*) or with the portal venous bed (*portal drainage*), although a metabolic advantage of one or the other technique is not clearly apparent from the clinical data. It has been recently suggested that portal drainage may provide an immunologic advantage to graft outcome (Sutherland et al, 2001).

Pancreatic Islet Cell Transplantation

Transplantation of isolated pancreatic islets offers the advantage of a minimally invasive procedure associated with very low incidence of adverse effects (Hering and Ricordi, 1999). Following islet infusion a dramatic reduction of insulin requirement is generally observed, and insulin independence can be achieved when an optimal islet mass has been implanted (Shapiro et al, 2000 and 2003; Goss et al, 2002; Markmann et al, 2003).

Transplantation of islets of Langerhans consists in the implantation of different degrees of purified endocrine pancreatic tissue into diabetic recipients. The protocols for the isolation and purification of islets of Langerhans are not yet completely standardized and differ slightly between centers. The *islet isolation* procedure consists of a mechanically enhanced enzymatic digestion of the pancreatic tissue that frees the islets from the surrounding connective and acinar tissue without destroying islet integrity (Ricordi, 1995). The subsequent *purification* step addresses the need to physically separate the islet tissue, which constitutes < 2% of the digest, from nonendocrine tissue (exocrine fragments, ductal and vascular tissues, and lymph nodes) (Ricordi, 1995). Islets are transplanted in the portal system and minimization of the volume of implanted tissue can prevent excessive ischemic insult to the liver and elevation of portal pressure, thereby decreasing the potential for procedure-related complications. After purification, islets can be transplanted immediately or cultured for a short period of time (usually 2 to 3 days) prior to implantation. Pretransplantation culture allows for the assessment of sterility and *in vitro* function of the islet preparation. Also, the culture period may provide a window of opportunity for manipulation of islets prior to implantation by means of emerging interventional approaches (modulation of immunogenicity, induction of cytoprotective molecules, gene therapy, immunoisolation, etc), and/or preconditioning the recipient (immunomodulation, immunosuppression, reduction of inflammation) to maximize both engraftment of the islets and their survival. Thanks to the availability of *minimally invasive interventional radiology techniques*, implantation of an islet graft consists in the cannulation of the portal vein *via* a transhepatic percutaneous access under ultrasound and angiographic guidance (Froud et al, 2004). This approach is associated with minimal surgical risk and low incidence of complications, it is quicker and less expensive than surgery, it is well tolerated by the patients (conscious sedation protocol), can be performed as outpatient procedure, and can be repeated in different occasions. The minimally invasive approach is generally offered to patients receiving solitary allogeneic islet grafts subsequent to a kidney transplant (*islets after kidney, IAK*), or to patients receiving *islet transplantation alone (ITA)*.

The *surgical approach* consists of the cannulation of a tributary of the portal vein (omental vein, branch of the middle colic vein, or inferior mesenteric vein) that requires laparotomy. This approach is preferred during a *simultaneous islet and kidney (SIK)* transplantation, when access to the portal system can be obtained during an open surgical procedure (Alejandro et al, 1997) or in selected cases (IAK and ITA) in which the percutaneous procedure may be contraindicated, including patients at high risk of bleedings, patients with hepatic hemangiomas, lack of an experienced interventional radiologist, or patient preference after inform consent. Alternative less invasive surgical procedures under evaluation include the use of laparoscopic access to infuse islets in the umbilical vein or islets implantation within the omental layers.

The main indication for *allogeneic islet transplantation* is T1DM (Brendel et al, 2001; Hering and Ricordi, 1999). Transplantation of islets of Langerhans can be performed in uremic patients as either SIK or IAK procedure, since chronic immunosuppression therapy is already implemented to sustain the function of the kidney graft. More recently, ITA has been introduced for the treatment of selected patients with brittle T1DM associated with hypoglycemic unawareness (absence of autonomic symptoms at glycemic levels < 54 mg/dL), severe metabolic lability (mean amplitude of glucose excursions > 11.1 mmol/L or 200 mg/dL), progressive secondary diabetes complications, and failure of intensive insulin therapy despite strict compliance (Robertson et al, 2003; Shapiro et al, 2000; Shapiro and Ricordi, 2004). In these patients the risk associated with metabolic lability and hypoglycemic unawareness (often life threatening) justifies that related to the transplantation procedure and chronic immunosuppression. A number of clinical trials of allogeneic ITA for patients with T1DM ongoing worldwide have shown that sustained insulin independence can be reproducibly achieved after islet transplantation in experienced centers (Shapiro et al, 2003; Shapiro and Ricordi, 2004). This is generally achieved after sequential infusion (Shapiro et al, 2000; Goss et al, 2002) or single infusion of pooled islet preparations (Markmann et al, 2003) obtained from more than one gland, and, in some cases, after the infusion of a single islet preparation (Hering et al, 2004; Shapiro and Ricordi, 2004). Insulin requirements are generally dramatically reduced after single islet transplantation, and improved glycemic metabolic control, with normalization of glycated hemoglobin and absence of hypoglycemic episodes is always observed even when exogenous insulin treatment is still required (such as in the case a suboptimal graft mass is implanted, or when partial loss of function is observed) (Brendel et al, 2001; Shapiro et al, 2003; Shapiro and

Ricordi, 2004) Success rates of ITA using a steroid-free immunosuppressive protocol are close to 90% insulin independence at 1 year, and approximately 80% at 2 years (Shapiro et al, 2003; Shapiro and Ricordi, 2004).

The need to transplant a large number of islets (> 12,000 islet equivalents per kg of body weight, in the recent successful clinical trials) to attain insulin independence may be consequent to multiple factors all contributing to the loss of viable insulin-producing cells (Pileggi et al, 2001). Brain death, donor characteristics, and isolation and purification procedures may dramatically influence both yield and quality of islets obtained from a cadaveric pancreas. Additionally, culture conditions, and nonspecific inflammation generated at the site of implant may affect the actual number of islets that will engraft and function after transplantation. Although the need for more than one islet preparation (therefore > 1 pancreatic gland per recipient) to restore normoglycemia may represent a drawback due to the shortage of organs for transplant, it is noteworthy that most centers performing islet isolations worldwide have mainly used "sub-optimal" pancreata that had been "discarded" by the pancreas transplantation surgeons for a number of reasons (fatty pancreas, technical problems, damaged glands, long ischemia, etc). Implementing fair allocation rules for cadaveric pancreata between whole pancreas and isolated islet programs may allow for the availability of optimal tissue for the isolation of islets for transplantation, which may render possible achieving insulin independence from a single islet preparation per recipient. Moreover, at the present time the use of pancreata for transplantation (either as whole organ or for islets) is still poor, and a large number of glands are, unfortunately, not used (Krieger et al, 2003).

Other indications for the transplantation of allogeneic islets include selected cases of pancreatectomy-induced diabetes (Hering and Ricordi, 1999). Patients with "insulin-requiring diabetes" secondary to cystic fibrosis (Cretin et al, 1998) and hemochromatosis (Brunicardi et al, 1995) may benefit of an islet graft combined with lung or liver transplantation. Islet transplantation for type 2 diabetes has been attempted in very few cases in pilot trials (Ricordi et al, 1997). Successful transplantation of allogeneic islets isolated from pancreatic grafts explanted for technical complications has been reported as a "rescue" procedure (Leone et al, 1998).

Transplantation of islets obtained from autologous pancreas (*islet autotransplantation*) removed for benign conditions has been performed for several years to prevent iatrogenic diabetes (Hering and Ricordi, 1999; Robertson et al, 2003). This procedure is mainly performed in patients undergoing total pancreatectomy to relive the pain associated with chronic pancreatitis, offering the perspective of a better quality of life and prevention of the occurrence of diabetes and its complications. Indeed, normoglycemia and insulin independence are observed in about 70% of the patients after intrahepatic islet autotransplantation when > 250,000 islets are implanted.

Increasing interest has been focused on islet isolation and transplantation in the recent years, following the unprecedented results of clinical trials (Brendel et al, 2001; Shapiro et al, 2003). The Food and Drug Administration regulates islet cell transplantation at the present time under the category of investigational new drug (Weber et al, 2002). Emerging evidence from the ongoing clinical trials supports the relevance of multidisciplinary expertise at the islet isolation and transplantation center (Shapiro et al, 2003; Shapiro and Ricordi, 2004). This includes the availability of adequate infrastructures and highly qualified personnel (endocrinology, transplant surgery, radiology, cell biology, immunology, administrative, and current Good Manufacturing Practice human islet cell processing facility and personnel). These important premises have been associated with the best results, not only in obtaining adequate islets from the donor pancreata, but also in assuring appropriate posttransplantation management (ie, metabolic and immunosuppression) of the recipients. Using specialized, experienced islet cell processing centers that distribute islet cell products to remote islet transplantation centers has also been demonstrated an effective strategy (Goss et al, 2002; Leone et al, 1998; Robertson et al, 2001). The possibility of having "regional centers" may improve the efficiency of use of cadaveric pancreata and may be of assistance to improve the success rate of clinical islet transplantation, while lowering the costs for islet preparation.

Conclusions

The success of β-cell replacement therapy through transplantation of the endocrine pancreas as either whole organ or isolated islets has been steadily increasing over the past decade. The shortage of organs and the need for chronic recipient immunosuppression remain major hurdles, limiting the applicability of allogeneic β-cells transplantation to a wider number of patients with insulin-dependent diabetes. As we better appreciate the complex phenomena involved in the immunobiology of transplantation, better tools to promote engraftment and survival of allogeneic tissues will become available for clinical testing. Implementation of methods to improve cadaveric organ donor preservation and storage may allow for optimization of pancreas use from marginal and/or from nonheart-beating donors, which are currently underused for whole pancreas and islet transplantation (Fraker et al, 2002; Markmann et al, 2003). Alternative sources for β-cells are under evaluation, such as *xenogeneic islets* and *stem cell*-derived insulin-producing cells, as they may provide an unlimited supply of tissue for transplantation.

Chronic immunosuppression is currently needed to prevent graft rejection and, possibly, recurrence of autoimmunity. Immunosuppressive drugs may have untoward effects, such as increased susceptibility to infection, neoplasms, and organ toxicity. In addition, some of the drugs currently available can be toxic to β-cells, resulting in chronic loss of graft function (Hering and Ricordi, 1999; Pileggi et al, 2001). A number of protocols for the induction of *immune tolerance* to transplanted tissues are under investigation in experimental animal models, and promising results have been reported that justify a cautious optimism for their potential clinical applicability in the near future.

Acknowledgements

This work was partially supported by the National Institute of Health and the Juvenile Diabetes Research Foundation International and from continuous support from the Diabetes Research Institute Foundation (Hollywood, FL).

Supplemental Reading

Alejandro R, Lehmann R, Ricordi C, et al. Long-term function (6 years) of islet allografts in type 1 diabetes. Diabetes 1997;46:1983–9.

Bahtiyar G, Shin JJ, Aytaman A, et al. Association of diabetes and hepatitis C infection: epidemiologic evidence and pathophysiologic insights. Curr Diab Rep 2004;4:194–8.

Brendel M, Hering BJ, Schultz AO, Bretzel RG. International Islet Transplant Registry. Newsletter #9 2001;8:4–20. <http://www.med.uni-giessen.de/itr/> (accessed Nov. 2, 2003).

Brunicardi FC, Atiya A, Stock P, et al. Clinical islet transplantation experience of the University of California Islet Transplant Consortium. Surgery 1995;118:967–71.

Cretin N, Buhler L, Fournier B, et al. Results of human islet allotransplantation in cystic fibrosis and type I diabetic patients. Transplant Proc 1998;30:315–6.

Fiorina P, Folli F, Maffi P, et al. Islet transplantation improves vascular diabetic complications in patients with diabetes who underwent kidney transplantation: a comparison between kidney-pancreas and kidney-alone transplantation. Transplantation 2003;75:1296–301.

Fioretto P, Steffes MW, Sutherland DE, et al. Reversal of lesions of diabetic nephropathy after pancreas transplantation. N Engl J Med 1998;339:69–75.

Fraker CA, Alejandro R, Ricordi C. Use of oxygenated perfluorocarbon toward making every pancreas count. Transplantation 2002;74:1811–2.

Friedman AL, Friedman EA. Pancreas transplantation for type 2 diabetes at U.S. Transplant centers. Diabetes Care 2002;25:1896.

Froud T, Yrizarry JM, Alejandro R, Ricordi C. Use of D-STAT to prevent bleeding following percutaneous transhepatic intraportal islet transplantation. Cell Transplant 2004;13:55–9.

Goss JA, Schock AP, Brunicardi FC, et al. Achievement of insulin independence in three consecutive type-1 diabetic patients via pancreatic islet transplantation using islets isolated at a remote islet isolation center. Transplantation 2002;74:1761–6.

Hering BJ, Kandaswamy R, Harmon J, et al. Transplantation of cultured islets from two-layer preserved pancreases in type 1 diabetes with anti-CD3 antibody. Am J Transplant 2004;4:390–401.

Hering BJ, Ricordi C. Results, research priorities, and reasons for optimism: islet transplantation for patients with type 1 diabetes. Graft 1999;2:12–27.

Herman WH, Eastman RC. The effects of treatment on the direct costs of diabetes. Diabetes Care 1998;21(Suppl3):C19–24.

International Pancreas Transplant Registry. <http://www.iptr.umn.edu/> (accessed Nov 2, 2003).

Kahn RC, Weir GC, editors. Joslin's diabetes mellitus, 13th ed. Philadelphia: Lea & Febiger; 1994.

Kendall DM, Sutherland DE, Najarian JS, et al. Effects of hemipancreatectomy on insulin secretion and glucose tolerance in healthy humans. N Engl J Med 1990;322:898–903.

Krieger NR, Odorico JS, Heisey DM, et al. Underutilization of pancreas donors. Transplantation 2003;75:1271–6.

Leone JP, Kendall DM, Reinsmoen N, et al. Immediate insulin-independence after retransplantation of islets prepared from an allograft pancreatectomy in a type 1 diabetic patient. Transplant Proc 1998;30:319.

Markmann JF, Deng S, Desai NM, et al. The use of non-heart-beating donors for isolated pancreatic islet transplantation. Transplantation 2003;75:1423–9.

Markmann JF, Deng S, Huang X, et al. Insulin independence following isolated islet transplantation and single islet infusions. Ann Surg 2003;237:741–9.

Pileggi A, Ricordi C, Alessiani M, Inverardi L. Factors influencing Islet of Langerhans graft function and monitoring. Clin Chim Acta 2001;310:3–16.

Ricordi C. Methods in cell transplantation. Austin: RG Landes Co; 1995.

Ricordi C, Alejandro R, Angelico MC, et al. Human islet allografts in patients with type 2 diabetes undergoing liver transplantation. Transplantation 1997;63:473–5.

Robertson RP, Davis C, Larsen J, et al. American Diabetes Association. Pancreas transplantation for patients with type 1 diabetes. Diabetes Care 2003;26:S120.

Robertson RP, Lanz KJ, Sutherland DE, Kendall DM. Prevention of diabetes for up to 13 years by autoislet transplantation after pancreatectomy for chronic pancreatitis. Diabetes 2001;50:47–50.

Sammartino C, Pham T, Panaro F, et al. Successful simultaneous pancreas kidney transplantation from living-related donor against positive cross-match. Am J Transplant 2004;4:140–3.

Shapiro AM, Lakey JR, Ryan EA, et al. Islet transplantation in seven patients with type 1 diabetes mellitus using a glucocorticoid-free immunosuppressive regimen. N Engl J Med 2000;343:230–8.

Shapiro AM, Ricordi C. Unraveling the secrets of single donor success in islet transplantation. Am J Transplant 2004;4:295–8.

Shapiro AM, Ricordi C, Hering B. Edmonton's islet success has indeed been replicated elsewhere. Lancet 2003;362:1242.

Sutherland DE, Gruessner RW, Dunn DL, et al. Lessons learned from more than 1,000 pancreas transplants at a single institution. Ann Surg 2001;233:463–501.

The Diabetes Control and Complications Trial Research Group. Effect of intensive therapy on residual beta-cell function in patients with type 1 diabetes in the diabetes control and complications trial. A randomized, controlled trial. Ann Intern Med 1998;128:517–23.

Watkins JG, Krebs A, Rossi RL. Pancreatic autotransplantation in chronic pancreatitis. World J Surg 2003;27:1235–40.

Weber DJ, McFarland RD, Irony I. Selected Food and Drug Administration review issues for regulation of allogeneic islets of Langerhans as somatic cell therapy. Transplantation 2002;74:1816–20.

Index

A

AA. *See* Alcoholics Anonymous (AA)
AAPC. *See* Attenuated adenomatous polyposis coli (AAPC)
Abdominal pain. *See also* Chronic abdominal pain
   chronic recurrent, 243–248
   with SCT, 287
Abdominal radiation, 579–582
   modalities, 579–580, 579t
   organ tolerances, 581t
   preoperative *vs.* postoperative, 580t
   role of, 581–582
   side effects, 580–581
   therapeutic intent, 579
   treatment sequence, 580
Abdominal rectal prolapse repair, 519–520
Abdominal wall defects
   incidence, 444
   inguinal hernia, 445
   laparoscopy, 445
   nomenclature, 444
   patient examination, 444–445
   prosthetic material, 445
   surgery, 445
   treatment, 444–445
Abdominal wall hernia
   with ascites, 660
Abdominal wall transplantation, 387
Abdominoperineal resection
   anorectal melanoma, 532
   rectal cancer, 572
Ablative therapy
   BE, 91–93
   selection of, 93–94
Abnormal illness behavior, 255
   management, 257–258
   therapeutic relationship, 257–258
Abnormal reflux
   monitoring, 69
Abscess
   anorectal, 530
   Crohn's disease of small bowel, 394–395
   horseshoe
      drainage of, 531f
   intersphincteric, 530
   perianal
      drainage, 479f
      inflammatory bowel disease, 479
   supralevator, 530
Absolute risk reduction (ARR), 2–3
   computation of, 3t
Acalculous cholecystitis. *See also* Acute acalculous cholecystitis
   chronic, 757

Acamprosate (Campral)
   for alcoholism, 229
ACER. *See* Average cost effectiveness ratio (ACER)
Acetaminophen
   inducing fulminant hepatic failure, 630
   inducing liver disease, 689, 692–693
Acetylcysteine (Mucomyst), 807
   for alcoholic liver disease, 669
   for fulminant hepatic failure, 630, 633
Acetyl p benzoquinoneimine
   for acetaminophen poisoning, 692
Achalasia, 109–110
   barium esophogram, 115
   diagnosis, 112–113
   followup, 117
   presentation, 112
   surgery, 114–115, 117
   treatment, 112–117, 113, 113t
Achlorhydria, 428
Acid back diffusion, 161
Acid peptic disorders
   smoking, 270–271
Acid secretion
   pathophysiologic consequences, 148
Acid suppressive therapy, 56t, 104
   bleeding peptic ulcer, 174–175
   NUD, 186
Aciphex. *See* Rabeprazole (Aciphex)
Actical
   for cholestasis, 290
   for erythropoietic protoporphyria, 730
   for VOD, 289
Acticon artificial bowel sphincter, 514f
Actonel
   for metabolic bone disease, 333
   for PBC, 703
Acupuncture
   for chronic abdominal pain, 254
Acute acalculous cholecystitis, 755–756, 755f
   diagnosis, 756
   etiology, 756
   presentation, 756
   treatment, 756
Acute appendicitis, 435–438
   classic patient, 435
   diagnosis, 435
   differential diagnosis, 435
   operative management, 437–438
   preoperative care, 437–438
   preoperative management, 436–437
   treatment, 436f
Acute arterial occlusion, 416–417

Acute benzodiazepine withdrawal, 20
Acute cholangitis
   with choledocholithiasis, 767–769
Acute cholestasis
   drug induced, 690t
Acute colonic pseudoobstruction, 503–505
   colonoscopic decompression, 505
   conservative management, 503–504
   interventional management, 504
   pharmacologic management, 504
   radiographs, 503
   spontaneous perforation, 503
Acute delta hepatitis, 614
Acute fatty liver of pregnancy (AFLP), 696–699, 697f
Acute gallstone pancreatitis
   simulations, 781, 783f
   TPN, 781
Acute gastric dilatation
   with eating disorders, 234
Acute graft versus host disease
   with diarrhea, 286–287
Acute hepatic failure
   pediatric liver transplantation, 651
Acute hepatitis
   drug induced, 690t
   prevention, 611–614
   treatment, 611–614
Acute hepatitis A, 611–612
Acute hepatitis B, 612–613
Acute hepatitis C, 613–614
   treatment, 614t
Acute hepatitis E, 614
Acute infectious diarrhea, 292–296
   diagnosis, 292
   pathogen specific therapy, 293–296
   treatment, 292–293, 294t
Acute intestinal ischemia
   diagnosis, 413t
   treatment, 415t, 416t
Acute liver failure (ALF), 611, 722
   hepatic encephalopathy, 664
   liver transplantation, 642
Acute pancreatitis, 777–783
   CT, 778f, 779t
   defined, 778t
   endoscopic therapy, 789–790
   etiology, 777, 777t
   pathogenesis, 777
   pharmacotherapy, 782
   postsimulations, 782, 783t
   prognosis, 777
   recurrence prevention, 782
   surgery, 782
   terminology, 777
   treatment, 778–779, 779–782, 779f
Acute Physiological and Chronic Health Evaluation (APACHE-II), 778
Acute porphyrias, 728–729
   diagnosis, 728
   treatment, 728–729
Acute self limiting colitis (ASLC), 448
Acute variceal bleeding
   endoscopic and pharmacologic treatment, 121

endoscopic therapy, 121
from nongastroesophageal sites, 123
pharmacologic treatment, 120–121
predictors of failure to control, 121–123
resuscitative measures, 120–121
treatment, 119–123, 119f
Acute viral hepatitis
   pediatric liver transplantation, 652
Acyclovir (Zocyrax)
   for fulminant hepatic failure, 634
   for Herpes, 535
   for viral esophagitis, 98
Adefovir dipivoxil
   for chronic hepatitis B, 618–619
Adenocarcinoma. See also Esophageal adenocarcinoma
   anal canal, 532
Adenomas, 550, 552f
   chronic gastritis, 180
   colonic
      smoking, 270
   gastric
      with CVID, 282
   pancreatic, 156
Adenosylmethionine
   for alcoholic liver disease, 668–669
   for pruritis of cholestasis, 710
Adjunct medications
   endoscopic sedation, 19
Adrenergic agents
   for secretory diarrhea, 427
Adrenocorticoids
   for microscopic colitis, 508
Adverse reactions to food
   functional disorders, 347
   management, 347–348, 347t
Advil, 143
AER. See Automated endoscope reprocessor (AER)
Aerobic exercise
   for fatigue of cholestasis, 711
   obesity, 216
AFAP. See Attenuated familial adenomatous polyposis (AFAP)
AFLP. See Acute fatty liver of pregnancy (AFLP)
AHA. See American Heart Association (AHA)
ALA dehydrase deficiency. See Aminolevulinic acid (ALA) dehydrase deficiency
Alagille syndrome
   pediatric liver transplantation, 651
Alanine aminotransferase (ALT), 605, 605t, 608f
   etiology, 607–608
Albendazole
   adverse effects, 314t
   for ascariasis, 311
   for Giardia lamblia, 310
   for hookworm, 311
   for human immunodeficiency virus (HIV), 277
   for intestinal helminths, 312t
   for intestinal protozoan parasites, 309t

for liver flukes, 310
   pregnancy, 313t
   for strongyloidiasis, 311
   for whipworm, 312
Albumin, 605, 609
Alcohol
   elevated liver enzymes, 607–608
   GERD, 60
   inducing chronic pancreatitis, 793f
Alcohol abuse
   with chronic pancreatitis, 796
   defined, 226–227, 227t
   liver transplantation, 640
Alcohol dependence
   treatment, 228–229
Alcoholic beverages
   alcohol content of, 665t
Alcoholic liver disease, 665–669
   calories, 667f
   cigarette smoking, 666
   diagnosis, 665–666
   drug therapy, 667–668
   lifestyle changes, 666–667
   nutrition therapy, 667
   obesity, 666–667
   treatment, 666–669, 666t
Alcoholics Anonymous (AA), 228–229
Alcoholism, 226–231
   defined, 226–227, 227t
   depression, 228
   with eating disorders, 237–238
   laboratory tests, 227–228
   medications for, 229
   psychological counseling, 228–229
   screening, 226–227
   structured program, 228–229
   treatment, 228–229
   withdrawal
      nutritional deficiencies and support, 230–231
   withdrawal seizures, 230
Alcohol withdrawal
   management of, 229–230
Alemtuzumab
   for transplantation, 387, 388
Alendronate (Fosamax)
   for metabolic bone disease, 333
ALF. See Acute liver failure (ALF)
Alkaline phosphatase, 605, 606t, 607–608
Allogeneic islet transplantation, 830–831
Allograft rejection
   pediatric liver transplantation, 653–654
Alosetron (Lotronex)
   for diabetic diarrhea, 422
   for IBS, 241
Alpers' disease
   pediatric liver transplantation, 652
Alpha 2 adrenergic agents
   for secretory diarrhea, 427
Alpha 2 agonist
   noncardiac surgery, 433
Alpha 1 antitrypsin deficiency, 808
   pediatric liver transplantation, 651
Alpha interferon
   for HBV in children, 625–626

for HCV in children, 627
  with ribavirin
    for HCV in children, 627
Alpha methyldopa
  for drug induced liver disease, 689
  inducing liver disease, 689
ALT. See Alanine aminotransferase (ALT)
AMA. See Antimitochondrial antibodies (AMA)
Amaranth
  with celiac disease, 369
Amebiasis, 308
American College of Cardiology (ACC)
  guidelines for perioperative cardiovascular evaluation, 430
American Dietetic Association
  National Center for Nutrition and Dietetics Consumer Nutrition Hotline, 369
American Heart Association (AHA)
  guidelines for perioperative cardiovascular evaluation, 430
American Joint Commission on Cancer
  TNM restaging, 30
  TNM staging
    colon cancer, 558t
Aminolevulinic acid (ALA) dehydrase deficiency, 728
Aminosalicylates
  for Crohn's colitis, 466
  for left sided colitis, 449–450
  mechanisms of action, 449t
Aminosalicylic acid (ASA)
  for microscopic colitis, 507
  for pediatric Crohn's disease, 397
  for UC, 454
Amitriptyline (Elavil)
  for FGID, 263, 263t
  for gastroparesis, 193
  for NUD, 186
Amoxicillin
  for *Helicobacter pylori,* 140
Amphotericin B
  for *Candida* esophagitis, 97
Ampullary adenoma, 770f
Ampullary tumors
  benign, 769–770
Amsterdam criteria, 547t
Amylase
  with eating disorders, 234
Anal anatomy, 476–477, 476f
Anal canal
  adenocarcinoma, 532
  anatomy of, 476–477
Anal cancer, 532
  smoking, 270
Anal fissure, 530
  lower gastrointestinal bleeding, 585
  surgical lateral sphincterotomy, 530
Anal mapping, 532
Anal stenosis, 533
  inflammatory bowel disease, 478
  self dilation, 533
  surgical sphincterotomy, 533
Anal transitional zone (ATZ), 459–460, 460f
Anaphylactic reactions, 349

Anaphylactoid reactions, 346
Ancylostoma duodenale, 311
  treatment, 312t
Anemia
  with celiac disease, 370
  Fanconi, 825
Anesthesiologists
  endoscopic sedation, 20
Angiodysplasia, 585, 588
Angiography
  obscure gastrointestinal bleeding, 359
Angiostrongyliasis costaricensis (anisakiasis), 311
Angiotensin II
  for portal hypertension, 678
Anisakiasis, 311
Ann Arbor staging
  PGL, 204
Anorectal abscess, 530
Anorectal disease, 530–535
  anal fissure, 530
  anal neoplasm, 532
  anal stenosis, 533
  anorectal abscess, 530
  Bowen's disease, 532
  fistula in ano, 530–532
  hidradenitis suppurativa, 533
  human immunodeficiency virus (HIV), 278–279
  Paget's disease, 532
  pruritus ani, 535
  rectal prolapse, 532
  STD, 534–535
Anorectal melanoma
  abdominoperineal resection, 532
Anorexia nervosa, 232–238. See also Eating disorders
  defined, 232
  management of, 234–236
  oral conditions, 45
Antacids
  for SRES, 162–163
Antegrade and retrograde dilatation procedure
  combined approach, 105
Anterior cingulate cortex (ACC), 261
Anthraquinone containing laxatives
  for constipation, 440
Antibiotic associated diarrhea
  Clostridium difficile, 302–305
Antibiotics
  for bacteremia, 104
  for Crohn's colitis, 466
  for Crohn's diseases perianal complications, 472–473
  for diabetic diarrhea, 422
  for hepatic encephalopathy, 663
  for pediatric Crohn's disease, 399
  pregnancy, 491
  for traveler's diarrhea, 98
Anticholinergics
  for IBS, 240t
Anticoagulants
  with NSAIDs, 144
Antidepressants
  for chronic abdominal pain, 252–253

for FGID, 261–265, 263t
for NUD, 186
Antiemetics
  for gastroparesis, 193–194
Antigenic structure modification
  for food allergy, 350
Antihistamines
  for left sided ulcerative colitis, 451
  for pruritis of cholestasis, 708–709
  for pruritus gravidarum, 696
Antiinflammatory therapy
  with active ulcers, 145
Antimitochondrial antibodies (AMA)
  PBC, 701
Antiparasitics
  adverse effects, 314t
  in children and pregnancy, 313t
Antireflux surgery, 57
  continued surveillance, 71
  for GERD, 69
  outcomes, 70
  side effects, 70
Antisecretory agents
  for PUD, 152t
  for traveler's diarrhea, 300
Antispasmodics
  for IBS, 240t
Antitrypsin deficiency, 808
  pediatric liver transplantation, 651
Anxiety disorders
  with Wilson's disease, 723
Anxiolysis
  continuum of depth, 17t
Anxiolytics
  for NUD, 186–187
Anzemet
  for gastroparesis, 193
AORN. See Association of Perioperative Registered Nurses (AORN)
Aortic aneurysm repair, 358
APACHE-II. See Acute Physiological and Chronic Health Evaluation (APACHE-II)
APC. See Argon plasma coagulation (APC)
APC I1307K mutation, 547t, 548
Aphthous stomatitis, 282
Appendicitis. See Acute appendicitis
Argon plasma coagulation (APC), 131, 577
  ablative treatment, 92t
  esophageal cancer, 132
  upper gastrointestinal bleeding, 171–172
Argon Plasma Coagulator
  BE, 38, 91–92
ARR. See Absolute risk reduction (ARR)
Arrhythmias, 19
Arterial catheterization, 599
Arterial embolism
  diagnosis, 413t
  treatment, 415t
Arterial occlusion
  acute, 416–417
Arterial thrombosis
  diagnosis, 413t
  treatment, 415t
Artificial anal sphincter
  fecal incontinence, 514
Artificial bowel sphincter

Acticon, 514f
Artificial nutritional support
  ethical issues, 200
ASA. See Aminosalicylic acid (ASA)
Asacol
  for Crohn's disease of small bowel, 391
  for microscopic colitis, 508
  for UC, 455–456
Ascariasis, 311
  treatment, 312t
Ascaris lumbricoides (Ascariasis), 311
  treatment, 312t
Ascites
  chylous
    with intestinal transplantation, 388
  complications, 656–660, 658–660
  diagnostic paracentesis, 656–657
  diet therapy, 657
  differentiation, 657t
  diuretic therapy, 657
  evaluation, 656–657
  fluid analysis, 656–657
  followup, 657–658
  history, 656
  pathogenesis, 656
  physical examination, 656
  sodium, 657
  treatment, 657–658
Ascitic fluid infection, 658–659, 659t
Ascitic fluid tests, 657t
ASLC. See Acute self limiting colitis (ASLC)
Aspartate aminotransferase (AST), 605, 605t
Aspiration
  with percutaneous endoscopic gastrostomy, 198
Aspiration pneumonia
  with achalasia, 113
Association of Perioperative Registered
    Nurses (AORN)
  endoscopic disinfection, 25
AST. See Aspartate aminotransferase (AST)
Asterixis
  with hepatic encephalopathy, 661
Asthma
  GERD, 66, 67t
Ataxia telangiectasia (AT), 281
  gastrointestinal manifestations, 283
Ativan
  for alcohol withdrawal, 230
Atropine sulfate (Lomotil). See
    Diphenoxylate with atropine sulfate
    (Lomotil)
Attenuated adenomatous polyposis coli
    (AAPC), 551, 552–553
Attenuated familial adenomatous polyposis
    (AFAP), 547t, 548
ATZ. See Anal transitional zone (ATZ)
AUDIT, 227
Aulin
  for nonsteroidal antiinflammatory drug
    (NSAID) induced small and large
    intestinal injury, 366
Autoimmune hepatitis
  elevated liver enzymes, 607–608
Automated endoscope reprocessor (AER),
  24

endoscope reprocessing, 27, 28, 28t
Autonomic neuropathy
  diabetic diarrhea, 420
Average cost effectiveness ratio (ACER), 15
Averaging out, 9
Axid
  for upper gastrointestinal bleeding, 153
Azathioprine (AZA)
  for Crohn's colitis, 468–469
  for Crohn's disease of small bowel, 392
  for Crohn's disease perianal complications, 473
  for liver disease during pregnancy,
    694–695
  metabolism of, 406f
  metabolite levels
    IBD, 406–409
  for pediatric Crohn's disease, 398
  pregnancy, 490, 491
  for UC, 44, 450–451
Azithromycin (Zithromax)
  for diarrhea, 295
  for intestinal protozoan parasites, 309t
  for traveler's diarrhea, 299t, 300
Azulfidine. See Sulfasalazine (Azulfidine)

B

Bacillus cereus, 294t, 295
Baclofen
  for GERD, 57
Bacteremia, 104
Bacterial esophagitis, 98
Bacterial overgrowth
  diabetic diarrhea, 422–423
  short bowel syndrome, 382
  with SRES, 165
Balantidiasis, 307–310
  treatment, 309t
Balantidium coli (Balantidiasis), 307–310
  treatment, 309t
Balloon dilatation
  for achalasia, 114, 116–117
  anastomotic and ileocolonic stenoses, 498t
  for postcholecystectomy syndrome, 776
Balloon dilators, 102–103
Balloon tamponade
  for acute variceal bleeding, 121, 122
Balneol
  for left sided ulcerative colitis, 451
Balsalazide (Colazal)
  for Crohn's disease of small bowel, 391
  for UC, 454, 456
Band ligation
  for acute variceal bleeding, 121, 122
Bannayan Riley Ruvalcaba syndrome, 555
Bariatric operations, 219–225
  complete malabsorption, 219
  gastric restriction, 219–220
  gastrointestinal bleeding, 224
  gastrointestinal complications, 223–225
  GERD, 224
  history of, 219–221
  intestinal obstruction, 224
  malabsorption, 224–225
  selective malabsorption, 220–221
  stomal problems, 223–224

  weight regain, 225
Bariatric surgery
  for nonalcoholic fatty liver disease, 672
Barium enema
  colorectal cancer screening, 543
Barrett's ablation
  photosensitizers, 92–93
Barrett's epithelium
  dysplastic, 92
  lasers, 91
Barrett's esophagus (BE), 38, 69, 86–88
  ablation with thermal electrocoagulation,
    90–91
  antireflux surgery, 86
  argon plasma coagulator, 91–92
  chemoprevention, 88
  EMR studies, 39t
  endoscopic ablation, 88
  GERD, 71
  laser therapy, 91
  with PDT, 92–93
  regression, 71
  surveillance, 88f
  treating GERD, 86
Bay12-9566
  for pancreatic cancer, 821
Bayes analysis, 8
BE. See Barrett's esophagus (BE)
Beclomethasone
  for GVHD, 286
  for UC, 450
BED. See Binge eating disorder (BED)
Beer
  GERD, 60
Behavioral disorders, 233
Belching reflex, 339
Belladonna with phenobarbital (Donnatal)
  for IBS, 240t
Benadryl
  endoscopic sedation, 19
Benign ampullary tumors, 769–770
Benign gastric outlet obstruction
  balloon dilatation, 495f
Benign strictures, 498–499
  intestinal and colonic
    endoscopy, 495t
Bentyl
  for functional abdominal pain syndrome,
    247
  for IBS, 240t
Benzodiazepines
  for alcohol withdrawal, 20, 230
  endoscopic sedation, 18, 19
  for pruritus gravidarum, 696
Benzoquinoneimine
  for acetaminophen poisoning, 692
Berger operation, 785
Best Evidence, 1
Beta blockers
  for acute variceal bleeding, 119, 122, 123
  for cystic fibrosis, 809
  noncardiac surgery, 430t, 432–433
  for portal hypertension, 676–677
Beta carotene deficiency, 712
Beta cell replacement
  type I diabetes mellitus, 828

Betaine
  for nonalcoholic fatty liver disease, 673
Bethanechol
  for GERD, 55
Bethesda criteria, 548t
Bichloroacetic acid
  for condylomata acuminata, 535
Biliary cirrhosis
  pediatric liver transplantation, 651
Biliary malabsorption
  diabetic diarrhea, 422
Biliary obstruction
  with chronic pancreatitis, 787
  with cystic fibrosis, 809
Biliary pain
  Milwaukee classification, 771t
  ROME II diagnostic criteria for, 771f
Biliary strictures
  with chronic pancreatitis, 787
  CT, 764
  endoscopy, 764
  EUS, 764
  MRCP, 764
  and neoplasms, 763–765
  with PSC, 717
Biliary tract disorders
  liver tests, 606t
Biliopancreatic diversion (BPD)
  duodenal switch, 223f
Bilirubin, 605–606
Bilirubin test, 606t
Binge eating disorder (BED), 214, 232–233
Biofeedback
  for chronic abdominal pain, 253
  for constipation, 442
Biologic therapy
  for food allergy, 350
Biopolymers
  injection/implantation, 80
Biopsy mapping
  stomach, 178
Bisacodyl
  for constipation, 439t, 441
  cost, 439t
Bismuth subsalicylate (Pepto Bismol)
  for acute infectious diarrhea, 293
  for microscopic colitis, 507
  for traveler's diarrhea, 299t
Bisoprolol
  noncardiac surgery, 433
Bisphosphonates
  for metabolic bone disease, 332t, 333
Bithionol
  adverse effects, 314t
  for intestinal helminths, 312t
  pregnancy, 313t
Blastocystis hominis, 307
  treatment, 309t
Bleeding peptic ulcer, 172–173
  acid suppression, 174–175
  future endoscopic therapies, 175
  PPI, 174–175
  prevalence, 168f
  recurrent, 175
  second look endoscopy, 175

Blood tests
  food allergy, 348–349
BMI. *See* Body mass index (BMI)
Body fat, 212
Body imaging tools
  pancreatic carcinoma detection, 31t
Body mass index (BMI), 212, 214
Body surface area (BSA), 741
Bone alkaline phosphatase
  metabolic bone disease, 327t
Bone metabolism
  and chronic inflammation, 333f
Bone mineral density, 331f
  disorders associated with low, 328t
  metabolic bone disease, 327t
Books
  CAM, 355
Botulinum toxin
  for achalasia, 109, 116
  for anal fissure, 530
  for constipation, 442
  for gastroparesis, 192
  for postcholecystectomy syndrome, 776
Bougie dilatation
  esophageal disruption, 103
Bowel
  absorptive capacity, 381
  adaptation, 381
  obstruction
    ileoanal pouch anastomosis controversies, 461
Bowen's disease, 532
Boyce's rule of threes, 101
BPD. *See* Biliopancreatic diversion (BPD)
Bradykinesia
  with Wilson's disease, 722
Bran
  for constipation, 439t
Breastfeeding
  UC, 455
Bruton's disease, 280
BSA. *See* Body surface area (BSA)
B subunit of cholera toxin (CTB), 301
Buckwheat seed
  with celiac disease, 368
Budd-Chiari syndrome, 683–684
  etiology, 683t
Budesonide (Entocort)
  for Crohn's colitis, 466
  for Crohn's disease of small bowel, 391
  for microscopic colitis, 508
  with osteoporosis, 331
  for pediatric Crohn's disease, 397
  vs. prednisone, 398t
  for UC, 450
Bulimia nervosa, 214, 232–238. *See also*
  Eating disorders
  defined, 232
  management of, 234–236
  oral conditions, 45
Bulk forming laxatives
  for constipation, 440
Buried bumper syndrome
  with percutaneous endoscopic gastrostomy, 198

Buspirone (Buspar)
  for FGID, 263t, 264
  for NUD, 187
Busulfan
  side effects, 286
Button's disease, 280

C
Caffeine
  food induced symptoms, 340, 341–342
CAGE questionnaire, 227, 227t
Calcitonin
  for PBC, 703
Calcium
  deficiency
    conditions leading to, 328–330
    Crohn's disease of small bowel, 395
  in foods, 374
  lactose intolerance, 374
  for PBC, 703
  recommended intake, 374
  for short bowel syndrome, 381
  supplements
    for metabolic bone disease, 334
Calcium channel blockers
  for achalasia, 113
  for secretory diarrhea, 428
  for unexplained chest pain, 111
Calcium polycarbophil
  for constipation, 439t
Calicivirus, 295
Calorie
  alcoholic liver disease, 667f
  assessment, 320
  needs, 320t
CAM. *See* Complementary and alternative
  medicine (CAM)
Campral
  for alcoholism, 229
Campylobacter, 294t
  traveler's diarrhea, 298
Campylobacter jejuni, 294
Campylobacter pylori
  patient to patient transmission, 24
Cancer cachexia
  enteral nutrition, 325
Candida albicans, 43, 96–97
Candidiasis
  with human immunodeficiency virus
    (HIV), 274
Capecitabine
  for colorectal carcinoma, 564
  for metastatic esophageal cancer, 129
Capsaisin
  food induced symptoms, 341–342
CAP System FEIA, 348
Carbamazepine
  for unexplained chest pain, 111
Carbohydrate deficient transferrin assay
  alcoholism, 228
Carbohydrates
  food induced symptoms, 340, 340t
Carbonated beverages
  with achalasia, 113
Carboplatin

for metastatic esophageal cancer, 129
Carcinoembryonic antigen (CEA), 557–558
Carcinoid syndrome
  secretory diarrhea, 428
Carcinoma
  with cystic fibrosis, 808
Cardia
  IM, 181
Cardiac arrhythmias, 19
  cardiovascular risk with major surgery, 432
Cardiovascular diseases
  COX 2 inhibitors, 143
  NSAID, 143
Cardiovascular risk
  with major surgery, 430–433, 430t
    noninvasive testing, 431–432
    perioperative management, 432–433
Caries
  with eating disorders, 233
Carnett's sign, 251
Carvedilol
  for portal hypertension, 677
Cascara
  for constipation, 439t, 440
  cost, 439t
  pregnancy, 443
Caspofungin
  for esophageal infections, 97
Castor oil
  pregnancy, 443
CBD stones. See Common bile duct (CBD) stones
CCK. See Cholecystokinin (CCK)
CE. See Complete eradication (CE)
CEA. See Carcinoembryonic antigen (CEA)
Cefixime
  for Whipple's disease, 317t
Cefotaxime
  for ascitic fluid infection, 659
Ceftriaxone (Rocephin)
  for gonorrhea, 534
  for Whipple's disease, 317t
Cefuroxime
  for acute pancreatitis, 781
Celebrex, 143
  for NSAID induced ulcers, 8
Celecoxib (Celebrex), 143
  for NSAID induced ulcers, 8
Celexa
  efficacy, 264
  for FGID, 263t
  side effects, 264
Celiac diet
  information sources, 369
Celiac disease, 345
  diabetic diarrhea, 420
  diet, 368t
  pharmalogic treatment, 369–370, 369t
  safe foods, 368–369
Celiac like conditions, 282
Celiac sprue, 367–370
  associated with low BMD, 328t
  diabetic diarrhea, 421
  diagnosis, 367

dietary treatment, 367–369
Cellcept
  for Crohn's disease of small bowel, 393
  for GVHD, 286
  side effects, 286
  for transplantation, 387
Centers for Disease Control and Prevention
  growth curves, 805f
Cephalosporin with vancomycin
  for bacterial esophagitis, 98
Cerebral edema
  with fulminant hepatic failure, 635–636
Cerebral toxicity
  for acute variceal bleeding, 121
Cerebral Whipple's disease, 318–319
Cervical osteophytes
  oropharyngeal dysphagia, 51
Cervical webs
  oropharyngeal dysphagia, 51
Cestodes, 311
Ceuximab
  for pancreatic cancer, 821
Chaga's disease, 99
Challenge
  adverse reactions to food, 347
Charcot's triad, 769
Chemical celiac splanchnicectomy
  for pancreatic and periampullary neoplasms, 816
Chemotherapy
  for metastatic esophageal cancer, 128–129
Chest pain
  esophageal
    etiology, 108
    GERD, 66, 67t
    pathophysiology, 108f
  unexplained
    treatment, 111
Child Pugh C, 122
Children
  antiparasitic drugs, 313t
  HBV, 625–627
  HCV, 627–628
  obesity, 213t
  viral hepatitis, 625–628
Childs Turcotte Pugh score, 638t
Chinese liver fluke, 310
  treatment, 312t
Chlamydia trachomatis, 534
Chloramphenicol
  for Whipple's disease, 317t
Chlordiazepoxide (Librium)
  for alcohol withdrawal, 230
Chlordioxipoxide (Librax)
  for IBS, 240t
Chloroquine
  for porphyria cutanea tarda, 729
Chlorpromazine
  for porphyria, 729
  for secretory diarrhea, 428
Cholangiocarcinoma, 717–718, 736–737
  pediatric liver transplantation, 652
Cholangitis
  acute
    with choledocholithiasis, 767–769

Cholecystectomy. See also Laparoscopic cholecystectomy
  open, 759–761
Cholecystitis, 753–757
  chronic, 756–757
    acalculous, 757
  CT, 753f
  diagnosis, 753–754
  presentation, 753
  with SCT, 287
  treatment, 754–755
Cholecystokinin (CCK), 147, 341
  with chronic pancreatitis, 796–797
  receptor antagonists
    for chronic pancreatitis, 800
Choledocholithiasis, 766–769
  complications, 767–769
  CT, 766
  CTC, 766
  EUS, 766
  imaging, 766
  MRCP, 766
  treatment, 766–767
Cholelithiasis, 713, 759–762
  ESWL, 761
  laparoscopic cholecystectomy, 760
  oral bile acid dissolution therapy, 761–762
  simulations with stone removal, 760–761
  surgery, 759–760
Cholera toxin
  B subunit, 301
Cholestasis
  acute
    drug induced, 690t
  chronic, 707–713
  cutaneous sequelae, 712–713
  drugs associated with, 290t
  fatigue of, 710–711
  intrahepatic of pregnancy, 695–696
  liver tests, 606t
  neonatal
    with cystic fibrosis, 808
  pruritis, 707–713
  with SCT, 290
  vitamin supplementation, 712, 713t
Cholestyramine, 712
  for Clostridium difficile diarrhea, 305
  for erythropoietic protoporphyria, 730
  for PBC, 703
  for pruritis of cholestasis, 707–708, 708, 708t
  for pruritus gravidarum, 696
  resin, 241t
  for secretory diarrhea, 428
  in white petroleum
    for left sided ulcerative colitis, 451
Chronic abdominal pain, 249–254, 784–786
  approach to, 250–251
  biology, 249–250
  ductal drainage operation, 785
  hard to control, 251
  management, 252–253
  morbidity, 784
  neural pathways, 249
  neurolytic blockade, 254

of no apparent cause, 251
pancreatic resection, 785–786
pharmacologic therapy, 252–253
preoperative imaging, 784–785
psychology, 249–250
rare causes, 251
referred pain, 250
sensitization, 249–250
surgery, 784
Chronic acalculous cholecystitis, 757
Chronic cholecystitis, 756–757
Chronic cholestasis, 707–713
Chronic gastritis, 140, 178–181
adenomas, 180
family history, 179
gastric biopsy mapping, 180
hyperplastic polyps, 180–181
Ménétrier's disease, 181
postoperative stomach, 181
Chronic graft versus host disease
with SCT, 287
Chronic hepatitis B, 616–620
diagnosis, 617
HCC, 617–619
liver biopsy, 617
natural history, 616–617
treatment, 617–618
treatment difficult issues, 619–620
viral characteristics, 616
Chronic hepatitis C, 621–624
baseline evaluation, 622–623
cirrhosis, 623
clinical implications, 621
diagnosis, 621–622
human immunodeficiency virus (HIV)
coinfection, 623
natural history, 621
recurrence after transplant, 623
treatment, 622–623
adverse effects, 623
Chronic immunodeficiency syndrome,
280–283
Chronic intestinal pseudoobstruction (CIP),
375–380
classification, 376t
clinical presentation, 376
diagnosis, 376–378, 377f
etiology, 375
familial visceral myopathy, 376
with food intolerance, 342
imaging studies, 377
impact, 375
laparotomy, 378
manometry, 378
plain abdominal radiography, 377
quality of life, 375
treatment, 378–380, 378t
wall biopsy, 378
Chronic megacolon
constipation, 443
Chronic pancreatitis, 251, 792f, 796–801
alcohol induced, 793f
celiac plexus block, 801
coexistent motility disturbances, 799
complications, 786–787

diagnosis, 797–798, 797t
diagnostic tests, 797t
endoscopic therapy, 791–795, 801
etiology, 796t
EUS, 798
exocrine secretion feedback control,
799–801
gene screening, 811
longitudinal pancreaticojejunostomy, 785t
mutation analysis, 810–811
pain, 798–799
pathogenesis, 796–797
patient counseling and monitoring, 811
presentation, 796
resection, 785t
surgery, 784–788, 801
treatment, 798
Chronic recurrent abdominal pain, 243–248
clinical presentation, 243
pathophysiology, 243
stress, 243–244
Chylous ascites
with intestinal transplantation, 388
Cidofovir
for viral esophagitis, 98
Cigarette smoking
alcoholic liver disease, 666
with PUD, 147
Cimetidine (Tagamet)
for OC with duodenal ulcer, 45
for OC with GERD, 45
for SRES, 163
for upper gastrointestinal bleeding, 153
CIP. See Chronic intestinal pseudoobstruction (CIP)
Ciprofloxacin
for acute pancreatitis, 781
for Crohn's colitis, 466
for Crohn's diseases perianal complications, 473
for diarrhea, 293, 294t
for diverticulitis, 601
for ileoanal pouch, 528
for nonsteroidal antiinflammatory drug
enteropathy, 365
for traveler's diarrhea, 299, 299t
Cirrhosis
pediatric liver transplantation, 650
treatment, 657–658
Cisapride (Propulsid)
for acute colonic pseudoobstruction, 504
for CIP, 379
for constipation, 441
for gastroparesis, 192
for GERD, 55
NUD, 186
promoting esophageal clearance, 109
Cisplatin
for anal neoplasm, 532
for esophageal cancer, 128
esophageal cancer injection therapy, 133
Cisplatinum
for metastatic esophageal cancer, 128–129
Citalopram (Celexa)
efficacy, 264

for FGID, 263t
side effects, 264
Citrucel
for acute infectious diarrhea, 293
for constipation, 439t, 440
CIWAr scale. See Clinical Institute
Withdrawal Assessment for Alcohol
(CIWAr) scale
Clarithromycin
for Helicobacter pylori, 140, 145
for human immunodeficiency virus
(HIV), 277
Classic syndrome, 255–256
Cleaning
endoscopic disinfection, 25
Clinical Institute Withdrawal Assessment
for Alcohol (CIWAr) scale, 230, 230t
Clinical questions
study design, 2f
Clobetasol, 43
Clonazepam
for porphyria, 729
Clonidine
for diabetic diarrhea, 421
for secretory diarrhea, 427
Clonorchis sinensis (Chinese liver fluke), 310
treatment, 312t
C-loop Wallstents, 496f, 497f
Clostridium difficile, 294t, 447
antibiotic associated diarrhea, 302–305
prevention, 305, 305t
Clostridium difficile colitis
antireflux surgery, 70
treatment, 305t
Clostridium difficile diarrhea, 304f
antimicrobial agents predisposing to, 302t
clinical manifestations, 303
diagnosis, 304
treatment, 304–305
Clostridium perfringens, 294t, 295
Clot busters, 168
CMV. See Cytomegalovirus (CMV)
Coagulation studies, 358
Cochrane Collaboration, 1
Codeine
for secretory diarrhea, 426
Cognitive behavioral therapy
for chronic abdominal pain, 253
Colace
for constipation, 440
Colazal
for UC, 454, 456
Colchicine
for alcoholic liver disease, 668
for constipation, 439t, 441
cost, 439t
for PBC, 704
Colesevalam
for pruritis of cholestasis, 707–708, 708
Colitis. See specific types
Collagenous colitis
with celiac disease, 370
Collagenous lymphocytic colitis, 507t
Colon
diverticular disease, 597–603

diverticulitis, 601–603
diverticulosis, 597–603
meal induced physiological changes, 339–340
radiation side effects, 581t, 582
Colon cancer, 557–562
  adjuvant therapy, 561
  American Joint Commission on Cancer TNM staging, 558t
  CAT, 558
  colon resection, 559
  diagnosis, 557–558
  followup, 561–562
  laparoscopic colectomy, 559–560
  left hemicolectomy, 560f
  lymphadenectomy, 560–561
  obstructing, 561
  perforated, 561
  PET, 558
  presentation, 557
  with PSC, 717
  right hemicolectomy, 559f
  sentinel lymph node mapping, 560–561
  sigmoid hemicolectomy, 560f
  staging, 558
  treatment, 558–559
Colonic adenomas
  smoking, 270
Colonic benign strictures
  endoscopy, 495t
Colonic bleeding
  etiology, 584t
Colonic Crohn's disease (Crohn's colitis)
  surgery, 405
Colonic neoplasia
  genetic counseling, 545–549
Colonic pseudoobstruction. *See* Acute colonic pseudoobstruction
Colonic stenoses
  malignant, 496t
  self expandable metallic stents, 499t
Colonic strictures, 494–501
  benign, 495
    endoscopy, 495t
  etiology, 494t, 495t
  malignant, 496–497
  management, 494–501
Colonoscopy
  colorectal cancer screening, 543–544
  infection, 23–24
Colorectal cancer
  abdominoperineal resection, 571
  adjuvant/neoadjuvant therapy, 572–573
  anterior resection, 571
  colonic J pouch, 572
  emergent cases, 572
  en bloc resection, 572
  laparoscopic resection, 572
  local recurrence, 573–574
  local staging, 570
  outcomes, 573–574
  preoperative *vs.* postoperative adjuvant radiation, 573t
  preparation for surgery, 570
  radical resection, 571–572

risk stratification, 542
  surgery, 570–572
  surveillance, 573
  TNM staging, 570t
  total mesorectal excision (TME), 571
Colorectal cancer screening, 541–544
  advanced adenoma, 541
  average risk population, 544
  barium enema, 543
  colonoscopy, 543–544
  flexible sigmoidoscopy, 543
  FOBT, 542
    with flexible sigmoidoscopy, 543
  objectives, 541–542
  options, 542–544
  three dimensional virtual colonoscopy, 543
Colorectal carcinoma, 563–567
  adjuvant chemotherapy, 565–566
  combination chemotherapy, 563–564
  forthcoming adjuvant trials, 566t
  monoclonal antibodies, 566–567
  postoperative adjuvant therapy randomized trials, 566t
  primary chemotherapy, 563–564
    adverse effects, 563
  regional chemotherapy, 565
Colorectal endoscopic mucosal resection
  articles, 36f
  studies, 41t
Colorectal polyps, 550
Colorectal prostheses, 499–500
Colorectum, 40
Colovesicle fistula
  contrast enema, 599f
Common bile duct (CBD) stones, 766, 767f, 768f
Common variable immunodeficiency (CVID), 281
  gastrointestinal manifestations, 281–282, 282t
  malignancy, 282–283
Compartment model, 8
Compazine
  for gastroparesis, 193
Complementary and alternative medicine (CAM), 352–355
  efficacy, 353
  information about, 355
  patient approach, 353–355
  safety, 353
  web sites, 355
Complete eradication (CE)
  of BE, 91
Complete malabsorption
  bariatric operations, 219
Compliance
  nurse advocate, 267
Complicated strictures, 100
Compression stockings, 570–572
Computed tomography (CT)
  application of, 4
  colonography
    screening, 4–7
  pancreatic carcinoma detection, 31t

severity index, 778
Concomitant chemoradiotherapy
  for esophageal cancer, 127
Condylomata acuminata, 535
Congestive heart failure
  cardiovascular risk with major surgery, 432
Conscious sedation, 17
  continuum of depth, 17t
Constipation, 439–443
  chronic megacolon, 443
  with cystic fibrosis, 807
  diagnosis, 442f
  with food intolerance, 342
  IBS, 240, 241, 443
    medications, 241t
  pregnancy, 443
  treatment, 442f
Conversion disorder, 256
Corn
  with celiac disease, 368
Corticosteroids
  for acetaminophen poisoning, 692
  for alcoholic liver disease, 667–668
  for Crohn's colitis, 466
  for Crohn's disease of small bowel, 391
  for liver disease during pregnancy, 694–695
  for pediatric Crohn's disease, 397
  pregnancy, 491
Cost
  genetic counseling, 546
Cost effectiveness analyses, 15
Cough
  GERD, 66, 67t
Courvoisier's sign, 763
Cowden's Syndrome, 555f
  oral conditions, 46
  risk and surveillance, 552t, 554
Cow's milk protein enteropathy, 345
COX2. *See* Cyclooxygenase 2 inhibitors (COX 2)
CPT-11
  for colorectal carcinoma, 564
  for metastatic esophageal cancer, 129
Cricopharyngeal bar, 52
Cricopharyngeal strictures
  oropharyngeal dysphagia, 51
Critically ill patients
  enteral nutrition for, 325
Crohn's colitis, 465–470
  clinical features, 465
  colorectal cancer, 542
  dysplasia surveillance programs, 486
  management, 465–470
  medical management, 466–467
  nutritional therapy, 466–467
  refractory disease, 468–469
  remission, 469
  steroid dependent disease, 468–469
  surgery, 469–470
  treatment algorithm, 467f
Crohn's disease
  annular stricture, 498f
  associated with low BMD, 328t

bowel resection, 404
colonoscopy, 402
colon resection, 405
fistula, 404, 404f
intraoperative decision making, 404
nutritional support, 403
oral conditions, 43–44
ostomy nurse, 403
pediatric
  future therapy, 399
  nutritional therapy, 399–400
  psychosocial therapy, 400
  therapy, 399t
  treatment, 397–400
perianal complications in, 471–475, 475t
  diagnosis, 471–472
  incidence, 471
  medical management, 472–475
  pathogenesis, 471
preoperative examination, 402–403
preoperative preparation, 402–403, 403t
radiology, 402
smoking, 271–272
surgery, 402–405
  indications for, 403t
Crohn's disease of small bowel, 390–396
abscesses, 394–395
clinical phenotypes, 390
complications, 394–396
fistulas, 394–395
induction therapy, 391–392
jejunoileitis, 394
maintenance therapy, 393
medical therapy, 390, 391t
NOD2, 390
nutritional deficiency, 395
nutritional therapy, 394
obstruction, 395
osteoporosis, 395
postresection, 393
steroid sparing therapy, 393–394
surgery, 394
Cryotherapy
hemorrhoids, 538
Cryptosporidiosis. *See Cryptosporidium parvum* (Cryptosporidiosis)
Cryptosporidium parvum
(Cryptosporidiosis), 294, 294t, 307–308
traveler's diarrhea, 298–299
treatment, 309t
CT. *See* Computed tomography (CT)
CTB. *See* B subunit of cholera toxin (CTB)
Cuffed tracheostomy, 53
Cuffitis
ileoanal pouch anastomosis controversies, 461
Cumulative cost over time
ratio, 15
CVID. *See* Common variable immunodeficiency (CVID)
Cyclooxygenase 2 inhibitors (COX 2), 143
for nonsteroidal antiinflammatory drug enteropathy, 365
for NSAID induced ulcers, 8
Cyclophosphamide
side effects, 286
Cyclospora cayetanensis (Cyclosporiasis), 294, 294t, 308
traveler's diarrhea, 298–299
treatment, 309t
Cyclosporiasis. *See Cyclospora cayetanensis* (Cyclosporiasis)
Cyclosporine
for Crohn's colitis, 468
for Crohn's disease of small bowel, 392
for Crohn's diseases perianal complications, 473–474
drug interactions, 97
with osteoporosis, 331–332
pediatric liver transplantation, 653
pregnancy, 491
for UC, 454, 455
Cystic fibrosis, 803–810
with chronic pancreatitis, 796
diabetes, 828–829
diagnosis, 806–807
differential diagnosis, 805t, 806t
gastrointestinal manifestations, 803t
GERD, 803
pediatric liver transplantation, 651
Cytomegalovirus (CMV)
colitis, 277
inducing fulminant hepatic failure, 630
with intestinal transplantation, 388
Cytotec. *See* Misoprostol (Cytotec)

D

Dairy
adverse reactions to food, 347
DALM. *See* Dysplasia associated lesion or mass (DALM)
DBPCFC, 349
Deceased donor liver procurement
liver transplantation, 644–645
Decision analysis
digestive disease management, 8–16
towards clinical application, 8–16
Decision trees, 8–10
costs or probabilities, 11
example, 11
for NSAID induced peptic ulcer treatment, 9
sensitivity analysis, 12
therapy success rates, 13
ulcer management, 13f
Decompression
with CIP, 379
Deep sedation
continuum of depth, 17t
Deferoxamine
for porphyria cutanea tarda, 729
Definitive resection
PGL, 208
Dehydration
mesenteric vascular ischemia, 413–414
for traveler's diarrhea, 300
Delayed gastric emptying
with pancreatic and periampullary neoplasms, 816
Delorme's operation

rectal prolapse, 521
Delta aminolevulinic acid dehydrase deficiency, 728
Delta hepatitis
acute, 614
Demerol. *See* Meperidine (Demerol)
Demerol (meperidine)
pregnancy, 492
Deodorized tincture of opium
for short bowel syndrome, 381
Depression
alcoholism, 228
with Wilson's disease, 723
Designated individual
monitoring, 21
Desipramine (Norpramin)
for FGID, 262, 263, 263t
for IBS, 240t
for spastic motor disorders, 111
Desoximetasone, 43
Desyrel
for chronic abdominal pain, 253
Dexamethasone
for pruritus gravidarum, 696
Diabetes
cystic fibrosis, 828–829
Diabetic diarrhea
autonomic neuropathy, 420
bacterial overgrowth, 422–423
biliary malabsorption, 422
celiac disease, 420
clinical examination, 420–421
fecal incontinence, 422
laboratory tests, 421
mechanisms, 420–421, 420t
nonpharmacologic treatment, 422–423
pancreatic insufficiency, 422
pharmacologic treatment, 422
tests, 420–421
treatment, 420–421, 420–424, 421–424, 422f
Diabetic gastroparesis, 193
Diagnosis
well-designed trial characteristics, 4t
Diarrhea, 276f. *See also* specific types
antireflux surgery, 70
with food intolerance, 342
IBS, 240
  medications, 241t
ileoanal pouch, 529
microscopic colitis, 506
with percutaneous endoscopic gastrostomy, 199
stem cell transplantation, 286–287
Diarrhea and wasting
human immunodeficiency virus (HIV), 275–276
Diazepam (Valium)
for alcohol withdrawal, 230
Diazepam (Valium) with meperidine
endoscopic sedation
patient controlled, 22
Dicyclomine (Bentyl)
for functional abdominal pain syndrome, 247

for IBS, 240t
Dientamoeba fragilis, 308
 treatment, 309t
Diet
 celiac disease, 368t
 with CIP, 378–379
 for microscopic colitis, 507
 obesity, 216–217
 overweight, 217
 severe obesity, 217
 for short bowel syndrome, 382–383
Dietary assessment
 obesity, 215–216
Dietary counseling
 for pediatric Crohn's disease, 400
Dietary fiber
 for constipation, 440
Dietary induced symptoms, 339–343
Dietary restrictions, 349–350
Diet therapy
 ascites, 657
 oral, 321
Dieulafoy's lesions, 169, 173, 173f
Diffuse type mucosal gastric cancer, 40
Difibrotide
 for VOD, 289
DiGeorge syndrome, 281
 gastrointestinal manifestations, 283
Dilatated esophagus
 barium study, 115f
Dilation
 goals, 101
Dilators
 types, 101
Dilinoleoylphosphatidylcholine
 for alcoholic liver disease, 669
Diloxanide furcate
 for intestinal protozoan parasites, 309t
Dimethyl sulfoxide (DMSO), 80
DIOS
 with cystic fibrosis, 806
Dipentum
 for Crohn's disease of small bowel, 391
 for UC, 454, 455–456
Diphenhydramine (Benadryl)
 endoscopic sedation, 19
Diphenoxylate with atropine sulfate (Lomotil), 241t
 for acute infectious diarrhea, 292
 for fecal incontinence, 512
 for secretory diarrhea, 426
 for short bowel syndrome, 381
Diphyllobothrium latum
 treatment, 312t
Diprovan. *See* Propofol (Diprovan)
Dipylidium canium
 treatment, 312t
Dipyridamole exercise thallium
 cardiovascular risk with major surgery, 431–432
Discrete event simulations, 8
Distal esophagus, 81f
 categorizing, 107f
Distal splenorenal shunt
 for acute variceal bleeding, 122

Distal subtotal gastrectomy
 PGL, 208
Disulfiram
 for alcoholism, 229
Diuretic abuse
 with eating disorders, 233, 234
Diuretics
 for ascites, 657
 for portal hypertension, 677
 secretory diarrhea, 429
Diverticular disease
 colon, 597–603
Diverticulitis
 colon, 601–603
 CT, 603t
 elective colon resection, 603
 treatment, 603f
Diverticulosis, 584–585
 colon, 597–603
  bleeding, 597–598
  complications, 597–598
  elective resection, 601–602
  etiology, 597
  infection, 598
  spasm, 597
  treatment, 598–603
D lactic acidosis
 short bowel syndrome, 382
DMSO. *See* Dimethyl sulfoxide (DMSO)
Dobutamine stress echocardiography (DSE)
 cardiovascular risk with major surgery, 431–432
Docetaxel
 for metastatic esophageal cancer, 129
Docusates (Colace, Surfak)
 for constipation, 440
Dolasetron (Anzemet)
 for gastroparesis, 193
Domperidone (Motilium)
 for CIP, 379
 for gastroparesis, 191
 for GERD, 56
 for nausea and vomiting, 288
 for NUD, 186
Donnatal
 with belladonna
  for IBS, 240t
 for IBS, 240t
 for pruritis of cholestasis, 709
Dopamine antagonists
 for gastroparesis, 190–191
Double blinded placebo food challenge (DBPCFC), 349
Doxepin (Sinequan)
 for FGID, 263t
Doxycycline
 for gonorrhea, 534
 for Whipple's disease, 317t
D-penicillamine
 for PBC, 704
Dronabinol (Marinol)
 for gastroparesis, 193
 for pruritis of cholestasis, 710
Droperidol
 endoscopic sedation, 19

Drug abuse
 liver transplantation, 640
Drug induced acute cholestasis, 690t
Drug induced acute hepatitis, 690t
Drug induced chronic liver disease, 690t
Drug induced liver disease, 689–693
 acute reactions, 689–690
 autoantibody targets, 691t
 clinical presentation, 689–690
 diagnosis, 691
 pathogenesis, 690–691
 risk factors, 691–692
 treatment, 692–693
Drug induced osteoporosis, 331–332
Drying
 endoscopic disinfection, 26
Dry mouth (xerostomia), 45
DSE. *See* Dobutamine stress echocardiography (DSE)
DT, 229–230
Dukoral, 301
Duodenal gastrinoma, 156
Duodenal polyps, 551–552
Duodenal switch
 BPD, 222
 with BPD, 222, 223f
Duodenal ulcer
 smoking, 271
Duodenum
 ECG, 40
Dynamic (interpersonal) psychotherapy
 for chronic abdominal pain, 253
Dysarthria
 with Wilson's disease, 722
Dysentery, 308
Dyspepsia
 defined, 183
Dysphagia, 40. *See also* Oropharyngeal dysphagia
 palliative management of, 134
 treatment, 109
 unexplained
  evaluation, 115
 with Wilson's disease, 722
Dysplasia associated lesion or mass (DALM), 487
Dysplasia surveillance programs, 485–489
 high risk patients, 486
 interpretation, 486
 intervals, 486, 486f
 polyps, 487–488
 pouches, 488–489
 protocol, 485–487
Dysplastic Barrett's epithelium, 92
 PDT, 93t
Dystonia
 with Wilson's disease, 722

E

Ear, nose, and throat disease
 GERD, 67
Early gastric cancer (EGC)
 lymph node metastasis rate, 36
Early satiety
 antireflux surgery, 70

Eating cues, 214
Eating disorders
  chronicity, 237
  gastrointestinal complications, 233–234
  gastrointestinal problems, 233
  history, 235t
  inpatient treatment, 236–237
  management of, 234–236
  oral conditions, 45
  outcomes, 237
  outpatient treatment, 236
  pharmacotherapy, 237
  psychiatric comorbidity, 237–238
  psychiatric treatment, 236–237
  referral, 235
  relapse, 237
  screening, 235
Eating disorders not otherwise specified (EDNOS), 232–233
Ebstein Barr virus (EBV)
  inducing fulminant hepatic failure, 630
EBV infection
  with intestinal transplantation, 388
ECL. See Enterchromaffin like (ECL) cells
Eclampsia
  pregnancy, 698
Ectopic varices, 123
Ectropion, 533
Eder Puestow dilators, 102
EDNOS. See Eating disorders not otherwise specified (EDNOS)
Effexor
  for chronic abdominal pain, 253
  efficacy, 264
  for FGID, 263t, 264
EGC. See Early gastric cancer (EGC)
EGD. See Esophagogastroduodenoscopy (EGD)
Elavil. See Amitriptyline (Elavil)
Electrical stimulation
  for chronic abdominal pain, 254
Electrocardiography
  monitoring, 21
Electrocoagulation
  esophageal cancer, 131
Electrolyte replacement
  secretory diarrhea, 425–426
Electrolytes
  for short bowel syndrome, 384
Elimination
  adverse reactions to food, 347
Elimination diet, 348, 348t
Embolic materials, 592t
Empiric antifungal therapy, 97
EMR. See Endoscopic mucosal resection (EMR)
EMRC. See Endoscopic mucosal resection cap assisted (EMRC)
Encephalitozoon intestinales (Microsporidiosis), 308
  treatment, 309t
Encephalopathy
  fulminant hepatic failure, 634–635
  grading scheme, 631t
EndoCinch System, 76–78, 83
  effect, 76–77
  morbidity, 84
  procedure, 76
  step wise sequence, 77f
Endoprosthesis
  for pancreatic and periampullary neoplasms, 816
Endorectal advancement flap, 481f
Endoscopes
  flexible gastrointestinal
    LCS reprocessing, 26t
  insufficient drying, 24
Endoscopically placed metallic stents
  PGL, 210
Endoscopic band ligation, 174
Endoscopic devices
  for GERD, 83–84
Endoscopic dilation
  for esophageal cancer palliation, 134
Endoscopic disinfection, 23–28
Endoscopic examination
  technique, 101–102
Endoscopic gastroesophageal reflux disease
  treatment trials, 82–83
Endoscopic hemoclipping, 172–173
Endoscopic mucosal resection (EMR), 36–41, 87
  articles, 36f
  colorectal, 36f
  studies, 41t
  complications, 41
  histopathologic assessment, 38
  indications, 36–37, 39t
  perforation risk, 41
  postprocedure, 38
  stenosis, 40
  techniques, 37–38, 37t
Endoscopic mucosal resection cap assisted (EMRC), 37
Endoscopic procedures
  pharmacology, 18
  vascular access, 18
Endoscopic reprocessing, 23–28
  cautionary reports, 23
  protocol breaches, 24
  stages, 23, 25–26
Endoscopic retrograde cholangiopancreatography (ERCP), 24, 715
  acute gallstone pancreatitis, 781
  pancreatic carcinoma detection, 31t
Endoscopic sclerotherapy
  for acute variceal bleeding, 121
Endoscopic sedation, 17–22
  dosing, 20
  future trends, 21–22
  monitoring, 20–21
  postprocedure, 21
  preprocedure evaluation, 17–18
Endoscopic submucosal injection of bovine collagen, 80
Endoscopic surveillance
  for BE, 87
Endoscopic suturing (plication), 76
  for bleeding peptic ulcer, 175
Endoscopic Suturing Device (ESD), 78f
  effect, 78
  procedure, 78
Endoscopic Suturing System, 76–78
  step wise sequence, 77f
Endoscopic therapy
  preparation, 167
Endoscopic ultrasonography (EUS), 29–35
  indications, 29–34
  pancreatic carcinoma detection, 31t
Endoscopy
  terminal drying, 24
  upper
    for GERD, 69
Endovascular intervention
  upper gastrointestinal bleeding, 174
End stage liver disease
  model, 639t
  pediatric liver transplantation, 650
End stage renal disease
  with PCT, 729
Enemas
  for constipation, 439t
Engerix-B, 613
Entamoeba dispar (Amebiasis), 308
Entamoeba histolytica, 294, 308
  traveler's diarrhea, 298–299
  treatment, 309t
Entamoeba infections
  asymptomatic, 308
Enteral access decisions, 321t
Enteral and parenteral nutrition, 320–325
Enteral feeding
  complications, 322t
Enteral formulas, 321–322, 322t
Enteral nutrition, 321
  for cancer, 325
  for critically ill patients, 325
  for IBD, 324
  for liver disease, 324
  with percutaneous endoscopic gastrostomy, 199–200
  for renal failure, 325
  SRES, 164
Enteral tube feedings
  complications, 322
Enteral Wallstent delivery system, 496f
Enterchromaffin like (ECL) cells, 148
Enteroaggretive *E. coli*
  traveler's diarrhea, 298
Enterobius vermicularis (pinworm), 311
  treatment, 312t
Enteroclysis
  obscure gastrointestinal bleeding, 358–359
Enterocolitis, 277
Enterocytozoan bienusi, 308
  treatment, 309t
Enterostomal therapy nurse, 570–572
Enterotoxigenic *E. coli* (ETEC)
  traveler's diarrhea, 297–298
Enterra, 194
Enteryx, 80, 83, 84
  catheter delivery system, 80f
Entocort. See Budesonide (Entocort)
ENT syndrome
  GERD treatment regimens, 67t

Enzyme therapy
  for chronic pancreatitis, 800
Eosinophilic colitis, 509
Eosinophilic gastroenteritis, 345–346
Eosinophils
  diurnal variation, 450
  IBD, 448
  left sided ulcerative colitis, 448
Epidermolysis bullosa, 103
Epinephrine
  esophageal cancer injection therapy, 133
  upper gastrointestinal bleeding, 170
Epstein Barr virus (EBV) infection
  with intestinal transplantation, 388
ERCP. See Endoscopic retrograde cholangiopancreatography (ERCP)
Erythromycin
  for acute colonic pseudoobstruction, 504
  for *Chlamydia trachomatis*, 534
  for CIP, 379–380
  for gastroparesis, 192
  for GERD, 56
  for nausea and vomiting, 288
  for PUD, 44
  for Whipple's disease, 317t
Erythropoietic protoporphyria, 730–731
Escherichia coli, 293–294, 294t
  traveler's diarrhea
    enteroaggrative, 298
    enterotoxigenic, 297–298
Escitalopram (Lexapro)
  for FGID, 263t
  side effects, 264
ESD. See Endoscopic Suturing Device (ESD)
Esomeprazole (Nexium)
  for ENT with GERD, 67
  for extraesophageal GERD, 67t
  for GERD, 54, 66
  vs. lansoprazole, 55f
  for SRES, 163, 164
  for upper gastrointestinal bleeding, 153
Esophageal adenocarcinoma, 86, 90
  esophageal resection, 87
  esophagectomy, 87
  prevention of, 87
  smoking, 270
  surveillance endoscopy, 87
Esophageal cancer, 29–31, 90, 125–130, 129f
  APC, 132
  combined modality therapy options, 128t
  CT, 126
  debulking, 131–136
  electrocoagulation, 131
  endoscopic view, 133f
  epidemiology, 125
  EUS, 126
  injection therapy, 133
  lasers, 131–132
  locally advanced
    treatment, 127
  management algorithm, 30f
  metastatic, 128–129
  neoadjuvant chemoradiotherapy, 30
  nutrition, 131
  palliation, 131–137

PDT, 132–133
performance status
  treating, 126
PET, 126
preoperative chemotherapy, 127
recurrent
  followup, 129–130
restaging, 30f
smoking, 270
staging, 29–30, 125–126
stent occlusions, 136
superficial, 38
surgical resection, 30
treatment aggressiveness, 126–127
trimodality approach, 127
Esophageal chest pain
  etiology, 108
Esophageal dilatation
  complications, 103–104
  dilators for, 100t
Esophageal disease
  ablative therapy, 90–94
  treatment, 96t
Esophageal endoprosthesis
  for esophageal cancer palliation, 134
Esophageal hypomotility
  treatment, 109
Esophageal infections, 96–99
Esophageal motor disorders, 107–111
  types, 107–108
Esophageal perforation, 103–104
Esophageal problems
  with eating disorders, 233–234
Esophageal strictures
  differential diagnosis, 100t
  management of, 100–105
  perforation rate, 103
  predilatation evaluation, 100
  recurrence, 104
  technical considerations, 100–101
Esophageal symptoms
  with SCT, 288
Esophageal ulcer
  idiopathic, 99
Esophageal varices
  with PBC, 703–704
Esophagectomy
  for esophageal cancer, 127
Esophagogastroduodenoscopy (EGD)
  SRES, 165
Esophagus, 38. See also Barrett's esophagus (BE)
  adenocarcinoma, 86
  dilatated
    barium study, 115f
  distal, 81f
    categorizing, 107f
  meal induced physiological changes, 339
Essential fatty acids, 805
Estrogen
  pregnancy, 696
ESWL. See Extracorporeal shock wave lithotripsy (ESWL)
ETEC. See Enterotoxigenic *E. coli* (ETEC)
Ethanol

esophageal cancer injection therapy, 133
Ethanolamine oleate, 170t
Ethical issues
  artificial nutritional support, 200
  PEG tube, 200
Ethylene vinyl alcohol copolymer, 80
EUS. See Endoscopic ultrasonography (EUS)
Evidence-based medicine, 1–4
  approach to diagnosis, 4–6
    likelihood ratios, 4–5
  approach to prognosis, 6–7
    statistics, 7
  approach to therapy, 1–4
    methodologic validity, 1–2
    statistical analysis, 2–4
  defined, 1
Exaggerated and factitious disease, 255–259
Excessive drainage
  with percutaneous endoscopic gastrostomy, 198–199
Exercise assessment
  obesity, 216
Exercise ECG stress testing
  cardiovascular risk with major surgery, 431
Exercise induced anaphylaxis
  food associated, 345
Exocrine pancreas
  SDS, 810
Expandable hydrogel prosthesis, 81–82
  effect, 81–82
  procedure, 81
Expandable metal stents
  esophageal use, 135f, 135t
Extended low Hartmann operation
  rectal cancer, 576–577
External hemorrhoids
  excision, 537
  treatment, 537
Extracorporeal shock wave lithotripsy (ESWL)
  cholelithiasis, 761
Extraesophageal gastroesophageal reflux disease
  management, 64–66, 65f, 67t
  therapeutic trials, 63–64
Extranodal marginal zone lymphomas of MALT type, 202

F

Factitious illness, 258–259
  clinical suspicion, 258
  discussing behavior, 258–259
  involving family, 259
  psychiatric admission, 259
  psychiatric collaboration, 258
Famciclovir
  for viral esophagitis, 98
Famethoxazole
  for *Isospora belli*, 310
Familial adenomatous polyposis (FAP), 40, 547t, 548, 551–552, 552f
  risk and surveillance, 552t
Familial pancreatic cancer, 825

Familial pancreatitis, 825
Family history
  chronic gastritis, 179
Family therapy
  for eating disorders, 236
  for pediatric Crohn's disease, 400
FAMMM syndrome, 825
Famotidine (Pepcid)
  for SRES, 163
  for upper gastrointestinal bleeding, 153
Fanconi anemia, 825
FAP. See Familial adenomatous polyposis (FAP)
FAPS. See Functional abdominal pain syndrome (FAPS)
Fasciolopsis buski, 310
  treatment, 312t
Fasciolopsis hepatica (sheep liver fluke)
  treatment, 312t
Fat
  food induced symptoms, 341, 341t
  malabsorption, 711–712
    with short bowel syndrome, 383
    soluble vitamins, 383–384
Fatigue
  of cholestasis, 710–711
  of liver disease
    treatment, 711t
  PBC, 702–703
Fecal elastase
  for chronic pancreatitis, 797
Fecal incontinence, 511–516
  anal canal bulking and obstructing agents, 515
  anorectal histologic function, 512
  artificial anal sphincter, 514
  biofeedback, 513
  cinedefecography, 512
  diabetic diarrhea, 422
  dynamic graciloplasty, 513–514
  electromyography, 512
  encirclement procedures, 513–514
  endoanal ultrasound, 511
  etiology, 511, 511t
  evaluation, 511
  medical management, 512–513
  neuromodulation, 514–515
  pudendal nerve terminal motor latency testing, 512
  radiofrequency energy delivery, 515
  severity and impact, 512
  sphincteroplasty, 513
  stoma, 515
  surgery, 513–515
  treatment, 512–515, 516f
Fecal occult blood tests (FOBT)
  colorectal cancer screening, 542
  with flexible sigmoidoscopy, 543
Feculent peritonitis, 602
Feeding
  pediatric liver transplantation, 654
Feeding tolerance
  assessment, 322
Feeding tube clogging
  with percutaneous endoscopic gastrostomy, 199
Fenfluramine challenge
  NUD, 186
Fentanyl
  endoscopic procedure sedation, 18–19
Ferguson hemorrhoidectomy, 539
Fertility, 490
FGID. See Functional gastrointestinal disorders (FGID)
FiberCon
  for acute infectious diarrhea, 293
  for constipation, 440
  for irritable bowel syndrome, 241
Fiber supplements
  for ileoanal pouch, 526
Fibrin glue
  for fistula in ano, 531
  inflammatory bowel disease fistulas, 481
  upper gastrointestinal bleeding, 170–171
Fibromyalgia, 264–265
Fibrosing colonopathy
  with cystic fibrosis, 807–808
Filgrastim
  for chronic hepatitis C, 623
Fine needle aspiration (FNA), 29
Fissures
  inflammatory bowel disease, 478
Fistula in ano, 530–532
  cutting seton technique, 531
  endorectal advancement flap, 531
  incontinence, 531
Fistulas. See also specific fistulas
  Crohn's disease, 404, 404f
  Crohn's disease of small bowel, 394–395
  inflammatory bowel disease, 479–482
Fistulotomy, 480f
5 nucleotidase, 605, 606t
FK506. See Tacrolimus (FK506)
Flagyl. See Metronidazole (Flagyl)
Flamingo Wallstent, 135
Flexible gastrointestinal endoscopes
  LCS reprocessing, 26t
Flexible sigmoidoscopy
  colorectal cancer screening, 543
  with FOBT
    colorectal cancer screening, 543
Flours
  with celiac disease, 369
FLR. See Future liver remnant (FLR)
Fluconazole
  for *Candida* esophagitis, 97
  preventing esophageal candidiasis, 99
Fluid and electrolyte replacement
  secretory diarrhea, 425–426
Flukes, 310–313
Flumazenil (Romazicon)
  endoscopic sedation, 19
Flumecinol
  for pruritus of cholestasis, 710
Fluocinonide, 43
Fluoroquinolones
  for traveler's diarrhea, 299
5-fluorouracil (5-FU)
  for esophageal cancer, 128
  for metastatic esophageal cancer, 128–129
Fluoxetine (Prozac)
  for chronic abdominal pain, 252
  for FGID, 263t
  side effects, 264
FNA. See Fine needle aspiration (FNA)
FOBT. See Fecal occult blood tests (FOBT)
Focal biliary fibrosis/cirrhosis
  with cystic fibrosis, 808–809
Folate
  deficiency during alcohol withdrawal, 230
Folinic acid
  for colorectal carcinoma, 563
Food
  immunologic reactions to, 344t
  nonimmune adverse reactions to, 346–347
  physiologic reactions to, 346–347
  pseudoallergic reactions to, 346
  psychological reactions to, 346
Food allergy, 344–351
  blood tests, 348–349
  classification, 344t
  differential diagnosis, 348
  prevention, 350
  testing, 348
  treatment, 349–350
Food Allergy and Anaphylaxis Network, 349
Food diary, 215
Food intake
  diagnostic algorithm, 275f
Food intolerance
  with functional syndromes, 342
  with motility disorders, 342
  with postsurgery syndrome, 342
Food protein induced enterocolitis syndrome (FPIES), 345
Fosamax
  for metabolic bone disease, 333
Foscarnet
  for viral esophagitis, 98
FPIES. See Food protein induced enterocolitis syndrome (FPIES)
Frey operation, 785
Fructose
  food induced symptoms, 340–341
5-FU
  for esophageal cancer, 128
  for metastatic esophageal cancer, 128–129
Full thickness plication system, 78–80, 79f
  effect, 79–80
  stepwise sequence, 79f
Fulminant hepatic failure, 629–637
  with cerebral edema, 635–636
  complications
    treatment, 633t
  diagnosis, 631–632
  encephalopathy, 634–635
  etiology, 629–630, 629t
  history, 631
  incidence, 629–630
  infection with, 636
  liver transplantation, 634
  physical examination, 631
  predicting prognosis, 632, 632t
  pregnancy, 634

renal failure with, 637
toxicology screen, 631
treatment, 632–637, 634t
with Wilson's disease, 721–722
Fumagillin
adverse effects, 314t
for intestinal protozoan parasites, 309t
pregnancy, 313t
Functional abdominal pain syndrome, 244–245
diagnosis, 245–246, 245t, 246t, 247t
hospitalization, 247
medications, 247
organic abdominal pain, 246
organic disorders, 244–245
outcome, 247–248
pain pattern, 244t
parents reinforcing pain behavior, 245t
personalities, 246
physical examination, 246
presentation, 246
questions for parents, 244t, 245t
questions for patients, 245t
reinforcement response, 245
treatment, 246–247
Functional abdominal pain syndrome (FAPS), 251
Functional dyspepsia, 183
consultation, 184
diagnosis, 184t
etiology, 183t
treatment, 184
Functional gastrointestinal disorders (FGID)
central pain modulating effects, 261
combination treatment, 264–265
lack of effective treatment, 261
psychological symptoms comorbidity, 260–261
psychotropic drugs, 260–265
psychotropic medications, 262t
Furazolidone
adverse effects, 314t
for *Giardia lamblia*, 310
pregnancy, 313t
Furosemide
for ascites, 657
Future liver remnant (FLR), 741

G

GABA B receptor agonists. *See* Gamma aminobutyric acid (GABA) B receptor agonists
Gabapentin (Neurontin)
for chronic abdominal pain, 253
for unexplained chest pain, 111
Gallbladder, 754f
radiation side effects, 581t, 582
Gallstone(s), 427
symptomatic treatment, 759t
VLCD, 217
Gallstone pancreatitis, 750
acute
simulations, 781, 783f

TPN, 781
with choledocholithiasis, 769
Gamma aminobutyric acid (GABA) B receptor agonists
GERD, 57
Gamma glutamyl transpeptidase (GGT), 605, 606t
alcoholism, 227–228
Ganciclovir
for CMV esophageal disease, 275
for fulminant hepatic failure, 634
for viral esophagitis, 98
Gardner's syndrome, 551
oral conditions, 46
Gas bloating
antireflux surgery, 70
Gastric acid secretion
dose dependent inhibition of, 153f
physiology, 148, 150f
Gastric adenomas
with CVID, 282
Gastric antral vascular ectasia (GAVE), 288
Gastric banding, 222, 225f
Gastric biopsy, 178
mapping, 178
chronic gastritis, 180
Gastric bypass, 218, 220–221
Gastric cancer, 207–210
computed tomography, 207
diagnosis, 207
endoscopic ultrasound, 207
preoperative workup, 207–208
risk factors, 207
surgery, 208–209, 208t
treatment, 208f
Gastric D cells, 148
Gastric dilatation
acute
with eating disorders, 234
Gastric distention, 59–60
Gastric malignancy
Helicobacter pylori, 139
Gastric mucosal defense, 148
Gastric outlet obstruction
benign
balloon dilatation, 495f
Gastric problems
with eating disorders, 234
Gastric restriction
bariatric operations, 219–220
Gastric varices, 123
Gastrinoma, 156–160
abdominal exploration, 158–159
clinical presentation, 156
diagnosis, 156–157, 157t
duodenal, 156
EUS, 157
forms, 156
preoperative localization, 157
prognosis, 159
site, 156
SRS, 157
surgery
controversies, 159–160
treatment, 157–158, 158f

tumor removal, 158
unresectable metastic, 159
Gastritis. *See also* Chronic gastritis
Helicobacter pylori, 202f
lymphocytic
with celiac disease, 370
Gastrocolocutaneous fistula
with percutaneous endoscopic gastrostomy, 198
Gastroduodenal artery, 169f
Gastroenteritis
eosinophilic, 345–346
Gastroesophageal junction (GEJ), 73–74
schema, 73f
Gastroesophageal reflux disease (GERD)
acid suppression, 64f
airway disease, 70–71
algorithm, 57f
bariatric operations, 224
control of, 71
daily PPI
treatment failure, 56
dietary measures, 59–60
endoscopic devices for, 74t
premarketing guidelines, 74t
endoscopic therapies, 73–84
factors in, 74t
endoscopic treatment trials, 82–83
extraesophageal
management, 64–66, 65f, 67t
therapeutic trials, 63–64
extraesophageal presentation, 63–67
H_2RA, 55
initial treatment, 54
lifestyle modifications, 55, 55t, 59–61
low suspicion, 66
medical therapy, 54–58
open label trials, 83–84
oral conditions, 45
patient assessment, 69
perioperative considerations, 69
pregnancy, 55
prevalence, 64f
safety issues, 83–84
smoking, 270
surgery, 57, 69–72
twice daily PPI, 56–57
Gastroesophageal variceal bleeding, 119
Gastrointestinal bleeding, 600f, 600t. *See also* Lower gastrointestinal bleeding; Obscure gastrointestinal bleeding; Upper gastrointestinal bleeding
acute pancreatitis, 780
heater probe, 171
multidisciplinary teams, 168
multipolar/bipolar electrocautery, 171
with SCT, 288
vasopressin, 590t
Gastrointestinal disease
smoking, 270–272
Gastrointestinal endoscopy
anesthesiology assistance guidelines, 20t
disease transmission, 24
exogenous infection risk during, 23–24
Gastrointestinal neoplasms

smoking cessation, 270
Gastrointestinal strictures
　upper, 494–500
Gastrointestinal stromal tumor (GIST), 35
　EUS diagnosis, 35f
Gastroparesis, 190–195
　diabetic, 193
　with food intolerance, 342
　for nausea and vomiting, 288
　nutrition restoration, 190
　prokinetics, 190–191
　treatment, 191f
Gastroplasties, 219–220, 220f
Gastroprotective agents, 144
Gatekeeper, 82f
Gatekeeper repair system, 83
GAVE. See Gastric antral vascular ectasia (GAVE)
GEJ. See Gastroesophageal junction (GEJ)
Gelatin, 174
Gemcitabine
　for pancreatic cancer, 821
General anesthesia
　continuum of depth, 17t
Genetic counseling
　colonic neoplasia, 545–549
　followup, 546
　psychosocial issues, 546
Genetic discrimination, 546
Genetic screening
　chronic pancreatitis, 811
Genetic testing
　appropriate use, 545
　flowchart, 546f
　strategy, 546
GERD. See Gastroesophageal reflux disease (GERD)
GGT. See Gamma glutamyl transpeptidase (GGT)
Gianturco Z stent, 135
Giardia, 282
　gastrointestinal manifestations, 283
Giardia lamblia (Giardiasis), 294, 294t, 310
　traveler's diarrhea, 298–299
　treatment, 309t
Giardiasis, 294, 294t, 310
　traveler's diarrhea, 298–299
　treatment, 309t
Gingivitis
　with human immunodeficiency virus (HIV), 274
GIST. See Gastrointestinal stromal tumor (GIST)
Glucocorticoids
　for left sided colitis, 450
　with osteoporosis, 331
　for secretory diarrhea, 427
Glutamine
　for diarrhea, 286
Gluten
　celiac sprue, 367–369
　in medications, 369
Glycerine
　for constipation, 439t
Glycogen acanthosis, 555f

Glycopyrrolate (Robinul)
　for IBS, 240t
Glypressin
　for acute variceal bleeding, 120
GM 611
　for gastroparesis, 192
Gonorrhea, 534
Gradual change
　obesity, 215
Graft *versus* host disease (GVHD), 286f
　acute
　　with diarrhea, 286–287
　chronic
　　with SCT, 287
　clinical presentations, 289
　with diarrhea, 286–287
　with intestinal transplantation, 388
　treatment, 286–287
Grains, 368t
Granisetron (Kytril)
　for gastroparesis, 193
Granulocytopenia, 98
Gravity
　GERD, 60–61
Group therapy
　for chronic abdominal pain, 253
　for eating disorders, 236
Growth
　pediatric liver transplantation, 651
GSH prodrugs
　for alcoholic liver disease, 669
Gut dysmotility
　diabetic diarrhea, 421
Gut immune system, 280
GVHD. See Graft *versus* host disease (GVHD)

H

HAART. See Highly active antiretroviral therapy (HAART)
Hairy leukoplakia
　with human immunodeficiency virus (HIV), 274
Halobetasol, 43
Halothane
　for drug induced liver disease, 689
Harm
　well-designed trial characteristics, 6t
Harmonic scalpel, 539
Hartmann procedure, 571
Hartmann resection, 602f
HAV. See Hepatitis A virus (HAV)
HAVRIX, 612
Hazardous drinkers
　nondependent
　　brief interventions, 228
Hazardous drinking
　defined, 226–227
　screening, 226–227
HBIG. See Hyperimmune globulin (HBIG)
HB surface antigen (HBsAg), 616
HBV. See Hepatitis B virus (HBV)
HCC. See Hepatocellular carcinoma (HCC)
HCV. See Hepatitis C virus (HCV)

HDGC. See Hereditary diffuse gastric cancer (HDGC)
Healing rate
　Markov model, 14
Health time, 15
Heart
　acute pancreatitis, 780
Heater probe
　gastrointestinal bleeding, 171
Helicobacter pylori, 178
　detecting, 138t
　diagnosis, 138–139
　eradication regimens, 140t
　eradication therapy, 204–205
　gastric malignancy, 139
　gastritis, 202f
　gastroduodenal disease, 138–141
　IM, 179
　NSAIDs, 139
　　threshold analysis, 11–13
　NUD, 140, 185, 186
　PGL, 203
　PUD, 138–139, 149
　smoking, 271
　treatment, 140
HELLP. See Hemolysis elevated liver enzymes low platelets syndrome (HELLP)
Helminthic infection, 310–313
Hematemasis, 358
Hematin, 728, 729
　for erythropoietic protoporphyria, 730
Hematologic malignancies, 98
Hemochromatosis. See Hereditary hemochromatosis
Hemodynamic monitoring, 21
Hemolysis elevated liver enzymes low platelets syndrome (HELLP), 697, 698–700, 698f, 699t
Hemorrhage
　with percutaneous endoscopic gastrostomy, 198
Hemorrhoidectomy
　Ferguson, 539
　stapled, 539
Hemorrhoids, 536–540
　anatomy and physiology, 536–537
　classification, 537
　cryotherapy, 538
　diagnosis, 536–537
　external
　　excision, 537
　　treatment, 537
　inflammatory bowel disease, 478
　injection sclerotherapy, 538
　IRC, 538
　lower gastrointestinal bleeding, 585
　mixed, 536f
　treatment, 537–538
　pathophysiology, 536
　and prolapse, 539, 539f
　rubber band ligation, 538
　surgery, 538–539
　thermal injury, 538
　treatment, 537

Hemosiderosis
  with SCT, 290
Hepatcarboxyl porphyrin, 729
Hepatic arterial thrombosis
  pediatric liver transplantation, 654
Hepatic encephalopathy, 661–664
  ALF, 664
  antibiotics, 663
  combination therapy, 663–664
  diagnosis, 661–662
  dietary recommendations, 663
  lactulose, 663
  precipitation factors, 662t
  severity assessment, 661t
  treatment, 662–664
Hepatic enzyme inducers
  for pruritis of cholestasis, 709
Hepatic failure
  acute
    pediatric liver transplantation, 651
Hepatic hydrothorax
  ascites, 659–660
Hepatic ischemia, 630
Hepatic metastases, 744–747
  assessment, 744–745
  CT, 744
  FDG, 745
  IOUS, 745
  liver resection, 745–746
    outcomes, 746
  local ablation, 746
  MR angiography, 744
  MRI, 744
  MRI cholangiography, 744
  PET, 745
  radiofrequency ablation, 746
  systemic chemotherapy, 745
  treatment, 745–746
Hepatic neoplasms, 732–737
Hepatic osteodystrophy
  associated with low BMD, 328t
  metabolic bone disease, 330
Hepatic sarcoma
  pediatric liver transplantation, 652
Hepatic sinusoid
  microvascular anatomy of, 682f
Hepatic steatosis, 289–290
  with cystic fibrosis, 808
Hepatic vein gradient, 289
Hepatic venoocclusive disease, 684–685
Hepatitis
  acute
    prevention, 611–614
  drugs associated with, 290t
Hepatitis A
  acute, 611–612
  immunization, 612t
  vaccines, 612t
Hepatitis A virus (HAV)
  inducing fulminant hepatic failure, 630
Hepatitis B. See also Chronic hepatitis B
  acute, 612–613
  immunization schedule, 613t
  with SCT, 290
Hepatitis B virus (HBV)

children
  treatment, 625–627
  inducing fulminant hepatic failure, 630
Hepatitis C. See also Chronic hepatitis C
  acute, 613–614
    treatment, 614t
  prognosis, 6–7
  with SCT, 290
Hepatitis C virus (HCV)
  children, 627–628
  nonalcoholic fatty liver disease, 671
Hepatitis E
  acute, 614
Hepatoblastoma
  pediatric liver transplantation, 651
Hepatocellular carcinoma (HCC), 625,
    732–736
  AJCC/UICC TNM, 740t
  chronic hepatitis B, 617–619
  defined, 732t
  diagnosis, 739–740
  etiology, 739
  hormonal therapy, 736
  intraarterial chemoembolization, 735–736
  liver transplantation, 642
  local ablation, 734–735, 734t
  microwave acetic acid injection, 735
  natural history, 739
  with PBC, 704
  pediatric liver transplantation, 651
  prevalence, 739
  prognosis, 739
  radiation, 736, 742
  radiofrequency ablation, 735
  staging, 739–740
  surgery, 734
  surgical resection
    candidate selection, 740–741
    optimization, 741
    techniques, 740–741, 741–742
  surveillance, 732f
  systemic chemotherapy, 736, 742–743
  treatment, 733–736, 736f, 739–743,
    740–743
Heptimax, 622
Hereditary cancer, 545
Hereditary colorectal cancer syndrome,
    547–549, 547t
Hereditary diffuse gastric cancer (HDGC),
    207
Hereditary hemochromatosis, 724–727
  blood iron studies, 725
  clinical features, 725
  diagnosis, 725–726
  family member screening, 726
  genetic testing, 725
  liver biopsy, 725–726
  liver disease, 727
  population screening, 726–727
  treatment, 726–727
Hereditary nonpolyposis colorectal cancer
    (HNPCC), 547–549, 547t, 825
Hereditary pancreatitis, 825
Hernia
  abdominal wall

  with ascites, 660
  hiatal, 72
  inguinal
    abdominal wall defects, 445
  paraesophageal, 72
Herpes, 535
Herpes simplex virus (HSV), 275
  inducing fulminant hepatic failure, 630
Heterophyes heterophyes, 310
HGD. See High grade dysplasia (HGD)
Hiatal hernia, 72
Hidradenitis suppurativa, 533
High grade dysplasia (HGD), 36
High level endoscopic disinfection, 25–26
Highly active antiretroviral therapy
    (HAART), 96
Hirschsprung's disease, 512
Histamine, 148
  reactions to, 346
Histamine 2 blockade
  for reflux, 234
Histamine 2 receptor antagonists (H2RA)
  for ENT with GERD, 67
  for GERD, 803
  for SRES, 163
HIV. See Human immunodeficiency virus
    (HIV)
HMG CoA. See Hydroxy 3 methyl glutaryl
    coenzyme A (HMG CoA)
HNPCC. See Hereditary nonpolyposis col-
    orectal cancer (HNPCC)
Hookworm, 311
  treatment, 312t
Hopkins scintigraphic scoring
  SOD, 775t
Hormonal therapy
  obscure gastrointestinal bleeding, 362
  for PBC, 703
Horseshoe abscess
  drainage of, 531f
Hospital hobo, 256
24 hours pH monitoring
  GERD, 69
House shape flap, 534f
H2RA. See Histamine 2 receptor antagonists
    (H2RA)
HSV. See Herpes simplex virus (HSV)
Human immunodeficiency virus (HIV)
  anorectal disease, 278–279
  diagnosis, 274–275, 276–377
  diarrhea and wasting, 275–276
  gastrointestinal complications, 274–279
  nutritional complications, 274–279
  nutritional management, 278
  oral and esophageal disease, 274–278
  treatment, 274–275, 277–278
  tumors, 278–279
Humatin. See Paromomycin (Humatin)
Hurst dilator, 101
Hycosyamine (Levsin)
  for IBS, 240t
Hydrocortisone
  for microscopic colitis, 508
Hydrogel prosthesis
  expandable, 81–82

Hydrostatic balloon dilatation, 102–103
Hydroxy 3 methyl glutaryl coenzyme A (HMG CoA)
   for nonalcoholic fatty liver disease, 672–673
Hydroxytryptamine agonists
   for gastroparesis, 192
Hydroxyzine
   for pruritis of cholestasis, 708–709
Hymenolepis nana
   treatment, 312t
Hyperamylasemia
   with eating disorders, 234
Hyperbilirubinemia, 808
Hypercholesterolemia, 711
   with PBC, 704
Hyperemesis gravidarum, 695
Hypergastrinemia
   differential diagnosis, 157t
Hyperglycemia
   with parenteral nutrition, 323
Hyperimmune globulin (HBIG), 612–613
Hyperlipidemic pancreatitis, 782
   with eating disorders, 234
Hypermotility, 108
   treatment, 109–111
Hyperpigmentation, 712–713
Hyperplastic polyposis
   risk and surveillance, 555
Hyperplastic polyps
   chronic gastritis, 180–181
Hypersecretion
   diabetic diarrhea, 421
Hypersensitivity, 108
Hypersensitivity drug induced liver disease, 689t
Hypertension
   cardiovascular risk with major surgery, 432
Hypnosis
   for chronic abdominal pain, 253
Hypnotherapy
   for NUD, 187
Hypoallergenic diet, 348
Hypochondriasis, 256
Hypoglycemia
   with fulminant hepatic failure, 633
Hypogonadism
   metabolic bone disease, 330
Hypokalemia, 428
Hypolipidemic agents
   for nonalcoholic fatty liver disease, 672–673
Hypomotility, 107
   treatment, 109
Hypopharyngeal diverticula, 52
   treatment, 52
Hyposensitivity, 108
Hypothyroidism
   with PBC, 702
Hypovolemia
   mesenteric vascular ischemia, 413–414
Hysteria, 256
Hysterical dysphagia, 46

I

IAS. *See* Internal anal sphincter (IAS)
Iatrogenic diabetes, 828–829
IBD. *See* Inflammatory bowel disease (IBD)
IBS. *See* Irritable bowel syndrome (IBS)
Ibuprofen (Advil), 143
ICAM. *See* Intracellular adhesion molecule (ICAM)
Idiopathic esophageal ulcer (IEU), 99
Idiopathic pancreatitis, 796
   obstructive etiologies, 789t
Idiopathic portal hypertension, 685
IEU. *See* Idiopathic esophageal ulcer (IEU)
Ig A deficiency. *See* Immunoglobulin (Ig) A deficiency
Ig E mediated food allergy syndrome. *See* Immunoglobulin (Ig) E mediated food allergy syndrome
IGLE. *See* Intraganglionic laminar endings (IGLE)
IHCP. *See* Intrahepatic cholestasis of pregnancy (IHCP)
Ileoanal pouch, 525–529
   acute pouchitis, 527
   adequate history, 525
   anastomotic leakage, 526
   approach after six months, 528t
   approach in first six months, 525t
   defective sphincteric continence, 526
   diarrhea, 529
   excessive bowel frequency, 527–529
   irritable pouch syndrome, 529
   outlet problems, 528
   pouch outlet obstruction, 526–527
   recurrent pouchitis, 528
Ileoanal pouch anastomosis, 457–463, 457f
   controversies, 459–460
      anastomotic issues, 459–460
      bowel obstruction, 461
      cuffitis, 461
      evacuation disorders, 461
      irritable pouch syndrome, 461–462
      long term followup, 462–463
      paradoxical puborectalis contraction, 461
      postoperative management, 462–463
      pouch construction, 459
      pouchitis, 461
      sepsis, 459–461
   indications, 459
IM. *See* Intestinal metaplasia (IM)
Imipenem
   for acute pancreatitis, 781
Imipramine (Tofranil)
   for FGID, 263, 263t
Immunization schedule
   hepatitis B, 613t
Immunodeficiencies
   classification, 280t
   classification and clinical presentation of, 280–281
Immunoglobulin (Ig) A deficiency, 280–281
   with CVID, 283
Immunoglobulin (Ig) E mediated food allergy syndrome, 344–345

Immunomodulation
   for UC, 450–451
Immunosuppression
   for PBC, 704
   pediatric liver transplantation, 653
Imodium. *See* Loperamide (Imodium)
Imodium
   for fecal incontinence, 512
Inborn errors of metabolism
   pediatric liver transplantation, 651
Incontinence. *See also* Fecal incontinence
   fistula in ano, 531
Indomethacin
   for secretory diarrhea, 427
Ineffective esophageal motility, 71–72
Infants
   lactose intolerance, 373–374
Infectious colitis
   lower gastrointestinal bleeding, 585
Infectious diarrhea
   acute, 292–296
      diagnosis, 292
      pathogen specific therapy, 293–296
      treatment, 292–293, 294t
   with SCT, 287
Inflammatory bowel disease (IBD), 282, 347, 715
   adverse reactions to food, 347
   anal stenosis, 478
   associated with low BMD, 328t
   azathioprine metabolite levels, 406–409
   clinical parameters, 409
   constipation, 443
   enteral nutrition for, 324
   eosinophils, 448
   fissures, 478
   fistulas, 479–482
      fecal diversion, 482
      fibrin glue, 481
      proctectomy, 482
      proximal disease, 482
      setons, 480
   with food intolerance, 342
   hemorrhoids, 478
   lower gastrointestinal bleeding, 585
   6-mercaptopurine (6-MP), 407
   NSAID induced small and large intestinal injury, 366
   oral conditions, 43
   perianal abscess, 479
   perianal disease, 476–482, 482
      classification, 477
      diagnosis, 477–478
      fistula activity, 477
      hemorrhoids, 478
      surgery, 478–479
   peripheral abnormalities, 261
   pregnancy, 490–492, 491t
   relapse, 448–449
   smoking, 271–272
   surveillance, 485f
Inflammatory cytokines
   metabolic bone disease, 329–330
Infliximab (Remicade)
   for Crohn's colitis, 468, 469

for Crohn's disease, 403
  pediatric, 398–399
  perianal complications, 474
  of small bowel, 392, 393
for GVHD, 286
pregnancy, 492
for UC, 454
Informed consent
  genetic counseling, 546
Infrared photocoagulation (IRC)
  hemorrhoids, 538
Inguinal hernia
  abdominal wall defects, 445
Inheritance, 490
Injection sclerotherapy
  hemorrhoids, 538
Injection therapy
  effect, 80
  esophageal cancer, 133
  procedure, 80
  upper gastrointestinal bleeding, 170
Insulated tip diathermic knife (IT knife)
  EMR, 37
Insulin resistance
  nonalcoholic fatty liver disease, 671
Insurance
  genetic counseling, 546
Interferon
  for chronic hepatitis B, 618
  for chronic hepatitis C, 622
  for HBV in children, 625–626
  for HCV in children, 627
  with ribavirin
    for HCV in children, 627
Internal anal sphincter (IAS)
  anatomy of, 476–477
  UC, 448
Internal hemorrhoids
  treatment, 537–538
Interpersonal psychotherapy
  for chronic abdominal pain, 253
Intersphincteric abscess, 530
Intestinal and multivisceral transplantation, 386–388
  candidate evaluation, 386
  donor selection, 387
  indications for, 386
  outcomes, 388–389
  postoperative complications, 388
  postoperative management, 387–388
  procedure, 387
  rejection, 387–388
Intestinal angioectasia
  obscure gastrointestinal bleeding, 360
Intestinal benign strictures
  endoscopy, 495t
Intestinal compression
  with chronic pancreatitis, 787
Intestinal failure
  parenteral nutrition for, 324
Intestinal flukes, 310
Intestinal helminths
  drug therapy, 312t
Intestinal ischemia
  acute

    diagnosis, 413t
    treatment, 415t, 416t
Intestinal metaplasia (IM), 178
  cardia/GEJ, 181
  distal to gastric cardia, 179
  H. pylori, 179
Intestinal obstruction
  bariatric operations, 224
  with chronic pancreatitis, 787
Intestinal parasites, 307–314
Intestinal protozoan parasites
  drug therapy for, 309t
Intestinal stenoses
  malignant, 496t
Intestinal strictures, 494–501
  benign, 495
    endoscopy, 495t
    etiology, 495t
  malignant, 496–497
  management, 494–501
Intracellular adhesion molecule (ICAM), 448
Intractable constipation, 441–442
  testing, 441
Intraductal papillary mucinous neoplasms (IPMN), 823–824
  surgery, 823–824
Intraganglionic laminar endings (IGLE), 74
Intrahepatic cholestasis of pregnancy (IHCP), 695–696
Intralesional steroid injections
  for esophageal strictures, 104
Intraoperative endoscopy
  obscure gastrointestinal bleeding, 360
Intraoperative ultrasonography (IOUS), 741–742
Intrasphincteric botulinum toxin injections
  for achalasia, 114
Intravenous erythromycin, 167
Intravenous foscarnet
  for viral esophagitis, 98
Intravenous (IV) gamma globulin
  for Clostridium difficile diarrhea, 304
Intravenous replacement
  secretory diarrhea, 426
Intravenous volume expanders
  SBP, 659
Intussusception
  with cystic fibrosis, 807
Investigational preoperative chemotherapy
  PGL, 208
Iodoquinol
  adverse effects, 314t
  for Balantidium coli, 307
  Blastocystis hominis, 307
  for Dientamoeba fragilis, 308
  for intestinal protozoan parasites, 309t
  pregnancy, 313t
Ionized calcium
  metabolic bone disease, 327t
IOUS. See Intraoperative ultrasonography (IOUS)
IPMN. See Intraductal papillary mucinous neoplasms (IPMN)
Irbesartan

    for portal hypertension, 678
IRC. See Infrared photocoagulation (IRC)
Irinotecan (CPT-11)
  for colorectal carcinoma, 564
  for metastatic esophageal cancer, 129
Iron overload, 724t
  with SCT, 290
Irritable bowel syndrome (IBS), 239–242, 260
  defined, 239
  diet, 239–240
  pain, 240
  pathophysiology, 239
  prognosis, 6
  psychological intervention, 241–242
  psychotropic medications, 240
  treatment, 239–240
Irritable pouch syndrome
  ileoanal pouch anastomosis controversies, 461–462
Ischemic colitis, 418
  diagnosis, 413t
  lower gastrointestinal bleeding, 585
  treatment, 415t
Islet autotransplantation, 831
ISMN. See Isosorbide mononitrate (ISMN)
Isolated hyperbilirubinemia, 607–608
Isolated intestinal transplantation, 387
Isoniazid
  for drug induced liver disease, 689
  inducing liver disease, 689
Isosorbide mononitrate (ISMN)
  for achalasia, 109
  for acute variceal bleeding, 121
  for portal hypertension, 677
Isospora belli (Isosporiasis), 294t, 310
  treatment, 309t
Isosporiasis, 294t, 310
  treatment, 309t
Isosporiasis, 277
IT knife. See Insulated tip diathermic knife (IT knife)
IV. See Intravenous (IV) gamma globulin
Ivermectin
  adverse effects, 314t
  for intestinal helminths, 312t
  pregnancy, 313t
  for strongyloidiasis, 311
IV gamma globulin
  for Clostridium difficile diarrhea, 304

J

Jejunoileal bypass, 219
Jejunoileitis
  Crohn's disease of small bowel, 394
Juvenile polyposis (JPS), 547t, 549, 554f
  risk and surveillance, 552t, 554

K

Kaposi's sarcoma
  with human immunodeficiency virus (HIV), 274
Ketaconazole
  for OC with GERD, 45
Kidneys. See also Renal failure

acute pancreatitis, 780
Killian's dehiscence, 52
Kytril
  for gastroparesis, 193

L

Laboratory testing abnormalities
  liver disorders associated with, 606t
Lactase persistence, 373
Lactic acidosis
  short bowel syndrome, 382
Lactobacillus
  for food allergy, 350
Lactobacillus GG
  for pediatric Crohn's disease, 400
Lactose
  food induced symptoms, 341
  in foods, 374
  hidden, 373t
Lactose intolerance, 346, 348, 372–374
  infants, 373–374
  management, 373–374
Lactose malabsorption
  with celiac disease, 370
Lactulose, 241t
  for constipation, 439t, 440
  cost, 439t
  for fulminant hepatic failure, 634
  hepatic encephalopathy, 663
  pregnancy, 443
Lactulose taper
  for constipation, 234
Lamivudine
  for chronic hepatitis B, 618
  for HBV in children, 626
Lanreotide
  for portal hypertension, 679
  for secretory diarrhea, 426
Lansoprazole (Prevacid)
  for ENT with GERD, 67
  for extraesophageal GERD, 67t
  for GERD, 54
  for SRES, 163
  for upper gastrointestinal bleeding, 153
Laparoscopic cholecystectomy, 748–752
  cholelithiasis, 760
  complications, 751–752
  evaluation, 748–749
  expanded indications, 749–751
  indications, 748–749
  outcomes, 751–752
  perioperative care, 749
  surgical technique, 749
Laparoscopic common bile duct exploration, 750
Laparoscopic myotomy
  for achalasia, 109
Laparoscopy
  for crohn's disease, 402
  PGL, 208
Lapband, 222
Large volume paracentesis
  tense ascites, 657
Lasers
  ablative treatment, 91t

esophageal cancer, 131–132
Laser thermocoagulation
  upper gastrointestinal bleeding, 172
Latex food allergy syndrome, 345
Latex fruit syndrome, 345
Laxatives
  abuse
    with eating disorders, 233, 234
  anthraquinone containing
    for constipation, 440
  bulk forming
    for constipation, 440
  for constipation, 439t
  cost of, 439t
  magnesium
    pregnancy, 443
  osmotic
    for constipation, 440
  secretory diarrhea, 429
  stimulant
    for constipation, 440
LCS. See Liquid chemical sterilant (LCS)
LDLT. See Living donor liver transplantation (LDLT)
Left sided ulcerative colitis, 447–452
  anorectal physiology, 448
  diagnosis, 447–449
  eosinophils, 448
  histology, 448
  inflammation
    treatment, 449–450
  modifying symptoms, 451–452
  pathophysiology, 447–449
  perineal dermatitis, 451
  refractory disease, 452
  relapse, 450
  SCFA, 451
  surgery, 451
Leiomyomas, 35
LES. See Lower esophageal sphincter (LES)
Leucovorin calcium
  for colorectal carcinoma, 563
  for *Isospora belli*, 310
Leuprolide acetate
  for gastroparesis, 193
Level of consciousness
  monitoring, 21
Levsin
  for IBS, 240t
Lexapro
  for FGID, 263t
  side effects, 264
LGD. See Low grade dysplasia (LGD)
Lhermitte Duclos disease, 555
Librax
  for IBS, 240t
Librium
  for alcohol withdrawal, 230
Lidocaine
  for OC with GERD, 45
Lifestyle
  alcoholic liver disease, 666–667
  obesity, 216
Ligasure, 539
Lignocaine

for pruritis of cholestasis, 710
Likelihood ratios
  computation of, 5t
Linear programming, 8
Lipid synthesis, 609
Lipomas, 35
Lipoprotein synthesis, 609
Liquid chemical sterilant (LCS), 24
  endoscope reprocessing procedure, 26–27, 26t
Lithotripsy, 768f
Liver. See also Hepatic
  radiation side effects, 581, 581t
  vascular anatomy of, 682
Liver biopsy, 605–610, 609–610
  chronic hepatitis B, 617
  PBC, 701
Liver disease. See also Drug induced liver disease
  with cystic fibrosis, 808
  diagnosis, 605f
  oral conditions, 46–47
  pregnancy, 695t
    liver disease, 694–700
  TPN, 673–674
Liver enzymes, 605–608
  interpretation, 607–608
Liver failure. See also Acute liver failure (ALF)
  drugs associated with, 290t
Liver flukes, 310
Liver function tests, 608–609
  drugs associated with abnormal, 290t
  with parenteral nutrition, 323
  with SCT, 288–289
Liver injury
  enzymes reflecting, 605t
Liver intestine transplantation, 387
Liver tests
  cholestasis, 606t
Liver transplantation, 638–642
  acute liver failure, 642
  aftercare, 640
  for alcoholic liver disease, 669
  alcohol or drug abuse, 640
  cholangiocarcinoma, 718
  comorbid conditions, 640
  for cystic fibrosis, 809
  deceased donor liver procurement, 644–645
  donor hepatectomy, 647
  donor selection, 646
  for erythropoietic protoporphyria, 730
  followup, 642
  fulminant hepatic failure, 634
  for HCC, 642, 733–734, 733t
  inadequate portal venous flow, 648
  LDLT, 640–641, 646–648
  liver graft implantation, 645–646
  liver graft surgical challenges, 648–649
  nonheart beating donor procurement, 645
  pediatric, 650–655
    indications for, 650–652, 650t
    postoperative, 654–655
    surgical innovations, 653–655

portal hypertension, 680
pretransplantation examination, 641
with PSC, 717
recipient liver graft implantation, 647–648
selection, 638–641
surgery, 644–649
survival rate, 122, 123
timing, 639
Living donor liver transplantation (LDLT), 640–641, 646–648
pediatric liver transplantation, 653
Lomotil. See Diphenoxylate with atropine sulfate (Lomotil)
Lonafarnib
for pancreatic cancer, 821
Loop gastric bypass, 220f
Loperamide (Imodium), 241t
for acute infectious diarrhea, 292
for ileoanal pouch, 526
for secretory diarrhea, 426
for short bowel syndrome, 381
for traveler's diarrhea, 299t, 300
Lorazepam (Ativan)
for alcohol withdrawal, 230
Losartan
for portal hypertension, 678
Lotronex
for diabetic diarrhea, 422
for IBS, 241
Lower esophageal sphincter (LES), 54, 59, 73–74
categorizing, 107f
relaxation
and sleep, 61
Lower gastrointestinal bleeding, 584–589
angiography, 587–588, 588–589
capsule enteroscopy, 587
clinical presentation, 584–586
colonoscopy, 587
diagnosis, 586–587
endoscopic therapy, 588
enteroscopy, 587
etiology, 584–586
nuclear bleeding scans, 587
surgery, 589
technical pitfalls, 595
transcatheter management, 593–595
indications, 593
nuclear medicine, 593
treatment, 586–587, 586t
Lower gastrointestinal tract
transcatheter embolotherapy, 594–595
complications, 595, 595t
provocative testing, 594–595
Low grade dysplasia (LGD)
with esophageal adenocarcinoma, 87
UC
dysplasia surveillance programs, 486
Lumitene
for erythropoietic protoporphyria, 730
Lungs
acute pancreatitis, 780
Lymph node dissection
PGL, 208–209
Lymph nodes

routine removal of, 160
Lymphocytic colitis
microscopic colitis, 506
Lymphocytic gastritis
with celiac disease, 370
Lymphoepithelial lesion, 203f

M

MAC. See Mycobacterium avium complex (MAC)
Magnesium
with diarrhea, 342
Magnesium citrate
for constipation, 439t, 440
cost, 439t
Magnesium hydroxide
cost, 439t
Magnesium laxatives
pregnancy, 443
Magnesium sulfate
for constipation, 439t, 440
Malabsorption, 711–712
associated with low BMD, 328t
bariatric operations, 224–225
complete
bariatric operations, 219
with cystic fibrosis, 804
selective
bariatric operations, 220–221
short bowel syndrome, 382
Malabsorption syndrome
oral conditions, 46
Maldigestion
with cystic fibrosis, 804
Malignant colon strictures, 499–500
Malignant sigmoid stricture, 500f
Malignant strictures
evaluation, 737f
Malingering, 256
Mallory Weiss tear, 173–174, 234
Maloney dilator, 101, 101f
MALT. See Mucosal associated lymphoid tissue (MALT)
Mannitol
food induced symptoms, 340
for fulminant hepatic failure, 636
Manometry
GERD, 69
Marimastat
for pancreatic cancer, 821
Marinol
for gastroparesis, 193
for pruritis of cholestasis, 710
Markov chain, 8, 14–15
average or cumulative amount of time, 14f
ulcer, 15f
ulcer natural history, 14f
MARS procedure
for pruritis of cholestasis, 708
Mast cells, 447
MCC. See Midcingulate cortex (MCC)
MCN. See Mucinous cystic neoplasms (MCN)
MCV. See Mean corpuscular volume (MCV)
Meal related physiological changes, 339–340

Meals
responses to, 339
Mean corpuscular volume (MCV)
alcoholism, 227–228
Mebendazole
adverse effects, 314t
for ascariasis, 311
for hookworm, 311
for intestinal helminths, 312t
for pinworms, 311
pregnancy, 313t
for whipworm, 312
Mechanical dilator, 100–101
Meckel's scan
obscure gastrointestinal bleeding, 359
Meconium ileus
with cystic fibrosis, 806
Medications
adjunct
endoscopic sedation, 19
elevated liver enzymes, 607–608
IBS, 240t
inducing fulminant hepatic failure, 629–630, 629t
pregnancy, 490–492
Megacolon
chronic
constipation, 443
Ménétrier's disease, 282
chronic gastritis, 181
MEN 1 gastrinoma
cure rates, 159t
MEN 1 syndrome, 149, 156
Meperidine
pregnancy, 492
Meperidine (Demerol)
for chronic abdominal pain, 252
for diverticulitis, 601
endoscopic sedation, 19
for GERD, 79
for porphyria, 729
Meperidine with diazepam (Valium)
endoscopic sedation
patient controlled, 22
6-mercaptopurine (6-MP)
for Crohn's colitis, 468–469
for Crohn's disease of small bowel, 392
for Crohn's diseases perianal complications, 473
IBD, 407
metabolism of, 406f
for pediatric Crohn's disease, 398
pharmacology of, 406–409
for UC, 450–452
Meropeneme
for Whipple's disease, 317t
Mesalamine (Pentasa)
for Crohn's colitis, 466
for Crohn's disease of small bowel, 391, 394
for ileoanal pouch, 528
for left sided colitis, 449
for left sided ulcerative colitis, 451–452
for microscopic colitis, 508
pregnancy, 490, 491

for UC, 454, 455–456
Mesenteric vascular ischemia, 411–418
   clinical factors predisposing to, 412t
   dehydration, 413–414
   diagnosis, 411–412
   early manifestations *vs.* necrosis, 412
   hypovolemia, 413–414
   metabolic acidosis, 414
   multisystem failure, 414
   pathogenesis, 411t
   sepsis, 414
   surgery
      timing, 414–416
   treatment, 412–414
Mesocaval shunt
   for acute variceal bleeding, 122
Metabolic acidosis
   mesenteric vascular ischemia, 414
Metabolic bone disease, 327–334
   bone tests, 327t
   diagnosis, 330f, 332–333
   mechanisms of, 332t
   treatment, 333–334
Metabolic idiosyncratic drug induced liver disease, 689t
Metagonimus yokogawai, 310
Metallic stents, 135
   expandable
      esophageal use, 135f
   for pancreatic and periampullary neoplasms, 816
Metallothionein
   for Wilson's disease, 721
Metamucil (Psyllium)
   for acute infectious diarrhea, 293
   for constipation, 439t, 440
Metamucil
   for left sided ulcerative colitis, 451
Metformin
   for insulin resistance, 672
Methotrexate
   for Crohn's colitis, 469
   for Crohn's disease of small bowel, 392, 393
   for Crohn's disease perianal complications, 473
   for fatigue, 702
   with metabolic bone disease, 332
   for microscopic colitis, 508
   for PBC, 704
   for pediatric Crohn's disease, 398
   pregnancy, 491
   toxicity
      with SCT, 290
   for UC, 450–451
Methoxamine
   for fecal incontinence, 513
Methscopolamine bromide (Pamine)
   for IBS, 240t
Methylcellulose (Citrucel)
   for acute infectious diarrhea, 293
   for constipation, 439t, 440
Methyldopa
   for drug induced liver disease, 689
   inducing liver disease, 689

Methylprednisone
   pediatric liver transplantation, 653
Metoclopramide
   for nausea and vomiting, 288
Metoclopramide (Reglan)
   for CIP, 379
   for gastroparesis, 190–191
   for GERD, 55
   NUD, 186
Metronidazole (Flagyl)
   for acute pancreatitis, 781
   adverse effects, 314t
   for ascitic fluid infection, 659
   for *Balantidium coli*, 307
   for *Blastocystis hominis*, 307
   for *Clostridium difficile* diarrhea, 304, 305
   for Crohn's colitis, 466
   for Crohn's diseases perianal complications, 472–473
   for diarrhea, 293, 294, 294t
   for *Dientamoeba fragilis*, 308
   for diverticulitis, 601
   for *Giardia*, 282
   for *Giardia lamblia*, 310
   for *Helicobacter pylori*, 140
   for intestinal protozoan parasites, 309t
   for nonsteroidal antiinflammatory drug enteropathy, 365
   pregnancy, 313t
   for short bowel syndrome, 382
   for traveler's diarrhea, 301
Micronutrients
   assessment, 320
   requirements, 321t
Microscopic colitis, 506–509
   colectomy, 509
   defined, 506
   diarrhea, 506
   ileostomy, 509
   lymphocytic colitis, 506
   medical management, 506–509
   mucosal lacerations, 506
   surgery, 509
Microsporidia, 294
Microsporidiosis, 308
   treatment, 309t
Midazolam
   endoscopic procedure sedation, 18
   for GERD, 79
   pregnancy, 492
Midcingulate cortex (MCC), 261
Migraine headaches, 346
   with gastroparesis, 193
Milk of magnesium, 241t
Milk thistle
   for alcoholic liver disease, 668
Milwaukee classification
   biliary pain, 771t
Mineral
   assessment, 320
   requirements, 321t
   supplements
      for short bowel syndrome, 383t, 384
Mineral oil
   for constipation, 440

Minimal sedation
   continuum of depth, 17t
Miralax
   for constipation, 441
Mirizzi syndrome, 766
Mirtazepine (Remcron)
   for chronic abdominal pain, 253
   for FGID, 263t, 264
Misoprostol (Cytotec), 144
   for constipation, 439t, 441
   cost, 439t
   for nonsteroidal antiinflammatory drug enteropathy, 365
   for SRES, 164
Mivazerol
   noncardiac surgery, 433
Mixed hemorrhoids, 536f
   treatment, 537–538
Moderation sedation, 17
   continuum of depth, 17t
   monitoring and resuscitation equipment, 18t
Molecular assays
   for pancreatic cancer, 826
Monosodium glutamate (MSG)
   reactions to, 346
Monte Carlo Markov Chain modeling, 8
Monte Carlo simulations, 8
Montgomery salivary bypass tubes, 136
Mood disorders
   with eating disorders, 237–238
Morphine
   for porphyria, 729
Mosapride
   for gastroparesis, 192
Motilin agonists
   for gastroparesis, 192
   NUD, 186
Motility dysfunction, 239
Motilium. *See* Domperidone (Motilium)
Motor disorders
   categorizing, 107f
6-MP. *See* 6-mercaptopurine (6-MP)
MSG. *See* Monosodium glutamate (MSG)
Mucinous cystic neoplasms (MCN), 823, 824
Mucomyst. *See* Acetylcysteine (Mucomyst)
Mucosal associated lymphoid tissue (MALT), 202
   lymphomas, 138, 139–140
   low grade, 202
Mucosal ischemia, 161
Mucosal lacerations
   microscopic colitis, 506
Multiple organ dysfunction syndrome
   organ involvement, 414t
Multiple sedating agents, 20
Multipolar/bipolar electrocautery
   gastrointestinal bleeding, 171
Multivisceral transplantation, 387. *See also* Intestinal and multivisceral transplantation
Munchausen syndrome, 256
Mutation analysis
   chronic pancreatitis, 810–811

Mycobacterial involvement
   of esophagus, 98
Mycobacterium avium complex (MAC), 98, 276
Mycobacterium tuberculosis, 98
Mycophenolate mofetil (Cellcept)
   for Crohn's disease of small bowel, 393
   for GVHD, 286
   side effects, 286
   for transplantation, 387
Myofascial trigger points, 251

N

N-acetyl cysteine (NAC)
   for alcoholic liver disease, 669
   for fulminant hepatic failure, 630, 633
N-acetyl p-benzoquinoneimine (NAPQI)
   for acetaminophen poisoning, 692
Nadalol
   for acute variceal bleeding, 122
   for portal hypertension, 676–677, 677
Nalmefene
   for alcoholism, 229
   for fatigue of cholestasis, 710
Naloxone (Narcan)
   endoscopic sedation, 19
   for pruritis of cholestasis, 709
Nalozone
   for pruritis of cholestasis, 708t
Naltrexone
   for alcoholism, 229
   for PBC, 703
   for pruritis of cholestasis, 708t, 709
NAPQI. *See* N-acetyl p-benzoquinoneimine (NAPQI)
Naprosen
   concomitant steroids, 144
   for NSAID induced ulcers, 8
Naproxen (Naprosen)
   concomitant steroids, 144
   for NSAID induced ulcers, 8
Narcan
   endoscopic sedation, 19
   for pruritis of cholestasis, 709
Narcotics
   for chronic abdominal pain, 252
   endoscopic procedure sedation, 18
Nasal calcium
   for metabolic bone disease, 333
Nasogastric aspirate (NGA)
   HRL, 167–168
National Center for Complementary and Alternative Medicine
   web sites, 355
National Center for Nutrition and Dietetics Consumer Nutrition Hotline
   American Dietetic Association, 369
Nausea
   with SCT, 288
N butyl 2 cyaocrylate
   for acute variceal bleeding, 121
Nd:YAG laser, 499f
Necator Americanus, 311
   treatment, 312t
Necrotizing fasciitis
   with percutaneous endoscopic gastrostomy, 198
Nefazadone (Serzone)
   for chronic abdominal pain, 253
Negative predictive value (NPV)
   computation of, 5t
Nematodes (roundworms), 311
Neonatal cholestasis
   with cystic fibrosis, 808
Neoral
   pediatric liver transplantation, 653
Neostigmine
   for acute colonic pseudoobstruction, 504
Neosynephrine
   for fulminant hepatic failure, 636
Neuroendocrine tumors
   secretory diarrhea, 425
Neurogenic dysphagia
   myotomy, 52
Neurontin
   for chronic abdominal pain, 253
   for unexplained chest pain, 111
Neutropenic enterocolitis (typhlitis)
   with SCT, 287–288
Nexium. *See* Esomeprazole (Nexium)
NGA. *See* Nasogastric aspirate (NGA)
NHL. *See* Non Hodgkin's lymphoma (NHL)
Niclosamide
   adverse effects, 314t
   for cestodes, 311
   for intestinal flukes, 310
   for intestinal helminths, 312t
   pregnancy, 313t
Nifedipine
   for achalasia, 109
   for postcholecystectomy syndrome, 776
Niftutimox
   for Chaga's disease, 99
Night time regurgitation
   with achalasia, 113
Nimesulide (Aulin)
   for nonsteroidal antiinflammatory drug (NSAID) induced small and large intestinal injury, 366
Nitazoxanide
   for intestinal protozoan parasites, 309t
   for traveler's diarrhea, 301
Nitinol stents
   for esophageal strictures, 104–105
Nitric ointment
   for anal fissure, 530
Nitroglycerin
   for portal hypertension, 678, 679
Nizatadine (Axid)
   for upper gastrointestinal bleeding, 153
NNT. *See* Number needed to treat (NNT)
Nociception, 250
NOD2
   Crohn's disease of small bowel, 390
Nodular lymphoid hyperplasia
   with CVID, 283
NOMI. *See* Nonocclusive mesenteric ischemia (NOMI)
Nomogram
   converting likelihood ratios into posttest probability, 5f
Nonacidic reflux
   GERD, 65–66
Nonalcoholic fatty liver disease, 671–674
   bariatric surgery, 672
   cytoprotective strategies, 673
   treatment, 671–672, 673t
Nonchemical sedation, 20
Noncirrhotic portal hypertension, 682–687
   defined, 682–683
   etiology, 683–684, 683t
   TIPS, 687, 687t
Nondependent hazardous drinkers
   brief interventions, 228
Nondysenteric colitis, 308
Nondysplastic Barrett's epithelium, 90
Non Hodgkin's lymphoma (NHL)
   with CVID, 282
Nonimmune adverse reactions to food, 346–347
Nonocclusive ischemia
   diagnosis, 413t
   treatment, 415t
Nonocclusive mesenteric ischemia (NOMI), 411–418
Nonsteroidal antiinflammatory drug (NSAID)
   associated dyspepsia
      treatment, 144–145
   enteropathy, 364–365
      diagnosis, 364–365
      treatment, 365–366
   gastrointestinal complications, 142–146
   Helicobacter pylori, 139
   hepatotoxicity, 606
   induced small and large intestinal injury, 364–366
      colonic complications, 366
      IBD, 366
   induced ulcer, 8–10
   PUD, 149
   risk estimation, 142–143, 142t
   risk reduction, 143
   risk stratification, 144t
   ulcerogenic potential, 142
   ulcers
      complications, 145
      with *H. pylori*, 147
      refractory, 147
Nonulcer dyspepsia (NUD)
   H. pylori, 140, 185
   psychological interventions, 187
   psychometric testing, 185
   threshold analysis, 12
   treatment, 183–187
Nonvariceal upper gastrointestinal bleeding (NVUGIB), 167
   patient resuscitation, 167
   selection for treatment, 168–169
   therapeutic endoscopy, 168
Norfloxacin
   for portal hypertension, 678
   for SBP, 659
Normal transit constipation, 442–443

Noroviruses, 295
Norpramin. *See* Desipramine (Norpramin)
Nortriptyline (Pamelor)
   for chronic abdominal pain, 253
   for FGID, 263, 263t
   for gastroparesis, 193
   for IBS, 240t
   for spastic disorders, 110–111
Norwalk virus, 295
Nosocomial pneumonia
   with SRES, 165
NPV. *See* Negative predictive value (NPV)
NSAID. *See* Nonsteroidal antiinflammatory drug (NSAID)
5 nucleotidase (5NT), 605, 606t
NUD. *See* Nonulcer dyspepsia (NUD)
Null hypothesis, 3
Number needed to treat (NNT), 3
   computation of, 3t
Nurse administered propofol, 21
Nurse advocate, 266–269
   clinic visit, 266
   compliance, 267
   outreach, 268
   patient education, 267
   position role, 266
   psychosocial issues, 267–268
   role impact, 268
   sexual and reproductive issues, 268
   telephone triage, 266–267
Nursing
   UC, 455
Nutrition
   acute pancreatitis, 781
   assessment, 320
   with cystic fibrosis, 804–805
   esophageal cancer, 131
   pediatric liver transplantation, 654
   requirements, 320–321
Nutritional therapy
   alcoholic liver disease, 667
   for Crohn's colitis, 466–467
NVUGIB. *See* Nonvariceal upper gastrointestinal bleeding (NVUGIB)

O

Obesity, 212–218
   alcoholic liver disease, 666–667
   assessment, 213–214
   behavioral assessment, 214
   children, 213t
   defined, 212–213
   diet, 216–217
   dietary assessment, 215–216
   drugs, 217–218
   epidemiology, 212
   exercise assessment, 216
   GERD, 60, 70
   medical risks, 212, 212t
   severe
     diet, 217
   suggestions, 215
   surgery, 217–218
   treatment, 213
   trivial, 213
Obscure gastrointestinal bleeding, 357–363
   angiography, 359
   diagnosis, 358–361, 358t
   enteroclysis, 358–359
   enteroscopy, 359–360
   etiology, 360–361
   hormonal therapy, 362
   intestinal angioectasia, 360
   proximal intestinal lesions causing, 358t
   radionucleotide studies, 359
   small bowel series, 358–359
   small bowel tumors, 362
   treatment, 360–361
Octacarboxyl porphyrin, 729
Octreotide
   for bleeding peptic ulcer, 175
   for chronic pancreatitis, 800
   for CIP, 380
   for Crohn's disease of small bowel, 395
   for diabetic diarrhea, 421
   for gastrinoma, 159
   for microscopic colitis, 508
   for portal hypertension, 679
   for secretory diarrhea, 426–427
OKT3
   pediatric liver transplantation, 653
Olsalazine (Dipentum)
   for Crohn's disease of small bowel, 391
   for UC, 454, 455–456
OLT. *See* Orthotopic liver transplantation (OLT)
Omeprazole (Prilosec)
   for ENT with GERD, 67
   for esophageal strictures, 104
   for extraesophageal GERD, 67t
   for GERD, 54, 66
   for SRES, 163
   for upper gastrointestinal bleeding, 153
Ondansetron (Zofran)
   for fatigue of cholestasis, 710, 711
   for fatigue of liver disease, 711t
   for gastroparesis, 193
   for porphyria, 729
   for pruritis of cholestasis, 708t, 709–710
One way sensitivity
   of ulcer management, 10f
One way sensitivity analysis, 10
Open cholecystectomy, 759–761
Open hemorrhoidectomy, 539
Operant interventions
   for chronic abdominal pain, 253
Opiate antagonists
   for alcoholism, 229
   for PBC, 703
   for pruritis of cholestasis, 709
Opiates
   endoscopic procedure sedation, 18
   for secretory diarrhea, 426
Opioid analgesics
   for chronic abdominal pain, 252
Opisthorchis viverrini (Southeast Asian liver fluke), 310
   treatment, 312t
Opium
   deodorized tincture of
     for short bowel syndrome, 381
   tincture of
     for secretory diarrhea, 426
Oprelvekin
   for chronic hepatitis C, 623
Oral bile acid dissolution therapy
   for cholelithiasis, 761–762
Oral conditions, 43–47
Oral diet therapy, 321
Oral lichenoid, 43
Oral problems
   with eating disorders, 233
Oral rehydration solutions (ORS)
   for acute infectious diarrhea, 292, 292t
   secretory diarrhea, 425–426
   for short bowel syndrome, 382–383
   for traveler's diarrhea, 300
Orlistat, 217–218
Oropharyngeal cancer
   smoking, 270
Oropharyngeal dysphagia, 49–53
   evaluation and classification, 49–51
   functional etiologies, 52
   hypopharyngeal diverticuli and cricopharyngeal bar, 51–52
   identifying underlying disease, 52
   intraluminal manometry, 51
   management algorithm, 50f
   patient history, 50–51
   patterns and manifestations, 49t
   physical examination, 51
   radiographic endoscopic examination, 51
   severe aspiration, 53
   surgery, 52
   swallowing therapy, 52–53
   treatment, 51–53
     structural etiologies, 51–52
   videofluoroscopy, 51
ORS. *See* Oral rehydration solutions (ORS)
Orthotopic liver transplantation (OLT)
   for HCC, 742
   refractory ascites, 658
Osler Weber Rendu, 686
Osmotic laxatives
   for constipation, 440
Osteocalcin
   metabolic bone disease, 327t
Osteomalacia
   Crohn's disease of small bowel, 395
Osteopenia
   Crohn's disease of small bowel, 395
Osteoporosis
   with celiac disease, 370
   Crohn's disease of small bowel, 395
   drug induced, 331–332
   with PBC, 703
   with PSC, 716–717
   smoking, 272
OTW balloons. *See* Over the wire (OTW) balloons
Outcomes research, 1
Outer external sphincter
   anatomy of, 476–477
Outlet dysfunction constipation, 441–442
Outreach

nurse advocate, 268
Over the wire (OTW) balloons, 101, 103
Overweight
  diet, 217
Oxaliplatin
  for colorectal carcinoma, 564–565, 564t
Oxamniquine
  adverse effects, 314t
  for intestinal helminths, 312t
  pregnancy, 313t
  for schistosomiasis, 310
Oxandrolone
  for alcoholic liver disease, 667
Oxazepam (Serax)
  for alcohol withdrawal, 230
Oxylates
  with short bowel syndrome, 383

P
PACAP. See Pituitary adenylate cyclase activating polypeptide (PACAP)
Paclitaxel
  for metastatic esophageal cancer, 129
Paget's disease, 532
Pain
  chronic pancreatitis, 798–799
  IBS, 240
PAK. See Pancreas after kidney (PAK)
Palliative chemotherapy
  PGL, 210
Palliative radiation therapy
  PGL, 210
Palliative sodium bicarbonate mouth rinse, 43
Palliative therapy
  cholangiocarcinoma, 718
  defined, 579
  esophageal cancer, 131–137
  pancreatic and periampullary neoplasms, 816
  rectal cancer, 575–578
Pamelor. See Nortriptyline (Pamelor)
Pamine
  for IBS, 240t
Pancreas
  radiation side effects, 581–582, 581t
  transplantation, 829–830
Pancreas after kidney (PAK), 829
Pancreas transplantation alone (PTA), 829
Pancreatic adenomas, 156
Pancreatic and periampullary neoplasms, 813–817
  distal lesions, 816
  incidence, 813
  palliation, 816
  postoperative results, 816
  presentation, 813
  survival, 816–817
  treatment, 814–815
  workup, 813–814
Pancreatic cancer, 31–36
  detection, 31
  diagnosis and staging algorithm, 33f
  EUS guided FNA, 31–32
  EUS M staging, 33–34

EUS N stage accuracy, 32t
EUS staging, 32
EUS T stage accuracy, 32t
EUS vs. helical CT, 32–33, 33t
future screening modalities, 826
risk of, 825t
smoking, 270
Pancreatic cancer therapy, 818–822
  for adjuvant disease, 818–820, 818t
  advanced, 821t
  current practice, 820
  inconclusive study results, 819–820
  locally advanced disease, 820–822
  metastatic disease, 821
  neoadjuvant therapy role, 820, 820t
Pancreatic disease
  pathologic examination, 804f
Pancreatic enzyme preparations, 798t, 800t
Pancreatic fistula
  with chronic pancreatitis, 786–787
Pancreatic gastrinomas, 156
Pancreatic insufficiency
  associated with low BMD, 328t
  diabetic diarrhea, 422
Pancreatic intraepithelial neoplasia (PanIN), 824–825
Pancreatic islet cell transplantation, 830–832
Pancreatic malignancy, 787
Pancreatic necrosis
  acute pancreatitis, 781
Pancreatic neoplasms, 813t
Pancreatic neoplastic cysts, 823–826
Pancreaticoduodenectomy (Whipple resection), 785, 814–815, 815f
Pancreatic precancerous lesions, 823–826
Pancreatic pseudocysts, 795
Pancreatic sphincterotomy, 790f
Pancreatic transplantation, 828–832
Pancreatitis, 794f. See also Acute pancreatitis; Chronic pancreatitis
  with eating disorders, 234
  endoscopic therapy, 789–795
  hereditary, 825
  idiopathic, 796
  parenteral nutrition for, 324
  with SCT, 288
Panhematin, 728
PanIN. See Pancreatic intraepithelial neoplasia (PanIN)
Pantoprazolen (Protonix)
  for GERD, 54
  for SRES, 163
Paradoxical puborectalis contraction
  ileoanal pouch anastomosis controversies, 461
Paraesophageal hernia, 72
Paraldehyde
  for porphyria, 729
Parathyroid hormone (PTH), 608
Paregoric
  for secretory diarrhea, 426
Parenteral nutrition, 322
  administration of, 323
  central venous catheter complications, 323
  compounding, 323

  for intestinal failure, 324
  metabolic complications, 323
  for pancreatitis, 324
  sample order, 323t
  vascular access devices, 323
Parietal cell vagotomy, 160
Parkinsonism
  with Wilson's disease, 722
Paromomycin (Humatin)
  adverse effects, 314t
  for Balantidium coli, 307
  for Cryptosporidium parvum, 307–308
  for diarrhea, 295
  for Giardia lamblia, 310
  for HIV, 277–279
  for intestinal protozoan parasites, 309t
  pregnancy, 313t
Parotid gland enlargement
  with eating disorders, 233
Paroxetine (Paxil)
  for chronic abdominal pain, 252
  efficacy, 263
  for fatigue of cholestasis, 710
  for FGID, 263t
  for NUD, 186
  side effects, 264
Paroxysmal nocturnal hemoglobinuria, 684
Partial (Toupet) fundoplication, 72
Passive smoking, 272
Patch testing, 349
Patient controlled sedation, 21–22
Patient counseling and monitoring
  chronic pancreatitis, 811
Patient education
  for eating disorders, 234
  genetic counseling, 545–546
  nurse advocate, 267
Patient management
  decision models, 8–16
Paxil. See Paroxetine (Paxil)
PBC. See Primary biliary cirrhosis (PBC)
PBG. See Porphobilinogen (PBG)
PCT. See Porphyria cutanea tarda (PCT)
PDT. See Photodynamic therapy (PDT)
Peanut allergy, 345
Pediatric Crohn's disease
  future therapy, 399
  nutritional therapy, 399–400
  psychosocial therapy, 400
  therapy, 399t
  treatment, 397–400
Pediatric liver transplantation, 650–655
  indications for, 650–652, 650t
  postoperative, 654–655
  surgical innovations, 653–655
Peer interaction
  for pediatric Crohn's disease, 400
PEG. See Percutaneous endoscopic gastrostomy (PEG)
PEG (Miralax)
  for constipation, 441
PEG-J
  with percutaneous endoscopic gastrostomy, 199
Pegylated interferon

for acute hepatitis C, 614
for chronic hepatitis B, 618
for chronic hepatitis C, 622, 623
for HCV in children, 627
PEJ tube
  with percutaneous endoscopic gastrostomy, 199
Penicillamine
  for liver disease during pregnancy, 694–695
  for PBC, 704
  for Wilson's disease, 721
Penicillin
  for fulminant hepatic failure, 633
Penicillin G
  for gonorrhea, 534
  for Whipple's disease, 317t
Penicillin VK
  for Whipple's disease, 317t
Pentasa. See Mesalamine (Pentasa)
Pentobarbital
  for fulminant hepatic failure, 636
Pentostatin
  for GVHD, 286
Pentoxifylline (PTX)
  for alcoholic liver disease, 668
Pepcid
  for SRES, 163
  for upper gastrointestinal bleeding, 153
Peptic ulcer disease (PUD), 8, 147–154, 168. See also Bleeding peptic ulcer
  clinical presentation, 148–150
  with cystic fibrosis, 804
  diagnosis, 149
  epidemiology, 147–148
  gastric analysis, 149–150
  H. pylori, 149
  NSAIDs, 149
  oral conditions, 44
  pharmacologic treatment, 152–153
  stress related, 148
  upper gastrointestinal bleeding
    natural history, 150
  ZE syndrome, 149
Pepto Bismol. See also Bismuth subsalicylate (Pepto Bismol)
  for Helicobacter pylori, 140
  for secretory diarrhea, 428
Percutaneous drainage
  for acute pancreatitis, 782
Percutaneous endoscopic gastrostomy, 196–200
  complications, 197–199
  contraindications for, 196
  enteral nutrition, 199–200
  indications for, 196
  introduce method, 197
  pull techniques, 197
  push method, 197
  techniques, 197
Percutaneous endoscopic gastrostomy (PEG)
  site metastasis, 198
  solutions
    for constipation, 440

tubes, 234
  ethical issues, 200
Percutaneous ethanol injection
  vs. radiofrequency ablation, 735t
Percutaneous liver biopsy, 609–610
Perendoscopic gastroesophageal reflux disease therapies, 74–75
Periampullary neoplasms, 813–817, 813t. See also Pancreatic and periampullary neoplasms
Perianal abscess
  drainage, 479f
  inflammatory bowel disease, 479
Perianal Crohn disease activity index, 477t
Perianal fistula, 480f
Perihilar ductal cholangiocarcinoma, 718
Perimolysis
  with eating disorders, 233
Perineal dermatitis
  left sided ulcerative colitis, 451
Perineal rectal prolapse repair, 520–521
Perineal rectosigmoidectomy, 521
Peritoneovenous shunt (PV)
  refractory ascites, 658
Peritonitis
  with percutaneous endoscopic gastrostomy, 198
Personality disorders
  with eating disorders, 237–238
Peutz-Jegher's Syndrome (PJS), 547t, 548–549, 825
  oral conditions, 46
  risk and surveillance, 552t, 553–554
PGL. See Primary gastric lymphoma (PGL)
Pharmacologic stress testing
  cardiovascular risk with major surgery, 431–432
Pharyngeal strictures
  oropharyngeal dysphagia, 51
Phenergan
  endoscopic sedation, 19
  for gastroparesis, 193
Phenobarbital (Donnatal)
  with belladonna
    for IBS, 240t
  for pruritis of cholestasis, 709
Phenylephrine gel
  for fecal incontinence, 513
pH monitoring
  24 hours
    GERD, 69
Phosphosoda
  pregnancy, 443
Photodynamic therapy (PDT), 131
  BE, 38
  BE ablation, 92–93
  cholangiocarcinoma, 718
  dysplastic Barrett's epithelium, 93t
  esophageal cancer, 132–133
  photosensitizers, 93t
Photosensitizers
  Barrett's ablation, 92–93
  PDT, 93t
Physical status
  ASA classification system, 18t

Phytonadione, 712
PI-IBS. See Postinfective IBS (PI-IBS)
Pinworm, 311
  treatment, 312t
Pioglitazone
  for insulin resistance, 672
Pituitary adenylate cyclase activating polypeptide (PACAP), 148
PJS. See Peutz-Jegher's Syndrome (PJS)
Plasmapheresis
  for pruritis of cholestasis, 708
Plexiglas implantation, 80–81
  procedure, 81
Plication, 76
  for bleeding peptic ulcer, 175
Plicator, 83
Plummer-Vinson syndrome
  oral conditions, 46
PMMA. See Polymethylmethacrylate (PMMA)
PMN. See Polymorphonuclear leukocyte (PMN)
Pneumatic compression devices, 570–572
Pneumatic dilatation
  for achalasia, 109
Pneumoperitoneum
  with percutaneous endoscopic gastrostomy, 199
Pneumostatic dilatation, 117
Polidocanol, 170t
  esophageal cancer injection therapy, 133
Polycarbophil (FiberCon)
  for acute infectious diarrhea, 293
Polyethylene glycol solution, 241t
  for constipation, 439t
  cost, 439t
Polyflex esophageal stent, 134, 134f
Polymethylmethacrylate (PMMA), 80–81
  effect, 81
Polymorphonuclear leukocyte (PMN), 656
Polypectomy
  criteria for, 571t
Polypoid lesions, 487f
Polyposis syndrome, 550–556
  extracolonic cancer
    risk and surveillance, 553t
  risk and surveillance, 552t
Polyps. See also specific polyps
  dysplasia surveillance programs, 487–488
Polytetrafluoroethylene, 80
Porphobilinogen (PBG), 728
Porphyria cutanea tarda (PCT), 729–730
  phlebotomy, 729
Porphyrias, 728–730
  acute, 728–729
    diagnosis, 728
    treatment, 728–729
Portal hypertension, 675–680
  endoscopic therapy, 677, 679
  etiology, 675–678, 675t
  future, 678
  idiopathic, 685
  liver transplantation, 680
  natural history, 676
  noncirrhotic, 682–687

pathophysiology, 675–678
TIPS, 679
transjugular intrahepatic portosystemic shunts, 678
variceal hemorrhage
prevention, 676–678, 677t, 679–680
TIPS, 680
treatment, 678–679
Portal pressure
measurement of, 682–683
Portal vein embolization (PVE), 741
Portal vein thrombosis, 685–686
etiology, 686t
Portocaval shunt
for acute variceal bleeding, 122
Positive predicted value (PPV)
computation of, 5t
Postcholecystectomy syndrome, 774–776
clinical classification, 775
diagnosis, 775
etiology, 774t
hepatobiliary scintigraphy, 775
sphincter manometry, 775–776
surgery, 776
symptoms, 774
treatment, 774, 776
Post endoscopic mucosal resection stenosis, 40
Postgastrectomy
associated with low BMD, 328t
Postinfective IBS (PI-IBS), 261
Postoperative stomach
chronic gastritis, 181
Postpartum weight gain, 213t
Posttransplantation lymphoproliferative disease (PTLD)
with intestinal transplantation, 388
pediatric liver transplantation, 654
Potatoes
with celiac disease, 368
Pouches
excessive or uncontrolled bowel movements with, 525–526
Pouchitis
ileoanal pouch anastomosis controversies, 461
smoking, 271
PPH. See Procedure for prolapse and hemorrhoids (PPH)
PPI. See Proton pump inhibitor (PPI)
PPV. See Positive predicted value (PPV)
Praziquantel
adverse effects, 314t
for cestodes, 311
for intestinal flukes, 310
for intestinal helminths, 312t
for liver flukes, 310
pregnancy, 313t
for schistosomiasis, 310
Prazosin
for portal hypertension, 678
Prednisone
vs. budesonide
for pediatric Crohn's disease, 398t
for Crohn's colitis, 466

for Crohn's disease of small bowel, 391
for IEU, 99
for UC, 450
Preeclampsia
pregnancy, 698
Pregnancy
anatomic changes, 694
antibiotics, 491
antiparasitic drugs, 313t
AZA, 490, 491t
cascara, 443
castor oil, 443
constipation, 443
corticosteroids, 491
cyclosporine, 491
delivery mode, 492
disease activity assessment, 492
eclampsia, 698
estrogen, 696
fulminant hepatic failure, 634
IBD, 490–492, 491
infliximab, 492
laboratory studies, 694
lactulose, 443
liver disease, 694–700, 695t
magnesium laxatives, 443
medications, 490–492
mesalamine, 490, 491
methotrexate, 491
normal changes, 694–695, 694t
outcome, 492
phosphosoda, 443
physical examination, 694
preeclampsia, 698
sorbitol, 443
sulfasalazine, 490, 491
toxemia, 698
UC, 455
Preoperative fasting
ASA guidelines for, 18
Prevacid. See Lansoprazole (Prevacid)
Prilosec. See Omeprazole (Prilosec)
Primary biliary cirrhosis (PBC), 701–705
diagnosis, 701–702
disease modifying agents, 704, 705t
natural history, 702
prevention, 702t
risk scores, 702
treatment, 702–705, 702t
Primary gastric lymphoma (PGL), 202–205
adjuvant therapy, 209, 209t
chemotherapy, 205
clinical presentation, 204
defined, 202
endoscopic ultrasound, 204
epidemiology, 202
followup, 209–210
H. pylori, 203
histopathology, 202–203
Kaplan Meier survival curve, 210f
molecular events, 203–204
neoadjuvant therapy, 209
outcome, 209–210
palliation, 205
palliative care, 210

pathogenesis, 203–204
radiation, 205
staging classification, 204, 204t
surgery, 205
treatment, 204–205
Primary immunodeficiencies
classification, 280–281, 280t
gastrointestinal manifestations, 281–283
Primary lactase deficiency, 372
Primary psychiatric illness, 255–256
Primary sclerosing cholangitis (PSC), 715–717
clinical manifestations, 715–716
diagnosis, 716
prognosis, 716
treatment, 716–717
Probenecid
for gonorrhea, 534
Probiotics
for diabetic diarrhea, 422
for food allergy, 350
for nonsteroidal antiinflammatory drug enteropathy, 365
for pediatric Crohn's disease, 400
Procedure for prolapse and hemorrhoids (PPH), 539, 539f
Prochlorperazine (Compazine)
for gastroparesis, 193
Proctectomy
inflammatory bowel disease fistulas, 482
Prognosis
well-designed trial characteristics, 7t
Prognosis studies
purpose, 6
Prokinetic agents
for CIP, 379–380
for constipation, 441
NUD, 186
Prolamins
celiac disease, 368
Prolapse and hemorrhoids, 539, 539f
Promethazine (Phenergan)
endoscopic sedation, 19
for gastroparesis, 193
Promotility agents, 55–56
Prophylactic total pancreatectomy
for pancreatic cancer, 826
Propofol (Diprovan)
with alfentanil
patient controlled endoscopic sedation, 22
endoscopic sedation, 20
for fulminant hepatic failure, 634
nurse administered, 21
pregnancy, 492
for pruritis of cholestasis, 710
Propranolol
for acute variceal bleeding, 122
for porphyria, 729
for portal hypertension, 676–677, 678
Propulsid. See Cisapride (Propulsid)
Propylthiouracil
for alcoholic liver disease, 668
Prospect theory, 8
Prostaglandin analogues

for constipation, 441
SRES, 164
Prostaglandin synthetase inhibitors
  for secretory diarrhrea, 427
Protein
  assessment, 320
  food induced symptoms, 341
  with hepatic encephalopathy, 663
  needs, 320t
Prothrombin time (PT), 605
Protonix
  for GERD, 54
  for upper gastrointestinal bleeding, 153
Proton pump inhibitor (PPI), 54
  bleeding peptic ulcer, 174–175
  for esophageal strictures, 104
  for GERD, 803
  for *Helicobacter pylori,* 140
  for nausea and vomiting, 288
  pharmacophysiology, 152
  for reflux, 234
  for SRES, 163
Protozoa, 307–310
  of esophagus, 99
  traveler's diarrhea, 298–299
Proximal gastrectomy
  PGL, 208
Proximal pancreatic duct stricture
  with acute pancreatitis, 782
Prozac. *See* Fluoxetine (Prozac)
Pruritus
  ani, 535
  of cholestasis, 707–713
    treatment, 707–711, 708t
  gravidarum, 696
  with PBC, 703
  with PSC, 716
PSC. *See* Primary sclerosing cholangitis (PSC)
Pseudoachalasia, 112
Pseudoallergic reactions to food, 346
Pseudocysts
  with acute pancreatitis, 782
  with chronic pancreatitis, 786
Pseudologica phantastica, 256
Pseudomembranous colitis, 303f
Pseudomonas aeruginosa, 24
Psychiatric illness, 257
  with Wilson's disease, 723
Psychological counseling
  alcoholism, 228–229
  for pediatric Crohn's disease, 400
Psychometric testing
  NUD, 185
Psychosis
  with Wilson's disease, 723
Psychosocial factors
  questions about, 184t
Psychotherapy
  for eating disorders, 236
Psychotropic medications
  FGID, 260–265
  IBS, 240
Psyllium (Metamucil)
  for acute infectious diarrhea, 293

for constipation, 439t, 440
PT. *See* Prothrombin time (PT)
PTA. *See* Pancreas transplantation alone (PTA)
PTH. *See* Parathyroid hormone (PTH)
PTLD. *See* Posttransplantation lymphoproliferative disease (PTLD)
PTX. *See* Pentoxifylline (PTX)
PubMed, 1
PUD. *See* Peptic ulcer disease (PUD)
Pulmonary hypertension
  pediatric liver transplantation, 652
Pulmonary wedge pressure, 120
Pulse oximetry, 21
Push dilator, 100–101
PV. *See* Peritoneovenous shunt (PV)
PVE. *See* Portal vein embolization (PVE)
Pyrantel pamoate
  adverse effects, 314t
  for ascariasis, 311
  for hookworm, 311
  for intestinal helminths, 312t
  for pinworms, 311
  pregnancy, 313t
Pyrimethamine
  for *Isospora belli,* 310

Q

Quackwatch
  web sites, 355
Quality adjusted life years (QALY), 15
Quality of life
  chronic intestinal pseudoobstruction, 375
  pediatric liver transplantation, 654–655
Quinacrine
  adverse effects, 314t
  for *Giardia lamblia,* 310
  for intestinal protozoan parasites, 309t

R

R115777
  for pancreatic cancer, 821
Rabeprazole (Aciphex)
  for GERD, 54
  for *Helicobacter pylori,* 140
  for SRES, 163
  for upper gastrointestinal bleeding, 153
Radiation induced rectal bleeding, 588
Radiation proctocolitis
  lower gastrointestinal bleeding, 585
Radiation therapy. *See also* Abdominal radiation
  palliative
    PGL, 210
Radical colorectal resection
  criteria for, 571t
Radioallergosorbent test (RAST), 348
Radiofrequency ablation
  vs. percutaneous ethanol injection, 735t
Radiofrequency (RF) thermal energy, 75, 76f
Radionucleotide studies
  obscure gastrointestinal bleeding, 359
RAIR. *See* Rectoanal inhibitory reflex (RAIR)
Ranitidine (Zantac)

for esophageal strictures, 104
for OC with duodenal ulcer, 45
for SRES, 163
for upper gastrointestinal bleeding, 153
RAST. *See* Radioallergosorbent test (RAST)
Receiver operation characteristics, 8
Recombinant human erythropoetin
  for chronic hepatitis C, 623
Recombivax-HB, 613
Rectal cancer, 34, 566
  chemotherapy, 577
  classification, 569–570
  colonoscopy, 569
  colostomy, 576
  curative intent management, 569–574
  digital examination, 569
  EUS accuracy, 34t
  history, 569
  invasive therapy, 576–577
  outcomes, 34f
  palliative therapy, 575–578
    clinical evaluation, 575–576
    goals, 575
    indications, 575
  preoperative examination, 569–570
  radiation therapy, 577
  rectal stenting, 576–577
  resection, 576
  rigid proctoscopy, 569
  surgery, 576
  treatment, 574t
Rectal intussusception
  treatment, 522t
Rectal prolapse, 518, 532, 533f
  anterior resection, 520
  Delorme's operation, 521
  epidemiology, 518
  etiology, 518
  laparoscopic prolapse repair, 520
  preoperative evaluation, 519
  recurrence rates, 519t
  resection rectopexy, 520
  Ripstein rectopexy, 520
  surgery, 519
    diagnosis, 522
    functional outcome, 521–522
    rectal intussusception, 521–522
    treatment, 522
  suture rectopexy, 520
  symptoms, 518–519
  Wells' rectopexy, 520
Rectal ulcers
  lower gastrointestinal bleeding, 585–586
Rectoanal inhibitory reflex (RAIR), 512
Rectovaginal fistula (RVF), 481
Rectum
  radiation side effects, 581t, 582
Recurrent gastrointestinal bleeding
  therapy to prevent, 1
Refeeding syndrome, 234, 235
  with parenteral nutrition, 323
Referred pain
  chronic abdominal pain, 250
Reflux Pyramid, 64f
Refractory ascites, 658

defined, 658
orthotopic liver transplantation, 658
peritoneovenous shunt, 658
serial LVP, 658
transjugular intrahepatic portosystemic shunt, 658
Refractory nonsteroidal antiinflammatory drug ulcers, 147
Refractory sprue
  with celiac disease, 370
Refractory strictures, 103
Reglan. See Metoclopramide (Reglan)
Rehydration
  for acute infectious diarrhea, 292
Relapse rate
  Markov model, 14
Relative risk reduction (RRR), 2, 3
  computation of, 3t
Relaxation techniques
  for chronic abdominal pain, 253
ReliefBand
  for gastroparesis, 193
Remcron
  for chronic abdominal pain, 253
  for FGID, 263t, 264
Remicade. See Infliximab (Remicade)
Renal failure
  COX 2 inhibitors, 143
  enteral nutrition for, 325
  with fulminant hepatic failure, 637
  NSAID, 143
Research Council for Complementary Medicine
  web sites, 355
Resection rectopexy
  rectal prolapse, 520
Respiratory depression, 18
Restraint
  obesity, 215
Reversal agents
  endoscopic sedation, 19
RF thermal energy. See Radiofrequency (RF) thermal energy
Ribavirin
  for acute hepatitis C, 614
  with alpha interferon
    for HCV in children, 627
  for chronic hepatitis C, 623
Rice
  with celiac disease, 368
Rifabutin
  for human immunodeficiency virus (HIV), 277
Rifampicin
  for PBC, 703
  for pruritis of cholestasis, 708t, 709
  for Whipple's disease, 317t
Rifaxamin
  for traveler's diarrhea, 300
Ripstein rectopexy
  rectal prolapse, 520
Risedronate (Actonel)
  for metabolic bone disease, 333
  for PBC, 703
Risk assessment

genetic counseling, 545
Robinul
  for IBS, 240t
Rocephin
  for gonorrhea, 534
  for Whipple's disease, 317t
Rofecoxib (Vioxx), 143
Romazicon
  endoscopic sedation, 19
ROME II diagnostic criteria for biliary pain, 771f
Rosiglitazone
  for insulin resistance, 672
Rotavirus, 295
Roundworms, 311
Roux en Y gastric bypass (RYGB), 221, 221f, 222
  GERD, 70
RRR. See Relative risk reduction (RRR)
Rubber band ligation
  hemorrhoids, 538
RVF. See Rectovaginal fistula (RVF)
RYGB. See Roux en Y gastric bypass (RYGB)

S

SAAG. See Serum ascites albumin gradient (SAAG)
Sacral nerve stimulation (SNS), 514, 515f
  for diabetic diarrhea, 422
SADD. See Short Alcohol Dependence Data Questionnaire (SADD)
S-adenosylmethionine (SAMe)
  for alcoholic liver disease, 668–669
  for pruritis of cholestasis, 710
Safety issues
  GERD, 83–84
Salicylates
  for pediatric Crohn's disease, 397–398
Salmonella, 293, 294t
  traveler's diarrhea, 298
Salvage therapy
  NVUGIB, 174
SAMe. See S-adenosylmethionine (SAMe)
Sandostatin
  for diarrhea, 286
Savary dilatation, 105
Savary dilatators, 101f, 102, 499
  technique, 102
SCFA enemas. See Short chain fatty acid (SCFA) enemas
Schistosoma japonicum, 310
  treatment, 312t
Schistosoma mansoni, 310
Schistosomiasis, 310, 686
SCID. See Severe combined immunodeficiency (SCID)
SCJ. See Squamocolumnar junction (SCJ)
Sclerosants, 170t
  upper gastrointestinal bleeding, 170
Sclerosing cholangitis
  smoking, 271
Sclerotherapy
  for acute variceal bleeding, 121, 122
SCL 90 R. See Symptom Checklist 90 R (SCL 90 R)

Scopinaro procedure, 220f, 221
Scopolamine patch
  for gastroparesis, 193
SDS. See Shwachman Diamond syndrome (SDS)
Secondary achalasia, 112
Secondary lactase deficiency, 373
Secretin hormone stimulation test
  for chronic pancreatitis, 797
Secretins
  chronic pancreatitis, 798
Secretory diarrhea, 425–429
  carcinoid syndrome, 428
  diuretics, 429
  factitious cause, 429
  fluid and electrolyte replacement, 425–426
  laxatives, 429
  neuroendocrine tumors, 425
  pharmacologic control, 426–427
  systemic mastocytosis, 428
  treatment, 425–429
  VIPomas, 428
Sedation
  continuum of depth, 17t
  levels, 17
Selective malabsorption
  bariatric operations, 220–221
Selective serotonin reuptake inhibitors (SSRI)
  for chronic abdominal pain, 252
  for FGID, 263–265, 263t
    dosage, 264
    efficacy, 263–264
    mechanism of action, 263
    side effects, 264
Self dilatation
  anal stenosis, 533
  esophageal strictures, 105
Self expandable metallic stents (SEMS), 134, 499, 500f
Senna
  for constipation, 439t
  cost, 439t
Sensitivity
  computation of, 5t
Sensitivity analysis, 10–11
  of ulcer management, 10f
Sensitization
  chronic abdominal pain, 249–250
Sepsis
  ileoanal pouch anastomosis controversies, 460–461
Serax
  for alcohol withdrawal, 230
Serotonin antagonists
  for fatigue of cholestasis, 710
  for pruritis of cholestasis, 709–710
Serotonin receptors
  for constipation, 441
Sertraline (Zoloft)
  for chronic abdominal pain, 252
  for FGID, 263t
  for NUD, 186
  for pruritis of cholestasis, 710
Serum aminotransferses, 697

Serum ascites albumin gradient (SAAG), 656
Serum IgG
   for hepatitis A, 611
Serzone
   for chronic abdominal pain, 253
Sessile colorectal polyps
   recurrence rate, 40
Setons
   inflammatory bowel disease fistulas, 480
Severe combined immunodeficiency (SCID), 281
   gastrointestinal manifestations, 283
Severe obesity
   diet, 217
Sexual and reproductive issues
   nurse advocate, 268
Sexually transmitted diseases, 534–535
Sheep liver fluke
   treatment, 312t
Shigella, 293, 294t
   traveler's diarrhea, 298
Short Alcohol Dependence Data Questionnaire (SADD), 227
Short bowel syndrome, 381–385
   absorption enhancement, 382–383
   bacterial overgrowth, 382
   complications, 384–385
   excessive fluid loss, 381–382
   malabsorption, 382
   surgery, 385
   TPN, 384–385
   treatment, 381–384
Short chain fatty acid (SCFA) enemas
   for UC, 451
Short Michigan Alcoholism Screening Test (S-MAST), 227
Shwachman Diamond syndrome (SDS)
   with cystic fibrosis, 809–810
   exocrine pancreas, 810
   hematology dysfunction, 810
   liver abnormalities, 810
   statue and skeletal phenotypes, 809–810
Sildenafil
   for gastroparesis, 192
Silent reflux
   sleep disorder, 61
Silibinin
   for fulminant hepatic failure, 633–634
Silymarin (milk thistle)
   for alcoholic liver disease, 668
Simple strictures, 100
Simultaneous kidney and pancreas (SKP), 829
Sinequan
   for FGID, 263t
Sinusoidal obstructive syndrome (SOS), 684–685
   medications for, 684t
Sjögren's syndrome
   with PBC, 703
Skin maceration
   with percutaneous endoscopic gastrostomy, 199
Skin prick tests, 348

SKP, 829
Sleeping position
   GERD, 61
Slow transit constipation, 441
   with outlet dysfunction constipation, 442–443
Small bowel. *See also* Crohn's disease of small bowel
   meal induced physiological changes, 339
   radiation side effects, 581t, 582
Small bowel series
   obscure gastrointestinal bleeding, 358–359
Small bowel transplantation
   with parenteral nutrition, 323
Small bowel tumors
   obscure gastrointestinal bleeding, 362
Small bowel ulceration
   etiology, 362t
Small intestinal bypass, 219
S-MAST. *See* Short Michigan Alcoholism Screening Test (S-MAST)
Smoking
   acid peptic disorders, 270–271
   cigarette
      alcoholic liver disease, 666
      with PUD, 147
   duodenal ulcer, 271
   gastrointestinal disease, 270–272
   GERD, 60, 270
   inflammatory bowel disease, 271–272
   passive, 272
Smoking cessation, 270, 272
   gastrointestinal neoplasms, 270
   weight gain after, 213t
SNS. *See* Sacral nerve stimulation (SNS)
SOD. *See* Sphincter of Oddi dysfunction (SOD)
Sodium
   ascites, 657
Sodium cromoglycate, 349
Sodium morrhuate
   esophageal cancer injection therapy, 133
Sodium tetradecyl sulfate, 170t
Solitary rectal ulcer syndrome (SRUS), 448, 522–523
Solumedrol
   for UC, 450
Somatization disorder, 256
Somatostatin
   for acute variceal bleeding, 120
   for bleeding peptic ulcer, 175
   for diarrhea, 286
   for gastroparesis, 192
   for portal hypertension, 678, 679
Sonde enteroscopy
   obscure gastrointestinal bleeding, 360
Sorbitol
   for constipation, 439t, 440
   cost, 439t
   food induced symptoms, 340
   pregnancy, 443
SOS. *See* Sinusoidal obstructive syndrome (SOS)
Southeast Asian liver fluke, 310
   treatment, 312t

Spastic disorders, 110–111
Spastic motor disorders
   treatment, 110f
Specificity
   computation of, 5t
Sphincter of Oddi dysfunction (SOD), 770–772, 772f, 774
   clinical evaluation, 771–772
   clinical presentation, 771
   epidemiology, 770
   Hopkins scintigraphic scoring, 775t
   post simulations pancreatitis, 772
Sphincteroplasty
   for diabetic diarrhea, 422
Spironolactone
   for ascites, 657
   for portal hypertension, 677
Splanchnic hypoperfusion, 161
S plasty, 534f
Splenic vein thrombosis, 685–686
Splenorenal shunt
   for acute variceal bleeding, 122
Split liver transplantation, 647
Squamocolumnar junction (SCJ), 75
Squamous cell carcinoma, 532, 533
SRES. *See* Stress related erosive syndrome (SRES)
SRUS. *See* Solitary rectal ulcer syndrome (SRUS)
SSRI. *See* Selective serotonin reuptake inhibitors (SSRI)
Staphylococcus aureus, 295
Stapled hemorrhoidectomy, 539
Starvation
   with eating disorders, 233
Stem cell transplantation
   complications
      clinical presentation, 286–287
   diarrhea, 286–287
   gastrointestinal complications, 285–291, 285f
   hepatic complications, 285–291, 285f
Stents. *See also* specific stents
   endoscopically placed metallic PGL, 210
   for postcholecystectomy syndrome, 776
   selection of, 134
Steroids
   for GVHD, 286
   for inflammatory arthritis, 145
   with NSAIDs, 144
   for UC, 455
Stimulant laxatives
   for constipation, 440
Stoma
   fecal incontinence, 515
Stomach. *See also* Gastric
   ECG, 40
   meal induced physiological changes, 339
   postoperative
      chronic gastritis, 181
   radiation side effects, 581, 581t
Stool softeners
   for constipation, 440

Strangulated prolapsed internal hemorrhoids, 538
Strangulation obstruction, 417
  diagnosis, 413t
  treatment, 415t
Streptococcus viridans, 104
Stress
  chronic recurrent abdominal pain, 243–244
Stress related erosive syndrome (SRES)
  actively bleeding
    treatment, 164–165
  complications, 165
  EGF, 165
  enteral nutrition, 164
  epidemiology, 161
  interventional therapy, 165
  natural history, 162
  pathophysiology, 161
  prophylactic therapy, 162
  prophylaxis, 165
  prostaglandin analogues, 164
  risk factors, 162, 165t
  treatment, 161–166, 162–163
Stress related peptic ulcer disease, 148
Stretta catheter, 75
Stretta System, 75, 76f
Strictures. See specific strictures
Strip biopsy, 37
Strongyloides stercoralis (strongyloidiasis), 311–312
  treatment, 312t
Sublingual nitroglycerin
  for chest pain, 116
Submucosal injection
  EMR, 38
Submucosal lesions, 34–35
  EUS diagnosis, 35f
Suck and ligate technique
  EMR, 37
Sucralfate
  for esophageal symptoms, 288
  for SRES, 163, 164
Sulfadiazine
  for Crohn's colitis, 466
  for *Isospora belli*, 310
Sulfasalazine (Azulfidine)
  for Crohn's disease of small bowel, 391
  for microscopic colitis, 507–508
  for nonsteroidal antiinflammatory drug enteropathy, 365
  pregnancy, 490, 491
  for UC, 44, 454, 455–456
Superficial esophageal cancer, 38, 39
Supplements, 321
  vitamin
    for short bowel syndrome, 383t
  vitamin D
    for metabolic bone disease, 334
  zinc
    for short bowel syndrome, 384
    for Wilson's disease, 721
Suprahyoid muscle strengthening, 53
Supralevator abscess, 530
Surfak

  for constipation, 440
Surgical lateral sphincterotomy
  anal fissure, 530
Surgical sphincterotomy
  anal stenosis, 533
Suture rectopexy
  rectal prolapse, 520
Swallowing
  antireflux surgery, 70
  mechanics, 49
Symptomatic gallstones
  treatment, 759t
Symptomatic nonacid reflux, 57
Symptom Checklist 90 R (SCL 90 R), 185, 185f
Symptoms
  related to food ingestion, 342–343
Syphilis, 535
Syrup of ipecac
  cardiotoxicity of, 233
Systematic review
  characteristics of, 5t
Systemic anaphylaxis, 344–345
Systemic mastocytosis
  secretory diarrhea, 428

T
TACE. See Transcatheter arterial chemoembolization (TACE)
Tachyphylaxis, 153
Tacrolimus (FK506)
  for Crohn's disease of small bowel, 393
  for Crohn's diseases perianal complications, 474
  with osteoporosis, 331–332
  pediatric liver transplantation, 653
  for transplantation, 388
Taenia saginata
  treatment, 312t
Taenia solium
  treatment, 312t
Tagamet. See Cimetidine (Tagamet)
Tapeworms, 311
  treatment, 312t
TCA. See Tricyclic antidepressants (TCA)
Technetium Tc99, 587
TEF. See Tracheoesophageal fistula (TEF)
Tegaserod (Zelnorm)
  for CIP, 380
  for constipation, 439t, 441
  cost, 439t
  for gastroparesis, 192
  for GERD, 55–56
  for IBS, 241
Telephone triage
  nurse advocate, 266–267
Temporary stents
  for esophageal strictures, 104–105
Tense ascites
  large volume paracentesis, 657
Teriparatide
  for metabolic bone disease, 334
Terlipressin
  for acute variceal bleeding, 120, 121
  for portal hypertension, 678

Tetracycline
  for *Balantidium coli,* 307
  for *Chlamydia trachomatis,* 534
  for *Helicobacter pylori,* 140
  for intestinal protozoan parasites, 309t
  for PUD, 44
  for short bowel syndrome, 382
Tetrathiomolybdate
  for Wilson's disease, 721
Thailand
  traveler's diarrhea, 300
Thalidomide
  for IEU, 99
Theobromine
  food induced symptoms, 340
Therapy
  cost difference, 10
  well designed trial characteristics, 3t
Thermal coagulation
  of Barrett's mucosa, 90–91
Thermal injury
  hemorrhoids, 538
Thiabendazole
  adverse effects, 314t
  for intestinal helminths, 312t
  for nematodes, 311
  pregnancy, 313t
  for strongyloidiasis, 311
Thiamine
  deficiency during alcohol withdrawal, 230
Thiazolidinediones (TZD)
  for insulin resistance, 672
Thioguanine
  for Crohn's colitis, 469
  metabolite levels, 407–409, 407t, 408f
Thiopental
  for fulminant hepatic failure, 636
Three dimensional virtual colonoscopy
  colorectal cancer screening, 543
Threshold analysis, 8, 11–13
  cost effectiveness ratio, 12
  cost involvement, 11–12
  estimating cost data, 12
  NUD, 12
  ulcer management, 13f
  of ulcer management, 11f
Thrombin
  upper gastrointestinal bleeding, 170
Through the scope (TTS) balloons, 101, 102f
  technique, 103
Timolol
  for portal hypertension, 677
Tincture of opium
  for secretory diarrhea, 426
Tinidazole
  adverse effects, 314t
  for *Giardia lamblia,* 310
  for intestinal protozoan parasites, 309t
  pregnancy, 313t
TIPS. See Transjugular intrahepatic portosystemic shunt (TIPS)
Tissue adhesive
  for acute variceal bleeding, 121

tLESrs. *See* Transient LES relaxations (tLESrs)
TNF alpha. *See* Tumor necrosis factor alpha (TNF alpha)
Tobacco
  gastrointestinal neoplasms, 270
Tocopherols, 712
Tofranil
  for FGID, 263, 263t
Total abdominal colectomy, 601
Total gastrectomy
  PGL, 208
Total parenteral nutrition (TPN)
  acute gallstone pancreatitis, 781
  associated cholestasis, 289–290
  with CIP, 379
  for human immunodeficiency virus (HIV), 275
  liver disease, 673–674
  short bowel syndrome, 384–385
Total vascular exclusion (TVE), 742
Toupet fundoplication, 72
Toxemia
  pregnancy, 698
Toxin mediated infectious diarrhea, 295–296
TPN. *See* Total parenteral nutrition (TPN)
Tracheoesophageal fistula (TEF), 98, 131
Traction diverticulum, 98
Tramadol (Ultram)
  for chronic abdominal pain, 252
Transcatheter arterial chemoembolization (TACE), 742
Transcatheter embolization, 588, 594t
Transhiatal esophagectomy
  for esophageal cancer, 128
Transient LES relaxations (tLESrs), 73–74
Transient pancreatic insufficiency
  with celiac disease, 370
Transjugular intrahepatic portosystemic shunt (TIPS)
  for acute variceal bleeding, 121
  for hepatic hydrothorax, 660
  portal hypertension, 678, 679
    variceal hemorrhage, 680
  refractory ascites, 658
Transjugular liver biopsy, 289
Trastuzimab
  for pancreatic cancer, 821
Traveler's diarrhea, 297–311
  attack rate, 297
  Campylobacter, 298
  Cryptosporidium parvum, 298–299
  Cyclospora cayetanensis, 298–299
  Entamoeba histolytica, 298–299
  enteroaggrative *E. coli*, 298
  enterotoxigenic *E. coli*, 297, 298, 298t
  epidemiology, 299
  etiology, 297, 298t
  Giardia lamblia, 298–299
  immunologically naive, 297
  persistent, 300–301
  prevention, 299–300, 299t
    dietary, 299
    with medication, 299–300

protozoa, 298–299
  Salmonella, 298
  sequelae, 301
  Shigella, 298
  treatment, 299t, 300–301
  vaccines, 301
  viruses, 298
Trazadone (Desyrel)
  for chronic abdominal pain, 253
Tree outcome, 9
Trematodes (flukes), 310–313
Triage
  telephone
    nurse advocate, 266–267
Triamcinolone, 43
Trichostrongylus, 312
  treatment, 312t
Trichuris trichiura (whipworm), 312
  treatment, 312t
Triclabendazole
  adverse effects, 314t
  for intestinal helminths, 312t
  for liver flukes, 310
Tricyclic antidepressants (TCA)
  for chronic abdominal pain, 252–253
  for FGID, 262–263
  for gastroparesis, 193
  for IBS, 240t
Trientine
  for liver disease during pregnancy, 694–695
  for Wilson's disease, 721
Trifluoroperazine
  for secretory diarrhea, 428
Triglycyl lysine vasopressin
  for acute variceal bleeding, 120
Trimethoprim sulfamethoxazole
  adverse effects, 314t
  Blastocystis hominis, 307
  for *Cyclospora cayetanensis*, 308
  for intestinal protozoan parasites, 309t
  for *Isospora belli*, 310
  for *Pneumocystis*, 99
  pregnancy, 313t
  for SBP, 659
  for traveler's diarrhea, 301
  for UC, 455
  for Whipple's disease, 317t
Trivial obesity, 213
TTS balloons. *See* Through the scope (TTS) balloons
Tube feedings
  advancement, 322
  with CIP, 379
Tumor necrosis factor alpha (TNF alpha)
  for alcoholic liver disease, 668
  for pediatric Crohn's disease, 397
Turcot's syndrome, 551
TVE. *See* Total vascular exclusion (TVE)
24 hours pH monitoring
  GERD, 69
Two way sensitivity, 10–11
  of ulcer management, 10f
Tygon polyvinyl endoprosthesis, 136
Type I diabetes mellitus

  beta cell replacement, 828
Typhlitis
  with SCT, 287–288
Tyrosine kinase inhibitors
  for metastatic esophageal cancer, 129
TZD. *See* Thiazolidinediones (TZD)

U

UC. *See* Ulcerative colitis (UC)
UDCA. *See* Ursodeoxycholic acid (UDCA)
Ulcerative colitis (UC), 453–456. *See also* Left sided ulcerative colitis
  associated with low BMD, 328t
  breastfeeding, 455
  colorectal cancer, 542
  distal disease therapy, 454
  dysplasia surveillance programs, 486
  extensive disease therapy, 454–455
  IAP, 454
  long term maintenance therapy, 455–456
  nursing, 455
  oral conditions, 44
  pregnancy, 455
  restorative proctocolectomy with ileal pouch anal anastomosis, 459–462
  sequential therapy, 453t
  smoking, 271
  subtotal colectomy and ileostomy, 458
  total colectomy and ileorectal anastomosis, 458
  total colectomy and ileostomy, 458
  total proctocolectomy (TPC) and ileostomy, 458
  treatment, 453–454
Ulcerative colitis ileal pouch anal anastomosis
  treatment, 528f
Ulcerative proctitis, 447–452
Ulcers. *See* specific ulcers
Ultraflex stent, 135, 136f, 501f
Ultram
  for chronic abdominal pain, 252
Ultrashort Barrett's, 181
Ultrasonography (US)
  pancreatic carcinoma detection, 31t
Undifferentiated mucosal cancer, 40
Unexplained chest pain
  treatment, 111
Unexplained dysphagia
  evaluation, 115
Unguided bougies, 101
United Network of Organ Sharing (UNOS), 732
UNOS. *See* United Network of Organ Sharing (UNOS)
Upper endoscopy
  for GERD, 69
Upper gastrointestinal bleeding, 167–176
  APC, 171–172
  Doppler ultrasound, 169
  endoscopic treatment, 150
  endovascular intervention, 174
  epinephrine, 170
  fibrin glue, 170–171
  injection therapy, 170

laser thermocoagulation, 172
nonvariceal, 167
pharmacologic treatment, 153–154
sclerosants, 170
technical pitfalls, 595
thermocoagulation, 171
thrombin, 170
transcatheter management, 590–593, 592t
  bridging bleeding site, 592
  complications, 593
  postgastric surgery, 592
  technique, 592
  vasoconstriction, 592
treatment, 150–151, 151f
Upper gastrointestinal strictures, 494–500
Ureteral stents, 603
Urine N telopeptide cross linked of type 1 collagen
  metabolic bone disease, 327t
Ursodeoxycholic acid (UDCA)
  for focal biliary fibrosis, 808
  for nonalcoholic fatty liver disease, 673
  for PBC, 704–705
  for pruritis of cholestasis, 710
  for pruritus gravidarum, 696
Ursodiol (Actigal)
  for cholestasis, 290
  for erythropoietic protoporphyria, 730
  for VOD, 289
US. See Ultrasonography (US)

V

Vaccines
  traveler's diarrhea, 301
Vagal mechanosensory mechanisms, 75
Valacyclovir
  for viral esophagitis, 98
Valium
  for alcohol withdrawal, 230
  endoscopic sedation
    patient controlled, 22
Valium with meperidine
  endoscopic sedation
    patient controlled, 22
Valvular heart disease
  cardiovascular risk with major surgery, 432
Vancomycin
  with cephalosporin
    for bacterial esophagitis, 98
  for *Clostridium difficile* diarrhea, 304, 305
Variceal bleeding. See Acute variceal bleeding
Varicella zoster virus (VZV)
  inducing fulminant hepatic failure, 630
Vasopressin
  for acute variceal bleeding, 120, 121
  gastrointestinal bleeding, 590t
  for portal hypertension, 679
VBG. See Vertical banded gastroplasty (VBG)
Venlafaxine (Effexor)
  for chronic abdominal pain, 253
  efficacy, 264
  for FGID, 263t, 264

Venoocclusive disease (VOD)
  clinical criteria, 289t
  with SCT, 289
Venous thrombosis, 417
  diagnosis, 413t
  treatment, 415t
Ventilatory function
  monitoring, 21
Verapamil
  for secretory diarrhea, 428
Verbal feedback, 20
Versed. See Midazolam
Vertical banded gastroplasty (VBG), 221–222, 221f
Very low calorie diet (VLCD), 217
Vibrio cholerae, 294t, 295–296
Vibrio fluvialis, 296
Vibrio hollisae, 296
Vibrio mimicus, 296
Vibrio parahemolyticus, 294t, 296
Vigorous achalasia, 112
Vioxx, 143
VIPomas
  secretory diarrhea, 428
Viral esophagitis, 97–98
Viral gastroenteritis, 295
Viral hepatitis
  acute
    pediatric liver transplantation, 652
  children, 625–628
Viral infection
  elevated liver enzymes, 607–608
  with SCT, 288
Viruses
  inducing fulminant hepatic failure, 630
Visceral hyperalgesia, 251
Visceral hypersensitivity
  IBS, 239
Vitamin(s)
  deficiency
    with PSC, 716
  requirements, 321t
  supplements
    for short bowel syndrome, 383t
Vitamin A deficiency, 712
Vitamin D
  deficiency, 712
    conditions leading to, 328–330
    Crohn's disease of small bowel, 395
  for PBC, 703
  supplements
    for metabolic bone disease, 334
  synthesis and metabolism, 329f
Vitamin E
  for alcoholic liver disease, 669
  for nonalcoholic fatty liver disease, 673
Vitamin K, 712
  for pruritus gravidarum, 696
VLCD. See Very low calorie diet (VLCD)
VOD. See Venoocclusive disease (VOD)
Vomiting
  with eating disorders, 233
  with SCT, 288
Voriconazole
  for esophageal infections, 97

VSL-3
  for ileoanal pouch, 528
VZV. See Varicella zoster virus (VZV)

W

Waist circumference, 214
Waiting line theory, 8
Walking
  obesity, 216
Wallstent II, 135
Warfarin
  noncardiac surgery, 432
WAS. See Wiskott Aldrich syndrome (WAS)
Water diarrhea, 428
Water soluble vitamins
  with short bowel syndrome, 384
WBC. See White blood cell (WBC)
WCE. See Wireless capsule endoscopy (WCE)
WDHA syndrome (water diarrhea, hypokalemia, achlorhydria) syndrome, 428
Web sites
  CAM, 355
  National Center for Complementary and Alternative Medicine, 355
  Quackwatch, 355
  Research Council for Complementary Medicine, 355
Weight control programs, 213t
Weight gain
  after smoking cessation, 213t
  postpartum, 213t
Weight loss
  with achalasia, 113
  GERD, 60
  maintenance, 218
  nonalcoholic fatty liver disease, 671
Weight regain
  bariatric operations, 225
Wells' rectopexy
  rectal prolapse, 520
Whipple resection, 785, 814–815, 815f
Whipple's disease, 316–319
  adjuvant therapy, 319
  antibiotics, 317–318, 317t
  cerebral, 318–319
  historical lessons, 316
  monitoring, 318
  primary nonresponders, 318
  staging, 316–317, 317t
  treatment, 316–318
Whipworm, 312
  treatment, 312t
White blood cell (WBC), 656
Wilson's disease, 720–723
  diagnosis, 720t
  with fulminant hepatic failure, 630–631
  hepatic disease, 721–722
  neurologic disease, 722–723
  prognosis, 723
  treatment, 722t
Wine
  GERD, 60
Wire guided polyvinyl dilators, 102

Wireless capsule endoscopy (WCE), 357
   contraindications to, 360t
   indications for, 360t
   obscure gastrointestinal bleeding, 360–361
Wiskott Aldrich syndrome (WAS), 281
   gastrointestinal manifestations, 283
Wound infection
   with percutaneous endoscopic gastrostomy, 198

X
Xerostomia, 45
XLA, 280
   gastrointestinal manifestations, 283

Y
Yersinia, 294t
Yo-yo dieting, 214

Z
Zantac. *See* Ranitidine (Zantac)
Zelnorm. *See* Tegaserod (Zelnorm)
Zenker's diverticulum, 52
ZE syndrome. *See* Zollinger Ellison (ZE) syndrome
Zinc supplements
   for short bowel syndrome, 384
   for Wilson's disease, 721
Zithromax. *See* Azithromycin (Zithromax)
Zocyrax
   for fulminant hepatic failure, 634
   for Herpes, 535
   for viral esophagitis, 98
Zofran. *See* Ondansetron (Zofran)
Zollinger Ellison (ZE) syndrome, 147, 156
   PUD, 149
Zoloft. *See* Sertraline (Zoloft)
Z stent, 135
   with antireflux valve, 135f

RC
801
.A38
2005

Advanced therapy in
gastroenterology and
liver disease.

35010000515658

$159.95

DATE			

Ask for CD at Circ Desk

SOUTH UNIVERSITY
709 MALL BLVD.
SAVANNAH, GA 31406

BAKER & TAYLOR